RHEUMATOLOGY SECRETS

RHEUMATOLOGY SECRETS

THIRD EDITION

STERLING G. WEST, MD, MACP, FACR
Professor of Medicine
Department of Medicine
Division of Rheumatology
University of Colorado School of Medicine
Aurora, Colorado

ELSEVIER

ELSEVIER

Reed Elsevier India Pvt. Ltd.
Registered Office: 818, 8th Floor, Indraprakash Building, 21, Barakhamba Road, New Delhi-110 001
Corporate Office: 14th Floor, Building No. 10B, DLF Cyber City, Phase II, Gurgaon-122 002, Haryana, India

---

Rheumatology Secrets, 3/e by Sterling G. West

Copyright © 2015 by Mosby, Inc., an imprint of Elsevier Inc. All rights reserved.
Copyright © 2002, 1996 by Mosby, Inc., an affiliate of Elsevier Inc. All rights reserved.
Chapters 37, 38, and 40 are in the public domain as the author, Dr.William R. Gilliland, is a U.S. Government Employee. The copyright line for Chapters 37, 38, and 40 is 2015, published by Elsevier Inc.

ISBN: 978-0-323-03700-6

This reprint of Rheumatology Secrets, 3/e by Sterling G. West was undertaken by Reed Elsevier India Pvt. Ltd. and is published by arrangement with Elsevier Inc.

Copyright © 2016 by Reed Elsevier India Pvt. Ltd.

Indian Reprint ISBN: 978-81-312-4531-6

First Reprinted in India 2016

All rights reserved. No part of this publication may be reproduced or transmitted in any form or by any means, electronic or mechanical, including photocopying, recording, or any information storage and retrieval system, without permission in writing from the publisher. Details on how to seek permission, further information about the Publisher's permissions policies and our arrangements with organizations such as the Copyright Clearance Center and the Copyright Licensing Agency, can be found at our website: www.elsevier.com/permissions.

This book and the individual contributions contained in it are protected under copyright by the Publisher (other than as may be noted herein).

Notices:

Knowledge and best practice in this field are constantly changing. As new research and experience broaden our understanding, changes in research methods, professional practices, or medical treatment may become necessary.

Practitioners and researchers must always rely on their own experience and knowledge in evaluating and using any information, methods, compounds, or experiments described herein. In using such information or methods they should be mindful of their own safety and the safety of others, including parties for whom they have a professional responsibility.

With respect to any drug or pharmaceutical products identified, readers are advised to check the most current information provided (i) on procedures featured or (ii) by the manufacturer of each product to be administered, to verify the recommended dose or formula, the method and duration of administration, and contraindications. It is the responsibility of practitioners, relying on their own experience and knowledge of their patients, to make diagnoses, to determine dosages and the best treatment for each individual patient, and to take all appropriate safety precautions.

To the fullest extent of the law, neither the Publisher nor the authors, contributors, or editors, assume any liability for any injury and/or damage to persons or property as a matter of product liability, negligence or otherwise, or from any use or operation of any methods, products, instructions, or ideas contained in the material herein.

Although all advertising material is expected to conform to ethical (medical) standards, inclusion in this publication does not constitute a guarantee or endorsement of the quality or value of such product or of the claims made of it by its manufacturer.

This reprint is licensed for sale in India, Bangladesh, Bhutan, Maldives, Nepal, Pakistan and Sri Lanka only. Circulation of this version outside these territories is unauthorized and illegal.

Online resources are not available with this reprint. To access any or all of these assets, the original edition must be purchased by the individual user.

Printed and bound in India at Rajkamal Electric Press, Kundli (Haryana).

To my wife, Brenda, my best friend

To my children, Dace and Matthew, the joys of my life

To my amazing grandchildren, Aidan, Eva, and Owen

Paras Medical Books Pvt. Ltd.
Door No. 3-6-291/4, Near Apollo Hospital
Lane Opp. to Hyderguda Petrol Pump,
Adjacent Lane to Bata Showroom
HYDERABAD-500 029. 040-32955558
helpdesk@parasmedicalbooks.com
www.parasredkart.com

PREFACE

In the past year, we have been extensively authorized, approved, inspected, renovated, elevated, visited, consulted, circularized, informed; and have completed so many forms, orders, questionnaires, and reports that no medical progress has been made.

Rudolf Virchow
Berlin, 1865

With all the regulatory changes, many physicians might agree with Virchow's lament. In Rheumatology, this has clearly not been the case. It has been a decade since the last edition of *Rheumatology Secrets*, and I am amazed with the advances that have occurred in both the science and treatment of the rheumatic diseases. Each chapter in the present edition has been extensively reviewed and updated to include those advancements through January 2014.

I have frequently been asked why the long delay between editions? For many years I had the privilege of serving on the American Board of Internal Medicine Certifying Examination Committee in Rheumatology. As many use the *Secrets* to study for board certification and recertification I wanted to avoid what I considered a possible conflict of interest. With my term on the committee ended it is a pleasure to be able to edit this book again.

As in the previous editions, *Rheumatology Secrets*, Third Edition, is presented in the Socratic question and answer format that is the hallmark of The *Secrets* Series. The chapters are organized into 15 sections, each with a common theme emphasized by an introductory quotation. Common and uncommon rheumatic disease problems that we encounter in clinical practice, discuss during teaching rounds, and find on board examinations are covered. Each chapter reviews basic immunology and pathophysiology, important disease manifestations, and practical management issues. The book also contains a wealth of mnemonics, lists, tables, figures, and illustrations to emphasize important points. Chapter 2 lists some of the top *Rheumatology Secrets* and I encourage readers to send me their top secrets. I hope that the reader will find *Rheumatology Secrets*, Third Edition, both enjoyable and useful in daily practice.

Sterling G. West, MD

CONTRIBUTORS

Venu Akuthota, MD, FAAPMR
Professor and Vice Chair,
Director, Spine Center
Department of Physical Medicine and Rehabilitation
University of Colorado School of Medicine
Aurora, Colorado

Ramon A. Arroyo, MD, FACP, FACR
Assistant Professor of Medicine
Department of Medicine
Uniformed Services University of the Health Sciences
Bethesda, Maryland;
Rheumatology Staff
San Antonio Military Medical Center
San Antonio, Texas

Daniel F. Battafarano, DO, MACP, FACR
Adjunct Professor of Medicine
University of Texas Health Science Center
San Antonio, Texas;
Associate Professor of Medicine
Uniformed Services University of Health Science
Bethesda, Maryland

Vance J. Bray, MD, FACP, FACR
Assistant Clinical Professor, Rheumatology
University of Colorado Denver School of Medicine
Denver Arthritis Clinic
Denver, Colorado

Christina M. Bright, MD, FACR
Rheumatologist
Bend Memorial Clinic
Bend, Oregon

Amy C. Cannella, MD, MS, FACP, FACR, RhUS
Assistant Professor of Internal Medicine
Rheumatology Fellowship Program Director
University of Nebraska Medical Center
Omaha, Nebraska

Puja Chitkara, MD, FACR
Consultant Rheumatologist
Center for Arthritis and Rheumatologic Excellence (CARE)
San Diego, California

Marc D. Cohen, MD, FACP, FACR
Clinical Emeritus Professor of Medicine
Mayo Clinic
Jacksonville, Florida;
Clinical Professor of Medicine
University of Colorado School of Medicine
Aurora, Colorado;
Clinical Emeritus Professor of Medicine
Mayo Clinic
Jacksonville, Florida

Carolyn Anne Coyle, MD, FACR
Staff Rheumatologist
St. Peter's Hospital
Helena, Montana

Randy Q. Cron, MD, PhD, FACR
Professor of Pediatrics & Medicine
Arthritis Foundation, Alabama Chapter, Endowed Chair;
Director, Division of Pediatric Rheumatology
Children's Hospital of Alabama/University of Alabama at Birmingham
Birmingham, Alabama

Kevin D. Deane, MD, PhD, FACR
Associate Professor of Medicine
Division of Rheumatology
University of Colorado School of Medicine
Aurora, Colorado

M. Kristen Demoruelle, MD, FACR
Assistant Professor of Medicine
Department of Medicine
Division of Rheumatology
University of Colorado School of Medicine
Aurora, Colorado;
National Jewish Health
Denver, Colorado

Gregory J. Dennis, MD, FACP, FACR
Global Product Development
PPD, Inc.
Rockville, Maryland

Esi Morgan DeWitt, MD, MSCE, FACR
Associate Professor of Medicine
Pediatric Rheumatology
University of Cincinnati College of Medicine
Division of Rheumatology
James M. Anderson Center for Health Systems Excellence
Cincinnati Children's Hospital Medical Center
Cincinnati, Ohio

Donald G. Eckhoff, MD, MS, FACS
Professor Orthopaedics
Department of Orthopaedics
University of Colorado School of Medicine
Denver, Colorado

Alan R. Erickson, MD, FACR
Assistant Professor of Medicine
Section of Rheumatology and Immunology
University of Nebraska Medical Center
Omaha, Nebraska

David R. Finger, MD, FACP, FACR
Rheumatology Department
Honolulu Kaiser Permanente
Honolulu, Hawaii

Aryeh Fischer, MD, FACR
Associate Professor of Medicine
National Jewish Health
University of Colorado School of Medicine
Aurora, Colorado

William R. Gilliland, MD, MHPE, FACP, FACR
Professor of Medicine,
Associate Dean for Medical Education
Uniformed Services University of the Health Sciences
Bethesda, Maryland

Karen E. Hansen, MD, MS, FACR
Associate Professor of Medicine
Division of Rheumatology
University of Wisconsin School of Medicine & Public Health
Madison, Wisconsin

Robert A. Hawkins, MD, FACP, FACR
Associate Professor of Medicine
Department of Medicine
Wright State University Boonshoft School of Medicine
Dayton, Ohio;
Kettering Medical Center
Kettering, Ohio

Kathryn Hobbs, MD, FACR
Clinical Professor of Medicine
University of Colorado School of Medicine
Denver Arthritis Clinic
Denver, Colorado

J. Roger Hollister, MD, FACR
Professor of Pediatrics
Department of Pediatrics
University of Colorado Health Sciences Center
Denver, Colorado

Edmund H. Hornstein, DO, FACR
Assistant Professor of Medicine,
Chief, Rheumatology Division
Berkshire Medical Center;
University of Massachusetts Medical School
Pittsfield, Massachusetts

Robert W. Janson, MD, FACP, FACR
Associate Professor of Medicine
University of Colorado School of Medicine;
Chief, Rheumatology Section
Denver Veterans Affairs Medical Center
Denver, Colorado

Mark Jarek, MD, FACP, FACR
Jarek Medical
Republic, Missouri

John K. Jenkins, MD, FACR
Professor of Medicine (Ret)
Arthritis and Osteoporosis Center
Billings, Montana

Jason R. Kolfenbach, MD, FACR
Assistant Professor of Medicine
Department of Medicine
Division of Rheumatology
University of Colorado Denver
Aurora, Colorado

James S. Louie, MD, FACP, MACR
Professor of Medicine
UCLA School of Medicine
Los Angeles, California

Mark Malyak, MD, FACR
Associate Clinical Professor of Medicine
Department of Medicine
Division of Rheumatology
University of Colorado Health Sciences Center;
Denver Arthritis Center
Denver, Colorado

Michael T. McDermott, MD, FACP
Professor of Medicine and Clinical Pharmacy
Division of Endocrinology
Metabolism and Diabetes
University of Colorado Denver School of Medicine;
University of Colorado Hospital and Denver Veterans Administration Medical Center
Denver, Colorado

Richard T. Meehan, MD, FACP, FACR
Professor of Medicine
National Jewish Health
Denver, Colorado

Frederick T. Murphy, DO, FACP, FACR
Adjunct Clinical Assistant Professor of Medicine
Division of Rheumatology
Department of Medicine
University of Pennsylvania School of Medicine
Philadelphia, Pennsylvania;
Altoona Arthritis & Osteoporosis Center
Altoona Center for Clinical Research
Duncansville, Pennsylvania

James R. O'Dell, MD, FACP, FACR
Bruce Professor of Internal Medicine, Rheumatology
University of Nebraska Medical Center
Omaha, Nebraska

Brian D. Petersen, MD
Associate Professor of Radiology and Orthopaedics,
Chief of Musculoskeletal Radiology
University of Colorado Denver
Aurora, Colorado

Dianna Quan, MD, FAAN, FANA
Professor of Neurology,
Director, Electromyography Laboratory
University of Colorado Denver
Aurora, Colorado

Julia J. Rhiannon, MD, MSW, FACR
Rheumatologist
Virginia Mason Medical Center
Seattle, Washington

James D. Singleton, MD, FACR
Assistant Clinical Professor of Medicine
University of Colorado School of Medicine
Aurora, Colorado;
South Denver Medicine Associates
Highlands Ranch, Colorado

Marcus H. Snow, MD, FACR
Clinical Assistant Professor
University of Nebraska Medical Center
Omaha, Nebraska

Robert T. Spencer, MD, FACR
Associate Clinical Professor of Medicine
Department of Medicine
Division of Rheumatology
University of Colorado School of Medicine
Aurora, Colorado;
Colorado Arthritis Center
Englewood, Colorado

Jennifer Stichman, MD, FACR
Instructor of Medicine
Divisions of Rheumatology and General Internal Medicine
University of Colorado School of Medicine
Aurora, Colorado;
Denver Health Medical Center
Denver, Colorado

Colin Strickland, MD
Assistant Professor of Radiology
Division of Musculoskeletal Radiology
University of Colorado School of Medicine
Aurora, Colorado

Christopher C. Striebich, MD, PhD, FACP, FACR
Associate Professor of Medicine
Department of Medicine
Division of Rheumatology
University of Colorado School of Medicine
Aurora, Colorado

Kim Nguyen Tyler, MD, FACR
Assistant Clinical Professor of Medicine
Division of Rheumatology
University of Colorado School of Medicine
Aurora, Colorado;
Denver Arthritis Clinic
Denver, Colorado

Korey R. Ullrich, MD, FACR
Affiliate Assistant Clinical Professor
Charles E Schmidt College of Medicine at FAU
Rheumatology Associates of South Florida
Boca Raton, Florida

Scott Vogelgesang, MD, FACP, FACR
Clinical Professor of Medicine
Division of Immunology/Rheumatology
University of Iowa Hospital and Clinics
Iowa City, Iowa

Sterling G. West, MD, MACP, FACR
Professor of Medicine
Department of Medicine
Division of Rheumatology
University of Colorado School of Medicine
Aurora, Colorado

JoAnn Zell, MD, FACR
Associate Professor of Medicine
National Jewish Health
Denver, Colorado;
Assistant Professor
University of Colorado School of Medicine
Aurora, Colorado

ACKNOWLEDGMENTS

As Editor, I want to thank:

All the contributors for their time and effort in writing their chapters

The staff at Elsevier for their patience and help, and for giving me the opportunity to edit *Rheumatology Secrets*

My patients, teachers, and students for what they have taught me.

Sterling G. West, MD

CONTENTS

I GENERAL CONCEPTS

CHAPTER 1 CLASSIFICATION AND HEALTH IMPACT OF THE RHEUMATIC DISEASES 3
Sterling G. West, MD

CHAPTER 2 TOP 100+ RHEUMATOLOGY SECRETS 7
Sterling G. West, MD

CHAPTER 3 ANATOMY AND PHYSIOLOGY OF THE MUSCULOSKELETAL SYSTEM 16
Sterling G. West, MD

CHAPTER 4 OVERVIEW OF THE IMMUNE RESPONSE, INFLAMMATION, AND AUTOIMMUNITY 24
Sterling G. West, MD

II EVALUATION OF THE PATIENT WITH RHEUMATIC SYMPTOMS

CHAPTER 5 HISTORY AND PHYSICAL EXAMINATION 41
Richard T. Meehan, MD

CHAPTER 6 LABORATORY EVALUATION 48
Kathryn Hobbs, MD

CHAPTER 7 ARTHROCENTESIS AND SYNOVIAL FLUID ANALYSIS 58
Robert T. Spencer, MD

CHAPTER 8 RADIOGRAPHIC AND IMAGING MODALITIES 63
Colin Strickland, MD

CHAPTER 9 SYNOVIAL BIOPSIES 76
Sterling G. West, MD

CHAPTER 10 ELECTROMYOGRAPHY AND NERVE CONDUCTION STUDIES 78
Dianna Quan, MD

CHAPTER 11 APPROACH FOR PATIENTS WITH MONOARTICULAR ARTHRITIS SYMPTOMS 82
Robert A. Hawkins, MD

CHAPTER 12 APPROACH FOR PATIENTS WITH POLYARTICULAR ARTHRITIS SYMPTOMS 86
Robert A. Hawkins, MD

CHAPTER 13 APPROACH FOR THE PATIENT WITH NEUROMUSCULAR SYMPTOMS 91
Robert A. Hawkins, MD

CHAPTER 14 PERIOPERATIVE MANAGEMENT OF PATIENTS WITH RHEUMATIC DISEASES 96
Kim Nguyen Tyler, MD and Kevin D. Deane, MD

III SYSTEMIC CONNECTIVE TISSUE DISEASES

CHAPTER 15 RHEUMATOID ARTHRITIS 107
Sterling G. West, MD and James R. O'Dell, MD

CHAPTER 16 SYSTEMIC LUPUS ERYTHEMATOSUS 119
Jennifer Stichman, MD and JoAnn Zell, MD

CHAPTER 17 DRUG-INDUCED LUPUS 137
Christopher C. Striebich, MD, PhD

CHAPTER 18 SYSTEMIC SCLEROSIS 141
Aryeh Fischer, MD

CHAPTER 19 SCLERODERMA MIMICS 154
Puja Chitkara, MD and Gregory J. Dennis, MD

CHAPTER 20 INFLAMMATORY MUSCLE DISEASE 158
Sterling G. West, MD and Robert T. Spencer, MD

CHAPTER 21 MIXED CONNECTIVE TISSUE DISEASE, OVERLAP SYNDROMES, AND UNDIFFERENTIATED CONNECTIVE TISSUE DISEASE 166
Vance J. Bray, MD

CHAPTER 22 SJÖGREN'S SYNDROME 171
Vance J. Bray, MD

CHAPTER 23 ANTIPHOSPHOLIPID ANTIBODY SYNDROME 179
Sterling G. West, MD and Karen E. Hansen, MD, MS

| CHAPTER 24 | ADULT-ONSET STILL'S DISEASE 189
Vance J. Bray, MD |

| CHAPTER 25 | POLYMYALGIA RHEUMATICA 193
James D. Singleton, MD |

IV The Vasculitides and Related Disorders

| CHAPTER 26 | APPROACH FOR PATIENTS WITH SUSPECTED VASCULITIS 201
Marc D. Cohen, MD |

| CHAPTER 27 | LARGE-VESSEL VASCULITIS: GIANT CELL ARTERITIS, TAKAYASU ARTERITIS, AND AORTITIS 208
Puja Chitkara, MD and Gregory J. Dennis, MD |

| CHAPTER 28 | MEDIUM-VESSEL VASCULITIDES: POLYARTERITIS NODOSA, THROMBOANGIITIS OBLITERANS, AND PRIMARY ANGIITIS OF THE CENTRAL NERVOUS SYSTEM 216
Ramon A. Arroyo, MD |

| CHAPTER 29 | ANTINEUTROPHIL CYTOPLASMIC ANTIBODY-ASSOCIATED VASCULITIS 224
Mark Malyak, MD |

| CHAPTER 30 | IMMUNE-COMPLEX–MEDIATED SMALL-VESSEL VASCULITIDES 236
Ramon A. Arroyo, MD |

| CHAPTER 31 | CRYOGLOBULINEMIA 241
Korey R. Ullrich, MD |

| CHAPTER 32 | BEHÇET'S DISEASE AND COGAN'S SYNDROME 248
Sterling G. West, MD |

| CHAPTER 33 | RELAPSING POLYCHONDRITIS 253
Marc D. Cohen, MD |

V Seronegative Spondyloarthropathies

| CHAPTER 34 | ANKYLOSING SPONDYLITIS 261
Robert W. Janson, MD |

| CHAPTER 35 | RHEUMATIC MANIFESTATIONS OF GASTROINTESTINAL AND HEPATOBILIARY DISEASES 268
Sterling G. West, MD |

| CHAPTER 36 | REACTIVE ARTHRITIS 276
Richard T. Meehan, MD |

| CHAPTER 37 | ARTHRITIS ASSOCIATED WITH PSORIASIS AND OTHER SKIN DISEASES 284
William R. Gilliland, MD, MHPE |

VI Arthritis Associated with Infectious Agents

| CHAPTER 38 | BACTERIAL SEPTIC ARTHRITIS, BURSITIS, AND OSTEOMYELITIS 291
William R. Gilliland, MD, MHPE |

| CHAPTER 39 | LYME DISEASE 300
John K. Jenkins, MD |

| CHAPTER 40 | MYCOBACTERIAL AND FUNGAL JOINT AND BONE DISEASES 307
William R. Gilliland, MD, MHPE |

| CHAPTER 41 | VIRAL ARTHRITIDES 313
Carolyn Anne Coyle, MD |

| CHAPTER 42 | HIV-ASSOCIATED RHEUMATIC SYNDROMES 319
Daniel F. Battafarano, DO |

| CHAPTER 43 | WHIPPLE'S DISEASE 325
Carolyn Anne Coyle, MD |

| CHAPTER 44 | ACUTE RHEUMATIC FEVER AND POSTSTREPTOCOCCAL ARTHRITIS 328
Carolyn Anne Coyle, MD |

VII Rheumatic Disorders Associated with Metabolic, Endocrine, and Hematologic Diseases

| CHAPTER 45 | GOUT 337
Robert W. Janson, MD |

| CHAPTER 46 | CALCIUM PYROPHOSPHATE DEPOSITION DISEASE 346
Frederick T. Murphy, DO |

| CHAPTER 47 | BASIC CALCIUM PHOSPHATE AND OTHER CRYSTALLINE DISEASES 352
Frederick T. Murphy, DO |

| CHAPTER 48 | ENDOCRINE-ASSOCIATED ARTHROPATHIES 357
Edmund H. Hornstein, DO |

| CHAPTER 49 | ARTHROPATHIES ASSOCIATED WITH HEMATOLOGIC DISEASES 365
Kevin D. Deane, MD, PhD |

| CHAPTER 50 | MALIGNANCY-ASSOCIATED RHEUMATIC DISORDERS   371
Daniel F. Battafarano, DO

VIII BONE AND CARTILAGE DISORDERS

| CHAPTER 51 | OSTEOARTHRITIS   381
Scott Vogelgesang, MD

| CHAPTER 52 | METABOLIC BONE DISEASE   393
Michael T. McDermott, MD

| CHAPTER 53 | PAGET'S DISEASE OF BONE   400
David R. Finger, MD

| CHAPTER 54 | OSTEONECROSIS   405
Robert T. Spencer, MD

IX HEREDITARY, CONGENITAL, AND INBORN ERRORS OF METABOLISM ASSOCIATED WITH RHEUMATIC SYNDROMES

| CHAPTER 55 | HERITABLE CONNECTIVE TISSUE DISEASES   413
John K. Jenkins, MD

| CHAPTER 56 | INBORN ERRORS OF METABOLISM AFFECTING CONNECTIVE TISSUE   420
Sterling G. West, MD

| CHAPTER 57 | STORAGE AND DEPOSITION DISEASES   424
Sterling G. West, MD

| CHAPTER 58 | RHEUMATOLOGIC MANIFESTATIONS OF THE PRIMARY IMMUNODEFICIENCY SYNDROMES   430
Sterling G. West, MD and Mark Malyak, MD

| CHAPTER 59 | BONE AND JOINT DYSPLASIAS   437
Edmund H. Hornstein, DO

X NONARTICULAR AND REGIONAL MUSCULOSKELETAL DISORDERS

| CHAPTER 60 | APPROACH FOR THE PATIENT WITH NECK AND LOW BACK PAIN   445
Richard T. Meehan, MD

| CHAPTER 61 | FIBROMYALGIA   452
Mark Malyak, MD

| CHAPTER 62 | REGIONAL MUSCULOSKELETAL DISORDERS   462
Scott Vogelgesang, MD

| CHAPTER 63 | SPORTS MEDICINE AND OCCUPATIONAL INJURIES   471
Donald G. Eckhoff, MD, MS

| CHAPTER 64 | ENTRAPMENT NEUROPATHIES   477
David R. Finger, MD

| CHAPTER 65 | COMPLEX REGIONAL PAIN SYNDROME   483
Julia J. Rhiannon, MD, MSW

XI NEOPLASMS AND TUMORLIKE LESIONS

| CHAPTER 66 | BENIGN AND MALIGNANT TUMORS OF JOINTS AND SYNOVIUM   493
Edmund H. Hornstein, DO

| CHAPTER 67 | COMMON BONY LESIONS: RADIOGRAPHIC FEATURES   497
Brian D. Petersen, MD

XII PEDIATRIC RHEUMATIC DISEASES

| CHAPTER 68 | APPROACH TO THE CHILD WITH JOINT PAIN   509
Esi Morgan DeWitt, MD, MSCE and Randy Q. Cron, MD, PhD

| CHAPTER 69 | JUVENILE IDIOPATHIC ARTHRITIS   516
J. Roger Hollister, MD

| CHAPTER 70 | JUVENILE SYSTEMIC CONNECTIVE TISSUE DISEASES   522
Esi Morgan DeWitt, MD, MSCE and Randy Q. Cron, MD, PhD

| CHAPTER 71 | KAWASAKI DISEASE   530
J. Roger Hollister, MD

XIII MISCELLANEOUS RHEUMATIC DISORDERS

| CHAPTER 72 | METABOLIC AND OTHER GENETIC MYOPATHIES   535
Ramon A. Arroyo, MD

| CHAPTER 73 | AMYLOIDOSIS   543
James D. Singleton, MD

| CHAPTER 74 | RAYNAUD'S PHENOMENON   549
Marc D. Cohen, MD

| CHAPTER 75 | AUTOIMMUNE EYE AND EAR DISORDERS   555
Korey R. Ullrich, MD

CHAPTER 76	RHEUMATIC SYNDROMES ASSOCIATED WITH SARCOIDOSIS 565 *Daniel F. Battafarano, DO, MACP*		CHAPTER 84	IMMUNOSUPPRESSIVE AND IMMUNOREGULATORY AGENTS 627 *Amy C. Cannella, MD and James R. O'Dell, MD*
CHAPTER 77	RHEUMATIC DISORDERS IN PATIENTS ON DIALYSIS 571 *Mark Jarek, MD*		CHAPTER 85	BIOLOGIC AGENTS 633 *Sterling G. West, MD*
CHAPTER 78	RHEUMATIC DISEASE AND THE PREGNANT PATIENT 577 *Sterling G. West, MD and Mark Jarek, MD*		CHAPTER 86	HYPOURICEMIC AGENTS AND COLCHICINE 645 *David R. Finger, MD*
CHAPTER 79	FAMILIAL AUTOINFLAMMATORY SYNDROMES 586 *M. Kristen Demoruelle, MD and Christina M. Bright, MD*		CHAPTER 87	BONE STRENGTHENING AGENTS 652 *Michael T. McDermott, MD*
			CHAPTER 88	REHABILITATIVE TECHNIQUES 661 *Venu Akuthota, MD*
CHAPTER 80	ODDS AND ENDS 592 *Sterling G. West, MD*		CHAPTER 89	SURGICAL TREATMENT AND RHEUMATIC DISEASES 668 *Donald G. Eckhoff, MD, MS*

XIV MANAGEMENT OF THE RHEUMATIC DISEASES

CHAPTER 81	NONSTEROIDAL ANTIINFLAMMATORY DRUGS 601 *Jason R. Kolfenbach, MD*

CHAPTER 90	DISABILITY 676 *Scott Vogelgesang, MD*

XV FINAL SECRETS

CHAPTER 82	GLUCOCORTICOIDS—SYSTEMIC AND INJECTABLE 612 *Puja Chitkara, MD and Gregory J. Dennis, MD*		CHAPTER 91	COMPLEMENTARY AND ALTERNATIVE MEDICINE 685 *Alan R. Erickson, MD*
CHAPTER 83	SYSTEMIC ANTIRHEUMATIC DRUGS 619 *Marcus H. Snow, MD and James R. O'Dell, MD*		CHAPTER 92	HISTORY, THE ARTS, AND RHEUMATIC DISEASES 692 *Sterling G. West, MD and James S. Louie, MD*

I
GENERAL CONCEPTS

The rheumatism is a common name for many aches and pains, which have yet no peculiar appellation, though owing to very different causes.

William Heberden (1710–1801)
Commentaries on the History and Cure of Diseases, Ch. 79

CLASSIFICATION AND HEALTH IMPACT OF THE RHEUMATIC DISEASES

Sterling G. West, MD

CHAPTER 1

The rheumatism is a common name for many aches and pains, which have yet no peculiar appellation, though owing to very different causes.

–William Heberden (1710-1801)
Commentaries on the History and Cure of Diseases, Chapter 79.

KEY POINTS

Approximately 30% of the U.S. population has arthritis and/or back pain.
One out of every five office visits to a primary care provider and 10% of all surgeries are for a musculoskeletal problem.
Arthritis/back pain is the second leading cause of acute disability, the number one cause of chronic disability, and most common reason for social security disability payments.

1. **What is rheumatology?**
   A medical science devoted to the study of rheumatic diseases and musculoskeletal disorders.

2. **What are the roots of rheumatology?**
   First century AD—The term *rheuma* first appears in the literature. Rheuma refers to "a substance that flows" and probably was derived from phlegm, an ancient primary humor, which was believed to originate from the brain and flow to various parts of the body causing ailments.
   1642—The word rheumatism is introduced into the literature by the French physician Dr. G. Baillou, who emphasized that arthritis could be a systemic disorder.
   1928—The American Committee for the Control of Rheumatism is established in the United States of America by Dr. R. Pemberton. Renamed American Association for the Study and Control of Rheumatic Disease (1934), then American Rheumatism Association (1937), and finally American College of Rheumatology (ACR) (1988).
   1940s—The terms rheumatology and rheumatologist are first coined by Drs. Hollander and Comroe, respectively.

3. **How many rheumatic/musculoskeletal disorders are there?**
   Over 120.

4. **How have these rheumatic/musculoskeletal disorders been classified over the years?**
   1904—Dr. Goldthwaite, an orthopedic surgeon, makes the first attempt to classify the arthritides. He had five categories: gout, infectious arthritis, hypertrophic arthritis (probably osteoarthritis), atrophic arthritis (probably rheumatoid arthritis), and chronic villous arthritis (probably traumatic arthritis).
   1964—American Rheumatism Association (ARA) classification.
   1983—The ARA classification is revised based on the ninth edition of the International Classification of Disease (ICD 9). ICD 10 is at present being developed and scheduled for implementation in October 2015.

5. **The 1983 ARA classification is overwhelming. Is there a simpler outline to remember?**
   Most of the rheumatic diseases can be grouped into 10 major categories:
   1. Systemic connective tissue diseases.
   2. Vasculitides and related disorders.
   3. Seronegative spondyloarthropathies.
   4. Arthritis associated with infectious agents.
   5. Rheumatic disorders associated with metabolic, endocrine, and hematologic disease.
   6. Bone and cartilage disorders.
   7. Hereditary, congenital, and inborn errors of metabolism associated with rheumatic syndromes.
   8. Nonarticular and regional musculoskeletal disorders.
   9. Neoplasms and tumor-like lesions.
   10. Miscellaneous rheumatic disorders.

Table 1-1. Estimated Prevalence of Rheumatic/Musculoskeletal Disorders in the U.S. Population

NUMBER OF PATIENTS	PREVALENCE (ADULTS)	
All Musculoskeletal Disorders	20% to 30%	60 to 90 million*
Arthropathies		
Osteoarthritis	12%	27 million
Rheumatoid arthritis	1%	1.5 million
Crystalline arthritis (gout)	4%	8.3 million
Spondyloarthropathies	0.25%	0.4 to 1 million
Connective Tissue Disease		
Polymyalgia rheumatica	<0.01%	0.3 to 0.7 million
Systemic lupus erythematosus	<0.01%	240,000
Systemic sclerosis	<0.01%	50,000
Back/neck pain: frequent	15%	33 million
Osteoporosis (>age 50 years)	10%	9 million
Soft tissue rheumatism	3% to 5%	5 to 10 million
Fibromyalgia	2%	3 to 5 million

*Overall, 45 to 50 million (1 in 5) adults have doctor-diagnosed arthritis and 300,000 children have arthritis with 50,000 having juvenile idiopathic arthritis.

6. **What is the origin and difference between a collagen vascular disease and a connective tissue disease?**

   1942—Dr. Klemperer introduces the term diffuse collagen disease based on his pathologic studies of systemic lupus erythematosus (SLE) and scleroderma.
   1946—Dr. Rich coins the term collagen vascular disease based on his pathologic studies in vasculitis, indicating that the primary lesion involved the vascular endothelium.
   1952—Dr. Ehrich suggests the term connective tissue diseases, which has gradually replaced the term collagen vascular diseases.
   In summary, the two terms are used synonymously, although the purist would say that the heritable collagen disorders (see Chapter 55) are the only true "diffuse collagen diseases."

7. **How common are rheumatic/musculoskeletal disorders in the general population?**

   Approximately 30% of the population has symptoms of a musculoskeletal condition. Only two thirds of these patients (i.e., 20% of the population) have symptoms severe enough to cause them to seek medical care. The prevalence of musculoskeletal disorders increases with the age of the patient population.

8. **What is the estimated prevalence for the various rheumatic/musculoskeletal disorders in the general population?**

   The estimated prevalence of rheumatic/musculoskeletal disorders in the U.S. population is shown in Table 1-1.

9. **What is the prevalence of autoimmune diseases in the general population?**

   Any organ system can be affected by autoimmunity. Presently there are over 70 autoimmune diseases. When analyzing the 30 most common, it is estimated that over 5% of the population have one or more autoimmune disease. Approximately 40% of these patients (i.e., 2% of the population) have an autoimmune rheumatic disease. Of all patients with an autoimmune rheumatic disease about half will have rheumatoid arthritis and half will have one of the other autoimmune rheumatic diseases (SLE, polymyositis, etc.).

10. **Which autoimmune diseases primarily affect women?**

    The various autoimmune diseases target women 75% of the time frequently during their reproductive years. Diseases suspected to be autoantibody-mediated (Th2 diseases) have the highest female predominance (Table 1-2).

11. **How often are one of the rheumatic/musculoskeletal disorders likely to be seen in an average primary care practice?**

    About 1 out of every 5 to 10 office visits to a primary care provider is for a musculoskeletal disorder. Interestingly, 66% of these patients are <65 years old. The most common problems are osteoarthritis, back pain, gout, fibromyalgia, and tendinitis/bursitis.

Table 1-2. The Female/Male Ratio of Autoimmune Diseases

DISEASE	FEMALE/MALE
Hashimoto's disease	9:1
Systemic lupus erythematosus	9:1
Sjögren's syndrome	9:1
Antiphospholipid syndrome	9:1
Mixed connective tissue disease	8:1
Graves' disease	7:1
Rheumatoid arthritis	4:1
Scleroderma	3:1
Multiple sclerosis	2:1
Polymyositis	2:1

Box 1-1. Morbidity and Mortality of Rheumatic/Musculoskeletal Diseases

Percent of Population
- Symptoms of arthritis—30%
- Symptoms requiring medical therapy—20%
- Disability due to arthritis—5% to 10%
- Totally disabled from arthritis—0.5%
- Mortality from rheumatic disease—0.02%

12. **How many rheumatologists are there in the United States of America?**
    In 2005, there were approximately 4900 adult rheumatologists and 260 pediatric rheumatologists, although not all are actively seeing patients. This number is projected to decrease over the next 10 years and helps explain why there is often a long delay to see a rheumatologist.

13. **Discuss the impact of the rheumatic/musculoskeletal diseases on the general population in terms of morbidity and mortality.**
    Arthritis/back pain is the second leading cause of acute disability (behind respiratory illness) and is the number one cause of chronic disability in the general population (Box 1-1). An estimated 45 to 50 million U.S. adults have doctor-diagnosed arthritis. Of these, 21 million (42%) have arthritis-attributable activity limitations, which equates into 9% of all U.S. adults have at least one limitation. Of working-age adults (aged 18 to 64 years) with doctor-diagnosed arthritis, 31% have arthritis-attributable work limitations. Because these are prime working years, musculoskeletal conditions cause significant loss of work productivity. Overall, a quarter (25%) of social security disability payments are related to rheumatologic disorders making it the leading cause of social security disability payments. Ten percent of all surgical procedures are for disabilities related to arthritis.

14. **What is the economic impact of rheumatic/musculoskeletal diseases?**
    In 2007, the Medical Expenditures Panel Survey reported that 91.3 million persons reported one or more musculoskeletal condition (including the 45 to 50 million adults with doctor-diagnosed arthritis). The aggregate direct medical costs were $620.9 billion and indirect costs due to lost earnings were $380 billion. The total costs are the equivalent of 7.3% of the gross domestic product (GDP).

BIBLIOGRAPHY

Benedek TG: A century of American rheumatology, Ann Intern Med 106:304–312, 1987.
Centers for Disease Control and Prevention: Racial/ethnic differences in the prevalence and impact of doctor diagnosed arthritis: United States 2002, Morb Mortal Wkly Rep 54:119–121, 2005.
Deal CL, Hooker R, Harrington T, et al: The United States rheumatology workforce: supply and demand, 2005–2025, Arthritis Rheum 56:722–729, 2007.
Decker JL: Glossary Subcommittee of the ARA Committee on Rheumatologic Practice: American Rheumatism Association nomenclature and classification of arthritis and rheumatism, Arthritis Rheum 26:1029–1032, 1983.
Helmick CG, Felson DT, Lawrence RC, et al: Estimates of the prevalence of arthritis and other rheumatic conditions in the United States. Part I, Arthritis Rheum 58:15–25, 2008.

Jacobson DL, Gange SJ, Rose NR, et al: Epidemiology and estimated population burden of selected autoimmune diseases in the United States, Clin Immunol Immunopathol 84:223–243, 1997.

Lawrence RC, Felson DT, Helmick CG, et al: Estimates of the prevalence of arthritis and other rheumatic conditions in the United States. Part II, Arthritis Rheum 58:26–35, 2008.

Reynolds MD: Origins of the concept of collagen–vascular diseases, Semin Arthritis Rheum 15:127–131, 1985.

Yelin E: Economic burden of rheumatic diseases. In Firestein GS, Budd RS, Gabriel SE, McInnes IB, O'Dell JR, editors: Kelley's textbook of rheumatology, ed 9, Philadelphia, 2013, Elsevier Saunders, pp 440-451.

FURTHER READING

www.aarda.org
www.usbjd.org
www.rheumatology.org
www.arthritis.org

TOP 100+ RHEUMATOLOGY SECRETS

Sterling G. West, MD

CHAPTER 2

A physician is judged by the three A's—ability, availability, and affability.

—Paul Reznihoff
Aphorism

Rheumatology can be confusing to many physicians during their housestaff training (and beyond!). Often the patient's presentation is not according to the "textbook." That is what makes rheumatology fun, that is, diagnosing unusual presentations of disease! In addition to having interesting diseases, we now have many more effective therapies compared to the last edition of *Rheumatology Secrets*. Although nothing in medicine is 100%, I have found the following useful and cost effective when evaluating a patient with a rheumatic/musculoskeletal problem:

1. **A good history and physical examination, coupled with knowledge of musculoskeletal anatomy, is the most important part of the evaluation of a patient with rheumatic symptoms.**
   You have to examine the patient! That means taking off their shoes and socks, examining their feet, and watching them walk if they have lower extremity (hip, knee, ankle, foot) complaints.

2. **Soft tissue rheumatism.**
   - Most shoulder pain is periarticular (i.e., a bursitis or tendinitis). *Rule out impingement in patients with recurrent shoulder tendinitis.*
   - Causes of olecranon or prepatellar bursitis: trauma, infection, gout, rheumatoid arthritis (RA).
   - Recalcitrant trochanteric bursitis: rule out leg length discrepancy, hallux rigidus with an abnormal gait, and lumbar radiculopathy.
   - Recalcitrant medial knee pain: rule out anserine bursitis.
   - Recalcitrant patellofemoral syndrome: rule out pes planus/hypermobility causing patellar maltracking.
   - Due to risk of rupture, do not inject corticosteroids for therapy of Achilles tendinitis/enthesitis. Use iontophoresis.

3. **Back pain.**
   - Patients with significant low back pain cannot do a sit-up.
   - Most back pain is nonsurgical.
   - Magnetic resonance imaging (MRI)/computed tomography (CT) scans of lumbar spine are abnormal in 30% of patients with *no* symptoms. Do not attribute a patient's symptoms to an abnormal radiograph.
   - Spinal Phalen's test is useful to diagnose spinal stenosis. Patients with spinal stenosis have more pain walking uphill due to spinal extension making the spinal canal smaller. Straight leg raise test and electromyography/nerve conduction velocities (EMG/NCV) are often normal or nonspecific.

4. **Do not order a laboratory test unless you know why you are ordering it and what you will do if it comes back abnormal.**

5. **Laboratory tests**
   - Laboratory tests should be used to confirm your clinical diagnosis not make it.
   - All patients with a positive rheumatoid factor do not have RA, and all patients with a positive antinuclear antibody do not have systemic lupus erythematosus (SLE).
   - Low complement (C3, C4) levels in a patient with systemic symptoms suggest an immune complex-mediated disease and narrows your diagnosis: SLE, cryoglobulinemia (types II and III), urticarial vasculitis (HepB and C1q autoantibodies), subacute bacterial endocarditis (SBE), poststreptococcal or membranoproliferative glomerulonephritis.
   - An undetectable (not just low) CH50 activity may indicate a disease associated with a hereditary complement component deficiency: autoimmune (C1, C4, C2), infection (C3), *Neisseria* infection (C5 to C8).
   - Separating iron deficiency from anemia of chronic disease is best done by measuring the ferritin level. In a patient with elevated C-reactive protein, a ferritin level of >100 ng/mL rules out iron deficiency.

6. **Failure to aspirate, prepare to litigate!**
   Patients with acute inflammatory monoarticular arthritis need a joint aspiration to rule out septic arthritis and crystalline arthropathy.
   - To lessen the pain associated with an aspiration or injection, have the patient do the Valsalva maneuver when inserting the needle.

- Joint aspiration is generally safe up to an INR of 4.5. However, if septic arthritis is possible, the joint should be aspirated regardless of the INR.

7. **The synovial fluid analysis is a liquid biopsy of the joint.**
   Send any aspirated synovial fluid for cell count, crystal examination, Gram stain, and culture. Never send it for uric acid or lactate dehydrogenase (LDH).
   - One can estimate the synovial fluid white blood cell (WBC) count by using the equation that one WBC per high powered field (HPF; 40×) equals 500 cells/μL. Thus, 6 WBCs/HPF estimates a synovial fluid WBC count of 3000 cells/μL, which is inflammatory.
   - Crystal mnemonic: **ABC = A**lignment **B**lue **C**alcium. If the long axis of the crystal is aligned with the first order red compensator and is blue then it is a calcium pyrophosphate crystal. Uric acid crystals are yellow when aligned.
   - If you cannot find uric acid crystals initially, let the slide dry for 3 hours and reexamine it.

8. **Most patients with chronic inflammatory monoarticular arthritis of >8 weeks' duration, whose evaluation has failed to define an etiology for the arthritis, need a synovial biopsy to rule out an unusual cause (indolent infection, etc.).**

9. **In response to the Choosing Wisely initiative of the ABIM, the American College of Rheumatology (ACR) recommended the following five tests/treatments *not* be done in adult rheumatology patients:**
   1. Do not test antinuclear antibody (ANA) subserologies (anti-dsDNA, anti-Sm, anti-RNP, anti-SS-B, anti-Scl-70) without a positive ANA and clinical suspicion of immune-mediated disease. Anti-SS-A may be an exception to this recommendation.
   2. Do not test for Lyme disease as a cause of musculoskeletal symptoms without an exposure history and appropriate examination findings.
   3. Do not perform an MRI of the peripheral joints to routinely monitor inflammatory arthritis.
   4. Do not prescribe biologics for RA before a trial of methotrexate (or other conventional nonbiologic disease-modifying antirheumatic drugs [DMARDs]).
   5. Do not routinely repeat dual-energy X-ray absorptiometry (DXA) scans more often than once every 2 years.

10. **In response to the Choosing Wisely initiative of the ABIM, the ACR recommended the following five tests/treatments *not* be done in pediatric rheumatology patients:**
    1. Do not order autoantibody panels without a positive ANA and evidence of a rheumatic disease.
    2. Do not test for Lyme disease as a cause of musculoskeletal symptoms without an exposure history and appropriate examination findings.
    3. Do not routinely perform surveillance joint radiographs to monitor juvenile idiopathic arthritis (JIA) disease activity.
    4. Do not perform methotrexate toxicity laboratory tests more than every 12 weeks on stable doses.
    5. Do not repeat a confirmed positive ANA in patients with established JIA or SLE.

11. **In response to the Choosing Wisely initiative of the ABIM, the American Association of Orthopedic Surgeons (AAOS) recommended the following treatments *not* be done in patients (only those that apply to rheumatology patients are listed):**
    - Do not use needle lavage for long-term relief in symptomatic osteoarthritis (OA) treatment.
    - Lateral wedge or neutral insoles do not improve pain or function in patients with knee OA.
    - Do not use glucosamine and chondroitin sulfate to treat patients with symptomatic knee OA.

12. **In response to the Choosing Wisely initiative of the ABIM, the North American Spine Society (NASS) recommended the following tests/treatments *not* be done in patients with back pain:**
    - Do not order MRI of the spine within the first 6 weeks in patients with nonspecific low back pain in the absence of red flags (trauma, use of corticosteroids, unexplained weight loss, progressive neurologic signs, age >50 years or <age 17 years, fever, IV drug abuse, pain unrelieved by bed rest, history of cancer).
    - Do not perform elective spinal injections without imaging guidance.
    - Do not order EMG/NCVs to determine the cause of neck and back pain without radicular symptoms.
    - Do not recommend bed rest for more than 48 hours when treating low back pain.

13. **A few other "do nots" in rheumatology:**
    - Except for anti-dsDNA, do not repeat ANA subserologies in patients with an established connective tissue disease (CTD) diagnosis.
    - Do not perform serial measurements of rheumatoid factor and anti-cyclic citrullinated peptide (CCP) in patients with documented seropositive RA or serial ANAs in patients with a documented positive ANA and a CTD diagnosis (e.g., SLE).
    - Do not order a human leukocyte antigen (HLA)-B27 unless you suspect an undifferentiated spondyloarthropathy based on history and examination but have nondiagnostic radiographs.
    - Do not check CH50 to follow lupus disease activity.
    - Do not order an MRI before ordering plain films in a patient presenting with joint or back pain.

- Do not use intraarticular hyaluronic acid injections for advanced knee OA (i.e., bone on bone).
- Do not treat low bone mass in patients at low risk for fracture (T score > −2.5, no history of fragility fracture, no steroids, low FRAX).
- Do not order serial yearly plain radiographs in a patient with good clinical (symptoms, examination, laboratory tests) control of their arthritis unless you are willing to change therapy for minor radiographic disease progression.

14. The innate immune system is critical to the activation of the adaptive immune system.
15. Joint effusion and limited range of motion are the most specific signs for arthritis.
16. True hip joint pain is in the groin. In a young patient who cannot flex their hip greater than 90°, rule out femoroacetabular impingement syndrome.
17. Feel both knees with the back of your hand for temperature differences and compare it to the lower extremity.
    The knee should be cooler than the skin over the tibia. If the knee is warmer then there is ongoing knee inflammation.
18. Osteoarthritis (OA).
    - Cracking knuckles does not cause OA.
    - Patients with arthritis can predict the weather due to changes in barometric pressure as weather fronts move in and out of an area.
    - Obesity is the major modifiable risk factor for OA.
    - The joints typically involved in primary OA are: distal interphalangeal joints (DIPs) (Heberden's nodes), proximal interphalangeal joints (PIPs) (Bouchard's nodes), first carpometacarpal (CMC), hips, knees, first metatarsophalangeal joint (MTP), the cervical and lumbosacral spine.
    - Patients with OA affecting joints not normally affected by primary OA (i.e., metacarpophalangeals, wrists, elbows, shoulder, ankles) need to be evaluated for secondary causes of OA (i.e., calcium pyrophosphate disease [CPPD], metabolic diseases, others).
    - Erosive OA is an inflammatory subset of OA (10% of patients) primarily affecting the hands (DIPs, PIPs, first CMC) and causing the "seagull" sign on radiographs. It is more disabling than primary OA.
19. Knee and hip osteoarthritis (OA).
    - Over 50% of patients over 65 years have radiographic knee OA but only 25% have symptoms. Do not rely on the radiograph to make the diagnosis of the cause of knee pain.
    - Recurrent, large, noninflammatory knee effusions are frequently due to an internal derangement (e.g., meniscal tear).
    - Nonsteroidal antiinflammatory drugs (NSAIDs) are better than acetaminophen if a patient has an effusion, which indicates more inflammation (wet OA).
    - Intraarticular corticosteroids also work and are cheaper than viscosupplementation (hyaluronic acid), especially in patients with a knee effusion.
    - Drain any knee effusion before giving viscosupplementation or corticosteroids.
    - Incidental and asymptomatic meniscal tears are common (>20%) in patients with knee OA. Meniscal repair and/or arthroscopic debridement and washout are not helpful unless there are signs of locking.
    - Femoroacetabular impingement is a common cause of hip pain in young patients who develop early OA.
20. Extraarticular manifestations are often the most important findings to make a diagnosis in a patient with polyarthritis.
21. Myopathies tend to cause proximal and symmetric weakness, whereas neuropathies cause distal and asymmetric weakness and atrophy of muscles.
22. Cardiac disease occurs 10 years earlier in patients with inflammatory rheumatic disease compared to normal individuals with the same cardiac risk factors.
    This must be considered during the preoperative evaluation.
23. In a patient with a known systemic rheumatic disease who presents with fever or multisystem complaints, rule out infection and possibly other nonrheumatic etiologies (clot, drug reaction, other illness [thrombotic thrombocytopenic purpura, hypothyroidism, sleep apnea, fibromyalgia, cancer]) before attributing the symptoms and signs to the underlying rheumatic disease.
    Clearly, infection causes death in rheumatic disease patients more often than the underlying rheumatic disease does.
24. RA is the most common inflammatory arthritis presenting with symmetric involvement of the small joints of the hands (MCPs, PIPs), wrists, and feet (MTPs).
    In a patient with a diagnosis of RA who is seronegative or only has large joint involvement, always reassess to make sure the patient does not have another diagnosis.

25. Seropositive RA patients are at risk for developing extraarticular disease manifestations.
    If a patient is seronegative the "extraarticular manifestation" is probably not due to RA.
26. Seronegative RA is a difficult diagnosis in patients without erosions on radiographs.
    Always consider CPPD in these patients.
27. Treat to target.
    Early therapy with the goal of low disease activity is essential to RA (and psoriatic arthritis) therapy.
    - It does not matter which disease activity measure you use (e.g., Clinical Disease Activity Index [CDAI], Routine Assessment of Patient Index Data 3 [RAPID3], etc.), just pick one and use it to document if your therapy is achieving low disease activity or remission.
28. The development of drug-induced autoantibodies (usually anti-histone) is much more common than the development of lupus-like disease due to a drug.
29. In a patient with SLE with worsening renal function, rule out over-the-counter NSAIDs.
    In a patient with photosensitivity, rule out NSAIDs and thiazide diuretics.
30. Systemic sclerosis.
    - New onset hypertension and schistocytes on blood smear in a diffuse systemic sclerosis patient heralds the onset of scleroderma renal crisis, especially in a patient who is anti-RNA polymerase III positive. Angiotensin-converting enzyme (ACE) inhibitors work better than angiotensin receptor blockers (ARBs).
    - A %forced vital capacity (FVC)/%DLCO ratio of >1.6 predicts pulmonary hypertension.
    - An FVC <70% and a high resolution CT scan of the lung showing >20% fibrosis predicts progression of scleroderma-related interstitial lung disease.
31. One should suspect a disease mimicking scleroderma in any patient with skin induration who lacks Raynaud's phenomenon, nailfold capillary abnormalities, sclerodactyly, and autoantibodies.
32. Patients with Raynaud's phenomenon are likely (>80%) to develop systemic sclerosis if they have abnormal nailfold capillaroscopy and positive scleroderma-associated antibodies.
33. Inflammatory myositis should be highly considered in all patients with proximal muscle weakness, an elevated creatine phosphokinase (CPK), an elevated MB fraction of total CPK (>2% of total), and an elevated aspartate aminotransferase (AST).
34. Skin ulcerations and anti-155/140 antibodies signal the presence of an underlying associated malignancy in a patient with dermatomyositis.
35. Steroid myopathy does not cause an elevated CPK.
36. Statins can cause myalgias without an elevated CPK, myalgias with an elevated CPK, and a necrotizing myopathy with anti-HMGCoA reductase antibodies.
    - Myalgias can be improved with coenzyme Q.
    - Hydrophilic statins (pravachol, rosuvastatin) cause less myopathy than lipophilic statins (simvastatin, etc.).
37. All patients with mixed connective tissue disease (MCTD) should have Raynaud's phenomenon and high titer antibodies only against U1-RNP.
38. Up to half of all patients presenting with a CTD will be undifferentiated and half of those will evolve into a defined CTD within 3 years.
    Patience and follow-up are important.
39. Sjögren's syndrome is the most common autoimmune disease in middle-aged women and should be considered in any patient with unexplained symptoms and a positive ANA.
40. One in five rule: 20% of deep venous thromboses, 20% of young adult (<50 years old) strokes, and 20% of recurrent miscarriages are due to the antiphospholipid antibody (aPLab) syndrome.
41. "Triple positive" (positive lupus anticoagulant, positive anticardiolipin antibodies, and positive anti-$\beta_2$glycoprotein I antibodies) aPLab patients are the most likely to have clots.
42. All patients with significantly positive aPLabs should have prophylactic anticoagulation if they undergo a surgical procedure and/or following pregnancy delivery even if they have never had a clot.
    Surgical release of tissue factor is the second hit in the "two hit" hypothesis for clots in aPLab positive patients.
    - Always have placenta assessed (clinically and/or pathologically) for evidence of damage in patients with aPLab regardless of pregnancy outcome. If placental damage is present, the patient needs anticoagulation during any future pregnancy.
43. Still's disease should be considered in any patient with a quotidian fever (decreases to normal or below once a day), rash, and joint pain.
    A ferritin level >1000 ng/mL supports the diagnosis.

44. Polymyalgia rheumatica (PMR) patients should respond completely to 20 mg daily of prednisone and normalize their **erythrocyte sedimentation rate (ESR)** within a month.
    The presence of fever or failure to respond to prednisone clinically and serologically suggests giant cell arteritis or another diagnosis such as lymphoma.

45. After ruling out infection and malignancy, consider vasculitis in any patient with multisystem disease who has an ESR >100 mm/hour and a C-reactive protein >10 times the upper limit of normal.
    - The primary vasculitides (i.e., not due to another disease) are not associated with positive serologies (ANA, rheumatoid factor (RF), low complements), neutropenia, or thrombocytopenia. If one of these are present, consider another diagnosis.

46. Giant cell arteritis (GCA) is the most common vasculitis in the elderly and jaw claudication is the most specific symptom.

47. Listen for subclavian bruits in all patients suspected of having GCA as it may be their only clinical finding.
    Large vessel involvement puts them at increased (17×) risk for aortic dissections and aneurysms.

48. Do not delay starting prednisone in a patient suspected to have GCA.
    It will not affect the temporal artery biopsy results for at least a week.

49. When the suspected diagnosis is primary vasculitis of the central nervous system (CNS), it probably is incorrect.
    Rule out other diseases with a brain biopsy.

50. Granulomatosis with polyangiitis (GPA or Wegener's) should be considered in any adult who develops otitis media.
    GPA predominantly affects the upper and lower respiratory tracts and kidneys and is associated with proteinase 3-antineutrophil cytoplasmic antibody (PR3-ANCA).

50. Microscopic polyangiitis should be considered in all patients presenting with pulmonary–renal syndrome and is associated with myeloperoxidase (MPO)-ANCA.

51. Skin biopsy in Henoch–Schonlein purpura (HSP) shows leukocytoclastic vasculitis with IgA deposition in vessel walls on direct immunofluorescence.
    HSP is the most common small vessel vasculitis in childhood.

52. Urticarial lesions lasting longer than 24 hours and resolving with hyperpigmentation are likely to be vasculitic.

53. Most patients with mixed cryoglobulinemia will present with palpable purpura, arthralgia, and weakness/myalgias (Meltzer's triad).
    A positive rheumatoid factor and low C4 ("poor man's cryo") level supports the diagnosis before the cryoglobulin screen has returned.

54. "Refractory" vasculitis is an infection until proven otherwise.

55. Behcet's disease is the only vasculitis that causes pulmonary aneurysms.

56. Many diseases, especially vasculitis and myelodysplastic syndromes, are associated with relapsing polychondritis.

57. Enthesitis is the hallmark of the seronegative spondyloarthropathies.

58. Even though HLA-B27 increases a person's risk of developing a spondyloarthropathy 50 times, only 1 out of every 50 (2%) HLA-B27 positive individuals without a family history will develop ankylosing spondylitis during their lifetime.
    If the person has a family history the risk increases to one in five (20%).
    - Nearly 50% of HLA-B27 positive patients with recurrent unilateral anterior uveitis have or will develop an underlying spondyloarthropathy.

59. A patient less than 40 years old with three out of four of the following has a high likelihood of having inflammatory back pain: (1) morning stiffness of at least 30 minutes; (2) improvement of back pain with exercise but not rest; (3) awakening because of back pain and stiffness during second half of the night only; and (4) alternating buttock pain.

60. Inflammatory arthritis is most likely to occur in Crohn's disease patients with extensive colonic involvement.
    These patients may present with prominent arthritis but few gastrointestinal symptoms.

61. Pancreatic cancer can release enzymes which cause fat necrosis resulting in a triad of lower extremity arthritis, tender nodules, and eosinophilia (Schmidt's triad).

62. Reactive arthritis is a sterile, inflammatory arthritis that is typically preceded by a gastrointestinal or genitourinary infection occurring 1 to 4 weeks previously.
    The arthritis can improve with prolonged antibiotics only if it is due to chlamydia.

63. Inflammation of the DIP joints and finger dactylitis are highly characteristic of psoriatic arthritis.
    - Differential diagnosis of DIP arthritis: psoraitic, OA, multicentric reticulohistiocytosis, and primary biliary cirrhosis. In a patient with OA who gets inflamed DIP–R/O gout.

64. Any patient with fever, arthralgias, and tenosynovitis should be evaluated for a disseminated gonococcal infection (DGI).
    The majority of females develop DGI within 1 week of onset of menses.

65. Suspect coinfection with babesia or anaplasma in any Lyme disease patient with hemolysis, neutropenia, and/or thromboctopenia.

66. The chest radiograph is normal in 50% of patients who have tuberculous septic arthritis, which most commonly presents as chronic inflammatory monoarticular arthritis involving the knee.
    The diagnosis of tuberculous arthritis is best confirmed by synovial biopsy and culture because synovial fluid acid fast bacilli (AFB) stain is positive in only 20%.

67. Parvovirus is the most common viral arthritis and should be considered in any patient presenting with fever, rash, and arthritis particularly if they have exposure to children.

68. Hepatitis C is the most common cause of cryoglobulinemia.
    Overall, 50% of hepatitis C patients have cryoglobulins, but only 5% develop cryoglobulinemic vasculitis.

69. Gout is the most common cause of inflammatory arthritis in men over age 40 years.
    It should not occur in premenopausal females.

70. Uric acid is less soluble in the cold.
    Consequently, gout occurs in the cooler distal joints and not in the spine or joints near the spine. If you do not get any fluid when you tap the first MTP joint, blow out the end of the needle onto a slide and examine the blood speck for uric acid crystals.

71. In a gouty patient, the goal for uric acid lowering medications is to decrease the uric acid to <6.0 mg/dL; in tophaceous disease to <5.0 mg/dL.

72. CPPD disease is a disease of the elderly with onset and increasing frequency after the age of 55 years.
    Only patients with familial mutations or metabolic abnormalities (e.g., hemochromatosis, hypophosphatasia, etc.) get CPPD before age 55 years.

73. CPPD should be considered in any elderly patient with a seronegative inflammatory or degenerative arthritis involving the MCPs, wrists, and shoulders.
    CPPD can mimic seronegative RA, PMR, and OA involving atypical joints.

74. The diabetic stiff hand syndrome is related to disease duration and therapy and predicts microvascular complications of diabetes.

75. Hypothyroidism (thyroid-stimulating hormone always >20 mIU/L with low free T4) should be ruled out in patients with muscle symptoms and an elevated creatine kinase.

76. If a fracture is suspected as a cause of hemarthrosis, evaluate the synovial fluid for fat droplets which indicates release of bone marrow elements through bony disruption.

77. When palmar fasciitis presents in a female, think ovarian carcinoma.

78. Leukocytoclastic vasculitis is the most common paraneoplastic vasculitis presentation especially in patients with myelodysplastic syndromes.

79. Osteoporosis.
    - The major risk factors for fragility fractures are low bone mass, advancing age, previous fragility fractures, corticosteroid use, and the propensity to fall. The best predictor of a future fall is a fall within the previous 6 months. Screen the patient with the "get up and go" test.
    - Each decrease of –1.0 T-score on DXA correlates with a 12% loss of bone. At a T-score of –2.5, the patient has lost 30% of their bone mass, which is when osteopenia can reliably be detected on plain radiographs.
    - Rule out vitamin D insufficiency in all patients with a low bone mass. Consider celiac disease in any Caucasian patient with a low vitamin D level even if they do not have diarrhea.
    - Pharmacological therapy should be initiated in patients who have had a fragility fracture, a bone mineral density T-score ≤–2.5, or a FRAX-derived 10-year risk of ≥3% for hip fractures and ≥20% for other major osteoporosis fractures.

- Vertebroplasty and kyphoplasty are most effective when done within 6 months of onset of a severely symptomatic vertebral compression fracture and in patients with vertebral edema pattern on MRI.
- Stress fracture should be considered when new onset lower extremity bone pain (tibia, fibula, metatarsal) is increased by the vibration of a tuning fork (128 Hz) (sensitivity and specificity >80%).

80. Musculoskeletal manifestations can be the presenting manifestation in up to 33% of patients with hemochromatosis.
Consider in any Caucasian male under age 40 years with "seronegative RA," degenerative changes of the second and third MCP joints, and/or hypogonadotrophic hypogonadism with low bone mass.

81. Primary fibromyalgia does not occur for the first time in patients after the age of 55 years, nor is it likely to be the correct diagnosis in patients with musculoskeletal pain who also have abnormal laboratory values.

82. Fibromyalgia is a chronic noninflammatory, nonautoimmune central afferent processing disorder leading to a diffuse pain syndrome as well as other symptoms.
Narcotics and corticosteroids should not be used for treatment.

83. Obstructive sleep apnea (ask if they snore even if they are nonobese), hypothyroidism, and vitamin D deficiency (25 OH vitamin D <5 ng/mL) should be ruled out in all fibromyalgia patients regardless of body size.
In patients with severe and refractory symptoms, ask about physical and/or sexual abuse.

84. Growing pains do not occur during the daytime.
A limp in a child is pathologic until proven otherwise.

85. Malignancy is more likely than systemic JIA in any child who has fever, painful arthritis, an elevated LDH, and/or a low platelet count.

86. Neck or back pain in a young child is never normal and demands an extensive workup.

87. ANA positivity, female sex, and age less than 6 years old increase the risk of chronic uveitis regardless of the JIA subgroup.

88. Inflammatory myositis in childhood is almost always dermatomyositis and not polymyositis, whereas scleroderma in childhood is most commonly linear scleroderma.

89. Consider Kawasaki disease in any child under age 5 years presenting with prolonged high fevers and conjunctivitis.
Intravenous immunoglobulin (IVIG) within 10 days of disease onset is the treatment of choice.

90. Muscle cramps, pain, or myoglobinuria brought on by exercise suggests a metabolic myopathy.
    - Muscle symptoms with short bursts of high-intensity exercise and the second wind phenomenon are characteristic of a glycogen storage disease. McArdle's disease and acid maltase deficiency are most common.
    - Muscle symptoms with prolonged low-intensity exercise and/or prolonged fasting suggests a defect in fatty acid oxidation. Carnitine palmitoyltransferase II (CPT II) deficiency is most common.
    - The most common metabolic myopathies associated with myoglobinuria are CPT II deficiency and McArdle's disease.
    - The most common myopathies that are confused with polymyositis are acid maltase deficiency and limb-girdle muscular dystrophy.
    - Children presenting with a muscle disease without rash almost always have a metabolic or genetic myopathy and not primary polymyositis.

91. Abdominal fat pad aspiration is the easiest and most sensitive method of obtaining tissue to examine for amyloid deposition (polarized microscopy of Congo red-stained tissue).

92. Uveitis is frequently a symptom of an underlying disease and not the primary diagnosis.

93. A patient with acute, inflammatory arthritis involving bilateral ankles should always be evaluated for sarcoidosis.
    - Erythema nodosum typically affects the anterior aspect of lower legs and never ulcerates. Subcutaneous nodules on the posterior aspect of calf or any that ulcerate should raise concern for vasculitis or infection.

94. SLE and Sjögren's patients who have anti-Ro (SS-A) and anti-La (SS-B) antibodies are at increased risk for having infants who develop the neonatal lupus syndrome and complete heart block.

95. Autoinflammatory syndromes are characterized by episodes of fever, rash, arthritis, peritonitis, eye inflammation, lack of autoantibodies, and elevated acute phase reactants in various combinations that normalize between flares.
The duration of flares differs between diseases: TRAPS > HIDS > FMF > MWS/FCAS. Inhibition of interleukin-1 is the treatment of choice.

96. **Medications.**
    - Always rule out a medication as the cause of musculoskeletal symptoms.
      — pANCA vasculitis: hydralazine, propylthiouracil, minocycline, cocaine (levamisole).
      — Fluoroquinolones: Achilles tendinitis and rupture.
      — Drug-induced lupus: hydralazine, minocycline, anti-tumor necrosis factor (TNF) agents, rifabutin, procainamide, and others.
    - All NSAIDs should be used with caution (if at all) in patients with underlying renal or cardiovascular disease.
    - All NSAIDs can cause photosensitivity. Piroxicam is most likely to cause small bowel webs.
    - NSAIDs can interfere with conception.
    - Cortisol (Solucortef) 20 mg = prednisone 5 mg = prednisolone 5 mg = medrol 4 mg (Solumedrol) = decadron 0.75 mg.
    - Avascular necrosis (AVN) from corticosteroids is the most common reason a physician is sued for a medication adverse effect. Record in the chart that you counseled the patient on the following risk: for each 20 mg of prednisone taken for over a month, the risk of AVN is 5% (e.g., a 60-mg dose for a month confers a risk of 15% for AVN). Patients with SLE, those that have aPLabs, and those that rapidly become cushingoid are most at risk.
    - Choice of DMARD therapy is based on disease severity, comorbidities, and fertility plans.
    - Methotrexate is the most effective anchor drug for all combination therapies. An increase of the mean corpuscular volume by 5 fL correlates with a good methotrexate effect.
    - Hydroxychloroquine is less effective in smokers, can cause dizziness, and requires the patient to have eye examinations.
    - Sulfasalazine can cause reversible azospermia.
    - Azathioprine is better used for maintenance of remission than for induction of remission. It should not be used in patients on allopurinol, febuxostat, or ampicillin (rash). It can cause resistance to coumadin effectiveness.
    - Live vaccines should not be given to patients on biologic agents. Check a tuberculosis skin test (PPD) and immunize patients before biologic therapy.
    - Stop anti-TNF agents if a patient has an open wound until it heals.
    - Infliximab is most commonly associated with mycobacterial and fungal infections. Abatacept and rituximab are least associated.
    - Tocilizumab may interfere with the effectiveness of birth control pills. Do not use in patients at risk for bowel perforations (history of diverticulitis).
    - Rituximab works best in seropositive RA patients who have germinal centers in their synovium. Always send synovial tissue at time of any joint surgery to see if germinal centers are present.
    - Allopurinol hypersensitivity syndrome is more common in Asian patients with kidney disease and the HLA-B*5801 gene.
    - Do not use colchicine in patients who are on cyclosporine/tacrolimus (causes myopathy), antifungals (e.g., ketoconazole), or HIV protease inhibitors. Do not use in patients on clarithromycin who have renal insufficiency.
    - Pegloticase should not be used in patients with G6PD deficiency.
    - Stop ACE inhibitors in patients with chronic regional pain syndrome; stop calcium channel blockers in patients with erythromelalgia.
    - Do not inject a joint or soft tissue area (tendon) with corticosteroids more than 3 to 4 times within a year and never within 2 months of a previous injection. If an injection does not last 4 months, find a different therapeutic approach instead of repeatedly injecting the joint, tendon area, or bursa.
    - Voriconazole can cause nodular hypertrophic osteoarthropathy.

97. **"ADEPTTS"** (Ambulation, Dressing, Eating, Personal hygiene, Transfers, Toileting, Sleeping/sexual activities) is a useful mnemonic to screen for a patient's functional limitations.

98. **Rehabilitative techniques.**
    - A properly fitted cane used in the contralateral hand can unweight a diseased hip by 25% to 40%.
    - Fatigue for more than 1 hour or soreness for more than 2 hours after exercise indicates too much exercise for that arthritic patient.
    - Up to heaven, down to hell. When a patient has a painful lower extremity joint, tell him/her to use the good leg to step up a stair (up to heaven) and use the painful leg to step down a stair (down to hell).

99. **Surgery.**
    - There are two indications for joint replacement surgery: (1) pain unresponsive to medical therapy and (2) loss of joint function. Therefore, inability to walk more than one block, stand longer than 20 to 30 minutes due to pain, or walk up stairs are indications for total hip and total knee replacement.
    - Lumbar spine surgery is most successful in patients with radicular symptoms confirmed by clinical examination, EMG, and MRI findings who have failed conservative therapy. Success of surgery decreases by 33% for each one that does not confirm the other.

- Stop anti-TNF agents for at least one administration cycle before major surgery and restart when staples/stitches are out.
- Take vitamin C 500 mg daily starting just before and for 50 days after carpal tunnel syndrome surgery to lessen the chance of developing chronic regional pain syndrome.

100. Most rheumatic disease patients are considering, have tried, or are presently using **complementary and alternative medicine (CAM) therapies.**
 Physicians should ask patients about CAM therapies and record them in the medical record because some interact with other medications or can cause bleeding during surgery.
 I am sure the readers of this book have other TOP SECRETS. Please send them to me (Sterling.west@ucdenver.edu) for inclusion in the next edition.

CHAPTER 3

ANATOMY AND PHYSIOLOGY OF THE MUSCULOSKELETAL SYSTEM

Sterling G. West, MD

KEY POINTS

1. Collagen is the most abundant protein in the body. Mutations of collagen types I and II can lead to musculoskeletal disorders.
2. Hyaline cartilage is the major cartilage of diarthroidial joints. It is avascular and aneural and composed mainly of type II collagen and aggrecan.
3. Synovial fluid is a selective transudate of plasma. It is made viscous by the secretion of hyaluronic acid by synoviocytes into the synovial fluid.
4. The Wnt/β-catenin signaling pathway is a critical pathway for osteoblast activation and bone mass regulation.
5. The RANKL/RANK/OPG signaling pathway is critical for osteoclast differentiation/activation and bone remodeling.

1. **Name two major functions of the musculoskeletal system.**
   Structural support and purposeful motion. The activities of the human body depend on the effective interaction between joints and the neuromuscular units that move them.

2. **Name the five components of the musculoskeletal system.**
   (1) Muscles, (2) tendons, (3) ligaments, (4) cartilage, (5) bone. All of these structures contribute to the formation of a functional and mobile joint.

3. **The different connective tissues differ in their composition of macromolecules. List the major macromolecular "building blocks" of connective tissue.**
   Collagen, elastin and adhesins, and proteoglycans.

COLLAGEN

4. **How many types of collagen are there? In which tissues is each type most commonly found?**
   The collagens are the most abundant body proteins and account for 20% to 30% of the total body mass. There are at least 29 different types of collagen. The most common ones are listed in Table 3-1 and can be divided into seven subclasses. The unique properties and organization of each collagen type enable that specific collagen to contribute to the function of the tissue of which it is the principal structural component. Abnormalities of collagen types can cause disease.

5. **Discuss the structural features common to all collagen molecules.**
   The definitive structural feature of all collagen molecules is the **triple helix**. This unique conformation is due to three polypeptide chains (α-chains) twisted around each other into a right-handed major helix. Extending from the amino and carboxyl terminal ends of both helical domains of the α-chains are nonhelical components called telopeptides. In the major interstitial collagens, the helical domains are continuous, whereas in the other collagen classes the helical domains may be interrupted by 1 to 12 nonhelical segments.
   The primary structure of the helical domain of the α-chain is characterized by the repeating triplet Gly–X–Y. X and Y can be any amino acid but are most frequently proline and hydroxyproline, respectively. Overall, approximately 25% of the residues in the triple helical domains consist of proline and hydroxyproline. Hydroxylysine is also commonly found. In the most abundant interstitial collagens (i.e., type I, II), the triple helical region contains about 1000 amino acid residues $(Gly–X–Y)_{333}$ (Figure 3-1).

6. **Identify the major collagen classes and the types of collagen included in each class.**
   - Fibril-forming (interstitial)—types I, II, III, V, XI. The most abundant collagen class, these collagens form the extracellular fabric of the major connective tissues. They have the same tensile strength as steel wire.
   - Fibril-associated collagens with interrupted triple helices (FACIT)—types IX, XII, XIV. XVI, XIX. These collagens are associated with the interstitial (fibrillar) collagens and occur in the same tissues.
   - Collagens with specialized structures or functions:
   Basement membrane collagen—type IV.
   Nonfibrillar collagens—types VI, VII, XIII, XV, XVII, XVIII.
   Short-chain collagens—types VIII, X.

Table 3-1. Collagen Types, Tissue Distribution, and Diseases Caused by Mutations

CLASSES	TISSUE DISTRIBUTION	DISEASE
Fibril-Forming (Interstitial) Collagens		
Type I	Bone, tendon, skin, joint capsule/synovium	OI, ED
Type II	Hyaline cartilage, disk, vitreous humor	CD, Stickler's
Type III	Blood vessels, skin, lung	ED (vascular)
Type V	Same as type I	ED (classical)
Type XI	Same as type II	SED, Stickler's
Network-Forming Collagens		
Type IV*	Basement membrane	Alport syndrome
Type VIII	Endothelium, Descemet's membrane	Corneal dystrophy
Type X	Growth plate cartilage	MD
FACIT Collagens		
Type IX	Same as type II, cornea	MED
Type XII	Same as type I	
Type XIV	Same as type I	
Type XVI	Several tissues	
Type XIX	Rhabdomyosarcoma cells	
Beaded Filament-Forming Collagen		
Type VI	Most connective tissues	Rare muscle diseases
Collagen of Anchoring Fibrils		
Type VII	Dermoepidermal, cornea, oral mucosa	Epidermolysis bullosa dystrophica
Collagen with a Transmembrane Domain		
Type XIII	Endomysium, placenta, meninges	
Type XVII*	Skin, hemidesmosomes, cornea	
Other Collagen		
Type XV	Many tissues, especially muscle	Knobloch syndrome
Type XVIII	Many tissues	

CD, Chondrodysplasia; ED, Ehlers–Danlos syndrome; OI, osteogenesis imperfecta; MD, metaphyseal dysplasia; MED, multiple epiphyseal dysplasia; SED, spondyloepiphyseal dysplasia.
*Goodpasture syndrome results from an autoimmune response against collagen type IV; bullous pemphigoid results from an autoimmune response against collagen type XVII.

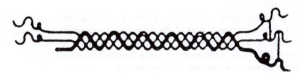

Figure 3-1. Diagram of interstitial (fibrillar) collagen molecule demonstrating triple helix configuration with terminal telopeptides.

7. How are the fibril-forming (interstitial) collagens synthesized?
   1. There are at least 30 distinct genes that encode the various collagen chains. In adults, collagen gene expression is subject to positive regulation (TGF-β) and negative regulation (IFN-γ and TNF-α). The collagen genes studied thus far contain coding sequences (exons) interrupted by large, noncoding sequences (introns). The DNA is transcribed to form a precursor mRNA, which is processed to functional mRNA by excising and splicing, which remove mRNA coded by introns. The processed mRNAs leave the nucleus and are transported to the polyribosomal apparatus in the rough endoplasmic reticulum for translation into polypeptide chains.
   2. The polypeptide chains are hydroxylated by prolyl hydroxylase and lysine hydroxylase. These enzymes require O_2, Fe^{2+}, α-ketoglutarate, and ascorbic acid (vitamin C) as cofactors. Hydroxyproline is critical to the stable formation of the triple helix. A decrease in hydroxyproline content as seen in scurvy (ascorbic acid deficiency) results in unstable molecules that lose their structures and are broken down by proteases.
   3. Glycosylation of hydroxylysine residues, which is important for secretion of procollagen monomers (molecules).
   4. Formation of interchain disulfide links, followed by procollagen triple-helix formation.

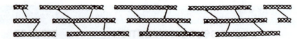

Figure 3-2. Self-assembly of collagen molecules into fibrils with cross-linking.

5. Secretion of procollagen into the extracellular space.
6. Proteolysis by procollagen peptidase of amino and carboxyl terminal telopeptides, resulting in conversion of procollagen to collagen.
7. Assembly of collagen monomers (molecules) into fibrils (microfibrils) by quarter-stagger shift, followed by cross-linking of fibrils.
8. End-to-end and lateral aggregation of fibrils to form collagen fiber.

Each collagen molecule is 300 nm in length and 1.5 nm in width and has five charged regions 68 nm apart. The charged regions align in a straight line when the fibrils are formed, even though the individual molecules themselves are staggered a quarter of their lengths in relation to each other. One can easily see that there are multiple steps where defects in collagen biosynthesis could result in abnormalities leading to disease (Figure 3-2; see also Chapter 55).

8. **Which enzymes are important in collagen degradation? How are they regulated?**
    The most important collagenolytic enzymes responsible for cleavage of type I collagen belong to the matrix metalloproteinase (MMP) group. The collagenases are secreted in latent form and, when activated, cleave the collagen molecule at a single specific site following a glycine residue located about three quarters of the distance from the amino terminal end (between residues 775 and 776 of the α1[I] chain). Gelatinases and stromelysins then degrade the unfolded fragments.
    Both α-macroglobulin and tissue inhibitors of metalloproteases (TIMP 1 to 4) are capable of inhibiting collagenase activity. It is likely that other collagen types have type-specific collagenases capable of degrading them. Serum procollagen peptides, urinary hydroxyproline, urinary pyridinoline/deoxypyridinoline cross-links, and serum C-telopeptides and urinary N-telopeptides are used as measures of collagen turnover.

ELASTIN AND ADHESINS

9. **What is elastin, and where is it located?**
    Elastin fibers are connective tissues that can stretch when hydrated and return to their original length after being stretched. They are synthesized by smooth muscle cells and less so by fibroblasts. They comprise a significant portion of the dry weight of ligaments (up to 70% to 80%), lungs, larger blood vessels such as aorta (30% to 60%), and skin (2% to 5%). Elastin is a polymer of tropoelastin monomers, which contain 850 amino acids, predominantly valine, proline, glycine, and alanine. When tropoelastin molecules associate to form a fiber, lysine residues cross-link by forming desmosine and isodesmosine, which are unique to elastin. Mutations in the elastin gene can cause **cutis laxa** and **supravalvular aortic stenosis**. Elastases, which are serine proteases, are capable of degrading elastase. Elastases are located in tissues, macrophages, leukocytes, and platelets. Such elastases may contribute to blood vessel wall damage and aneurysm formation in the vasculitides. Urinary desmosine levels are used as a measure of elastin degradation.

10. **What are fibrillin-1 and fibrillin-2?**
    These fibrillins are large glycoproteins coded for by a gene located on chromosome 15 (fibrillin-1) and chromosome 5 (fibrillin-2). They function as part of the microfibrillar proteins, which are associated with an elastin core. Fibrillin can also be found as isolated bundles of microfibrils in skin, blood vessels, and several other tissues. Abnormalities in fibrillin-1 are thought to cause Marfan's syndrome (see also Chapter 55), whereas abnormalities in fibrillin-2 cause contractural arachnodactyly.

11. **List the important adhesins (cell-binding glycoproteins) that can be present in intracellular matrices and basement membranes.**
    Fibronectin—connective tissue.
    Laminin—basement membrane.
    Chondroadherin—cartilage.
    Osteoadherin—bone.
    These glycoproteins have specific adhesive and other important properties. They bind cells by attaching to integrins on cells. Some have the classical arginine–glycine–aspartic acid (RGD) cell-binding sequence.

PROTEOGLYCANS

12. **How do a proteoglycan and a glycosaminoglycan differ?**
    Proteoglycans are glycoproteins that contain one or more sulfated glycosaminoglycan (GAG) chains. They are classified according to their core protein, which is coded for by distinct genes.
    GAGs are usually classified into five types: chondroitin sulfate, dermatan sulfate, heparan sulfate, heparin, and keratan sulfate. GAGs make up part of the proteoglycans.

13. **How are proteoglycans distributed?**
    Proteoglycans are synthesized by all connective tissue cells. They can remain associated with these cells on their cell surface (syndecan, betaglycan), intracellularly (serglycin), or in the basement membrane (perlecan). These cell-associated proteoglycans commonly contain heparin/heparan sulfate or chondroitin sulfate as their major GAGs. Alternatively, proteoglycans can be secreted into the extracellular matrix (aggrecan, decorin, biglycan, fibromodulin, lumican). These matrix proteoglycans usually contain chondroitin sulfate, dermatan sulfate, or keratan sulfate as their major GAGs. Decorin helps bind type II collagen fibers together in cartilage, whereas fibromodulin and lumican bind type II collagen to type IX.

14. **How are proteoglycans metabolized in the body?**
    Proteoglycans are degraded by proteinases, which release the GAGs. The GAGs are taken up by cells by endocytosis, where they are degraded in lysosomes by a series of glycosidases and sulfatases. Defects in these degradative enzymes can lead to diseases called **mucopolysaccharidoses**.

MUSCULOSKELETAL SYSTEM

15. **Discuss the classification of joints.**
    - **Synarthrosis:** suture lines of the skull where adjoining cranial plates are separated by thin fibrous tissue.
    - **Amphiarthroses:** adjacent bones are bound by flexible fibrocartilage that permits limited motion to occur. Examples include the pubic symphysis, part of the sacroiliac joint, and intervertebral discs.
    - **Diarthroses** (synovial joints): these are the most common and most mobile joints. All have a synovial lining. They are subclassified into ball and socket (hip), hinge (interphalangeal), saddle (first carpometacarpal), and plane (patellofemoral) joints.

16. **What major tissues comprise a diarthroidal (synovial) joint?**
    A diarthroidal joint consists of **hyaline cartilage** covering the surfaces of two or more opposing bones. These articular tissues are surrounded by a **capsule** that is lined by **synovium**. Some joints contain **menisci**, which are made of fibrocartilage. Note that the joint cavity is a potential space. The pressure within normal joints is negative (−5.7 cm H_2O) compared with ambient atmospheric pressure.

17. **Describe the microanatomy of normal synovium.**
    Normal synovium contains synovial lining cells that are one to three cells deep. Synovium lines all intracapsular structures except the contact areas of articular cartilage. The synovial lining cells reside in a matrix rich in type I collagen and proteoglycans.
    There are two main types of synovial lining cells, but these can be differentiated only by electron microscopy. **Type A** cells are macrophage-like and have primarily a phagocytic function. **Type B** cells are fibroblast-like and produce hyaluronate, which accounts for the increased viscosity of synovial fluid.
    Other cells found in the synovium include antigen-presenting cells called dendritic cells and mast cells. The synovium does not have a limiting basement membrane. Synovial tissue also contains fat and lymphatic vessels, fenestrated microvessels, and nerve fibers derived from the capsule and periarticular tissues.

18. **Why is synovial fluid viscous?**
    Hyaluronic acid, synthesized by synovial lining cells (type B), is secreted into the synovial fluid, making the fluid viscous. Synovial means "like egg white," which describes the normal viscosity of synovial fluid.

19. **What are the physical characteristics of normal synovial fluid from the knee joint?**
    Color—colorless and transparent.
    Amount—thin film covering surfaces of synovium and cartilage within joint space.
    Cell count—<200/mm^3 with <25% neutrophils.
    Protein—1.3 to 1.7 g/dl (20% of normal plasma protein).
    Glucose—within 20 mg/dl of the serum glucose level after 6 hours of fasting.
    Temperature—32° C (peripheral joints are cooler than core body temperature).
    String sign (measure of viscosity)—1 to 2 inches (2.5-5 cm).
    pH—7.4.

20. **What is the function, structure, and composition of articular cartilage?**
    Articular cartilage is **avascular** and **aneural**. It serves as a load-bearing connective tissue that can absorb impact and withstand shearing forces. Its ability to do this relates to the unique composition and structure of its extracellular matrix.
    Normal cartilage is composed of a sparse population of specialized cells called **chondrocytes** that are responsible for the synthesis and replenishment of extracellular matrix. This matrix consists mainly of collagen and proteoglycans. Most of the collagen is type II (>90%), which makes up 50% to 60% of the *dry* weight of cartilage. Collagen forms a fiber network that provides shape and form to the cartilage tissue.
    Proteoglycans comprise the second largest portion of articular cartilage. The proteoglycan monomers (aggrecan) are large (MW=2 to 3 million) and contain mostly keratan sulfate and chondroitin sulfate GAGs. The proteoglycans are arranged into supramolecular aggregates consisting of a central hyaluronic acid filament to which multiple proteoglycan monomers are noncovalently attached and stabilized by a link protein.

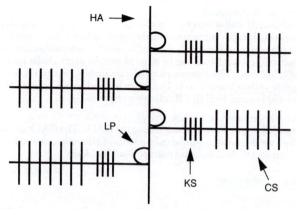

Figure 3-3. Diagram of a proteoglycan aggregate in articular cartilage. Hyaluronate (HA) is the backbone of the aggregate. Proteoglycan monomers (aggrecan) arise at intervals from either side of the hyaluronate core. CS, Chondroitin sulfate; KS, keratin sulfate; LP, link protein.

The entire structure looks like a large "bottle brush" and has a MW of 200 million (Figure 3-3). These proteoglycans are stuffed into the collagen framework. The negative charge of the proteoglycans causes them to spread out until the elastic forces are balanced by the tensile forces of the collagen. Note that other collagens (types V, VI, IX, X, XI), proteins (chondroadherin, others), and lipid are also present in cartilage. Water is the most abundant component of articular cartilage and accounts for 80% of the tissue wet weight. Water is held in cartilage by its interaction with matrix proteoglycan aggregates.

21. **What are the four zones of cartilage?**
    The different molecular components of cartilage are highly organized into a structure that varies with the depth of cartilage. From top to bottom, these four zones include:
    1. **Superficial (tangential) zone (10%)**—smallest zone. Collagen fibers are thin and are oriented horizontally to subchondral bone. Low GAG content. This zone is called the **lamina splendens**.
    2. **Middle (transitional) zone (50%)**—largest zone. Collagen fibers are thicker and start to be arranged into radial bundles. High proteoglycan and water content.
    3. **Deep (radial) zone (20%)**—largest collagen fibers arranged radially (perpendicular) to subchondral bone. Many chondrocytes.
    4. **Calcified zone**—separates cartilage from subchondral bone. Collagen fibers penetrate into this zone and anchor the cartilage to the bone.

22. **Cartilage does not have a blood supply; therefore how do chondrocytes obtain nutrition?**
    Adult cartilage is avascular, and chondrocytes obtain nutrients through diffusion. The nutrients are derived from the synovial fluid. Diffusion is facilitated during joint loading. With joint loading, some of the water in the cartilage is squeezed out into the synovial space. When the joint is unloaded, the hydrophilic properties of the cartilage proteoglycans cause the water to be sucked back into the cartilage. As the water returns to the cartilage, diffusion of nutrients from the synovial fluid is facilitated.

23. **If cartilage is not innervated, why do patients with osteoarthritis have pain?**
    Patients experience pain due to irritation of the subchondral bone, which is exposed as the cartilage degenerates. Additionally, accumulation of synovial fluid can cause pain through distention of the innervated joint capsule and synovium. Mild synovial inflammation also causes pain.

24. **Describe the lubrication of diarthroidal joints.**
    Diarthroidal (synovial) joints serve as mechanical bearings with coefficients of friction lower than the friction an ice skate generates as it glides over ice. Their three major sources of lubrication are:
    - Hydrodynamic lubrication: loading of the articular cartilage causes compression that forces water out of the cartilage. This fluid forms an aqueous layer that separates and protects the opposing cartilage surfaces.
    - Boundary layer lubrication: a small glycoprotein called **lubricin**, which is produced by synovial lining cells, binds to articular cartilage where it retains a protective layer of water molecules.
    - Hyaluronic acid: produced by synovial lining cells, this molecule lubricates the contact surface between synovium and cartilage. It does not contribute to cartilage on cartilage lubrication.

25. **Discuss the normal matrix turnover of articular cartilage.**
    In normal articular cartilage, chondrocytes rarely divide. Chondrocytes synthesize and replace the extracellular matrix components. Proteoglycans have a faster turnover rate ($t_{1/2}$ of weeks) compared with collagen ($t_{1/2}$ of years). The degradation of these macromolecules is accomplished by proteolytic enzymes. MMPs, such as the

secreted collagenase MMP-13 and the membrane-anchored MMP-14, are most important in collagen type II breakdown. Two aggrecanases (ADAMTS 4 and 5) are metalloproteinases that degrade aggrecan, the major proteoglycan in cartilage, between the Glu^{373} and Ala^{374} bond. Gelatinases (MMP-2, MMP-9) and stromelysins (MMP-3, MMP-10) further degrade the collagen and proteoglycan fragments. Cytokines such as interleukin-1 and tumor necrosis factor-α (TNF-α) can upregulate the degradative process, whereas transforming growth factor-β and insulin-like growth factor-1 have an anabolic effect on chondrocyte metabolism. Assays using monoclonal antibodies to measure type II collagen and proteoglycans (keratan sulfate, COMP) in bodily fluids have been used to detect cartilage breakdown.

26. **What is the difference between a ligament and a tendon?**
   A **ligament** is a specialized form of connective tissue, which attaches one bone to another. It frequently reinforces the joint capsule and provides stability to the joint. A **tendon** attaches a muscle to a bone. Both are comprised mostly of type I collagen.

27. **What is a bursa?**
   A **bursa** is a closed sac lined with mesenchymal cells. Bursae facilitate gliding of one tissue over another. There are approximately 160 in the body which form during embryogenesis. Trauma, overuse, and inflammation may lead to formation of new bursae or enlargement of existing ones.

28. **How many bones are there in the skeleton? Discuss the types and composition of bone.**
   - The human skeleton (from the Greek, *skeletos*, "dried up") consists of 206 bones (126 appendicular bones, 74 axial bones, and 6 ossicles).
   - Bone is a mineralized connective tissue. It is comprised of two subtypes: **cortical** (or compact) bone and **cancellous** (or trabecular) bone. Cortical bone comprises 80% of the skeleton and is increased in long bone shafts. Cancellous bone is in contact with bone marrow cells and is enriched in the vertebral bodies, pelvis, and proximal ends of femora, all of which are subject to osteoporosis and fractures. Bone remodeling normally replaces 25% of the trabecular bone and 3% of the cortical bone each year.
   - Bone is comprised mainly of type I collagen and contains three cell types: **osteoclasts**, which resorb mineralized bone; **osteoblasts**, which synthesize the proteins of the bone matrix; and **osteocytes**, which are probably osteoblasts that have secreted bone matrix and become buried within it. Osteocytes communicate with each other through a canalicular system and play a role in response to mechanical loading. The skeleton contains 99% of the total calcium, 80% to 85% of the total phosphorus, and 66% of the total magnesium in the body.

29. **Which pathway regulates bone metabolism though osteoblast signaling?**
   The **Wnt/β-catenin** signaling pathway (Figure 3-4) is a critical component of bone mass regulation and is required for bones to respond to mechanical loading. The Wnt signaling cascade is triggered upon binding of members of the Wnt family of lipid-modified proteins (more than 12) to a coreceptor complex comprising low-density lipoprotein receptor-related proteins 5 or 6 (LRP 5 or 6) and frizzled protein (Frz). Activation of this receptor complex leads to activation of Dishevelled (Dsh). Dsh then inactivates GSK-3β. This prevents GSK-3β from phosphorylating β-catenin which, when phosphorylated, is targeted for ubiquitination and proteosomal degradation. Thus β-catenin is able to accumulate in the cytoplasm. Upon reaching a certain concentration, the β-catenin translocates to the nucleus where it combines with the Tcf/Lef family of transcription factors, which regulate the expression of specific osteoblastic genes necessary for bone formation. There are three extracellular proteins that regulate Wnt binding. One is secreted frizzled protein which binds and neutralizes Wnt protein. The other two are sclerostin (Scler) and dickkopf (Dkk-1) proteins which are produced by osteocytes and bind to LRP5/6 and prevent Wnt signaling through these receptors. Notably LRP5 mutations have been associated with both low and high bone mass. Sclerostin mutations have been linked to **osteosclerosis** (van Buchem syndrome) because of their inability to block Wnt signaling. Monoclonal antibodies against sclerostin are being tested as a therapy for osteoporosis.

30. **Which pathway regulates bone metabolism through osteoclast signaling?**
   The RANKL/RANK/OPG signaling pathway involves members of the TNF superfamily and is a critical pathway for the regulation of osteoclast activation and bone remodeling (Figure 3-5). **RANKL** (receptor activator of NF-κB ligand) is a cell membrane-bound ligand (can also be secreted) on osteoblasts, activated T cells, and other cells. It binds **RANK** on osteoclast precursors, which causes the osteoclast to differentiate and become activated. In most cases, RANKL is also assisted by macrophage colony-stimulated factor (M-CSF) as a cofactor for osteoclast differentiation. **Osteoprotegerin** (OPG) is a soluble, regulatory cytokine secreted by osteoblasts that competitively binds RANKL and prevents its binding to RANK, thus inhibiting osteoclastogenesis. Expression of RANKL on osteoblasts is stimulated through vitamin D receptor (1,25 OH vitamin D_3), protein kinase A (PGE_2, parathyroid hormone), and gp 130 (IL-11). Cytokines (IL-1, IL-7, IL-17, TNF-α, M-CSF) and glucocorticoids also upregulate RANKL expression while downregulating OPG production. The periarticular osteoporosis and erosions seen on radiographs of individuals with inflammatory arthritis may be through local production of PGE_2 and interleukins (TNF-α, IL-1), causing upregulation of RANKL on osteoblasts and T cells leading to osteoclast activation. Conversely, blocking RANKL (i.e., denosumab) is a therapy for osteoporosis. Genetic disorders due to mutations in this signaling pathway have been reported. Activating mutations of RANK cause diseases characterized by bone deformities, dental defects, and deafness. An inactivating mutation of OPG is associated with juvenile Paget's disease.

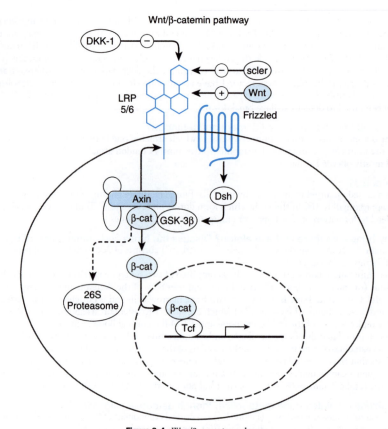

Figure 3-4. Wnt/β-catenin pathway.

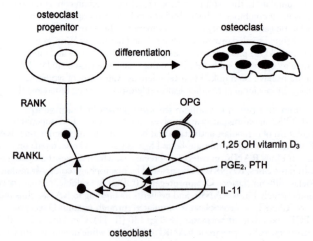

Figure 3-5. RANKL–RANK-OPG system.

31. **How many muscles are in the human body?**
    Approximately 640. Muscles constitute up to 40% of the adult body mass.

32. **Discuss the morphology of muscle.**
    - Skeletal muscle consists of cells called **fibers**. Fibers are grouped into **fascicles**.
    - Muscle fibers are part of **motor units** that consist of a lower motor neuron originating from a spinal cord anterior horn cell and all the muscle fibers it innervates. All muscle fibers within a motor unit are of the same type. Different fibers within a single fascicle are innervated by different motor neurons.
    - Muscle fibers are divided into three types based on their metabolism and response to stimuli: types 1, 2a, and 2b. Fiber type can be altered by reinnervation with a different motor neuron type, physical training (controversial), or disease processes. However, heredity is the most important determinant of fiber type distribution. On average, muscle contains 40% type 1 and 60% type 2 fibers.
    - Each muscle fiber is surrounded by a plasma membrane called a **sarcolemma**. Fibers contain **myofilaments** called actin, troponin, tropomyosin, and myosin, which are contractile proteins. The myofilaments are bathed in sarcoplasm and organized into **fibrils**, which are enveloped by the sarcoplasmic reticulum. Communication between the sarcolemma and sarcoplasmic reticulum occurs through a channel network called the **T-tubule system**.

33. **Describe the characteristics of the three types of muscle fibers.**
    - **Type 1** (slow twitch, oxidative fibers) (red fiber): respond to electrical stimuli slowly. Fatigue-resistant with repeated stimulation. Many mitochondria and higher lipid content. Endurance training (long-distance running) enhances metabolism of these fibers.
    - **Type 2a** (fast twitch, oxidative-glycolytic fibers): properties intermediate between type 1 and type 2b.
    - **Type 2b** (fast twitch, glycolytic fibers) (white fiber): respond rapidly and with greater force of contraction but fatigue rapidly. These fibers contain more glycogen and have higher myophosphorylase and myoadenylate deaminase activity. Strength training (weight-lifting, sprinters, jumpers) leads to hypertrophy of these fibers.

34. **How does muscle contraction and relaxation occur?**
    Muscle contraction occurs by shortening of myofilaments within muscle fibers. Stimulation causes an **action potential** to be transmitted along the sarcolemma, then through the T-tubule system to the sarcoplasmic reticulum. This causes release of calcium into the sarcoplasm. As the calcium concentration increases, **actin** is released from a state of inhibition, allowing actin-myosin cross-linkage and shortening of the myofilaments. The muscle fiber shortens until calcium is actively pumped back into the sarcoplasmic reticulum, which breaks the cross-links causing the fiber to relax. ATP, electrolytes (Na, K, Ca, Mg) and three ATPase proteins contribute to normal fiber contraction and relaxation. (See also Chapter 72.)

BIBLIOGRAPHY

Baron R, Rawadi G: Minireview: targeting the Wnt/β catenin pathway to regulate bone formation in the adult skeleton, Endocrinology 148:2635–2643, 2007.
Goldring SR, Goldring MB: Biology of the normal joint. In Firestein GS, Budd RS, Gabriel SE, McInnes IB, O'Dell JR, editors: Kelley's textbook of rheumatology, ed 9, Philadelphia, 2013, Elsevier Saunders. 2013, pp 1-19.
Goldring MB: Cartilage and chondrocytes. In Firestein GS, Budd RS, Gabriel SE, McInnes IB, O'Dell JR, editors: Kelley's textbook of rheumatology, ed 9, Philadelphia, 2013, Elsevier Saunders. 2013, pp 33-60.
Kearns AE, Sundeep K, Kostenuik PJ: Receptor activator of nuclear factor κβ ligand and osteoprotegerin regulation of bone remodeling in health and disease, Endocrine Rev 29:155–192, 2008.
Miller MS, Palmer BM, Toth MJ, et al: Muscle: anatomy, physiology, and biochemistry. In Firestein GS, Budd RS, Gabriel SE, McInnes IB, O'Dell JR, editors: Kelley's textbook of rheumatology, ed 9, Philadelphia, 2013, Elsevier Saunders. 2013, pp 67-78.
Okada Y: Proteinases and matrix degradation. In Firestein GS, Budd RS, Gabriel SE, McInnes IB, O'Dell JR, editors: Kelley's textbook of rheumatology, ed 9, Philadelphia, 2013, Elsevier Saunders. 2013, pp 97-116.
Schett G: Biology, physiology, and morphology of bone. In Firestein GS, Budd RS, Gabriel SE, McInnes IB, O'Dell JR, editors: Kelley's textbook of rheumatology, ed 9, Philadelphia, 2013, Elsevier Saunders. 2013, pp 61-66.

CHAPTER 4: OVERVIEW OF THE IMMUNE RESPONSE, INFLAMMATION, AND AUTOIMMUNITY

Sterling G. West, MD

The origin of all science is in the desire to know causes.
William Hazlitt, 1829

Science has been seriously retarded by the study of what is not worth knowing, and what is not knowable.
Johann Wolfgang von Goethe, 1825

KEY POINTS

1. The innate immune system (IIS) is the first line of defense and recognizes specific molecular components found only in microbial pathogens.
2. The IIS is necessary to activate and instruct the adaptive immune system (AIS).
3. T cell activation requires two signals: (1) contact of T cell receptor (TCR) with the major histocompatibility complex (MHC)–peptide complex and (2) engagement of costimulatory molecules.
4. T cells are critical for both humoral and cellular adaptive immunity.
5. Autoimmunity results when there is loss of tolerance to self-antigens.

1. **What are the two broad categories of immunity involved in host defense?**
   The categories of immunity are given in Table 4-1.

INNATE IMMUNITY

2. **What is the function of the innate immune system? How is it activated?**
   Innate immunity is present from birth, genetically determined, and not permanently altered by exposure to a foreign antigen. The IIS is phylogenetically older than the adaptive (specific/acquired) immune system. Because clonal expansion of lymphocytes in the adaptive immune system takes 3 to 5 days to differentiate into effector cells, there needs to be a system capable of controlling a pathogen during that time so that it does not damage the host. The effector mechanism of the IIS is activated immediately (20 to 30 minutes) and can rapidly control the replication of the infecting pathogens until the lymphocytes can deal with it. Furthermore, the IIS can interact with and control the adaptive immune responses.
   Alarmins are endogenous molecules that are constitutively available and passively released from necrotic cells upon infection or tissue injury. They are also secreted by stimulated leukocytes and epithelia. Once released they activate the IIS through **pattern-recognition receptors (PRRs)** such as Toll-like receptors (TLR2 and TLR4). Alarmins activate and recruit antigen-presenting cells (APCs) including dendritic cells (DCs). Examples of alarmins are:
   - High-mobility group protein B1 (HMGB1): can be released from any cell type. Proinflammatory when bound to other **danger-associated molecular patterns (DAMPs)** and **pathogen-associated molecular patterns (PAMPs).**
   - S100A8/A9/A12: released by epithelial cells and phagocytes causing inflammation with increased neutrophil adhesion, migration, and release from bone marrow. Some antibacterial activity.
   - Heat shock proteins (HSP60, HSP70): autoantigens stimulating pathways to suppress inflammation.
   - Antimicrobial peptides (AMPs): the main AMPs are **β-defensins** and **cathelicidin.** They are secreted by epithelial cells to form a microbial shield when the physical barriers (skin and mucous membranes) become injured. The AMPs integrate into the outer cell membranes of invading microbes to form pores that disrupt the integrity of the microbes. AMPs serve as chemoattractants for innate (neutrophils, DCs) and adaptive (lymphocytes) immune cells. AMPs can govern the composition of commensal microbes that colonize body surfaces. Abnormal AMP production may contribute to diseases such as psoriasis and Crohn's disease.

3. **What are the mechanisms that the innate immune system uses to recognize that an invading pathogen is foreign?**
   The strategy of the IIS is to recognize and interact with a few highly conserved structural motifs specific to microbes. These structures are called PAMPs, and the receptors of the IIS that recognize them are called PRRs. PAMPs are produced only by microbial pathogens and not by the host. Examples of PAMPs include bacterial lipopolysaccharides, peptidoglycan, mannans, flagellin, and bacterial and viral DNA/RNA.

Table 4-1. Categories of Immunity

	INNATE (NATURAL) IMMUNITY	ADAPTIVE (SPECIFIC/ACQUIRED) IMMUNITY
Physical barriers	Skin, mucous membranes	Mucosal immune systems
Circulating factors	Complement, CRP, MBL	Antibody
Cells	Macrophages, neutrophils, NK cells, dendritic cells, eosinophils, basophils, mast cells	Lymphocytes
Cell derived mediators	Monokines, chemokines, and interferons	Lymphokines (interleukins)

CRP, C-reactive protein; MBL, mannose-binding lectin; NK, natural killer.

4. **Name the pattern-recognition receptors that recognize pathogen-associated molecular patterns.**
   There are two broad categories of PRRs:
   - Secreted and circulating PRRs. These include the following:
     - **Collectins**—these are secreted collagen-like proteins that bind to carbohydrate or lipids in microbial cell walls and can be antimicrobial or activate the complement system. **Mannan-binding lectin (MBL)** is synthesized in the liver and secreted into the serum as part of the acute phase response. It binds to microbial carbohydrates to initiate the lectin pathway of complement activation (see Question 26). The MBL has mannose-associated serine proteases (MASP-2) that function like C1r and C1s to activate the classical complement pathway. MBL deficiency is associated with frequent infections.
     - **Lectins**—these are proteins that bind to microbial carbohydrates. In addition to MBL, this group include **ficolins** 1/2/3 and **galectins.** MBL and ficolins can bind to microbes and activate complement through the lectin pathway. Galectins can disrupt microbial membranes in the absence of complement.
     - **Pentraxins**—this group includes **C-reactive protein** (CRP), serum amyloid P, and pentraxin-3 (PTX3). All have a pentraxin domain with five subunits and are secreted as part of the acute phase response due to proinflammatory cytokines such as interleukin-6 (IL-6). **CRP** can fix C1q and activate complement to opsonize the organism for phagocytic clearance. PTX3 binds endothelial P-selectin to decrease neutrophil recruitment and suppress inflammation.
   - **Cell associated PRRs.** These include the following:
     - **TLRs**—there are at least 10 human TLRs. Some (TLR1, TLR2, TLR4, TLR5, and TLR6) are on cell surfaces (especially cells of the IIS) and recognize many of the PAMPs of foreign microbes. Each TLR is stimulated by a different PAMP (TLR1, TLR2, TLR6–lipoprotein; TLR4–lipopolysaccharide; TLR5–flagellin). In addition, they also recognize DAMPs that are endogenous molecules (alarmins) released by dead and necrotic cells. Stimulation of TLRs by the corresponding PAMPs or DAMPs initiates signaling cascades leading to activation of transcription factors (AP-1, NF-κB, IRFs). This results in induction of inflammatory and immune response genes with subsequent production of interferons (IFNs), proinflammatory cytokines (IL-1, IL-6, TNF), chemokines (IL-8), and other effector cytokines that attract more innate immune cells and direct the adaptive immune response.
     - **PRRs linked to phagocytosis**—macrophages have **scavenger receptors** and the **mannose receptor** binds bacteria and fungi, respectively, and facilitates phagocytic clearance, cytokine release, and activation of immune cells. **Dectin-1** is a lectin receptor on host cells that binds glucans on fungi. Mutations can lead to recurrent mucocutaneous fungal infections. The **formyl peptide receptor** on host cells binds N-formylmethionine from bacteria leading to the release of chemoattractants and facilitates phagocytosis.
     - **Intracellular PRRs**—includes some TLRs, **NOD-like receptors (NLRs)**, and RIG-I-like receptors (RLRs). TLR3, TLR7, TLR8, TLR9, and TLR10 reside inside the cell in endolysosomes. The endolysosomes contain bacterial and viral breakdown products, including nucleic acid, which bind to their corresponding TLR (TLR3–viral dsRNA; TLR7/8–ssRNA; TLR9–CpG-DNA) leading to production of IFNs and proinflammatory cytokines. NLRs include NOD1, NOD2, CARDs, NALPs, and NAIPs. Activation of NLRs leads to formation of an intracellular complex called the inflammasome, which contributes to the processing and secretion of IL-1 and IL-18. Urate crystals and peptidoglycans are examples of PAMPs that activate NLRs. Polymorphisms of the NOD2 gene are associated with Crohn's disease. **RIG-I-like receptors (RLRs)** include RIG1, MDA5, and LGP2. RLRs react with double-stranded RNA (dsRNA) and mediate production of type 1 IFNs.

5. **What cells are important in the innate immune system?**
   - **Phagocytes:** contain PRRs and are critical effector cells of the IIS.
     - **Neutrophils**—first cells recruited to sites of inflammation by a variety of chemotactic signals (e.g., AMPs, N-formyl bacterial oligopeptide, C5a, leukotriene B4, IL-8). Neutrophils use at least two mechanisms to neutralize an invading microbe:
       - Neutrophils phagocytose the invading microbe opsonized by the IIS. The phagosome containing the microbe merges with intracellular granules with microbicidal peptides, proteases, and highly reactive oxidizing agents generated by NADPH oxidase resulting in microbial death. Note that even in the

absence of infection, billions of neutrophils normally leave the bone marrow, circulate, enter tissues, and die each day. When they die they undergo apoptosis and are processed by macrophages so that they do not release their toxic constituents into normal tissues (efferocytosis). The macrophages that phagocytize the apoptotic neutrophils release antiinflammatory cytokines to maintain homeostasis.
- Neutrophil extracellular traps (NETs): upon activation neutrophils release granule (azurophilic, specific) proteins and histones that are bound to DNA that bind and kill microbes (bacteria, fungi) extracellularly independent of phagocytic uptake.
* **Monocytes and macrophages**—monocytes are the circulating precursors of macrophages. Macrophages are specific to tissues (e.g., Kupffer cells in the liver) and contain PRRs. Macrophages digest microbes and present them to lymphocytes to initiate the adaptive immune response. Macrophages secrete over 100 proteins including cytokines (both proinflammatory and antiinflammatory) that mediate inflammation.
* **Natural killer (NK) cells**: are potent cytotoxic cells whose targets are not MHC-restricted. They make up 5% to 10% of the recirculating lymphocyte population, express CD16 and CD56 cell surface markers, and look like large granular lymphocytes. They express PRRs and respond to viral infections and tumors. NK cells have killer cell immunoglobulin (Ig)-like receptors (KIRs), which recognize MHC class I molecules. Cells that are infected with viruses or are malignant downregulate their MHC class I receptors and upregulate stress ligands, signaling NK cells to induce apoptosis of the abnormal cell. NK cells have granules with perforins and granzymes, which are released upon NK cell activation to kill the target cell. Activated NK cells also secrete IFN-γ in addition to other cytokines. Dendritic cells recruit and activate NK cells by secreting type I IFNs, IL-12, and IL-18.
* **Other cells exhibiting PRRs**: epithelial cells express PRRs and can react to infection and secrete AMPs and IL-8 (CXCL8), which are neutrophil chemoattractants. Mast cells have PRRs and release tumor necrosis factor (TNF)-α and IL-8. They also make inflammatory mediators [histamine, leukotrienes, platelet-activating factor (PAF)], proteases (tryptase, chymase), and defensins. Platelets express PRRs and can produce cytokines recruiting leukocytes to sites of tissue damage. They also release microparticles that may modulate the immune response. Eosinophils are specialized leukocytes whose granules contain numerous toxic products, including major basic protein, eosinophil peroxidase, and eosinophil cationic protein. These products are especially toxic to helminths. Activated eosinophils also produce large quantities of leukotriene C4 (LTC_4) and transforming growth factor (TGF)-β that promote increased venular permeability and fibroblast-dependent fibrosis, respectively.
* **Dendritic cells**: are "professional" APCs. They serve as a link between the IIS and the AIS. They are located in tissues in contact with the external environment including the skin and mucous membranes of the respiratory, gastrointestinal (GI), and genitourinary (GU) tracts. They are also in lymphoid tissues and in most solid organs. There are two major types of DCs: **myeloid DCs** (mDCs) and **plasmacytoid DCs** (pDCs). Most mDCs are derived from monocytes and a few from lymphoid cells. They display TLR2 and TLR4. The major cytokine that mDCs produce is IL-12 and it is the most important cell needed to activate naïve T cells. Plasmacytoid DCs resemble plasma cells and comprise <1% of peripheral blood mononuclear cells. They display TLR7 and TLR9. They rapidly secrete large amounts of type I IFN (IFN-α and IFN-β) following viral stimulation. They can induce Th1-type and Th2-type AIS responses.

6. **What are the important endothelial adhesion molecules involved in the influx of neutrophils and mononuclear cells into a damaged or infected tissue?**
The important endothelial adhesion molecules involved in the influx of neutrophils and mononuclear cells into a damaged or infected tissue are given in Table 4-2.

Table 4-2. Important Endothelial Adhesion Molecules Involved in the Influx of Neutrophils and Mononuclear Cells Into a Damaged or Infected Tissue*

TIME TO ACTIVATION	LEUKOCYTE	ACTIVATED ENDOTHELIUM
<2 h	L-selectin PSGL-1 (unactivated neutrophil/monos)	CD34, GlyCAM-1, MADCAM-1, P-selectin (Weibel–Palade bodies)
<4 h	ESL-1	E-selectin (ELAM-1)
<12 h	LFA-1 (CD11a/CD18) (activated neutrophil/monos)	ICAM-1 (CD54)
<24 h	Mac-1 (CD11b/CD18) (activated neutrophils/monos) PECAM1 (activated neutrophils/monos)	ICAM-1 Endothelial PECAM1
<48 h	VLA-4 (CD49d/CD29) (lymphocytes, monocytes, adhesion molecules)	VCAM-1 (CD106)

*Note that CD34, PSGL-1, and ESL-1 all contain sialylated carbohydrate determinants related to Sialyl Lewis (CD15). Platelet endothelial adhesion molecules (PECAMs) are concentrated at endothelial junctions and are critical for transmigration of cells. The time to adhesion molecule activation explains why neutrophils and monocytes/macrophages enter the inflammatory site first (acute inflammation) and lymphocytes enter later (chronic inflammation).

7. **Name the four cardinal signs of inflammation. What are the underlying mechanisms responsible for the signs of inflammation?**
   1. Erythema (rubor).
   2. Warmth (calor).
   3. Swelling (tumor).
   4. Pain (dolor).

   Local arteriolar dilation produces erythema and warmth. Permeability increases in the postcapillary venules, allowing vascular fluid to leak into the surrounding tissue to produce swelling (edema). Pain is a result of the action of numerous inflammatory mediators and inflammatory cell derived products on local nerves. **Note that these symptoms and signs are the result of innate immune system activation.**

8. **What are the major classes of inflammatory mediators that facilitate inflammation during the innate immune system response?**

VASOACTIVE MEDIATORS	CHEMOTACTIC FACTORS
Histamine	Complement products (C3a, C5a)
Arachidonic acid products	Leukotriene B_4
—Prostaglandins	Platelet-activating factor (PAF)
—Leukotrienes	Chemokines (IL-8, other CXCLs)
Platelet-activating factor (PAF)	**Proinflammatory cytokines**
Kinins	Interleukins 1 and 6
Enzymes	Tumor necrosis factor
Tryptase	Interferons
Chymase	

9. **How are prostaglandins and leukotrienes formed?**

   Unlike histamine (which is a preformed and stored mediator), prostaglandins (PGs) and leukotrienes require active synthesis. The initial source molecule is arachidonic acid (an omega-6 polyunsaturated free fatty acid), which is liberated from cell membrane phospholipids by cytoplasmic phospholipase A_2 that is bound to the cell membrane. Once formed, arachidonic acid can be metabolized by either of two enzyme pathways (see Figure 4-1):
   - Cyclooxygenase pathway—results in PGs. The amount and type of PG made by a cell or tissue is determined by the expression levels of COX-1, COX-2, and cell specific terminal synthase enzymes (e.g., platelets only make thromboxane A_2 because platelets contain only COX-1 and thromboxane synthase).
   - Lipoxygenase pathway—results in leukotrienes and hydroxyeicosatetraenoic acids.

   Once formed, PGs are exported from cells by the multidrug resistance-associated protein family of efflux transporters. The PG actions are mediated by binding to G-protein-coupled receptors. There are at least nine receptors mediating various PG effects.

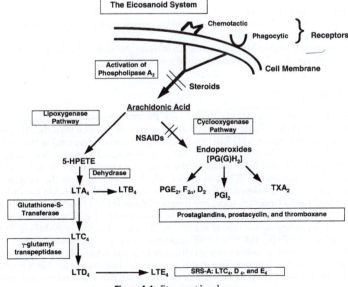

Figure 4-1. Eicosanoid pathways.

10. **How do prostaglandins and leukotrienes promote inflammation?**
PGs (especially PGD_2) induce local vasodilation and increased vascular permeability. PGE_2 is the most abundant PG at sites of inflammation and can have both proinflammatory and antiinflammatory effects depending on the receptor it activates. LTs fall into the following classes: LTC_4, LTD_4, and LTE_4 induce smooth muscle contraction, bronchoconstriction, and mucous secretion. They were once collectively called slow reacting substance of anaphylaxis (SRS-A). LTB_4 has none of the above properties but is a potent chemotactic factor for neutrophils. Note that omega-3 polyunsaturated free fatty acids from dietary sources can serve as substrates for COX and lipoxygenase leading to the generation of resolvins and protectins, which are antiinflammatory.

11. **Describe the initial events in chronological order resulting in an inflammatory response against a microbial pathogen.**
    - The invading microbe breaches the epithelial physical barrier. Antimicrobial proteins (defensins, cathelicidin) are secreted by epithelial cells.
    - Innate immune system responds—the alternate complement pathway is activated by C3 and factor B binding to the microbial membrane. The classical complement pathway is activated by the CRP and MBL pathway.
    - N-Formylmethionyl peptides from the microbe stimulate seven α-helical transmembrane receptors on neutrophils and macrophages. These peptides are chemoattractants and activators of the neutrophils, and thus they upregulate integrins for binding to endothelium and produce reactive oxygen intermediates to kill microbes.
    - Local macrophages phagocytize the microbe by mannose and scavenger receptors and complement receptors as a result of the complement opsonized microbe. Other plasma proteins and natural antibodies can also opsonize the microbe to facilitate phagocytosis.
    - Activation of macrophage TLRs by PAMPs and DAMPs signal cytokine (IL-1, IL-6, IL-8, TNF) release.
    - Prostaglandins and leukotrienes are released in response to cytokines (IL-1, TNF-α) and other stimuli. IL-6 stimulates the liver to synthesize more acute phase proteins (CRP, fibrinogen, α1 antitrypsin, α2 macroglobulin, haptoglobin, serum amyloid A). The acute phase response causes elevated erythrocyte sedimentation rate (ESR) and CRP and decreased albumin.
    - Interleukin-1 and TNF upregulate endothelial cell adhesion molecules to facilitate the influx of neutrophils, monocytes, and lymphocytes into the area.
    - Complement activation products (C3a, C5a), IL-8, LTB_4, and PAF are chemoattractants for neutrophils and circulating monocytes. Monocytes enter the inflammatory site and become macrophages.
    - Neutrophils phagocytize microbes. Specific granules filled with degradative enzymes (lysozyme, collagenase, elastase) and azurophilic granules (lysosomes) destroy the phagocytized microbe. Neutrophils die at the inflammatory site, contributing to inflammation.
    - Monocytes and macrophages become dominant effector cells 24 to 48 hours into inflammation. Phagocytize opsonized microbes and release further inflammatory and antiinflammatory mediators.
    - Inflammatory mediators released throughout this process contribute to cardinal signs of inflammation.
    PGE_2: vasodilation (redness, warmth), increased vascular permeability (swelling), and increased pain sensitivity to bradykinin.
    Prostacyclin (PGI_2): vasodilation.
    Thromboxane A_2: platelet activation.
    Platelet-activating factor: vasodilation, increased vascular permeability, platelet activation.
    Bradykinin: activate nerve fibers (pain).
    - APCs present antigen bound to MHC molecules to activate the acquired (adaptive) immune system (T and B lymphocytes). Occurs 3 to 5 days after microbial invasion.

ADAPTIVE IMMUNITY

12. **How does the innate immune system interact with the acquired immune system?**
If the IIS cannot completely handle the invading foreign antigen or microbe then the AIS is stimulated to respond. Pattern recognition receptors (PRRs) on APCs (e.g., mannose receptors) of the IIS bind pathogens, which are endocytosed. The most important APCs are immature DCs in the skin, lung, and mucous membranes that become activated by internalizing the antigen and by the cytokine milieu caused by the IIS. The activated DC upregulates CCR7 on its surface, which causes it to leave the local area and migrate toward the chemokine CCL21 produced by the lymphoid tissues. Note that the AIS can only be activated in organized lymphoid tissues (mucosal-associated lymphoid tissue [MALT], lymph node, spleen, etc.). The phagocytized pathogen is processed in the DCs/APCs and presented to T cells in the context of MHC class I or class II molecules depending on the type of antigen. Furthermore, binding of PAMPs to TLRs/PRRs signals the APC to upregulate CD80 (B7-1)/CD86 (B7-2) and other costimulatory molecules (e.g., CD40) on the surface of the APC. Note that unlike other somatic cells, only DCs and other APCs constitutively express MHC class II molecules and have the necessary costimulatory molecules to activate the AIS. Only when the APC presents both the MHC class II (or I) molecule with the antigen to the TCR and the costimulatory molecules

CD80 (B7-1)/CD86 (B7-2) to CD28 on the T cell, can the T cell be activated resulting in stimulation of the AIS (two signal model). The activated T cells then regulate the activities of B cells, other T cells, and other cells participating in the immune response. Note that self-antigens are not recognized by TLRs/PRRs of the innate immune system and therefore do not induce the mandatory costimulatory molecules (second signal) on APCs needed to activate the AIS. This mechanism ensures that only pathogen-specific T cells are activated.

13. **Which cells are specialized antigen-presenting cells? Where are they found?**
    Antigen presenting cells are given in Table 4-3.

14. **What is the major histocompatibility complex (MHC) and what does it do?**
    The **MHC** is located on the short arm of chromosome 6 in a region stretching approximately four million base pairs and encodes the **human leukocyte antigens (HLAs)**. Within the MHC, there are three major regions that encode for three different classes of proteins that have traditionally been defined—MHC classes I, II, and III (see Figure 4-2).
    The role of the MHC HLA class I and HLA class II molecules on APCs is to enable presentation of peptide antigens to T cells. There are over 1100 common and well-documented polymorphisms of HLA class I and class II molecules that are found in the population. For the MHC class I region, over 200 alleles have been identified for the HLA-A locus, over 300 for the HLA-B locus, and over 100 for the HLA-C locus. Other class I genes (HLA-E, HLA-F, HLA-G) have limited function and polymorphisms. For the MHC class II region,

Table 4-3. Antigen Presenting Cells

CELL TYPE	LOCATION
Macrophages	
Histiocyte	Connective tissue
Monocyte	Blood
Alveolar macrophage	Lung
Kupffer cell	Liver
Microglia	Central nervous system
Mesangial	Kidney
Osteoclast	Bone
Dendritic cells	Lymphoid, mucous membranes, solid organs
Langerhans cells	Skin (dendritic cell)
B lymphocytes	Lymph nodes

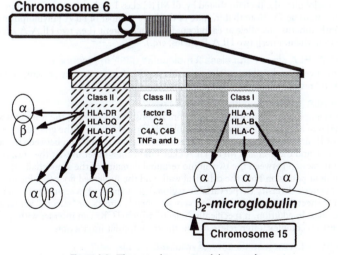

Figure 4-2. The major histocompatibility complex.

Table 4-4. Function of MHC Class I and Class II Molecules

	MHC HLA CLASS I	MHC HLA CLASS II
Cellular distribution	All nucleated cells and platelets	Certain immune system cells, particularly if they serve as "professional" antigen presenting cells: —B cells —Monocytes/macrophages —Dendritic cells —Thymic epithelial cells Some activated T cells Some cells in which MHC class II expression can be induced, particularly during chronic inflammatory processes: —Endothelial cells —Synovial cells
Antigen size	8 to 13 amino acids in length	13 to 25 amino acids in length
Antigen type	Antigenic peptide fragment endogenous to the cytoplasm or nucleus of the cell that is expressing the MHC molecule (e.g., endogenous or "self"-peptides; peptides of obligate intracellular pathogens such as viruses and chlamydia; tumor antigens)	Antigenic peptide fragment present in lysosomal compartments as a result of phagocytosis or receptor-mediated endocytosis (e.g., exogenous or foreign infectious material [bacteria])
T cell recognition	$CD8^+$ T cell	$CD4^+$ T cell
Resultant T cell response	Cell mediated killing or suppression of the MHC class I-presenting cell	T cell coordinated phagocytic and/or antibody response to eradicate the antigen that was presented

HLA, Human leukocyte antigen; MHC, major histocompatibility complex.

over 250 alleles for the HLA-DRβ locus, 50 for the DQ locus, and 60 for the DP locus have been identified. Other genes in the class II region that are involved in peptide processing include peptide sizing (proteosome subunits [LMP1 and LMP2]), peptide transport (TAP1 and TAP2), and peptide loading onto class II molecules (DMA, DMB, DO/DN). The remainder of the MHC complex stretches between the class I and class II regions and encodes various proteins that are not capable of presenting antigen. However, many of these MHC class III proteins are involved in the regulation of the immune response, and some have rheumatic disease associations. These include C2, C4A and C4B, and factor B of the complement system; TNF-α and lymphotoxin; and some of the heat shock proteins. Both MHC HLA class I and class II molecules are dimers. Although the MHC encodes both the α- and β-chains of the class II molecules, it encodes only the MHC HLA class I α-chain. β₂-microglobulin, the β-chain shared by all MHC class I molecules, is encoded by a relatively invariant allele on chromosome 15. Note that in spite of the large number of HLA polymorphisms, each individual only codominantly inherits one allele at each locus from each parent (i.e., two HLA-A alleles [one from the father and one from the mother]; two HLA-B alleles, etc.).

15. **How do the MHC HLA class I and class II molecules differ in function?**
    They differ in their cellular distribution, the antigenic peptide fragments they present, and the type of T cell that recognizes and responds to the complex they present (see Table 4-4).

16. **How does the HLA protein bind its peptide antigen?**
    Each peptide-binding site has a similar configuration. It consists of a groove, the walls of which are α-helical structures. A series of antiparallel strands of the molecule form the floor of the groove, a β-pleated sheet. In MHC HLA class II molecules, this configuration is formed by the interaction between the amino termini of both the α-chain and the β-chain. MHC HLA class I molecules differ in that the antigen-binding site is formed by the interaction between the two amino terminal domains of the same chain, the α-chain. The antigen binds at points on both the α-helical walls and the β-pleated floor (see Figure 4-3). The three areas of greatest genetic diversity (**hypervariable regions**) are expressed in segments of each of the α-helices and the β-pleated sheet. This genetic variation very specifically affects, or "selects," which antigens can bind to specific molecules. In addition, it specifically "selects" which TCRs can interact with specific combinations of the MHC–antigen complex, often referred to as the trimolecular interaction.

17. **How do the MHC HLA molecules control what the T cells see?**
    They do this in two ways. First, the sequence of amino acids in an MHC HLA molecule determines which antigenic peptide fragments can bind to that molecule. Only those "selected" antigenic peptides that can

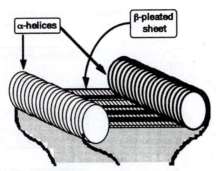

Figure 4-3. The antigen-binding site.

bind to one of an individual's HLA molecules have the potential to be specifically recognized. Second, not all T cells can see all the MHC HLA molecules. The peptides presented in the context of MHC HLA class I molecules can only be seen by T cells that have CD8 molecules associated with their TCR, whereas the peptides presented in the context of MHC HLA class II molecules can only be seen by T cells that have CD4 molecules associated with their TCR.

18. **What are the two main types of lymphocytes? How are they differentiated? What are their subtypes?**
    - **T lymphocytes**, or T cells, are thymus-derived and express the TCR–CD3 complex on their surface. They can be separated from other lymphocytes by use of monoclonal antibodies that recognize CD3, a component of the TCR that transduces the TCR signal across the lymphocyte membrane. The majority of circulating lymphocytes in the bloodstream are T cells with α–β TCR. To generate the necessary diversity the TCR β-chain genes on chromosome 7 contains four segments (V, D, J, C), whereas the α-chain genes on chromosome 14 contain three segments (V, D, C). Each segment has several members to choose from (50 to 100 V, 15 D, 6 to 60 J, 1 to 2 C). During the process of TCR gene rearrangement as well as the addition of additional nucleotides (N-region), the combination of the two TCR chains yields >10^8 possible combinations. The T cell then undergoes thymic selection to select cells that will not react to self-antigens.
    - **CD4$^+$ T cells**: Th1 (T helper cell, type 1), Th2, Th17, Tregs (regulatory T cells), Tfh (follicular helper T cells).
    - **CD8$^+$ T cells**: cytotoxic T lymphocytes.
    - **Natural killer T cells.**
    - **γ–δ T cells**: express γ–δ TCR and most are double negative (lack CD4 and CD8). They make up 2% to 3% of circulating T cells and are primarily found in the skin and the gut epithelium. These TCRs cannot recognize antigen in context with MHC. They can recognize antigen directly or in association with MHC class I-like molecules such as CD1 (binds glycolipid antigens) and MICA/MICB in the gut. Heat shock proteins can directly activate these cells. They interact with alkyl phosphates found in mycobacteria and are expanded during certain infections.
    - **B lymphocytes**, or B cells, are Bone marrow-derived antibody-secreting cells that express surface immunoglobulin (e.g., B cell receptor) on their surfaces. There are several subpopulations of B cells.
        - **B1**—develop earliest during ontogeny. Most express CD5. They are the source of "natural" antibodies and do not require T cell help. These antibodies are low affinity, IgM, and polyreactive, recognizing both common pathogens and autoantigens. They are predominantly located in peritoneal and pleural cavities.
        - **B2**—develop later in ontogeny and lack the CD5 surface marker. Before encountering antigen, mature B2 cells coexpress IgM and IgD antibodies on their surfaces. With antigen stimulation and T cell help, they secrete highly specific antibody (IgM, IgG, IgA, or IgE) within the secondary lymphoid tissue. Follicular B cells can freely circulate and are organized into the primary follicles of B cell zones focused around follicular DCs in the white pulp of the spleen and the cortical areas of peripheral lymph nodes. They comprise 95% of B cells in lymph nodes and the spleen. Marginal zone B cells are noncirculating B cells that are located in the marginal zone of the spleen. Memory B cells are CD27$^+$, constitute 1% of the total B cell population, and can be long-lived (years) with continued antigen stimulation.
        - **Bregs (B10)**—subsets are found within the B1 and B2 populations. They secrete IL-10 to modulate the immune response.

19. **Specific adaptive immune responses can be differentiated into two major categories based on whether B or T cells are primarily involved. What are these two categories?**
    1. **Humoral immunity** refers to immune responses involving antibody that is produced by mature B cells and plasma cells (terminally differentiated B cells). This is important for defense against bacteria, especially those with a polysaccharide capsule (e.g., *Pneumococcus*, *Haemophilus influenzae*).

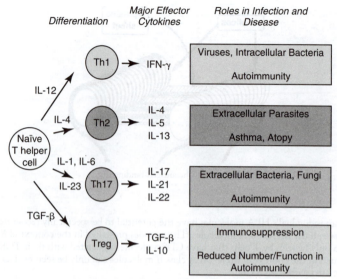

Figure 4-4. Human CD4+ T helper differentiation pathways and roles in normal immunity and disease.

2. **Cellular immunity** is mediated by T cells that secrete cytokines and signal effector cells to direct an overall cell mediated immune response. This is important for defense against viruses, parasites, fungi, and mycobacteria.

20. Describe how CD4+ T cells are activated.
    - DCs capture and process antigen from peripheral sites. They migrate to lymph nodes displaying the processed antigenic peptide in context with MHC.
    - Naïve T cells continually recirculate through the blood, spleen, lymph nodes, and MALT in search of DCs displaying a complementary MHC–peptide complex that can engage its TCR.
    - If the naïve T cell TCR binds the HLA class II–peptide complex on the APC without engaging any costimulatory molecules, it becomes anergic or undergoes apoptosis. However, if a naïve T cell TCR binds the HLA class II–peptide complex on the APC and the T cell is activated, then the T cell expresses CD40L, which binds to CD40 on the DC/APC. This induces expression of CD80/CD86 on the DC/APC, which binds to CD28 on the T cell triggering production of IL-2, which binds to the IL-2 receptor on the T cell causing a positive feedback loop resulting in T cell proliferation.
    - Naïve T cells are activated to become one of the four distinct subpopulations of CD4+ T cells based on the cytokines produced by DCs/APCs in response to the antigen they are processing. The type of CD4+ T cell can be identified based on the cytokines it secretes (see Figure 4-4.).
       - **Th1** responses promote production of opsonizing antibodies (IgG1) and induction of cellular cytotoxicity and macrophage activation. This is important against pathogens that replicate intracellularly (viruses, intracellular bacteria).
       - **Th2** responses promote IgE and IgG4 production and stimulate eosinophil development. This is important for helminth infections.
       - **Th17** responses are important for defense against chronic infections with extracellular bacteria and fungi. This may be part of the IIS.
       - **Tregs** (CD4+, CD25+, FOXP3) are important for the establishment and maintenance of tolerance and suppression of immune response.
    - The activated T cell proliferates and its progeny travel throughout the body until they reach where the antigen has invaded. They are restimulated by local APCs and release their cytokines (see Figure 4-4) that contribute to augmenting the immune response by activating monocytes/macrophages.
    - Some activated T cells undergo further interactions with B cells in the lymphoid tissue inducing a humoral immune response.
    - Some activated T cells become long-lived memory T cells. Memory T cells are activated more easily and rapidly in a secondary immune response.

21. Describe how B cells can be stimulated to produce a humoral antibody response.
    - Thymus-independent antigens: type 1 (mitogens) and type 2 (bacterial polysaccharides) antigens have repeating structures that enable them to cross-link surface immunoglobulin (i.e., B cell receptor) causing B cell activation that results in a predominantly IgM response.

- Thymus-dependent antigens: the majority of protein and glycoprotein antigens require T cell help to mount a humoral response against them. The steps for this to occur are:
  - Naïve T cells recognize antigen associated with MHC HLA class II molecules on DCs/APCs. The CD4+ T helper cell is activated and can provide help to a B cell for antibody production.
  - The B cell through its immunoglobulin receptor binds and internalizes the antigenic peptide it is specific for. This antigen is often provided by follicular dendritic cells (FDCs) that present antigen–antibody complexes on their surface to B cells entering into the primary lymphoid follicles in secondary lymphoid organs (lymph nodes, spleen, MALT). The B cell processes the antigen and puts it on its surface in association with its MHC HLA class II molecules. The CD4+ T helper cell TCR will bind to this HLA class II–antigenic peptide complex. A second signal is then provided by CD40 on B cells binding to CD40L on activated CD4+ T helper cells. Other costimulatory activating pathways also exist (BAFF/BLYS, TACI, APRIL, etc.). Note that if a second signal is not provided the B cell becomes anergic. Additionally, Tfh cells (CD4+, CXCR5+) are antigen-experienced T cells found in the B cell follicles. They mediate antigen-specific naïve and memory B cell activation, which triggers germinal center formation through the Tfh cell secretion of IL-21 and IL-4.
  - Within germinal centers the activated B cell differentiates into centroblasts, which divide and become centrocytes. Somatic mutation of Ig V genes takes place during cell division. Each cycle of division leads to the selection of cells with Ig receptors with the highest affinity for the antigen (**affinity maturation**). Centrocytes with the highest affinity/specificity immunoglobulin receptors on their surfaces have their receptors cross-linked by antigen complexed on FDCs and are selected to differentiate into plasma cells or memory B cells. The CD40–CD40L costimulation is critical for immunoglobulin class-switching, antibody affinity maturation, and memory B cell formation.
  - In the primary immune response there is first an IgM response occurring 4 to 10 days after antigen exposure. With clonal expansion there is immunoglobulin class-switching to IgG and other isotypes. In the secondary immune response, memory B cells that actively circulate from the blood to the lymph in search of antigenic stimulation can mount a much quicker (1 to 3 days) humoral response with the production of isotypes other than IgM. Memory B cells require less antigen and less T cell help than naïve B cells due to the high affinity surface Ig receptors for their specific antigen.
  - One activated B cell can generate up to 4000 plasma cells which can produce up to 10^{12} antibody molecules/day.

22. **Describe the structure of an immunoglobulin. How is antibody diversity generated?**
Unlike TCRs that can only respond to linear antigenic peptides bound to a HLA molecule, immunoglobulins (antibodies) can bind to linear and bound antigens as well as soluble antigens and conformational antigenic determinants. The number of antigenic determinants (epitopes) that antibodies need to be able to bind is in the billions. An immunoglobulin is composed of four polypeptide chains: two identical heavy (H) and two identical light (L) chains. Each chain has a constant (C) and variable (V) domain. There are five different H-chain constant regions (isotypes): IgM (μ), IgG (γ), IgA (α), IgE (ε), and IgD (δ) coded for on chromosome 4. The H-chain constant region determines the ability of the immunoglobulin to fix complement and to bind to Fc receptors. The H-chain variable region is coded for on chromosome 14. Light chains are designated kappa (κ) and lambda (λ) and coded for by chromosomes 2 and 22, respectively. Kappa chains are used more often (65%) than lambda chains.
To generate the necessary diversity, the H-chain V region genes contains three segments (V_H, D_H, J_H), whereas each of the L-chain genes contain two (V_κ, J_κ or V_λ, J_λ). Each segment has several members to choose from (38 to 46 V_H, 23 D_H, 9 J_H), (31 to 35 V_κ, 5 J_κ), (29 to 32 V_λ, 4 to 5 J_λ). During the process of V(D)J recombination in the absence of the antigen, the random combination of gene segments orchestrated by RAG-1/RAG-2 generates a diverse immunoglobulin repertoire. Nongermline encoded sequences (N additions) can also be added to increase diversity further. The antigen-binding regions are formed by pairing the variable domains of the L-chain to the variable region of the H-chain. Within the variable region of the immunoglobulin molecule are discrete regions, called complementary determining regions (CDRs) that contact the antigen specifically. Both the H-chain and L-chain contain three of these regions. The structure of the CDRs of an immunoglobulin is called the idiotype. The minimal antigenic determinant recognized by the CDRs is called the antigenic epitope. This process of generating immunoglobulin diversity occurs during B cell maturation and is antigen-independent. After the B cell responds to the antigen, the B cell receptor and immunoglobulins produced can undergo somatic mutation to increase the specificity of the antibody-binding site for the antigen.

23. **Name the five major classes of antibodies. What specific role does each play in humoral immunity?**
The mnemonic is GAMED:
G—IgG—Highest concentration in serum (70% of total immunoglobulins) and excellent penetration into tissues. Can cross the placenta by week 16 of pregnancy. Fixes complement. Four subtypes: IgG1 and IgG3 respond to protein antigens; IgG2 is the main response against polysaccharide antigens; IgG4 arises against nematodes and can dampen chronic inflammation.

A—**IgA**—Despite its low concentration in serum, more IgA is produced than any other immunoglobulin isotypes. Most IgA exists as secretory IgA (SIgA) in mucosal cavities and milk. There are two subclasses: IgA1 is a monomer in serum and IgA2 is a dimer/polymeric and is the most important antibody for host defense at mucosal surfaces (sites of antigen entry). Dimer/polymeric IgA2 contains a J-chain. This complex is produced locally by plasma cells, captured by a receptor on the basolateral surface of epithelial cells, transported to the apical side, and cleaved from the receptor. The IgA is released into secretions associated with a secretory component. This form (secretory IgA) is more resistant to enzymatic degradation.

M—**IgM**—The first class of antibody made in the primary response to antigen. Pentameric form vigorously fixes complement and is very important in host defense against blood-borne antigens. IgM also associates with a J-chain, which allows its active transport to mucosal surfaces. A monomeric form of IgM complexed with Igα and Igβ on the surface of naïve B cells and serves as the B cell receptor.

E—**IgE**—Binds to the surface of mast cells and basophils by high-affinity IgE Fc receptor (FcεR1). Cross-linking of IgE by antigen binding results in the release of the granular contents of the cell (primarily histamine). Important in allergic diseases and host defense against parasites.

D—**IgD**—Found primarily as a membrane immunoglobulin on the surface of naïve B cells. B cells with IgD on their surface are more resistant to being tolerized.

24. How does an antibody participate in immune and inflammatory responses?

There are three main ways in which an antibody is immunologically active:
1. An antibody can coat and neutralize invading organisms, not allowing the organism access to the host.
2. Two classes of antibody (IgM and IgG) activate ("fix") complement by the classical pathway, resulting in cell chemotaxis, increased vascular permeability, and target cell lysis.
3. An antibody coats foreign particles (opsonization), increasing the efficiency of phagocytosis by cells that contain surface immunoglobulin (Fc) receptors (neutrophils and macrophages). Complement activation can also opsonize foreign particles facilitating removal through complement receptors.

25. What is the role of complement in the immune response?

- Complement components have immunological activity both individually and in an activation cascade leading to a polymer formed by C5b, C6, C7, C8, and C9 (the **membrane attack complex**, or MAC), which results in lysis of target cell membranes (see Figure 4-5).
- Early classical complement component split products (especially C3b, C4b) act as opsonins and assist in the phagocytosis of bacterial particles by neutrophils and macrophages. C3b/C4b bind to CR1 on peripheral cells to assist in immune adherence; C3d binds to CR2 on B cells to help signal the B cell for antigen processing; and iC3b binds to CR3/CR4 on myeloid cells to assist in phagocytosis.
- Certain complement split products (C3a and C5a) are chemotactic for phagocytic neutrophils and also act as "anaphylatoxins," which directly stimulate mast cells and basophils to release histamine resulting in increased vascular permeability and augment inflammation.

Deficiency of early complement components is associated with increased pyogenic infections (C3 deficiency) and an increased incidence of autoimmune diseases (C1, C4, and C2 deficiency), possibly owing to impaired clearance of immune complexes. The MAC appears especially important in host defense against *Neisseria* infection. Deficiency of any one of the terminal complement components can result in recurrent infections with *Neisseria*.

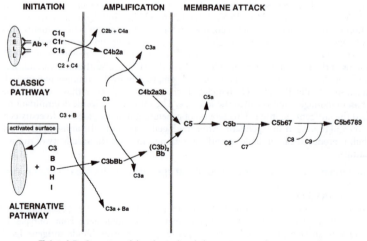

Figure 4-5. Overview of the classical and alternative complement cascades.

26. What activates the complement system?

The complement system can be activated by three pathways:
- **Classical**—IgM and IgG binding to antigen-forming immune complexes that can bind C1q-activating C1r and C1s to cleave C4. Other proteins including CRP (binds C1q), serum amyloid P, and C4 nephritic factor can activate this pathway. This is important in the AIS.
- **Alternative**—activated by lipopolysaccharide on microbial cell surfaces in the absence of an antibody. C3b binds to the target cell surface. Factor B (structurally similar to C2) is cleaved by factor D to Bb. This binds to the cell surface forming C3bBb, which functions to cleave more C3 molecules. This is part of the IIS. IgA complexes and the C3 nephritic factor can also activate this pathway.
- **Lectin**—Mannose binding lectin (MBL) is secreted by the liver and binds to microbial ligands. MBL resembles C1q and activates mannose-associated serine proteases (MASP-2) that are similar to C1r and C1s and can cleave C4 and C2, resulting in complement activation. Note this is important in the IIS.

27. How are cytotoxic T lymphocytes activated? How about natural killer T cells?

Most cytotoxic (killer) T lymphocytes (CTLs) are $CD8^+$ T cells. They are activated by DCs/APCs in lymphoid tissues. However, the APC has to be activated by an antigen-specific $CD4^+$ T cell before the APC can activate the naïve $CD8^+$ T cell to become an effector CTL. Antigens that replicate (e.g., viruses) intracellularly are processed and presented on the surface of cells in association with MHC-encoded HLA class I molecules. Notably, all cells including APCs contain HLA class I molecules on their surface. After being activated, CTLs divide and circulate to find infected/abnormal cells to kill. The CTL ($CD8^+$) TCR specific for the antigen binds the HLA class I molecule containing the foreign peptide. Several other adhesion molecules also contribute to this interaction (e.g., CD2 [LFA-2]–CD58 [LFA-3]). Cytotoxicity occurs by:
- Granule exocytosis: granules containing granzymes from the CTL enter the target cell through pores in its membrane created by perforin. These proteases can cause apoptosis of the target cells.
- Fas ligand (FasL)-induced apoptosis: FasL on the CTL binds to Fas (CD95) on the target cell causing apoptosis.

CTLs can secrete cytokines (IFN-γ) and recruit macrophages into the area to augment the immune response. One CTL can lyse multiple cells.

Natural killer T (NKT) cells are T cells that share properties of T cells (express αβ TCR) and NK cells (express CD16, CD56, CD161, and granzyme production), but are different from CTL and NK cells. They constitute 0.1% of all peripheral blood T cells. Most NKT cells are restricted to recognizing self and foreign lipids and glycolipids presented by CD1d molecules on target cells. Upon activation, NKT cells make IFN-γ, IL-4, granulocyte macrophage colony-stimulating factor (GM-CSF), and other cytokines (IL-2, TNF-α, etc.). They are important in the defense against mycobacterial infections.

28. What pathways lead to cellular apoptosis?

Multiple triggers can lead to a cell undergoing apoptosis by one of two major pathways:
- Death receptors (Fas [CD95], TNFR1, DR4/5)—these receptors all have a homologous intracellular region "death domain." These death domains bind to adaptor proteins (Fas and DR4/5 binds to FADD, TNFR1 to TRADD). These adaptor proteins can activate the cysteine protease, procaspase 8. This can be inhibited by FLIP. The activated caspase 8 activates the executioner caspases (3, 6, and 7), which in turn activate an endonuclease called caspase-activated DNAse as well as others. These endonucleases cleave DNA causing fragmentation and cell death. Caspases also activate proteases that act on actin microfilaments leading to blebbing of the membrane.
- Mitochondria—cellular stress causes Bax, Bak, and/or Bid to bind to mitochondria. This displaces Bcl-2 and Bcl-x, which are normally on the outer mitochondrial membrane and inhibit apoptosis. When this happens, cytochrome c is released from the mitochondria. Cytochrome c activates the adaptor protein, Apaf-1, which is in the cytosol. Apaf-1 activates procaspase 9, which activates caspases 3 and 7 causing apoptosis (see above). Akt inhibits this pathway. Many tumors have chronically activated Akt, so the tumor cell does not undergo apoptosis.
- Others—(1) cytotoxic cells (T and NK cells) inject granzyme B, which activates caspases 3 and 7. (2) DNA damage is detected by p53, resulting in the activation of apoptosis.

29. Describe the differences between apoptosis, necrosis, and autophagy.

- Apoptosis: ten million cells a day undergo program cell death (apoptosis) in a healthy individual. The mechanism is necessary to control tissue size and homeostasis without inciting inflammation. The two pathways leading to apoptosis are listed in Question 28. During apoptosis the chromatin condenses, cells shrink, and cell membranes form blebs that become apoptotic bodies containing organelles. The cell membrane is inverted and the phosphatidylserine in the membrane signals macrophages to phagocytose the apoptotic bodies causing them to release antiinflammatory cytokines. Binding of C1q, collectins, and MBL to apoptotic cells can facilitate their clearance.
- Necrosis: the cell swells and the plasma membrane ruptures releasing intracellular contents. This contributes to an inflammatory response.
- Autophagy: this is a degradation pathway for cellular components without killing the cell. Autophagosomes take in impaired organelles and unwanted cellular components and deliver them to lysosomes for degradation and recycling without causing apoptosis.

30. How is the immune response turned off after it is activated?

Once the immune response has been activated it is important to restore immune homeostasis. This is done through a variety of mechanisms:
- Negative regulation of the innate immune response:
  - Efferocytosis: activation of macrophages induces not only the secretion of proinflammatory molecules but also antiinflammatory mediators (IL-10, TGF-β, and PGE_2) that downregulate macrophage and DC function. In addition, macrophage ingestion of apoptotic cells (efferocytosis) that they identify by phosphatidylserine on the outer surface of the apoptotic cell results in release of antiinflammatory mediators.
- Negative regulation of the adaptive cellular immune response:
  - CTLA-4: after activation, T cells increase expression of CTLA-4, which has higher affinity for CD80/CD86 than CD28 leading to loss of costimulation. This results in cessation of T cell proliferation and cytokine production.
  - Activation-induced cell death: the signals that activate T cells also result in the upregulation of Fas and TNFR2 on their surface. When Fas binds to FasL on another cell or TNF-α binds to TNFR1, the activated T cell undergoes apoptosis.
  - Treg suppression: regulatory T cells release IL-10 and TGF-β, which suppress the immune response. Other suppressor T cells also exist (Tr1, Th3, $CD8^+CD28^+$).
  - Breg suppression: regulatory B cells (B10) release IL-10, which suppress T cells and DCs. Other subsets of Bregs exist.
- Negative regulation of the adaptive humoral immune response:
  - IgG binds the antigen and eliminates it so it no longer serves as an inducer of the immune response.
  - IgG binds antigen-forming immune complexes. These immune complexes can bind to FcγRII on B cells, which suppresses them.
  - Antiidiotype antibodies may neutralize the antibody being made by binding to its idiotypic determinants.
- Regulation of complement cascade: C1 inhibitor (C1INH) binds C1r/C1s preventing C1 activation. C3 convertase (C4b2a and C3bBb) and C5 convertase (C4b2a3b and C3bBbC3b) are regulated by serum inhibitors (C4-binding protein and factor H) and membrane-bound factors [decay accelerating factor (DAF) and membrane cofactor protein (MCP)]. C4b-binding protein inactivates C4b and the classical pathway and factor H inactivates C3b and the alternative pathway by serving as cofactors for factor I-mediated cleavage of C4b and C3b, respectively. DAF causes release of C2a or Bb from cell surfaces leaving C4b and C3b to bind to MCP, which serves as a cofactor for factor I-mediated cleavage of C4b/C3b halting the classical and alternative complement cascades. Complete deficiency and loss-of-function polymorphisms of factors H and I result in dysregulated complement activation and the atypical hemolytic uremic syndrome. Other complement regulatory proteins (vitronectin, CD59) block fluid phase and membrane-bound MAC. Note that all these regulatory proteins bind to glycosaminoglycans specific to host cells and not on microbes, therefore protecting host cells while allowing complement-mediated destruction of pathogens.

31. Using the classification developed by Gel and Coombs, immune responses causing immunopathology can be segregated into four main types. Name them.

Type I—IgE-mediated immediate hypersensitivity (e.g., allergic rhinitis or hayfever).
Type II—Antibody-mediated tissue injury (e.g., autoimmune hemolytic anemia).
Type III—Immune complex (antigen–antibody) formation (e.g., serum sickness, Arthus skin reaction).
Type IV—Delayed-type hypersensitivity (e.g., immune response to mycobacterial antigens, purified protein derivative [PPD] skin test).

A fifth type has been added where antibodies bind to a receptor causing overstimulation [e.g., the thyroid-stimulating immunoglobulin binds to the thyrotropin receptor mimicking TSH in Graves' disease].

AUTOIMMUNITY

32. What is tolerance?

Tolerance is the term used to describe the phenomenon of **antigen-specific unresponsiveness**. In other words, the immune system encounters certain antigens to which it is programmed specifically to not respond and, therefore, not eradicate.

33. Is tolerance innate or acquired?

The phenomenon of tolerance is present in both the IIS and the AIS. We are protected from the IIS by specific mechanisms that block its activities, such as membrane complement regulatory proteins that protect self tissues from the alternative complement pathway. The AIS "learns" to be tolerant of some specific antigens, such as self tissues, just as it learns to be "intolerant" of many foreign antigens. When discussing autoimmune disorders, we often narrow our perspective to the tolerance of **autoantigens**, such as an individual's own nucleoproteins or cell surface molecules, by the AIS. However, the phenomenon of tolerance is not limited to autoantigens. In fact, tolerance to **exogenous antigens**, such as dietary proteins, is just as crucial for the survival of an individual as "self-tolerance."

34. What are the main pathogenetic mechanisms used to develop and maintain tolerance to self-antigens?

Most autoimmune diseases require the presence of self-reactive $CD4^+$ T lymphocytes that have lost their tolerance to self-antigens. Mechanisms to maintain tolerance are:

- Central tolerance:
  - Thymic selection of T cells: during this process the autoimmune regulator (AIRE) gene is responsible for orchestrating intrathymic presentation of self-antigens bound to MHC HLA class I and class II molecules. Those T cells that react to strongly with the MHC–self-antigen complexes are deleted (clonal deletion). This is particularly important for such antigens as major blood groups and MHC. T cells capable of reacting to other self-antigens may not be deleted and can gain access to the periphery.
  - Receptor editing of B cell receptors: this process occurs during B cell maturation in the bone marrow. B cells that too strongly interact with self-antigens undergo death by apoptosis. To avoid apoptosis, receptor editing modifies the sequence of light chain (more than heavy chain) V and J genes so that the B cell receptor has a different specificity and will not recognize the self-antigen. Some estimate that 20% to 50% of B cells that come from the bone marrow have had receptor editing of their B cell receptor. There is some evidence that TCRs may also undergo receptor editing.
- Peripheral tolerance:
  - Clonal anergy: self-reactive T cells that encounter self-antigens presented by HLA molecules in the periphery may not receive the necessary second costimulatory signals. These T cells may be tolerized to the antigen and remain unresponsive. This anergic state may be terminated if costimulatory signals are upregulated during a nonspecific infection, tissue injury, or inflammatory state involving the IIS.
  - Immunologic ignorance: self-reactive T cells may not have a TCR that reacts well enough with the MHC/peptide complex to become activated. This anergic state may be breached if the antigen is changed in some manner such as during an infection.
  - Regulatory T and B cells: some Tregs suppress self-reactive T cells by cell-to-cell contact of membrane-bound molecules such as CTLA-4. Other Tregs are induced and exert suppressive effects by secreting cytokines, IL-10, and TGF-β. Some Bregs (e.g., B10 cells) secrete IL-10.
  - Idiotype network theory: a network of antibodies exists naturally or an antiidiotypic antibody directed against the self-reactive antibody idiotype can be generated, which are capable of neutralizing self-reactive antibodies.

35. What is autoimmunity?

The term **autoimmunity** is commonly employed to describe conditions in which self-tolerance is broken and an individual becomes the victim of his or her own immune response. Just like immunity to foreign antigens, autoimmune disorders are antigen-driven processes that are characterized by specificity, high affinity, and memory. However, an autoimmune process involves the recognition of an antigen by the immune system, either foreign or self, that is then followed by an assault on its own self-antigens (i.e., autoantigens). Typically, these processes develop in an individual who previously displayed tolerance to the same antigens that are now targeted by the immune response. Therefore, most autoimmune processes are better described not simply as an absence of tolerance but as a **loss of previously established tolerance**. Clinically, autoimmunity can be divided into two categories:

- Organ-specific autoimmunity: defined as an immune response against a single autoantigen or a restricted group of autoantigens within a given organ (e.g., myasthenia gravis [antibodies to the acetylcholine receptor]).
- Systemic autoimmunity: defined as an immune response against multiple autoantigens resulting in clinical manifestations in multiple organs (e.g., systemic lupus erythematosus).

36. What are the stages of an autoimmune disease?

Autoimmune diseases generally follow three stages. The first is thought of as the combination of genes that confer a genetic risk. Some genes contribute significant risk (e.g., HLA), whereas most genes (e.g., PTPN22, STAT4) confer a modest risk (usually 2-fold to 3-fold), but in aggregate the risk is very high in the setting of a combination of disease-promoting polymorphisms and the "right" environmental exposure. Epigenetics (DNA methylation, histone modifications, microRNAs) also contribute to the genetic predisposition. The second is the development of autoimmune phenomena such as autoantibodies produced by B cells that have lost self-tolerance (and presumably driven by autoimmune T cells) but in a state wherein the individual still does not exhibit symptoms because the target organs have not yet become damaged to a sufficient level. The third stage is the development of clinical symptoms that impair quality of life and require treatment. Although most autoimmune diseases are detected and treated only in the third phase, ongoing work in several diseases is expected to allow the detection of a "preclinical" disease state in which specific preventive therapies could be used.

37. Describe the mechanisms that may be involved in the pathogenesis of autoimmune disease.

Several mechanisms have been hypothesized. All are operative only in a genetically predisposed host who has most likely had one or more environmental exposures that over time start the autoimmune process. The environmental trigger or triggers are usually not identifiable because they may have occurred years before the

first clinical symptom develops (see Question 36). More than one of the following possible mechanisms may contribute to the development of autoimmunity:
- Superantigens: these are foreign antigens, particularly of bacterial or viral origin, that are capable of binding to the TCR (typically the V region of the β-chain) and the MHC class II molecule outside the antigen-binding groove and, in turn, bind the two together. These types of antigens are not as restricted in their effects as typical antigens. In the case of T cells, superantigens do not need to be processed and subsequently presented in the antigen-binding cleft of MHC molecules in order to stimulate T cell activation. B cell superantigens also exist that bind to regions of surface immunoglobulin that are common to various subtypes and cause polyclonal B cell activation without the need for T cell help.
- T–B cell discordance with abnormal receptor-mediated feedback and suppression: T cells responding normally to a foreign antigen release cytokines to augment the immune response. Self-reactive B cells in proximity are stimulated by the cytokine milieu. If these autoreactive B cells have defective receptors that do not respond to inhibitory signals needed to maintain self-tolerance then they will survive, contribute to the inflammation, and become self-perpetuating. Additionally, abnormal Treg and Breg suppressive function can contribute to this autoimmune process.
- Molecular mimicry: an exogenous antigen may share structural similarities with a host antigen. Antibodies produced against this antigen can bind the host antigen causing amplification of the immune response.
- Cytokine dysregulation: IIS activation releases cytokines that activate the AIS. Excessive or defective cytokine production could result in an aberrant immune response and/or activation of anergic self-reactive T cells.
- Defective apoptosis: accelerated apoptosis of cells with increased release of self-antigens and/or defective presentation of apoptotic cell antigens to lymphocytes could lead to abnormal lymphocyte activation including self-reactive T and B cells.
- Epitope spreading: occurs when the immune reaction changes from targeting the primary epitope to also targeting other epitopes.
- Cryptic epitope exposure: the innate immune response is activated by an invading pathogen. The inflammatory response causes tissue damage with release of self-antigens whose epitopes the immune system has not previously developed tolerance to. The AIS is recruited and continually stimulated by exposure to the new self-antigen released by the host tissue.

38. **What is the difference between an autoinflammatory disease and an autoimmune disease?**
Autoinflammatory diseases (e.g., Familial Mediterranean fever, see Chapter 79) are diseases that have a chronic inflammatory response due to a defect in a component or regulation of the IIS. Autoimmune diseases (e.g., systemic lupus erythematosus) typically involve self-reactive $CD4^+$ T lymphocytes and abnormalities in the regulation of the AIS.

BIBLIOGRAPHY

Amulic B, Cazalet C, Hayes GL, et al: Neutrophil function: from mechanisms to disease, Annu Rev Immunol 30:459–489, 2012.
Chan JK, Roth J, Oppenheim JJ, et al: Alarmins: awaiting a clinical response, J Clin Invest 122:2711–2719, 2012.
Devitt A, Marshall LJ: The innate immune system and the clearance of apoptotic cells, J Leukoc Biol 90:447–457, 2011.
Kaplan MJ, Radic M: Neutrophil extracellular traps: double-edged swords of innate immunity, J Immunol 189:2689, 2012.
Kuballa P, Notte WM, Castoreno A, et al: Autophagy and the immune system, Annu Rev Immunol 30:611–646, 2012.
Lu Q: The critical importance of epigenetics in autoimmunity, J Autoimmunity 41:1–5, 2013.
Nurieva R, Liu X, Dong C: Molecular mechanisms of T-cell tolerance, Immunol Rev 241:133–144, 2011.
Parish IA, Heath WR: Too dangerous to ignore: self-tolerance and the control of ignorant autoreactive T cells, Immunol Cell Biol 86:146, 2008.
Ricklin D, Hajishengallis G, Yang K, et al: Complement: a key system for immune surveillance and homeostasis, Nat Immunol 11:785, 2010.
Robinson MW, Hutchinson AT, Donnelly S: Antimicrobial peptides: utility players in innate immunity, Front Immunol 3:325, 2012.
Sharpe AH: Mechanisms of costimulation, Immunol Rev 229:5, 2009.
Steinman RM, Hemmi H: Dendritic cells: translating innate to adaptive immunity, Curr Top Microbiol Immunol 311:17, 2006.
Takeuchi O, Akira S: Pattern recognition receptors and inflammation, Cell 140:805, 2010.

II

EVALUATION OF THE PATIENT WITH RHEUMATIC SYMPTOMS

Specialism is a natural and necessary result of the growth of accurate knowledge, inseparably connected with the multiplication and perfection of instruments of precision. It has its drawbacks, absurdities even . . . . A few years ago a recent graduate and ex-hospital intern asked me, apparently seriously, to give him the name of a specialist in rheumatism. We can afford to laugh at these things . . .

Frederick Shattuck, 1897
Professor of Medicine
Harvard Medical School

HISTORY AND PHYSICAL EXAMINATION

Richard T. Meehan, MD

CHAPTER 5

Specialism is a natural and necessary result of the growth of accurate knowledge, inseparably connected with the multiplication and perfection of instruments of precision. It has its drawbacks, absurdities even....A few years ago a recent graduate and ex-hospital intern asked me, apparently seriously, to give him the name of a specialist in rheumatism. We can afford to laugh at these things...
—Frederick Shattuck, 1897
Professor of Medicine
Harvard Medical School

KEY POINTS

1. A good history and physical examination evaluating for both articular and extraarticular features are the most important components in establishing a correct diagnosis of a rheumatic disorder.
2. If musculoskeletal pain is reproduced with direct palpation of a localized area and worsened by resistive maneuvers then the source of pain is most likely periarticular (bursa or tendon).
3. The cardinal signs of musculoskeletal inflammation are pain, swelling, erythema, warmth, and limitation of motion. Of these, a joint effusion and limitation of motion are the most indicative of a true arthritis.

---

1. **What should your history include when interviewing a patient for connective tissue disease?**
   A chronological history of symptom progression should include which joints have been involved (pain and or swelling) and identify any precipitating factors such as new drugs, recent infections, diet, activity, or recent trauma. Determine responsiveness to prior therapeutic modalities. Has the joint involvement been episodic, additive, mono-, oligo-, or polyarticular and/or in a symmetrical distribution? Identify any constitutional symptoms that suggest systemic illness, vasculitis, or paraneoplastic disease such as fever, weight loss, or fatigue. A complete review of systems is necessary to determine which organ systems may be involved such as: skin (malar rash, photosensitivity, alopecia, sclerodactyly, Raynaud's disease, digital ulcers, psoriasis, mucosal ulceration, purpura, nodules, ulcerations, genital lesions, or sicca symptoms), cardio-respiratory (dyspnea, cough, hemoptysis, pleurisy or pericardial pain, edema, or pulmonary emboli), gastrointestinal (reflux, dysphagia, abdominal pain, diarrhea, hematochezia, or jaundice), renal (prior proteinuria, or nephrolithiasis), hematologic (leukopenia, thrombocytopenia, anemia, fetal loss, deep vein thrombosis or pulmonary embolism, or abnormal serologies), neurologic symptoms (neuropathies, weakness, transient ischemic attack, strokes seizures, psychosis, cognitive deficits, or temporal headaches). Also determine if there is underlying depression or risk factors for human immunodeficiency virus, hepatitis B or C. Ask about functional losses including how their symptoms interfere with activities of daily living and ability to do their job. Finally ask about family history including various arthritides and other autoimmune diseases that tend to cluster in families.

2. **What historical symptoms enable you to categorize a rheumatic disorder as inflammatory or mechanical (degenerative)? (Table 5-1)**

3. **List the five cardinal signs of inflammation.**
   Swelling (*tumor*)
   Warmth (*calor*)
   Erythema (*rubor*)
   Tenderness (*dolor*)
   Loss of function (*functio laesa*)

4. **In a patient with inflammatory arthritis, what history is useful in assessing disease activity?**
   Duration of morning stiffness, night pain, joint swelling, or new joint involvement are more helpful than the severity of pain, which is too subjective.

5. **Which signs of inflammation are suggestive of acute synovitis in a joint?**
   In the absence of corticosteroids, most joints affected by an inflammatory arthritis exhibit synovial distention, warmth, and limitation of range. The best indicator of synovitis is a distended joint capsule especially

Table 5-1.

FEATURE	INFLAMMATORY	MECHANICAL
Morning stiffness	>1 h	≤30 min
Fatigue	Significant	Minimal
Activity	May improve symptoms	May worsen symptoms
Rest	May worsen symptoms	May improve symptoms
Systemic involvement	Yes	No
Corticosteroid responsiveness	Yes	No

if accompanied by warmth. Swelling due to joint effusions may occur in the noninflammatory arthritides (e.g., osteoarthritis). Most inflamed joints are not typically erythematous, with the exception of acute septic and crystalline arthritis. If you encounter red, hot joints, particularly in a monoarticular distribution, your first thought should be, "Where's the needle?" This is needed in order to perform a joint aspiration.

6. **How much pressure should you apply when palpating a joint for synovitis?**

    A good "rule of thumb" is to palpate with enough pressure to blanche your distal thumbnail (4 kg/cm^2). This standardizes the joint exam and ensures that adequate pressure is being applied to detect synovitis. Obviously, with overtly inflamed joints, this degree of pressure may be excessive. The tender points characteristic of fibromyalgia may be similarly palpated.

7. **How do you determine if joint pain is originating from intra-articular or extra-articular structures?**

    "Stressing" a joint is easily accomplished by gentle passive range of motion of the joint by the examiner. In contrast, pain during attempted active ROM (performed by the patient) against a joint held immobile by the examiner suggests pathology in the surrounding tendons. Local tenderness by direct palpation of periarticular structures such as bursae may also indicate that the origin of pain is extra-articular.

8. **Describe the STWL system for recording the degree of arthritic involvement of a joint.**

    The STWL system records the degree of **swelling, tenderness, warmth,** and **limitation** of motion in a joint based on a quantitative estimate of severity. A score of 0 (normal), 1 (mild), 2 (moderate), or 3 (severe) can be assigned to the S, T, and W categories. Limitation of motion is scored as 0 (normal), 1 (25% loss of motion), 2 (50% loss), 3 (75% loss), or 4 (ankylosis) or report the ROM of a joint in degrees. For example, Rt. 2nd MCP S2T2W1L2 means the right second MCP joint has moderate synovitis, moderate tenderness, mild warmth, and a 50% loss of normal range of motion. An evaluation of joint instability should also be performed and deformities described such as swan-neck, ulnar drift, genu varus, etc.

9. **What is crepitus? What does it signify?**

    Crepitus is an audible or palpable "grating" sensation felt during joint motion. The **fine** crepitus of inflamed synovium is of uniform intensity and perceptible only with a stethoscope. In contrast, **coarse** crepitus is easily detected, of variable intensity, and transmitted from damaged cartilage and/or bone. Crepitus may be elicited by compressing a joint throughout its range of motion.

10. **Which joints are included in a joint count? (Table 5-2)**

11. **How do tender points and trigger points differ? (Table 5-3)**

12. **Define photosensitivity and photophobia.**

    Photosensitivity refers to the development of a **rash following less than 30 minutes of sun exposure** (typically ultraviolet-B light). This feature is noted among 30% to 60% of patients with cutaneous lupus (discoid, or subacute cutaneous lupus), systemic lupus erythematosus, and dermatomyositis. Photophobia indicates **ocular sensitivity** to light and is commonly found in patients with uveitis.

13. **What rheumatic disorders, other than rheumatoid arthritis, may exhibit subcutaneous nodules? (Box 5-1)**

14. **What historical or physical features are essential for the diagnosis of Raynaud's phenomenon?**

    Raynaud's phenomenon is a reversible, vasospastic disorder characterized by transient, stress-induced (e.g., cold temperature) ischemia of the digits, nose-tip, and/or ears. As a result of vasospastic alterations in blood flow, a triphasic color response is usually observed. The initial color is **white** (ischemic pallor), then **blue** (congestive cyanosis), and finally **red** (reactive hyperemia). The diagnosis of Raynaud's phenomenon best correlates with the initial "dead-white" pallor of ischemia. It should involve primarily the fingers and not the entire hand.

Table 5-2.

Peripheral Joints	
Hand	Foot
Distal interphalangeal (DIP)	Interphalangeal
Proximal interphalangeal (PIP)	Metatarsophalangeal (MTP)
Metacarpophalangeal (MCP)	Talocalcaneal (subtalar)
Thumb carpometacarpal (CMC)	Ankle
Wrist	Knee
Elbow	
Axial Joints	
Shoulder	Spine
Glenohumeral	Cervical
Acromioclavicular	Thoracic
Sternoclavicular	Lumbar
Hip	Temporomandibular
Sacroiliac	

Table 5-3.

FEATURE	TENDER POINT	TRIGGER POINT
Disorder	Fibromyalgia	Myofascial pain syndrome
Distribution	Widespread	Regional
Abnormal tissue	No	±
Tenderness	Focal	Focal
Referred Pain	No	Yes

15. **Describe the examination of a patient with suspected median nerve entrapment of the wrist (carpal tunnel syndrome).**
Thenar atrophy is a reliable sign of carpal tunnel syndrome (CTS) but occurs only as a consequence of chronic disease with damage to the motor nerve. Acute or subacute CTS symptoms are typically sensory (the median nerve supplies sensory innervation to the palmar surface of the thumb, index finger, middle finger, and radial half of the ring finger). Its symptoms may be reproduced by the provocation tests. **Tinel's test** is best performed with the wrist in extension. The full width of the transverse carpal ligament is then percussed using a broad-headed, reflex hammer or the examiner's long finger. In contrast, **Phalen's test** is performed by gently positioning the wrist at full volar flexion for 60 seconds. Nerve conduction velocity studies are useful in confirming the clinical diagnosis of CTS.

16. **In the examination of an arthritic hand, what features enable you to differentiate rheumatoid arthritis from osteoarthritis? (Table 5-4)**

17. **What is Finkelstein's test?**
Finkelstein's test is a useful adjunct to direct palpation in the clinical diagnosis of wrist **tenosynovitis (deQuervain's)**. The test is initially performed by asking the patient to make a fist enclosing the thumb. While stabilizing the patient's forearm, the examiner gently bends the fist toward the ulnar styloid. If extreme discomfort occurs at the "anatomic snuffbox," de Quervain's tenosynovitis of the **abductor pollicis longus** and **extensor pollicis brevis** tendons is present. Occasionally crepitus may also be felt or heard with the stethoscope.

18. **How do you diagnose "tennis elbow" (lateral epicondylitis)?**
In addition to direct palpation, tennis elbow may be diagnosed by stressing the wrist extensor muscles at their origin, the lateral epicondyle. This provocation maneuver requires the patient to form a fist and maintain the wrist in extension. The examiner then flexes the wrist against resistance, while supporting the patient's forearm. Pain arising from the lateral epicondyle confirms the diagnosis. Patients also report grabbing and lifting a full milk carton reproduces the pain.

Box 5-1.

Systemic lupus erythematosus
Rheumatic fever
Tophaceous gout
Juvenile chronic arthritis
Limited scleroderma (calcinosis)
Erythema nodosum
Multicentric reticulohistiocytosis
Sarcoidosis
Vasculitis
Panniculitis
Type II hyperlipoproteinemia
Lupus profundus

Table 5-4.

FEATURE	RHEUMATOID ARTHRITIS	OSTEOARTHRITIS*
Symmetry	Yes	Occasional
Synovitis	Yes	Rarely†
Nodules	Yes	No
Digital infarcts	Seldom	No
Bony hypertrophy	No	Yes
Joint involvement		
DIP	No	Heberden's nodes
PIP	Yes	Bouchard's nodes
MCP	Yes	No‡
CMC	No	Thumb
Wrist	Yes	No§
Deformities	Swan neck	DIP or PIP angulation
	Boutonniere	
	Subluxation	
	Ulnar drift	

*Osteoarthritis may occur secondary to any inflammatory arthritis.
†Synovitis can occur in inflammatory erosive osteoarthritis.
‡Osteoarthritis of the index and middle finger MCP joints may be a feature of hemochromatosis.
§Osteoarthritis of the wrist may occur secondary to trauma or crystalline arthritis.

19. **When examining a swollen, inflamed elbow, how can you differentiate olecranon bursitis from true arthritis?**
Differentiation may be difficult as a result of swelling, pain, and limitation of range (extension and flexion). Rotation of the forearm, with the elbow flexed at 90 degrees, is one maneuver that can help differentiate the two disorders. True arthritis of the elbow will inhibit pronation and supination of the radiohumeral joint, whereas in olecranon bursitis, the joint moves freely. Synovitis usually distends the normal sulcus of the ulnar groove not over the tip of the olecranon. Full extension of the elbow exacerbates true arthritis, whereas it does not affect olecranon bursitis.

20. **In the evaluation of shoulder pain, what single maneuver can best differentiate glenohumeral joint involvement from that of the periarticular tissues?**
Significant glenohumeral joint pathology can usually be excluded if **passive external rotation** of the shoulder is unrestricted and pain free.

21. **What are the best maneuvers to quickly assess shoulder function?**
Ask the patient to raise their hands over their head by fully abducting both shoulders with palms up (NFL touchdown sign). From this position ask them to clasp their fingers together behind their head while keeping their elbows back. Next to test abduction and external rotation, ask the patient to reach behind his head and touch/scratch the superior medial edge of the opposite scapula (Apley "Scratch" Test). Finally, to test internal rotation and adduction have the patient put their hands at their sides and then reach behind their back and try to touch the inferior angle of the opposite scapula. If the patient can perform these maneuvers the shoulder function is normal.

22. How do you test for rotator cuff/supraspinatus tendinitis?

Have the patient abduct their outstretched arm to 90 degrees with the shoulder in 30 degrees of forward flexion and internally rotated such that their thumb is pointing down. The examiner pushes down on the arm while the patient resists. This will cause pain if rotator cuff/supraspinatus tendonitis is present. A patient with a complete rotator cuff tear will not be able to hold the arm up even without pressure being applied by the examiner.

23. What does shoulder impingement mean and how do you test for it?

This multifactorial disorder represents a continuum of degenerative, inflammatory, and attrition of the structures in the subacromial space (SITS muscles [supraspinatous, infraspinatous, teres minor, and subscapularis], subdeltoid bursae, capsule, and bicipital tendon). Pain occurs during passive and active shoulder abduction between an arc of 70 and 120 degrees. Impingement commonly occurs following weakness or destruction of the rotator cuff muscles, the function of which are to stabilize the humeral head against the shallow glenoid fossa. Active abduction by the large deltoid muscle would force the humeral head to migrate superiorly into the narrow subacromial space were it not for the counter force applied by intact rotator cuff muscles. Impingement is tested for by forward flexion of the arm to 90 degrees followed by internal rotation of the glenohumeral joint while the elbow is flexed at 90 degrees (like emptying out a beer can).

24. What are Speed's test and Yergason's maneuver?

These are tests for bicipital tendinitis of the shoulder:
- **Speed's test**—anterior pain in bicipital groove with resisted elevation of the humerus while the elbow and forearm are fully extended forward.
- **Yergason's maneuver**—pain in bicipital groove with resisted supination of the forearm with elbow flexed to 90 degrees and held at patient's side.

Recurrent bicipital tendinitis (and/or rotator cuff tendinitis) should prompt an evaluation for impingement syndrome (see Chapter 62).

25. How do you perform *Adson's test* to evaluate for vascular compromise in thoracic outlet syndrome?

While the examiner palpates the radial pulse, the patient's arm is abducted, extended, and externally rotated. The patient is then asked to look *toward* the side being tested and inhale deeply. Diminution or loss of the radial pulse with development of a new supraclavicular bruit is suggestive of significant subclavian artery compression.

26. When a patient has true hip joint pathology, where is the pain usually reported and how is the hip joint examined?

Despite misconceptions of the lay public, true hip pain is felt in the **groin** region in 90% of cases. In contrast, pain in the lateral hip region or buttock is usually referred from the lumbar spine or trochanteric bursa. Hip pain may occasionally radiate from the groin to the anteromedial thigh, greater trochanter, buttock, and knee. Assessment of hip mobility may help differentiate hip pathology from other causes of groin pain (e.g., adductor tendinitis). The origin of the hip joint as the source of pain can be confirmed by one of two maneuvers: Reproducing the pain during passive external or internal rotation of the hip in the seated position, or rotating the lower leg while the subject is supine with the knee in extension using the hip joint as a pivot (log roll). ROM of the hip can best be assessed while supine by hip flexion (with the knee flexed), whereas abduction and adduction should be assessed with the knee extended. Hip extension requires the patient to position the ipsilateral pelvis off the examining table so the lower leg can be extended posteriorly. In hip disease, the motion lost first is internal rotation.

The **Patrick** test (**FABER** maneuver) is done with the patient lying supine and the examiner flexes, **ab**ducts, and externally **r**otates the patient's leg so that the foot is on top of the opposite knee (forms a "4"). The examiner lowers the leg toward the examining table while applying pressure to the opposite anterior superior iliac crest. If there is a difference between the two legs, the test indicates hip disease (groin pain) or sacroiliitis (sacroiliac joint pain).

27. What does a positive Trendelenburg's test indicate?

A positive Trendelenburg's test reveals weakness of the **gluteus medius** muscle, which may indicate hip joint pathology. The test is performed by observing the patient from behind as he or she stands on one leg. Normally, gluteus medius contraction of the ipsilateral, weight-bearing limb will elevate or allow the contralateral pelvis to remain level. In contrast, a weakened gluteus medius muscle cannot support the contralateral pelvis, and thus it will drop. Neurogenic causes (i.e., L5 nerve root compression) of gluteus medius weakness should also be excluded.

28. Why examine a patient for leg-length inequality, and how is this measured?

Leg-length discrepancy is associated with several "mechanical disorders," such as chronic back pain, trochanteric bursitis, and degenerative hip disease. **True** leg-length discrepancy reflects measurable differences (congenital or acquired) of both limbs using the anterior, superior iliac spines and lateral malleoli as landmarks. **Apparent** or functional leg-length discrepancy is primarily a measure of "pelvic tilt" typically induced by scoliosis or hip contractures. This apparent inequality is determined in the supine position by measuring the distance from the umbilicus to each medial malleoli. True leg-length measurement is usually *equal* in disorders of apparent leg-length discrepancy. Correction of significant inequality (≥1 cm) with a simple shoe lift can be therapeutic.

29. **Describe the physical findings of a patient with meralgia paresthetica.**
Meralgia paresthetica (lateral femoral cutaneous nerve entrapment syndrome) results from compression of the lateral femoral cutaneous sensory nerve as it passes under the inguinal ligament medial to the anterior pelvic brim. Typical symptoms include burning dysesthesias and pain over the anterolateral thigh, unaffected by hip rotation or straight leg raising. In some patients, these symptoms may be elicited by performing **Tinel's test** at the site of entrapment.

30. **How do you diagnose trochanteric bursitis?**
The diagnosis of trochanteric bursitis is best made by direct palpation of the soft tissues overlying the greater trochanter of the femur. Trochanteric bursa pain may also be elicited by hip abduction, flexion, and external rotation and relieved by lidocaine injection.

31. **What is the Ober test?**
The Ober test evaluates the iliotibial band for contracture. The patient lies on the side with the lower leg flexed at the hip and knee. The examiner abducts and extends the upper leg with the knee flexed at 90 degrees. The examiner slowly lowers the limb with the muscles relaxed. A positive test result occurs if the leg does not fall back to the level of the table top. This indicates iliotibial band tightness, which can lead to altered gait causing low back pain, recurrent trochanteric bursitis, and lateral knee pain due to "snapping" of the iliotibial band over the lateral femoral condyle causing iliotibial bursitis.

32. **When examining a swollen knee, how can you tell if it is inflamed?**
In the absence of erythema, **warmth** may be the best indicator of inflammation in a swollen knee. Knee temperature as determined by feeling with the back of your hand is generally cooler than the quadriceps muscles or pretibial skin in normal individuals. Thus, if comparative palpation reveals the anterior knee skin to be warmer than these regions or the contralateral knee, inflammation is likely.

33. **When examining a swollen knee, how can you determine if an effusion is present?**
In addition to comparing the symmetry of the medial knee region to the unaffected knee, the patellar **bulge** test is most useful when evaluating minimal effusions. To perform this maneuver, the supine patient should relax the quadriceps muscle and have the supported knee flexed to 10 degrees. The examiner's palm is used to "milk" a potential effusion from the *medial* knee to the suprapatellar or lateral compartment. A reverse, similar maneuver is then performed on the lateral side. If rapid filling of the *medial* patellar fossa occurs, the bulge test is positive.

34. **What is the patellofemoral compression test?**
This test is used to evaluate damage (e.g., osteoarthritis) to the retropatellar surface. With the knee in flexion, the examiner compresses the patella against the femoral condyles. The patient is then asked to extend the knee forcefully, thus contracting the quadriceps muscle. With quadriceps contraction, the patella will be displaced proximally against the femur. If this maneuver produces pain, the test is positive. Patients usually report that squatting or stair climbing reproduces their pain.

35. **How do you differentiate prepatellar bursitis from knee arthritis?**
A typical feature of acute inflammatory arthritis of the knee is loss of extension as a result of pain with an associated effusion. In prepatellar bursitis, the swelling tends to be localized anteriorly over the patella and pain is increased during knee flexion and direct palpation. Thus, if an inflamed knee demonstrates full extension without pain and a negative bulge sign, the disease is likely to be extraarticular.

36. **When evaluating an unstable knee, how do you perform Lachman's test?**
Lachman's test is a type of drawer test used to evaluate the integrity of the anterior cruciate ligament. It is best performed by holding the knee in 15 to 20 degrees of flexion. While stabilizing the thigh with one hand, the examiner uses the other hand to pull the tibia forward. A mild "give," or forward subluxation, is suggestive of anterior cruciate laxity or tear. Congenital laxity (hypermobility) must be excluded by comparison of both knees.

37. **Where is the pes anserine bursa?**
The pes anserine ("goose foot") bursa is on the medial side of the knee between the aponeurosis of the hamstring's insertion and the medial collateral ligament, approximately 5 cm below the anteromedial joint line. It is a common cause of medial knee pain and frequently mistaken for osteoarthritis of the knee. Reproduction of pain by direct palpation with resolution of the pain after a lidocaine injection confirms the diagnosis.

38. **Describe the ankle joint examination.**
The ankle is a hinge joint. Palpation for synovitis is best done over the anterior (not lateral) aspect of the joint. When the ankle is at the normal position of rest (right angle between foot and leg), the ankle normally has 20 degrees of dorsiflexion and 45 degrees of plantar flexion. Subtalar (talocalcaneal) joint motion is tested

by the examiner grasping the calcaneus with a hand and inverting (25 degrees) and everting (15 degrees) the foot while the ankle joint is held motionless. Muscular strength is assessed by the patient walking on his toes and heels.

39. **List some common causes of heel pain.**
    - Achilles tendonitis—insertional or noninsertional. Usually due to overuse or overpronation of foot.
    - Preadventitial Achilles bursitis—pump bump. Usually due to rubbing from shoe wear on a calcaneus that has Haglund's deformity.
    - Retrocalcaneal bursitis—inflammation of bursa between Achilles tendon and calcaneus.
    - Calcaneal stress fracture.
    - Plantar fasciitis—pain along medial plantar aspect of heel. Pain worse on first getting out of bed in morning with weight stretching plantar fascia. Not due to heel spurs.

40. **What type of patient usually gets posterior tibialis tendonitis (PTT)?**
    PTT dysfunction occurs commonly in women aged 45 to 65 years old. It is associated with flatfoot deformity, obesity, and rheumatoid arthritis. Pain and swelling occur along medial aspect of ankle. Patients cannot stand on their toes owing to pain and/or weakness.

41. **How should the foot be examined?**
    With shoes and socks off! The foot is usually neglected in the physical examination but can be a source of lower extremity pain. Have the patient stand and put weight on his feet to see if there is excessive pronation (flat feet) or a high-arched cavus deformity. Check the range of motion of the *metatarsophalangeal* (MTP) joints. The range of motion for functional ambulation is 65 to 75 degrees of dorsiflexion for first MTP joint and 60 degrees for lesser MTP joints. Have the patient ambulate in his bare feet. Foot deformity, ankle instability, and lack of range of motion of the toes (particularly the first MTP) can result in gait abnormalities that can contribute to ankle, knee, hip, and low back pain.

42. **Name and describe five abnormal gaits.**
    - **Antalgic**—the patient remains on the painful extremity for as short a time as possible during the stance phase of gait. This is known as a "gait of pain" and usually indicates pain in knee, ankle, or foot.
    - **Coxalgic**—a patient with hip pain will lean toward the painful hip during the midstance phase to place the center of gravity over the hip. This lessens the stress on the hip and lessens pain.
    - **Trendelenburg**—a patient with a weak gluteus medius muscle will lurch toward the involved side to place the center of gravity over the hip. This can be seen in an L5 radiculopathy. This "gait of weakness" is similar to the coxalgic gait in appearance but is due to weakness and not pain.
    - **Steppage**—a loss of ankle dorsiflexion (foot drop) such as seen with peroneal nerve injuries will cause the patient to flex the hip excessively and bend the knee during the midswing phase so the toe doesn't scrape the floor. Often there is a loud slap as the foot then hits the floor at the end of the swing phase.
    - **Simian**—a patient with spinal stenosis will often walk flexed forward to lessen the stenosis of the spinal canal. This gait has this name because it is suggestive of a gorilla walking.

BIBLIOGRAPHY

American College of Rheumatology Ad Hoc Committee on Clinical Guidelines: Guidelines for the initial evaluation of the adult patient with acute musculoskeletal symptoms, Arthritis Rheum 39:1, 1996.
Hoppenfeld S: Physical examination of the spine and extremities, New York, CT, 1976, Applelon-Century-Crofts.
Polley HF, Hunder GG: Rheumatologic interviewing and physical examination of the joints, ed 2, Philadelphia, 1978, WB Saunders.
Robinson DB, El-Gabalawy HS: Evaluation of the patient: history and physical examination. In Klippel JH, et al: Primer on the rheumatic diseases, ed 13, New York, 2008, Springer.
Simms RW: Field guide to soft tissue pain: diagnosis and management, Lippincott, 2000, Williams & Wilkins.

CHAPTER 6

LABORATORY EVALUATION

Kathryn Hobbs, MD

KEY POINTS

1. Screening tests for inflammation include C-reactive protein (CRP; most rapid onset), erythrocyte sedimentation rate (ESR), and serum protein electrophoresis (SPEP; most inclusive).
2. A positive antinuclear antibody (ANA) test is not diagnostic of systemic lupus erythematosus (SLE) and can be found in normal individuals and in patients with various other autoimmune and inflammatory diseases.
3. Rheumatoid factor and anti-cyclic citrullinated peptide (anti-CCP) antibodies are equally sensitive in rheumatoid arthritis (RA) patients, but anti-CCP is more specific.
4. A positive anti-neutrophil cytoplasmic antibodies (ANCA) test with anti-PR3 or anti-MPO specificity supports the clinical diagnosis of a systemic necrotizing vasculitis.
5. Low complement (C3, C4) levels suggest an immune complex-mediated disease, whereas undetectable CH50 activity may indicate a disease associated with a hereditary complement component deficiency.

1. **What is the ESR? How is it measured, and what influences its result?**
The Westergren ESR is a measurement of the distance in millimeters that red blood cells (RBCs) fall within a specified tube over 1 hour. The ESR is an indirect measurement of alterations in acute-phase reactants and quantitative immunoglobulins. Acute-phase reactants are a heterogeneous group of proteins (fibrinogen, haptoglobin, C-reactive protein, alpha-1-antitrypsin, and others) that are synthesized in the liver in response to inflammation. Interleukin-6 (IL-6), an inflammatory cytokine, is an important mediator that stimulates the production of acute-phase reactants. Any condition that causes either a rise in the concentration of these asymmetrically charged acute-phase proteins or hypergammaglobulinemia (polyclonal or monoclonal) will cause an elevation of the ESR by increasing the dielectric constant of the plasma. This dissipates inter-RBC repulsive forces, and leads to closer aggregation of RBCs (i.e., rouleaux formation), which causes them to fall faster, increasing the result of the ESR. Aging, female sex, obesity, pregnancy, and possibly race are noninflammatory conditions that can elevate the sedimentation rate. Alterations in number, size, or shape of erythrocytes may physically interfere with rouleaux formation affecting the ESR. Normal ranges of values therefore vary with patient characteristics. The 2012 Medicare National Limitation Amount cost for test was: $5.00 plus $3.00 for venipuncture.
Pearl: A rough rule of thumb for the age-adjusted upper limit of normal for ESR (mm/h) is:

$$Male = age/2; Female = (age+10)/2$$

2. **What causes an extremely high or extremely low ESR?**
   1. Markedly elevated ESR (>100 mm/h)
   - Infection, bacterial (35%)
   - Connective tissue disease: giant cell arteritis, polymyalgia rheumatica, SLE, other vasculitides (25%)
   - Malignancy: lymphomas, myeloma, others (15%)
   - Other causes (25%)
   2. Markedly low ESR (0 mm/h)
   - Afibrinogenemia/dysfibrinogenemia
   - Agammaglobulinemia
   - Extreme polycythemia (hematocrit >65%)
   - Increased plasma viscosity

3. **Describe an approach to the evaluation of an elevated ESR.**
   a. Complete history and physical examination and routine screening laboratories (complete blood count, chemistries, liver enzymes, urinalysis). Make sure that routine health care maintenance is up-to-date. Repeat ESR to ensure it is still elevated and there was no laboratory error.
   b. If there is no clear association after step a, consider the following:
   - Review the medical record to compare with any previously obtained ESR data to determine how long the ESR may have been elevated.

- Check SPEP, fibrinogen, and CRP for evidence of acute-phase response, as well as to rule out myeloma or polyclonal gammopathy.
   c. If still no obvious explanation, recheck the ESR in 1–3 months. Up to 80% of patients will normalize. Follow patient for development of other symptoms or signs of disease if ESR remains elevated.

4. **What is the CRP?**
   CRP is a pentameric protein comprised of five identical, noncovalently linked 23-kD subunits arranged in cyclic symmetry in a single plane. It is present in trace concentrations in the plasma of all humans, and it has been highly conserved over hundreds of millions of years of evolution. Although its exact function is unknown, it shows important recognition and activation properties. Ligands recognized by CRP include phosphatidylcholine as well as other phospholipids and some histone proteins. CRP is able to activate the classic complement pathway, and it can bind to and modulate the behavior of phagocytic cells in both pro- and antiinflammatory ways. CRP is produced as an acute-phase reactant by the liver in response to IL-6 and other cytokines. Elevation occurs within 4 hours of tissue injury and peaks within 24 to 72 hours. In the absence of inflammatory stimuli, it falls rapidly, with a half-life of about 18 hours. A normal value is typically, <0.5 to 1.0 mg/dl (<5.0 to 10.0 mg/l) depending on the laboratory. CRP is measured by immunoassay or nephelometry, and the Medicare test cost is $7.28.
   Pearl: A rough rule of thumb for the age-adjusted upper limit of normal for CRP (mg/dL) is:

   $$\text{Male} = \text{age}/50; \quad \text{Female} = (\text{age}+30)/50$$

   Pearl: Levels >8 to 10 mg/dL (>80 to 100 mg/L) should suggest bacterial infection, systemic vasculitis, acute polyarticular crystal disease, or widely metastatic cancer.

5. **When should you order a CRP instead of an ESR?**
   Both tests measure components of the acute-phase response and are useful in measuring generalized inflammation. The ESR is affected by multiple variables and, as such, is somewhat imprecise. Nevertheless, it is inexpensive and easy to perform. The CRP test measures a specific acute-phase reactant, and thus it is more specific. It rises more quickly and falls more quickly than the ESR, which tends to remain elevated for a longer time (decreases by 50% in 1 week) after inflammation subsides. Note that hypergammaglobulinemia causes a persistently elevated ESR preventing it from ever becoming normal whereas CRP is not affected by immunoglobulin levels.

6. **What is the most sensitive test for detecting inflammatory change?**
   Although serum protein electrophoresis is the most expensive test (Medicare cost=$31.46), it directly quantifies the acute-phase response. Inflammation is followed by characteristic protein alterations that are reflected on high-resolution electrophoresis. The typical pattern includes increases in immunoglobulins as well as increases in the α-1 zone (e.g. α-1 antitrypsin, others) and α-2 zone (e.g., α-2 macroglobulin, haptoglobin) and the β area (fibrinogen, CRP). Decreases (negative acute phase reactants) are seen in prealbumin, albumin, and the β zone (transferrin).

7. **How are antinuclear antibodies measured?**
   The major method currently in use is the indirect immunofluorescence (IIF) technique. Permeabilized cells are fixed to a microscope slide and incubated with the patient's serum, allowing ANAs to bind to the cell nuclei. After washing, a fluoresceinated second antibody is added, which binds to the patient's antibodies (which are bound to the nucleus). Cells are visualized through a fluorescence microscope to detect nuclear fluorescence. The amount of ANAs in a patient's serum is determined by diluting the patient's serum before adding the serum to the fixed cells—the greater the dilution (titer) at which nuclear fluorescence is detected, the greater the amount of ANAs present in the patient's serum.
   Most laboratories now use HEp-2 cells (a proliferating cell line derived from a human epithelial tumor cell line) for the substrate to detect ANAs. This is because rapidly growing and dividing cells contain a larger array and higher concentration of nuclear antigens (such as SS-A and centromere antigens). Recently, enzyme-linked immunoassay methods (ELISA) and multiplex bead assays have become available for the detection of ANAs. These assays vary among manufacturers but are less expensive than ANAs done using fluorescence microscopy. The Medicare cost for an ANA screening test is $17.00.

8. **What is an LE cell?**
   The LE cell (lupus erythematosus cell) was used as the major method of measuring ANAs in the 1950s and 1960s. In this test, a bare nucleus stripped of cytoplasm is incubated with the patient's serum, allowing ANAs to bind to the nucleus. Normal polymorphonuclear leukocytes (PMNs) are then added, and if sufficient antibodies have been bound to the nucleus, the nucleus is opsonized and the PMNs engulf the nuclear material. A PMN containing phagocytosed nuclear material is known as an LE cell. This test is time consuming, relatively insensitive in detecting ANAs (50% to 60%), and is difficult to interpret. The ANA detected by IIF and other techniques therefore have replaced it.

9. **At what point is an ANA test considered positive?**
   A positive ANA is arbitrarily defined as that level of antinuclear antibodies that exceeds the level seen in 95% of the normal population. Each laboratory must determine the level that it considers positive, and this level may vary significantly among labs. In most laboratories where HEp-2 cells are used as substrate to detect an ANA, clinically significant titers are usually ≥1:160.

10. **Can a positive ANA occur in a normal healthy individual?**
    Yes. The frequency depends on ANA titer and patient characteristics:
    - ANA 1:40: 20% to 30% of healthy individuals can be positive
    - ANA 1:80: 10% to 15% positive
    - ANA 1:160: 5% positive
    - ANA 1:320: 3% positive
    - Healthy relative of an SLE patient: 5% to 25% positive (usually low titers)
    - Elderly (>age 70): up to 70% positive at ANA titer 1:40

11. **Can a patient with SLE ever be ANA negative?**
    Yes, but very rarely. Very few patients (<1%) with active, untreated SLE will have a negative ANA. These patients usually have one of the following:
    1. Hereditary early complement component deficiency (C2,C4). These patients usually have low titer ANAs.
    2. Antibodies only to the nuclear antigen SS-A (Ro) and are ANA negative because:
       - The substrate used in the fluorescent ANA test did not contain sufficient SS-A antigen to allow detection of those antibodies. Although such patients are ANA negative on rodent tissue substrates, they are almost always positive when HEp-2 substrate is used, OR
       - The antibody is directed only against the 52 kDa SS-A/Ro protein which is only located in the cytoplasm and not against the 60 kDa SS-A/Ro protein located in the nucleus.
    3. A very few cases of SLE may have antibodies restricted to cytoplasmic constituents (ribosomes, ribosomal P, and others).
    4. Rarely, SLE patients (up to 10% to 15%) will become ANA negative with treatment and their disease becomes inactive.
    5. Rarely, SLE patients with severe proteinuria may be ANA negative due to antibody loss in the proteinuria. ANA becomes positive with a decrease in proteinuria with therapy.
    6. SLE patients with end-stage renal disease on chronic dialysis can become ANA negative.
    7. Technical factors and prozone effect can sometimes be responsible for a negative ANA.

12. **What medical conditions are associated with a positive ANA? (Table 6-1)**
    Pearl: A positive ANA in a person with a single autoimmune clinical manifestation such as discoid lupus, Raynaud's disease, or idiopathic thrombocytopenia purpura increases their risk for developing other manifestations of a connective tissue disease in the future.

Table 6-1.

CONDITION	% ANA POSITIVE
SLE	99-100
Drug-induced lupus	100
Mixed connective tissue disease	100
Autoimmune liver disease (hepatitis, cholangitis)	100
Systemic sclerosis (limited and diffuse subsets)	80-95
Oligoarticular juvenile idiopathic arthritis (uveitis)	70-80
Polymyositis/dermatomyositis	40-80
Primary Sjögren's syndrome	40-80
Antiphospholipid antibody syndrome	40-50
Rheumatoid arthritis	30-50
Autoimmune thyroid disease (Hashimoto's disease, Graves' disease)	30-50
Primary pulmonary hypertension	40
Multiple sclerosis	25
Neoplasia (especially lymphoma)	15-25
Chronic Infections (SBE, TB, mononucleosis)	Varies

SBE, Subacute bacterial endocarditis; SLE, systemic lupus erythematosus; TB, tuberculosis.

13. **Can the ANA titer be used to follow disease activity in patients with SLE or other autoimmune diseases?**
    No. There is no evidence that variations in ANA titer (level) as measured by screening ANAs correlate with disease activity.

14. **What is the significance of the pattern of ANA?**
    ANA patterns refer to the patterns of nuclear fluorescence observed under fluorescence microscopy. Certain patterns of fluorescence are associated with certain nuclear antigens are associated with specific diseases (Box 6-1).
    Patterns of staining provide a clue to the category of nuclear antigens involved and are dependent upon the type of substrate used, and to a certain extent, the experience of the technician. Reliance on ANA patterns has largely been replaced by identification of specific antinuclear antibodies through the ANA profile (see Question 16).
    Pearl: An ANA-positive patient with an autoimmune disease frequently will not have one of the specific autoantibodies listed above detected. This is because of the 100 to 150 ANAs against specific autoantigens that have been described, only about 10 of the most common are routinely tested for (Figure 6-1).

15. **Is the ANA a good screening test for SLE or another autoimmune disease?**
    No. Simple mathematics indicate that if 5% of the normal American population is ANA positive, then 12.5 million normal individuals have a positive ANA. In contrast, even if 100% of SLE patients are ANA positive, because the prevalence of SLE is only approximately 1/1000, there are only 250,000 individuals with SLE who are ANA positive. Thus, if the entire population were screened for ANA, more normal individuals would be detected who are ANA positive than SLE individuals (i.e., 50 to 1). The clinical value of an ANA test is tremendously enhanced by ordering an ANA when there is a reasonable pretest probability (i.e., clinical suspicion) of an autoimmune disease. Alternatively, a negative ANA (or 1:40 titer) makes it highly unlikely that the patient has SLE, mixed connective tissue disease (MCTD), Sjögren's syndrome, or systemic sclerosis.

16. **Which diseases are associated with the different antibodies measured in the ANA profile? (Table 6-2)**

17. **In some diseases, antibodies against cytoplasmic antigens can be more helpful diagnostically than antibodies against nuclear antigens. Which diseases? (Table 6-3)**
    Patients with these diseases frequently lack antibodies to nuclear antigens and hence are often ANA negative. Consequently, the specific anticytoplasmic antibody should be ordered when these diseases are suspected.

18. **Which of the ANAs measured in the ANA profile are useful to follow disease activity?**
    Antibodies to double-stranded (dsDNA) often parallel disease activity in SLE. High titers of antibody to dsDNA are associated with lupus nephritis, and increases in dsDNA antibody levels are frequently predictive of a flare of lupus activity. Other antibodies included in the ANA profile are markers of disease subsets but do not fluctuate with disease activity. The Medicare cost for testing for anti-dsDNA antibodies is $19.33.

Box 6-1.

Homogenous (diffuse)
— DNA-histone (nucleosome)	SLE, drug-induced LE, other diseases
— Mi-2	Dermatomyositis (15-20%)

Rim (peripheral)
— dsDNA	SLE

Speckled
— SS-A (Ro)	SLE, SCLE, primary Sjögren's syndrome, systemic sclerosis (SSc), other diseases
— SS-B (La)	SLE, primary Sjögren's syndrome, SCLE
— RNP	MCTD, SSc, SLE
— Sm	SLE
— Ku	SLE, PM/SSc overlap

Nucleolar
— Topoisomerase I (Scl-70)	Systemic sclerosis (diffuse type) (20-30%)
— RNAP I, II, III	Systemic sclerosis (diffuse type) (4-20%)
— Fibrillarin (U3-RNP)	Systemic sclerosis (diffuse type) (8%)
— TH/TO	Systemic sclerosis (limited type) (5%)
— PM-Scl (PM-1)	Polymyositis overlap (1%)

Centromere (kinetochore)
— CENP	Limited scleroderma (CREST)

52   II EVALUATION OF THE PATIENT WITH RHEUMATIC SYMPTOMS

19. What syndromes are associated with antibodies to SS-A (Ro)?
Antibodies to SS-A/Ro may target one or both of two cellular proteins with different molecular weights (52 kDa and 60 kDa) and cellular locations. The 52-kDa protein is an interferon-inducible protein located in the cytoplasm. It functions as an E3 ubiquitin ligase that adds ubiquitin to several proteins involved in the inflammatory and immune response resulting in their accelerated degradation. The 60-kDa protein binds to small

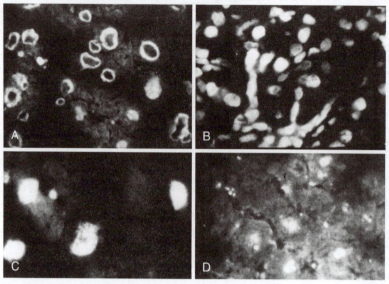

Figure 6-1. Patterns of ANA fluorescence. **A**, Rim (peripheral); **B**, homogenous (diffuse); **C**, speckled; **D**, nucleolar. (© 2014 American College of Rheumatology. Used with permission.)

Table 6-2.

	dsDNA	RNP	SM	SS-A	SS-B	CENTROMERE (CENP)
SLE	70-80%	30%	30%	40%	15%	Rare
Rheumatoid arthritis	(-)	(-)	(-)	5%	Rare	(-)
Mixed connective tissue disease	(-)	100% (high titer)	(-)	Rare	Rare	Rare
Diffuse systemic sclerosis	(-)	20% (low titer)	(-)	10-20%	Rare	10-15%
Limited systemic sclerosis (CREST)	(-)	(-)	(-)	(-)	(-)	60-90%
Primary Sjögren's syndrome	(-)	Rare	(-)	75%	40-50%	(-)

Table 6-3. Autoimmune Diseases Associated with Anticytoplasmic Antibodies

DISEASE	CYTOPLASMIC ANTIGEN	FREQUENCY
Polymyositis	tRNA synthetase (anti-Jo-1, others)	20-40%
	Signal recognition particle	4%
SLE	Ribosomal P	5-10%
Granulomatosis with polyangiitis (Wegener's)	Serine proteinase-3 (seen only in neutrophils)	90%
Microscopic polyangiitis (+ other vasculitides)	Myeloperoxidase, others (seen only in neutrophils)	70%
Primary biliary cirrhosis	Mitochondria	80%

noncoding RNAs located in the nucleus. It functions as an RNA chaperone that binds to defective cellular and viral RNAs to hasten their degradation. Diseases associated with these antibodies include:
1. SLE
2. Primary Sjögren's syndrome
3. Subacute cutaneous lupus (SCLE) (a variant of lupus characterized by prominent photosensitivity and rash)
4. Neonatal lupus
5. Congenital heart block
6. Undifferentiated connective tissue disease (UCTD)
7. Other diseases: primary biliary cirrhosis (30%), anti-tRNA synthetase polymyositis (19%), systemic sclerosis (10% to 20%)

Notably some diseases have antibodies directed preferentially against one of the two SS-A/Ro proteins. Antibodies primarily against 52-kDa SS-A/Ro are seen in patients with anti-tRNA polymyositis and in patients with systemic sclerosis. Patients with the other autoimmune diseases listed above typically have antibodies against both the 52-kDa and 60-kDa SS-A/Ro proteins.

20. **What is the significance of antibodies to ribonuclear protein?**
Antibodies to ribonuclear protein (RNP) produce a speckled pattern on immunofluorescent ANA, reflective of the focal distribution of their target; the spliceosomal snRNPs in the nucleus involved in premessener RNA splicing. These antibodies are seen in a number of autoimmune diseases, including SLE, systemic sclerosis, and MCTD. The presence of very high levels of anti-RNP is highly suggestive of MCTD, a syndrome of overlapping disease manifestations with features of systemic sclerosis, SLE, and polymyositis. Patients with anti-RNP antibodies are more likely to have Raynaud's disease, pulmonary hypertension, myositis, and esophageal dysmotility.

21. **What is the significance of an ANA with a nucleolar or centromere pattern?**
The patient either has or will develop systemic sclerosis. The nucleolar pattern is seen in patients with diffuse disease, limited disease with anti-TH/TO, or polymyositis overlap (anti-PM-Scl). Limited systemic sclerosis (CREST) is associated with anticentromere antibodies.

22. **Describe how the ANA pattern and antigen specificity are used in the diagnosis of the connective tissue diseases (Figure 6-2).**

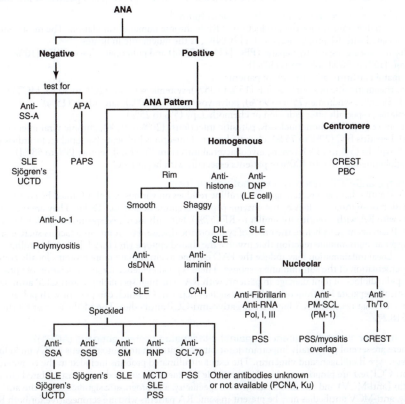

Figure 6-2. APA, Antiphospholipid antibodies (lupus anticoagulant, anticardiolipin antibodies); CAH, chronic active hepatitis; DIL, drug-induced lupus; MCTD, mixed connective tissue disease; PAPS, primary antiphospholipid antibody syndrome; PSS, progressive systemic sclerosis (scleroderma); RNA Pol, RNA polymerase; SCL-70, topoisomerase I; UCTD, undifferentiated connective tissue disease.

23. **How would you evaluate an unexplained positive ANA in a patient with nonspecific arthralgias?**
    1. History and physical examination: look for signs of a connective tissue disease and particularly occult Sjögren's syndrome.
    2. Obtain an ANA profile: ANA titers ≥1:160 or the presence of disease-specific autoantibodies usually indicates the ANA is significant.
    3. Obtain additional studies looking for evidence of immune hyperactivity and/or organ involvement:
       - CBC: Look for anemia of chronic disease, neutropenia, and thrombocytopenia.
       - Liver enzymes: If elevated, consider autoimmune hepatitis.
       - C3, C4: Look for hypocomplementemia.
       - SPEP: Look for polyclonal gammopathy.
       - RF, ESR, VDRL (false-positive), PTT (lupus anticoagulant).
       - Electrolytes, creatinine, urinalysis for completeness.

    If any of the above are abnormal, the ANA may be indicative of an evolving autoimmune disease, and the patient will need to be followed closely. Note that a history of Hashimoto's thyroiditis can be associated with a positive ANA with negative specific autoantibodies.

24. **What are rheumatoid factors, and how are they measured?**
    Rheumatoid factor (RF) is the general term used to describe an autoantibody directed against antigenic determinants on the Fc fragment of immunoglobulin G. RF may be of any isotype: IgM, IgG, IgA, or IgE. IgM RF is the only one routinely measured by clinical laboratories, using nephelometry, ELISA, and latex agglutination techniques. RF has a sensitivity in RA of 50% to 80%, with specificity from 80% to 90%. RA patients who are RF positive tend to have more aggressive joint disease and are at increased risk to develop extraarticular manifestations. Disease activity of rheumatoid arthritis is best determined by clinical assessment and not by RF titer. Teleologically, RFs probably developed in humans as a mechanism to help remove immune complexes from the circulation. Therefore, many conditions associated with chronic inflammation are also associated with RF positivity. The Medicare cost for an RF test is $8.00.

    RF can be positive in normal individuals but usually at low titer (<50 International Units, <1:160). Males and females are affected equally. Age affects the frequency of a positive RF in normal individuals with 2% to 4% (20 to 60 years old), 5% (60 to 70 years) and 10% to 25% (>70 years) positive at low titers.

25. **What are the causes of a positive rheumatoid factor?**
    The common denominator for the production of RF is chronic immune stimulation. The most common diseases associated with RF production are: CHRONIC, as the mnemonic indicates:

    CH Chronic disease, especially hepatic (PBC [45% to 70%]) and pulmonary diseases (IPF [10% to 50%], silicosis [30% to 50%], asbestosis [30%])
    R Rheumatoid arthritis, 50% to 85% of patients
    O Other rheumatic diseases, such as SLE (15% to 35%), systemic sclerosis (20% to 30%), MCTD (50% to 60%), Sjögren's syndrome (75% to 95%), polymyositis (5% to 10%), sarcoidosis (15%)
    N Neoplasms, especially after radiation or chemotherapy (5% to 25%)
    I Infections (e.g., AIDS, mononucleosis, parasitic infections) (20% to 90%), chronic viral infections (15% to 65%), hepatitis B/C (20% to 75%), chronic bacterial infections [subacute bacterial endocarditis (25% to 50%), syphilis (5% to 13%), others, mycobacterial infections (TB [8%], leprosy [5% to 58%])
    C Cryoglobulinemia, 40% to 100% of patients especially with hepatitis C

26. **What is the anti-CCP antibody and what does it test?**
    Anti-CCP antibodies are directed against citrulline residues on various proteins formed by posttranslational deimination of arginine residues by the enzyme peptidylarginine deiminase (PAD). They are often found in patients with RA with a sensitivity similar to RF (67%), but with increased specificity (95%). Both RF and anti-CCP can occur years before the onset of symptomatic disease. Environmental factors such as smoking may trigger an autoimmune reaction that involve the shared epitope (in HLA-DR4) and citrulline-modified peptides. Local inflammation may induce the PAD enzyme to citrullinate more proteins locally contributing to the perpetuation of the autoimmune response. There is good evidence for an association of anti-CCP with more rapid radiological joint damage in patients with RA. The high specificity of anti-CCP antibodies helps to diagnostically separate RA from other diseases such as hepatitis C, which can present with polyarthralgias and a positive RF that resembles RA but have negative anti-CCP antibodies. The Medicare cost for the anti-CCP test is $18.22.

27. **Are there other antibodies directed against citrullinated protein antigens (ACPA)?**
    Yes. There are several potentially important joint-targeted citrullinated autoantigens in RA including fibrin, α-enolase, type II collagen, and vimentin. The exact citrullinated proteins included in the commercially available anti-CCP test are proprietary. Another available test measures antibodies against mutated citrullinated vimentin (anti-MCV) and has similar sensitivity, specificity, and prognostic significance as the anti-CCP test. Notably, anti-MCV antibodies may be present in some RA patients who are seronegative for both RF and anti-CCP.

28. **What are anti-neutrophil cytoplasmic antibodies?**
 Anti-neutrophil cytoplasmic antibodies (ANCAs) are antibodies directed against specific antigens present in the cytoplasm of neutrophils. There are three different types of indirect immunofluorescence staining patterns for ANCAs using ethanol-fixed neutrophils as substrate:
 - C-ANCA pattern: diffuse cytoplasmic staining on immunofluorescence. The most common antibodies causing this pattern are directed against serine proteinase-3 (PR3). Less commonly the target antigen is bactericidal/permeability-increasing protein (BPI) or others.
 - P-ANCA pattern: perinuclear staining pattern around the nucleus. The most important antibody causing this pattern is directed against myeloperoxidase (MPO). Other antigen targets include elastase, cathepsin G, lactoferrin, lysozyme, and azurocidin.
 - Atypical ANCA pattern: snow-drift staining pattern around the nucleus often confused with the P-ANCA pattern. Usually seen in patients with inflammatory bowel disease, connective tissue diseases, or autoimmune hepatitis.

29. **Which diseases are associated with ANCAs?**
 Patients who are ANCA positive should have ELISA testing for specific antibodies directed against PR3 and MPO which are the most relative autoantibodies associated with an underlying systemic necrotizing vasculitis. Other disease associations with C-ANCA and P-ANCA are typically negative for anti-PR3 and anti-MPO antibodies:
 C-ANCA (PR3 positive): granulomatosis with polyangiitis (Wegener's), microscopic polyangiitis (usually P-ANCA), Churg-Strauss vasculitis (rare).
 P-ANCA (MPO positive): microscopic polyangiitis, Churg-Strauss vasculitis, pauci-immune glomerulonephritis (renal-limited vasculitis), Goodpasture's syndrome, drug-induced syndromes (hydralazine, PTU, minocycline, and others).
 P-ANCA (MPO negative): autoimmune gastrointestinal disorders (ulcerative colitis, primary sclerosing cholangitis, autoimmune hepatitis), rheumatic diseases (RA, SLE, many others), cystic fibrosis, HIV infection, certain other acute and chronic infectious or neoplastic diseases (rare).
 Anti-HNE: antibodies against human neutrophil elastase are commonly seen in ANCA positive disease associated with cocaine cut with levamisole. The ANCA staining pattern is atypical or perinuclear but can be cytoplasmic or have multiple patterns.
 Pearl: If C-ANCA is not against PR3 or P-ANCA is not against MPO, look for causes other than vasculitis for the positive ANCA.

30. **Do ANCA titers fluctuate with disease activity?**
 This is controversial. In granulomatosis and polyangiitis (Wegener's), a rising titer of C-ANCA can correlate with disease activity (in 60% of cases) and has been used to predict flares of disease. However, because this relationship is inconsistent, a rising C-ANCA titer should not be used as the sole basis for changes in therapy. There is little evidence that P-ANCA titers fluctuate with disease activity. The Medicare cost for the ANCA test is $21.19.

31. **What are the causes of decreased circulating complement components?**
 Serum complement may be decreased as a result of:
 1. Decreased production, owing to either a hereditary deficiency or liver disease (complement components are synthesized in the liver).
 2. Increased consumption (proteolysis) as a result of complement activation. A major cause of complement consumption is increased levels of circulating immune complexes, which activate the classic complement pathway.

32. **What clinical conditions are associated with hereditary complement deficiencies? (Table 6-4)**

33. **Can a patient with active inflammation involving circulating immune complexes have a normal complement level?**
 Yes. The serum level of complement components represents a balance between consumption and production. Complement components are acute-phase reactants, therefore their production by the liver increases with inflammatory states. If increased production keeps pace with consumption, the result will be a normal level of complement. Clinically, this means that although a decreased level of complement (C3, C4) is confirmatory evidence for complement consumption, normal complement levels cannot exclude complement consumption.

34. **What diseases are associated with decreased levels of complement (not hereditary deficiency)?**
 Rheumatic diseases
 - SLE
 - Systemic vasculitis (especially polyarteritis nodosa, urticarial vasculitis)
 - Cryoglobulinemia (types II and III)
 - Rheumatoid arthritis with extra-articular manifestations (rare)

 Infectious diseases
 - Subacute bacterial endocarditis
 - Bacterial sepsis (pneumococcal, gram-negative)
 - Viremias (especially hepatitis B)

Table 6-4.

COMPLEMENT COMPONENTS	DISEASE
Early (C1, C2, C4)	SLE-like disease
	Glomerulonephritis
Mid (C3, C4)	Recurrent pyogenic infections
	SLE-like disease
Terminal (C5-C9)	Recurrent infections (especially gonococci and meningococci)
Regulatory proteins	HAE (C1INH), aHUS (Factor H), AMD (Factor H), PNH (DAF/CD59)

- Parasitemias
Glomerulonephritis
- Post-streptococcal
- Membranoproliferative

35. **What complement components should one order?**
    - Complement components, **C3** and **C4**, measured by nephelometry. Low levels of both C3 and C4 indicates classic complement pathway activation usually by immune complexes. Alternative complement pathway activation is indicated by low levels of C3 with normal C4. A normal C3 but low C4 suggests heterozygous C4 deficiency or low level complement pathway activation (C1 INH deficiency etc.). The Medicare cost for a C3/C4 test is $17.00 each.
    - **CH50**, total hemolytic complement assay, requires all components of the complement pathway to be present. It is a good screen for complement deficiency. A CH50 level of 0 or "unmeasurable" is suggestive of a hereditary (and homozygous) complement deficiency. It is not a good disease activity marker because in active inflammation its level can be either low, normal, or high, reflecting the end result of balance between production and consumption of the complement components. The Medicare cost for a CH50 test is $28.78.

36. **How do you separate iron deficiency anemia from the anemia of chronic disease in a patient with a chronic inflammatory disease like rheumatoid arthritis?**
    In patients with uncomplicated iron deficiency anemia (IDA), measurement of iron status with serum level of iron (low), percent iron saturation (low), TIBC (high), and ferritin (low) are adequate. However, in patients with inflammatory disease, the TIBC and ferritin can be normal as a result of the acute phase response. Thus, to separate IDA from the anemia of chronic disease (ACD), the gold standard is a bone marrow biopsy. However, studies have shown that a serum ferritin greater than 100 µg/L excludes iron deficiency in patients with an active inflammatory disease as indicated by an elevated ESR/CRP. Likewise, a serum ferritin less than 50 to 60 µg/L, particularly when associated with an elevated serum transferrin receptor level, is highly specific for IDA in patients with rheumatoid arthritis. The Medicare cost for a ferritin test is $19.30.

37. **Other than an elevated ESR, CRP, and ACD, what additional tests suggest systemic inflammation?**
    Patients with a systemic inflammatory disease such as vasculitis frequently have reactive thrombocytosis, mild elevation of hepatic alkaline phosphatase, and low albumin. The low albumin is due to hepatic synthesis of acute-phase reactants (CRP, etc.) at the expense of albumin. Thus, the low albumin is not due to malnutrition, which is frequently postulated but incorrect.

38. **What is the Vectra-DA Test? What is the IdentRA test?**
    The Vectra-DA test is a multi-biomarker test which measures rheumatoid arthritis disease activity. This test measures 12 immune, endothelial, bone, cartilage, and metabolic protein biomarkers (VCAM-1, EGF, VEGF-A, IL-6, TNF-RI, MMP-1, MMP-3, YKL-40, leptin, resistin, SAA, CRP) that reflect the underlying biology of RA. Serum concentrations of the biomarkers are integrated into a proprietary algorithm that generates a single score from 1 to 100 that classifies disease activity as high (>44), moderate (29 to 43), low (25 to 28), or remission (<25). Recent studies report good correlation with other clinical disease activity measures (DAS28, CDAI, SDAI). The cost of the test for private insurance is "several hundred dollars." Medicare recently approved this test for coverage but the cost has not been released.
    The IdentRA is an ELISA test that detects the presence and amount of the 14-3-3η (eta) protein. This protein is one of seven isoforms of the 14-3-3 protein family which are ubiquitous intracellular chaperones that regulate communication pathways involved in inflammation. Patients with rheumatoid arthritis and

erosive psoriatic arthritis have high levels in the synovial fluid. The protein is thought to be secreted by synovial fibroblasts and synovial macrophages. In conjunction with rheumatoid factor and anti-CCP antibodies, this test may also help identify those patients with early undifferentiated inflammatory arthritis who are most likely to evolve into rheumatoid arthritis and/or develop erosive arthritis. Therefore it has both diagnostic and prognostic properties that may guide therapeutic decisions.

Bibliography

Bang H, Egerer K, Gauliard A, et al: Mutation and citrullination modifies vimentin to a novel autoantigen for rheumatoid arthritis, Arthritis Rheum 56:2503–2511, 2007.
Bultink IEM, Lems WF, Vande Stadt RJ: Ferritin and serum transferrin receptor predict iron deficiency in anemic patients with rheumatoid arthritis, Arthritis Rheum 44:979–981, 2001.
Curtis JR, van der Helm-van Mil AH, Knevel R, et al: Validation of a novel multibiomarker test to assess rheumatoid arthritis disease activity, Arthritis Care Res 64:1794–1803, 2012.
Gabay C, Kushner I: Acute phase proteins and other systemic responses to inflammation, N Engl J Med 340:448–454, 1999.
Kavanaugh A, Tomar R, Reveille J, et al: Guidelines for clinical use of the antinuclear antibody test and tests for specific autoantibodies to nuclear antigens, Arch Pathol Lab Med 124:71–81, 2000.
Mandl L, Solomon DH, Smith EL: Using ANCA testing to diagnose vasculitis: can test ordering guidelines improve diagnostic accuracy? Arch Int Med 162:1509–1514, 2002.
Miller A, Green M, Robinson B: Simple rule for calculating a normal erythrocyte sedimentation rate, Br Med J 286:266, 1983.
Satoh M, Vazquez-Del Mercado M, Chan EK: Clinical interpretation of antinuclear antibody tests in systemic rheumatic diseases, Mod Rheumatol 19:219–228, 2009.
Shmerling RH, Delbanco TL: The rheumatoid factor: an analysis of clinical utility, Am J Med 91:528–534, 1991.
Shmerling RH: Diagnostic tests for rheumatic disease: clinical utility revisited, So Med J 98:704, 2005.
Shmerling RH: Testing for anti-cyclic citrullinated peptide antibodies, Arch Int Med 169:9–14, 2009.
Solomon DH, Kavanaugh AJ, Schur PH: Evidenced-based guidelines for the use of immunologic tests: antinuclear antibody testing, Arthritis Rheum 47:434–444, 2002.
Sox HC, Liang MH: The erythrocyte sedimentation rate: guidelines for rational use, Ann Intern Med 104:515–523, 1986.
Walport MJ: Complement, N Engl J Med 344:1058, 2001. and 1104.
Wener MH, Daum PR, McQuillan GM: The influence of age, sex, and race on the upper reference limit of serum C-reactive protein concentration, J Rheumatol 27:2351–2359, 2000.

CHAPTER 7
ARTHROCENTESIS AND SYNOVIAL FLUID ANALYSIS

Robert T. Spencer, MD

KEY POINTS

1. Aspirate any monoarticular inflammatory arthritis.
2. The synovial fluid analysis should be viewed as a liquid biopsy of the joint.
3. The most important tests to send synovial fluid for are cell count, crystal examination, Gram stain, and culture.
4. The synovial fluid analysis can tell you if the arthritis is noninflammatory, inflammatory, hemarthrosis, crystalline, or infectious.

1. **When should arthrocentesis be performed?**
   Without doubt, the single most important reason to perform arthrocentesis is to check for joint infection. Timely identification and treatment of a patient with septic arthritis are of paramount importance to a favorable clinical outcome. In addition, arthrocentesis is generally indicated to gain diagnostic information through synovial fluid analysis in the patient with a monoarticular or polyarticular arthropathy of unclear etiology characterized by joint pain and swelling.

2. **When is arthrocentesis contraindicated?**
   When the clinical indication for obtaining synovial fluid is strong, such as in the patient with suspected septic arthritis, there is no absolute contraindication to joint aspiration. Relative contraindications include **bleeding diatheses**, such as hemophilia, anticoagulation therapy, or thrombocytopenia; however, these conditions can be frequently treated or reversed before arthrocentesis. **Cellulitis** overlying a swollen joint can make the approach to the joint space difficult, but this rarely precludes the ability to perform the procedure.

3. **How safe is arthrocentesis in patients on warfarin (Coumadin)?**
   Although hemarthrosis has been reported following joint aspiration in anticoagulated patients, it appears to be uncommon. A recent study found no hemorrhagic complications in patients on Coumadin with an international normalized ratio of <4.5. Using the smallest needle necessary for the procedure and applying prolonged pressure following the arthrocentesis are recommended.

4. **What techniques should be used when performing an arthrocentesis of the knee to rule out a septic joint?**
   The procedure should be performed using an **aseptic technique**. A topical antiseptic should be applied to the area. Nonsterile gloves should always be worn as part of universal precautions. Sterile gloves should be used if palpation of the area is foreseen subsequent to antiseptic preparation and before placement of the needle. A 25-gauge needle should be used to administer a local anesthetic (e.g., 1% lidocaine). The aspiration itself should be performed using an 18-gauge, 1.5-inch needle, when possible, and a 10-mL to 30-mL syringe. Aspiration techniques for individual joints are described elsewhere.

5. **What precautions should be done if the patient is "allergic" to povidone–iodine, lidocaine, or latex?**
   - Patients with topical iodine reactions can have their skin cleansed with chlorhexadine or pHisoHex followed by an alcohol pad.
   - True "caine" allergy is extremely rare. Many of the symptoms that occur during dental procedures are due to the epinephrine or preservatives (parabens) in the lidocaine (Xylocaine) and not an IgE-mediated reaction. To be absolutely sure, skin testing and subcutaneous incremental challenge would have to be done. This is usually not practical; therefore, options include numbing the area with a skin refrigerant (ethyl chloride, Frigiderm) only or using a local anesthetic from the benzoic acid ester group that does not cross-react with lidocaine such as chloroprocaine (Nesacaine). Note that a patient with a procaine (Novocain) reaction can use lidocaine (Xylocaine).
   - Most latex allergies are minor local reactions. However, some patients can have a severe latex allergy. In these patients, arthrocentesis must be performed using latex-free gloves and syringes. The rubber stopper on the top of the lidocaine must be removed because sticking a needle through this can result in latex protein being introduced into the lidocaine.

6. **What are the potential complications of arthrocentesis?**
   - Infection (risk <1 in 10,000).
   - Bleeding/hemarthrosis.
   - Vasovagal syncope.
   - Pain.
   - Cartilage injury.

7. **Where does normal synovial fluid come from?**
   The synovial fluid is a selective transudate of plasma. Large molecules such as clotting factors are excluded and therefore normal synovial fluid does not clot spontaneously. Synovial fluid is viscous like an egg yolk (synovial is derived from *ovum*, Latin for egg). The increased viscosity is due to hyaluronic acid produced by fibroblast-derived type B synoviocytes and contributes to the lubricating function of the fluid. With inflammation, cells with their degradative enzymes enter the joint cavity breaking down the hyaluronans causing the synovial fluid to become less viscous. In addition clotting factors gain entry causing the synovial fluid to clot spontaneously.

8. **What studies should be performed for synovial fluid analysis?**
   Because the single most important determination of synovial fluid analysis is for the presence of infection, **Gram stain** and **culture** should be performed on samples from joints with even relatively low suspicion for infection. Determining **total leukocyte count** and **differential** helps in differentiating between noninflammatory and inflammatory joint conditions. Lastly, **polarized microscopy** should be done to evaluate for the presence of pathological crystals. Chemistry determinations, such as glucose and total protein, are unlikely to yield helpful information beyond that obtained by the previous studies, and therefore they should not be routinely ordered. Normal synovial fluid glucose is within 20 mg% of the serum value unless inflammation or infection is present. Normal synovial fluid protein averages around 2 mg% (33% of the serum total protein) and increases with inflammation. Lactate dehydrogenase, uric acid, pH, electrolytes, and immunological studies are of no value and should not be ordered.

9. **What if no synovial fluid is obtained (a "dry tap")?**
   Even if no fluid is aspirated into the syringe, frequently one or two drops of fluid and/or blood can be found within the needle and its hub. This amount is sufficient for culture, in which case the syringe with a capped needle should be submitted to the microbiology laboratory. If one extra drop can be spared, it can be placed on a microscope slide with a coverslip for estimated cell count (1 white blood cell [WBC]/40× objective=500 WBCs) and polarized microscopy. When microscopy is completed, the coverslip can be removed and the specimen may then serve as a smear for Gram stain. The specimen remaining on the coverslip may be an adequate smear on which to perform a Wright stain, allowing determination of leukocyte differential. Thus, two drops of fluid can yield the same important diagnostic information as that obtained from a larger specimen, with the exception of a leukocyte count. The lesson to be learned from this is that when a "dry tap" is encountered, the needle and syringe should not be reflexively discarded!

10. **What are some causes of "dry taps"?**
    Inability to obtain synovial fluid from a joint with an obvious effusion can be from:
    - Synovial fluid too thick to aspirate through the lumen of a needle.
    - Obstruction of the needle lumen with debris such as rice bodies (infarcted pieces of synovium in synovial fluid) or thick fibrin.
    - Chronically inflamed synovium can undergo fat replacement and become markedly thickened (lipoma arborescens), so that the needle never makes it into the effusion.
    - In the knee, a medial plica or medial fat pad (especially in obese patients) may block the needle. In this case, aspirate from the lateral aspect of the knee.
    - Poor technique and not getting into the joint with a needle.

11. **Within what time frame should synovial fluid analysis occur?**
    Synovial fluid should be analyzed as soon as possible after the fluid is drawn. If it is delayed more than 6 hours, results may be spuriously altered. Problems that can arise include:
    - Decrease in leukocyte count (due to cell disruption).
    - Decrease in number of crystals (primarily calcium pyrophosphate dihydrate).
    - Appearance of artifactual crystals.

12. **How may synovial fluid WBC count be estimated by "wet drop" examination?**
    At the time polarized microscopy is performed, the synovial fluid WBC count can be easily estimated. The finding of 2 or fewer WBCs per high-power field (40× high dry objective) confidently suggests a noninflammatory fluid (<2000 WBCs/mm^3). If greater than 4 WBCs per high-power field are seen, there is a significant chance the synovial fluid is inflammatory and formal determination of the WBC count should be ordered. The rule of thumb is that 1 WBC seen at 40× objective estimates 500 cells in total WBC count. For example, if you observe 10 WBCs in a 40× field the estimated cell count would be 5000/mm^3.

Table 7-1. Synovial Fluid Classification

FLUID TYPE	APPEARANCE	Total WBC COUNT/mm^3	% PMNs
Normal	Clear, viscous, pale yellow	0 to 200	<10%
Group 1 (noninflammatory)	Clear to slightly turbid	200 to 2000	<20%
Group 2 (inflammatory)	Slightly turbid	2000 to 50,000	20% to 75%
Group 3 (pyarthrosis)	Turbid to very turbid	>50,000 to 100,000	>75%

PMN, Polymorphonuclear cell; WBC, white blood cell (leukocyte).

Box 7-1. Rheumatic Disorders with Group 2 (Inflammatory) Synovial Fluid

Rheumatoid arthritis
Gout
Pseudogout
Psoriatic arthritis
Ankylosing spondylitis
Reactive arthritis
Juvenile idiopathic arthritis
Rheumatic fever
Systemic lupus erythematosus
Polymyalgia rheumatica
Giant cell arteritis
Granulomatosis with polyangiitis
Hypersensitivity vasculitis
Polyarteritis nodosa
Familial Mediterranean fever
Sarcoidosis
Infectious arthritis
   Viral (hepatitis B, rubella, HIV, parvovirus, others)
   Bacterial (gonococci)
   Fungal
   Mycobacterial
   Spirochetal (Lyme disease, syphilis)
Subacute bacterial endocarditis
Palimic rheumatism

13. **Describe the classification based on synovial fluid analysis.**
    Synovial fluid classification is given in Table 7-1.

14. **Name some causes of noninflammatory (group 1) joint effusions.**
    Osteoarthritis, joint trauma, mechanical derangement, pigmented villonodular synovitis, and avascular necrosis.

15. **Group 2 (inflammatory) synovial fluid is typical for which rheumatic disorders?**
    Typical rheumatic disorders for group 2 (inflammatory) synovial fluid are given in Box 7-1.

16. **Other than joint sepsis, which conditions are associated with a group 3 fluid (pyarthrosis)?**
    When a group 3 fluid is discovered, septic arthritis must be assumed until proved otherwise by synovial fluid culture. A few disorders may cause noninfectious pyarthrosis, sometimes referred to as joint **pseudosepsis**.
    - Gout.
    - Reactive arthritis.
    - Rheumatoid arthritis.

17. **How does the synovial fluid WBC differential help in diagnosing an inflammatory arthritis?**
    - Neutrophil predominance: most inflammatory synovial fluids. Septic arthritis and crystalline arthropathies have >90% to 95% polymorphonuclear cells (PMNs).
      - Ragocytes are neutrophils that have ingested immune complexes: consider rheumatoid arthritis, septic, and crystalline.
    - Lymphocyte predominance (>70%): consider systemic lupus erythematosus and mycobacterial infections.
    - Macrophage predominance (>80%): consider spondyloarthropathies, "Milwaukee shoulder."
      - Lipid-laden macrophages: traumatic, pancreatic disease.
    - Monocyte predominance (>80%): consider viral arthritis, serum sickness, spondyloarthropathies.
    - Eosinophil predominance: hypereosinophilia syndrome, parasitic arthritides, arthrography (dye), therapeutic radiation, metastatic adenocarcinoma, idiopathic.
    - Mast cells present: consider spondyloarthropathies and systemic mastocytosis.

18. **List some causes of a hemarthrosis (see Chapter 49).**
    - Trauma
    - Bleeding diatheses
    - Tumors
    - Pigmented villonodular synovitis
    - Hemangiomas
    - Scurvy
    - Iatrogenic (postprocedure)
    - Arteriovenous fistula
    - Intense inflammatory disease
    - Charcot's joint

Pearl: fat/lipid droplets (look like bubbles) in bloody synovial fluid (may have tomato soup appearance) should suggest subchondral fracture if the joint has been traumatized or avascular necrosis.

19. **Compare the polarized light microscopic findings of synovial fluid from a joint with gout and one with pseudogout.**

    A comparison of polarized light microscopic findings of synovial fluid from a joint with gout and pseudogout is given in Table 7-2.

    Pearl: for the crystal color, use the mnemonic ABC (Alignment, Blue, Calcium). If the crystal aligned with the red-plate compensator is blue, it is calcium pyrophosphate dihydrate. Urate crystals are the opposite, being yellow when parallel to the compensator. Crystals within WBCs are more indicative of a crystalline arthropathy than free-floating crystals. Note that hydroxyapatite crystals are too small to see with polarized light (Figure 7-1).

20. **Are there any "tricks" that can be done to increase the yield of finding uric acid crystals in a patient who clinically has gout?**

    Rarely, you may encounter a patient who clinically has gout but you cannot find crystals on synovial fluid examination. Some "tricks" that have been tried are to centrifuge the fluid and examine the centrifugate for crystals. Another is to cool the fluid in the refrigerator, although this usually does not work. Finally, putting fluid on a microscope slide and allowing it to dry for 2 to 3 hours may allow overhydrated uric acid crystals to dehydrate and be drawn toward each other to form spherules that are easier to see.

21. **What special stains can be done on the cytocentrifuge preparation to help establish the diagnosis?**
    - Wright stain.
      - LE cell: PMN with ingested homogeneous nuclear material.
      - Reiter's cell: large macrophage with ingested PMNs (cytophagocytic mononuclear cells).
      - Hydroxyapatite crystals in PMNs.
      - Charcot–Leyden crystals in eosinophils.

Table 7-2. A Comparison of Polarized Light Microscopic Findings of Synovial Fluid from a Joint With Gout and a Joint with Pseudogout

	GOUT	PSEUDOGOUT
Crystal	Urate	Calcium pyrophosphate dihydrate
Shape	Needle	Rhomboid or rectangular
Birefringence	Negative	Positive
Color of crystals parallel to axis of red-plate compensator	Yellow	Blue

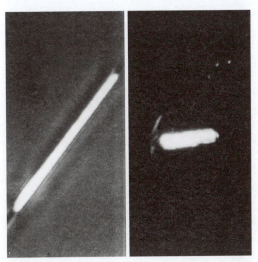

Figure 7-1. **Left,** Urate crystal of gout, showing needle shape. **Right,** Calcium pyrophosphate dihydrate crystal of pseudogout, showing rhomboid shape.

- Alizarin Red S: stains calcium crystals (hydroxyapatite and calcium pyrophosphate dihydrate).
- Oil Red O/Sudan Black: stains for fat globules.
- Congo Red: stains amyloid fragments.

BIBLIOGRAPHY

Clayburne G, Daniel DG, Schumacher HR: Estimated synovial fluid leukocyte numbers on wet drop preparations as a potential substitute for actual leukocyte counts, J Rheumatol 19:60, 1992.

El-Gabalawy HS: Synovial fluid analysis, synovial biopsy, and synovial pathology. In Firestein GS, Budd RS, Gabriel SE, McInnes IB, O'Dell JR, editors: Kelley's textbook of rheumatology, ed 9, Philadelphia, 2013, Saunders Elsevier.

Fiechtner JJ, Simkin PA: Urate spherulites in gouty synovia, JAMA 245:1533–1536, 1981.

Fye KH: Arthrocentesis, synovial fluid analysis, and synovial biopsy. In Klippel JH, Stone JH, Crofford LEJ, White PH, editors: Primer on the rheumatic diseases, ed 13, Atlanta, 2007, Springer.

Gatter RA, Andrews RP, Cooley DA, et al: American College of Rheumatology guidelines for performing office synovial fluid examinations, J Clin Rheumatol 1:194–200, 1995.

Kerolus G, Clayburne G, Schumacher HR: Is it mandatory to examine synovial fluids promptly after arthrocentesis? Arthritis Rheum 32:271, 1989.

Roberts WN, Hayes CW, Breitbach SA, et al: Dry taps and what to do about them: a pictorial essay on failed arthrocentesis of the knee, Am J Med 100:461, 1996.

Shmerling RH, Delbanco TL, Tosteson AN, et al: Synovial fluid tests: what should be ordered? JAMA 264:1009, 1990.

Swan A, Amer H, Dieppe P: The value of synovial fluid assays in the diagnosis of joint disease, Ann Rheum Dis 62:493–498, 2002.

Thumboo J, O'Duffy JD: A prospective study of the safety of joint and soft tissue aspirations and injections in patients taking warfarin sodium, Arthritis Rheum 41:736, 1998.

RADIOGRAPHIC AND IMAGING MODALITIES

Colin Strickland, MD

CHAPTER 8

> **KEY POINTS**
> 1. Inflammatory arthritis causes periarticular osteoporosis, marginal erosions, and uniform joint space narrowing.
> 2. Noninflammatory, degenerative arthritis causes sclerosis, osteophytes, nonuniform joint space narrowing, and cysts.
> 3. Chronic tophaceous gout typically causes erosions with a sclerotic margin and overhanging edge in peripheral small joints.
> 4. Sacroiliitis, best seen on a modified AP Ferguson view of the sacrum, is the radiological hallmark of an inflammatory axial arthropathy.

1. **Is there a pattern approach to interpreting a plain radiograph for arthritis?**
   In assessing a skeletal radiograph, a pattern approach using ABCDES can be very helpful:
   A—Alignment. Rheumatoid arthritis (RA) and systemic lupus erythematosus (SLE) are characterized by deformities such as ulnar deviation at metacarpophalangeal (MCP) joints.
   —Ankylosis. Seronegative spondyloarthropathies frequently cause ankylosis. Previous surgery or infection is an additional cause.
   B—Bone mineralization. **Periarticular** osteopenia is typical of RA or infection and is rare in crystalline arthropathy, seronegative spondyloarthropathies, and degenerative joint disease.
   —Bone formation. Reactive bone formation (periostitis) is the hallmark of seronegative spondyloarthropathies. Osteophytosis is seen in degenerative joint disease and calcium pyrophosphate deposition disease (CPPD) and can be present in any end-stage arthritis.
   C—Calcifications. Soft tissue calcific densities may be seen in gouty tophi, SLE, or scleroderma. Cartilage calcification is typical of CPPD, although this finding may also be seen in patients with degenerative joint disease.
   —Cartilage space. Symmetric and uniform cartilage or joint-space narrowing is typical of inflammatory disease. Focal or nonuniform joint-space loss in the area of maximal stress in weight-bearing joints is the hallmark of osteoarthritis.
   D—Distribution of joints. For example, RA usually has symmetric distribution of affected joints, whereas seronegative spondyloarthropathies are asymmetric. Also, target sites of involvement may permit differentiation of arthritides.
   —Deformities. Swan neck or boutonniere deformities of the hands are typical of RA.
   E—Erosions. In addition to their presence or absence, the character of erosions may be diagnostic, such as overhanging edges and sclerotic margins in gout. Marginal erosions are more suggestive of an inflammatory arthropathy such as RA.
   S—Soft tissue and nails. Look for distribution of soft tissue swelling, nail hypertrophy in psoriasis, and sclerodactyly in scleroderma.
   —Speed of development of changes. Septic arthritis will rapidly destroy the affected joint.
   Pearl: when obtaining radiographs on patients with arthritis, always order weight-bearing radiographs to evaluate joint-space narrowing in lower extremity joints (i.e., hip, knee, ankles).

2. **Describe the radiographic features of an inflammatory arthritis (synovial-based diseases).**
   1. Soft tissue swelling.
   2. Periarticular osteopenia.
   3. Uniform loss of cartilage (i.e., diffuse joint-space narrowing best seen in weight-bearing joints).
   4. Bony erosion in "bare" areas.
   Synovial inflammation causes soft tissue swelling. The inflammation also results in hyperemia, which, coupled with the inflammatory mediators released (such as prostaglandin E_2), causes periarticular (juxtaarticular) osteopenia. With chronicity, inflammatory arthritis may lead to more diffuse osteoporosis (due to disuse and other factors) of the joints due to pain. As the inflammation leads to synovial hypertrophy and pannus formation, the pannus erodes into the bone. These erosions occur first in the marginal "bare areas" where synovium abuts bone that does not possess protective cartilage (Figure 8-1). The pannus ultimately extends over the

cartilaginous surface and/or erodes through the bone to the undersurface of the cartilage. Cartilage destruction results either by enzymatic action of the inflamed synovium and/or by interference with normal cartilage nutrition. Owing to its generalized nature, this cartilage destruction is radiographically seen as uniform or symmetric, diffuse joint-space narrowing observed best in weight-bearing joints. It is important to remember that some findings of degenerative arthritis may be superimposed on those of an inflammatory nature, particularly in long-standing cases.

3. **What is the "bare area"? Why do the earliest erosions begin here?**
In synovial articulations, hyaline articular cartilage covers the ends of both bones. The articular capsule envelopes the joint cavity and is composed of an outer fibrous capsule and a thin inner synovial membrane. The synovial membrane typically does not extend over cartilaginous surfaces but lines the nonarticular portion of the synovial joint and also covers the intracapsular bone surfaces that are not covered by cartilage. These unprotected bony areas occur at the peripheral aspect of the joint and are referred to as "bare areas" (Figure 8-2).

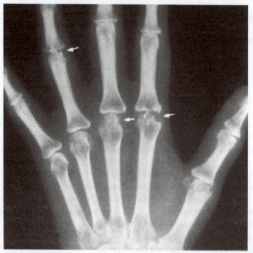

Figure 8-1. Radiograph of a hand showing periarticular osteopenia and bony erosions (arrows) compatible with inflammatory arthritis in this patient with rheumatoid arthritis.

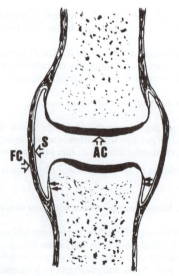

Figure 8-2. Diagram of a typical synovial joint. Small black arrows point to "bare areas," where the bone is exposed to synovium without protective cartilage covering. AC, Articular cartilage; FC, fibrous capsule; S, synovium.

In these areas, the bone does not have a protective cartilage covering. Consequently, the inflamed synovial pannus, which occurs in inflammatory arthritides such as RA, comes in direct contact with bone, resulting in marginal erosions. These "bare areas" are where you should look for the earliest evidence of erosions. Specialized views including the Norgaard view (ball catcher's view) of the hands will pick up the earliest erosive changes in inflammatory peripheral arthritis, whereas the AP Ferguson view of the sacroiliac joints demonstrates the earliest changes in inflammatory axial arthropathy. With progression of the disease, the pannus proliferates to cover the cartilage surfaces, resulting in cartilage destruction (joint-space narrowing) and more diffuse bony erosions.

4. **List the rheumatic disease categories that typically cause radiographic features of inflammatory arthritis.**
   - Rheumatoid arthritis (adult and juvenile)
   - Septic arthritis
   - Seronegative spondyloarthropathies
   - Connective tissue diseases

5. **Describe the radiographic features of noninflammatory, degenerative arthritis (cartilage-based diseases).**
   1. Sclerosis/osteophytes.
   2. Nonuniform loss of cartilage (focal joint-space narrowing in area of maximal stress in weight-bearing joints).
   3. Cysts/geodes.

   The causes of degenerative arthritis are multifactorial. However, the primary problem and end result is cartilage degeneration. As the cartilage degenerates, the joint space narrows. However, in contrast to uniform, diffuse narrowing seen with inflammatory arthritides, the noninflammatory, degenerative arthritides tend to have nonuniform, focal joint-space narrowing, being most pronounced in the area of the joint where stresses are more concentrated (e.g., superolateral aspect of the hip, medial compartment of the knee) (Figure 8-3).

   Following cartilage loss, subchondral bone becomes sclerotic or eburnated, owing to trabecular compression and reactive bone deposition. With denudation of the cartilage, synovial fluid can be forced into the underlying bone, forming subchondral cysts or geodes with sclerotic margins. As an attempted reparative process, the remaining cartilage undergoes endochondral ossification to develop osteophytes. Such osteophytes commonly occur first at margins or nonstressed aspects of the joint (e.g., medial and lateral aspects of the distal femur and proximal tibia of the knee).

6. **List the rheumatic disease categories that typically cause radiographic features of noninflammatory arthritis.**
   - Degenerative joint disease (e.g., primary osteoarthritis and secondary causes of osteoarthritis, such as traumatic arthritis, congenital bone diseases, others).
   - Metabolic or endocrine diseases (e.g., diseases associated with calcium pyrophosphate deposition, ochronosis, acromegaly) may demonstrate findings best characterized as degenerative, although the distribution or specific features (such as extensive chondrocalcinosis in CPPD) may allow for more definitive characterization.

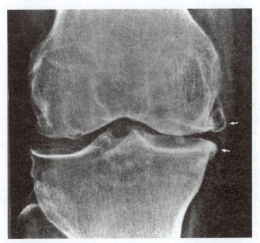

Figure 8-3. Knee radiograph demonstrating osteophytes (*arrows*) and medial joint-space narrowing consistent with degenerative arthritis.

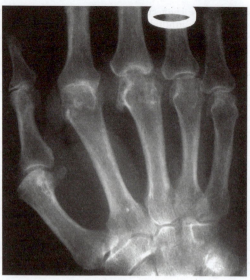

Figure 8-4. Hand radiograph with degenerative features including joint-space narrowing and osteophyte formation. The severity of disease specifically at the index and long finger metacarpophalangeal (MCP) joints suggests the diagnosis of hemochomatosis.

7. **What are the typical sites of joint involvement in primary (idiopathic) osteoarthritis compared with secondary causes of noninflammatory, degenerative arthritis?**

   Primary (idiopathic) osteoarthritis can cause noninflammatory, degenerative arthritic changes in the following joints:
   - Hands.
     - Distal interphalangeal joints (DIPs).
     - Proximal interphalangeal joints (PIPs).
     - First carpometacarpal joint (CMC) of the thumb.
   - Acromioclavicular joint of the shoulder.
   - Cervical, thoracic, and lumbosacral spine.
   - Hips—subchondral cysts (Eggars' cysts) in superior acetabulum are characteristic.
   - Knees—patellofemoral, medial, and lateral compartments.
   - Feet.
     - First metatarsophalangeal (MTP) joint.

   Secondary causes of degenerative arthritis can result in noninflammatory, degenerative changes in any joint (not just those for primary disease). Consequently, if a patient has degenerative changes in any of the following joints, you must consider secondary causes of osteoarthritis:
   - Hands.
     - MCPs (Figure 8-4).
   - Wrist.
   - Elbow.
   - Glenohumeral joint of shoulder.
   - Ankle.
   - Feet, other than first MTP.

   If the degenerative changes involve only one joint, consider traumatic arthritis. If multiple joints are involved, consider a metabolic or endocrine disorder that has caused the cartilage to degenerate in several joints. Note that the end stage of an underlying inflammatory arthritis that has destroyed the cartilage can result in degenerative changes superimposed on the inflammatory radiographic features.

8. **Describe the radiographic features of chronic gouty arthritis.**
   - Erosions with sclerotic margins and an overhanging edge (Figure 8-5). These are caused by tophaceous deposits in the synovium slowly expanding into the bone. The bone reacts and forms a sclerotic margin around the erosion.
   - Relative preservation of joint space until late in disease.
   - Relative lack of periarticular osteopenia for the degree of erosion seen.
   - Nodules in soft tissue (i.e., tophi) near involved joints. Unlike rheumatoid nodules, tophi can become radiopaque.

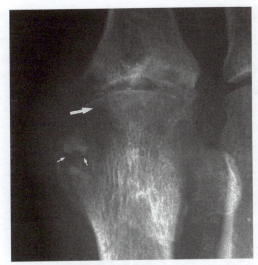

Figure 8-5. Radiograph of foot showing gouty erosions of first MTP with the characteristic overhanging edge (*arrow*). Note calcium in tophi (*small arrows*). MTP, Metatarsophalangeal.

9. **What other diseases can give radiographic features similar to those of chronic gouty arthritis?**
   - *Mycobacterium tuberculosis* and some chronic fungal infections.
   - Pigmented villonodular synovitis.
   - Amyloidosis.
   - Multicentric reticulohistiocytosis.
   - Synovial osteochondromatosis.

10. **Compare the radiographic features of inflammatory and noninflammatory spinal arthritis.**
    Inflammatory spinal arthritis is typically related to either infection or a seronegative spondyloarthropathy. Hematogenous spread of infection usually results in osteomyelitis originating near the endplate regions with subsequent spread to the intervertebral disc. The typical radiographic appearance of osteomyelitis is disc-space narrowing with poorly defined cortical endplates and destruction of the adjacent vertebrae (Figure 8-6). Although this appearance is very suggestive of infection, other inflammatory arthropathies, such as RA (cervical spine), seronegative spondyloarthropathies, and CPPD, can rarely give a similar appearance.
    Ankylosing spondylitis (AS) is associated with squared anterior vertebral bodies with sclerotic anterior corners, syndesmophytes (ossification of the annulus fibrosus), discovertebral erosions (Andersson lesions), and vertebral and apophyseal fusion (Figure 8-6). Psoriatic or chronic reactive arthritis may cause spinal changes similar to AS; however, more typical is the presence of large bulky nonmarginal paravertebral ossifications near the thoracolumbar junction. Radiographic sacroiliitis will also be present in patients with spondyloarthropathy who have inflammatory spinal disease (see Chapters 34 to 37).
    Noninflammatory lumbar arthritis is characterized by disc-space narrowing and vacuum phenomenon, osteophytosis, and bony sclerosis in the absence of sacroiliitis (Figure 8-6 and Table 8-1). Degenerative diseases of the vertebral column can affect cartilaginous joints (discovertebral junction), synovial joints such as apophyses, or ligaments (enthesopathy). Typically, dehydration of the disc results in cartilage fissuring, with subsequent diminution in height and vacuum phenomenon (gas within the disc), and ultimately bony sclerosis (intervertebral osteochondrosis). Osteophytosis (spondylosis deformans) is generally believed to be initiated by annulus fibrosus disruption. Ligamentous degeneration also occurs; ligamentum flavum hypertrophy may contribute to spinal stenosis, whereas ossification of the anterior longitudinal ligament is characteristic of diffuse idiopathic skeletal hyperostosis (DISH) (see Chapter 51).

11. **What is the difference between an osteophyte and a syndesmophyte?**
    The differences between an osteophyte and a syndesmophyte are given in Table 8-2.

12. **What rheumatic disease categories typically have unique radiographic features and are difficult to categorize using the inflammatory, noninflammatory, or gout-like patterns of radiographic changes?**
    - Collagen vascular disease (e.g., scleroderma, SLE).
    - Endocrine arthropathies (e.g., hyperparathyroidism, acromegaly, hyperthyroidism).
    - Miscellaneous (sickle cell disease, hemophilia, Paget's disease, avascular necrosis, Charcot joints, sarcoidosis, hypertrophic osteoarthropathy).
    - Primary articular disorders (e.g., synovial osteochondromatosis).

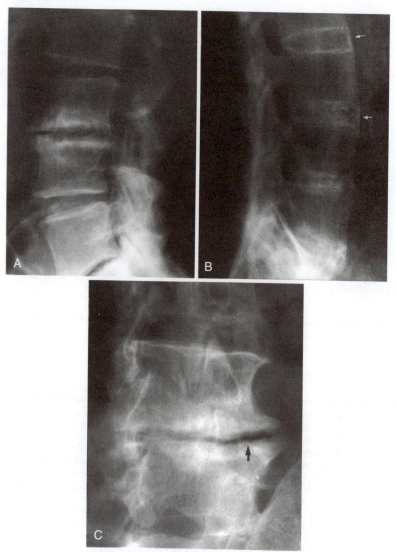

Figure 8-6. A, Lateral radiograph of the lumbar spine demonstrating osteomyelitis at L3 to L4 with erosive/destructive changes of the adjoining cortical endplates. **B,** Lateral radiograph of the lumbar spine demonstrating ankylosing spondylitis with anterior squaring of vertebrae and syndesmophytes (*arrows*). **C,** Oblique radiograph of the lumbar spine showing degenerative disc disease, vacuum sign (*arrow*), and osteophytes.

Table 8-1. Radiographic Features of Inflammatory versus Noninflammatory Spinal Arthritis

	INFLAMMATORY		NONINFLAMMATORY
	Infection	Spondyloarthropathy	
Sacroiliac joints	Erosions	Erosions	Normal
Vertebral bodies	Irregular, eroded endplates	Squaring ± erosions	Sclerosis
Disc space	Narrowed	Variable	Narrowed, vacuum
	One site	Multiple sites	Multiple sites
Syndesmophytes	−	+	−
Osteophytes	−	−	+
Osteopenia	+	+	−
Soft tissue mass	+	−	−

Table 8-2. Differences Between an Osteophyte and a Syndesmophyte

FEATURE	OSTEOPHYTE	SYNDESMOPHYTE
Disorder	Osteoarthritis	Spondyloarthropathy*
Vertebral involvement	Lower cervical Lumbar Cervical	Lower thoracic Upper lumbar
Vertebral orientation	Horizontal	Vertical
Pathogenesis	Endochondral ossification calcification "Bony spurs"	Outer annulus fibrosus "Vertebral bridging"
Complications	Radiculopathy Vertebrobasilar ischemia	Ankylosis —"Bamboo spine" —Fracture

*Includes ankylosing spondylitis, psoriatic arthritis, chronic reactive arthritis, and inflammatory bowel disease arthritis.

13. List the most common diseases associated with the following radiographic changes seen in the hands.
    Extensive arthritis of multiple DIP joints:
    - Primary osteoarthritis. Especially erosive OA.
    - Psoriatic arthritis.
    - Multicentric reticulohistiocytosis.
    First CMC joint arthritis:
    - Primary osteoarthritis.
    Second and third MCP joint arthritis:
    - Hemochromatosis—hook-like osteophytes involving all the MCPs (second to fifth).
    - CPPD—involves primarily second and third MCPs.
    - Acromegaly (initially widened joint spaces, later osteoarthritic changes).
    - Rheumatoid arthritis or psoriatic arthritis if erosive changes.
    Arthritis mutilans of the hands (or feet):
    - Psoriatic arthritis
    - Rheumatoid arthritis
    - Chronic gouty arthritis
    - Multicentric reticulohistiocytosis

14. Outline the approach to the radiographic diagnosis of a patient with peripheral arthritis.
    The approach to the radiographic diagnosis of a patient with peripheral arthritis is outlined in Figure 8-7.

15. List the most common diseases associated with the following radiographic changes seen in the upper extremity and shoulder.
    Radioulnar joint arthritis:
    - RA.
    - Juvenile idiopathic arthritis.
    - CPPD.
    Swan neck and/or ulnar deviation deformities:
    - RA if erosive changes and nonreversible deformities.
    - SLE if nonerosive and reversible deformities.
    Elbow nodules in soft tissue:
    - RA
    - Tophaceous gout (particularly if it contains calcium deposits).
    - Scleroderma-associated calcium deposits.
    "Penciling" of clavicle distal end:
    - RA.
    - Post-traumatic osteolysis.
    - Hyperparathyroidism.

16. Outline an approach to the radiographic diagnosis of a patient with arthritis of the back.
    The approach to the radiographic diagnosis of a patient with arthritis of the back is outlined in Figure 8-8.

17. List the most common diseases associated with the following radiographic changes seen in the feet.
    Destructive arthritis of great-toe interphalangeal joint:
    - Chronic reactive arthritis.
    - Psoriatic arthritis.
    - Gout and RA, less commonly.

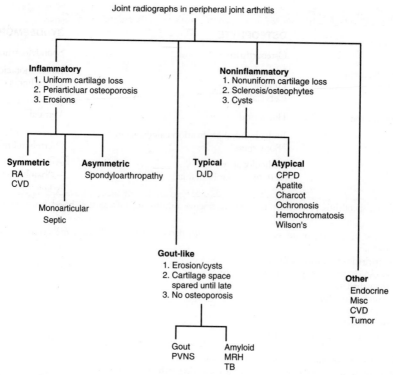

Figure 8-7. The approach to the radiographic diagnosis of a patient with peripheral arthritis. CPPD, Calcium pyrophosphate deposition disease; CVD, collagen vascular disease; DJD, degenerative joint disease; MRH, multicentric reticulohistiocytosis; PVNS, pigmented villonodular synovitis; TB, tuberculosis.

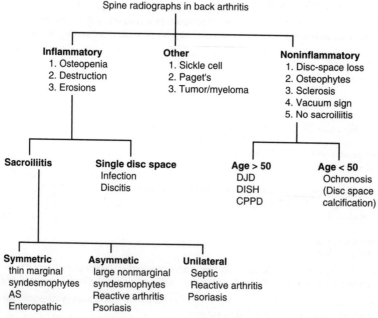

Figure 8-8. The approach to the radiographic diagnosis of a patient with arthritis of the back. AS, Ankylosing spondylitis; DISH, diffuse idiopathic skeletal hyperostosis.

Destructive arthritis at great-toe MTP joint:
- RA.
- Chronic gouty arthritis.
- Chronic reactive and psoriatic arthritis, less commonly.
- Primary osteoarthritis if noninflammatory degenerative changes.

MTP joint erosive arthritis:
- Chronic reactive or psoriatic if asymmetric distribution.
- RA if symmetric distribution.

Calcaneal spurs:
- Traction spurs (noninflammatory)—blunted spur with well-corticated margin.
- Seronegative spondyloarthropathies (inflammatory spurs)— pointed spur with poorly corticated margin and/or erosions.

18. **List the most common diseases associated with the following radiographic changes seen in the spine.**
    Vacuum disc sign:
    - Degenerative disc disease (presence of gas makes infection unlikely).

    Disc space calcification at multiple levels:
    - Ochronosis if the patient is young (<30 years).
    - CPPD and others.

    Sacroiliitis:
    - Ankylosing spondylitis (usually symmetric sacroiliitis).
    - Enteropathic spondyloarthropathy (usually symmetric sacroiliitis).
    - Chronic reactive arthritis (frequently asymmetric sacroiliitis).
    - Psoriatic arthritis (frequently asymmetric sacroiliitis).
    - Infection (unilateral sacroiliitis).
    - Diffuse idiopathic skeletal hyperostosis (DISH) may demonstrate abnormality of the sacroiliac joints with large osteophytic sclerosis at the junction of upper 1/3 and lower 2/3 of sacroiliac joints.

    Syndesmophytes:
    - Ankylosing spondylitis and enteropathic arthritis (thin, marginal bilateral syndesmophytes).
    - Chronic reactive and psoriatic arthritis (large, nonmarginal, asymmetric syndesmophytes).
    - Do not be fooled by DISH with its calcification of the anterior longitudinal ligament (sacroiliac joints will be normal).
    - **Ossification of posterior longitudinal ligament (OPLL)**—usually C3 to C4. Can cause spinal stenosis. Frequently in Asian patients.

19. **List the most common diseases associated with the following radiographic changes:**
    Chondrocalcinosis:
    - Idiopathic CPPD.
    - Osteoarthritis.
    - Hyperparathyroidism.
    - Hemochromatosis.

    Erosions (hallmark of inflammatory synovial-based arthritis):
    - RA or juvenile idiopathic arthritis.
    - Seronegative spondyloarthropathies.
    - Chronic gouty arthritis.
    - Septic (infectious) arthritis.
    - Others (SLE rarely, mixed connective tissue disease, multicentric reticulohistiocytosis, pigmented villonodular synovitis, amyloidosis).

    Isolated patellofemoral degenerative arthritis:
    - CPPD.

20. **Give the characteristic radiographic features of the different arthritides.**
    Rheumatoid arthritis—symmetric, erosive arthritis, uniform joint-space narrowing (especially weight-bearing joints). Most common sites are small joints of the hands and feet (MCPs, PIPs, wrists, MTPs) and cervical spine. Soft tissue nodules that do not calcify. Swan neck deformities and ulnar deviation.
    Juvenile idiopathic arthritis—periarticular osteoporosis, but joint-space narrowing and erosions typically absent until late. Periosteal reaction and **bony fusion** (carpus, facets in cervical spine) may distinguish it from RA. Overgrowth of bone at the margins of a joint suggests juvenile idiopathic arthritis.
    Ankylosing spondylitis—bilateral, symmetric sacroiliitis with ankylosis. **Bilateral, thin, marginal** syndesmophytes in the spine may cause spinal fusion (bamboo spine). Peripheral arthropathy affects large axial joints (shoulders, hips).
    Chronic reactive arthritis (formerly Reiter's syndrome)—can be bilateral or **unilateral, asymmetric sacroiliitis**. Peripherally, there is a predilection for **lower extremities** (especially the interphalangeal joint of great toe), with erosions and fluffy periostitis. Enthesopathy with erosions and calcifications at tendon insertions into calcaneus. Frequently, asymmetric joint involvement. **Large, asymmetric, nonmarginal** (jug-handle) bridging syndesmophytes.

Psoriatic arthritis—axial arthropathy similar to chronic reactive arthritis. Peripherally, it has an upper extremity predilection; DIP or PIP fusion. "Pencil-in-cup" deformity. Enthesopathy and periostitis. Erosions of several joints of a single digit (MCP, PIP, and DIP of one finger). Frequently, asymmetric joint involvement. Acroosteolysis. Jug-handle (chunky) bridging syndesmophytes in the spine.

Gout—erosions with overhanging edge and sclerotic margins. Preserved joint space. Soft tissue tophi that can contain calcium.

CPPD—osteoarthritic changes at sites **atypical for degenerative joint disease** (MCPs, elbow, radiocarpal, ankle, shoulder). Large osseous cysts associated with joint space loss.

Degenerative joint disease (primary osteoarthritis)—nonuniform joint-space narrowing, sclerosis, **osteophytosis**, cysts. Most common sites include the DIPs, PIPs, thumb CMC, knees, hips, acromioclavicular joint, and spine.

Neuropathic joint (Charcot arthropathy)—destruction, disorganization, density (i.e., sclerosis), debris, dislocation (**the five Ds**).

SLE—reversible swan neck and ulnar deviation deformity and subluxation, but absence of erosions.

Scleroderma—tapered, atrophic soft tissues (**sclerodactyly**) with soft tissue calcifications. Acroosteolysis of terminal phalanges.

Hemochromatosis—chondrocalcinosis. **Degenerative changes at MCPs** with "hook-like" spurs. Cystic changes of radiocarpal joint of the wrist.

Ochronosis—**vertebral disc calcification**, chondrocalcinosis, osteoarthritis in multiple joints (especially spine) at a young age.

Acromegaly—**widened joint and disc spaces**. Large spurs at bases of distal phalanges (**spade phalanges**).

Hyperparathyroidism—**subperiosteal resorption** at the radial side of middle phalanges. Soft tissue calcifications, chondrocalcinosis, "salt and pepper" skull, ligament and tendon ruptures.

Avascular necrosis—**crescent sign** of subchondral sclerosis and lucency. Hips and shoulders are most commonly affected.

Hypertrophic osteoarthropathy (periosteal reaction)—intrathoracic pathology such as primary lung cancer. Less likely causes include thyroid acropachy, voriconazole, or pachydermoperiostosis. Other causes of periosteal reaction venous stasis and infection.

21. **What are TR and TE time parameters and how do they relate to magnetic resonance imaging?**
    Magnetic resonance imaging (MRI) functions by submitting tissue to a strong magnetic field and then disturbing that magnetization in tissue by use of radiofrequency (RF) pulses. Return of an RF signal from tissue is then detected and used to construct an image. TR is the time of repetition parameter, or time between 90 degree radiofrequency pulses. TE is the time to echo, or time between the 90 degree pulse and the time when the signal from tissue is recorded. Modulation of the TR and TE parameters determines how much T1 and T2 weighting any given image displays. The TR and TE also determine how long a sequence takes to acquire (from seconds to minutes) and how much heating of tissue occurs.

22. **What is the difference between T1-weighted and T2-weighted images on MRI?**
    T1 or T2 weighting typically refers to spin echo MR sequences. **T1-weighted images** are short TR (300 to 1000 ms) and short TE (10 to 30 ms) and provide excellent anatomical detail. In contrast, **T2-weighted images** are long TR (1800 to 2500 ms) and long TE (40 to 90 ms), sensitive for detecting fluid and edema. An intermediate-weighted sequence or **proton density** sequence combines T1 and T2 weighting by having a long TR (>T1) and short TE (<T2). This technique has some advantages of both T1-weighted and T2-weighted sequences and is commonly used in musculoskeletal imaging.
    Two other sequences commonly used are gradient echo and STIR (short tau [T1] inversion recovery). **Gradient echo** sequences can be either T1-weighted or T2-weighted and permit very rapid acquisition with thin-section, high-quality images. **STIR** is effectively a fat-suppression technique, very sensitive in detection of fluid or edema. These images greatly aid in the detection of subtle marrow and soft tissue disease such as muscle tears. Gadolinium is a paramagnetic element used as a contrast agent in MRI. It adds to the cost of MRI but depicts areas of increased blood flow on T1-weighted images, which is helpful in the detection of early erosions and in distinguishing between effusion and synovial inflammation. Gadolinium should be avoided in patients with significant renal insufficiency (glomerular filtration rate < 30mL/min) due to risk of nephrogenic systemic fibrosis.

23. **Describe the appearances of the various tissues on T1-weighted and T2-weighted MR images.**
    Details of the appearances of various tissues on T1-weighted and T2-weighted MR images are outlined in Table 8-3.

24. **In which clinical situations is a computed tomography scan superior to MRI and vice versa?**
    Radiographs should be obtained before a computed tomography (CT) scan or MRI when evaluating musculoskeletal disorders. Radiographs depict subtle calcifications and collections of gas that may be very difficult to detect with MRI alone. A CT scan is mainly useful to detect bony abnormalities but causes high radiation exposure. It is mainly used when a patient cannot have an MRI (pacemaker, etc.). MRI has no ionizing radiation and can demonstrate soft tissue and bony changes long before radiographs.

A CT scan is preferred over MRI in:
Acute trauma (complex fractures)
Tarsal coalition
Intraarticular osteocartilaginous loose bodies

An MRI scan is preferred over CT in:
Cervical spine disease or instability
Spinal stenosis or disc disease
Internal derangement of the knee
Rotator cuff tears and tendinosis
Avascular necrosis
Osteomyelitis
Soft tissue tumors or skeletal muscle pathology
Pigmented villonodular synovitis
Inflammatory sacroiliitis
Synovitis and tenosynovitis

25. **What is a dual energy CT scan?**

    Dual energy CT scan (DECT scan) is a CT scanner that has two X-ray tubes capable of producing different energies (80 and 140 kV). A software algorithm has been developed to detect uric acid deposits, which have a lower attenuation value than calcium (bone). By color coding the different attenuation values (uric acid vs calcium), the uric acid deposits can be demonstrated.

26. **What imaging features are typically seen in infections of bones or joint spaces?**

    In acute osteomyelitis, the earliest radiographic abnormality is **soft tissue swelling** with obliteration of normal tissue planes (Figure 8-9). Hyperemia results in osteopenia, and bone destruction or periostitis may not be visualized for 7 to 14 days. MRI is much more sensitive for detection of early osteomyelitis. MRI is particularly helpful in defining the full extent of osteomyelitis, particularly when amputation is a therapeutic option. Subacute osteomyelitis is frequently referred to as a **Brodie's abscess**, usually in the metaphysis of tubular bones. A well-marginated **lucent defect** (commonly elongated) is seen surrounded by a thick band of sclerosis. With chronic osteomyelitis, radiodense spicules of necrotic bone, referred to as **sequestra**, may be seen within the lucent defect.

Table 8-3. Details of the Appearances of Various Tissues on T1-Weighted and T2-Weighted MR Images

STRUCTURE	T1 INTENSITY	T2 INTENSITY
Fat, fatty marrow	High	High
Hyaline cartilage	Intermediate	Intermediate
Muscle	Intermediate	Intermediate
Fluid, edema	Low	High
Neoplasm	Low	High
Cortical bone	Very low	Very low
Tendon, ligaments	Very low	Very low

High signal appears white on MRI; low signal appears black on MRI.

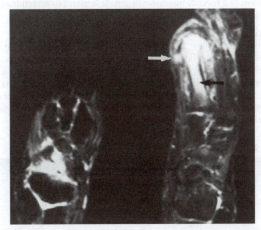

Figure 8-9. An STIR MR image depicts high-signal edema (*black arrow*) corresponding to osteomyelitis involving the entirety of the first metatarsal. Focus of high signal in the adjacent soft tissues represents an abscess (*white arrow*). MR, Magnetic resonance; STIR, short tau [T1] inversion recovery.

27. What are some of the potential uses for ultrasound in the evaluation of musculoskeletal conditions?

Ultrasound is good at detecting abnormalities of superficial structures. High-frequency transducers offer high spatial resolution.

Potential indications include:
- Tendon pathology—tears and inflammation in tendons such as the posterior tibial tendon, Achilles tendon, shoulder, or finger tendons are well demonstrated. Fluid in the tendon sheath is also well visualized.
- Enthesitis— can detect inflammatory enthesitis in peripheral areas.
- Soft tissue masses—non-radioopaque foreign bodies are often invisible on radiographs but are well demonstrated by ultrasound.
- Joint and bursal inflammation—synovitis and effusions of superficial joints are well shown. Can show "double contour" sign in patients with gouty arthritis and hyperechoic chondral deposits in chondrocalcinosis. Can be used to follow disease activity and structural progression.
- Guide articular and periarticular aspiration and/or injections.
- Parotid and submandibular glands— can detect changes compatible with Sjögren's syndrome.
- Nerve entrapment— diagnose median nerve, ulnar nerve, and posterior tibial nerve entrapment.

Pitfalls of ultrasound imaging include:
- Operator dependence—the accuracy of ultrasound is highly affected by the level of training and experience of the user. Certain structures such as the metacarpal head may demonstrate a normal defect that simulates an erosion. Radiographs are needed for comparison and confirmation.
- Deep central portions of joints are obscured—cartilage and meniscal injuries are usually not visible.

28. What role does nuclear medicine have in musculoskeletal imaging?

- **Bone scintigraphy** (also known as bone scan) is routinely performed with ^{99m}Tc-labeled diphosphonates, which are adsorbed onto the surface of the bone proportional to the local osteoblastic activity and skeletal vascularity. Bone scans are therefore sensitive in detecting bone abnormalities but somewhat nonspecific, as tumor, trauma, infection, or other pathology can all cause increased tracer uptake. Bone scintigraphy is the screening examination of choice for the evaluation of bony metastatic disease and Paget's disease, as it images the entire skeleton. Bone scans will commonly detect metastatic disease or osteomyelitis, whereas plain radiographs are still normal, because up to 50% of bone must be decalcified for plain film detection of tumor or infection versus a tiny amount for bone scintigraphy. Bone scintigraphy can also detect stress fractures earlier than plain radiographs.

  In arthritis, MRI and ultrasonography have replaced bone scintigraphy. Other common indications for bone scanning are in the evaluation of chronic regional pain syndrome or metabolic bone disease.

- **Single-photon emission computed tomography** (SPECT) allows increased sensitivity and specificity when assessing spinal pathology. It is frequently combined with conventional CT scanning to map an abnormality on the bone scan to an exact anatomical site (facet joint, pars intraarticularis, or vertebral body).

- **Positron emission tomography** (PET) typically uses ^{18}F-fluorodeoxyglucose (^{18}F-FDG), which goes to sites of increased glucose utilization to map metabolically active tissue in bone and soft tissue. A PET/CT scan provides precise anatomical location of the metabolically active lesion. In rheumatic diseases, it is useful in the diagnosis and management of large vessel vasculitis, osteomyelitis, and sarcoidosis. It may be the test of choice for the evaluation of a fever of unknown origin. It is useful to screen for occult malignancy in older patients with inflammatory myositis.

29. What is a three phase bone scan?

A three phase scan evaluates blood flow to a particular area of the musculoskeletal system during the first two phases of imaging (20 to 30 minutes following injection) and then bony uptake in the delayed third phase (2 to 4 hours later) (Table 8-4). Areas of increased blood flow will have increased activity in the first two phases of imaging, whereas areas of bony remodeling will have increased uptake and thus activity in the third (delayed imaging) phase. Bone scans are highly sensitive to abnormalities of the bone (including fracture, infection, tumor, and arthritis), but are nonspecific. They also allow the entire skeleton to be imaged, which makes the technique useful in the detection of metastatic lesions.

Table 8-4. Three Phase Bone Scan

	CELLULITIS	SYNOVITIS	OSTEOMYELITIS*
First phase	+	+	+
Second phase	+	+	+
Third phase	−	+	+

*During the third phase, tracer uptake for osteomyelitis is more localized on one side of the joint, whereas synovitis is more diffuse.

30. **Is there any role for arthrography in the evaluation of musculoskeletal problems?**
    Arthrography is almost exclusively performed in conjunction with MRI or CT. In the knee, arthrograms are rarely performed, except in cases of previous meniscectomy. Arthrography still plays a role in the evaluation of the shoulder, wrist, ankle, and hip when the evaluation of cartilage or certain soft tissue structures (such as labrum) is required. Aspiration of a joint is certainly indicated in a patient with a painful hip or knee prosthesis, to differentiate infection from aseptic loosening.

31. **What is the radiation exposure to an individual undergoing one of these techniques?**
    The conversion for radiation units is as follows:
    - 1 Sievert (Sv)=1 Gray (Gy)=100 Rem=100 Rad

    The acceptable radiation exposure is:
    - General public=5 mSv/year
    - Occupational exposure for radiation worker=50 mSv/year

    The average background radiation exposure a person is exposed to is:
    - Natural background=3 mSv/year
    - Roundtrip flight from New York to Los Angeles=0.030 mSv

    The average radiation exposure for a radiological procedures is:
    - Mammography—0.5 mSv   Dual-energy X-ray absorptiometry (DXA)—0.001 mSv
    - Chest X-ray—0.02 mSv   Head CT scan—2 mSv
    - Lumbar spine X-ray—1.25 mSv   Ultrasound—0 (although heating of tissue and other effects may occur)
    - Bone scan—6.3 mSv   MRI—0 (although heating of tissue and other effects may occur)
    - Upper gastrointestinal (UGI) series—6 mSv
    - Barium enema—8 mSv (with fluoroscopy)

32. **What are the relative costs of the radiographic procedures used in musculoskeletal imaging of a specific joint (e.g., the shoulder)?**
    Plain radiograph—$120   DXA scan—$200
    Ultrasound—$230   CT scan—$1000
    Arthrography—$450   MRI scan—$1500 to $1800
    Bone scan—$800   PET scan—$3500 to $5000
    Note that the average Medicare reimbursement for each imaging procedure is approximately 25% of the above listed costs.

Acknowledgment
The author and editor wish to thank Dr. Kevin Rak for his contribution to this chapter in the previous edition.

BIBLIOGRAPHY
Brower AC, Flaming DJ, editors: Arthritis in black and white, ed 2, Philadelphia, 1997, Elsevier Saunders.
Hendrick RE, Dodd GD, Fullerton DG, et al: The University of Colorado Radiology Adult Dose-Risk Smartcard, J Am Coll Radiol 9:290–292, 2012.
Jacobson JA: Fundamentals of musculoskeletal ultrasound, Philadelphia, 2007, Elsevier Saunders.
McAlindon T, Kisson E, Nazarian L, et al: American College of Rheumatology report on reasonable use of musculoskeletal ultrasonography in rheumatology clinical practice, Arthritis Care Res 64:1625–1640, 2012.
Mettler FA, Guiberteau MJ: Essentials of nuclear medicine imaging, Philadelphia, 2007, Elsevier Saunders.
Resnick D, Kransdorf MJ: Bone and joint imaging, Philadelphia, 2005, Elsevier Saunders.
Rowbotham EL, Grainger AJ: Rheumatoid arthritis; ultrasound vs MRI, Am J Roentgenol 197:541–546, 2011.
Troum OM, Pimienta O, Olech E: Magnetic resonance imaging applications in early rheumatoid arthritis diagnosis and management, Rheum Dis Clin North America 38:277–297, 2012.

CHAPTER 9

SYNOVIAL BIOPSIES

Sterling G. West, MD

> **KEY POINTS**
>
> 1. The single most important indication for a synovial biopsy is to help establish a diagnosis in a patient with chronic inflammatory monoarticular arthritis.

1. **What are the indications to perform a synovial biopsy?**
   The main indication for a synovial biopsy is chronic (>6 to 8 weeks), nontraumatic, inflammatory (synovial fluid white blood cell count >2000 cells/mm^3) arthritis limited to one or two joints in which the diagnosis has not been made by history, physical examination, laboratory studies, or synovial fluid analysis with culture (including both fungi and mycobacteria).

2. **What diseases can be diagnosed with a synovial biopsy?**
   The diseases that can be diagnosed with a synovial biopsy are given in Box 9-1.

3. **Does a synovial biopsy help in the diagnosis of a systemic connective tissue disease such as rheumatoid arthritis?**
   No. Although a biopsy of the synovium in a patient with rheumatoid arthritis may be compatible with the diagnosis, it is not pathognomonic. Clearly, spondyloarthropathy can produce synovial biopsies that look very much like those obtained from patients with rheumatoid arthritis although prominent plasma cell infiltration suggests rheumatoid arthritis. In the future, synovial biopsies with histological and molecular analysis may better predict what biological therapy a patient is most likely to respond to.

4. **How can synovial tissue be obtained?**
   Table 9-1 shows how synovial tissue can be obtained.

5. **List the advantages and disadvantages of the different methods of synovial biopsy.**
   A comparison of synovial biopsy techniques is given in Table 9-2.
   An ultrasound-guided forceps biopsy has advantages/disadvantages similar to a needle biopsy but can indirectly visualize the best site to biopsy, which lessens sampling error.

6. **Which joints can be biopsied with a closed-biopsy needle?**
   Usually large joints, most commonly the knee. Smaller joints can be biopsied also but require a special needle.

> **Box 9-1.** Diseases That Can Be Diagnosed With a Synovial Biopsy
>
> - **Chronic infections**
>   Fungal arthritis
>   Mycobacterial arthritis
>   Spirochetal arthritis (Lyme disease, syphilis)
>   Whipple's disease
>   Chlamydia
> - **Other systemic diseases**
>   Plant thorn and foreign body
>   Camptodactyly-arthropathy-coxa vara-pericarditis syndrome
>   Chronic sarcoidosis
> - **Infiltrative/deposition diseases***
>   Multicentric reticulohistiocytosis
>   Amyloidosis
>
> Pancreatic fat necrosis
> Ochronosis
> Hemochromatosis
> Crystal-induced arthritis
>
> - **Tumors**
>   Pigmented villonodular synovitis
>   Synovial osteochondromatosis
>   Synovial cell sarcoma
>   Leukemia/lymphoma
>   Metastatic disease to the joint

*Synovial biopsy is usually not necessary in these diseases.

Table 9-1. How Synovial Tissue Can Be Obtained

METHOD	SIZE OF HOLE
Closed-needle biopsy	14-gauge needle
(Parker Pearson or Tru-Cut needle)	(1.6 mm)
Ultrasound-guided forceps biopsy	1.6 mm
Needle arthroscopy +/– ultrasound	1.8 to 2.7 mm
Arthroscopy	4 to 5 mm
Open surgical biopsy	Several inches

Table 9-2. Comparison of Synovial Biopsy Techniques

	ADVANTAGES	DISADVANTAGES
Needle biopsy	Least expensive Least traumatic One skin incision	Small biopsy specimens Sampling error
Needle arthroscopic biopsy	Minimally invasive Direct visualization	Two skin incisions Moderately expensive
Arthroscopic biopsy	Direct visualization Large biopsy specimen	Expensive Invasive
Open surgical biopsy	Direct visualization Large biopsy specimen Best if suspected tumor or foreign body Can be done on any joint	Expensive Most invasive Longest postoperative recovery time

7. **How many specimens must be obtained by a closed-biopsy needle to minimize sampling error?**
   Five to eight specimens from multiple locations in the joint being biopsied reduces sampling error and leads to biopsy specimen variability of less than 10%.

8. **What is the complication rate for obtaining a synovial biopsy by arthroscopy?**
   The total complication rate for arthroscopy by a needle or large bore method is similar: 15/1000 arthroscopies. This includes temporary joint swelling in 10%, hemarthrosis in 0.9%, deep vein thrombosis in 0.2%, and joint infection in 0.1% of cases.

9. **Who invented arthroscopy?**
   1918—Japanese physician, Dr. Takagi, performed the first knee arthroscopy with a cystoscope.
   1930s—German rheumatologist, Dr. Vaupel, proposed the use of arthroscopy to follow the course of arthritis.
   1957—Dr. M. Watanabe performed the first partial meniscectomy through an arthroscope.
   1969—Dr. N. Matsui performed the first arthroscopic synovectomy.

BIBLIOGRAPHY

Gerlag D, Tak PP: Synovial biopsy, Best Pract Res Clin Rheumatol 19:387–400, 2005.
Gerlag DM, Tak PP: How useful are synovial biopsies for the diagnosis of rheumatic diseases? Nat Clin Pract Rheumatol 3:248–249, 2007.
Gibson T, Fagg N, Highton J, et al: The diagnostic value of synovial biopsy in patients with arthritis of unknown cause, Br J Rheumatol 24:232–241, 1985.
Schumacher HR, Chen LX, Pessler F: Synovial biopsy in the evaluation of nonrheumatic systemic diseases causing arthritis, Curr Opin Rheumatol 20:61–65, 2008.

CHAPTER 10

ELECTROMYOGRAPHY AND NERVE CONDUCTION STUDIES

Dianna Quan, MD

KEY POINTS

1. Nerve conduction studies (NCS) and needle electromyography (EMG) are the most useful diagnostic tests in determining the presence, type, severity, and chronicity of a suspected neuromuscular disorder.
2. Although the information collected during NCS and needle EMG testing is more objective and quantitative than that obtained in a standard clinical examination, there are many important technical factors that contribute to the collection of accurate data. Selection of a reputable or accredited laboratory and experienced electrodiagnostic consultant will help to ensure the most accurate data collection and reliable interpretation.
3. Sensory NCS are the most useful way to distinguish preganglionic from postganglionic processes that cause numbness.

1. What is EMG?
EMG is a term used in two ways:
- EMG is used as a general description of the combination of NCS and needle EMG testing.
- More specifically, EMG is used to describe the needle electrode recording performed to assess the function of motor units.

2. What is NCS?
NCS may be performed on either sensory or motor nerves. From the skin surface, a brief electrical stimulus is applied to the nerve of interest and the electrical signal evoked is recorded distally from another point on the nerve, in the case of a sensory nerve, or from the innervated muscle in the case of a motor nerve. The evoked responses are known as the sensory nerve action potential (SNAP) and compound motor action potential (CMAP). Characteristics of the evoked action potentials such as amplitude, onset latency, and conduction velocity provide information about axon and myelin components of the tested nerve.

3. Name some other types of electrodiagnostic tests.
- **Repetitive stimulation studies** are utilized to evaluate the neuromuscular junction (e.g., in myasthenia gravis).
- **Somatosensory evoked potentials** are used to evaluate conduction within the spinal cord and brain.
- Other less frequently used tests include **single-fiber EMG**, **motor-evoked potentials**, and **nerve root stimulation**.

4. What is a motor unit?
A motor unit includes the **motor neuron** found within the anterior horn of the spinal cord, its **axon**, the **neuromuscular junction**, and the associated **muscle fibers** supplied by the axon. The electrodiagnostic physician can utilize a combination of needle EMG, NCS, repetitive stimulation, and other electrophysiologic tests to assess individual components of the motor unit.

5. What are the clinical indications for ordering an EMG?
An EMG should be ordered to determine the localization and severity of a suspected neuromuscular disorder. NCS and needle EMG are almost always performed together in reputable laboratories. Testing can distinguish between neurogenic (nerve- or neuron-related) disorders, myopathic (muscle-related) disorders, and neuromuscular junction disorders. In neurogenic conditions, testing is often able to distinguish between disorders primarily affecting myelin (i.e., demyelinating neuropathies) and axonal or neuronal disorders. EMG is generally not useful in assessing brain or spinal cord disease. To obtain the most useful information from the test, the requesting physician should indicate any clinical question or concern as specifically as possible. It is not usually necessary to request particular procedures (e.g., NCS, repetitive stimulation, needle EMG) because a qualified electrodiagnostic consultant can decide what is needed to answer the clinical question.

6. What are some common nerve disorders?
Functionally, the peripheral nervous system starts in the vicinity of the spinal neural foramen, where sensory and motor fibers join. At its most proximal level, peripheral nervous system injury in the form of **radiculopathy** is caused by compression of the nerve root by a herniated disc or bony fragment. **Plexus involvement** by disease or injury may occur in the upper (brachial plexus) or lower extremity (lumbar or lumbosacral plexopathy).

Peripheral nerve conditions can be acquired or congenital. Congenital problems include hereditary sensory and motor neuropathies (e.g., Charcot–Marie–Tooth disease). Acquired peripheral neuropathies can stem from conditions such as diabetes, toxins (medications or other exogenous substances), and metabolic disturbances.

Focal neural entrapment can be seen in carpal tunnel syndrome, cubital tunnel syndrome, and tarsal tunnel syndrome, to name just a few examples.

7. **Describe three main types of nerve injury.**
   Nerve injuries can be described according to a gradient that was originally defined by Seddon:
   1. **Neurapraxia** is functional loss of conduction without an anatomic change in the axon, usually because of focal demyelination. With remyelination, conduction returns to normal.
   2. In **axonotmesis**, axonal continuity is lost. This loss leads to wallerian degeneration in the distal segment. Recovery, which is frequently incomplete, occurs as a result of axonal regrowth at a rate of 1 to 3 mm/day in otherwise healthy individuals.
   3. **Neurotmesis** results from separation of the entire nerve, including its supporting connective tissue. Regeneration frequently does not occur. Nerves with this degree of trauma may need surgical attention for recovery to occur.

8. **Do these types of nerve injuries occur together?**
   Neurapraxia and axonotmesis commonly occur as a result of the same injury. When compression is relieved from the involved segment of nerve, two periods of healing typically occur. One is relatively immediate, ranging from hours to weeks, as the neurapraxia resolves. A second period of healing, ranging from weeks to months, may occur as a result of axonal regrowth.

9. **What is an innervation ratio?**
   For each motor axon, there are a variable number of associated terminal axons and muscle fibers. Depending on the specific requirement for control, the ratio may be quite low or extremely high. The innervation ratio of the extraocular muscles is typically 1:3 owing to the fine control required for binocular vision. Conversely, the innervation ratio of the gastrocnemius can be as high as 1:2000 because most movements involving the plantar flexors of the ankle are relatively large motions requiring more force than accuracy.

10. **Describe the components of a needle EMG evaluation.**
    Insertional/Spontaneous Activity: An EMG needle inserted into normal muscle should evoke brief electrical discharges by muscle fibers. Increased or prolonged electrical activity may indicate abnormalities of the muscle fibers or the nerves supplying them. Fibrillations, positive sharp waves, and complex repetitive discharges (CRDs) are electrical signals that represent abnormal spontaneous firing of muscle fibers due to nerve or muscle damage. There should be no spontaneous activity in a healthy relaxed muscle.

    Motor Unit Analysis: When a patient slightly contracts a muscle, **motor unit action potentials** (MUAPs) can be recorded. The parameters of interest include the amplitude, duration, number of phases, and firing pattern of the MUAPs. Assessment of these parameters occurs in real time and is generally subjective. The quality of the interpretation depends on the skill and experience of the electromyographer, technical recording conditions, and patient cooperation.

    Recruitment: When a patient contracts a muscle more forcefully, a large number of MUAPs can be recorded. The fullness of this pattern of MUAPs reflects the underlying health of the motor units and the ability of the patient to recruit available motor units. In myopathic conditions, recruitment may be early because myopathic motor units generate less force than healthy ones do. In neurogenic conditions, recruitment may be reduced due to axon or neuron loss.

11. **How do fasciculations, fibrillations, and positive sharp waves differ on needle EMG recordings?**
    A **fasciculation** potential is an involuntary firing of an entire motor unit, that is, a single motor neuron and all its innervated muscle fibers. This is seen as a large electrical spike on needle EMG recordings for a relaxed muscle. It is sometimes clinically visible in the patient as a brief, irregular muscle twitch. This can often be seen in normal individuals, but in excess may be a sign of a motor nerve or motor neuron disorder.

    A **fibrillation** potential is an involuntary contraction of a single muscle fiber that usually indicates that denervation or muscle damage has occurred. Unlike a fasciculation, a fibrillation usually does not cause clinically visible muscle movement.

    Positive sharp wave potentials are similar to fibrillation potentials in that they represent abnormal firing by a muscle fiber due to nerve or muscle damage. They are identified by their initial positive deflection from the baseline, as opposed to the initial negative deflection of a fibrillation potential.

12. **How do normal EMG findings compare with the findings seen in a denervated muscle (neurogenic disorder)?**
    Table 10-1 compares EMG findings for normal and denervated muscles. Note that fibrillations and positive sharp waves are not seen in denervated muscles until 7 to 14 days after the onset of axonal degeneration. Full reinnervation of denervated muscle, resulting in large, polyphasic MUAPs, may take 3 to 4 months or more. In patients with reinnervation after nerve injury, muscles may be clinically strong and yet yield very abnormal needle EMG results.

Table 10-1. EMG Findings for Normal and Denervated Muscles

EMG FINDINGS	NORMAL	ACUTE DENERVATION	CHRONIC DENERVATION/REINNERVATION
Spontaneous activity	None	Fibrillations, positive sharp waves	None
MUAP morphology	Normal	Normal	Large amplitude, long duration, variable increased polyphasia
Recruitment	Normal or full recruitment	Reduced recruitment	Reduced recruitment

EMG, Electromyography; MUAP, motor unit action potential.

Table 10-2. EMG Findings for Normal Muscle and Myopathic Disorders

EMG FINDINGS	NORMAL MUSCLE	MYOPATHY
Spontaneous activity	None	Variable fibrillations, positive sharp waves
MUAP morphology	Normal	Small amplitude, short duration, increased polyphasia
Recruitment	Normal	Early recruitment

EMG, Electromyography; MUAP, motor unit action potential.

13. **How do normal EMG findings compare with the findings seen in myopathic disorders?**
    The weaker a patient with myopathy is, the more likely it is that needle EMG findings will be abnormal. In patients with very mild weakness or those with steroid myopathy, the needle EMG recording may appear normal (Table 10-2).

14. **Is nerve conduction velocity the same throughout the length of a nerve?**
    Nerve conduction velocities vary among nerves and along their lengths. Normally, proximal nerve conduction is faster than distal nerve conduction as a result of the increased temperature and larger diameter of the proximal nerve segments. For example, median nerve conduction velocity from the wrist to the palm should be faster than from the palm to the finger.

15. **Why is temperature recorded during the course of an electrodiagnostic examination?**
    Nerve conduction velocity decreases by 1.5 to 2.5 m/s for every 1° C decrease in temperature in both sensory and motor nerves. These changes can be significant. Failure to warm the limb to a standard temperature, usually 30° C for the leg and 32° C for the arm, can result in false-positive studies, leading to a misdiagnosis.

16. **What are the H-reflex and F-wave? How are they clinically useful?**
    The **H-reflex** is the electrical counterpart of the ankle jerk and gives information on the S1 afferent–efferent reflex arc. The H-reflex may be abnormal in neuropathies, S1 radiculopathies, and sciatic mononeuropathies. The **F-wave** is a delayed motor potential recorded by stimulating a motor nerve in the distal extremity. As the electrical impulse travels backward along the nerve to the spinal cord, a small population of anterior horn cells is stimulated, resulting in small motor action potentials that can be recorded from the associated muscle. Abnormal F-waves can indicate proximal nerve disease such as radiculopathy and plexopathy. Absent F-waves are also an early finding in Guillain–Barré syndrome.

17. **How is the sensory portion of the peripheral nervous system tested?**
    Sensory nerve conduction studies are the primary means used to test the integrity of the sensory nerves. The amplitude of the sensory nerve action potential (SNAP), its point of onset, and its peak can be compared with standardized normal values and with those from the opposite extremity. Sensory nerve conduction studies are only abnormal in lesions distal to the dorsal root ganglia, where sensory neurons reside. Abnormal SNAPs can be an important way of distinguishing between peripheral neuropathies or plexopathies and radiculopathies, where SNAPs are usually normal, even when a patient complains of numbness. Using the complementary information obtained from needle EMG examination, an electromyographer can further localize the lesion to a particular spinal nerve root, portion of the plexus, or peripheral nerve.

18. **How can a demyelinating peripheral neuropathy and an axonal peripheral neuropathy be differentiated by NCS and needle EMG?**
    Axonal loss and demyelination rarely occur in strict isolation, but some electrodiagnostic features may indicate relatively more damage to myelin versus axons. The features of **demyelinating neuropathies** include moderate to severe slowing of conduction velocity, temporal dispersion of evoked sensory or motor action potentials, conduction block, and prolonged distal latencies. **Axonal neuropathies** show milder slowing of

Table 10-3. Nerve Abnormalities and Possible Differential Diagnoses

PERIPHERAL NERVE SYNDROME	DIFFERENTIAL DIAGNOSIS
Carpal tunnel syndrome	C6 to C7 radiculopathy
	Other areas of median nerve entrapment
Ulnar entrapment at the elbow	C8 radiculopathy
	Brachial plexus lesion
Radial nerve palsy	C7 radiculopathy
Suprascapular nerve lesion	C5 to C6 radiculopathy
Peroneal nerve palsy	L4 to L5 radiculopathy
Femoral nerve lesion	L3 to L4 radiculopathy

nerve conduction, with generally low sensory and motor amplitudes on NCS. Needle EMG shows denervation abnormalities early in axonal neuropathies and only later in demyelinating neuropathies, when axons are secondarily affected.

19. **Which systemic diseases predominantly cause a demyelinating peripheral neuropathy and an axonal peripheral neuropathy?**
In most rheumatologic conditions in which neuropathy is present, the axons are primarily affected, although myelin is rarely completely normal. Demyelination may predominate in a few disorders such as Guillain–Barré syndrome, which involves acutely chronic inflammatory demyelinating polyneuropathy, multifocal motor neuropathy, anti-MAG (myelin-associated glycoprotein) antibody syndrome, and other paraproteinemias, and some hereditary neuropathies such as Charcot–Marie–Tooth disease type Ia.

20. **How is EMG/NCS used in diagnosing carpal tunnel syndrome and ulnar nerve entrapment at the elbow (cubital tunnel syndrome)?**
Carpal tunnel syndrome (CTS) or compressive median neuropathy at the wrist is the most common entrapment neuropathy, affecting 1% of the population. CTS may show slowing of segmental nerve conduction across the wrist. The latency of sensory nerve action potentials of the median nerve is delayed most often, but with increasing severity, motor latencies can be affected. Denervation of the thenar muscles seen on needle EMG indicates moderate to severe CTS. Clinical correlation is recommended for mild CTS because sometimes NCS/EMG studies are normal despite classic symptoms of hand pain/numbness in a median nerve distribution or NCS studies may be abnormal in an asymptomatic individual.

In cubital tunnel syndrome, the ulnar nerve is compressed at the elbow, resulting in slowing of motor or sensory nerve conduction. Needle EMG examination may identify denervation in the ulnar-innervated muscles of the hand and forearm. The ulnar nerve can also be compressed at the wrist.

21. **List a few nerve abnormalities that can be differentiated from common peripheral nerve syndromes via EMG/NCS.**
Table 10-3 lists abnormalities to consider in the differential diagnosis of peripheral nerve syndrome.

Acknowledgment
The editor and author wish to thank Dr. Cliff Gronseth for his contributions to this chapter in the previous edition.

BIBLIOGRAPHY
Aminoff MJ: Electrodiagnosis in clinical neurology, ed 5, New York, 2005, Churchill Livingstone. 2005.
Dumitru D: Electrodiagnostic medicine, ed 2, Philadelphia, 2001, Hanley & Belfus.
Kimura J: Electrodiagnosis in diseases of nerve and muscle: principles and practice, ed 3, New York, 2001, Oxford University Press.
Preston DC, Shapiro BE: Electromyography and neuromuscular disorders: clinical–electrophysiologic correlations, ed 2, Boston, 2005, Butterworth–Heinemann.

CHAPTER 11: APPROACH FOR PATIENTS WITH MONOARTICULAR ARTHRITIS SYMPTOMS

Robert A. Hawkins, MD

KEY POINTS

1. Most common diagnoses in acute monoarticular arthritis: crystalline, septic, osteoarthritis, trauma.
2. Most important diagnostic test in acute monoarticular arthritis: synovial fluid analysis and culture.
3. Most important diagnoses to rule out in chronic monoarticular arthritis: indolent infection, tumor.
4. Best diagnostic tests in chronic monoarticular arthritis: synovial fluid analysis, radiography, magnetic resonance imaging, arthroscopy with synovial biopsy and culture.

---

1. **What conditions can be mistaken for a monoarticular process?**
   Several common inflammatory processes occur in the soft tissues around, but not in, the joints. These conditions can be painful and may mimic arthritis. Examples include rotator cuff tendonitis of the shoulder, olecranon bursitis of the elbow, and prepatellar bursitis of the knee. It is important to distinguish these disorders from true joint disease because their management is often quite different from that of monoarticular arthritis. A careful history and physical examination usually allow correct identification of the affected region (see Chapter 62).

2. **What diseases commonly present with monoarthritis?**
   Box 11-1 lists diseases that commonly present with monoarthritis.

3. **What polyarticular diseases occasionally present with a monoarticular onset?**
   Rheumatoid arthritis, reactive arthritis, juvenile idiopathic arthritis, psoriatic arthritis, viral arthritis, enteropathic arthritis, sarcoid arthritis, Whipple disease.

4. **What is the most critical diagnosis to consider in a patient with monoarticular arthritis symptoms?**
   Joint infection, which is one of the few rheumatologic emergencies. A septic joint must be diagnosed quickly and managed aggressively. Bacterial infections, especially those due to gram-positive organisms, can destroy the joint cartilage within a few days. Prompt and proper treatment of the septic joint will usually leave it without permanent structural damage. In addition, because a septic joint is usually the result of hematogenous spread of infection from another body site, early recognition of the joint process allows more timely diagnosis and treatment of the primary infection. When evaluating a patient with acute monoarticular arthritis, a good rule of thumb is to assume that the joint is infected until proven otherwise.

Box 11-1. Diseases that Commonly Present with Monoarthritis

Septic diseases
  Bacterial
  Mycobacterial
  Lyme disease
  Fungal
Crystal deposition diseases
  Gout
  Calcium pyrophosphate dihydrate deposition disease (pseudogout)
  Hydroxyapatite deposition disease
  Calcium oxalate deposition disease
Traumatic
  Fracture
  Internal derangement
  Hemarthrosis

Other diseases
  Osteoarthritis
  Juvenile idiopathic arthritis
  Coagulopathy
  Avascular necrosis of bone
  Foreign-body synovitis
  Pigmented villonodular synovitis
  Palindromic rheumatism

5. **What seven questions should you ask when obtaining a history from a patient with monoarticular arthritis?**
   1. Did the pain come on over several hours or 1 to 2 days? (Consider infection, crystal deposition diseases, inflammatory arthritis syndromes, and palindromic rheumatism.)
   2. Did the pain come on insidiously over weeks? (Consider indolent infections, osteoarthritis, and tumor.)
   3. Is there a history of intravenous drug abuse or recent infection of any kind? (Consider infection.)
   4. Has the patient ever experienced previous acute attacks of joint pain and swelling? (Consider crystal deposition diseases and other inflammatory joint syndromes.)
   5. Has the patient had symptoms, such as a skin rash, low-back pain, diarrhea, urethral discharge, conjunctivitis, or mouth sores? (Consider reactive arthritis, psoriatic arthritis, or enteropathic arthritis.)
   6. Is there a history of a bleeding diathesis or use of anticoagulants? (Consider hemarthrosis.)
   7. Has the patient been treated with a prolonged course of glucocorticoids? (Consider infection, avascular necrosis, and fragility fracture.)

6. **Is the age of the patient useful in differential diagnosis?**
   Patient age is extremely useful in differential diagnosis. With the exception of infection (which occurs in all age groups), some joint diseases presenting as monoarthritis are more likely to occur at certain ages.
   - In children, consider congenital dysplasia of the hip, slipped capital femoral epiphysis, or a monoarticular presentation of juvenile inflammatory arthritis.
   - In young adults, consider seronegative spondyloarthropathy, rheumatoid arthritis, or internal derangement of the joint. A septic joint in this age group is often due to gonococcal infection.
   - Older adults are more likely to have crystalline arthritis, osteoarthritis, osteonecrosis, or internal derangement of the joint. A septic joint in such individuals is less likely to be due to gonococcal organisms.

7. **Is fever a useful sign?**
   Fever is a useful sign but it can be misleading. Fever is often present in infectious arthritis, but it may be absent. Fever, however, can also be a feature of acute attacks of gout and calcium pyrophosphate dihydrate deposition (CPPD) disease, rheumatoid arthritis, juvenile inflammatory arthritis, sarcoidosis, and reactive arthritis. Many clinicians have been fooled by a gout attack masquerading as cellulitis or a septic joint.

8. **What are the most likely diagnoses in hospitalized patients who develop acute monoarticular arthritis following admission for another medical or surgical disease?**
   Acute gout, pseudogout, and infection are by far the most common causes of acute attacks of such monoarthritis. These patients are often middle-aged or elderly, which is the primary age range for crystalline arthropathies. In addition, they often have hospitalization-related risk factors known to provoke gout or pseudogout attacks: trauma, surgery, hemorrhage, infection, or medical stress such as renal failure, myocardial infarction, and stroke. Clinicians must be especially careful to exclude infection in such hospitalized patients.

9. **What is the single most useful diagnostic study in the initial evaluation of monoarthritis?**
   Synovial fluid analysis.

10. **List the most common indications for arthrocentesis and synovial fluid analysis.**
    1. **Suspicion of infection.** As little as 2 mL of fluid is sufficient for a Gram stain, culture, and white blood cell (WBC) count and differential.
    2. **Suspicion of crystal-induced arthritis.** The sensitivity of polarizing microscopy in identifying birefringent crystals approaches 90% in acute gout and 70% in acute pseudogout.
    3. **Suspicion of hemarthrosis.** Bloody joint fluid is characteristic of traumatic arthritis, clotting disorder, and pigmented villonodular synovitis.
    4. **Differentiating inflammatory from noninflammatory arthritis.** The degree of elevation of synovial fluid WBC count is useful in narrowing the list of possible diagnoses (see Chapter 7).

11. **What other diagnostic studies are useful in the initial evaluation of monoarthritis?**
    1. *Radiograph of the joint*: Although frequently normal, a radiograph may disclose important information. It may help in diagnosing an unsuspected fracture, osteonecrosis, osteoarthritis, or a juxtaarticular bone tumor. The presence of chondrocalcinosis, a radiologic feature of CPPD disease, increases suspicion for a pseudogout attack. Tumor, chronic fungal or mycobacterial infection, and other indolent destructive processes may be revealed. A contralateral joint radiograph for comparison may be useful, especially in children.
    2. *Complete blood count*: Leukocytosis supports the possibility of infection.

12. **What other diagnostic studies are useful in *selected patients* in the initial evaluation of monoarthritis?**
    1. *Cultures of blood, urine*, or other possible primary sites of infection: mandatory when a septic joint is being considered.
    2. *Serum prothrombin and partial thromboplastin time*: useful if the patient is receiving anticoagulation or if a coagulation disorder is suspected.

3. *Erythrocyte sedimentation rate or C-reactive protein*: although results are often nonspecific, significant elevation may suggest an inflammatory process.
4. *Serum uric acid levels*: notoriously unreliable in making or excluding a diagnosis of gout. These levels may be spuriously elevated in acute inflammatory conditions, or acutely diminished in a true gout attack.
5. *Serologic tests for antinuclear antibodies (ANA) and rheumatoid factor*: these tests are rarely if ever indicated. However, ANA may be positive in the oligoarticular form of juvenile idiopathic arthritis.

13. If infection cannot be adequately ruled out by initial diagnostic studies, what should you do?
The patient should be hospitalized and treated presumptively for a septic joint until culture results become available. This is usually indicated in a patient with synovial fluid findings suggestive of a highly inflammatory process (synovial fluid WBC count >50,000 /mL) but with a negative synovial fluid Gram stain and no obvious primary source of infection. To lessen confusion regarding response to therapy, antiinflammatory drugs should be withheld during this period.

14. Is a diagnosis always established by the end of the first week of onset of acute monoarticular arthritis?
No, many patients defy initial attempts at diagnosis despite appropriate evaluation. A few achieve spontaneous remission, leaving the physician frustrated about the diagnosis but relieved. Many patients, however, continue to have symptoms.

15. The initial evaluation is unrevealing and the arthritis persists. What should be done?
If the initial evaluation was carefully accomplished, a period of watchful waiting is often useful at this time. As noted previously, some processes resolve spontaneously. Others become polyarticular, and the differential diagnosis will change to reflect the new joint involvement. New findings, such as the skin rash of psoriasis, occasionally emerge to aid in diagnosis. In a small number of patients, the monoarthritis persists and further evaluation for chronic monoarticular arthritis must be undertaken.

16. What is the definition of chronic monoarticular arthritis? Why is it useful to consider this as a category separate from acute monoarticular arthritis?
Chronic monoarticular arthritis can be arbitrarily defined as **symptoms persisting within a single joint for more than 6 weeks**. The differential diagnosis shifts away from some important and common causes of acute arthritis, such as pyogenic infection and acute crystal deposition diseases. In patients with inflammatory synovial fluid, the likelihood of chronic inflammatory syndromes, such as mycobacterial or fungal septic arthritis, or a seronegative spondyloarthropathy increases. In patients with a noninflammatory process, a structural abnormality or internal derangement is a possibility.

17. Name the most likely causes of chronic monoarticular arthritis.
Table 11-1 lists the most likely causes of chronic monoarthritis.

18. What six questions should you ask when obtaining a history from a patient with chronic monoarticular arthritis?
1. Is there a history of tuberculosis or a positive tuberculin skin test? (Consider mycobacterial disease.)
2. Is the patient a farmer, gardener, or floral worker? (Consider sporotrichosis.)
3. If the knee is involved, has the joint been damaged in the past? Does it ever lock in flexion? (Consider internal derangement and osteoarthritis.)
4. Has the patient ever experienced previous acute attacks of joint pain and swelling that resolved spontaneously in any joint? (Consider inflammatory joint syndromes.)
5. Has the patient recently been treated with a prolonged course of corticosteroids for any reason? (Consider osteonecrosis.)
6. Has the patient had symptoms such as a skin rash, low-back pain, diarrhea, urethritis, or uveitis? (Consider the spondyloarthropathies.)

Table 11-1. Inflammatory and Noninflammatory Causes of Chronic Monoarthritis

INFLAMMATORY	NONINFLAMMATORY
Mycobacterial infection	Osteoarthritis
Fungal infection	Internal derangement of the knee
Lyme arthritis	Avascular necrosis of bone
Monoarticular presentation of rheumatoid arthritis	Pigmented villonodular synovitis
Seronegative spondyloarthropathies	Synovial chondromatosis
Sarcoid arthritis	Synovioma
Foreign-body synovitis	

19. **What physical findings are useful in the differential diagnosis of chronic monoarticular arthritis?**
    1. Extraarticular features of the spondyloarthropathies, such as skin rashes (psoriasis, keratoderma blennorrhagicum), oral ulcers, urethral discharge, conjunctivitis, and uveitis.
    2. Erythema nodosa, a feature of sarcoidosis and inflammatory bowel syndrome.
    3. A positive McMurray maneuver in a knee examination, suggesting internal derangement.

20. **In evaluating chronic monoarthritis, what initial studies should be obtained?**
    1. *Radiograph of the joint*: radiographs are often revealing in chronic arthritis. Chronic infections by mycobacteria and fungi often cause radiographically detectable abnormalities. Osteoarthritis, avascular necrosis of bone, and other causes of noninflammatory chronic arthritis also have characteristic radiographic appearances. Radiographs of the contralateral joint for comparison may be helpful.
    2. *Synovial fluid analysis*, when possible: this analysis is useful in dividing possible causes of the joint process into the two broad diagnostic categories of inflammatory and noninflammatory arthritis. A bloody synovial effusion points to pigmented villonodular synovitis, synovial chondromatosis, or synovioma. Cultures of synovial fluid may demonstrate mycobacterial or fungal infection.

21. **In evaluating chronic monoarthritis, what initial studies are indicated in selected patients?**
    1. *Erythrocyte sedimentation rate or C-reactive protein*: although results are often nonspecific, significant elevation may suggest an inflammatory process.
    2. *Radiograph of sacroiliac joints*: this may demonstrate asymptomatic sacroiliitis in young patients presenting with chronic monoarticular arthritis as an initial manifestation of a spondyloarthropathy.
    3. *Chest radiograph*: to detect evidence of a prior mycobacterial disease, or pulmonary sarcoidosis.
    4. *Skin test reaction to tuberculin*: a negative test is useful in excluding mycobacterial infection.
    5. *Serologic tests for Lyme disease* (Borrelia burgdorferi), *rheumatoid factor, anti-cyclic citrullinated peptide antibody, antinuclear antibody, and human leukocyte antigen B27*.

22. **Are other diagnostic studies useful in evaluation of chronic monoarthritis?**
    1. Arthroscopy: Arthroscopy allows direct visualization of many important articular structures and provides the opportunity for synovial biopsy in all large and some medium-sized joints. It is particularly useful for diagnosing internal derangement of the knee.
    2. Synovial biopsy: Microscopic evaluation with culture of synovial tissue is useful in the diagnosis of benign and malignant tumor, fungal and mycobacterial infection, and foreign-body synovitis.
    3. Magnetic resonance imaging of the joint: Useful in diagnosing avascular necrosis of bone, internal derangement of the knee, osteomyelitis, and destruction of periarticular bone. Can pick up most abnormalities seen on a bone scan.
    4. Bone scan: Can evaluate for avascular necrosis of bone, stress fracture, osteoid osteomas, bone metastases, bone sarcomas, and osteomyelitis.
    5. Universal primer: Synovial fluid can be sent to identify bacteria, fungi, and mycobacterial infections that cannot be grown in culture. The 16S rDNA sequence is a gene encoding small subunit ribosomal RNA. This gene contains conserved sequences of DNA common to all bacteria and divergent sequences unique to each bacterial species. When a small piece of this sequence is used as a primer in a polymerase chain reaction (PCR) assay, it acts as a universal primer for nonselective amplification of any bacterial DNA in the patient's synovial fluid. Once the DNA has been amplified, the PCR product is then stained with ethidium bromide and visualized by electrophoresis on an agarose gel. If bacterial DNA is identified, it can then be directly sequenced to identify the bacterial species.

23. **How often is a specific diagnosis made in patients with chronic monoarthritis?**
    Appropriate evaluation yields a diagnosis in approximately two-thirds of patients. Fortunately, the most serious and treatable diseases yield to diagnosis if a carefully reasoned clinical approach is taken.

BIBLIOGRAPHY

American College of Rheumatology Ad Hoc Committee on Clinical Guidelines: Guidelines for the initial evaluation of the adult patient with acute musculoskeletal symptoms, Arthritis Rheum 39:1–8, 1996.

Deane K, West SG: Differential diagnosis of monoarticular arthritis. In Wortmann R, editor: Crystal-induced arthropathies, New York, 2006, Taylor & Francis.

Golbus J: Monoarticular arthritis. In Firestein GS, Budd RC, Harris Jr ED, McInnes IB, Ruddy S, Sergent JS, editors: Kelley's textbook of rheumatology, ed 8, Philadelphia, 2009, Saunders.

Hubscher O: Pattern recognition in arthritis. In Hochberg MC, Silman AJ, Smolen JS, Weinblatt ME, Weisman MH, editors: Rheumatology, ed 5, Philadelphia, 2011, Mosby.

Mohana-Borges AVR, Chung CB, Resnick D: Monoarticular arthritis, Radiol Clin N Am 42:135–139, 2004.

Schumacher HR, Habre W, Meador R, Hsia EC: Predictive factors in early arthritis: long-term follow-up, Semin Arthritis Rheum 33:264–272, 2004.

Swan A, Amer H, Dieppe P: The value of synovial fluid assays in the diagnosis of joint disease: a literature survey, Ann Rheum Dis 61:493–498, 2002.

CHAPTER 12

APPROACH FOR PATIENTS WITH POLYARTICULAR ARTHRITIS SYMPTOMS

Robert A. Hawkins, MD

KEY POINTS

1. The history and physical examination, not laboratory testing, are the best tools for diagnosis.
2. The two most common causes of polyarthritis are osteoarthritis and rheumatoid arthritis.
3. The extraarticular features (such as the malar rash of systemic lupus erythematosus, SLE) are often key to diagnosing polyarticular syndromes.
4. Laboratory tests are most useful in confirming a diagnosis based on the history and physical examination.

1. What are the most important tools that the clinician can use on a patient with polyarticular arthritis symptoms?

A careful history and physical examination. Laboratory testing and radiographic or other imaging studies provide definitive answers in only a few instances. Tests are often most useful in confirming the suspected diagnosis or in providing prognostic information. When confronted with a patient with polyarticular symptoms, an inexperienced clinician often will slight the most important, the history and physical examination, opting instead for "shotgun" laboratory testing. Although tests such as rheumatoid factor, uric acid, antistreptolysin O titers, and antinuclear antibodies may be indicated in many instances, the history and physical examination will reveal 75% of the information required for diagnosis.

2. How are the many diseases causing polyarticular arthritis symptoms classified?

No single classification scheme can be used to differentiate the wide variety of diseases presenting with polyarthritis symptoms. In most instances, the clinician uses several variables in combination to reduce the number of diagnostic possibilities. These variables include:
- Acuteness of onset of the process
- Degree of inflammation of the joints
- Temporal pattern of joint involvement
- Distribution of joint involvement
- Age and sex of the patient
- Extraarticular features

3. Which diseases commonly present with acute polyarthritis symptoms?

Table 12-1 lists diseases for which patients commonly present with acute polyarthritis symptoms.

4. Which diseases commonly present with chronic (persisting for >6 weeks) polyarthritis symptoms?

Box 12-1 lists diseases for which patients commonly present with chronic polyarthritis symptoms.

Despite a long list of diseases causing polyarthritis, over 75% of patients with inflammatory arthritis will have rheumatoid arthritis (30%), crystalline arthritis, psoriatic arthritis, reactive arthritis, or sarcoidosis. The vast majority of patients with noninflammatory polyarthritis will have osteoarthritis.

5. How do polyarthritis, polyarthralgias, and diffuse aches and pains differ?

Polyarthritis is definite inflammation (swelling, tenderness, warmth) of more than four joints demonstrated by physical examination. A patient with two to four involved joints is said to have pauci- or oligoarticular arthritis. The acute polyarticular diseases (see Question 3) and chronic inflammatory diseases (see Question 4) commonly present with polyarthritis.

Polyarthralgia is defined as pain in more than four joints without demonstrable inflammation by physical examination. The chronic noninflammatory arthritides commonly present with polyarthralgias.

Diffuse aches and pains are poorly localized symptoms originating in joints, bones, muscles, or other soft tissues. A joint examination does not reveal inflammation. Polymyalgia rheumatica, fibromyalgia, SLE, polymyositis, and hypothyroidism commonly present with these symptoms.

6. Describe the three characteristic temporal patterns of joint involvement in polyarthritis.

1. **Migratory pattern**: Symptoms are present in certain joints for a few days and then remit, only to reappear in other joints. Rheumatic fever, early gonococcal arthritis, early Lyme disease, and acute childhood leukemia are examples.

Table 12-1. Diseases with Acute Polyarthritis Symptoms

INFECTION	OTHER INFLAMMATORY CONDITIONS
Gonococcal	Rheumatoid arthritis
Meningococcal	Polyarticular and systemic JIA
Lyme	Acute sarcoid arthritis
Acute rheumatic fever	Systemic lupus erythematosus
Infective endocarditis	Reactive arthritis
Viral (especially rubella, hepatitis B and C, parvovirus, Epstein–Barr, HIV)	Psoriatic arthritis
	Polyarticular gout

Box 12-1. Diseases with Chronic Polyarthritis Symptoms

Inflammatory
Rheumatoid arthritis
Systemic lupus erythematosus
Polyarticular gout
Juvenile idiopathic arthritis
Systemic sclerosis
Chronic CPPD
Psoriatic arthritis
Polymyalgia rheumatic
Vasculitis
Reactive arthritis
Enteropathic arthritis
Sarcoid arthritis

Noninflammatory
Osteoarthritis
Chronic CPPD
Fibromyalgia
Hemochromatosis
Benign hypermobility syndrome

2. **Additive pattern**: Symptoms begin in some joints and persist, with subsequent involvement of other joints. This pattern is common in rheumatoid arthritis, SLE, and other polyarticular syndromes.
3. **Intermittent pattern**: This pattern is typified by repetitive attacks of acute polyarthritis with remission between attacks. A prolonged observation may be necessary to establish this phenomenon. Polyarticular crystal-induced diseases, psoriatic arthritis, reactive arthritis, palindromic rheumatism, familial Mediterranean fever, and Whipple disease may present in this manner. Rheumatoid arthritis, RS3PE, SLE, sarcoidosis, and Still disease can also present episodically early in their disease course.

7. **How is the distribution of joint involvement helpful in the differential diagnosis of polyarthritis?**
Different diseases characteristically affect different joints. Knowledge of the typical joints involved in each disease is a cornerstone of diagnosis in polyarthritis. In practice, knowledge of which joints are spared in each form of arthritis is also quite useful (Table 12-2).

8. **Name the two most common causes of chronic polyarthritis.**
   1. Osteoarthritis: The prevalence of osteoarthritis rises steeply with age. Between 10% and 20% of people of 40 years of age have evidence of osteoarthritis, and 75% of women over age 65 years have osteoarthritis. This very high prevalence makes osteoarthritis the single most likely diagnosis in older patients complaining of polyarticular pain who have noninflammatory signs and symptoms.
   2. Rheumatoid arthritis: **The prevalence in U.S. whites is approximately 1%, making it the most common chronic inflammatory joint disease.**

9. **What are the most likely diagnoses in women aged 25 to 50 years who present with chronic polyarticular symptoms?**
Osteoarthritis, rheumatoid arthritis, SLE, fibromyalgia, and benign hypermobility syndrome.

10. **What are the most likely diagnoses in men aged 25 to 50 years who present with chronic oligoarticular or polyarticular symptoms?**
Gonococcal arthritis, reactive arthritis, ankylosing spondylitis, osteoarthritis, and hemochromatosis.

11. **What are the most likely diagnoses in patients over age 50 years presenting with chronic polyarticular symptoms?**
Osteoarthritis, rheumatoid arthritis, calcium pyrophosphate dihydrate deposition (CPPD) disease, polymyalgia rheumatica, and paraneoplastic polyarthritis.

Table 12-2. Distribution of Joint Involvement in Polyarthritis

DISEASE	JOINTS COMMONLY INVOLVED	JOINTS COMMONLY SPARED
Gonococcal arthritis	Knee, wrist, ankle, hand IP	Axial
Lyme arthritis	Knee, shoulder, wrist, elbow	Axial
Rheumatoid arthritis	Wrist, MCP, PIP, elbow, glenohumeral, cervical spine, hip, knee, ankle, tarsal, MTP	DIP, thoracolumbar spine
Osteoarthritis	First CMC, DIP, PIP, cervical spine, thoracolumbar spine, hip, knee, first MTP, toe IP	MCP, wrist, elbow, glenoshoulder, ankle, tarsal
Reactive arthritis	Knee, ankle, tarsal, MTP, first toe IP, elbow, axial	Hip
Psoriatic arthritis	Knee, ankle, MTP, first toe IP, wrist, MCP, hand IP, axial	
Enteropathic arthritis	Knee, ankle, elbow, shoulder, MCP, PIP, wrist, axial	
Polyarticular gout	First MTP, instep, heel, ankle, knee	Axial
CPPD disease	Knee, wrist, shoulder, ankle, MCP, hand IP, hip, elbow	Axial
Sarcoid arthritis	Ankle, knee	Axial
Hemochromatosis	MCP, wrist, ankle, knee, hip, feet, shoulder	

CMC, Carpometacarpal; DIP, distal interphalangeal; IP, Interphalangeal; MCP, metacarpophalangeal; MTP, metatarsophalangeal; PIP, proximal interphalangeal;

12. **What is morning stiffness? How is it useful in sorting out the causes of polyarticular symptoms?**
Morning stiffness refers to the amount of time it takes for patients with polyarthritis to "limber up" after arising in the morning. It is useful in differentiating inflammatory from noninflammatory arthritis. In inflammatory arthritis, morning stiffness lasts >1 hour. In untreated rheumatoid arthritis, it averages 3.5 hours and tends to parallel the degree of joint inflammation. By contrast, noninflammatory processes, such as osteoarthritis, may produce transient morning stiffness that lasts <15 minutes.

13. **List possible causes of fever and polyarthritis.**
Infectious arthritis: septic arthritis, bacterial endocarditis, Lyme disease, viral arthritis.
Reactive arthritis: enteric infections, Reiter syndrome, rheumatic fever, inflammatory bowel disease.
Systemic rheumatic diseases: rheumatoid arthritis, SLE, Still disease, systemic vasculitis.
Crystal-induced arthritis: gout, pseudogout.
Miscellaneous disease: malignancy, familial Mediterranean fever, sarcoidosis, dermatomyositis, Behçet disease, Henoch–Schönlein purpura, Kawasaki disease, erythema nodosum, erythema multiforme, Whipple disease, relapsing polychondritis.

14. **Define tenosynovitis. How is its presence useful in the differential diagnosis of polyarticular symptoms?**
Tenosynovitis is inflammation of the synovial-lined sheaths surrounding tendons in the wrists, hands, ankles, and feet. Physical examination usually reveals tenderness and swelling along the track of the involved tendon *between* the joints. It is a characteristic feature of rheumatoid arthritis, gout, reactive arthritis, gonococcal arthritis, and tuberculous and fungal arthritis. It is distinctly uncommon in other causes of polyarticular disease.

15. **List skin lesions that can be useful in the diagnosis of acute or chronic polyarthritis.**
    - Erythema chronicum migrans (Lyme arthritis)
    - Erythema nodosum (sarcoid arthritis, enteric arthritis)
    - Psoriatic plaques (psoriatic arthritis)
    - Keratoderma blennorrhagicum (reactive arthritis)
    - Erythema marginatum (acute rheumatic fever)
    - Palpable purpura (vasculitis)
    - Livedo reticularis (vasculitis)
    - Vesicopustular lesions or hemorrhagic papules (gonococcal arthritis)
    - Butterfly rash, discoid lupus, or photosensitive rash (SLE)
    - Thickening of the skin (systemic sclerosis)
    - Heliotrope rash on eyelids, upper chest, and extensor aspects of joints (dermatomyositis)
    - Gottron papules overlying the extensor aspects of the MCP and IP joints of the hands (dermatomyositis)

Table 12-3. Extraarticular Organ Involvement in Polyarticular Rheumatic Diseases								
DISEASE	LUNG	PLEURA	PERICARDIUM	HEART MUSCLE	HEART VALVE	KIDNEY	GI TRACT	LIVER
Acute rheumatic fever		X	X	X	X			
Viral arthritis								X
Bacterial endocarditis					X	X		
Rheumatoid arthritis	X	X	X	X	X			
SLE	X	X	X	X	X	X		
Systemic sclerosis	X	X	X	X		X	X	X
Polymyositis/dermatomyositis	X	X	X	X				
Reactive arthritis						X		X
Enteropathic arthritis							X	X
Polyarticular gout						X		
Sarcoid arthritis	X							X
Vasculitis	X					X		
Polymyalgia rheumatica								X
Hemochromatosis				X				X

- Gray/brown skin hyperpigmentation (hemochromatosis)
- Periungual nodules (multicentric reticulohistiocytosis)

16. **Which rheumatic diseases should be considered in a patient with Raynaud phenomenon and polyarticular symptoms?**
    - Mixed connective tissue disease (prevalence >90%)
    - Progressive systemic sclerosis (prevalence of 90%)
    - SLE (prevalence of 20%)
    - Polymyositis/dermatomyositis (prevalence of 20% to 40%)
    - Vasculitis (variable prevalence, depending on the particular syndrome)

17. **What other systemic features are seen in diseases causing polyarthritis?**
    Table 12-3 lists other systemic features observed in diseases causing polyarthritis.

18. **Which tests are most useful in evaluating a patient with chronic polyarticular symptoms?**
    Complete blood count, creatinine, urinalysis, liver-associated enzymes, erythrocyte sedimentation rate (ESR) or C-reactive protein (CRP), antinuclear antibody (ANA), rheumatoid factor, anti-cyclic citrullinated peptide (CCP) antibody, and radiographs. In some patients consider serum uric acid, thyroid stimulating hormone (TSH), iron studies, HLA-B27 antigen and synovial fluid analysis.

19. **What is the significance of a positive ANA in a patient with chronic polyarticular symptoms?**
    A patient with polyarthralgia or polyarthritis who has a significantly elevated ANA titer (≥1:320) often will have one of the following diseases: SLE (including drug-induced lupus), rheumatoid arthritis, Sjögren's syndrome, polymyositis, systemic sclerosis, or mixed connective tissue disease.
    The history and physical examination should be directed toward the clinical findings in these diseases. A careful medication history may reveal that the patient has received drugs that can cause drug-induced lupus (see Chapter 17). Finally, it must be stressed that a positive ANA is a feature of several other chronic diseases and can also be found in normal healthy individuals, although usually in low titer (see Chapter 6).

20. **Why should a rheumatoid factor not be ordered in the evaluation of patients with acute polyarticular symptoms?**
    Rheumatoid factor (RF) has low sensitivity and specificity for rheumatoid arthritis in patients with acute polyarticular symptoms. Serum RF is frequently positive in acute infectious syndromes caused by hepatitis B,

Epstein–Barr, influenza, and other viruses but disappears as the viral syndrome resolves. Although RF will eventually become positive in 75% to 85% of patients with rheumatoid arthritis, it is positive in early rheumatoid arthritis in only 50% to 70% of patients (see Chapter 6).

21. Which chronic polyarticular diseases are most likely to be associated with low serum complement levels?

SLE and some of the vasculitis syndromes. Low serum complement levels (C3, C4, and total hemolytic complement) usually suggest the presence of an immune complex disease. In SLE, cryoglobulinemia (especially hepatitis C), and some diseases associated with vasculitis (infective endocarditis, urticarial vasculitis), immune complexes often activate the complement cascade, resulting in consumption of individual complement components. In many instances, the liver is unable to produce these components as rapidly as they are consumed, resulting in a fall in serum levels.

22. When should arthrocentesis for synovial fluid analysis be considered in the evaluation of polyarthritis?

When the diagnosis has not been established and joint fluid can be obtained. Both of these requirements need to be met. For example, a patient with obvious osteoarthritis established on the basis of history, physical examination, and radiographs does not require a diagnostic aspiration in an uncomplicated knee effusion. If it can be obtained, synovial fluid analysis can be useful in the diagnosis of bacterial joint infection and crystal-induced arthritis. Even if a specific diagnosis is not forthcoming, synovial fluid analysis reduces the list of diagnostic possibilities by categorizing the process as either inflammatory or noninflammatory.

23. Should radiographs of affected joints always be obtained?

Radiographs need not always be obtained. As a general rule, patients with acute polyarticular arthritis will not benefit from joint radiographs. Radiographs are most valuable in evaluating chronic arthritis that has been relatively long-standing and that has resulted in characteristic changes in joints. Osteoarthritis, chronic rheumatoid arthritis, psoriatic arthritis, gout, CPPD disease, systemic sclerosis, and sarcoidosis all have specific appearances on radiographs that are very useful in diagnosis. However, it should be remembered that osteoarthritis is so common that it may coexist with other arthritis syndromes, and that radiographic changes may be a mixture of both types of arthritis in a given patient.

24. Why should the rheumatologist think in "geologic" time?

Because many chronic polyarthritis diseases require months or years to diagnose, tremendous patience is often required. This prolonged but necessary period of observation often seems like "geologic" time to many patients, who may expect an immediate diagnosis. The characteristics of chronic polyarticular diseases require this extraordinary degree of patience, in that:
- Many present insidiously with few objective findings for prolonged times.
- Many initially masquerade as other diseases before finally settling into their usual pattern.
- Characteristic laboratory abnormalities may require months or years to develop.
- Joint symptoms may precede the extraarticular features of the disease by months or years.
- Joint radiographs may not show characteristic changes of arthritis for months or years.

BIBLIOGRAPHY

Cush JJ, Dao KH: Polyarticular arthritis. In Firestein GS, Budd RS, Gabriel SE, McInnes IB, O'Dell JR, editors: Kelley's textbook of rheumatology, ed 9, Philadelphia, 2013, Saunders.

El-Gabalawy HS, Duray P, Goldbach-Mansky R: Evaluating patients with arthritis of recent onset: studies in pathogenesis and prognosis, JAMA 284(18):2368–2373, 2000.

Hubscher O: Pattern recognition in arthritis. In Hochberg MC, Silman AJ, Smolen JS, Weinblatt ME, Weisman MH, editors: Rheumatology, ed 5, Philadelphia, 2011, Mosby.

Jansen LM, et al: One year outcome of undifferentiated polyarthritis, Ann Rheum Dis 61:700–703, 2002.

West S: Polyarticular joint disease. In Klippel JH, Stone JH, Crofford LJ, White PH, editors: Primer on the rheumatic diseases, ed 13, Atlanta, 2008, Springer.

CHAPTER 13

APPROACH FOR THE PATIENT WITH NEUROMUSCULAR SYMPTOMS

Robert A. Hawkins, MD

> **KEY POINTS**
> 1. Myopathies tend to be proximal and symmetrical in location.
> 2. Neurologic lesions tend to be distal and asymmetric in location.
> 3. The statin drugs are the most common cause of drug-induced myopathy and usually present as myalgia.
> 4. "Strokes in young folks" should raise diagnostic suspicion for a rheumatic cause.

1. **Discuss the relationship between rheumatic diseases and neuromuscular disease.**
    Many primary rheumatic diseases, such as systemic lupus erythematosus, rheumatoid arthritis, and systemic vasculitis, are frequently complicated by neurologic or myopathic disease. Chronic synovitis, joint contractures, and deformities seen in rheumatoid arthritis lead to muscle atrophy and weakness. Other rheumatic diseases such as polymyositis are dominated by immune-mediated inflammation of muscle, and the differential diagnosis of myopathy is quite broad. Neuromuscular manifestations of rheumatic diseases may present as early and dominant findings, or as late complications of well-established diseases. They may also be complications of therapy for rheumatic diseases, as with the use of glucocorticoids.

2. **What are the cardinal symptoms of neuromuscular lesions?**
    Weakness and/or **pain** are the most common symptoms reported by patients. Weakness should be differentiated from fatigue and malaise. Fatigue differs from weakness in that fatigue is a loss of strength with activity that recovers with rest. Malaise is a subjective feeling of weakness without objective findings.

3. **Many patients complain of weakness. What is the best way to determine the cause of weakness in a given patient?**
    The first step is to exclude **systemic causes** of fatigue or weakness, such as cardiopulmonary disease, anemia, hypothyroidism, malignancy, sleep apnea, or depression. Many of these patients have malaise rather than weakness, and their examination usually fails to reveal true muscle weakness if they give their best effort. The carefully directed history and physical examination, combined with focused laboratory testing, are usually effective in eliminating these causes of weakness (Box 13-1).

4. **Once systemic causes of weakness have been excluded, what is the next step?**
    The neuromuscular causes of weakness should be considered. A very useful method of categorizing neuromuscular diseases is by their customary level of anatomic involvement, beginning with the spinal cord and proceeding distally through nerve roots, peripheral nerves, neuromuscular junctions, and muscle (Box 13-2).

5. **Many patients complain of pain. What historical features are most useful in the differential diagnosis of pain?**
    Pure spinal cord lesions are not painful, although occasionally painful flexor muscle spasms will occur. Nerve root compression commonly produces pain and paresthesias in the affected nerve distribution. Peripheral nerve disease is often manifested by numbness and paresthesias. Motor neuron diseases (i.e., Guillain–Barré syndrome) cause weakness. Neuromuscular junction lesions are not painful.
    Myopathies may or may not be painful. In categorizing them, the following concepts are useful:
    - Inflammatory myopathies are usually dominated by weakness, not pain. The exception to this rule is when the inflammatory myopathy has a fulminant onset, when pain may be a dominant feature.
    - Muscle pain on exertion is suggestive of vascular insufficiency or diseases of muscle metabolism.

> **Box 13-1. Common Systemic Causes of Weakness or Fatigue**
>
> | | | |
> |---|---|---|
> | Cardiopulmonary disease | Hypo- or hyperthyroidism | Malignancy |
> | Anemia | Sleep apnea | Depression |
> | Chronic infection | Poor physical conditioning | Chronic inflammatory disease |

6. **How does the distribution of weakness or pain aid in differentiating neurologic from muscular lesions?**
   Myopathies tend to cause *proximal* and *symmetrical* (bilateral) weakness or pain involving the shoulder girdle and hip girdle. If present, pain may be reported as aching or cramping.
   Peripheral neuropathies, as a rule, cause *distal* (hands and feet) weakness and/or pain.
   Nerve root compression causes asymmetric weakness and pain that may be either proximal or distal, depending on the level of the involved nerve root.
   Spinal cord lesions usually are associated with a distinct sensory level described as a tightness bilaterally around the trunk or abdomen. Distal spastic weakness, often with loss of bowel and bladder sphincter function, is also a feature of spinal cord disease.

7. **How does the temporal pattern of weakness or pain aid in diagnosis?**
   1. **Abrupt onset** of weakness is characteristic of Guillain–Barré syndrome, poliomyelitis, and hypokalemic periodic paralysis.
   2. **Intermittent** weakness may occur with myasthenia gravis, the rare causes of metabolic myopathy, and hypokalemic periodic paralysis.
   3. **Gradual onset** of weakness or pain is typical of most muscle diseases, including inflammatory myopathies, the muscular dystrophies, and endocrine myopathies, as well as most neuropathies. It may also occur with myasthenia gravis.

8. **What is meant by fatigability? How is it useful in diagnosing neuromuscular disease?**
   Fatigability is defined as progressive weakness of muscle with repetitive use, followed by recovery of strength after a brief period of rest. It is a classic finding in myasthenia gravis. Eaton–Lambert syndrome is often referred to as reverse myasthenia gravis, owing to the paradoxical increase in muscle strength observed with repetitive muscle contraction.

9. **How does the family history aid in diagnosis?**
   Many of the muscular dystrophy syndromes have strong patterns of inheritance (Table 13-1).

10. **Name three hormones whose deficiency or excess is associated with myopathy.**
    Thyroxine, T4 (hypothyroidism or hyperthyroidism)
    Cortisol (Addison's disease or Cushing's disease)
    Parathyroid hormone (hypoparathyroidism or hyperparathyroidism)

11. **Which drugs are most commonly responsible for neuromuscular symptoms?**
    Corticosteroids, chloroquine, alcohol, D-penicillamine, statins, emetine, hydroxychloroquine, colchicine, cocaine, fibrates, zidovudine, amiodarone, interferon α, antifungals.

12. **What toxins should be sought in the evaluation of neuromuscular symptoms?**
    - **Organophosphates**: these are used in pesticides, petroleum additives, and modifiers of plastic. Their toxicity affects peripheral nerves. Eventually, pyramidal tract signs and spasticity may develop.

Box 13-2. Diseases Affecting Neuromuscular Structures, by Level of Anatomic Involvement

Spinal Cord	Nerve Root	Peripheral Nerve	Neuromuscular Junction	Muscle
Amyotrophic lateral sclerosis	Herniated nucleus Pulposus	Vasculitis	Myasthenia gravis Syndrome	Polymyositis
Transverse myelitis	Cervical spondylosis	Guillain–Barré syndrome		Hypothyroidism
Vasculitis	Lumbar spondylosis	Collagen vascular diseases		Hyperthyroidism
Collagen vascular diseases		Nerve compression		Muscular dystrophy
		Amyloidosis		Corticosteroid use
				Vasculitis
				Collagen vascular diseases

Table 13-1. Muscular Dystrophy Syndromes Inheritance Patterns

MUSCULAR DYSTROPHY SYNDROME	PATTERN OF INHERITANCE
Duchenne muscular dystrophy	X-linked
Limb-girdle muscular dystrophy	Autosomal recessive or dominant
Facioscapulohumeral muscular dystrophy	Autosomal dominant
Myotonic dystrophy	Autosomal dominant
Peroneal muscular atrophy (Charcot–Marie–Tooth disease)	Autosomal dominant

- **Lead**: lead toxicity can result in encephalopathy and psychiatric problems (children), abdominal pain, and peripheral neuropathy appearing in the hands before the feet (adults).
- **Thallium**: this toxin is used in rodenticides and industrial processes. Patients present with a sensory and autonomic neuropathy. Alopecia usually develops at the onset of symptoms.
- **Arsenic, mercury**: these toxins from electrical and chemical industries, and industrial solvents containing aliphatic compounds, can also cause neuromuscular symptoms.

13. What are the key elements of a physical examination in the evaluation of neuromuscular symptoms? (Table 13-2)

14. What is Gower's sign?
A patient attempts to rise from a seated position by climbing up his legs with his hands. It is seen in patients with proximal lower extremity muscular weakness due to myopathy.

15. How is muscle weakness graded by the physical examiner?
The most commonly accepted scale is the Medical Research Council Grading System. Because there is a wide range of muscle strength between grades 5 and 4, it is common to assign intermediate values such as 5− or 4+ to many muscle groups in the examination (Table 13-3).

16. How are deep tendon reflexes graded by the physical examiner? (Table 13-4)

17. How can alterations in deep tendon reflexes aid in differentiation of neuromuscular diseases?
- Spinal cord lesions (above L2) and upper motor neuron disease usually produce exaggerated deep tendon reflexes and pathologic plantar reflexes.

Table 13-2. Key Elements of the Physical Examination

SYSTEM	EXAMINE FOR
General	Cardiopulmonary disease, infection, thyroid disease, malignancy
Joints	Synovitis, deformities, contractures
Muscles	Muscle bulk, tenderness, weakness, fasciculations
Neurologic	Sensory abnormalities, deep tendon reflexes, weakness

Table 13-3. Manual Grading of Muscle Strength

GRADE	DEGREE OF STRENGTH
5	Normal strength
4	Muscle contraction possible against gravity plus some examiner resistance
3	Muscle contraction possible against gravity only
2	Muscle contraction possible only with gravity removed
1	Flicker of muscle contraction observed but without movement of extremity
0	No contraction

Table 13-4. Grading of Deep Tendon Reflexes

GRADE	STRENGTH OF CONTRACTION
4	Clonus
3	Exaggerated
2	Normal
1	Present but depressed
0	Absent

> **Box 13-3.** Screening Tests for Neuromuscular Diseases
>
> Complete blood count
> Serum electrolytes, calcium, magnesium, phosphorus
> Serum muscle enzymes
> Erythrocyte sedimentation rate (ESR)
> Serum liver enzyme tests
> Serum renal function tests
> Serum 25-hydroxyvitamin D level
> Thyroid function tests
> Chest radiograph
> Electrocardiogram

Table 13-5. Clinical Utility of Serum Muscle Enzymes

SERUM ENZYME	CLINICAL UTILITY
Creatine kinase (CK)	Most sensitive and specific for muscle disease
Aldolase	Elevated in muscle, liver, and erythrocyte diseases
Lactic dehydrogenase	Elevated in muscle, liver, erythrocyte, and other diseases
Aspartate aminotransferase (AST)	Most specific for inflammatory muscle disease

- Nerve root and peripheral nerve lesions usually produce depressed or absent reflexes.
- Primary muscle diseases do not usually *present* with altered deep tendon reflexes. Late in the disease process, however, substantial muscle atrophy may cause reduction or loss of the reflex.
- Hyperthyroidism produces exaggerated tendon reflexes.
- Hypothyroidism produces depressed deep tendon reflexes with a slow relaxation phase.
- Many people over the age of 60 years experience a natural loss of their ankle reflexes.

18. **Which screening laboratory tests can evaluate for systemic causes of neuromuscular symptoms? (Box 13-3)**

19. **Which serum enzymes are elevated in muscle disease? (Table 13-5)**

20. **What are other causes of elevation of serum creatine kinase besides myopathy?**
    Intramuscular injections
    Muscle crush injuries
    Recent strenuous exercise
    Myocardial infarction
    Race (healthy black individuals may have significantly higher creatine kinase [CK] levels than the "normal" values derived from the entire population).

21. **Are additional specific tests useful in the evaluation of neuromuscular symptoms? (Table 13-6)**

22. **What is mononeuritis multiplex?**
    Mononeuritis multiplex is a pattern of motor and sensory involvement of multiple individual peripheral nerves that is a classic neurologic presentation of systemic vasculitis. First, one peripheral nerve becomes involved (usually with burning dysesthesias), followed by other individual nerves, often with motor dysfunction as well. The patchy nature of nerve involvement reflects the patchy vasculitis of the vasa nervorum, which is the underlying cause of the neuropathy. It can also be present in diabetes mellitus, sarcoidosis, lead neuropathy, and Wartenburg's relapsing sensory neuritis.

23. **What are the most common causes of proximal shoulder girdle and hip girdle aches, pains, and/or weakness? How are they differentiated?**
    Six diseases are responsible for >90% of diffuse, proximal aches or weakness. The first step is to decide which is the dominant clinical finding: pain or weakness. To determine if true weakness is present, the examiner should ask the patient to ignore any pain that may occur during muscle strength testing so that a true measure of muscle strength can be determined. Although patients with fibromyalgia syndrome and polymyalgia rheumatica may complain of weakness in addition to pain, they are not truly weak on physical examination (Table 13-7).

24. **What are critical illness polyneuropathy (CIP) and critical illness myopathy (CIM)?**
    These are a group of neuromuscular disorders commonly affecting patients with critical illnesses. CIP is most likely to occur in patients with severe sepsis, multiple organ dysfunction, and those receiving prolonged mechanical ventilation. Manifestations include limb muscle weakness, reduced or absent deep tendon reflexes, loss of distal sensation, and respiratory insufficiency due to phrenic nerve involvement. Critical illness myopathy most commonly occurs in patients who have received IV glucocorticoids in the ICU setting. Patients have severe muscle weakness, preserved reflexes/sensation, and difficulty weaning off a ventilator. Half of the patients have an elevated CK. Clinical presentation, serum CK levels, electrodiagnostic testing, and muscle biopsy findings can separate patients with CIP from those with CIM. However, it is not uncommon for both conditions to coexist in the same individual. Treatment is supportive care, limiting the use of glucocorticoids and paralytics, and nutritional support. Patients usually take weeks to months to recover their strength.

Table 13-6. Additional Diagnostic Tests in Neuromuscular Disease Evaluation

SPECIFIC TEST	SUSPECTED DISEASE PROCESSES
Serum antinuclear antibodies	Inflammatory myopathy, vasculitis
Serum antisynthetase antibodies	Inflammatory myopathy +/− interstitial lung disease
Serum rheumatoid factor	Inflammatory myopathy, vasculitis
Serum complement assay	Inflammatory myopathy, vasculitis
Serum cryoglobulins	Vasculitis
Hepatitis B surface antigen and hepatitis C antibody	Vasculitis
Antineutrophil cytoplasmic antibodies	Vasculitis
Acetylcholine receptor antibodies	Myasthenia gravis
Serum parathyroid hormone	Parathyroid disease
Electromyography and nerve conduction tests	Disease of nerve roots, peripheral nerves, or myopathies
Muscle biopsy	Inflammatory or metabolic myopathies, vasculitis
Nerve biopsy	Vasculitis
Magnetic resonance scan	Spinal cord, nerve root, and myopathic processes

Table 13-7. Common Causes of Proximal Muscle Pain and/or Weakness

DISEASE	PAIN	WEAKNESS	ESR	SERUM CK	SERUM T4
Fibromyalgia	Yes	No	Normal	Normal	Normal
Polymyalgia rheumatic	Yes	No	Marked elevation	Normal	Normal
Polymyositis	Usually none	Yes	Usually normal	Elevated	Normal
Corticosteroid myopathy	No	Yes	Normal	Normal	Normal
Hyperthyroidism	No	Yes	Normal	Normal	Elevated
Hypothyroidism	Yes	No	Normal	Elevated	Depressed

CK, Creatine kinase; ESR, erythrocyte sedimentation rate; T4, thyroxine.

Box 13-4. Rheumatologic Causes of Strokes in Young Patients

Systemic lupus erythematosus
Antiphospholipid antibody syndrome
Takayasu's arteritis
Isolated angiitis of the CNS
Polyarteritis nodosa
Wegener's granulomatosis

25. **What is the diagnostic significance of "strokes in young folks"? What rheumatic syndromes should be considered in the differential diagnosis of cerebrovascular disease?**
    Most cerebrovascular disease occurs in patients over age 50 as a result of long-standing hypertension, atherosclerosis, and cardiac emboli. When ischemic cerebrovascular disease occurs in patients under age 50, the possibility of several rheumatic syndromes should be especially considered (Box 13-4).

BIBLIOGRAPHY

Alshekhlee A, Kaminksi HJ, Ruff RL: Neuromuscular manifestations of endocrine disorders, Neurol Clin 20:35–58, v-vi. 2002.
Baer AN: Metabolic, drug-induced, and other non-inflammatory myopathies. In Hochberg MC, Silman AJ, Smolen JS, Weinblatt E, Weisman MH, editors: Rheumatology, ed 5, Philadelphia, 2011, Mosby Elsevier.
Bolton CF: Neuromuscular manifestations of critical illness, Muscle Nerve 32:140, 2005.
Dalakas MC: Muscle biopsy findings in inflammatory myopathies, Rheum Dis Clin North Am 28:779–798, 2002.
Neal RC, Ferdinand KC, Ycas J, et al: Relationship of ethnic origin, gender, and age to blood creatine kinase levels, Am J Med 122:73–78, 2009.
Nirmalananthan N, Holton JL, Hanna MG: Is it really myositis? A consideration of the differential diagnosis, Curr Opin Rheumatol 16:684–691, 2004.
Schulze M, et al: MRI findings in inflammatory muscle diseases and their noninflammatory mimics, AJR 192:1708–1716, 2009.

CHAPTER 14

PERIOPERATIVE MANAGEMENT OF PATIENTS WITH RHEUMATIC DISEASES

Kim Nguyen Tyler, MD and Kevin D. Deane, MD

KEY POINTS

1. Careful preoperative evaluation is essential. Remember the ABCDE'S.
2. Subclinical cardiovascular disease (CVD) is common in patients with longstanding inflammatory rheumatic disease and should be screened for before major surgery.
3. Prophylaxis for deep venous thrombosis (DVT) must be instituted early and continued during the postoperative period.
4. An acutely painful, swollen joint in the postoperative period must be aspirated and evaluated for both infection and crystals.

1. **Why is it important for rheumatic disease patients to be evaluated perioperatively?**
    Patients with rheumatic diseases can have unique problems because of their underlying rheumatic disease, complications of medical therapy including immunosuppression, and limitations in functional status. The perioperative evaluation can identify factors that may contribute to surgical risk so that appropriate action can be taken to avoid complications.

2. **List the essential items to review in the perioperative evaluation of a patient with a rheumatic disease.**
    A comprehensive evaluation should include the "ABCDE'S":
    A—adjust medications
    B—bacterial prophylaxis
    C—cervical spine disease, cardiovascular risk
    D—DVT prophylaxis
    E—evaluate extent and activity of disease; maximize disease control
    S—stress-dose steroid coverage

3. **How are patients with rheumatic diseases "cleared" for surgery?**
    The term "clearance" was used at a time when the goal of the preoperative assessment was to crudely divide patients into those able to tolerate surgery ("cleared") and those unable to tolerate surgery. The term is archaic because today patients are rarely excluded from being considered for an operative procedure on the basis of their underlying medical conditions; however, because of a variety of factors, patients with rheumatic diseases may be at increased risk for complications. A more appropriate goal of the preoperative assessment is risk stratification, with identification of potential perioperative problems whose risk can be reduced.

4. **List three important issues to address in the preoperative history and physical examination of patients with rheumatic diseases.**
    - **Cardiovascular risk**: patients with inflammatory rheumatic diseases are at increased cardiovascular risk. Many are elderly and/or physically impaired. Determining cardiovascular risk may be more difficult because they are not physically active. A preoperative pharmacologic stress test may be needed to adequately assess the risk of a perioperative myocardial infarction. Based on specific criteria, perioperative beta blockers may be indicated.
    - **Cervical spine disease**: any neck pain, particularly with occipital radiation, needs radiographic evaluation. Some patients can have an unstable cervical spine without significant neck pain. A good rule of thumb is to get a cervical spine radiograph on any rheumatoid arthritis (RA) patient with longstanding disease (>10 years) and/or hand deformities even if they do not have neck symptoms.
    - **Occult infections**: patients should be examined for carious teeth, skin infections (look at the feet), and asymptomatic bacteriuria, cystitis, and pharyngitis, which may serve as sources of infection for total joint arthroplasties. Patients with an enlarged prostate are at increased risk of catheter-induced postoperative urinary tract infections.

5. **What laboratory tests are routinely required for patients with rheumatic diseases scheduled for elective surgery?**
    There is no consensus on preoperative screening, however, a complete blood count, blood urea nitrogen, creatinine, glucose, coagulation studies, urinalysis, chest radiograph, and electrocardiogram are commonly

Table 14-1. Potential Preoperative Evaluations	
TEST	**ORDER IN A PATIENT WITH**
Liver function tests	NSAID, methotrexate, leflunomide use
Prothrombin time/partial thromboplastin time	Liver disease or bleeding disorder Antiphospholipid antibody syndrome
Electrocardiogram	Age >40 yr, abnormal cardiac examination Coronary disease or risk factors (patients with RA or SLE may have silent vascular disease)
Bleeding time	Controversial, but may be assessed in recent NSAID users Often requested before renal biopsy
Chest x-ray	Longstanding inflammatory arthritis Acute pulmonary symptoms, abnormal examination Pulmonary disease or CVD Thoracic surgery Age >60 yr
Pulmonary function tests/arterial blood gases	Same as chest x-ray
Cervical spine x-ray, flexion and extension views	RA, juvenile idiopathic arthritis, ankylosing spondylitis

CVD, Cardiovascular disease; *NSAID*, nonsteroidal antiinflammatory drug; *RA*, rheumatoid arthritis; *SLE*, systemic lupus erythematosus.

obtained for each patient. A urine culture may be done before a total joint arthroplasty to eliminate a source for infection. Other tests may include those listed in Table 14-1.

6. **Are patients with rheumatic diseases at increased risk for perioperative complications compared with other patients?**
   Patients with rheumatic diseases may have a higher incidence of postoperative wound infections and impaired wound healing than nonrheumatic patients, usually because of medications used to treat their diseases. Accelerated CVD may be seen in patients with chronic inflammatory disease such as RA and systemic lupus erythematosus (SLE) as a result of disease activity or medications, and CVD may be asymptomatic if severe joint disease limits activity. As such, there should be a low threshold for CVD evaluation in patients with inflammatory rheumatic diseases.

7. **Should patients with active synovitis undergo elective surgery?**
   Usually no. Postoperatively, patients with active synovitis may have significant pain from their arthritis, which can impair functional status, impede progress with rehabilitation, and prolong hospitalization. Patients with active synovial disease and its consequent disability should have the inflammation controlled as much as possible before elective surgical procedures. If a patient does have active disease in the perioperative period and systemic corticosteroids or disease-modifying antirheumatic drugs (DMARDs) are inadvisable, intraarticular corticosteroids may be considered.

8. **Why is it important to evaluate patients with RA for cervical spine disease before surgery?**
   Although cervical spine disease in RA is likely to decrease in frequency as a result of the use of effective medications, instability of the cervical spine may still be present in patients with RA. In particular, cervical spine **atlantoaxial subluxation** can occur owing to inflammation and weakening of the transverse ligament, which holds the odontoid process of C2 against the anterior arch of C1. Manipulation of the neck during intubation and transport of the patient, especially extreme flexion or extension, can cause compression of the spinal cord by the odontoid process. Most anesthesiologists advocate preoperative flexion and extension c-spine radiographs for RA patients with the following risk factors (C-SPINE) because significant cervical spine disease may be present but asymptomatic:
   C—corticosteroid use
   S—seropositive RA
   P—peripheral joint destruction
   I—involvement of cervical nerves (paresthesias, neck pain, weakness)
   N—nodules (rheumatoid)
   E—established disease (present >10 years)

9. **How is atlanto-axial (C1–C2) instability diagnosed? How are they managed?**
   Instability of C1–C2 is diagnosed when the odontoid process is found to be displaced >3 mm from its normal position against the anterior arch of the atlas in the lateral flexion and extension radiographs. This indicates

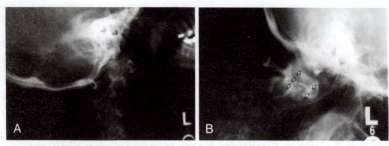

Figure 14-1. Atlanto-axial instability. Arrows show wide separation of the odontoid process of C2 from the anterior arch of C1 in a patient with severe RA. **A,** Extension view. **B,** Flexion view.

that the transverse ligament has been compromised. There is more concern when the displacement is greater than 7 to 8 mm because it is likely that the alar ligaments are destroyed, increasing the chance for spinal cord compromise.

Symptomatic patients should have surgical stabilization performed before other elective surgery. Patients with asymptomatic or mild disease may be considered for intubation with fiber optic assistance to minimize the extremes of motion associated with routine intubation. A soft cervical collar worn throughout the perioperative period will serve as a visual reminder that these patients should be handled with care, but it does not offer support to an unstable spine (Figure 14-1).

10. What is cricoarytenoid disease? How can it impact on anesthetic complications?

The cricoarytenoid (CA) joint is a true diarthrodial articulation and is subject to the same destructive changes that occur in other small joints in patients with RA. The degree of CA disease correlates with peripheral joint disease. Symptoms of CA involvement include tracheal pain, dysphonia, stridor, dyspnea, and dysarthria. Other patients can have minor symptoms related to synovitis but over time develop fibrous replacement of the normal cartilage and ankylosis across the joint space. The diagnosis of CA disease may be clinically silent until attempts at endotracheal intubation by standard techniques result in trauma to the adducted vocal cords, with subsequent edema, inflammation, and airway obstruction. Perioperative fiber optic laryngoscopy is recommended for all patients with symptoms of CA disease. Treatment includes systemic or locally injected corticosteroids. Intubation under fiberscopic guidance is also recommended at the time of surgery. Patients with severe CA disease should be considered for elective tracheostomy if the vocal cords are found to be chronically adducted.

11. Should aspirin and nonsteroidal antiinflammatory drugs be discontinued preoperatively in rheumatic disease patients?

Patients treated with aspirin (ASA) and acetylsalicylate-containing medications may be at risk for increased surgical bleeding, because these drugs impair platelet aggregation for the life of the platelet (7 to 10 days). ASA should be discontinued 7 to 10 days before planned surgery except in patients at high risk for myocardial infarction, thrombotic transient ischemic attacks, or stroke.

Traditional nonsteroidal antiinflammatory drugs (NSAIDs) have a mixture of cyclooxygenase-1 (COX-1) and COX-2 inhibiting action and decrease platelet aggregation, but unlike aspirin, their effects are reversible with discontinuation of the medicine. NSAIDs have also been associated with more frequent episodes of gastrointestinal bleeding when given perioperatively. These agents should be held preoperatively for a time equal to three to five half-lives of the drug to allow return of normal platelet function, and they may be restarted 2 to 3 days postoperatively provided the patient is stable. If an NSAID is needed in the perioperative period but side effects are a concern, an option is to switch from a longer acting NSAID to one with a shorter half-life (Table 14-2). Because there has been recent concern regarding the cardiovascular safety of COX-2 specific inhibitors, they should be used cautiously if at all in the perioperative period. If NSAIDs for control of pain/inflammation are contra-indicated in the perioperative period, other agents may be used as appropriate including acetaminophen, prednisone, or other non-NSAID pain medications (e.g., tramadol, narcotic analgesics).

Celecoxib is a highly selective COX-2 inhibitor and salsalate is a nonacetylated salicylate. Both of these should have minimal if any effect on platelet function. However, many surgeons stop these medications to lessen cardiovascular risks. Patients with dyspepsia from their NSAIDs or prior history of peptic ulcer disease should receive prophylactic H-2 blocker therapy postoperatively.

PEARL: Ask about nonprescription drugs and supplements. Many rheumatic disease patients may take complementary and alternative medicine (CAM) therapies that can affect platelet function (ginkgo, ginger, etc.) or interact with anesthesia.

12. How does the normal adrenal gland respond to surgery?

In a baseline state, the adrenal gland secretes the equivalent of 20 to 30 mg of cortisol (e.g., hydrocortisone; equivalent to 5 to 7.5 mg prednisone) per day, but with major stress or general anesthesia, it may increase

Table 14-2. Half-Lives of Selected NSAIDS

NSAID	Half-life (Hours)	Five Half-lives (Days)
Ibuprofen	1.6-1.9	1
Diclofenac	2	1
Indomethacin	4.5	1
Etodolac	6-7	2
Sulindac	8-16	4
Celecoxib	11	4
Naproxen	12-15	4
Nabumetone	24-29	7
Piroxicam	30	7

NSAID, Nonsteroidal antiinflammatory drug.

tenfold up to 200 to 300 mg of cortisol (50 to 75 mg of prednisone) per day. Cortisol levels typically peak within 24 hours of the time of surgical incision and return to normal after 72 hours if no other factors contribute to perioperative stress.

13. What causes exogenous corticosteroid-related perioperative adrenal insufficiency?

The administration of exogenous corticosteroids can interfere with the normal function of the hypothalamic–pituitary–adrenal (HPA) axis and blunt endogenous cortisol excretion. With stress, the adrenal output blunted by exogenous corticosteroids may become inadequate to support physiologic demands, which include vascular tone and maintenance of blood pressure. The following patients are at risk for corticosteroid-related adrenal insufficiency:
- Patients with features of Cushing's syndrome (moon facies, buffalo-hump, etc.)
- Patients on a prednisone dose (or equivalent of another corticosteroid) of: ≥20 mg daily for ≥5 days or >5 mg daily for ≥30 days

If there is any question about whether adrenal insufficiency may occur, an adrenal stimulation test should be performed or the patient should receive stress-dose steroids empirically. Patients who become adrenally insufficient during stress (infection, trauma, etc.) usually become hypotensive (systolic <90 mm/Hg) in spite of fluid resuscitation. These patients should be placed on intravenous hydrocortisone 100 mg every 8 hours with subsequent tapering once the stress resolves. Tapering is best done by lowering the dose and not the frequency (i.e., every 8 hours) of hydrocortisone.

14. How can patients at risk of adrenal insufficiency be tested preoperatively?

The cosyntropin stimulation test is a simple and reliable method to evaluate the ability of the adrenal gland to respond to stress. After the baseline cortisol level has been obtained, 250 μg of cosyntropin (an adrenocorticotropic hormone [ACTH] analog) is injected intravenously or intramuscularly, and the cortisol level is measured after 30 and 60 minutes. Patients with a normal HPA axis should be able to double their baseline cortisol level and demonstrate a stimulated value of >20 μg/dL at either 30 or 60 minutes.

15. How are stress-dose steroids given?

Because the complications of adrenal insufficiency can be life-threatening, the risks of perioperative corticosteroids are perceived to be low, and the cost of the ACTH stimulation test is high (>$200), many providers provide perioperative stress-dosing of corticosteroids routinely without testing in any patient at risk for exogenous corticosteroid-induced adrenal insufficiency. However, prolonged high-dose steroids in a surgical setting leads to increased risk of infection and poor wound healing and clinically appropriate rapid tapers need to be performed in the postoperative setting. Hydrocortisone (Solu-Cortef) is the corticosteroid of choice for stress-dosing regimens because it has a more rapid onset of action than other agents. Elaborate tapering schedules are not required unless postoperative complications prolong stress after surgery. Patients on oral steroids preoperatively may typically resume their normal daily oral dose (1 mg prednisone=4 mg hydrocortisone) if stable postoperatively and taking oral medications well. Some data suggest that in many patients on corticosteroids, perioperative stress-dosing is not necessary, especially if the patient is undergoing a minor procedure and is monitored closely in the perioperative period. However, the anesthetic agent etomidate (Amidate) may interfere with adrenal corticosteroid synthesis; as such, if this agent is used for anesthesia, stress-dose steroids should be used. If a provider chooses to provide stress-dosing, there are multiple approaches but the regimens shown in Table 14-3 are generally accepted.

Table 14-3. Perioperative Regimens for Stress-Dose Corticosteroid Administration

Level of Surgical Stress	Surgical Procedure	Stress-Dose Steroids
Superficial procedure	Skin biopsy	Continue daily dose of corticosteroids
Minor	Procedures under local anesthesia and <1 h Colonoscopy Cataract surgery Carpal tunnel release Tenosynovectomy Knee arthroscopy Most minor podiatry/orthopedic foot procedures (hammer toe correction, toe fusion)	Hydrocortisone 25 mg IV on call to operating room (OR), resume daily oral dosing of corticosteroids afterwards
Moderate	Unilateral total joint replacement Complex foot reconstruction Lower extremity vascular surgery Uncomplicated appendectomy, gall bladder removal	Hydrocortisone 50 to 100 mg IV on call to OR, then taper down over 1 to 2 days to preoperative daily oral dose
Major	Multiple trauma Colon resection Bilateral joint replacement Revision arthroplasty Multiple level spinal fusion Any surgery requiring cardiopulmonary bypass	Hydrocortisone 100 mg IV on call to OR, then 100 mg IV every 8 h for 24 h postoperatively, then 50 mg IV every 8 h the next day, then 100 mg as a single dose on third postoperative day, then usual daily dose on fourth postoperative day

Caveats: (1) Patients must be monitored carefully for signs of adrenal insufficiency (hypotension) in the perioperative period and stress-dosing may need to be adjusted; (2) resumption of daily oral dosing of corticosteroids is dependent on oral intake postoperatively and may be delayed if nil per os (NPO) status is prolonged (e.g., with abdominal surgery, nausea). Also, if postoperative hypotension develops, patient should be assessed for etiologies other than adrenal insufficiency including volume depletion, cardiovascular disease (CVD), pulmonary embolus, and infection.

16. **Name the two most common organisms to infect a prosthetic joint at the time of surgery.**
    Coagulase-negative staphylococci
    Staphylococcus aureus

17. **What is standard antibiotic prophylaxis for prosthetic joint surgery?**
    The goal of perioperative antibiotics is to reduce organism burden and prevent postoperative infection. For joint replacement surgery, typically cefazolin is used, dosed at 1 g IV within 60 minutes of incision, then every 8 hours for 1 day postoperatively. Vancomycin, 1 g IV every 12 hours (or renal dosing), may be used in patients who are allergic to penicillin. There are no data to support the use of prophylactic antibiotics for >24 hours postoperatively. Other measures to reduce postoperative infection include skin cleansing preoperatively with agents such as chlorhexidine.

18. **Should patients who have prosthetic joints be prescribed antibiotic prophylaxis before undergoing dental procedures?**
    There is not yet a consensus among orthopedic surgeons, dentists, infectious disease physicians, and primary care providers as to the utility of antibiotic prophylaxis during dental procedures in patients with prosthetic joints, and there are little controlled data to guide therapy. Until better data becomes available, the American Academy of Orthopaedic Surgeons (AAOS) recommends prophylaxis for the following patients with total large joint (hip, knee, shoulder) arthroplasties:
    - All patients who have had an arthroplasty within the last 2 years.
    - All high-risk patients: previous prosthetic joint infection, malignancy, immunosuppressed (drug-induced, HIV, other), insulin-dependent diabetes, RA, SLE, previous native joint infection, hemophilia, and malnourishment.

    Antibiotics prescribed for these select patients may provide benefit without excess risk. In the absence of good data, amoxicillin (2 g), cephradine (2 g), cephalexin (2 g), or clindamycin (600 mg) for the penicillin-allergic patient, dosed once orally 1 hour before the procedure, may be rational choices for higher risk patients. Antibiotic prophylaxis is not necessary for patients who only have had small joint (e.g., metacarpophalangeal joint, MCP) replacements, pins, plates, or screws.

19. **Should patients with antiphospholipid antibodies be given antibiotic prophylaxis before dental, urologic, and gastrointestinal procedures?**
    There is concern that patients with antiphospholipid antibodies may have valvular disease predisposing them to endocarditis. Certainly, if valvular disease is known to be present, antibiotic prophylaxis should be used. However, if antiphospholipid antibodies are present but there is no known valvular disease, clinical judgment must be used.

20. **What are the options for DVT prophylaxis in patients undergoing joint replacement procedures?**
    DVT risk varies with the procedure, with hip replacement being higher risk than knee replacement. Guidelines in this area are changing as new therapies are developed, but the following are options for DVT prophylaxis:
    - Warfarin, with dose adjustment to reach a target prothrombin time of 16–18 seconds (international normalized ratio [INR] 2–3) for at least 10 days after the procedure. Continuing warfarin for up to 42 days postoperatively may be associated with decreased DVT in patients after hip surgery. Dosing for longer than 10 days after knee replacement surgery has not been shown to be beneficial.
    - Heparin (unfractionated) 5000 units subcutaneously before surgery, then 5000 units every 8 hours after surgery, adjusted by sliding scale every day to maintain the adjusted partial thromboplastin time within 4 seconds of the upper limit of normal. Time and expense of administration of this agent limit its usefulness.
    - Pneumatic compression devices, worn on the lower extremities at all times starting the morning of surgery, until the patient is ambulatory or discharged. Compression stockings only offer minimal protection against DVT and are not recommended as a single therapy.
    - Low molecular weight heparins (LMWHs) may be used for prophylaxis (check product recommendations for prophylactic dosage). The best efficacy is achieved by starting dosing preoperatively and continuing dosing for at least 10 days postoperatively. In hip replacement surgery, continued DVT prophylaxis with LMWHs up to 42 days postoperatively has been shown to decrease the incidence of DVT without significantly increasing bleeding episodes.
    - Fondaparinux (synthetic heparin) preoperatively and continued for 10 to 42 days postoperatively.
    - Hirudin and lepirudin are used in Europe for DVT prophylaxis in patients that cannot tolerate standard heparin (heparin-associated thrombocytopenia) but are only approved in the United States for treatment of heparin-associated thrombocytopenia.
    - Aspirin (325 mg/day) can modestly decrease the incidence of DVT, but is associated with an increased risk of bleeding and is not routinely recommended for perioperative DVT prophylaxis.
    - Dextran IV can be used although its efficacy is less than LMWH or warfarin in preventing DVT.

21. **Should DMARDs be stopped before elective surgery?**
    There are mixed conclusions regarding methotrexate (MTX) and other DMARDs and increased risk for postoperative complications including wound infection and poor wound healing. Most of the studies related to this issue included small numbers of patients and a low mean dose of MTX (10 mg) weekly. Practically, many rheumatologists discontinue methotrexate the week of surgery, with resumption of MTX once the patient is doing well postoperatively (usually within 1 week; i.e., hold a total of two doses of MTX). Most experts will continue hydroxychloroquine. There are limited data regarding perioperative use of other DMARDs and recommendations are predominantly based on expert opinion. A reasonable approach is to stop DMARDs one to two half-lives before surgery and resume them approximately 1 week after surgery provided there are no infectious or wound healing complications. Careful consideration must also be made regarding those postoperative complications that may affect metabolism and/or clearance of the DMARDs (e.g., renal or hepatic insufficiency, concomitant anticoagulation, or antibiotics) (Table 14-4).

22. **What about the use of anti-TNF alpha agents or other biologics in the perioperative period?**
    Studies evaluating the use of biologic agents in the perioperative period are limited, and there are conflicting results regarding increased rates of infection and delayed wound healing. Taking into account the different half-lives of these medications, it is prudent to stop them for at least two half-lives before surgery, and resume these agents postoperatively only once the patient is doing well from a surgical standpoint (see Table 14-5 for two calculated half-lives). There are limited data regarding perioperative complications with the other biologic agents, such as abatacept, anakinra, tocilizumab, tofacitinib, and rituximab. Regarding rituximab, one should be aware of potential hypogammaglobulinemia in those patients who have received repeated cycles of rituximab. With regard to other biologics, a good rule of thumb is to stop them at least two half-lives before surgery and restart afterwards after external wound healing is complete (usually 4 weeks).

23. **A patient with RA is found to have a swollen, warm, and tender knee on postoperative day 4 after a cholecystectomy. Should the patient have an arthrocentesis performed?**
    Yes. An acutely inflamed joint postoperatively should always be aspirated to exclude a septic joint. Do not assume that the symptoms are due to a flare of RA, especially if the involved joint seems inflamed out of proportion to the rest of the patient's disease activity. Keep in mind that patients with RA may have "pseudoseptic arthritis," where synovial fluid white blood cell (WBC) count is >50,000/mm^3, mimicking infection.

Such "pseudoseptic" arthritis may be due to rebound autoimmune-mediated inflammation in a patient whose immunosuppression has been held perioperatively.

24. **A patient with chronic tophaceous gout has the acute onset of left knee pain and swelling postoperatively. Aspiration reveals negatively birefringent needle-shaped crystals. Can you be certain of the diagnosis of acute gouty arthritis?**
Not yet. In patients with chronic gout, uric acid crystals can be seen on synovial fluid aspirated from an asymptomatic joint—in this case, their presence is not diagnostic. Sepsis and gout can also occur simultaneously, so evaluation for infection (gram stain, culture) is mandatory.

25. **What predisposes patients to perioperative gout attacks?**
Dehydration
Increased uric acid production as a result of adenosine triphosphate breakdown (energy utilization) during surgery
Medicines (diuretics, heparin, cyclosporine)
Minor trauma to the joint during surgery and transport
Infections

Table 14-4. Perioperative Management of DMARDS

DMARD	Half-life	Perioperative Recommendation*
Methotrexate	3-12 h	Stop during week of surgery and for 1 week postoperatively (total two doses, controversial)
Hydroxychloroquine	30-50 days	Continue throughout surgery
Leflunomide	14 days	Stop 2 weeks preoperatively; resume 3 days after surgery
Sulfasalazine	10 h	Stop for 1 day preoperatively; resume 3 days after surgery
Azathioprine (or 6-mercaptopurine)	3 h	Stop 1 day before surgery; resume 3 days after surgery
Mycophenolate mofetil	18 h	Stop 3 days preoperatively; resume 3 days after surgery

DMARD, Disease-modifying antirheumatic drug.
*Caveat: medication should be resumed postoperatively once the patient is doing well (wound without infection and healing well, patient taking oral medications, no new renal/hepatic insufficiency).

Table 14-5. Two Half-Lives of Selected Biologic Agents

Biologic Agent	Two Half-lives (Days)
Etanercept	7
Adalimumab	20
Infliximab	20
Golimumab	30
Certolizumab	30
Abatacept	25
Tocilizumab	16-25
Rituximab	40
Anakinra	0.50
Tofacitinib	0.50
Ustekinumab	40-60
Belimumab	40
Apremilast	1

Hyperalimentation
Surgical stress
Cessation of prophylactic medications (allopurinol, colchicine)
Preoperative serum uric acid level ≥9 mg/dL

26. **What are the options for treating patients with acute gouty arthritis postoperatively if they are unable to take oral agents?**
    - Indomethacin or another NSAID per nasogastric tube or suppositories per rectum. These agents may be contraindicated if the patient is at risk for surgical bleeding or gastric ulcer disease. Intramuscular ketorolac 30 to 60 mg is another option if NSAID use is appropriate.
    - Intravenous colchicine has been used in the past for patients unable to take oral medicines, however, given its toxicities (bone marrow, neuromuscular, gastrointestinal), IV use of this agent should be avoided.
    - ACTH, 20 units intravenously (slow), or 40 units intramuscularly (rarely used because of cost and availability).
    - Triamcinolone acetonide, 40 to 60 mg per day intramuscularly for one to two doses. This may be the safest option in many cases.
    - Methylprednisolone 20 to 60 mg IV daily for several days, and then replace with oral prednisone, tapering when appropriate.
    - Corticosteroid preparation injected into the joint (if you are sure it is not infected).

27. **What special considerations should be made in the perioperative management of patients with antiphospholipid syndrome?**
    It is essential to minimize the amount of time without anticoagulation and avoid the use of vitamin K, which can complicate the resumption of therapeutic warfarin use. Another important concept is to minimize all aspects of Virchow's triad (hypercoagulability, stasis, and endothelial injury). Examples of this include using external pneumatic compression devices in the operating room and postoperatively, setting the blood pressure cuffs to inflate less frequently, avoiding tourniquets, encouraging ambulation as soon as possible after surgery, and limiting intravascular line placement and removing them as soon as they are no longer needed.

28. **What is the perioperative approach to those patients who are antiphospholipid antibody positive without a history of blood clots?**
    This is a controversial issue with experts on both sides of the argument. The fear is that surgery and its postoperative issues can tip a person with a potential predisposition to clot into a hypercoagulable state and thereby suffer thrombosis postoperatively. There seems to be general consensus to use standard approaches to perioperative DVT prophylaxis, as performed in the general population; however, the controversy is whether or not to continue prophylactic anticoagulation after discharge and for how long. Some experts advocate the continuation of prophylactic doses of LMWHs or therapeutic warfarin for 1 to 6 weeks postoperatively.

29. **What other disease-specific precautions should be considered in rheumatic diseases other than RA?**
    - **Sjögren's syndrome:** use lubricating gel and artificial tears during anesthesia to prevent corneal abrasion. Do not give pilocarpine preoperatively to avoid bronchospasm and bradycardia. Minimize the use of anticholinergic drugs during the perioperative period. Dryness may increase the risk of pneumonia.
    - **Juvenile idiopathic arthritis:** micrognathia may make intubation difficult. Cervical spine instability can occur.
    - **Ankylosing spondylitis:** cervical spine immobility may make intubation difficult. Restrictive chest excursion may increase the risk of pneumonia. Heterotopic ossification can complicate total hip arthroplasty.
    - **Psoriatic arthritis:** skin disease can flare at the surgical site (Koebner's phenomenon).
    - **SLE:** treat with intravenous immunoglobulin (IVIG) if the patient has severe thrombocytopenia and is in need of emergency surgery. There is increased cardiovascular risk.
    - **Systemic sclerosis:** poor venous access if sclerodermatous skin; risk of aspiration increased (esophageal dysmotility); postoperative ileus increased; arterial vasospasm increased in all organs including heart and kidneys; increased risk of scleroderma renal crisis if not hydrated. Increased risk of adverse outcome if have pulmonary hypertension. Increased cardiac arrhythmia risk.

Acknowledgment

The authors and editor would like to thank Dr. Kimberly May for her contribution to the previous edition of this chapter.

BIBLIOGRAPHY

American Academy of Orthopaedic Surgeons (AAOS): Prevention of orthopaedic implant infection in patients undergoing dental procedures. May 2014. www.aaos.org/research/guidelines/PUDP/dental_guideline.asp.
American Academy of Orthopaedic Surgeons (AAOS): Preventing thromboembolic disease. May 2014. www.aaos.org/research/guidelines/VTE/VTE_guideline.asp.
Axelrod L: Perioperative management of patients treated with glucocorticoids, Endocrinol Metab Clin North Am 32:367–383, 2003.
Coursin DB, Wood KE: Corticosteroid supplementation for adrenal insufficiency, JAMA 287:236–240, 2002.

Erkan D, et al: Perioperative medical management of antiphospholipid syndrome: hospital for special surgery experience, review of literature, and recommendations, J Rheumatol 29:843–849, 2002.

Geerts WH, Pineo GF, Heit JA, et al: Prevention of venous thromboembolism: the Seventh ACCP Conference on Antithrombotic and Thrombolytic Therapy, Chest 126(suppl 3):338S–400S, 2004.

Kolen ER, Schmidt MH: Rheumatoid arthritis of the cervical spine, Semin Neurol 22:179–186, 2002.

Lockhart PB, Loven B, Brennan MT, et al: The evidence base for the efficacy of antibiotic prophylaxis in dental practice, J Am Dent Assoc 138:458–474, 2007.

MacKenzie CR, Sharrock NE: Perioperative medical considerations in patients with rheumatoid arthritis, Rheum Dis Clin North Am 24:1–17, 1998.

Maradit-Kremers H, Crowson CS, Nicola PJ, et al: Increased unrecognized coronary heart disease and sudden deaths in rheumatoid arthritis: a population-based cohort study, Arthritis Rheum 52:402–411, 2005.

Marik PE, Varon J: Requirement of perioperative stress doses of corticosteroids: a systematic review of the literature, Arch Surg 143:1222–1226, 2008.

Mushtaq S, Goodman SM, Scanzello CR: Perioperative management of biologic agents used in the treatment of rheumatoid arthritis, Am J Ther 18:426, 2011.

Nierman E, Zakrzewski K: Recognition and management of preoperative risk, Rheum Dis Clin North Am 25:585–622, 1999.

Papadimitraki ED, Kyrmizakis DE, Kritikos I, et al: Ear-nose-throat manifestations of autoimmune rheumatic diseases, Clin Exp Rheumatol 22:485–494, 2004.

Saag K, et al: American College of Rheumatology 2008 recommendations for the use of nonbiologic and biologic disease-modifying antirheumatic drugs in rheumatoid arthritis, Arthritis Rheum 59:762–784, 2008.

Scanzello CR, et al: Perioperative management of medications used in the treatment of rheumatoid arthritis, HSS J 2:141–147, 2006.

Visser K, Katchamart W, Loza E, et al: Multinational evidence-based recommendations for the use of methotrexate in rheumatic disorders with a focus on rheumatoid arthritis, Ann Rheum Dis 68:1086, 2009.

Wortmann RL: Treatment of acute gouty arthritis: one physician's approach and where this management stands relative to developments in the field, Curr Rheumatol Rep 6:235–239, 2004.

III
SYSTEMIC CONNECTIVE TISSUE DISEASES

The wolf, I'm afraid, is inside tearing up the place.
Letter to Sister Mariella Gable from Flannery O'Connor,
a sufferer of systemic lupus erythematosus, July 5, 1964

[P.S.] Prayers requested. I am sick of being sick.
Letter to Louise Abbot from Flannery O'Connor, May 28, 1964

RHEUMATOID ARTHRITIS

Sterling G. West, MD and James R. O'Dell, MD

KEY POINTS

1. Rheumatoid arthritis (RA) is the most common chronic inflammatory arthritis.
2. Symmetric synovitis of the small joints of the hands (metacarpophalangeal joints [MCPs], proximal interphalangeal joints [PIPs]) and wrists is the classic initial pattern.
3. RA patients with extraarticular manifestations should be seropositive.
4. Early and aggressive therapy should target low disease activity for optimal outcomes.
5. RA patients have accelerated atherosclerosis warranting aggressive risk factor modification.

1. What is rheumatoid arthritis?

RA is a chronic, systemic, inflammatory disorder of unknown etiology that is characterized by its pattern of diarthrodial joint involvement. Its primary site of pathology is the synovium of the joints. The synovial tissues become inflamed and proliferate, forming **pannus** that invades bone, cartilage, and ligaments and leads to damage and deformities. Rheumatoid factor (RF), anticitrullinated protein antibodies (ACPAs), and extraarticular manifestations commonly accompany the joint disease, but arthritis represents the major manifestation.

2. What is the etiology and pathogenesis of RA?

Despite extensive research, the cause of RA remains unknown. It is thought to be multifactorial, with genetic factors (human leucocyte antigen [HLA] genes and others) and environmental factors (smoking, silica, and others) playing important roles. Notably, autoantibodies (RF, ACPAs) can be found in the sera years before the development of clinical symptoms. This suggests that initiating events incite a complex interaction between the innate and adaptive immune systems, which breaks tolerance and leads to autoreactivity. Over time, a critical immune threshold is breached resulting in clinical symptoms and tissue damage.

Genetic factors: twin studies show that the concordance rate for RA in monozygotic twins is 12% to 15% and in fraternal twins is 2% to 3% compared to 1% in the general population. This suggests that genetic factors account for 60% of an individual's susceptibility to RA. The major histocompatibility complex (MHC) region coding for certain HLA-DR genes account for 30% to 40% of this genetic predisposition. The susceptibility to RA is mainly associated with the third hypervariable region of DRβ chains from amino acids 70 to 74 (QKRAA). This **susceptibility** or **shared epitope** is found on HLA-DR4 (*0401,*0404) and, to a lesser extent, HLA-DR1 (*0101) and DR14 (*1402) β chains and is associated with a fourfold to fivefold increased risk of developing RA. However, this association is not found in all ethnic/racial groups (i.e., African-Americans) and HLA-DR4 positivity occurs in 20% to 30% of the general population, most of whom do not develop RA. Therefore, other factors must be present for the disease to develop. Over 30 genetic loci outside the MHC have been associated with an increased risk (5% of genetic risk) of developing RA. Most loci increase the odds ratio of developing RA only 1.2-fold to twofold, but this varies among ethnicities. Polymorphisms of PTPN22, TRAF1-C5, STAT4, TNFAIP3, and PADI4 (Asians) are well established. Epigenetic factors (histone modification, DNA methylation) are also likely to be important.

Environmental factors: smoking is the best characterized environmental risk factor and increases the odds ratio for developing RA 12-fold in susceptible monozygotic twins, 2.5-fold in dizygotic twins, and 1.8-fold in smokers (>20 pack-yrs). This risk persists for 10 to 20 years after a person quits smoking. **Bacteria** in the microbiomes of the mouth, lung, and gut may also be contributory. Smoking can alter microbiomes in the mouth and lung whereas diet and antibiotics can alter gut flora. *Porphyromonos gingivalis* in patients with chronic periodontitis can express PAD enzymes that can citrullinate proteins through the posttranslational modification of arginine to citrulline. Smoking can upregulate PAD enzymes in the lung resulting in protein citrullination. A similar process occurs with upregulation of myeloperoxidase that carbamylates proteins through modification of lysine to homocitrulline. Citrullinated and carbamylated proteins are neoantigens that cause a heightened immune response when presented to the immune system by HLA-DR molecules containing the shared epitope. ACPAs and anticarbamylated antibodies generated during this immune response can bind citrullinated and carbamylated proteins locally or form immune complexes that can deposit in tissue. Additionally, an altered microbiome at any site can stimulate the innate immune system through Toll-like receptors. Finally **viruses** (Epstein–Barr virus [EBV], parvovirus B19 [Parvo B19]) have been associated with triggering RA but none have been consistently implicated. In summary, a single environmental trigger for RA is highly unlikely.

Box 15-1. The 2010 ACR/EULAR Classification Criteria for RA

1. Joint involvement (swollen or tender joint on examination or synovitis on ultrasound/MRI)	**(0 to 5 points max)**
• One medium to large joint (shoulders, elbows, hips, knees, ankles)	0
• 2 to 10 medium to large joints	1
• 1 to 3 small joints (MCP, PIP, 2 to 5 MTP, or wrist with or without large joint involvement)	2
• 4 to 10 small joints (with or without large joint involvement)	3
• >10 joints (at least one small joint involved)	5
2. Serology	**(0 to 3 points max)**
• Negative RF and negative ACPA	0
• Low positive RF **or** low positive ACPA (<3 times the normal upper limit)	2
• High positive RF **or** high positive ACPA (>3 times the normal upper limit)	3
3. Acute phase reactants	**(0 to 1 points max)**
• Normal CRP and normal ESR	0
• Abnormal CRP **or** abnormal ESR	1
4. Duration of symptoms	**(0 to 1 points max)**
• <6 weeks	0
• ≥6 weeks	1

From Aletaha D, Neogi T, Silman AJ et al: 2010 rheumatoid arthritis classification criteria: an American College of Rheumatology/European League Against Rheumatism collaborative initiative, Ann Rheum Dis 69:1580-1588, 2010.

ACPA, Anticitrullinated protein antibody; *ACR/EULAR*, American College of Rheumatology/European League Against Rheumatism; *CRP*, C-reactive protein; *ESR*, erythrocyte sedimentation rate; *MCP*, metacarpophalangeal joint; *MRI*, magnetic resonance imaging; *MTP*, metatarsophalangeal joint; *PIP*, proximal interphalangeal joint; *RA*, rheumatoid arthritis; *RF*, rheumatoid factor.

Initiation of clinical disease: the mechanism of initiation of clinical synovitis is unknown. Certainly immune complexes (ACPAs and RF) could deposit in synovial postcapillary venules inciting vasculitis or tissue inflammation through complement activation. Tissue inflammation can increase vascular permeability with influx of more inflammatory cells and antibodies (including ACPAs). Inflammation can upregulate PAD enzymes and myeloperoxidase causing citrullination and carbamylation of synovial proteins and cartilage proteins. Binding of ACPAs can lead to chondrocyte damage and release of degraded collagen and proteoglycan neoepitopes from cartilage.

Perpetuation of clinical disease: RA is thought to be perpetuated by activation of the adaptive immune system with the innate immune system acting as a persistent adjuvant. Neoepitopes created by synovial inflammation and cartilage injury can be taken up by an influx of dendritic cells into the synovium. Dendritic cells from the genetically predisposed host present the neoantigens to T lymphocytes in both the synovial tissue and draining lymph nodes. Epitope spreading may occur with breakage of tolerance and an immune response to native antigens. T-cells, macrophages, synovial fibroblasts, and B cells are activated in different combinations to produce proinflammatory cytokines that play a key role in the perpetuation of chronic synovitis and tissue destruction. Activation of local osteoclasts can facilitate development of bony erosions.

3. **List the new ACR/EULAR criteria for the classification of RA (Box 15-1).**
According to the American College of Rheumatology (ACR)/European League Against Rheumatism (EULAR) criteria, to be classified as having RA, a patient must satisfy ≥6 out of 10 points. The criteria demonstrate 82% sensitivity and 61% specificity for RA when compared with control subjects with non-RA rheumatic disease.
PEARL: Most patients with RA have **symmetric polyarthritis** involving the small joints of the hands (MCPs, PIPs), wrists, and frequently the feet (metatarsophalangeals [MTPs]). In clinical practice, the diagnosis of RA should be questioned in patients who do not have a symmetric small joint arthritis and in those who are seronegative.

4. **What other diseases should be excluded before making the diagnosis of RA?**

COMMON DISEASES

Seronegative spondyloarthropathies, calcium pyrophosphate deposition disease, connective tissue diseases (systemic lupus erythematosus [SLE], scleroderma, polymyositis, vasculitis, mixed connective tissue disease [MCTD], polymyalgia rheumatica), osteoarthritis, viral infection (EBV, human immunodeficiency virus [HIV], hepatitis B, parvovirus, rubella, hepatitis C), polyarticular gout, fibromyalgia, Parkinson's disease, reactive arthritis.

UNCOMMON DISEASES

Hypothyroidism, relapsing polychondritis, subacute bacterial endocarditis, rheumatic fever, hemochromatosis, sarcoidosis, hypertrophic osteoarthropathy, Lyme disease, hyperlipoproteinemias (types II, IV), amyloid arthropathy, hemoglobinopathies (sickle cell disease), malignancy and paraneoplastic syndrome, Behçet's disease.

RARE DISEASES

Familial Mediterranean fever, Whipple's disease, multicentric reticulohistiocytosis, angioimmunoblastic lymphadenopathy, remitting seronegative symmetrical synovitis with pitting edema (RS3PE).

PEARL: A clinician should consider a diagnosis *other than* RA particularly in patients who have an asymmetric arthritis, migrating pattern, predominantly large-joint arthritis, distal interphalangeal (DIP) joint involvement, rash, back disease, renal disease, RF-negative status, leukopenia, hypocomplementemia, or no erosions on radiographs after many months of disease.

5. **Discuss the epidemiologic characteristics of RA.**
   - Race—worldwide, all races. Native Americans (Algonquian and Pima Indians) have higher prevalence.
   - Sex distribution—females > males 2-3:1
   - Age—women 40 to 60 years, men are older
   - Occurs in about 1% of adults in the United States. The prevalence increases with age.

6. **Describe the various ways RA can present.**
   - Typical patterns of onset (90% of patients)

   Insidious (55% to 65%): onset with arthritic symptoms of pain, swelling, and stiffness, with the number of joints increasing over weeks to months.
   Subacute (15% to 20%): similar to insidious onset but more systemic symptoms.
   Acute (10%): severe onset, some have fever.
   - Variant patterns of onset (10% of patients)

   Palindromic (episodic) pattern: usually involves one joint and resolves within a couple of days. After an asymptomatic period, a flare in the same or another joint occurs. Over time, 33% to 50% evolve into RA involving more joints persistently. Seropositive patients and those with elevated acute phase reactants are more likely to progress to RA. Antimalarial therapy decreases the frequency of attacks and progression to RA.

   Insidious onset of elderly (>65 years): present with severe pain and stiffness of limb girdle joints often with diffuse swelling of hands, wrists, and forearms. May be difficult to differentiate from polymyalgia rheumatica and RS3PE.

   Arthritis robustus: typically seen in men. Patients have bulky, proliferative synovitis causing joint erosions and deformities but the patient experiences little pain or disability.

   Rheumatoid nodulosis: patients with recurrent pain/swelling in different joints, subcutaneous nodules, and subchondral bone cysts on radiographs.

7. **Which joints are commonly affected in RA? (Box 15-2)**

   The joints most commonly involved *first* are the MCPs, PIPs, wrists, and MTPs. Larger joints generally become symptomatic after small joints. Patients may start out with only a few joints involved (oligoarticular onset) but progress to involvement of multiple joints (polyarticular) in a symmetric distribution within a few weeks to months.

   Involvement of the thoracolumbar, sacroiliac, or hand DIP joints is very rare in RA and should suggest another diagnosis, such as a seronegative spondyloarthropathy (sacroiliac joints), psoriatic arthritis (DIP joints), or osteoarthritis (lumbar spine, DIP joints) (Figure 15-1).

8. **What clinical and laboratory findings predict a patient with early undifferentiated arthritis will develop RA?**

   Some patients present with early (<3 to 6 months) undifferentiated arthritis that does not meet the criteria for RA. Over time, 33% of these patients progress to RA, 33% are eventually diagnosed with another type of inflammatory arthritis, and 33% undergo spontaneous remission. The best predictors that a patient will progress to RA are: (1) higher number of joints involved (mean ≥7 joints); (2) positive anticyclic citrullinated peptides (anti-CCP) antibodies; (3) positive RF. Older age, female sex, prolonged morning stiffness (>90 min), and an elevated C-reactive protein (CRP) also contributed to the risk of developing RA.

Box 15-2. The Most Common Joints Involved During the Course of RA			
MCP	90% to 95%	Ankle/subtalar	50% to 60%
PIP	75% to 90%	Cervical spine (esp. C1–C2)	40% to 50%
Wrist	75% to 80%	Elbow	40% to 50%
Knee	60% to 80%	Hip	20% to 40%
Shoulder	50% to 70%	Temporomandibular	10% to 30%
MTP	50% to 60%		

MCP, Metacarpophalangeal joint; *MTP*, metatarsophalangeal joint; *PIP*, proximal interphalangeal joint; *RA*, of rheumatoid arthritis.

9. What is pannus?

The synovium is the primary site for the inflammatory process in RA. The inflammatory infiltrate consists of mononuclear cells, primarily CD4+ T lymphocytes (30% to 50% of cells), as well as activated macrophages, B cells (5% of cells), plasma cells (some making RF), and dendritic cells that can lead to an organizational structure that resembles a lymph node. Notably, unlike the synovial fluid, few if any polymorphonuclear leukocytes (PMNs) are found in the synovium. The inflammatory cytokine milieu causes the synovial lining cells (macrophage-like and fibroblast-like synoviocytes) to proliferate. The inflamed synovium becomes thickened, boggy, and edematous and develops villous projections. This proliferative synovium is called **pannus**, and it is capable of invading bone and cartilage, causing destruction of the joint. One of the most important cells in the pannus contributing to cartilage destruction is the fibroblast-like synoviocyte, which has tumor-like characteristics capable of tissue invasion.

10. What are the common deformities of the hand in RA (Figure 15-2)?

Fusiform swelling—synovitis of PIP joints, causing them to appear spindle-shaped.

Boutonnière deformity—flexion of the PIP and hyperextension of the DIP joint, caused by weakening of the central slip of the extrinsic extensor tendon and a palmar displacement of the lateral bands. This deformity resembles a knuckle being pushed through a buttonhole.

Swan-neck deformity—results from contraction of the flexors (intrinsic muscles) of the MCPs, resulting in flexion contracture of the MCP joint, hyperextension of PIP, and flexion of the DIP joint.

Ulnar deviation of fingers—with subluxation of MCP joints. This results from weakening of the extensor carpi ulnaris leading to radial deviation of the wrist causing all finger tendons to pull the fingers ulnarly with power grasp.

Hitchhiker thumb—hyperextension of IP joint with flexion of MCP and exaggerated adduction of first metacarpus. Causes inability to pinch.

"Piano key" ulnar head—secondary to destruction of ulnar collateral ligament leading to a floating ulnar styloid.

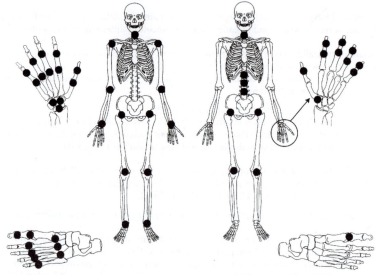

Figure 15-1. Joint distribution of rheumatoid arthritis (RA; *left*) and osteoarthritis (OA; *right*).

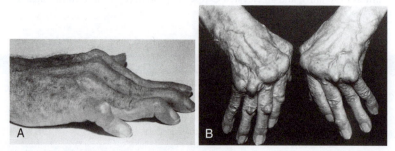

Figure 15-2. **A**, Swan neck (second to fourth fingers) and boutonnière (fifth finger) deformities. **B**, Ulnar deviation of fingers (note rheumatoid nodules). (© 2014 American College of Rheumatology. Used with permission.)

11. **Does RA affect the feet?**
    Yes, over 33% of patients develop significant foot deformities. The most common deformity is **claw toe or hammer toe**. This is caused by inflammation of the MTP joints leading to subluxation of the metatarsal heads. When this problem occurs, the patient has difficulty fitting his or her toes into the shoe because the tops of the toes rub on the shoe box, resulting in callous or ulcer formation. Additionally, because the soft tissue pad that normally sits underneath the metatarsal heads is displaced, the heads of the metatarsal bones are no longer cushioned and become very painful to walk on, frequently resulting in calluses on the inferior surface of the foot. Patients commonly complain that it feels as though they are walking on pebbles or stones. Arthritic involvement of the tarsal joint and subtalar joint can result in flattening of the arch of the foot and hindfoot valgus deformity.

12. **Describe the radiographic features of RA.**
    The mnemonic **ABCDE'S** is a convenient way to remember these:
    A—*Alignment*, abnormal; no ankylosis
    B—*Bones*—periarticular (juxta-articular) osteoporosis; no periostitis or osteophytes
    C—*Cartilage*—uniform (symmetric) joint-space loss in weight-bearing joints; no cartilage or soft tissue calcification
    D—*Deformities* (swan neck, ulnar deviation, boutonnière) with symmetrical *distribution*
    E—*Erosions*, marginal
    S—*Soft-tissue swelling*; nodules without calcification
    The radiographic changes in RA take months to develop. Juxta-articular osteopenia is seen early in the course of the disease, followed later by more diffuse osteopenia. Joint erosions typically occur at the margins of small joints. Later, joint-space narrowing and deformities develop. The earliest erosions occur in the hands (2, 3, 5 MCPs) before the feet in a third of patients; the feet (1, 5 MTPs) before the hands in a third of patients; and in both hands and feet at the same time in a third of patients. Magnetic resonance imaging (MRI) will show 40% more erosions than conventional radiography (Figure 15-3).

13. **Compare the radiographic features of RA with those of osteoarthritis (OA) (Table 15-1).**

14. **What are the typical features of the synovial fluid in RA?**
    The synovial fluid is inflammatory, with white blood cell (WBC) counts typically between 5000 and 50,000/mm³. Rarely, synovial fluid WBC count can exceed 100,000/mm³ (pseudoseptic) but infection must always be ruled out. Generally the differential shows a predominance (>50%) of PMNs. The protein level is elevated, and the glucose level may be low compared with serum values (40% to 60% of serum glucose). There are no crystals in the fluid, and cultures are negative. Unfortunately, there are no specific findings in the synovial fluid that allow a definitive diagnosis of RA.

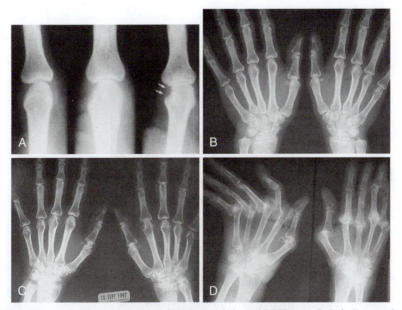

Figure 15-3. A, Progressive marginal erosions *(arrows)* of a metacarpophalangeal (MCP) joint. B, Early rheumatoid arthritis (RA) with symmetrical joint space narrowing and juxta-articular osteoporosis. C, The same patient, 5 years later, with significant marginal erosions and severe wrist involvement. D, Severe RA with destruction of MCP joints, subluxation of MCP joints *(left)* leading to ulnar deviation, and marked wrist involvement. (A, *Copyright 2014 American College of Rheumatology. Used with permission.*)

15. How is the cervical spine involved in RA?

The cervical spine is involved in 30% to 50% of RA patients, with C1–C2 the most commonly involved level. Arthritic involvement of the cervical spine can lead to instability with potential impingement of the spinal cord; thus it is important for the clinician to obtain radiographs of the cervical spine before surgical procedures requiring intubation. It is important to note that cervical spine disease parallels peripheral joint disease. The earliest and most frequent symptom of subluxation is pain radiating to the occiput. Pain, neurologic involvement, and death are the main concerns with subluxation. The patterns of cervical spine involvement include:

- **C1–C2 subluxation** (60% to 65% of patients)—the most common C1–C2 (atlantoaxial) subluxation is **anterior**, resulting in >3 mm between the arch of C1 and the odontoid of C2. This is caused by synovial proliferation around the articulation of the odontoid process with the anterior arch of C1, leading to stretching and rupture of the transverse and alar ligaments, which keep the odontoid in contact with the arch of C1. The risk of spinal cord compression is greatest when the anterior atlanto-odontoid interval is ≥9 mm or the posterior atlanto-odontoid interval is ≤14 mm. **Lateral** (rotary) and **posterior** atlantoaxial subluxations can also occur.
- **C1–C2 impaction** (20% to 25% of patients)—destruction between the occipitoatlantal and atlantoaxial joint articulations between C1 and C2, causing a cephalad movement of the odontoid into the foramen magnum, which may impinge on the brainstem. Overall, it has the worst prognosis neurologically, especially when the odontoid is ≥5 mm above Ranawat's line.
- **Subaxial involvement** (10% to 15% of patients)—involvement of typically C2–C3 and C3–C4 facets and intervertebral disks. This can lead to "stair-stepping" with one vertebrae subluxing forward on the lower vertebrae. Translation of more than 3.5 mm of one vertebra on the other is usually clinically relevant. Subaxial disease usually occurs later than other forms of cervical involvement (Figure 15-4).

Table 15-1. Radiographs in RA and OA

	RA	OA
Sclerosis	±	++++
Osteophytes	±	++++
Osteopenia	+++	0
Symmetry	+++	+
Erosions	+++	0
Cysts	++	++
Narrowing	+++	+++

OA, Osteoarthritis; RA, rheumatoid arthritis.

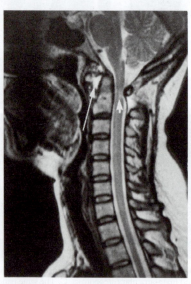

Figure 15-4. Magnetic resonance imaging (MRI) of the cervical spine demonstrating pannus formation of the C1–C2 articulation (long arrow) and impingement of the odontoid on the spinal cord (arrow).

16. **What are the typical laboratory findings in RA patients?**
    - **CBC:** anemia of chronic disease and thrombocytosis correlate with active disease. The WBC count and the differential should be normal unless the patient has Felty's syndrome or another disease.
    - **Chemistries:** normal renal, hepatic, and uric acid tests. Albumin may be low in active disease because it is a negative acute phase reactant.
    - **Urinalysis:** normal.
    - **Erythrocyte sedimentation rate (ESR):** usually elevated. Can be normal in patients with early limited disease. ESR can be elevated as a result of inflammation and hypergammaglobulinemia.
    - **CRP:** usually elevated. Better to follow disease activity than ESR because it is not influenced by hypergammaglobulinemia.
    - **Rheumatoid factor (RF):** positive in 70% to 80% with a specificity of 86% for RA. RF positivity is associated with more severe disease, with extraarticular manifestations including subcutaneous nodules, and with increased mortality. The RF titer does not correlate with disease activity so it does not have to be repeated. Note that several diseases with arthritis that can mimic RA can have a positive RF such as hepatitis C (40%), SLE (20%), Sjögren's syndrome (70%), and subacute bacterial endocarditis.
    - **Anti-CCP:** positive in 57% to 66%. It has a high specificity for RA (93% to 97%) although it has been reported in patients with psoriatic arthritis with symmetric arthritis (10%) and in patients with tuberculosis (TB). Anti-CCP is positive in 10% to 15% of seronegative (RF−) RA patients. Anti-CCP-positive RA patients have more severe and erosive disease.
    - **Antinuclear antibodies (ANA):** positive in 30%. However, they are not directed against any specific antigens (e.g., SS-A, SS-B, RNP, Sm, dsDNA). ANA-positive patients tend to have more severe disease and a poorer prognosis than RA patients who are ANA-negative. Many have secondary Sjögren's syndrome. Middle-aged women with seronegative (RF−) RA are frequently ANA-positive.
    - **ANCA:** usually negative. If it is positive, it should not have specificity against PR3 or myeloperoxidase.
    - **Complement (C3, C4, CH50):** normal or elevated. If it is low, consider a disease other than RA.

17. **List some of the extraarticular manifestations of RA.**

General	*Cardiac*
Fever	Pericarditis
Lymphadenopathy	Myocarditis
Weight loss	Coronary vasculitis
Fatigue	Nodules on valves

Dermatologic	*Neuromuscular*
Palmar erythema	Entrapment neuropathy
Subcutaneous nodules	Peripheral neuropathy
Vasculitis	Mononeuritis multiplex

Ocular	*Hematologic*
Episcleritis	Felty's syndrome
Scleritis	Large granular lymphocyte syndrome
Choroid and retinal nodules	Lymphomas

Pulmonary	*Others*
Pleuritis	Sjögren's syndrome
Nodules	Amyloidosis
Interstitial lung disease	Osteoporosis
Bronchiolitis obliterans	Atherosclerosis
Arteritis	

18. **Which patients with RA are most likely to get extraarticular manifestations?**
    Patients who are RF-positive, HLA-DR4-positive, and males are more likely to have extraarticular manifestations. It is important for clinicians to rule out other causes (infection, malignancy, medications, etc.) for an extraarticular manifestation before ascribing it to RA, *especially if the patient is RF-negative*.

19. **How commonly do fever and lymphadenopathy occur in RA patients?**
    They are uncommon and generally seen only in those patients with severely active disease. Infection and lymphoreticular malignancy should always be considered in an RA patient with these symptoms.

20. **What are rheumatoid nodules? Where are they found?**
    Rheumatoid nodules are subcutaneous nodules that have the characteristic histology of a central area of fibrinoid necrosis surrounded by a zone of palisades of elongated histiocytes and a peripheral layer of cellular

connective tissue. They occur in about 20% to 35% of RA patients, who typically are RF-positive and have severe disease. They tend to occur on the extensor surface of the forearms, in the olecranon bursa, over joints, and over pressure points such as sacrum, occiput, and heel. They frequently develop and enlarge when the patient's RA is active and may resolve when disease activity is controlled. Methotrexate therapy can rarely cause increased nodulosis in some RA patients, even when the disease is well controlled. Nodules caused by methotrexate tend to be multiple small nodules on the finger pads.

21. **Which diseases should be considered in a patient with subcutaneous nodules and arthritis?**
Rheumatoid arthritis, xanthoma, gout (tophi), SLE (rare), amyloidosis, rheumatic fever (rare), sarcoidosis, multicentric reticulohistiocytosis, leprosy.

22. **Which cutaneous disorder can cause lesions that pathologically are similar to rheumatoid nodules?**
Granuloma annulare lesions have been called "benign" rheumatoid nodules. Patients with granuloma annulare do not have arthritis and are RF-negative. These lesions are more common in childhood.

23. **What are the ocular manifestations of RA?**
Both episcleritis and scleritis can occur in less than 1% of RA patients. If scleral inflammation persists, scleral thinning and scleromalacia perforans can occur. Corneal melt is a rare but severe and blinding manifestation. Sicca symptoms of dry eyes frequently accompany coexistent Sjögren's syndrome.

24. **Discuss the pulmonary manifestations of RA.**
Pleural disease: pleurisy and pleural effusions can occasionally be the first manifestations of RA. Pleural effusions are characterized as cellular exudates with high protein and lactate dehydrogenase levels, a low glucose level (resulting from a defect in the transport of glucose across the pleura), and frequently a low pH (suggesting an infection). TB must be ruled out in patients at risk.
Nodules: rheumatoid nodules in the lung may be solitary or multiple and can cavitate or resolve spontaneously. *Caplan's syndrome* involves multiple rheumatoid nodules occurring in the lungs of RA patients who are coal miners. In patients at risk (smokers), lung cancer needs to be ruled out.
Interstitial pulmonary fibrosis (IPF): fibrosing alveolitis occurs commonly in RA patients but is symptomatic and progressive in <10%. Patients can have progressive dyspnea, Velcro rales, and fibrosis primarily in the lower lobes on chest radiography. Rapidly progressive IPF is called *Hamman-Rich syndrome*. Rarely, IPF can antedate the onset of arthritis.
Bronchiolitis obliterans (BO): also called constrictive bronchiolitis. Patients have dyspnea, hyperinflated chest x-ray, and small airway obstruction on pulmonary function tests. This condition can be rapidly fatal.
Cryptogenic organizing pneumonia (COP): also known as bronchiolitis obliterans with organizing pneumonia (BOOP). COP and **nonspecific interstitial pneumonitis (NSIP)** can occur and are more responsive to corticosteroid therapy than BO or IPF, respectively.

25. **What are the clinical consequences of the cardiac manifestations of RA?**

Pericarditis	Pain (1% of RA patients)
	Tamponade (rare)
	Constriction (uncommon)
Nodules	Conduction abnormalities
	Valvular problems
Coronary arteritis	Myocardial infarction
Myocarditis	Congestive heart failure

Pericarditis is the most common cardiac manifestation of RA and is present in up to 50% of patients at autopsy. It usually manifests as asymptomatic pericardial effusions, which may be detected by echocardiography in about 30% of patients. These effusions are rarely large enough to cause tamponade but may result in constrictive pericarditis late in the course of the disease. Constrictive pericarditis must be treated with a pericardiectomy because it is fibrous and unresponsive to immunosuppressive medications. RA may also cause nodules to form in and around the heart, leading to conduction defects and, occasionally, valvular insufficiency.

26. **Which types of vasculitis occur in RA patients?**
Vasculitis most commonly occurs in RA patients with long-standing disease, significant joint involvement, high-titer RF, and nodules. The types of vasculitis are:
- **Leukocytoclastic vasculitis**—usually presents as palpable purpura and results from inflammation of postcapillary venules.
- **Small arteriolar vasculitis**—presents as small infarcts of digital pulp/nailfolds (rarely gangrene) and frequently is associated with a mild distal sensory neuropathy caused by vasculitis of vasa nervorum.
- **Medium-vessel vasculitis**—can resemble polyarteritis nodosa with visceral arteritis, mononeuritis multiplex, and livedo reticularis.
- **Pyoderma gangrenosum**

27. **What three findings make up the classic triad of Felty's syndrome?**
Felty's syndrome is **RA** in combination with **splenomegaly** and **leukopenia**. Felty's syndrome is seen in 1% of RA patients who have RF, subcutaneous nodules, and other extraarticular manifestations. Most (95%) of patients are HLA-DR4- and RF-positive. Articular disease parallels those of RF-positive patients, but Felty's syndrome patients have more extraarticular manifestations. The leukopenia is generally a neutropenia (<2000/mm^3); thrombocytopenia may occur. The major complications of Felty's syndrome include bacterial infections (twentyfold increase compared with other RA patients) and chronic nonhealing ulcers. Severe bacterial infections correlate with the neutrophil counts of <1000/mm^3. Patients with Felty's syndrome also have a thirteenfold increased risk of developing nonHodgkin's lymphoma. Some patients develop nodular regenerative hyperplasia of the liver with portal hypertension and varices that can bleed.

Treatment is the same as for RA patients with joint disease. With control of the RA, leukopenia may improve. Granulocyte colony stimulating factor (G-CSF) has been used and shown effective at increasing WBC counts and decreasing infections in some patients (neutrophils <1000/mm^3). However, G-CSF can cause increased arthritis and vasculitis in some Felty's patients when the WBC count is raised. Splenectomy is reserved for patients with severe, recurrent bacterial infections or chronic nonhealing leg ulcers who are not responsive or tolerant to drug therapy. Unfortunately, neutropenia recurs in 25% of patients who undergo splenectomy.

28. **What other clinical problems occur with increased frequency in RA patients?**
    Atherosclerosis—RA patients develop atherosclerosis 10 years earlier compared to patients who do not have RA but have the same traditional cardiovascular risk factors.
    Sjögren's syndrome—up to 20% to 30% of RA patients develop secondary Sjögren's syndrome with dry eyes and dry mouth. They are frequently ANA-positive but typically do not have the anti-SS-A or anti-SS-B antibodies commonly seen in primary Sjögren's syndrome.
    Amyloidosis—RA patients rarely develop amyloid A (AA)-associated amyloidosis. This occurs in long-standing, poorly controlled RA and usually presents as nephrotic syndrome.
    Osteoporosis—seen in the majority of RA patients and related to disease activity, immobility, and medications. Insufficiency fractures of the spine, sacrum, and other areas are common in long-standing disease.
    Entrapment neuropathy—median nerve (carpal tunnel), posterior tibial nerve (tarsal tunnel), ulnar nerve (cubital tunnel), and posterior interosseous branch of the radial nerve are most commonly involved.
    Laryngeal manifestations—cricoarytenoid arthritis can present as pain, dysphagia, hoarseness, and, rarely, stridor.
    Ossicles of ear—tinnitus and decreased hearing.
    Renal and gastrointestinal involvement—rare. Usually abnormalities are attributable to nonsteroidal antiinflammatory drugs (NSAIDs) causing renal insufficiency or gastric ulcers with hemorrhage.
    Large granular lymphocyte (LGL) syndrome—a syndrome of neutropenia, splenomegaly, susceptibility to infections, and large granular lymphocytes bearing CD2, 3, 8, 16, and 57 surface phenotypes in the peripheral blood smear. These cells have natural killer and antibody-dependent cell-mediated cytotoxicity activity. It is now recognized that when this syndrome occurs in RA patients, it is a subset of Felty's syndrome. Approximately a third of Felty's patients have significant clonal expansions of these cells on their peripheral smear, and these patients are HLA-DR4-positive, similar to Felty's patients without LGL expansion.

29. **Are patients with RA at increased risk for joint infections?**
Unfortunately, yes. Joint infections tend to occur in abnormal joints, and RA patients have lots of these. Patients are also at increased risk secondary to immunosuppressive medication. Any time an RA patient presents with one or two joints that are swollen, red, and hot, out of proportion to the other joints, the clinician should suspect infection. In addition, following joint replacement surgeries, an infected artificial joint is a constant concern. The most common infecting organism is *Staphylococcus aureus*.

30. **Do any markers help predict if an RA patient will have severe disease and a poor prognosis?**
RF and anti-CCP positivity and poor functional status (high health assessment questionnaire [HAQ] score >1) at presentation are the best predictors of subsequent disability and joint damage. Other factors include:
    1. Generalized polyarthritis involving both small and large joints (>13 to 20 total joints)
    2. Extraarticular disease, especially nodules and vasculitis
    3. Persistently elevated ESR or CRP
    4. ANA positivity (if also RF-positive)
    5. Radiographic erosions within 2 years of disease onset
    6. HLA-DR4 genetic marker
    7. Education level <11th grade (frequently have a manual labor job contributing to joint damage)

31. **What are the most important goals for treatment of RA?**
    - Begin treatment early: the best results are seen when RA patients are started on therapy within 3 to 6 months of synovitis onset.
    - Treat to a target of low disease activity or remission.

32. What instruments are used to measure RA disease activity?

There are several validated instruments that can be used to measure disease activity. Each uses various combinations of tender and swollen joint count (TJC, SJC), patient global assessment of disease (PtGA), physician global assessment of disease (PhGA), patient pain, CRP or ESR, and the multidimensional health assessment questionnaire (MDHAQ). The most important thing is that disease activity is measured; the type of instrument used is of less importance. The instruments commonly used are shown in Table 15-2.

Disease activity score in 28 joints (DAS28): calculate using the DAS calculator (www.das-score.nl).
Components: TJC, SJC, ESR, PtGA.
Simplified disease activity index (SDAI): TJC (0-28) + SJC (0-28) + PtGA (0-10) + PhGA (0-10) + CRP (mg/dL)
Clinical disease activity index (CDAI): TJC (0-28) + SJC (0-28) + PtGA (0-10) + PhGA (0-10)
Routine assessment of patient index data (RAPID3): MDHAQ (0-10) + patient pain (0-10) + PtGA (0-10)

33. Discuss the management principles for the initial treatment of RA.

Current strategies include early aggressive treatment with one or more disease-modifying antirheumatic drugs (DMARDs; see Chapter 83 and 84) and/or biologic agents (see Chapter 85) in addition to symptomatic therapy with NSAIDs, low-dose prednisone, physical therapy (see Chapter 88), occupational therapy, rest, and patient education. Methotrexate has been the most effective antirheumatic drug used and can induce low disease activity as monotherapy in about 30% of patients. Therapy should be advanced in patients who fail to respond to an adequate dose (15 to 25 mg/wk) of methotrexate. This can be the addition of synthetic DMARDs to methotrexate referred to as triple therapy (methotrexate, sulfasalazine, hydroxychloroquine). Patients intolerant to methotrexate may have leflunomide or, less commonly, azathioprine substituted. Patients who are compliant with triple therapy achieve low disease activity in 40% to 50% of patients without an increase in toxicity.

Patients who fail to respond to triple therapy within 6 months and/or RA patients with poor prognostic signs (see question #31) should receive a biologic agent (tumor necrosis factor [TNF] inhibitors abatacept, tocilizumab, or tofacitinib) usually in combination with methotrexate. Tocilizumab and tofacitinib can each be used as monotherapy or in combination with methotrexate. Patients on their first biologic agent can achieve low disease activity in 40% to 50% of cases. RA patients who fail to respond to an initial biologic agent should be switched to another biologic agent with a different mode of action. Patients who fail their first TNF inhibitor can try one alternative TNF inhibitor but if unsuccessful should not be tried on additional TNF antagonists. Rituximab is typically reserved for seropositive RA patients who have failed one or more biologic agents including at least one TNF inhibitor.

Special attention should be given to preventative therapy including immunizations (flu, pneumovax), cardiovascular disease (smoking, HBP, lipids), and osteoporosis (calcium, vitamin D, antiresorptives).

34. What is the long-term prognosis for RA patients?

RA is clearly a disease that shortens survival and produces significant disability. Over 33% of RA patients who were working at the time of onset of their disease will leave the workforce within 5 years. In addition, the standardized mortality ratio is 2:1 to 2.5:1 compared with people of the same sex and age without RA. Overall, RA shortens the lifespan of patients by 5 to 10 years. Aggressive DMARD/biologic therapy appears to reduce disability (30%), joint replacement surgery (50%), and mortality. However, it will take another 10 to 20 years to define the full extent that an aggressive "treat to a target" strategy benefits RA patients. A few patients who are treated very early (<3 months) and aggressively (methotrexate with or without a biologic) and enter disease remission may be able to have therapy decreased or withdrawn. This is more likely if they are seronegative.

35. What causes the increased mortality in RA patients?

- **Cardiovascular**—42%. Frequency is increased twofold over the general population.
- **Infections** (especially pneumonias)—9%. Increased fivefold over the general population.

Table 15-2. Classification of Disease Activity

INSTRUMENT (SCORE RANGE)	REMISSION	LOW DISEASE ACTIVITY	MODERATE DISEASE ACTIVITY	SEVERE DISEASE ACTIVITY
DAS28 (0-9.4)	≤2.6	≤2.6	>3.2 to ≤5.1	>5.1
SDAI (0-86)	≤3.3	≤11	>11 to ≤26	>26
CDAI (0-76)	≤2.8	≤10	>10 to ≤22	>22
RAPID3 (0-30)	≤1	<6	≥6 to ≤12	>12

CDAI, Clinical disease activity index; *DAS28*, disease activity score in 28 joints; *RAPID3*, routine assessment of patient index data; *SDAI*, simplified disease activity index.

- **Cancer and lymphoproliferative malignancies**—14%. Lymphoma and leukemia are increased two to three times the rate of the general population. Lung cancer is increased 1.5 to 3.5 times the general population. Melanoma may be increased. Other solid tumors are not increased in RA.
- **Others**—including renal disease as a result of amyloidosis, gastrointestinal hemorrhage resulting from NSAIDs (4%), and RA complications (5%). With the treatments available today, fewer deaths are attributable to RA complications such as vasculitis, atlanto-axial subluxation, rheumatoid involvement of lungs and heart, and medication toxicities.

36. What is "seronegative" RA?
It is a term to identify patients who are thought to have RA but are RF-negative and anti-CCP-negative. Although called "seronegative," some of these patients have a positive ANA (without antibodies against any specific antigen) whereas other patients may have antibodies against mutated citrullinated vimentin (anti-MCV). In general, RA patients who are seronegative have a better prognosis, fewer extraarticular manifestations, and better survival. Additionally, a number of these patients over time will, in fact, be found to have some other disease. Thus, when dealing with seronegative RA patients, the clinician should always look for the possibility of psoriatic arthritis, lupus arthritis, calcium pyrophosphate crystal deposition disease, gout, hemochromatosis, or another form of arthritis other than RA.

37. What is the RS3PE syndrome?
A syndrome characterized by the acute severe onset of symmetrical synovitis of the small joints of the hands, wrists, and flexor tendon sheaths accompanied by pitting edema of the dorsum of the hand ("boxing-glove" hand). Other joints may be involved. This syndrome affects mostly elderly (mean age 70 years) white men (M/F ratio 4:1). All patients are RF-negative. Symptoms do not respond to NSAIDs but are very sensitive to low-dose prednisone and hydroxychloroquine. Bony erosions do not occur. The disease predictably remits in <36 months and, unlike RA, does not recur after withdrawal of medications. Severe hand pitting edema has also been reported in polymyalgia rheumatica and as a paraneoplastic syndrome.

Acknowledgments
The authors would like to thank Dr. Jennifer Elliott and Dr. Annemarie Whiddon for their contributions to the previous editions of this chapter.

Bibliography

Anderson JK, Caplan L, Yazdany J, et al: Rheumatoid arthritis disease activity measures: American College of Rheumatology recommendations for use in clinical practice, Arthritis Care Res (Hoboken) 64:640–647, 2012.

Arend WP, Firestein GS: Pre-rheumatoid arthritis: predisposition and transition to clinical synovitis, Nat Rev Rheumatol 8:573–586, 2012.

Breeveld FC, Weisman MH, Kavanaugh AF, et al: A multicenter, randomized, double-blind clinical trial of combination therapy with adalimumab plus methotrexate versus methotrexate alone or adalimumab alone in patients with early, aggressive rheumatoid arthritis who had not had previous methotrexate treatment, Arthritis Rheum 54:26–37, 2006.

Cohen S, Emery P, Greenwald M, et al: Rituximab for rheumatoid arthritis refractory to anti-tumor necrosis factor therapy, Arthritis Rheum 54:2793–2806, 2006.

Emery P, Keystone E, Tony HP, et al: IL-6 receptor inhibition with tocilizumab improves treatment outcomes in patients with rheumatoid arthritis refractory to anti-tumor necrosis factor biologicals: results from a 24 week multicenter randomized placebo-controlled trials, Ann Rheum Dis 67:1516–1523, 2008.

Erickson AR, Mikuls TR: Switching anti-TNF-alpha agents: what is the evidence? Curr Rheumatol Rep 9:416–420, 2007.

Friedwald VE, Ganz P, Kremer JM, et al: Rheumatoid arthritis and atherosclerotic cardiovascular disease, Am J Cardiol 106:442–447, 2010.

Genovese MC, Becker JC, Schiff M, et al: Abatacept for rheumatoid arthritis refractory to tumor necrosis factor alpha inhibition, N Engl J Med 15:1114–1123, 2005.

Grigor C, Capell H, Stirling A, et al: Effect of a treatment strategy of tight control for rheumatoid arthritis (the TICORA study): a single-blind randomized controlled trial, Lancet 364:263–269, 2004.

Kirwan JR: The effect of glucocorticoids on joint destruction in rheumatoid arthritis, N Engl J Med 333:142–146, 1995.

Klarenbeek N, et al: The impact of four dynamic, gold-steered treatment strategies on the 5-year outcomes of rheumatoid arthritis patients in the BeSt study, Ann Rheum Dis 70:1039–1046, 2011.

Landewé RBM, Boers M, Verhoeven AC, et al: COBRA combination therapy in patients with early rheumatoid arthritis: long-term structural benefits of a brief intervention, Arthritis Rheum 46:347–356, 2002.

McCarty DJ, O'Duffy JD, Pearson L, et al: Remitting seronegative symmetrical synovitis with pitting edema (RS3PE) syndrome, JAMA 254:2763–2767, 1985.

McInnes IB, O'Dell JR: State-of-the-art: rheumatoid arthritis, Ann Rheum Dis 69:1898–1906, 2010.

Moreland L, O'Dell J, Paulus HE, et al: A randomized comparative effectiveness study of oral triple therapy versus etanercept plus methotrexate in early aggressive rheumatoid arthritis, Arthritis Rheum 64:2824–2835, 2012.

Nannin C, Ryu JH, Matteson EL: Lung disease in rheumatoid arthritis, Curr Opin Rheumatol 20:340–346, 2008.

O'Dell J, Haire C, Erikson N, et al: Treatment of rheumatoid arthritis with methotrexate alone, sulfasalazine and hydroxychloroquine, or a combination of all three medications, N Engl J Med 334:1287–1291, 1996.

Scott DL: Prognostic factors in early rheumatoid arthritis, Rheum 39(suppl):24–29, 2000.

Singh JA, Furst DE, Bharat A, et al: 2012 update of the 2008 American College of Rheumatology recommendations for the use of disease-modifying antirheumatic drugs and biologic agents in the treatment of rheumatoid arthritis, Arthritis Care Res (Hoboken) 64:625–639, 2012.

Van der Heijde D, Klareskog L, Rodriguez-Valverde V, et al: Comparison of etanercept and methotrexate, alone and combined, in the treatment of rheumatoid arthritis: two-year clinical and radiographic results from the TEMPO study, a double-blind, randomized trial, Arthritis Rheum 54:1063–1074, 2006.

van Dongen H, van Aken J, Lard LR, et al: Efficacy of methotrexate treatment in patients with probable rheumatoid arthritis: a double-blind, randomized, placebo-controlled trial, Arthritis Rheum 56:1424–1432, 2007.

Van Vollenhoven RF, Geborek P, et al: Conventional combination treatment versus biological treatment in methotrexate refractory early rheumatoid arthritis; 2 year follow-up of the randomized, non-blinded, parallel-group Swefot trial, Lancet 379:1712–1720, 2012.

Whiting PF, Smidt N, Sterne JAC, et al: Systemic review: accuracy of anti-citrullinated peptide antibodies for diagnosing rheumatoid arthritis, Ann Int Med 152:456–464, 2010.

Wolfe F, Michaud K: The loss of health status in rheumatoid arthritis and the effect of biologic-therapy: a longitudinal study, Arthritis Res Ther 12:R35, 2010.

Further Reading

www.rheumatology.org
www.arthritis.org

SYSTEMIC LUPUS ERYTHEMATOSUS

Jennifer Stichman, MD and JoAnn Zell, MD

CHAPTER 16

KEY POINTS

1. Lupus is a chronic autoimmune disease characterized by the production of autoantibodies, which deposit within tissues and fix complement leading to systemic inflammation.
2. Lupus typically affects women of childbearing age and is also more common in certain ethnic minority groups such as African Americans, Asians, and Hispanics.
3. Lupus is a heterogeneous disease with a continuum of disease activity. For example, some patients can have predominant skin and joint involvement, whereas others can present with organ-threatening diseases such as nephritis or diffuse alveolar hemorrhage.

1. **Who is the typical patient with systemic lupus erythematosus?**
   The typical patient is a female between the ages of 15 and 45 years suggesting that sex hormones influence the probability of developing or expressing systemic lupus erythematosus (SLE), a conclusion that is supported by studies in animal models of lupus. The prevalence is three to four times higher in non-Caucasian individuals (African American, Asian, Hispanic) (Table 16-1).

2. **Describe the new Systemic Lupus International Collaborating Clinics criteria used in the classification of SLE.**
   The criteria listed below are proposed to replace the American College of Rheumatology (ACR) classification criteria for SLE. Any person who satisfies four or more of the following clinical and immunological criteria including at least one clinical criterion and one immunological criterion, OR any person who has biopsy-proven lupus nephritis in the presence of antinuclear antibodies (ANAs) or anti-double-stranded (ds) DNA antibodies is considered to have SLE for the purposes of clinical studies (97% sensitivity and 84% specificity) (Table 16-2).

3. **How do the criteria for the classification of SLE relate to making a diagnosis of SLE?**
   Although these criteria are extremely helpful when considering the diagnosis of SLE for an individual patient, it should be emphasized that these criteria were designed for research purposes and not diagnosis. In particular for mild cases and patients with early disease, the classification criteria may not be sensitive enough to make the diagnosis. For example, a patient with a classic malar rash and a high titer positive ANA may in fact be developing SLE and yet would not satisfy the classification criteria. Similarly, a patient with glomerulonephritis, elevated anti-DNA antibodies, and a positive ANA almost certainly has SLE but would only have three criteria listed above.

4. **What is the evidence that heredity is important in the development of SLE?**
   The best evidence that SLE is genetically determined is from studies of familial aggregation (i.e., an increased frequency of persons with SLE in the same family). For example, an identical twin of a patient with SLE has a 25% to 50% chance of developing the disease, but this risk is 10 times less if the affected twin was nonidentical (risk ~2% to 5%). Still, this latter risk is much greater than that in the general population (~1 in 1000 for white females). First degree relatives with a family history of SLE have a 6-fold higher risk of developing SLE and a 4-fold higher risk of developing a non-SLE autoimmune disease (20% to 25%) or have a positive ANA (30%). Population-based studies have shown that susceptibility to SLE, similar to other autoimmune diseases in humans, is linked to particular class II genes of the major histocompatibility complex (HLA) in humans (HLA-DR2 and HLA-DR3 increase relative risk 2 to 3 times), which may allow more efficient presentation of self-antigens to self-reactive T and B cells. In addition, early complement component (C1q, C2, C4) deficiencies increase the risk 5 to 10 times, presumably owing to altered clearance of apoptotic debris allowing accumulation of more self-antigen for induction of self-reactive T cells as well as more type I interferon (IFN)-α production. However, unlike the

Table 16-1. Demographics of SLE by Age of Onset			
AGE OF ONSET	<16 years	16 to 55 years	>55 years
% OF SLE DIAGNOSES	20%	65%	15%
FEMALE/MALE RATIO	8:1	10 to 15:1	3:1

Table 16-2. Systemic Lupus International Collaborating Clinics Classification Criteria for SLE (2012)

CRITERION	DEFINITION*	FREQUENCY†
Clinical Criteria		
1. ACLE	Malar rash, bullous lupus, TEN variant, maculopapular, photosensitive, subacute cutaneous lupus	60% to 70%
2. CCLE	Classic discoid, hypertrophic, lupus panniculitis/profundus, mucosal, lupus erythematosus tumidus, chilblains lupus, discoid/lichen panus overlap	15% to 30%
3. Alopecia	Nonscarring, diffuse hair thinning or visible broken hairs	30% to 50%
4. Oral ulcers	Oral (palate, buccal, tongue) or nasal ulceration	15% to 45%
5. Synovitis	Arthritis involving two or more peripheral joints, characterized by tenderness, swelling, or effusion and morning stiffness >30 min	90%
6. Serositis	Pleuritis: convincing history of pleuritic pain for >1 day or pleural rub or evidence of pleural effusion, orPericarditis documented by ECG or rub or evidence of pericardial effusion	30% to 60% 10% to 40%
7. Renal disorder	Persistent proteinuria ≥0.5 g/day (24 h urine or urine protein/Cr ratio) Or Red blood cell casts	40% to 60%
8. Neurological disorder	Seizures, psychosis, myelitis, mononeuritis multiplex, peripheral or cranial neuropathy, acute confusional state	15% to 20%
9. Hemolytic anemia	Direct Coombs positive	5% to 10%
10. Leukopenia	Leukopenia <4000 mm^3 at least once, or Lymphopenia <1000/mm^3 at least once	15% to 20% 15% to 20%
11. Thrombocytopenia	Platelets <100,000/mm^3	15% to 20%
Immunological Criteria		
1. ANA	Level above laboratory reference range	98%
2. Anti-dsDNA	Level above laboratory reference range (or >2-fold ELISA reference range)	60% to 70%
3. Anti-Sm	Presence of antibody to Sm nuclear antigen	20% to 30%
4. Antiphospholipid antibody positivity as determined by any of the following: - Positive test for lupus anticoagulant - False positive test result for rapid plasma regain - Medium-titer or high-titer anticardiolipin antibody level (IgG, IgM, or IgA) - Positive test result for anti-β-glycoprotein I (IgG, IgM, or IgA)		30% to 50%
5. Low complement	Low C3, low C4, or low CH_{50}	55% to 60%
6. Direct Coombs test	In the absence of hemolytic anemia	10% to 30%

ACLE, Acute cutaneous lupus erythematosus; CCLE, chronic cutaneous lupus erythematosus; ds, double-stranded.
*Other causes for clinical and immunological manifestations must be ruled out before attributing them to SLE.
†Frequency, chance of occurrence at any time during the patient's illness.

large genetic risk conferred by certain HLA alleles and complement deficiencies, genome-wide association studies have identified a number of other genetic risk loci, each of which confers a modest risk (odds ratio < 2×) and may differ between racial groups. These risk alleles are involved in functional immune pathways linked to SLE:
- Aberrant clearance of nucleic acid-containing cellular debris and immune complexes: C-reactive protein (CRP), Fc γ receptors IIa, IIIa, ITGAM, complement deficiencies (C1q, C2, C4).
- Excessive innate immune activation involving Toll-like receptors and type I IFNs: IRF5, IRF7, TNFAIP3, TREX1.
- Abnormal T and B cell activation: STAT4, PTPN22, PCDCD1, BLK, BANK1, multiple others.

In summary, SLE is polygenetic which helps explain its varied disease manifestations. The genetic risk loci vary between patients with different clinical and serological manifestations and may differ between ethnic groups.

5. What is the laboratory hallmark of SLE?

ANA. Greater than 98% of patients with SLE demonstrate elevated serum levels of ANA, which is considered to be the laboratory hallmark of this disease. This test, however, is not specific for SLE and only a small percentage (5%) of people with a positive ANA will actually develop SLE. However, an ANA positive patient who has only one of the autoimmune manifestations associated with SLE (discoid, idiopathic thrombocytopenic purpura [ITP], anti-dsDNA, etc.), the percentage who develop SLE is over 80%. Alternatively, a patient who is ANA negative is unlikely to have or develop SLE.

6. How is a screening test for ANA usually performed in a clinical laboratory?

An **indirect immunofluorescence test** is the most widely accepted and studied assay used to detect ANA. The patient's serum is diluted and then layered onto a slide on which either tissue or cells (HEp2 most commonly) have been fixed. After any unbound antibodies are washed off, a fluorescein-tagged antibody reagent directed to human immunoglobulin is added as a secondary reagent. Any antibodies (from the patient) bound to the nucleus will be stained, and the nucleus will fluoresce when viewed under a fluorescence microscope. The results are registered as positive or negative and the strength of a positive reaction at a particular serum dilution. In many laboratories, the highest dilution of serum giving a positive reaction is commonly recorded as the test result. Serum dilutions begin at approximately 1:40. A dilution of at least 1:160 is required to consider a test significantly positive because >10% of the population can have a low titer ANA. Some laboratories perform ANAs using the less accurate ELISA method of testing.

The laboratory also reports a pattern of nuclear staining (rim, diffuse, speckled, or nucleolar). The peripheral or rim pattern (corresponding to autoantibodies to deoxynucleoproteins) is the most specific pattern for SLE, whereas a speckled pattern, which is the most common pattern in both SLE and other diseases, is the least specific. A nucleolar pattern should raise suspicion for scleroderma. Patterns currently have less significance because a positive test is usually followed with an ANA profile, which tests for specific types of autoantibodies including those highly specific for SLE (Figure 16-1).

7. Which ANAs are most specific for the diagnosis of SLE?

The screening ANA test is fairly nonspecific in that patients with other rheumatic diseases (Sjögren's syndrome, mixed connective tissue disease, scleroderma, rheumatoid arthritis, polymyositis), other types of

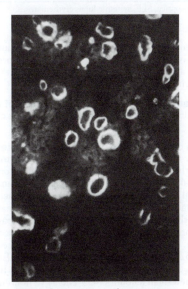

Figure 16-1. Indirect immunofluorescence test demonstrating a positive rim pattern.

Table 16-3. Autoantibodies in SLE and Some of Their Clinical Associations

TARGET	CLINICAL ASSOCIATIONS	FREQUENCY
dsDNA	High diagnostic specificity for SLE Correlation with disease activity (especially activity of lupus nephritis)	50% to 70%
Histones (H1, H2A, H2B, H3, H4)	SLE and drug-induced lupus	70% to 100%
Sm (SnRNP* core proteins B, B', D, E)	High diagnostic specificity for SLE No correlation with disease activity	20% to 30%
U1-RNP* (SnRNP specific proteins A, C, 70-kDa)	Mixed connective tissue disease/related overlap syndrome (when not accompanied by anti-Sm antibodies)	30% to 35%
Ro/SS-A (60-kDa and 52-kDa proteins)	Neonatal lupus (especially if anti-52-kDa) Photosensitivity, Sjögren's syndrome Subacute cutaneous lupus NMO spectrum disorder (myelitis, optic neuritis)	30%
La/SS-B (48-kDa protein)	Neonatal lupus (with anti-SS-A/Ro) Sjögren's syndrome Associated with anti-SS-A/Ro	15%
Ribosomal P proteins	High diagnostic specificity for SLE Cytoplasmic staining Psychiatric disease	15%
Phospholipids (β2-glycoprotein 1)	Inhibition of in vitro coagulation tests (lupus anticoagulant) Thrombosis Recurrent abortions/fetal wasting Neurological disease (focal presentations) Thrombocytopenia	30% to 50%
Cell Surface Antigens		
Red blood cells	Hemolytic anemia	5% to 10%
Platelets	Thrombocytopenia	10% to 30%
Lymphocytes	Lymphopenia	20% to 80%
Neuronal cells	Neurological disease (diffuse presentations)	30% to 80%

ds, Double-stranded; *NMO*, neuromyelitis optica; *SLE*, systemic lupus erythematosus.
*Ribonucleoprotein.

inflammatory disorders (autoimmune hepatitis, hepatitis C, lymphoma, autoimmune thyroid), or on certain drugs (hydralazine, etc.) may also be positive. Certain ANAs are more specific for the diagnosis of SLE, especially antibodies to dsDNA and to the Sm antigen. The higher the levels of antibodies to these nuclear antigens, the greater the specificity for SLE.

8. **List the most common autoantibodies found in SLE and some of their major clinical associations.**
   The most common autoantibodies found in SLE and some of their major clinical associations are listed in Table 16-3.

9. **Describe five different types of mucocutaneous lesions associated with SLE.**
   1. **Malar or butterfly rash.** The malar rash typifies one of the acute photosensitive rashes in SLE and indicates that the patient has active systemic disease. The rash extends from the cheeks over the bridge of the nose and spares the nasolabial folds. It can be flat but is usually erythematous and raised with papules and/or plaques. These lesions heal without scarring. Other causes of red face must be excluded, including rosacea, seborrhea, contact dermatitis, atopic dermatitis, and actinic dermatitis.
   2. **Acute cutaneous lupus erythematosus.** Many of the acute maculopapular rashes in SLE are related to photosensitivity and therefore are more likely to occur in sun-exposed areas. These rashes have similar characteristics to malar rash, including healing without scarring. Occasionally the rash can blister. UV-B (290 to 320 nm) > UV-A (320 to 400 nm) light is a problem for SLE patients. Sunscreens block UV-B and short-wave UV-A light. Only clothing blocks long-wave UV-A light. Glass blocks UV-B but not UV-A. Florescent lights emit a small amount of UV energy (8 hours of exposure to fluorescent lights is equal to 1 minute of sunlight exposure during summer). Other causes of photosensitivity include polymorphous

light eruption and phototoxic medications (nonsteroidal antiinflammatory drugs [NSAIDs], hydrochlorthiazide, etc.).
3. **Subacute cutaneous lupus erythematosus (SCLE).** These raised erythematous lesions occur in 10% of SLE patients, are commonly related to sun exposure, and are frequently associated with antibodies to Ro/SS-A. A rash occurs on the chest, back, and outer arms but tends to spare midfacial areas. The lesions are symmetric, nonfixed, and can be annular or serpiginous or psoriaform with central areas of scaling. These lesions usually heal without scarring but can leave areas of depigmentation, which can be especially prominent in dark-skinned individuals. May have negative lupus band test on biopsy. This rash can resemble tinea corporis, which can be excluded by a scraping by a dermatologist. It often responds well to hydroxycholorquine. There are several medications associated with triggering SCLE, most commonly hydrochlorothiazide, angiotensin-converting enzyme (ACE) inhibitors, calcium channel blockers, leflunomide, etanercept, and terbenafine.
4. **Discoid lupus erythematosus (DLE).** These lesions may begin as erythematous papules or plaques and evolve into larger, coin-shaped (discoid), chronic lesions with central areas of epithelial thinning and atrophy and with follicular plugging and damage. Lesions can expand with active erythematous inflammation at the periphery, leaving depressed central scarring, depigmentation, and patches of alopecia. Discoid lesions frequently leave scars after healing. The most affected skin areas include the face (85%), scalp (50%), ears (50%), neck, and extensor surfaces of the arms. Approximately 15% to 30% of patients with SLE demonstrate discoid disease at some time in their disease course. On biopsy, discoid lesions typically have inflammation around skin appendages (hair follicles, etc.) and vacuolization at the dermal–epidermal junction (*interface dermatitis*). On direct immunofluorescence, reactants (IgG, IgM, C3 > IgA, fibrin) can be seen at the dermal–epidermal junction (*lupus band test*).
   - There are many patients who only have discoid lupus lesions without other manifestations of SLE. Only 10% of patients with DLE who are ANA negative will later develop SLE, whereas over 80% who are ANA positive will eventually develop lupus within an average of 5 years. Other markers that predict progression to SLE are lesions above and below the waist and cytopenias.
5. **Oral/nasal ulcerations.** These lesions are typically seen on the hard palate or lower nasal septum and may be painless. One usually sees denudation of the epithelial area. This manifestation can represent an active systemic disease. Lesions on the lips or vermillion border that are painful should raise the question of herpes simplex. Other causes of oral ulcers include benign aphthous ulcers and fungal infection.

Less common rashes include bullous lesions, palpable purpura secondary to small vessel vasculitis, urticaria that may also be related to small vessel vasculitis due to antibodies against C1q, lobular panniculitis with subcutaneous nodules (lupus profundus), and livedo reticularis frequently associated with antiphospholipid antibodies (Figure 16-2).

10. Which type of hand rash strongly suggests the diagnosis of SLE?
The hand rash shown in Figure 16-3, A is almost pathognomonic for SLE. There are erythematous lesions over the dorsum of the hands and fingers, affecting the skin *between* the joints. In contrast, Figure 16-3, B shows lesions *over* the metacarpophalangeal (MCP) and proximal interphalangeal (PIP) joints, and this rash (Gottron's papules) is characteristic of dermatomyositis.

11. Name three causes of alopecia in the setting of SLE.
1. Active systemic disease can result in diffuse alopecia (telogen effluvium), which is reversible once disease activity is controlled.
2. Discoid disease results in patchy hair loss corresponding to the distribution of discoid skin lesions. This hair loss is permanent because the hair follicles are damaged by inflammation. Treatment includes intralesional steroids, hydroxycholorquine, or topical tacrolimus.
3. Drugs such as cyclophosphamide can result in diffuse hair loss, which is reversible after therapy is discontinued and disease activity decreases.

12. What therapies are recommended for skin lesions occurring in SLE patients?

GENERAL
- Avoid sun: clothing, UV-A and UV-B sunscreens (SPF 30 or equivalent <u>without</u> paraaminobenzoic acid), avoid the hot part of the day with most UV-B light (10 AM-4 PM), camouflage cosmetics.
- Smoking cessation, which can improve antimalarial efficacy.
- Avoid skin trauma: tattoos, skin piercing.
- Thiazides, NSAIDs, and sulfa-containing drugs may exacerbate skin disease.

ROUTINE THERAPY
- Topical steroids, intralesional steroids (for DLE).
  - Facial lesions: low to medium potency nonfluorinated (hydrocortisone, desonide).
  - Trunk/arm lesions: medium potency fluorinated (betamethasone valerate, triamcinolone acetonide).
  - Hypertrophic lesions: high potency fluorinated (betamethasone diproprionate, clobetasol). Only use 2 weeks.

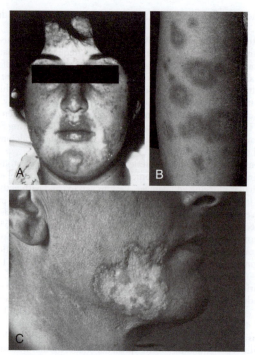

Figure 16-2. Rashes associated with SLE. **A**, Malar rash. **B**, Subacute cutaneous. **C**, Discoid. (**A**, Copyright 2014 American College of Rheumatology. Used with permission.) (**B**, Fitzpatrick J, Morelli J: Dermatology secrets plus, ed 4, Philadelphia, 2010, Elsevier Mosby, Figure 22-2, A.) (**C**, From Ferri F: Ferri's clinical advisor 2014, Philadelphia, 2013, Elsevier Mosby, Figure 1-283.)

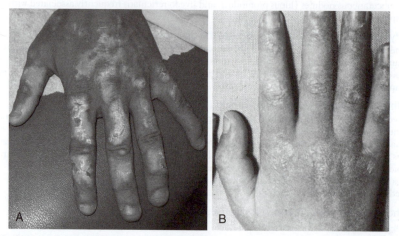

Figure 16-3. Hand rash. (**A**, Copyright 2014 American College of Rheumatology. Used with permission.) (**B**, From Firestein G, Budd R, Gabriel SE et al: Kelley's textbook of rheumatology, ed 9, Philadelphia, 2012, Elsevier Saunders, Figure 80-4.)

- Hydroxychloroquine: may take 3 months to see effect. Works best for tumid LE > SCLE > DLE.
- Oral corticosteroids.
- Dapsone: treatment of choice for bullous lesions.
- Topical tacrolimus: 0.1% cream BID for 3 weeks as an alternative to topical steroids.

ADVANCED THERAPY FOR RESISTANT CAUSES

- Subacute cutaneous lupus—mycophenolate mofetil, retinoids, or cyclosporine.
- Discoid lesions—chloroquine ± quinacrine, thalidomide, or cyclosporine. Rituximab does not work.

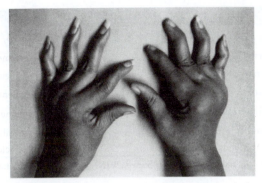

Figure 16-4. Swan-neck deformities in systemic lupus erythematosus, which are reversible.

- Lupus profundus—dapsone.
- Chronic lesions over >50% of body—tacrolimus, mycophenolate mofetil.
- Vasculitis—may need systemic immunosuppressives.
  - Hyperkeratotic lesions—oral retinoids.
  - Belimumab takes 4 to 6 months to help skin lesions.

13. You are caring for a patient with SLE who has arthritis and complains of severe joint pains. What is the likelihood that this patient will develop severe hand deformities?

The typical arthritis associated with SLE is rarely erosive or destructive of bone and therefore is very different from rheumatoid arthritis. Pain and tenderness are worse than the degree of swelling. Tenosynovitis is seen in 10% of patients. Joint deformities can occur and when present are categorized as follows:
- Nonerosive arthropathy (Jaccoud arthritis): seen in 10% to 35% of patients. MCP subluxation, ulnar deviation, and swan neck deformities are due to lax joint capsules, tendons, and ligaments. Deformities can be reversible early but later become fixed. Antibodies to mutated citrullinated vimentin, anti-dsDNA antibodies, and low complement levels are commonly seen.
- Erosive, symmetric polyarthritis (Rhupus): patients resemble *rheumatoid arthritis* with fixed deformities (Figure 16-4) associated with radiographic erosions and a positive rheumatoid factor (65%). Anti-cyclic citrullinated peptide antibodies are negative.

14. What are the best approaches for therapy in an SLE patient with arthritis who has no evidence of internal organ involvement?

The first line of therapy is NSAIDs. Cyclooxygenase-2 (Cox-2) specific inhibitors may be used but may also contribute to thrombotic risk in patients with antiphospholipid antibodies. Celecoxib is sulfa based and may lead to rashes. Antimalarial drugs, usually given in the form of low doses of daily oral hydroxychloroquine (200 mg twice a day, 6.5 mg/kg of ideal body weight per day), can also provide remarkable benefits including decreased risk of flares and decreased risk of developing end-organ damage.

15. Identify six manifestations of lupus that warrant high-dose corticosteroid therapy.

The most common problems that warrant this therapy include:
1. Severe lupus nephritis.
2. Central nervous system (CNS) lupus with severe manifestations (including transverse myelitis).
3. Autoimmune thrombocytopenia with extremely low platelet counts (e.g., <30,000/mm^3).
4. Autoimmune hemolytic anemia.
5. Acute pneumonitis caused by SLE.
6. Diffuse alveolar hemorrhage.

Additional problems that may warrant aggressive corticosteroid therapy (with doses ≥1 mg/kg/day in an adult) include severe vasculitis with visceral organ involvement, serious complications that result from serositis (pleuritis, pericarditis, or peritonitis), and the macrophage activation syndrome. It is important to emphasize that several problems in SLE should <u>not</u> be treated with high doses of corticosteroids (>60 mg/day) (i.e., lupus arthritis, skin rashes, etc.).

16. What are the indications for a renal biopsy in an SLE patient?

- Increasing serum creatinine without a compelling alternative cause (e.g., hypovolemia, medication, etc.).
- Confirmed proteinuria of ≥1 g per 24 hours.
- Proteinuria ≥0.5 g/day plus hematuria or cellular casts.

17. How do we classify renal biopsies for lupus nephritis?

There have been multiple classification schemes over the years. Originally we used the World Health Organization (WHO) classification, which was developed in 1974 and then revised in 1982, 1987, and 1995. In 2004,

Table 16-4. Pathologic Classifications Used for SLE Renal Biopsies

CLASS	ISN/RPS (2004)	WHO (1974, 1982, 1995)
I	Minimal mesangial lupus nephritis	Normal glomeruli
II	Mesangial proliferative lupus nephritis	Pure mesangial alterations
III	Focal lupus nephritis	Focal segmental glomerulonephritis
IV	Diffuse lupus nephritis (IV-S) or global lupus nephritis (IV-G)	Diffuse glomerulonephritis
V	Membranous lupus nephritis	Diffuse membranous glomerulonephritis
VI	Advanced sclerosing lupus nephritis	Advanced sclerosing glomerulonephritis

ISN/RPS, The Society of Nephrology and Renal Pathology Society; WHO, World Health Organization.

the Society of Nephrology and Renal Pathology Society (ISN/RPS) again revised the classification process. The new schema, somewhat similar to the WHO classification, separates class IV disease into segmental (IV-S) and global disease (IV-G) and adds subclassifications that designate "active" lesions (A), "chronic" lesions(C), or both (A/C) for class III and class IV lesions. The main classifications are given in Table 16-4. The characterization of the histological pattern seen on renal biopsy is used to determine the severity of disease and prognosis in a patient with lupus nephritis. Most importantly, it can be used to exclude other forms of glomerular damage such as antiphospholipid antibody syndrome in a patient with hematuria or the presence of scar (nonactive disease) in a patient with persistent proteinuria. However, it has been emphasized that knowledge of the histological type of renal disease may add little clinically useful information over and above what is already known from clinical laboratory studies (urinalysis, protein excretion, and especially renal function studies).

When interpreting histological findings in lupus nephritis, keep in mind that the renal biopsy is only a reflection of what is currently going on in the kidney and that change from one pathological class to another over time is well documented in patients with lupus nephritis and can occur in up to 40% of patients on therapy.

18. **Describe the key histological findings of the various pathological forms of lupus nephritis and their clinical implications.**

    Minimal mesangial nephritis (class I) is characterized by immune deposits in the mesangium that are best seen by immunofluorescence and electron microscopy. Biopsies are normal on light microscopy.

    Mesangial proliferative lupus nephritis (class II) is characterized by mesangial hypercellularity and mesangial immune deposits. These deposits rarely involve the peripheral capillary walls. Any sign of scar, crescents, or subendothelial deposits should suggest a higher class. Patients with mesangial nephritis usually demonstrate little clinical evidence of renal involvement, with normal or near-normal urinalysis and renal function, and rarely require any treatment for their renal disease.

    Focal proliferative glomerulonephritis (class III) is characterized by segmental lesions that involve <50% of glomeruli. Immune complex deposits are often also present in the subendothelium and mesangial space. Segmental endocapillary and mesangial hypercellularity is often seen. Patients with this pattern usually demonstrate proteinuria and hematuria, but severe (nephrotic range) proteinuria or progressive loss of renal function is less common than with diffuse disease. Focal proliferative nephritis should be viewed on a continuum with diffuse disease because the lesions are qualitatively similar but less extensive.

    Diffuse lupus nephritis (class IV) is seen in most SLE patients who progress to renal failure. Diffuse lupus nephritis is characterized by involvement of >50% of the glomeruli, with generalized hypercellularity of mesangial and endothelial cells. This class is now separated into two subclasses: either class IV-S, which describes segmental lesions in >50% of glomeruli or IV-G, which describes global glomerular lesions in >50% of glomeruli. The prognosis of class IV-S and class IV-G may differ. Inflammatory cellular infiltrates and areas of necrosis are common. These changes may ultimately lead to obliteration of the capillary loops and sclerosis. Regions of basement membrane thickening are also present. Immunofluorescence microscopy demonstrates extensive deposition with IgG, IgM, IgA, C3, and C1q (*full house pattern*) in the deposits. Electron microscopy shows immune complex deposits in both subendothelial and subepithelial distributions, although subepithelial lesions should involve less than 50% of glomeruli. The pathology report should also describe the activity and chronicity of the lesion. Clinically, patients almost always have proteinuria (frequently nephrotic), cellular casts, and hematuria and, not infrequently, decreased renal function. Hypertension is common. Hypocomplementemia and elevated anti-dsDNA antibodies are usually seen.

    Membranous lupus nephritis (class V) is characterized by the presence of granular global or segmental subepithelial immune deposits seen by immunofluorescence or electron microscopy. Subendothelial deposits should warrant a consideration for class III or class IV disease. Clinically, patients who have pure membranous disease frequently have extensive proteinuria but only minimal hematuria or renal functional abnormalities.

Table 16-5. Pathologic Features of Chronicity and Activity in Lupus Nephritis

CHRONICITY	ACTIVITY
Glomerular sclerosis	Cellular proliferation
Fibrous crescents	Fibrinoid necrosis
Fibrous adhesions	Cellular crescents
Interstitial fibrosis	Hyaline thrombi

Complement and anti-dsDNA antibody levels may be normal. Membranous disease can also be observed as a transition stage after treatment for proliferative glomerulonephritis.

Advanced sclerosing lupus nephritis (class VI) demonstrates ≥90% global glomerulosclerosis that is thought to be due to lupus nephritis. There should be no evidence of ongoing active glomerular disease.

19. **What is the importance of evaluating biopsies for the extent of activity or chronicity?**
Historically on a renal biopsy report, pathologists would provide a calculated score to represent disease activity and disease chronicity. However, more recent literature shows mixed predictive value of using such a score and these calculations are no longer universally used. However, the identification of histological changes that represent chronicity and activity are thought to be helpful in contributing to the overall description of the renal biopsy. Evidence of fibrosis indicates chronic scarring disease, which may be less likely to respond to therapy (Table 16-5).

20. **Which serological tests are most useful when following a patient with lupus nephritis?**
Only one ANA has been shown to correlate with the activity of lupus nephritis, antibodies to dsDNA. Therefore, serial monitoring should be limited to tests that specifically quantitate anti-dsDNA antibodies. In addition, patients with active lupus nephritis have decreased levels of complement components (e.g., C3 and C4) as well as total hemolytic complement (CH_{50}), which also correlate with the activity of renal disease. It should be noted that many SLE patients have partial C4 deficiency and therefore may always have a low C4 level. It should also be emphasized that many patients with high levels of anti-dsDNA antibodies and low complement levels never develop nephritis. Alternatively, glomerulonephritis can occur in an SLE patient who has normal complement levels and no elevation of anti-dsDNA antibodies (especially membranous lupus nephritis).

21. **What are the proposed mechanisms by which anti-dsDNA antibodies cause glomerulonephritis in SLE?**
Anti-dsDNA antibodies do not appear to mediate renal damage in SLE through the deposition of circulating immune complexes as once proposed. Even in patients with active glomerulonephritis or animal models with actively increasing amounts of anti-dsDNA antibodies in the glomerulus, DNA–anti-dsDNA complexes have been difficult to demonstrate in the circulation. Thus, two alternative theories have been proposed to explain the pathogenic mechanisms of these antibodies.
In the first hypothesis, DNA–anti-dsDNA complexes are proposed to form in the glomerulus (in situ complex formation) rather than being deposited from the blood. Evidence supports a model in which DNA, chromatin, or other cellular components first bind to the glomerulus and are then recognized and bound by anti-dsDNA antibodies. It is of interest that increased amounts of circulating DNA have been detected in the blood of patients with SLE. The circulating nuclear material, resembling nucleosomes, could thus become the planted renal target for a subset of pathogenic anti-dsDNA antibodies.
In an alternative model, the subset of pathogenic anti-DNA antibodies have been hypothesized to cross-react with glomerular antigens that are not DNA in origin. This model is supported by data showing that anti-dsDNA antibodies do contain other specificities and can bind to different glomerular structures.
The activation of complement components through the classical pathway, with amplification by the alternative pathway, appears to be involved in the pathogenesis of glomerular damage. Complement activation may cause direct damage as well as recruit inflammatory cells to the sites of immune complexes. Based on this scheme, IgG anti-dsDNA antibodies that are complement-fixing are likely to be more pathogenic.

22. **Which patients with severe lupus nephritis are more likely to progress to end-stage renal disease?**
Most studies show that African-American and Hispanic patients are more likely to develop end-stage renal disease (ESRD). Note that these studies treated patients primarily with cyclophosphamide before it was known that African-American and Hispanic SLE patients respond better to mycophenolate mofetil therapy than to cyclophosphamide. Other features, which have been suggested, include lower socioeconomic status, poor compliance with medications, and comorbidities such as hypertension and diabetes. Failure to normalize the serum creatinine and decrease proteinuria to <1 g/day within 6 months of starting therapy is associated with a poorer long-term renal prognosis. A serum creatinine that fails to decrease to <2 mg/dL with therapy is at increased risk of progressing to ESRD. Previous data using the WHO classification scheme found that evidence of high activity (cellular crescents) and chronicity (interstitial fibrosis) on renal biopsy correlates with a poorer prognosis.

23. What is the first line of therapy for patients with severe lupus nephritis?

- Adjunctive therapies:
  - Hydroxychloroquine.
  - ACE inhibitor or angiotensin-receptor blocker (ARB) if proteinuria ≥0.5 g per 24 hours.
  - Control blood pressure: should be ≤130/80.
  - Statin therapy if low-density lipoprotein (LDL) cholesterol >100 mg/dL.
  - Stop smoking.
  - Counsel against pregnancy while nephritis is active or creatinine >2 mg/dL.
- Induction therapy
  - Class III/class IV lupus nephritis.
  - IV pulse methylprednisolone (500 mg to 1 g) daily × 3 days followed by prednisone 1 mg/kg/day (crescents on biopsy) or 0.5 mg/kg/day (no crescents) tapered after a few weeks to lowest effective dose

  plus
  - Mycophenolate mofetil (MMF) 2 to 3 g/day for 6 months (preferred to cyclophosphamide in African-American and Hispanic patients), *or*
  - Cyclophosphamide (CYC): high dose IV (500 to 1000 mg/m^2 monthly × 6 doses) or low dose IV (500 mg every 2 weeks × 6 doses).

  Note: patients who fail to improve on MMF are switched to CYC. Patients who fail CYC are switched to MMF. Patients who fail to respond to both are candidates for rituximab or calcineurin inhibitors (cyclosporin, tacrolimus).
  - Class V lupus nephritis.
  - Oral prednisone 0.5 mg/kg/day for 6 months, *plus*
  - Mycophenolate mofetil (MMF) 2 to 3 g/day for 6 months.

  Note: patients who fail to improve on MMF are switched to high dose IV cyclophosphamide for 6 months.

24. Is there an optimal dosing regimen for cyclophosphamide (Cytoxan)?

Previously, cyclophosphamide was given as a daily oral dose or a prolonged (18 to 24 months) course of intravenous dosing. Newer data have shown that IV dosing is not inferior to oral and is associated with fewer side effects, notably bladder damage and hemorrhagic cystitis. There is also accumulating data that low-dose cyclophosphamide followed by maintenance therapy is equivalent in efficacy to higher-dose regimens. Low-dose therapy ("Euro-Lupus" protocol) is associated with fewer serious infections and less infertility but has mostly been studied in white Europeans. Studies in other nonwhite groups are ongoing. IV dosing regimens result in a lower total cyclophosphamide exposure, which is important when considering effects on fertility. Note that the risk of premature ovarian failure correlates with the cumulative dose of cyclophosphamide and the age of the patient.

The current recommended IV regimens are either:
1. High dose: monthly boluses of 0.5 to 1.0 g/m^2 IV with vigorous hydration × 6 months.
2. Low dose (Euro-Lupus protocol): 500 mg IV every 2 weeks × 6 doses.

25. Describe a protocol for using monthly IV cyclophosphamide.

There are many different protocols that can be used. The following is one example:

BEFORE CYCLOPHOSPHAMIDE

- Premedication 15 to 30 minutes before cyclophosphamide—dexamethasone 10 mg, lorazepam 1 mg, and ondansetron (Zofran) 8 mg or ganisetron (Kytril) 1 mg in 100 mL normal saline IV.
- Mesna (25% of cyclophosphamide dose in milligrams) in 250 mL normal saline.

CYCLOPHOSPHAMIDE INFUSION

- Cyclophosphamide 0.5 to 1.0 g/m^2 of body surface area in 1000 mL normal saline for initial dose. If creatinine clearance is less than 35 to 40 mL/min, then start the initial dose at 0.50 g/m^2 of body surface area. If on dialysis give 0.4 to 0.5 g/m^2 8 to 10 hours before dialysis.
- Subsequent monthly doses depend on white blood cell (WBC) counts at 10 to 14 days post-cyclophosphamide. If nadir <3000/mm^3, reduce dose by 0.25 g/m^2.
  If nadir >4000/mm^3, dose can be increased if necessary to maximum of 1 g/m^2.
- Consider the use of gonadotropin-releasing hormone (GnRH; Lupron) 3.75 mg IM 10 days before each of the monthly cyclophomide dose or testosterone supplementation for men to prevent premature gonadal failure from longstanding therapy (data are limited).

POST-CYCLOPHOSPHAMIDE INFUSION

- Mesna (25% of cyclophosphamide dose in milligrams) in 250 mL normal saline.
- Compazine SR 15 mg BID or compazine 10 mg TID for 2 to 3 days.

DOSE INTERVAL FOR CYCLOPHOSPHAMIDE

- Monthly for 6 doses, *then*
- Maintenance with azathioprine or mycophenolate mofetil.

26. **Which cytotoxic agents are most frequently used for maintenance therapy in treatment of lupus nephritis?**
   As noted above, IV cyclophosphamide in varying regimens and mycophenolate mofetil are most commonly used for induction therapy. Maintenance therapy is typically oral azathioprine (2 mg/kg/day) (or 6-mercaptopurine if nausea on azathioprine) or MMF (1 to 2 g/day). Each of these drugs are given in association with a dose of prednisone required to control extrarenal manifestations, and prednisone is tapered over time. Maintenance therapy is recommended for at least 3 years. Rituximab has also been used in maintenance therapy when patients fail or cannot tolerate MMF or azathioprine. Calcineurin inhibitors (cyclosporin, tacrolimus) have also been used for maintenance therapy and in patients with refractory disease.

27. **A 30-year-old woman with severe nephritis and end-stage renal failure is referred for further evaluation and treatment. The patient, who has been on dialysis for nearly 5 years, is being considered for transplantation but is afraid that her lupus will destroy the donor kidney. She asks for your opinion.**
   Approximately 10% to 20% of patients with severe lupus nephritis will progress over a 10-year follow-up period to ESRD. Lupus nephritis accounts for up to 1% to 2% of cases of end-stage renal failure requiring dialysis or transplantation. For unclear reasons, SLE patients with progressive renal failure and those on dialysis frequently demonstrate a decrease in nonrenal clinical manifestations of active SLE as well as a decrease in serological markers of active disease. In SLE patients with absent or minimal disease activity, the clinical course and survival (80% to 90% 5-year survival) on dialysis compare favorably with those of other patient groups. There is some evidence that transplantation before initiation of dialysis may result in improved allograft and patient survival. SLE patients appear to be excellent candidates for transplantation (a living donor is better than a cadaveric donor), and the recurrence of active lupus nephritis in the transplant is unusual (2% to 3%). Furthermore, even in patients with recurrent nephritis, it is unlikely to lead to allograft loss. Retrospective analysis has reported that lupus patients have a similar incidence of graft survival rates as compared with nonlupus patients; however, the presence of antiphospholipid antibodies may decrease the rate of allograft survival.

28. **List the manifestations of CNS involvement in SLE.**
   CNS involvement can be either diffuse or focal. Manifestations of diffuse disease include intractable headaches, generalized seizures, aseptic meningitis, acute confusional state, cognitive dysfunction, psychiatric disease (especially psychosis and severe depression), and coma. Manifestations of focal disease include stroke syndromes such as hemiparesis, focal seizures, movement disorders such as chorea, and transverse myelitis.

29. **Name five types of autoantibodies that have been associated with CNS involvement in SLE.**
    1. Serum antiphospholipid antibodies associated with focal neurological manifestations in CNS lupus.
    2. Cerebrospinal fluid antineuronal antibodies associated with diffuse manifestations of CNS lupus.
    3. Serum antibodies to ribosomal P proteins (antiribosomal P antibodies) associated with psychiatric problems (severe depression and psychosis) in SLE.
    4. N-Methyl-d-aspartate receptor (NMDAR) antibodies are a subset of dsDNA antibodies that appear to cross-react with the glutamate receptor and are associated with cognitive dysfunction in SLE.
    5. Antiaquaporin 4/neuromyelitis optica (NMO) antibodies are associated with longitudinal transverse myelitis with or without optic neuritis. Most patients have anti-SS-A/Ro antibodies and secondary Sjögren's syndrome.

30. **How does SLE cause CNS involvement?**
   CNS lupus (also referred to as *neuropsychiatric lupus erythematosus*) with **diffuse** manifestations appears to be primarily caused by autoantibodies directed to neuronal cells or their products. These autoantibodies are hypothesized to affect neuronal function in a generalized manner. Studies suggest that increased levels of inflammatory cytokines, induction of nitric oxide production, oxidative stress, and excitatory amino acid toxicity also may contribute to diffuse CNS dysfunction in SLE. Patients with acute encephalopathy frequently demonstrate elevated levels of antineuronal antibodies or other evidence of autoantibody production in the cerebrospinal fluid. As in multiple sclerosis, elevated levels of IgG (IgG index) and oligoclonal bands are markers of abnormal autoantibody production within the CNS and are frequently present in CNS lupus with diffuse manifestations. In patients with diffuse CNS lupus who present with primarily psychiatric disease, serum antiribosomal P antibodies appear to be a helpful diagnostic marker.
   CNS lupus with **focal** manifestations is most likely to be related to intravascular occlusion. Magnetic resonance imaging (MRI), which is much more sensitive than computed tomography (CT) scanning, almost always shows abnormalities characteristic of ischemic damage in these patients. Furthermore, these patients frequently demonstrate significantly elevated serum levels of antiphospholipid antibodies, which are associated with intravascular occlusion. Less commonly, evidence of vasculitis is apparent. Cardiac emboli should always be ruled out with an echocardiogram (transesophageal more sensitive than transthoracic).

31. **A 40-year-old woman with severe lupus nephritis has been treated with 60 mg of prednisone for the past 2 weeks but now seems disoriented and demonstrates bizarre behavior with delusional thinking. Describe the appropriate evaluation and treatment.**
   The differential diagnosis for the change in behavior in this patient should include CNS lupus, prednisone-induced psychosis, and a separate problem such as infection, medication effect, or metabolic disturbance.

First, the patient should be examined carefully, especially for evidence of active lupus, encephalopathy (i.e., decreased intellectual function), and any additional neurological (especially focal) deficits. Any focal neurological findings would strongly suggest that the change in behavior was not directly caused by the high doses of prednisone.

Laboratory tests should exclude the possibility of a new metabolic problem and determine the activity of nephritis and/or other organ involvement. Studies directed at the CNS should include MRI, electroencephalogram (which should be normal in steroid-induced psychosis), and lumbar puncture (for standard tests such as cell count, protein level, and culture). In a patient on high doses of steroids, the possibility of infection must be considered and excluded. In addition, analysis of the cerebrospinal fluid should include tests for increased CNS IgG production (IgG index), oligoclonal bands, and antineuronal antibodies. Serological tests should include antiribosomal P antibodies as well as studies for the systemic activity of disease (C3/C4 levels, anti-dsDNA antibodies). Note that patients with CNS lupus usually have clinical and serological evidence of active lupus.

If the evaluation is negative, the most likely cause for the change in behavior is steroid-induced psychosis, and the appropriate treatment would be to decrease the dose. In contrast, evidence for CNS lupus would warrant therapy directed at the pathogenic process. This might include increasing the dose of steroids and/or adding a cytotoxic drug.

32. In what ways can the heart be involved in SLE?

Pericarditis (40% to 50% of patients, most asymptomatic).
  Myocarditis—rare. Presents as congestive heart failure or unexplained tachycardia.
  Vasculitis (coronary).
  Secondary atherosclerotic coronary artery disease and myocardial infarction.
  Secondary hypertensive disease.
Valvular disease—possibly more frequent in patients with antiphospholipid antibodies. However, anticoagulation does not prevent valve destruction. Valvular thickening mainly of aortic and mitral valves. Libman–Sacks verrucae occur most commonly on ventricular side of posterior leaflet of mitral valve. May cause embolic stroke. Increased risk of developing subacute bacterial endocarditis (SBE).

33. In what ways can the lung be involved in SLE?

- Pleuritis—should be bilateral. CRP frequently elevated. If unilateral need to rule out infection (tuberculosis, fungal, bacterial).
- Acute lupus pneumonitis with or without pulmonary hemorrhage (2%)—associated with antiphospholipid antibodies.
- Chronic interstitial lung disease and pulmonary fibrosis (rare)—usually only in patients with previous lupus pneumonitis.
- Pulmonary hypertension— rule out secondary causes (pulmonary emboli, sleep apnea).
- Pulmonary embolism, especially in patients with antiphospholipid antibodies.
- "Shrinking lung syndrome"—decreased lung volumes without parenchymal disease. Due to diaphragmatic myopathy, phrenic neuropathy, or pleural fibrosis.
- Secondary infection—always consider in patient with "tree and bud" pattern on high-resolution CT scan. Rule out chronic aspiration.
- Bronchiolitis obliterans with organizing pneumonia: rare.

34. In what ways can the gastrointestinal tract be involved in SLE?

- Esophageal dysmotility: usually involves upper third of esophagus in patients with myositis.
- Pancreatitis: usually due to gallstones, alcohol, or hypertriglyceridemia. Can be due to medications (azathioprine). If due to lupus, the patient has a very active disease.
- Serositis: only occurs in patients with active systemic disease. Rare to get ascites. Need to rule out infection.
- Mesenteric vasculitis.
- Hepatitis: usually due to medications or other nonlupus cause. If due to lupus, patients do not have antismooth muscle or anti-liver-kidney microsome antibodies.
- Intestinal pseudoobstruction.
- Protein-losing enteropathy (PLE): consider in patients with severely low albumin but no proteinuria. Most patients have diarrhea. Diagnosis made by measuring transferrin in stool. Stool should have no transferrin unless there is a PLE.

PEARL: A gastrointestinal manifestation (serositis, vasculitis, and pancreatitis) is unlikely to be due to SLE unless the patient has evidence of active SLE in other organs and abnormal serologies.

35. The hematocrit in a patient with SLE has been dropping over the last several months to a steady level of 31%. Red blood cell indices are otherwise normal, as is the rest of the complete blood count. Recent medications have included prednisone (5 mg/day) and intermittent low doses of NSAIDs. What is the most likely cause for anemia in this patient?

The most likely cause is the so-called **anemia of chronic disease**, secondary to the persistent inflammation that occurs in SLE. The mechanisms of this type of anemia mostly relate to decreased production of red blood cells (RBCs) as well as slightly decreased RBC survival. There is an inability for iron to be handled normally by the reticuloendothelial system, and blood tests frequently disclose a low serum iron concentration as well as a low total iron-binding capacity. Ferritin is frequently elevated. Note that a ferritin level >100 ng/mL rules out iron deficiency in a patient with an active inflammatory disease.

The evaluation in this patient should rule out the possibility of an autoimmune hemolytic anemia. This should include a reticulocyte count to determine (in conjunction with a stable hematocrit) whether there is active destruction of RBCs, lactate dehydrogenase, haptoglobin, bilirubin, and test for autoantibodies to RBCs (direct Coombs test). Note, however, that many more SLE patients will have a positive Coombs test than a hemolytic anemia. The patient should also be evaluated for the possibility of gastrointestinal blood loss and iron deficiency related to the continued use of NSAIDs.

It is important to determine that the patient has the anemia of a chronic disease because it implies ongoing inflammation, prompting careful follow-up of the patient. Patients demonstrating this form of anemia are more likely to demonstrate flares of lupus activity in the near future.

36. **A patient with SLE has a low WBC count of 2500/mm^3 (70% neutrophils, 20% lymphocytes, 10% monocytes). Her prednisone has been tapered to 5 mg/day, and there are no clinical manifestations of active disease. A review of systems and physical examination are negative, except for a mild malar rash. Laboratory tests show no evidence for lupus nephritis or other internal organ involvement. How do you evaluate and treat this leukopenia?**

This degree of leukopenia, which includes both a neutropenia and lymphopenia, is not uncommon in SLE. A medication adverse effect should be excluded. Once that is done no further evaluation or treatment is necessary. It is not associated with an increased risk of infection. It does imply continued disease activity, so the patient needs to be followed carefully. Some physicians would start hydroxychloroquine in an attempt to lessen the chance for a future lupus flare.

37. **A 25-year-old woman with SLE has had difficulty with severe thrombocytopenia. Previous bone marrow biopsies showed increased numbers of megakaryocytes and no other abnormalities. Past therapy with high doses of corticosteroids has been successful in raising the platelet count to normal levels, but tapering to 20 mg/day has resulted in a progressive decline in platelet counts to <20,000/mm^3. The patient is taking no other medications, and her physical examination and other laboratory evaluation are normal. Discuss the options for therapy in this patient.**

Treatment is recommended for platelet counts <30,000/ mm^3. There are several therapeutic options to consider in this patient with autoimmune thrombocytopenia. One consideration would be **splenectomy**. If the patient had idiopathic thrombocytopenic purpura (ITP) without SLE, this would probably be recommended. However, the value of splenectomy in lupus-related thrombocytopenia has been debated, and its use is controversial. Some studies (retrospective and anecdotal) have suggested a high rate of failure in maintaining adequate platelet counts long term. Other reports (small case series) maintain that splenectomy is as valuable a long-term therapy in SLE as it is in ITP. Considering that the patient has no other severe problems from SLE and is a young woman, splenectomy would be a reasonable option.

Rituximab may be considered in patients who have failed steroids, and possible use as a first-line agent is currently under investigation. Rituximab can induce a durable response, but the rate of response at >1 year is only 18% to 35%. **Thrombopoietin receptor agonists** (romiplostim) are also considered in patients who have failed steroids; however, they are expensive ($55,000/year) and thrombocytopenia usually recurs when they are stopped. A variety of agents have been used as second-line agents. One option is the addition of an **immunosuppressive** or **cytotoxic drug** such as azathioprine (up to 2.5 mg/kg/day) or mycophenolate mofetil. This addition may decrease platelet destruction and allow the prednisone dose to be tapered. Azathioprine and mycophenolate are less toxic than cyclophosphamide and would be preferred in this setting. Cyclosporine A, vincristine, and dapsone have also been used as second-line agents. Another option is **danazol**, an androgen that increases platelet counts and allows the steroid dose to be decreased. Doses of 800 mg/day may be necessary, and the androgenic side effects in a young female may be troubling.

On a separate note, high-dose **intravenous immunoglobulin** (IVIG) 2 g/kg (400 mg/kg/day × 5 days) has been a very effective therapy to raise platelet counts acutely. This treatment can be used in preparation for splenectomy or if the patient showed signs of bleeding. Because of its cost, however, repeated treatments with IVIG are not a reasonable long-term therapeutic option. For Rh-positive nonsplenectomized patients anti-D is another possible first-line agent.

38. **A 25-year-old woman with SLE presents with fever, altered mental status, worsening renal function, hemolytic anemia, and thrombocytopenia. What is your next step?**

This patient has the five major manifestations of acute **thrombotic thrombocytopenic purpura** (TTP). Patients with SLE can develop TTP, which can be misdiagnosed as a flare of SLE. Making the correct diagnosis is essential so appropriate therapy can be instituted. The quickest way is to examine the peripheral blood smear for schistocytes, which will confirm a microangiopathic hemolytic anemia seen in TTP and rule out the Coombs positive autoimmune hemolytic anemia seen in SLE.

The etiology of TTP occurring in SLE may be similar to idiopathic TTP. Acute TTP has been found to be from an IgG autoantibody against the metalloproteinase (ADAMTS13) responsible for the cleavage of large multimers of von Willebrand factor into smaller units. This allows for the accumulation of unusually large multimers of von Willebrand factors secreted by endothelial cells into the plasma. These multimers bind to platelet glycoprotein receptors, causing platelet adhesion and microthrombi. The treatment of acute thrombotic thrombocytopenic purpura (TTP) in SLE patients includes plasmapheresis to remove the autoantibody and large multimers of von Willebrand factor, followed by fresh frozen plasma to replace the metalloproteinase. Antiplatelet agents, corticosteroids, and/or immunosuppressive drugs have been used but are not as effective as plasmapheresis and plasma replacement. Corticosteroids and immunosuppressives may be needed to prevent recurrence of TTP by suppressing autoantibody formation.

39. What is the lupus anticoagulant? What are its clinical associations?

Lupus anticoagulant refers to a subset of autoantibodies to phospholipids that interfere with certain clotting tests. It is usually picked up by an abnormally elevated partial thromboplastin time (PTT) and can be further demonstrated by specific clotting studies, such as the Russell viper venom test. Antiphospholipid antibodies can also be detected by an ELISA test for anticardiolipin and/or β2 glycoprotein I antibodies.

The term lupus anticoagulant is truly a misnomer, because the major clinical association of antiphospholipid antibodies is thrombosis (not bleeding), and these autoantibodies can occur in the absence of SLE. Patients who develop disease manifestations but do not have another autoimmune disease have the **primary antiphospholipid antibody syndrome** (see Chapter 23). Complications associated with antiphospholipid antibodies include arterial and venous thrombosis, miscarriage and fetal wastage, thrombocytopenia, livedo reticularis, and autoimmune hemolytic anemia. Antiphospholipid antibodies and their complications are a major issue in the care of patients with SLE.

40. A 25-year-old woman with severe SLE on prednisone and azathioprine complains of progressive right hip pain located in the groin for the past month. She denies fever and chills. She has good range of motion of the hip with some pain. What is your next step?

Although septic arthritis is always a concern, this presentation is worrisome for osteonecrosis of the hip (see Chapter 54). Patients with SLE are more prone to develop osteonecrosis than patients with other disease states treated with corticosteroids. Patients who become cushingoid on steroids, who have antiphospholipid antibodies, and those treated with >20 mg/day of prednisone are at increased risk. The femoral head and knee are more commonly involved than other joint areas. Evaluation should start with a radiograph followed by MRI. Both hips should be done even if only one is symptomatic, because the contralateral femoral head is involved in 50% of cases. In patients with >25% of the femoral head involved and without bony collapse, core decompression should be considered. All patients put on corticosteroids should be warned about this complication and documented in the chart, because this is a major cause of malpractice claims.

41. Discuss some of the management principles other than immunosuppression used in the treatment of SLE patients.

- Avoid possible disease triggers—sulfa-containing antibiotics, sun, high estrogen birth control pills (BCPs), alfalfa sprouts, and echinacea.
- Prevent atherosclerosis—control blood pressure (target 130/80), hyperlipidemia (target LDL cholesterol <100), stop smoking, check for and treat elevated homocysteine levels.
- Prevent osteoporosis—calcium (1000 mg), vitamin D (800 international unit), lower corticosteroid dosage, bisphosphonates if on ≥20 mg of prednisone per day for ≥3 months. Rule out low testosterone in males with SLE.
- Immunizations—human papilloma virus (HPV; patients less than 26 years old), influenza, hepatitis B (if at risk), and pneumococcal vaccines (SLE patients at risk due to functional hyposplenism and complement deficiencies). Patients on immunosuppressive agents and/or prednisone ≥20 mg/day may not mount a satisfactory immune response. Patients should not be given live attenuated vaccines (measles, mumps, rubella, polio, BCG, herpes zoster, smallpox, intranasal influenza vaccine, and yellow fever) if on prednisone >20 mg/day or immunosuppressive agents. However, patients on low-dose azathioprine (<3 mg/kg/day) or methotrexate (<0.4 mg/kg/week) can receive live attenuated vaccines. Immunization does not cause flares in SLE.
- Prevent infections—SBE prophylaxis (in patients with antiphospholipid antibodies and heart murmur), PPD or interferon gamma release assay (if starting >15 mg/day prednisone or a biologic), *Pneumocystis jirovecii* prophylaxis if on cyclophosphamide and/or glucocorticoids (prednisone >15 to 20 mg/day).
- Prevent progression of renal disease in patients with nephritis—avoid NSAIDs, control blood pressure (target 130/80), limit proteinuria (use ACE inhibitors or angiotensin receptor blockers).
- Prevent clots in patients with antiphospholipid antibodies (not on warfarin)—use of hydroxychloroquine, avoid unnecessary surgeries and vascular catheterizations, treat infections promptly, avoid Cox-2 specific inhibitors, avoid exogenous estrogen.
- Treat fatigue—rule out hypothyroidism, metabolic disturbances, myopathy, anemia, depression, and sleep apnea. Eliminate drugs that can cause fatigue. Antimalarials, modafinil, and didehydroepiandrosterone (prasterone 200 mg daily) can help fatigue.
- Cancer screens—skin, cervical, anal, breast, colon, bladder, lymphoma.

42. Can patients with SLE receive exogenous estrogens?

Because SLE is primarily a disease of premenopausal females and thought to have strong hormonal ties, there has been the concern that exogenous estrogen should be avoided as this may cause an increase in disease activity. However, patients with SLE are often females of childbearing age, and research has shown that patients with SLE should avoid pregnancy when active disease is present due to the risk of poor outcomes. Similarly, many SLE patients are treated with teratogenic medications, which are contraindicated in pregnancy. For these reasons, adequate birth control measures should be used when appropriate. In 2005 the SELENA trial showed that patients with mild to moderate SLE could be safely treated with BCPs without a significant risk of disease flare. It should be noted that in this study, patients with antiphospholipid antibodies were excluded as these patients are at significant risk for thrombosis. Patients with severe disease, especially renal impairment, were also excluded from this trial. Progesterone-containing intrauterine device (IUD) and progesterone-only BCPs are probably safe in patients with SLE, even those with antiphospholipid antibodies and do not seem to promote flare of disease. Unfortunately, prolonged use of progesterone-only therapy can lead to bone loss. (See Chapter 78 for issues related to birth control and pregnancy in SLE patients.)

Hormone replacement therapy (HRT) has also been a concern for patients with lupus. In recent years, studies have shown an increase in thrombotic events for all women taking HRT, but this has been of particular concern for patients with SLE who may have an increased baseline risk thrombosis, even without the presence of antiphospholipid antibodies. Studies show that HRT does not seem to cause significant disease flares; however, the risk of thrombosis was increased, especially for patients with antiphospholipid antibodies.

RECOMMENDATIONS

- BCPs are probably safe in patients with mild to moderate disease. Do not use in patients with antiphospholipid antibodies, a history of thrombosis, significant renal disease, or significant migraine disease. Use the lowest effective dose of estrogen.
- Selective estrogen receptor modulators (SERMs) such as raloxifene have not shown an increase in disease flare but should be avoided in patients with history of clot or significant risk factors for clot.
- Consider a progesterone implant device, progesterone-containing IUD, or progesterone-only BCPs in a patient with antiphospholipid antibodies.
- Weigh risks and benefits of HRT and do not use in patients with thrombotic risk. If needed, use lowest effective dose for shortest interval possible.

43. Outline a treatment approach for an SLE patient with increasing symptoms.

- Rule out a cause other than SLE for the patient's symptoms: rule out infection (see Question 49); rule out thrombosis (antiphospholipid antibodies, TTP); rule out drug side effect; rule out another disease (hypothyroidism, fibromyalgia, sleep apnea, etc.).
- Mild disease (fatigue, arthritis, rash, serositis):
  - NSAIDs: may cause worsening renal function, photosensitivity, aseptic meningitis (especially ibuprofen).
  - Hydroxychloroquine: needs eye examination yearly.
  - Low-dose prednisone (<20 mg/day): taper to lowest effective dose.
  - Methotrexate: can use leflunomide if methotrexate not tolerated.
- Moderate disease (severe minor symptoms unresponsive to standard therapy especially in patients with low complement and high anti-dsDNA antibodies):
  - Mycophenolate mofetil or azathioprine.
  - Belimumab.
  - Prednisone (20 to 40 mg/day): taper to lowest effective dose.
- Severe disease (nephritis, CNS, pneumonitis, vasculitis, severe cytopenias):
  - High-dose prednisone (>60 mg/day) including pulse methylprednisolone (1 g/day × 3 to 5 days) if needed.
  - Cytotoxic medications: induction therapy with cyclophosphamide or MMF followed by maintenance therapy with azathioprine, MMF, or calcineurin inhibitors (cyclosporin, tacrolimus).
  - Biologics: rituximab can be considered.
- Additional therapies: plasmapheresis (diffuse alveolar hemorrhage, TTP, anti-NMO spectrum disorder), IVIG (autoimmune cytopenias, antiphospholipid antibody syndrome), stem cell transplant (refractory SLE).

44. How does the erythrocyte sedimentation rate, CRP, and WBC count help in following disease activity in SLE? Help distinguish infection?

Unlike rheumatoid arthritis, the erythrocyte sedimentation rate (ESR) and CRP are not helpful in following disease activity in SLE. The ESR remains elevated even when the disease is controlled, usually owing to a persistent polyclonal gammopathy. By contrast, CRP usually does not rise much even during disease flare unless there is a systemic vasculitis, significant serositis, or associated infection. An SLE patient with fever and an elevated CRP should have an infection aggressively sought out and treated. Note when an SLE patient "flares," the WBC count frequently goes down. When an SLE patient becomes infected, the WBC count may rise to the "normal" range if the patient is usually leukopenic. A WBC differential showing a "left shift" with bands or metamyelocytes is also concerning for infection. Any febrile SLE patient with a high WBC count should be investigated for an infection and may be empirically treated with antibiotics until cultures return. Complement levels can also help differentiate between infection, where they become elevated, and an SLE flare during which they are typically low. An elevated procalcitonin level may be predictive of a bacterial or fungal infection in a febrile SLE patient.

45. What is the utility of following serological tests to assess disease activity and predict disease flares?

Hypocomplementemia (low C3) and elevated anti-dsDNA antibodies correlate with disease activity in most but not all SLE patients. However, some patients can flare their disease while maintaining a normal C3 and anti-dsDNA antibody level. The value of following complement and anti-dsDNA antibody levels serially and increasing the prednisone dose to prevent flares if the patient becomes more serologically active is controversial. Recent data support that individual patients act differently but usually fall into one of three patterns: (1) some patients flare without changing their serologies; (2) some patients flare only after they become more serologically active; and (3) some patients who are serologically active may never flare and may even improve their serologies. Therefore, the clinician needs to establish the serological pattern for each patient and treat accordingly. Only patients who demonstrate that they flare when their serologies become more active should receive prophylactic increases in their prednisone dose to prevent a flare.

46. What biological therapies have been evaluated for use in SLE?

- **Belimumab** (10 mg/kg IV monthly) is a monoclonal antibody that inhibits the B lymphocyte stimulator (BLyS), which modulates B cell growth and survival. It has been shown to improve disease activity and enable a decrease in steroid dosage in patients who fail standard-of-care therapy. Notably, patients with renal disease and severe active CNS disease were excluded from the trials. Patients are more likely to respond if they are serologically active (low complements, high anti-dsDNA antibody levels). Autoimmune cytopenias are less likely to respond to therapy. The number of B cells decreases 50% while on this therapy. Average annual cost is $35,000/year.
- **Rituximab** (1 g on days 1 and 15 or 375 mg/m^2 weekly × 4 doses) is an anti-CD20 monoclonal antibody that has been shown to be efficacious in severe refractory SLE in open label studies. Although randomized trials did not show benefit, rituximab continues to be used in patients who have failed multiple therapies, and in specific settings such as catastrophic antiphospholipid antibody syndrome. B cells are completely depleted by this therapy. Average cost for one course (two 1-g doses) of therapy is $14,200. Some investigators advocate combining with cyclophosphamide (15 mg/kg on days 1 and 15) for its immunomodulating effects in addition to B cell depletion.
- Other biologics including tumor necrosis factor inhibitors, abatacept, and tocilizumab have had mixed or negative results when used in SLE patients. Type I IFNs (IFN-α) have been implicated in the pathogenesis of SLE. The serum levels of IFN-α are high in a subset of SLE patients and correlate with disease activity. *Antiinterferon monoclonal antibodies* are currently under investigation. Other B cell targeted therapies are currently under investigation. *Epratuzumab* is a humanized monoclonal antibody that binds CD22 on B cell surfaces and modulates B cell function. Clinical trials are in progress.

47. What disease activity indices are used in SLE? What is the Systemic Lupus International Collaborating Clinics/American College of Rheumatology Damage Index?

- Disease activity indices: several have been proposed with the most common listed as follows:
  - British Isles Lupus Activity Group (BILAG-2004): the index is based on the physician's intent to treat. The index contains 97 items including clinical and laboratory variables in 9 organ systems. The index scores disease activity over the preceding 28 days by grading each organ system as A through E based on the presence of certain defined features. A severe flare is defined as a new BILAG A (requires prednisone >20 mg/day or immunosuppressive) in any organ system or two new BILAG B. A moderate flare is defined as one new BILAG B (requires prednisone <20 mg/day, hydroxychloroquine, NSAIDs) in an organ system. Remission is the resolution of all BILAG A and B scores. The BILAG index is used in clinical trials and requires training to apply accurately.
  - SLE Disease Activity Index (SLEDAI): this global index is a weighted scale based on the presence of 24 clinical and immunological descriptors in 9 organ systems. The score assigned to each descriptor varies between 1 and 8 based on severity with a total possible score of 105. Manifestations are scored if present over the previous 10 days. A score >20 indicates severely active disease. A severe flare is defined as an increase in score >12 points (or need to increase prednisone >0.5 mg/kg/day and/or add an immunosuppressive), whereas a mild/moderate flare is defined as an increase in score >3 to 4 points (or need to increase prednisone but <0.5 mg/kg/day and/or add hydroxychloroquine/NSAIDs). Clinically meaningful improvement is defined as a decrease in SLEDAI by 4 points. Variations of this index are the SELENA-SLEDAI and SLEDAI-2K. This index is used in clinical trials as well as in clinical practice.
  - The Systemic Lupus International Collaborating Clinics/American College of Rheumatology (SLICC/ACR) Damage Index: this index describes the accumulation of damage that has occurred since the onset of lupus in 12 different systems. It includes 41 items that may have resulted from previous lupus activity

leading to organ failure (e.g., renal failure), disease therapy (e.g., steroid-induced diabetes), or intercurrent illness (e.g., cancer, surgery) not attributable to lupus. Items must be present at least 6 months. Scores range from 0 to 49 with most patients being less than 10. Increase accrual of damage over time is associated with increased mortality.

48. What is the role of stem cell transplantation in SLE?

Hematopoietic stem cell transplantation (HSCT) has been utilized in the past 10 years in SLE to eliminate autoreactive lymphocytes and replace them with undifferentiated cells. In one study of 50 patients with severe SLE who underwent nonmyeloablative stem cell transplant, there was a 50% chance of 5-year disease-free survival. Other studies report a high incidence of treatment-related complications such as infection. Studies of both autologous transplant and mesenchymal stem cell transplant are currently ongoing. HSCT should be reserved for patients with refractory life-threatening disease.

49. What are the four most common causes of death in patients with SLE? The most common morbidities?

The overall 10-year survival is 85% to 90%. However, mortality is increased three times compared to a healthy, age-matched population. Some have emphasized the bimodal pattern of mortality in SLE. Death early in the disease is generally a reflection of active lupus or its treatment (infection), whereas death late in disease is due to atherosclerosis and malignancy. The most common causes of death are:

- **Infection:** accounts for 25% of all deaths. All infections (bacterial, fungal, TB, nontuberculous mycobacterial, viral) are increased mostly related to the complications of immunosuppressive therapy, especially to prolonged use of high-dose corticosteroids. For each increase of prednisone by 10 mg/day, the risk of serious infection increases 11-fold.
- **Active SLE:** accounts for 35% of deaths especially during first 5 years of disease. Lupus nephritis with renal failure, CNS lupus, vasculitis, and pneumonitis are the most lethal.
- **Cardiovascular disease:** accounts for 30% to 40% of deaths particularly after 10 years of disease. The risk of coronary artery disease is increased 2-fold to 8-fold in SLE patients. Factors playing a role in the coronary artery disease of SLE patients include corticosteroid therapy, hyperlipidemia from renal disease, proinflammatory high-density lipoprotein, hypertension, smoking, coagulation abnormalities, obesity, and vasculopathy from immune injury.
- **Malignancy:** accounts for 5% to 10% of all deaths. The overall standardized incidence ratio (SIR) is 1.15. HPV-related malignancies (cervical cancer) are increased (SIR 5) due to patient exposure to immunosuppressive medications. Patients should be offered the HPV vaccine if under age 26 years and should have annual PAP tests including testing for HPV DNA if at risk. Hematological malignancies (SIR 2.75) and lymphoma (SIR 3.64) are increased 5-fold. Lung cancer is increased (SIR 1.4) in smokers. Squamous cell skin cancers can arise in discoid lesions.

The most common morbidities (SLE damage index) seen in SLE patients are renal failure (20%), neuropsychiatric deficits, disfiguring skin lesions, and medication side effects.

BIBLIOGRAPHY

ACR Ad Hoc Committee on Neuropsychiatric Lupus Nomenclature: The American College of Rheumatology nomenclature and case definitions for neuropsychiatric lupus syndromes, Arthritis Rheum 42:599, 1999.

Burt RK, Traynor A, Statkute L, et al: Nonmyeloablative hematopoietic stem cell transplantation for systemic lupus erythematosus, JAMA 295:527–535, 2006.

Chelamcharla M, Javaid B, Baird BC, et al: The outcome of renal transplantation among systemic lupus erythematosus patients, Nephrol Dial Transplant 22:3623–3630, 2007.

Cohen D, Berger SP, Steup-Beekman GM, et al: Diagnosis and management of the antiphospholipid antibody syndrome, BMJ 340:c2541, 2010.

Collins E, Gilkeson G: Hematopoetic and mesenchymal stem cell transplantation in the treatment of refractory systemic lupus erythematosus–Where are we now? Clin Immunol 148:328–334, 2013.

Deng Y, Tsao BP: Genetic susceptibility to systemic lupus erythematosus in the genomic era, Nat Rev Rheumatol 6:683–692, 2010.

Grossman JM: Lupus arthritis, Best Pract Res Clin Rheumatol 23:495–506, 2009.

Hahn BH, Grossman JM: American College of Rheumatology guidelines for screening and management of lupus nephritis, Arthritis Care Res 64:797–808, 2012.

Hepburn AL, Narat S, Mason JC: The management of peripheral blood cytopenias in systemic lupus erythematosus, Rheumatology 49:2243–2254, 2010.

Hogan J, Appel GB: Update on the treatment of lupus nephritis, Curr Opin Nephrol Hypertension 22:224–230, 2013.

Izmirly PM, Buyon JP: Neonatal lupus syndromes, Rheum Clin N Am 33:267–285, 2007.

Karrar A, Sequeira W, Block JA: Coronary artery disease in systemic lupus erythematosus: a review of the literature, Semin Arthritis Rheum 30:436–443, 2001.

Liu LL, Jiang Y, Wang LN, et al: Efficacy and safety of mycophenolate mofetil versus cyclophosphamide for induction therapy of lupus nephritis: a meta-analysis of randomized controlled trials, Drugs 72:1521–1533, 2012.

Liu Z, Davidson A: Taming lupus—a new understanding of pathogenesis is leading to clinical advances, Nature Med 18:871–882, 2012.

Mok CC, Lau CS, Wong RWS: Use of exogenous estrogens in systemic lupus erythematosus, Semin Arthritis Rheum 30:426–435, 2001.

Neunert C, Lim W, Crowther M, et al: The American Society of Hematology 2011 evidence-based practice guideline for immune thrombocytopenia, Blood 117:4190–4207, 2011.

Petri M, Kim MY, Kalunian KC, et al: Combined oral contraceptives in women with systemic lupus erythematosus, N Engl J Med 353:2550–2558, 2005.

Petri M, Orbai AM, Alarcon GS, et al: Derivation and validation of the Systemic Lupus International Collaborating Clinics Classification Criteria for systemic lupus erythematosus, Arthritis Rheum 64:2677–2686, 2012.

Rahman A, Isenberg DA: Systemic lupus erythematosus, N Engl J Med 358:929–939, 2008.

Roman MJ, Salmon JE: Prevalence and correlates of accelerated atherosclerosis in systemic lupus erythematosus, N Engl J Med 349:2399–2406, 2003.

Ruiz-Irastorza G, Ramos-Casals M, Brito-Zeron P, et al: Clinical efficacy and side effects of antimalarials in systemic lupus erythematosus: a systemic review, Ann Rheum Dis 69:20–28, 2010.

Solomon DH, Kavanaugh AJ, Schur PH, American College of Rheumatology Ad Hoc Committee on Immunologic Testing Guidelines: Evidence based guidelines for the use of immunologic tests: antinuclear antibody testing, Arthritis Rheum 47:434–444, 2002.

Tseng CE, Buyon JP, Kim M, et al: The effect of moderate-dose corticosteroids in preventing flares in patients with serologically active, but clinically stable, systemic lupus erythematosus: findings of a prospective, randomized, double-blind, placebo-controlled trial, Arthritis Rheum 54:267–285, 2006.

Wallace DJ, Hahn BH, editors: Dubois' lupus erythematosus, ed 8, Philadelphia, 2013, Elsevier Saunders.

Weening JJ, D'Agati VD, Schwartz MM, et al: The classification of glomerulonephritis in systemic lupus erythematosus revisited, J Am Soc Nephrol 15:241–250, 2004.

Further Reading

www.lupus.org

DRUG-INDUCED LUPUS

Christopher C. Striebich, MD, PhD

KEY POINTS

1. The development of drug-induced autoantibodies is much more common than the development of lupus-like disease.
2. The classic autoantibody present in most cases of drug-induced lupus is an IgG antibody directed against histones.
3. The cornerstone of therapy in drug-induced lupus (DIL) is the discontinuation of the offending drug.
4. The use of drugs associated with DIL is not contraindicated in the treatment of patients with systemic lupus erythematosus (SLE), if their use is clinically indicated.

1. What is DIL and who gets it?
DIL is a lupus-like illness that occurs in some individuals after exposure to a causative drug for a few weeks to more than a year. Unlike idiopathic SLE, it occurs more commonly in older individuals (>age 50 years) and Caucasians and equally in males and females, reflecting the group of patients most likely to take these medications. Exceptions to this are DIL caused by minocycline and terbinafine, which occurs mostly in young women.

2. Name 10 drugs definitely associated with antinuclear antibody production and manifestations of lupus-like disease. What is the risk of developing DIL with each?
The names of 10 drugs definitely associated with antinuclear antibody (ANA) production and manifestations of lupus-like disease are listed in Table 17-1.

3. What are the clinical manifestations of DIL, and how do they differ from those of idiopathic SLE?
Patients with DIL can develop a variety of systemic signs and symptoms that typically come on abruptly. Similar to SLE, these include fever and/or other constitutional symptoms (50%), arthritis/arthralgias (80% to 95%), myalgias, serositis (50% with procainamide, 25% with quinidine, unusual with others), hepatomegaly (5% to 25%), and erythematous papular rashes (20%), but not discoid lesions or malar erythema (2%). Some patients may develop pulmonary infiltrates (procainamide). More severe manifestations of SLE, such as cytopenias, nephritis, and central nervous system (CNS) involvement are very rare in DIL, as are the presence of anti-double-stranded (ds) DNA antibodies and hypocomplementemia. Notably antitumor necrosis factor (anti-TNF) agents and interferon-α can induce anti-dsDNA antibodies but rarely cause symptomatic DIL.

4. List other drugs for which there is more than anecdotal evidence for lupus-inducing potential.
A variety of drugs have been associated with causing DIL and can be categorized as follows:
- **Definite:** procainamide, hydralazine, penicillamine, quinidine, isoniazid, minocycline, diltiazem (subacute cutaneous lupus rash), anti-TNF-α agents, interferon-α, methyldopa, chlorpromazine, and practolol.
- **Probable:** anticonvulsants (mephenytoin, phenytoin, carbamazepine, others), propylthiouracil, β-adrenergic blocking agents, sulfasalazine, antimicrobials (sulfonamides, nitrofurantoin), lithium, captopril, docetaxel, captopril, hydrochlorthiazide, glyburide, amiodarone, and interferon-γ. DIL has also been reported in patients receiving rifampin or rifabutin for treatment of a mycobacterial infection, particularly if they are also receiving clarithromycin or ciprofloxacin. This suggests that altered metabolism of rifampin/rifabutin by these medications induced DIL.
- **Possible:** statins, valproate, gemfibrozil, griseofulvin, others.

5. How do the clinical manifestations of procainamide-induced lupus differ from those of hydralazine-induced lupus?
Although both groups of patients commonly have fever, myalgias, and arthralgias/arthritis, and rarely manifest severe lupus nephritis or CNS involvement, patients with procainamide-induced disease are more likely to have pleuritis and/or pericarditis, and patients with hydralazine-induced disease are more likely to have rashes.

6. Which autoantibodies are most commonly seen in DIL? How do these compare with the autoantibodies seen in idiopathic SLE?
- **ANA:** As in SLE, virtually all patients with DIL will have a positive ANA; however, the spectrum of ANAs in DIL is much more limited than that seen in SLE. Notably, offending drugs are more likely to cause a positive ANA than symptomatic DIL. For example, procainamide causes a positive ANA in 90% of patients on the drug for over 2 years, but only 33% develop DIL.

III SYSTEMIC CONNECTIVE TISSUE DISEASES

Table 17-1. The Names of 10 Drugs Definitely Associated With Antinuclear Antibody Production and Manifestations of Lupus-Like Disease

HIGH (>5%)	MODERATE	LOW (<1%)
Procainamide (15% to 20%)	Quinidine	Isoniazid
Hydralazine (7% to 13%)	D-Penicillamine	Methyldopa
		Chlorpromazine
		Minocycline (5/10,000 patients)
		Anti-TNF-α agents (2/1000 patients)
		Terbinafine

- **Antihistone antibodies:** these are the most common of autoantibody specificity in DIL but frequency and specificity vary between drugs. Most patients (95%) with symptomatic drug-induced disease due to procainamide, hydralazine, chlorpromazine, and quinidine demonstrate elevated levels of IgG antihistone antibodies. Alternatively, patients who develop DIL due to minocycline, propylthiouracil, and statins have antihistone antibodies in fewer than 40% of patients. Antibodies to histones are also frequent in idiopathic SLE, detectable in 50% to 80% of patients, depending on disease activity.
- **Other autoantibodies against nuclear antigens:** antibodies to dsDNA are highly specific for idiopathic SLE and rarely found in DIL, with the exception of DIL due to anti-TNF agents or interferon-α. Antibodies to Sm, RNP, Ro/SS-A, and La/SS-B are common in idiopathic SLE but are unusual or do not persist in DIL.
- **Antiphospholipid antibodies:** can be seen in both DIL and idiopathic SLE. In DIL they occur most commonly with three drugs (chlorpromazine, procainamide, quinidine), tend to be IgM, and are rarely associated with thrombosis.

7. Is testing for antihistone antibodies clinically useful to distinguish drug-induced disease from idiopathic SLE in a patient taking either procainamide or hydralazine?

Testing for antihistone antibodies can occasionally be useful in situations in which the diagnosis of DIL is being considered. As discussed, nearly all patients (95%) with symptomatic procainamide-induced or hydralazine-induced lupus demonstrate elevated serum levels of IgG antihistone antibodies. Thus, a negative test would make this diagnosis unlikely. However, a positive test for antihistone antibodies has much less diagnostic value because 50% to 80% of patients with active SLE also have a positive test. Furthermore, some patients taking either procainamide or hydralazine will have a positive test but not symptoms of lupus-like disease. Asymptomatic patients tend to have IgM and not IgG antihistone antibodies. In most cases in which drug-induced lupus is being considered, performing an ANA test and if positive (usually in a homogeneous pattern) taking the patient off the offending agent may be the most cost-effective approach to the situation.

8. Contrast the type of antihistone antibodies found in DIL versus idiopathic SLE.

In certain specialized research laboratories, the specificity of antihistone antibodies for individual histones (i.e., H1, H2A, H2B, H3, and H4), histone complexes, or intrahistone epitopes can be distinguished. Overall, antihistone antibodies in DIL tend to be much more focused on certain histone complexes compared with SLE. For example, in procainamide-induced lupus (and most other causes of DIL), the onset of symptomatic disease has been associated with the production of IgG antibodies to the H2A–H2B–DNA complex. Although this complex is also a target in approximately 15% of patients with SLE, autoantibodies in idiopathic SLE are frequently directed to other individual histones (H1 and H2B) and other histone complexes. In hydralazine-induced disease, the major target is the H3–H4 complex. In contrast to procainamide-induced lupus and SLE, the autoantibodies induced by hydralazine appear to be directed more to determinants hidden within chromatin rather than exposed on the surface.

9. Are antineutrophil cytoplasmic antibodies ever seen in DIL?

Up to 80% to 85% of patients with minocycline-induced lupus can have a positive perinuclear antineutrophil cytoplasmic antibody (pANCA) with or without specificity for myeloperoxidase (anti-MPO). Propylthiouracil (PTU) and hydralazine can both cause DIL with an associated pANCA. However, both PTU and hydralazine therapy can also cause a positive pANCA usually with anti-MPO specificity that is associated with a more severe pauci-immune vasculitis with a necrotizing glomerulonephritis and possible pulmonary involvement (see Chapter 29). Notably, 15% to 20% of idiopathic SLE patients can have a positive ANCA.

10. What percentage of patients taking procainamide, hydralazine, or isoniazid develops a positive ANA? What percentage develops DIL?

Nearly 75% of patients receiving procainamide therapy will develop a positive ANA test within the first year of treatment, and over 90% develop a positive ANA by 2 years, yet only 33% develop DIL. In contrast, 30% to 50% of patients taking hydralazine will demonstrate a positive test after a year of drug therapy with 10% developing DIL, especially if they are slow acetylators. Finally, 15% of patients on isoniazid develop a positive ANA but few develop symptoms of DIL. Therefore, it is important to note that many more patients will demonstrate a positive ANA test than develop DIL, and the presence of a positive test is not a valid reason for stopping the medication.

11. **Do similar genetic factors predispose patients to develop DIL and SLE?**
The genetic risk factors in DIL and idiopathic SLE appear to be rather separate. The major risk for procainamide-induced or hydralazine-induced lupus appears to be acetylator phenotype. Metabolism of these drugs involves the hepatic enzyme N-acetyltransferase, which catalyzes the acetylation of amine or hydrazine groups. The rate at which this reaction takes place is under genetic control. Approximately 50% of the U.S. Caucasian population are fast acetylators, with the rest being slow acetylators. The slow acetylators, when treated with procainamide or hydralazine, develop ANA earlier and at higher titers and are more likely to develop symptomatic disease compared with fast acetylators. It should also be noted that N-acetylprocainamide, despite its chemical similarity to procainamide and its similar drug action, has not been associated with drug-induced ANA production or DIL. In idiopathic SLE, acetylator phenotype does not appear to be involved in genetic susceptibility. Instead, HLA class II genes, complement deficiencies, and multiple other genes are important in the complex genetic basis of SLE (see Chapter 16). HLA-DR4 and null gene for C4 may contribute to the risk of developing hydralazine-induced DIL.

12. **What hypotheses have been proposed for pathogenetic mechanisms causing DIL?**
- Genetic—slow acetylator status (see Question 11).
- Epigenetic—procainamide and hydralazine can decrease T cell DNA methylation leading to overexpression of LFA-1.
- Biotransformation—procainamide and hydralazine can serve as substrates for myeloperoxidase in activated neutrophils. The reactive metabolite, procainamide hydroxylamine (PAHA) can affect the immune system.
- Drugs acting as haptens or agonists for drug-specific T cells.

13. **Is the use of procainamide or other drugs associated with DIL contraindicated in patients with SLE? Can they exacerbate disease activity?**
No. The population at risk for developing DIL is very different compared with that developing SLE. There is no evidence that drugs capable of causing DIL will change or worsen disease activity in a patient with SLE. However, if an alternative drug is available, it may be prudent to use it so that there will not be any confusion if the SLE patient has a disease flare in the future. This is especially true for minocycline, which should be avoided if possible.

14. **What are the characteristic clinical features of minocycline-induced lupus?**
There have been multiple cases of DIL affecting young individuals (females > males, ages 14 to 31 years) after an average of 30 months (range 6 to 72 months) of minocycline use for acne in doses of 50 to 200 mg/day. All patients have arthritis/arthralgias and most have a positive ANA (92%). Fever (38%), rash (20% to 30%), pleuritis/pneumonitis (10%), hepatitis (50% with elevated liver-associated enzymes), and anticardiolipin antibodies (33%) can be seen. Interestingly, only 10% to 15% have antihistone antibodies but 67% to 85% have a positive pANCA with or without anti-MPO specificity.

15. **What drugs have been associated with causing subacute cutaneous lupus erythematosus?**
Diltiazem, terbinafine, hydrochlorothiazide, angiotensin-converting enzyme inhibitors, anti-TNF agents, statins, and various agents to treat malignancies (docetaxel) are among the drugs that have been reported to cause subacute cutaneous lupus erythematosus (SCLE). In addition to having a positive ANA, these patients frequently also have a positive anti-SSA (Ro) antibody, and thus more closely resemble idiopathic SCLE. However, the cutaneous eruption in drug-induced SCLE is more widespread in distribution and may be bullous or vasculitic. In addition, the anti-SSA(Ro) antibody will disappear in 75% of patients with drug-induced SCLE after the drug is stopped and the rash resolves.

16. **Therapeutic use of interferon-α and inhibitors of TNF-α (anti-TNF-α) have been associated with the development of SLE. How are these cases similar to classic DIL and how do they differ?**
As in other causes of DIL, autoimmunity due to the use of biologic therapies is more likely to cause the formation of lupus-associated autoantibodies than to cause true SLE. In contrast to classic DIL, the formation of anti-dsDNA antibodies is commonly seen. Patients taking interferon-α are more likely to develop typical lupus manifestations such as oral ulcers, alopecia, and nephritis, and frequently require corticosteroids or other lupus therapies to treat the disease. Anti-TNF agents causes ANAs in 13% to 83% of patients and anti-DNA antibodies in 3% to 32% of patients, but symptomatic DIL occurs in only 2 out of 1000 patients and resolves within 5 half-lives of stopping the drug.

17. **What is the treatment of DIL?**
The first and most important intervention is to discontinue the offending drug. Nonsteroidal antiinflammatory drugs will often help control symptoms such as arthralgias, as the disease gradually resolves after the drug has been stopped. Patients with more severe signs and symptoms, especially those with pericarditis or pleuritis, often require a short course of corticosteroids to control their disease. In more prolonged cases, antimalarials can be used. More toxic agents, such as azathioprine or cyclophosphamide, are almost never required in the

treatment of DIL although they may be needed in drug-induced ANCA vasculitis. Overall, the prognosis of DIL is good and symptoms resolve with stopping the offending drug. Notably, the positive ANA may persist for a prolonged time (>1 year) even after symptoms resolve.

Acknowledgment

The author and editor wish to thank Dr. Brian L. Kotzin for his contributions to this chapter in previous editions.

BIBLIOGRAPHY

Borchers AT, Keen CL, Gershwin ME: Drug-induced lupus, Ann NY Acad Sci 1108:166, 2007.
Callen JP: Drug-induced subacute cutaneous lupus erythematosus, Lupus 19:1107, 2010.
De Bandt M, Sibilia J, Le Loet X, et al: Systemic lupus erythematosus induced by anti-tumour necrosis factor alpha therapy: a French national survey, Arthritis Res Ther 7:R545–R551, 2005.
Dlott JS, Roubey RA: Drug-induced lupus anticoagulant and antiphospholipid antibodies, Curr Rheumatol Rep 14:71–78, 2012.
Gota C, Calabrese L: Induction of clinical autoimmune disease by therapeutic interferon-α, Autoimmunity 36:511–518, 2003.
Lawson TM, Amos N, Bulgen D, et al: Minocycline-induced lupus: clinical features and response to rechallenge, Rheumatology 40:329–335, 2001.
Mor A, Pillinger MH, Wortmann RL, et al: Drug-induced arthritic and connective tissue disorders, Semin Arthritis Rheum 38:249, 2008.
Patel D, Richardson B: Drug-induced lupus: etiology, pathogenesis, and clinical aspects. In Wallace DJ, Hahn BH, editors: Dubois' lupus erythematosus and related syndromes, ed 8, Philadelphia, 2013, Elsevier Saunders.
Rubin RL: Drug-induced lupus, Toxicology 209:135–147, 2005.

FURTHER READING

www.lupus.org/education/brochures/drug.html

CHAPTER 18

SYSTEMIC SCLEROSIS

Aryeh Fischer, MD

KEY POINTS

1. It is important to distinguish localized scleroderma (e.g., morphea) from the systemic form (systemic sclerosis) because localized disease does not have internal or systemic manifestations.
2. Nearly all patients with systemic sclerosis develop Raynaud's phenomenon and nearly all have gastroesophageal reflux disease.
3. Distinguishing the limited form versus diffuse form of systemic sclerosis and identifying disease-specific autoantibodies is important because these factors often impact the pace of the disease and pattern of internal organ involvement.
4. Because interstitial lung disease and pulmonary arterial hypertension are the main cause of mortality, vigilant screening assessments for their presence are indicated in all patients with systemic sclerosis because early detection and intervention strategies may favorably impact the natural history of the disease.
5. Scleroderma renal crisis, often heralded by an acute rise in blood pressure, is associated with early diffuse systemic sclerosis, and requires rapid recognition and initiation of angiotensin-converting enzyme inhibitor therapy.

1. **What is systemic sclerosis?**
    Systemic sclerosis (SSc, scleroderma) is a rare and potentially devastating connective tissue disease characterized by autoimmunity, vasculopathy, and fibrosis. Almost all patients with SSc have skin thickening, Raynaud's phenomenon, and esophageal reflux or dysmotility. More than 90% are antinuclear antibody (ANA) positive. Lung involvement – either with interstitial lung disease or pulmonary arterial hypertension (PAH) – is the leading cause of mortality in scleroderma.

2. **Describe the classification scheme of scleroderma.**
    It is crucial to distinguish the *localized* forms of scleroderma from the *generalized* (systemic) forms of the disease (Figure 18-1).
    - **Localized scleroderma:** cutaneous changes consisting of dermal fibrosis *without* internal organ involvement. The two types of localized scleroderma are:
        1. **Morphea:** single or multiple plaques commonly on the trunk.
        2. **Linear scleroderma:** bands of skin thickening commonly on the legs or arms but sometimes on the face (*en coup de sabre*) that typically follow a linear path.
    - **Generalized scleroderma = systemic sclerosis.**
        1. **Limited cutaneous systemic sclerosis (lcSSc, limited scleroderma):** patients with lcSSc have skin thickening limited to the neck, face, or distal aspects of upper and lower extremities (below the elbows and knees). Limited scleroderma patients may not come to clinical attention until many years after symptom onset. They often describe long-standing Raynaud's phenomenon, gastroesophageal reflux disease (GERD) and may have telangiectasia, skin calcifications (calcinosis), and digital edema or sclerodactyly as their only skin manifestations. Renal crisis is exceedingly rare in lcSSc. Among those with lcSSc, the presence of anti-Scl-70 (antitopoisomerase) antibody is associated with a high risk for the development of progressive interstitial lung disease (ILD), and the presence of **anticentromere antibody** is associated with a particularly high risk for PAH. Interestingly, those with a positive nucleolar staining ANA and negative anti-Scl-70 (referred to as "isolated" nucleolar ANA) are at high risk for both ILD and PAH and are frequently anti-Th/To positive (Figure 18-2).
        2. **Diffuse cutaneous systemic sclerosis (dcSSc, diffuse scleroderma):** patients with diffuse scleroderma have skin thickening proximal to the elbows, knees or trunk, excluding the face and neck. In contrast to limited scleroderma, patients with dcSSc usually present relatively acutely. Common presenting symptoms include puffy hands, Raynaud's phenomenon, arthritis, carpal tunnel symptoms (due to surrounding edema or inflammation), fatigue, and rapidly progressive skin thickening. Diffuse patients often have the onset of Raynaud's phenomenon within a year of developing SSc. Patients with diffuse disease are much more likely to develop scleroderma renal crisis. All patients with dcSSc are at high risk for progressive ILD particularly within the first 5 years of disease onset and are also at risk for the later development of PAH (Figure 18-3).

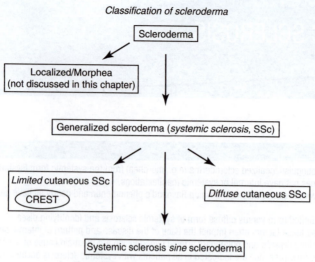

Figure 18-1. Classification of scleroderma.

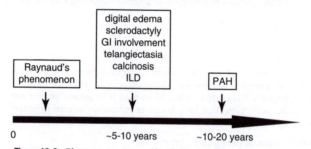

Figure 18-2. Classic presentation of limited cutaneous systemic sclerosis.

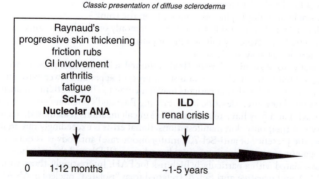

Figure 18-3. Classic presentation of diffuse scleroderma.

3. **Systemic sclerosis sine scleroderma:** patients with internal manifestations of SSc – along with a scleroderma specific antibody (such as a nucleolar pattern ANA, anticentromere antibody, anti-Scl-70 antibody, or anti-RNA polymerase III antibody) – without evidence of skin thickening, are characterized as having systemic sclerosis sine scleroderma (ssSSc). Examples of ssSSc include patients with:
   - Raynaud's phenomenon, digital edema, ILD, and a positive anti-Scl-70 antibody.
   - Raynaud's phenomenon, GERD, PAH, and a positive anticentromere antibody.
   - Raynaud's phenomenon, renal crisis, and a positive anti-RNA polymerase III antibody.

	ACA	Th/To	U1-RNP (MCTD)	PmScl	U3-RNP (FIBRILLARIN)	Scl-70 (TOPOISO-MERASE I)	RNA Pol 3
SSc subset (% of patients)	Limited (50% to 90%)	Limited (4% to 16%)	Limited (100% MCTD)	Limited (3%)	Diffuse (7%)	Diffuse (20% to 30%)	Diffuse (25%)
Lungs	PAH	ILD + PAH	PAH	ILD Myositis	ILD + PAH	ILD	—
Kidneys	—	—	—	—	SRC	SRC	SRC

Table 18-1. Predominant Features Associated With SSc-Specific Autoantibodies

Adapted from Steen VD, Lucas M, Fertig N et al: *Pulmonary arterial hypertension and severe pulmonary fibrosis in systemic sclerosis patients with a nucleolar antibody,* J Rheumatol 34:2230–2235, 2007.
ILD, Interstitial lung disease; MCTD, mixed connective tissue disease; PAH, pulmonary arterial hypertension; SRC, scleroderma renal crisis; SSc, systemic sclerosis.

3. **What is CREST?**
   CREST is a term that refers to a subgroup of patients with lcSSc. The term is derived from the clinical manifestations of:
   C—Calcinosis.
   R—Raynaud's phenomenon.
   E—Esophageal dysmotility.
   S—Sclerodactyly.
   T—Telangiectasia.
   The term *limited cutaneous* SSc is preferable because the CREST phenotype describes only a narrow part of the spectrum of scleroderma. Use of the term CREST is discouraged as it may be misleading and may give the wrong impression that it is distinct from SSc. Rather than CREST, the term limited SSc is preferred.

4. **Why does classification matter?**
   Knowledge of skin type (limited vs. diffuse) and the autoantibody profile of a scleroderma patient is fundamental to their care. As demonstrated above, the limited and diffuse scleroderma phenotypes "behave" very differently. Furthermore, specific autoantibodies are associated with certain internal organ manifestations (Table 18-1). For example:
   - Patients with lcSSc and a positive anticentromere antibody are at highest risk of developing PAH and yet rarely develop progressive ILD or renal crisis.
   - Patients with dcSSc and a positive RNA–polymerase III antibody are at highest risk for the development of renal crisis and yet rarely develop PAH.
   - Patients with lcSSc or ssSSc and a positive anti-Scl-70 antibody are at high risk for developing progressive ILD and yet rarely get renal crisis.

5. **What are the new American College of Rheumatology/European League Against Rheumatism classification criteria for SSc?**
   The new American College of Rheumatology/European League Against Rheumatism (ACR/EULAR) classification criteria for systemic sclerosis are outlined in Table 18-2.

6. **Who gets SSc?**
   SSc is most commonly seen in women (female/male = 4:1) between the ages of 35 and 64 years. Scleroderma occurs at a younger age in African-American women than in European-American women and is more likely to be dcSSc. Notably, Choctaw Native Americans residing in Oklahoma have the highest reported disease prevalence in the United States.

7. **What is the cause of SSc?**
   Unknown. The etiology of SSc may involve a complex interplay among a genetically susceptible host, sex-related factors, and external triggers. Pathophysiological mechanisms that may play a role in disease development include endothelial disruption, platelet activation, fibroblast proliferation, fetal microchimerism, and increased transforming growth factor-β. Some environmental factors, particularly silica dust, have been associated with an increased risk of disease.

8. **Are there effective treatments for SSc?**
   Yes. Although SSc can be a very difficult disease to manage, and there is no treatment for the underlying "scleroderma" per se, there are therapies that can help manage some of the specific disease manifestations. In particular, therapeutic options exist for Raynaud's phenomenon, esophageal reflux and dysmotility, renal crisis, PAH, and ILD.

Table 18-2. The New American College of Rheumatology/European League Against Rheumatism (ACR/EULAR) Classification Criteria for Systemic Sclerosis

ITEMS	SUBITEMS	WEIGHT
Skin thickening of fingers of both hands extending proximal to metacarpophalangeal (MCP) joints		9
Skin thickening of fingers (only count the highest score)	Puffy fingers Whole finger, distal to MCP	2 4
Fingertip lesions (only count the highest score)	Digital tip ulcers Pitting scars	2 3
Telangiectasia		2
Abnormal nailfold capillaries		2
Pulmonary arterial hypertension and/or interstitial lung disease (maximum score of 2)		2
Raynaud's phenomenon		3
Scleroderma-related antibodies (any of anticentromere, antitopoisomerase I [anti-Scl-70], anti-RNA polymerase III) (maximum score of 3)		3

Patients with a total score of 9 or more are classified as having definite systemic sclerosis with sensitivity of 91% and specificity of 92%.

Table 18-3. A Comparison of Organ System Involvement in Diffuse and Limited Systemic Sclerosis

ORGAN SYSTEM INVOLVEMENT	DIFFUSE (%)	LIMITED (%)
Skin thickening	100	95
Telangiectasia	30	80
Calcinosis	5	45
Raynaud's phenomenon	85 to 95	95
Arthralgias or arthritis	80	60
Tendon friction rubs	65	5
Myopathy	20	10
Esophageal hypomotility	75	75
Pulmonary fibrosis	35 to 59	25 to 35
Congestive heart failure	10	1
Renal crisis	15	1

9. **What are the main causes of mortality in SSc?**
   Before the introduction of angiotensin-converting enzyme (ACE) inhibitors, scleroderma renal crisis had been the leading cause of SSc-related mortality, but over the past 30 years PAH and ILD have been the leading causes of death in SSc.

10. **Compare and contrast organ system involvement in diffuse and limited SSc.**
    A comparison of organ system involvement in diffuse and limited SSc is outlined in Table 18-3.

11. **How is the skin affected in SSc?**
    The hallmark of scleroderma (*sclero* = thick, *derma* = skin) is thickened skin, thought to be due to the excessive production of normal type I collagen by a subset of fibroblasts along with the accumulation of glycosaminoglycan and fibronectin in the extracellular matrix. There is loss of sweat glands and hair loss in areas of tight skin. Although patients seem to have areas of involved and uninvolved skin, as based on the presence of procollagen-1 and adherence molecules, all skin tends to be abnormal. Skin thickening begins on the fingers and hands

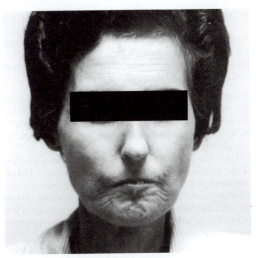

Figure 18-4. Scleroderma patient demonstrating tightened facial skin. Note exaggerated radial furrowing about the lips (tobacco pouch sign).

in virtually all cases of SSc. When skin thickening begins elsewhere, morphea, eosinophilic fasciitis, or another scleroderma mimic (see Chapter 19) should be considered. The progression of skin tightening is fairly variable. The **modified Rodnan skin score** has been used clinically and in trials to document skin involvement. The score is calculated by examining 17 areas and each area is graded from 0 (no involvement) to 3 (severe involvement) for a total possible score of 51. Skin scores over 15 to 20 and rapid progression (within the first year) indicate more severe disease. Most patients' skin, with no therapy, softens or atrophies over 3 to 10 years. Internal organ involvement does not mimic skin improvement and may worsen over time (Figure 18-4).

12. **How is skin thickening treated?**
    As a secondary outcome in the Scleroderma Lung Study, oral cyclophosphamide was shown to have a positive impact on the skin thickening of SSc. No other medication has been proven to be effective for skin thickening. Anecdotally, intravenous cyclophosphamide can also be very effective in this capacity. Although not proven in studies, some patients also note softening of their skin with mycophenolate mofetil or methotrexate use. Furthermore, low-dose prednisone (<15 mg/day) along with benzodiazepines can provide relief of the pruritus and pain that is associated with the acute phase of skin thickening that many patients with dcSSc experience.

13. **What is Raynaud's phenomenon?**
    Raynaud's phenomenon, frequently the first symptom of SSc, is an episodic self-limited and reversible vasomotor disturbance manifested as color changes bilaterally in the fingers, toes, and sometimes ears, nose, tongue, and lips. The color changes are **pallor**, **cyanosis**, and then **erythema** (white, blue, and then red) that occur sequentially and in response to environmental cold, emotional stress, or spontaneously. There does not need to be a three-color change to diagnose Raynaud's phenomenon; episodic pallor or cyanosis that reverses to erythema or normal skin color may be all that is seen. Patients may describe symptoms of numbness, tingling, or pain on recovery (also see Chapter 74).

14. **In a patient with new-onset Raynaud's phenomenon, what findings would suggest early SSc?**
    - Positive nucleolar staining ANA, anticentromere, or anti-Scl-70 antibody.
    - Nailfold capillary abnormalities of capillary drop out or dilatation (see Chapter 74).
    - Tendon friction rubs.
    - Digital edema or puffy hands.
    - Dilated, patulous esophagus (esophageal hypomotility).

15. **At the onset of SSc, how might the timing of the onset of Raynaud's phenomenon and skin thickening help suggest if the patient will develop the diffuse versus the limited form of SSc? How do the nailfold capillary abnormalities change as SSc progresses?**
    If the Raynaud's phenomenon precedes any skin changes by more than 1 year, the patient most likely will develop lcSSc. If the Raynaud's phenomenon occurs simultaneously with skin thickening, the patient will most likely develop dcSSc.
    There are three patterns of microvascular changes seen on nailfold capillaroscopy (NFC) as patients with SSc progress. Monitoring of NFC helps to identify disease progression as loss of capillary density is correlated with development of pulmonary hypertension and digital ulcers:

- Early pattern: few giant capillaries, few capillary microhemorrhages, no loss of capillaries, and preserved capillary distribution.
- Active pattern: frequent giant capillaries, frequent capillary microhemorrhages, moderate loss of capillaries, and mild disorganization of capillary architecture.
- Late pattern: giant capillaries and microhemorrhages are nearly absent, severe loss of capillaries, capillary ramification due to neoangiogenesis, and disorganized capillaries.

16. How is Raynaud's phenomenon treated? How are digital ulcers treated?

First, keep hands *and* body warm. Many patients carry gloves at all times. When going to cold places, patients may bring exothermic reaction bags (chemical heat packs), which can be obtained at sporting goods, hardware, and other stores. Repeated soaking in warm water sometimes helps. Cigarette smoking exacerbates Raynaud's phenomenon and should be avoided.

Various prescription vasodilators can be used. Calcium channel blockers are the first choice. Nifedipine, diltiazem, and amlodopine can be effective, but verapamil does not work. The dose of these drugs is increased until the desired effect is obtained or the patient cannot tolerate the side effects. Antiadrenergic agents such as prazosin, doxazosin, methyldopa, and reserpine and ACE inhibitors are also used as vasodilators but appear to be less effective than the calcium channel blockers for the management of Raynaud's phenomenon. More recently, good results have been obtained with angiotensin II receptor antagonists such as losartan, valsartan, or irbesartan. Topical nitroglycerin ointment applied sparingly over the affected area for 20 minutes three times a day can be helpful, but commonly the patient has an accompanying headache. A half an aspirin a day to inhibit platelet activation is also recommended. Niacin is also used starting at 50 mg twice a day and working up to 500 mg BID to TID. The limiting factor is the flushing that niacin can cause. Slow-release preparations of niacin may mitigate the flushing sensation and are often better tolerated. Pentoxyfylline is sometimes also effective. In severe cases of Raynaud's phenomenon, full anticoagulation with warfarin can be used. PAH-specific therapies are helpful for Raynaud's phenomenon but are not FDA approved for this indication. In particular, the off-label use of phosphodiesterase inhibitors (sildenafil and tadalafil), or endothelin receptor antagonists (bosentan and ambrisentan), can be helpful for more refractory Raynaud's phenomenon.

Digital ulcers occur in 30% to 40% of patients. All the therapies listed above have been used in an attempt to accelerate healing and prevent recurrence. A recent trial showed that bosentan can reduce the likelihood of digital ulcer recurrence. For cases of digit-threatening ischemia, intravenous prostacyclin can be instituted – but requires a several day inpatient hospitalization and can be difficult to get covered by insurance. Alternative modalities that can be tried in refractory cases also include digital sympathectomy and hyperbaric oxygen treatment to expedite digital ulcer healing (also see Chapter 74).

17. What is calcinosis?

Calcinosis consists of cutaneous deposits of basic calcium phosphate that characteristically occur in the hands (especially over the proximal interphalangeal joints and fingertips), periarticular tissue, and over bony prominences (especially the extensor surface of the elbows and knees) but can occur virtually anywhere on the body. The deposits of calcium are firm, irregular, and generally nontender, ranging in diameter from 1 mm to several centimeters. They can become inflamed, infected, or ulcerated or may discharge a chalky white material. Calcinosis can be persistent for years. It is extremely difficult to treat, and no therapy is consistently successful. Therapies used have included warfarin (1 to 2.5 mg/day, in an attempt to inhibit the vitamin K-dependent Gla matrix protein), topical sodium thiosulfate, aluminum hydroxide, diltiazem, probenecid, and high doses of bisphosphonates. All have limited success. Surgical resection should be considered a last resort option.

18. What are telangiectasia?

Telangiectasia are dilated venules, capillaries, and arterioles. In SSc they tend to be *matte* telangiectasia, which are oval or polygonal macules 2 to 7 mm in diameter found on the hands, face, lips, and oral mucosa. They are seen more commonly with limited SSc. Telangiectasia are usually harmless but can be a cosmetic problem. They may disappear spontaneously over time. Laser therapy has been used to remove them with some success, but commonly they will return. When they occur in the gastrointestinal (GI) mucosa (called "watermelon stomach" or gastric antral vascular ectasia), they can bleed, leading to iron deficiency anemia.

19. What are the GI manifestations of SSc?

Upper GI tract: GERD (heartburn), hypomotility, dysphagia, nausea, stricture formation, and risk of Barrett's esophagus (10% to 15%). It is important to note that cough due to aspiration is a common symptom associated with GERD. Calcium channel blockers used to treat Raynaud's phenomenon can make GERD worse in some patients.

Lower GI tract: hypomotility, bloating, nausea, small bowel bacterial overgrowth (manifested by fluctuating constipation and diarrhea), malabsorption, loss of rectal sphincter tone with resultant fecal incontinence. Calcium channel blockers used to treat Raynaud's phenomenon can make constipation worse in some patients.

20. Discuss the pathophysiologic progression of GI involvement in SSc.

Although no longitudinal studies have been done to document the anatomic progression in the GI system, there is good circumstantial evidence to suggest an orderly series of steps leading to progressive dysfunction.

First, there is neural dysfunction thought to be due to arteriolar changes of the vasa nervorum leading to dysmotility. Second, there is smooth muscle atrophy. Third, there is fibrosis of the smooth muscle.

21. **How is esophageal dysmotility assessed in patients with SSc?**
    Esophageal dysmotility is documented by manometry, barium esophagram, or by a routine upper GI series with barium swallow. Practically speaking, manometry, although the most sensitive, is so uncomfortable that it is rarely performed. A dilated, patulous esophagus is a frequent incidental finding noted on thoracic computed tomography scans of patients with SSc. Endoscopy is used to assess reflux esophagitis, candidiasis, Barrett's esophagus, and strictures of the lower esophageal area. Patients who develop Barrett's esophagitis are at risk for developing adenocarcinoma and will need surveillance endoscopies every 1 to 2 years depending on presence of dysplasia.

22. **How is esophageal dysmotility treated in SSc patients?**
    Treatment is designed to decrease complications of acid reflux, such as esophagitis, stricture, or nocturnal aspiration of stomach contents. The head of the bed should be elevated 4 to 6 inches; adding more pillows to sleep on may only make matters worse by decreasing the stomach area. The patient should not eat for 2 to 3 hours before bedtime. The acid content in the stomach should be decreased in the evening with antacids, H_2 blockers, or, for progressive problems, with the use of proton pump inhibitors. Motility agents such as metoclopramide (5 to 10 mg) or erythromycin (motilin receptor agonist) (250 mg) before meals are sometimes helpful early in the disease, but as the GI smooth muscles fibrose these agents become ineffective. Domperidone (Motilium) can be an effective promotility drug but is not FDA approved. **Both domperidone and erythromycin can cause a prolonged QT interval.** For more refractory cases of GI dysmotility, cisapride or injectable octreotide may be tried. Endoscopic injection of botox into the pyloric sphincter has been used for resistant cases of GERD.

23. **What is a "watermelon stomach"?**
    Watermelon stomach is a descriptive term for gastric antral venous ectasia ("GAVE") and is the result of extensive and prominent telangiectasia involving the gastric mucosal surface. This can be a cause of chronic iron deficiency anemia and acute upper GI bleeding in scleroderma. Laser treatment or argon plasma coagulation are effective treatments for GAVE.

24. **Patients with SSc may have small and large bowel involvement. What symptoms and signs do these patients have?**
    Involvement of the small intestine (17% to 57% of patients) and colon (10% to 50%) is common. The major manifestations are due to diminished peristalsis with resulting stasis and dilatation. The diminished peristalsis can lead to bacterial overgrowth (33% to 40% of patients) (hydrogen breath test, high folate, $\geq 10^5$ organisms/mL jejunal fluid). Later, malabsorption can be a major problem (low albumin, low B_6/B_{12}/folate/25-OH vitamin D, high fecal fat, low D-xylose absorption test, low β carotene, high international normalized ratio due to low vitamin K). Patients may report abdominal distention and pain due to dilated bowel, obstructive symptoms from intestinal pseudoobstruction, or diarrhea from bacterial overgrowth or malabsorption. If malabsorption becomes severe, the patient may have signs of vitamin deficiencies or electrolyte abnormalities.
    Patients with large bowel involvement, which frequently affects the anorectum, can lead to debilitating fecal incontinence. This may be due to a neuropathy more than sphincter atrophy/fibrosis. Atrophy and thinning of the muscular wall in the colon can lead to "wide mouth" diverticulae. It should be emphasized that barium studies are relatively contraindicated in SSc patients with poor GI motility, owing to the risk of barium impaction. Rectal prolapse has also been reported (Figure 18-5).

25. **How are small and large bowel problems managed in these patients?**
    Stimulation of gut motility with domperidone, metoclopramide, or erythromycin can be given a half an hour before meals to stimulate gut motility. Cisapride or injectable octreotide may help in severe or refractory cases. Fiber may help colonic dysmotility but may make small bowel problems worse. Fiber is worth an empiric trial. Diarrhea is treated initially as if it were due to bacterial overgrowth. An antibiotic is given that can partially decrease gut flora, such as metronidazole (250 mg TID), amoxicillin–clavulanic acid (500 mg TID), ciprofloxacin (250 mg BID), norfloxacin (400 mg BID), or rifamixin (1200 mg daily) for 10 days. In most cases, this stops the diarrhea. In patients with relapse, longer antibiotic regimens can be used. Agents that slow intestinal motility, such as paregoric or loperamide, should be avoided. If diarrhea persists, a malabsorption work-up should be pursued. Most patients with malabsorption can be treated with supplemental vitamins, minerals, and predigested liquid food supplements. A rare patient will need total parenteral nutrition.
    Fecal incontinence is treated with biofeedback, sacral nerve stimulation, and/or surgical repair. Rectal prolapse includes management of constipation and possibly surgical correction.

26. **What baseline cardiopulmonary testing is recommended in SSc?**
    - Thoracic high-resolution computed tomography (HRCT) scan (chest X-ray is inadequate).
    - Complete pulmonary function tests (PFTs) (lung volumes, spirometry, and diffusing capacity for carbon monoxide).
    - Echocardiography.

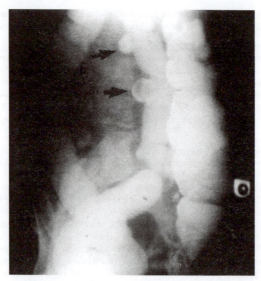

Figure 18-5. Barium enema in a systemic sclerosis patient, demonstrating wide mouth diverticulae *(arrows)*.

27. What types of lung disease do SSc patients get?
ILD and PAH are the two most common types of lung involvement identified in SSc and are the leading causes of SSc-associated mortality. Clinically significant airways or pleural disease is rare in SSc.

28. What is the most common ILD pattern seen in SSc?
Fibrotic nonspecific interstitial pneumonia (F-NSIP), identified in ~75% of cases, followed by usual interstitial pneumonia (UIP), identified in ~25% of cases, are by far the two most common ILD patterns identified in SSc. HRCT evidence of GERD with aspiration (centrilobular nodularity) is a frequent finding in patients with SSc.

29. Which scleroderma patients are at particularly high risk for developing ILD?
All SSc patients are at risk for the development of ILD. When assessed by thoracic HRCT, nearly all patients with SSc have evidence of bibasilar ILD. Clinically significant ILD warranting therapy, as determined by the presence of symptoms, restrictive defect on pulmonary function testing, or extensive disease by HRCT, is identified in only ~20% of patients with SSc.

Clinically significant ILD is most often identified within the first 3 years of disease onset. Patients at highest risk for clinically significant ILD are those with:
- Diffuse scleroderma.
- Positive anti-Scl-70 antibody (irrespective of skin involvement).
- Positive "isolated" nucleolar staining ANA – that is a nucleolar staining ANA with a negative anti-Scl-70. (Irrespective of skin involvement.) These patients frequently have anti-U3 RNP or anti-Th/To giving them a marked increased risk for severe ILD and PAH.

30. Does the presence of SSc–ILD require treatment?
Not necessarily. ILD requires treatment only when it is "clinically significant" or progressive in nature. The ILD assessment includes assessment of breathlessness, thoracic HRCT, and complete PFTs (lung volumes, spirometry, and diffusing capacity for carbon monoxide).

31. How are PFTs and the thoracic HRCT scan useful in the evaluation of SSc patients?
Serial assessment of the forced vital capacity (FVC) and diffusing capacity for carbon monoxide (DLco) allows for objective quantification of ventilatory capacity and gas exchange, respectively. These parameters are useful in assessing the degree of respiratory impairment due to ILD and may also provide clues about coexistent PAH. They are especially helpful when trying to assess for disease progression and response to therapy. Patients who decline ≥10% of predicted FVC or ≥15% of DLco are considered to have progressive disease by PFTs. In patients with SSc–ILD, pulmonary physiology appears to be a stronger predictor of survival than underlying histopathologic pattern.

Important information relevant to SSc–ILD can also be obtained by HRCT imaging including the pattern and extent of ILD, and on serial scanning, an assessment of disease progression, and the evaluation of extraparenchymal abnormalities. In most cases of SSc–ILD, a specific radiologic pattern (e.g., UIP or NSIP) can be determined with a high degree of confidence. Patients with >20% of their lung affected by ILD have a poor prognosis (5YS = 60%).

32. When should a patient with SSc–ILD undergo surgical lung biopsy?
A surgical lung biopsy is often indicated in those patients with an atypical or unclassifiable radiologic pattern. Because it is well established that NSIP and UIP are the most common types of ILD encountered in SSc, and because histopathology has not been shown to impact prognosis in SSc–ILD, surgical lung biopsy is typically NOT indicated when the HRCT is consistent with either pattern.

33. What is the drug of choice for SSc–ILD?
Based on the prospective placebo-controlled Scleroderma Lung Study trial, cyclophosphamide is the drug of choice for SSc. It can be given monthly IV or daily oral. However, the initial enthusiasm for cyclophosphamide in SSc–ILD has been tempered by (1) the modest degree of benefits (2.5% improvement in FVC) and (2) the lack of a sustained benefit in lung function after the drug was discontinued (benefits accrued over 18 months). Recently, mycophenolate mofetil has been reported to be a promising therapy for SSc–ILD. It is being studied in a head-to-head comparison with oral cyclophosphamide in Scleroderma Lung Study II. Mycophenolate mofetil appears to have an antifibrotic effect.

34. Discuss the frequency of PAH and its impact on survival in SSc.
The prevalence of right catheter confirmed SSc–PAH is estimated to be 10% to 15%. The presence of PAH in a scleroderma patient has a devastating impact on survival, and before the availability of PAH-specific therapies, the 5-year survival was 10% for scleroderma patients with PAH compared to 80% for scleroderma without PAH. The presence of advanced disease (functional class III to class IV) portends a particularly poor outcome. Over the past 10 years, multiple PAH-specific therapies have become available and their implementation has led to clinical improvement and an overall improved prognosis in patients with SSc–PAH when compared to historical controls.

35. What are the types of pulmonary hypertension?
The terminology and clinical classification of pulmonary hypertension (PH) is complicated. The current classification scheme divides PH into five distinct clinical groups:
Group 1—PAH.
Group 2—PH associated with left-heart disease (pulmonary venous hypertension, PVH).
Group 3—PH associated with chronic hypoxia (e.g., PH-associated with ILD).
Group 4—chronic thromboembolic associated PH.
Group 5—PH with unclear or multifactorial mechanisms (e.g., sarcoidosis, lymphangioleiomyomatosis).

36. What types of PH are seen in SSc?
Scleroderma patients most often have PAH (group 1) but can also commonly have other types of PH; particularly PVH (group 2) or PH-associated with ILD (PH–ILD, group 3). Because PAH-specific therapies are currently only approved for patients with *pulmonary arterial hypertension* (group 1), distinguishing whether a patient has PAH rather than an alternative category of PH is very important.
A diagnosis of PAH **absolutely** requires cardiac hemodynamic assessment via right-heart catheterization (RHC), and is defined by a mean pulmonary artery pressure (mPAP) ≥25 mmHg and pulmonary capillary wedge pressure (PCWP) of ≤15 mmHg.
In PVH, the elevated pulmonary pressures are a result of either systolic or diastolic dysfunction as confirmed by low cardiac output or an increased PCWP >15 mmHg on RHC. With PH–ILD, the elevated pulmonary pressures are considered to be a result of chronic hypoxia secondary to underlying lung disease. It is often a challenge to determine the degree of ILD necessary to cause secondary PH.

37. What are the presenting symptoms and signs of PAH?
Dyspnea and fatigue are the two most common symptoms of PAH, and yet they are both ubiquitous and unreliable among patients with scleroderma. Patients often underreport such symptoms, and providers have a difficult time reliably quantifying their severity or progression. It is important for ALL scleroderma patients to undergo PAH screening – *including patients who do not report dyspnea*.
There are few signs of early PAH on physical examination but there are several important physical examination findings that suggest the presence of advanced PAH (i.e., features of right-heart dysfunction, including lower extremity edema, the murmur of tricuspid regurgitation, jugular venous distension, hepatomegaly, or right-ventricular heave).

38. What are some "PAH risk factors" in scleroderma?
- Limited cutaneous scleroderma (especially >3 years).
- Duration of Raynaud's phenomenon >8 years.
- Anticentromere antibody positivity.
- Isolated nucleolar pattern ANA positivity.
- Extensive telangiectasia.
- DLco% <60% in the absence of extensive ILD.
- FVC%/DLco% ratio >1.6.

Table 18-4. Features Associated With Presence of PAH in Scleroderma

SYMPTOMS	**RECENT ONSET EXERTIONAL DYSPNEA**
Physical examination findings	Evidence of right-heart compromise (e.g., lower extremity edema, the murmur of tricuspid regurgitation, jugular venous distension, hepatomegaly, or right-ventricular heave)
Echocardiographic findings	RVSP > 40 mmHg TR jet > 2.8 m/s RV dilation/hypokinesis RA dilation Pericardial effusion
PFT parameters	DLco% <60% in absence of extensive ILD FVC%/DLco% >1.6
Other features	Elevated BNP or pro-NT BNP Oxygen desaturation with exercise

Adapted from Fischer A, Bull TM, Steen VD et al: Practical approach to screening for scleroderma-associated pulmonary arterial hypertension, Arthritis Care Res (Hoboken) 64:303-310, 2012.

BNP, B Type natriuretic peptide; DLco, diffusing capacity for carbon monoxide; FVC, forced vital capacity; ILD, interstitial lung disease; NT, N-terminal; PFT, pulmonary function test; RA, rheumatoid arthritis; RVSP, right ventricle systolic pressure; TR, tricuspid regurgitation.

39. What specific clinical, echocardiographic, PFT findings, and biomarkers suggest PAH in a patient with SSc?

Features associated with the presence of PAH in scleroderma are outlined in Table 18-4.

- The best predictor for the development of PAH in scleroderma is a declining DLco. The DLco is usually very low – <50% to 60% predicted – at the time of diagnosis of SSc–PAH and this is generally in the absence of significant ILD.
- All scleroderma patients should have a baseline set of complete PFTs including DLco and these should be repeated yearly in most patients. Restrictive physiology (i.e., reductions in total lung capacity or FVC) is seen with ILD, whereas disproportionate reductions in the DLco are more commonly seen with PAH. A disproportionate decline in the DLco relative to the FVC – as demonstrated by a FVC%/DLco% ratio >1.6 – is a strong predictor of the later development of PAH.

For those at high risk for ILD progression (e.g., diffuse cutaneous SSc or those with a positive anti-Scl-70 or isolated nucleolar ANA), one may choose to obtain PFTs even more frequently. A 6-minute walk test (6MWT) can identify exercise intolerance and hypoxemia, but it is not useful as a screening tool for SSc–PAH because it is neither specific nor sensitive for PAH.

- A transthoracic echocardiogram is the best noninvasive assessment for the presence of PH. A baseline echocardiogram is recommended in all SSc patients and should be repeated yearly. Asymptomatic and low-risk patients (DLco>70%) may only require an echocardiogram at 2-year intervals, but should have an annual clinical assessment that include PFTs with DLco. Notably, there are significant limitations to its role as a screening tool for SSc–PAH. Echocardiographic estimates of the right-heart side of the heart are limited by technical issues (body habitus, etc.) and up to 15% of patients do not have a visible tricuspid regurgitation (TR) jet, thereby not allowing for right ventricle systolic pressure (RVSP) estimation.
- Elevated B type natriuretic peptide (BNP) and N-terminal (NT) pro-BNP are surrogate biomarkers for myocardial disease, and are frequently elevated in patients with SSc–PAH. They may be useful as an adjunctive component of the SSc–PAH screening tool, with a caveat that early patients – without significant right-heart failure – will have normal values. Both proteins reflect generalized cardiac dysfunction (including left-heart failure) and are not specific for PAH. However, recent data do suggest that among those with SSc–PAH, high levels of BNP or NT pro-BNP are associated with a worse prognosis.

40. What is the "gold standard" test for confirming PAH?

RHC is the gold standard test for the diagnosis of PH – and is absolutely required to confirm a diagnosis of PAH. It has an overall complication rate of 1.1%, mainly related to venous access problems. If any patient with scleroderma has unexplained dyspnea with an echocardiogram showing an estimated RVSP >40 mmHg, or evidence of right-ventricular dilatation or hypokinesis, an RHC should be strongly considered. However, as mentioned above, the RVSP is not always reliable or available, so the practitioner often needs to consider other factors to decide whether to proceed with an RHC. An RHC should also be strongly considered in a scleroderma patient with any "PAH risk factors" – and particularly those with a disproportionately low DLco of <60% or FVC%/DLco% ratio >1.6, with unexplained dyspnea, findings of right-heart compromise on physical examination, oxygen desaturation on exercise, right-heart abnormalities on echocardiogram, an elevated BNP, or pro-NT BNP – even with a *normal* estimated RVSP. An echocardiogram with an estimated RVSP <40

Table 18-5. Decision Algorithm for Screening and Performing an RHC in Scleroderma*

	LOW RISK	MILD RISK	MODERATE RISK	HIGH RISK
Dyspnea, or Raynaud's phenomenon duration >8 years, positive anticentromere or isolated nucleolar ANA	No	Yes	Yes	Yes
DLco (without extensive emphysema or ILD)	>70%	>70%	<70%	60%
FVC%/DLco%	<1.6	<1.6	>1.6	>1.6
RVSP	<35 mmHg	<35 mmHg	>35 mmHg	>40 mmHg
Next step	Repeat PFTs annually, Repeat echo in 2 to 3 years	Repeat PFTs annually, Repeat echo annually	Consider repeat echo in 3 to 6 months or proceed to RHC	Proceed to RHC

Adapted from Fischer A, Bull TM, Steen VD et al: Practical approach to screening for scleroderma-associated pulmonary arterial hypertension, Arthritis Care Res (Hoboken) 64:303-310, 2012.
ANA, Antinuclear antibody; DLco, diffusing capacity for carbon monoxide; FVC, forced vital capacity; ILD, interstitial lung disease; PFT, pulmonary function test; RHC, right-heart catheterization; RVSP, right ventricle systolic pressure.
*The presence of echocardiographic features of right-ventricular hypokinesis or dilatation or an increased B type natriuretic peptide (BNP) or N-terminal pro-BNP in a dyspneic scleroderma patient should lead to RHC irrespective of the estimated RVSP.

mmHg – without any other PAH-suggestive features – should reassure the practitioner that the pulmonary artery pressures are normal.

As part of the standard RHC procedure, acute vasodilator testing via catheter-infused adenosine, nitric oxide, or prostacyclin may be performed. Even though current guidelines recommend that patients with idiopathic PAH undergo vasoreactivity testing as part of their initial RHC, no such consensus exists for SSc–PAH. Because vasoreactivity is so uncommon in scleroderma, the lack of its availability as part of the RHC should not preclude performing an RHC (Table 18-5).

41. Are there effective PAH therapies?
Yes. Conventional therapy for PAH typically includes treatment with calcium channel blockers, fluid/volume control (diuretics, fluid restriction, low salt diet), and supplemental oxygen. Although chronic anticoagulation with warfarin is a common adjunctive therapy for idiopathic PAH, it is controversial whether to use chronic warfarin as a component of PAH therapy in SSc due to the increased risk of bleeding in SSc patients relative to idiopathic PAH patients.

The biggest change in PAH therapy has been with the advent of PAH-specific therapies and these agents may be used as monotherapy or in combination. There are three separate categories of PAH-specific therapies, each representing a novel pathophysiologic pathway: prostacyclins (inhaled [iloprost], subcutaneous or intravenous [epoprostenol, treprostinil]), endothelin receptor antagonists (oral [bosentan, ambrisentan, macitentan]), or phosphodiesterase 5 inhibitors, which increases local nitric oxide(oral [sildenafil, tadalafil]). The presence of multiple available therapies has also made the management of SSc–PAH increasingly more complex and collaboration with PAH-treating providers is recommended.

42. What types of heart disease occur with SSc?
Myocardial, pericardial, or conduction system disease are all potential cardiac complications associated with SSc. Diastolic dysfunction is one of the more common cardiac manifestations of SSc and can lead to pulmonary venous hypertension. Pericardial effusions are almost always asymptomatic, are associated with the presence of PH, and do not require specific intervention. Cardiovascular disease including coronary disease is increased (hazard ratio [HR] 3.2×).

43. What is scleroderma renal crisis?
Renal failure, one of the most feared complications of SSc, may present as acute renal crisis, after prolonged hypertension, and less commonly as normotensive renal failure.

Scleroderma renal crisis (SRC) occurs in up to 10% of the entire SSc population and in 20% to 25% of patients with dcSSc. Renal crisis usually occurs in the patient with diffuse scleroderma and may be the presenting manifestation. Generally, renal crisis occurs early in the course of the disease, with a mean onset of 3.2 years, and more often in the autumn and winter months. Prognosis for recovery is poor with 40% to 50% requiring chronic dialysis. Overall 5-year mortality is 30% to 50%.

SRC is the abrupt onset of arterial hypertension (>150/90) (although 10% are normotensive), appearance of grade III (flame-shaped hemorrhages and/or cotton wool exudates) or grade IV (papilledema) retinopathy, and the rapid deterioration of renal function (within a month). Pericardial effusion is frequently present.

Abnormal laboratory tests include elevated renal function tests, consumptive thrombocytopenia, microangiopathic hemolysis (**schistocytes**) (50%), elevated renin levels (twice the upper limit of normal or greater), and normal or only mildly decreased ADAMTS13 levels (>20% of normal).

44. Which therapeutic intervention has helped avoid renal failure in patients with SSc?

The use of ACE inhibitors has dramatically changed the incidence and outcome of renal involvement in SSc. The diastolic blood pressure should be kept below 90 mmHg in all patients with SSc. Captopril and enalapril are the most studied ACE inhibitors in scleroderma, but probably any of the ACE inhibitors are effective. Angiotensin II receptor antagonists are not effective in preventing or treating SRC. Recently, some experts have suggested that routine use of ACE inhibitors may prevent early identification of SRC in some patients by modulating hypertension as an early sign of SRC. In these patients, they present in renal failure without having an elevated blood pressure (controversial).

45. What are some risk factors for SRC?

- Early diffuse scleroderma (first 1 to 4 years after diagnosis).
- Tendon friction rubs.
- Corticosteroid (prednisone > 20 mg/day or prolonged low dose) or cyclosporine use.
- Anti-RNA polymerase III antibody (60%).

46. How is SRC treated? What are the poor prognostic signs?

Patients with SRC should be hospitalized. They should be put on a short-acting ACE inhibitor with the goal of decreasing systolic blood pressure by 20 mmHg within the first 24 hours. Hypotension should be avoided. The ACE inhibitor should then be maximized to normalize the blood pressure. Up to 30% of patients will not respond to ACE inhibitors. These patients should have calcium channel blockers and/or angiotensin receptor blockers added to their regimen. Endothelin receptor antagonists and prostacyclins have also been tried. Poor prognostic factors include: (1) male, (2) initial creatinine > 3 mg/dL, (3) normotensive at onset, and (4) cardiac involvement with myocarditis or arrhythmias. Up to 75% will require dialysis within the first 24 months with half of those recovering enough renal function to stop dialysis. Therefore, kidney transplantation should be delayed at least 24 months.

47. Describe the bone and articular involvement in SSc.

Bone involvement is usually demonstrated by resorption of bone. Acrosclerosis with osteolysis is common. Resorption of ribs, mandible, acromion, radius, and ulna have been reported. Arthralgias and morning stiffness are relatively common, but erosive arthritis is rare. Hand deformities and ankylosis are seen, but these are attributed to the tethering effects of skin thickening instead of joint involvement. Tendon sheaths can become inflamed and fibrinous, mimicking arthritis. Tendon friction rubs can be palpated typically over the wrists, ankles, and knees and found mainly in patients with diffuse SSc patients (50% to 65%). Friction rubs are due to fibrin deposition in the synovial sheath of the tendon and/or increased thickness of the tendon retinacula (Figure 18-6).

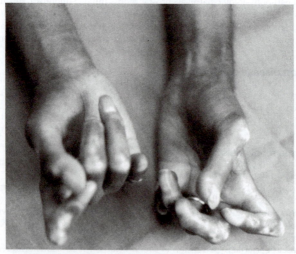

Figure 18-6. Articular and cutaneous involvement in systemic sclerosis. The skin is taut and thickened, leading to deformity and limited motility of the fingers. Note sclerodactyly and digital ulcerations.

48. **Discuss the three types of muscle abnormalities seen in SSc.**
    1. Mild proximal weakness due to a noninflammatory benign myopathy. On histology, this myopathy looks normal or shows muscle fiber type 2 atrophy. This pattern of fiber loss is seen with inactivity and corticosteroid use. The muscle enzymes are typically normal.
    2. Mild elevation of muscles enzymes with waxing and waning of symptoms. Muscle biopsy reveals interstitial fibrosis and fiber atrophy. Minimal inflammatory cell infiltration is noted. Should not be treated with corticosteroids.
    3. Inflammatory type of myopathy with elevated muscle enzymes (as seen with polymyositis). These patients are considered to have an overlap syndrome, and many fit the definition of mixed connective tissue disease. Needs to be treated with immunosuppressive therapy.

49. **What is the role of stem cell transplant in the therapy of SSc?**
    Anecdotally, hematopoietic stem cell transplantation (HSCT) has been reported to be effective in early (<4 years) SSc patients with poor prognostic signs (dcSSc, skin score >15 to 20, internal organ [lung, kidney] involvement). Two large multicenter trials (Scleroderma: Cyclophosphamide or Transplantation [SCOT] and Autologous Stem cell Transplantation International Scleroderma trial [ASTIS]) are ongoing to examine the effectiveness and toxicity of this therapy. Initial results show that patients who received HSCT had a greater mortality within the first 4 months, especially if they were past or current smokers. Among nonsmokers, HSCT had a 90% event-free survival rate compared to 60% if they received conventional intravenous cyclophosphamide therapy.

BIBLIOGRAPHY

Bouros D, Wells AU, Nicholson AG, et al: Histopathologic subsets of fibrosing alveolitis in patients with systemic sclerosis and their relationship to outcome, Am J Respir Crit Care Med 165:1581–1586, 2002.

Chang B, Schachna L, White B, et al: Natural history of mild-moderate pulmonary hypertension and the risk factors for severe pulmonary hypertension in scleroderma, J Rheumatol 33:269–274, 2006.

Christmann RB, Wells AU, Capelozzi VL, et al: Gastroesophageal reflux incites interstitial lung disease in systemic sclerosis: radiologic, histopathologic, and treatment evidence, Semin Arthritis Rheum 40:241–249, 2010.

Coghlan JG, Pope J, Denton CP, et al: Assessment of endpoints in pulmonary arterial hypertension associated with connective tissue disease, Curr Opin Pulm Med 16(Suppl 1):S27–S34, 2010.

Condliffe R, Kiely DG, Peacock AJ, et al: Connective tissue disease-pulmonary arterial hypertension in the modern treatment era, Am J Respir Crit Care Med 179:151–157, 2009.

Cuoma G, Zappia M, Iudici M, et al: The origin of tendon friction rubs in patients with systemic sclerosis: a sonographic explanation, Arthritis Rheum 64:1291–1293, 2012.

Cutolo M, Pizzorni C, Sulli A: Capillaroscopy, Best Pract Res Clin Rheumatol 22:1093–1108, 2008.

Fischer A, Bull TM, Steen VD, et al: Practical approach to screening for scleroderma-associated pulmonary arterial hypertension, Arthritis Care Res (Hoboken) 64:303–310, 2012.

Goh NS, Desai SR, Veeraraghavan S, et al: Interstitial lung disease in systemic sclerosis: a simple staging system, Am J Respir Crit Care Med 177:1248–1254, 2008.

Gyger G, Baron M: Gastrointestinal manifestations of scleroderma: recent progress in evaluation, pathogenesis, and management, Curr Rheumatol Rep 14:22–29, 2012.

Hoogen F, Khanna D, Fransen J, et al: 2013 Classification criteria for systemic sclerosis, Arthritis Rheum 65:2737–2747, 2013.

Hoyles RK, Ellis RW, Wellsbury J, et al: A multicenter, prospective, randomized, double-blind, placebo-controlled trial of corticosteroids and intravenous cyclophosphamide followed by oral azathioprine for the treatment of pulmonary fibrosis in scleroderma, Arthritis Rheum 54:3962–3970, 2006.

Mathai SC, Hummers LK, Champion HC, et al: Survival in pulmonary hypertension associated with the scleroderma spectrum of diseases: impact of interstitial lung disease, Arthritis Rheum 60:569–577, 2009.

Poormoghim H, Lucas M, Fertig N, et al: Systemic sclerosis sine scleroderma: demographic, clinical, and serologic features and survival in forty-eight patients, Arthritis Rheum 43:444–451, 2000.

Pope J, Harding S, Khimdas S, et al: Agreement with guidelines from a large database for management of systemic sclerosis: results from the Canadian Scleroderma Research Group, J Rheumatol 39:524–531, 2012.

Steen VD, Costantino JP, Shapiro AP, et al: Outcome of renal crisis in systemic sclerosis: relation to availability of angiotensin converting enzyme (ACE) inhibitors, Ann Intern Med 113:352–357, 1990.

Steen VD, Lucas M, Fertig N, et al: Pulmonary arterial hypertension and severe pulmonary fibrosis in systemic sclerosis patients with a nucleolar antibody, J Rheumatol 34:2230–2235, 2007.

Steen VD, Medsger TA: Changes in causes of death in systemic sclerosis, 1972-2002, Ann Rheum Dis 66:940–944, 2007.

Steen VD, Medsger TA: Epidemiology and natural history of systemic sclerosis, Rheum Dis Clin North Am 16:641–654, 1990.

Steen VD: Autoantibodies in systemic sclerosis, Semin Arthritis Rheum 35:35–42, 2005.

Tashkin DP, Elashoff R, Clements PJ, et al: Cyclophosphamide versus placebo in scleroderma lung disease, N Engl J Med 354:2655–2666, 2006.

Tashkin DP, Elashoff R, Clements PJ, et al: Effects of 1-year treatment with cyclophosphamide on outcomes at 2 years in scleroderma lung disease, Am J Respir Crit Care Med 176:1026–1034, 2007.

White B: Interstitial lung disease in scleroderma, Rheum Dis Clin North Am 29:371–390, 2003.

Williams MH, Das C, Handler CE, et al: Systemic sclerosis associated pulmonary hypertension: improved survival in the current era, Heart 92:926–932, 2006.

FURTHER READING

http://www.scleroderma.org

CHAPTER 19
SCLERODERMA MIMICS
Puja Chitkara, MD and Gregory J. Dennis, MD

KEY POINTS

1. One should suspect a disease mimicking scleroderma in any patient with skin induration who lacks Raynaud's, nailfold capillary abnormalities, sclerodactyly, and autoantibodies.
2. Scleredema and scleromyxedema can both be associated with a monoclonal paraprotein.
3. Eosinophilia may be absent at the time of clinical presentation of eosinophilic fasciitis.
4. Histologic confirmation of eosinophilic fasciitis requires a full thickness biopsy of skin, subcutis, fascia, and muscle.
5. Patients with severe kidney disease are at risk to develop nephrogenic systemic fibrosis (NSF) if exposed to gadolinium-containing contrast agents.

1. **What clinical characteristics separate conditions that mimic scleroderma from systemic sclerosis?**
   - Lack of Raynaud's phenomenon.
   - Lack of nailfold capillary abnormalities including dilatation and dropout.
   - Lack of calcinosis.
   - Lack of sclerodactyly or involvement of skin of the fingers.
   - Lack of autoantibody formation.

2. **List some of the diseases associated with skin abnormalities that may mimic the scleroderma seen in systemic sclerosis.**
   - Localized scleroderma syndromes.
     - Morphea.
     - Linear scleroderma.
   - Scleredema.
   - Scleromyxedema.
   - Eosinophilic syndromes.
     - Eosinophilic–myalgia syndrome.
     - Eosinophilic fasciitis.
     - Toxic oil syndrome.
   - Nephrogenic fibrosing neuropathy.
   - Chronic graft-versus-host disease.
   - Metabolic diseases.
     - Diabetic cheiroarthropathy (see Chapter 48).
     - Porphyria cutanea tarda.
     - Others (phenylketonuria, Werner syndrome, acromegaly).
   - Others.
     - POEMS.
     - Pachydermoperiostosis.
     - Complex regional pain syndrome (late stage) (see Chapter 65).

MORPHEA AND LINEAR SCLERODERMA

3. **What are the characteristics of localized scleroderma syndromes?**
   - **Morphea:** more common in Caucasians and adults. Can occur anywhere but spares the hands and fingers, is not associated with Raynaud's, and does not affect internal organs, which separates it from scleroderma clinically. Phototherapy is used for therapy. There are three subtypes:
     - Circumscribed: focal skin and subcutaneous fibrosis. Lesions are shiny and lack hair and exocrine glands similar to scleroderma. Borrelia infection should be excluded.
     - Generalized: defined as four or more lesions (>3 cm in size) that become confluent in two or more anatomical sites.
     - Pansclerotic: generalized involvement including the face, trunk, and extremities. Increased risk of cutaneous squamous cell cancers.

- **Linear scleroderma** (also known as linear morphea): more common in Caucasians and children. Affects a unilateral limb or rarely the scalp and face (en coup de sabre form). Can extend beyond skin to fascia, muscle, and bone leading to tissue atrophy. Not associated with Raynaud's or internal organ involvement but some patients have arthritis (10% to 15%). Neurologic symptoms and ocular disease can occur in the en coup de sabre form. Autoantibodies, such as antitopoisomerase II (not I), can be seen but are nonspecific. Methotrexate with or without systemic steroids is an effective therapy.

SCLEREDEMA AND SCLEROMYXEDEMA

4. What is scleredema?
Scleredema is characterized by firm, nonpitting skin edema ("woody") with normal epidermis that typically begins on the neck and upper back and spreads to the shoulders and trunk. The face and extremities are less commonly involved. The hands and feet are spared. Biopsies show normal epidermis but thickened dermis with deposition of acid mucopolysaccharides between collagen bundles. There are three types based on the underlying cause:
- Type I: scleredema adultorum of Buschke and scleredema neonatorum follow an infection or febrile illness with resolution occurring in months to years.
- Type II: scleredema with no preceding febrile illness and a slow, progressive course. Frequently develops a paraproteinemia (usually IgG or IgA). Rarely associated with another cancer.
- Type III: scleredema diabeticorum occurs in association with poorly controlled diabetes mellitus (type I or type II).

Unfortunately, there is no consistently effective therapy for any of these. Tamoxifen has been effective in case reports.

5. What is scleromyxedema?
Scleromyxedema (papular mucinosis) is characterized by a widespread eruption of small, nonpruritic, waxy papules on the face, neck, upper trunk, distal forearms, and hands but sparing the palms. Over 80% of individuals have an IgG monoclonal protein (usually IgG lambda) with 10% developing myeloma. Thyroid studies are normal. Skin biopsies show normal epidermis, mucin deposition in the dermis, fibroblast proliferation, and fibrosis. The pathophysiology is unknown but fibroblasts from these patients appear to be stimulated to produce large amounts of mucin. Mucin deposition can occur around blood vessels in visceral organs including esophagus, muscles, heart, nerves, and lungs leading to dysfunction. Joint pain and contractures can occur. Therapy is similar to that used in multiple myeloma, although the disease can progress even with eradication of the monoclonal paraprotein. Intravenous immunoglobulin has been used with success.

EOSINOPHILIC FASCIITIS (DIFFUSE FASCIITIS WITH EOSINOPHILIA)

6. Is eosinophilic fasciitis associated with ingestion of chemicals?
First described in 1974 by Dr. Lawrence Shulman, no association with the ingestion of chemicals has been convincingly demonstrated. Strenuous physical exertion may precede its onset in up to 50% of patients. Notably, two similar conditions, *eosinophilic–myalgia syndrome* (EMS) in the United States and *toxic oil syndrome* in Spain have been related to toxic exposures, L-tryptophan and aniline denatured rapeseed oil, respectively.

7. What are the three stages of eosinophilic fasciitis?
- Stage I: pitting and edema. There is usually simultaneous involvement in all affected areas. The most frequent pattern includes involvement of both the arms and legs in a symmetrical fashion with sparing of the fingers and toes. The proximal areas of the extremities are generally more affected than the distal. Raynaud's does not occur.
- Stage II: the initial manifestations of eosinophilic fasciitis (EF) are often followed by the development of severe induration of the skin and subcutaneous tissues of the affected areas. The skin becomes taut and woody with a coarse orange-peel appearance (*peau d'orange*). The groove sign is an indentation caused by retraction of the subcutaneous tissues along the tract of superficial veins and is best seen with elevation of the extremity. Although the induration often remains confined to the extremities, it may variably affect extensive areas of the trunk and face. A low-grade myositis with normal creatine phosphokinase (CPK) can occur.
- Stage III: because of involvement of the fascia, carpal tunnel syndrome is an early feature in many patients. Flexion contractures of the digits and extremities may occur as a consequence of the fascial involvement. Muscle atrophy can be prominent. Sclerodactyly and nailfold capillary abnormalities do not occur.

8. What laboratory and radiographic abnormalities usually occur in patients with EF?
Peripheral eosinophilia is present in 80% but not all cases. An elevated erythrocyte sedimentation rate, high C-reactive protein, and a polyclonal hypergammaglobulinemia are usually present. Aldolase can be elevated whereas CPK is normal in a significant number of patients. Magnetic resonance imaging (MRI) shows fascial thickening and enhancement of the fascia with gadolinium.

9. Is eosinophilia uniformly present throughout the course of a patient with EF illness?

No. Eosinophilia is often present only during the early stages of a patient's illness and tends to decline later in the illness. The degree of eosinophilia does not closely parallel disease activity and resolves quickly with corticosteroid therapy.

10. Is there any reason to expect hematologic abnormalities to be associated with EF?

The pathogenesis of these conditions is thought to involve autoimmune mechanisms. Hematologic problems have been significantly appreciated. Those described in a small number of patients include thrombocytopenia, aplastic anemia, myelodysplasia, and leukemia. These complications may occur at any time during the course of EF and do not correlate with the severity of disease.

11. How is the diagnosis of EF confirmed histologically?

Histologically, the diagnosis is best confirmed by performing a deep wedge en-bloc full thickness biopsy of an involved area. The biopsy should be deep enough to acquire skin, subcutis, fascia, and muscle for study. Although inflammation and fibrosis are generally found in all layers (except for the epidermis which is normal), they are usually most intense in the fascia. The inflammatory infiltrate consists of abundant lymphocytes, plasma cells, and histiocytes. Eosinophilic infiltration can be seen, especially early in the disease process, but is variably present.

12. Describe the course of illness in patients with EF.

If untreated, fascial inflammation will lead to joint contractures in 85% of patients. In addition, the skin that is initially indurated frequently may become bound down and develop a *peau d'orange* appearance. In some patients, the illness is self-limited with spontaneous improvement. Occasionally, complete remission can occur even after 2 or more years. Young age at onset and trunk involvement are poor prognostic signs.

13. Are any therapies effective in patients with EF?

High-dose prednisone (20 to 60 mg/day) often results in marked and rapid improvement in the eosinophilia and gradual improvement in the fasciitis and contractures. Hydroxychloroquine and methotrexate are most often used for treatment-resistant cases. Physical therapy to minimize flexion contractures is important. Strenuous physical exercise should be avoided.

NEPHROGENIC SYSTEMIC FIBROSIS

14. What is NSF?

NSF is a progressive fibrosing disorder occurring in patients with end-stage renal disease who have received gadolinium-containing contrast during an MRI procedure. Most patients are dialysis-dependent or have a glomerular filtration rate <15 mL/min (stage 5 chronic kidney disease). Some patients have developed NSF with less severe kidney disease.

15. Describe the typical course of a patient with NSF.

NSF occurs within days to weeks of an at-risk patient receiving gadolinium-containing contrast during MRI. Cutaneous features first involve lower extremities and extend proximally. The face is not involved. Patients first experience itching or burning followed by development of papules and plaques. The skin may develop a *peau d'orange* appearance and "cobblestone" texture over the upper arms, back, and thighs. The skin is very indurated and may develop hyperpigmentation. Flexion deformities of fingers, elbows, and knees are commonly disabling. Fibrosis of any visceral organ can occur and may be symptomatic. Raynaud's does not occur.

16. What are the characteristic laboratory abnormalities and histologic features in a patient with NSF?

There are no diagnostic laboratory tests. A paraproteinemia or scleroderma-associated autoantibodies are not present. Therefore, the diagnosis is made by clinical evaluation and confirmed by a deep skin biopsy. This biopsy shows increased number of dermal fibroblasts, increased dermal collagen, increased mucin deposition, no inflammatory cells, and increased CD34+ fibrocytes and CD68+ monocytes–macrophages from the circulation. Gadolinium has been demonstrated in the tissue by mass spectrometry.

17. Describe the therapy and prognosis of NSF.

There is no effective therapy. Early renal transplantation has helped some patients. Thalidomide and oral imatinib mesylate have been anecdotally reported as being effective. Patients with NSF have a three times increased mortality. Therefore, the best therapy is prevention. Patients with stage 4 and stage 5 chronic kidney disease should not receive gadolinium-containing contrast during MRI.

BIBLIOGRAPHY

Antic M, Lautenschlager S, Itin PH, et al: Eosinophilic fasciitis 30 years after what do we really know? Report of 11 patients and review of the literature, Dermatology 213:93–101, 2006.
Bardin T, Richette P: Nephrogenic systemic fibrosis, Curr Opin Rheumatol 22:54–58, 2010.
Boin F, Hummers LK: Scleroderma-like fibrosing disorders, Rheum Dis Clin North Am 34:199–220, 2008.

Cokonis Georgakis CD, Falasca G, Georgakis A, et al: Scleromyxedema, Clin Dermatol 24:493–497, 2006.
Cuffy MC, Singh M, Formica R, et al: Renal transplantation for nephrogenic systemic fibrosis: a case report and review of the literature, Nephrol Dialysis Transplant 26:1099–1101, 2011.
Endo Y, Tamura A, Matsushima Y, et al: Eosinophilic fasciitis: report of two cases and a systemic review of the literature dealing with clinical variables that predict outcome, Clin Rheumatol 26:1445–1451, 2007.
Fett N, Werth VP: Update on morphea: part I. Epidemiology, clinical presentation, and pathogenesis, J Am Acad Dermatol 64:217–228, 2011.
Fett N, Werth VP: Update on morphea: part II. Outcome measures and treatment, J Am Acad Dermatol 64:231–242, 2011.
Nashel J, Steen V: Scleroderma mimics, Curr Rheumatol Rep 14:39–46, 2012.
Shulman LE: Diffuse fasciitis with eosinophilia: a new syndrome, Arthritis Rheum 20:133, 1977.
Sullivan EA, Kamb ML, Jones JL, et al: The natural history of eosinophilia–myalgia syndrome in a tryptophan-exposed cohort in South Carolina, Arch Intern Med 156:973–979, 1996.
Zulian F, Athreya BH, Laxer R, et al: Juvenile localized scleroderma: clinical and epidemiological features in 750 children. An international study, Rheumatology 45:614–620, 2006.
Zulian F, Martini G, Vallongo C, et al: Methotrexate therapy in juvenile localized scleroderma: a randomized, double-blind, placebo-controlled trial, Arthritis Rheum 63:1998–2006, 2011.

Further Reading

http://www.icnfdr.org/

CHAPTER 20
INFLAMMATORY MUSCLE DISEASE
Sterling G. West, MD and Robert T. Spencer, MD

KEY POINTS

1. Polymyositis (PM) and dermatomyositis (DM) are characterized by proximal muscle weakness, elevated muscle enzymes, and abnormal electromyogram.
2. The typical skin manifestations of DM include heliotrope rash, Gottron's papules, and abnormal nailfold capillaries. Skin ulcerations and anti-155/140 antibodies signal the presence of an associated underlying malignancy.
3. Myositis-specific autoantibodies can predict extramuscular manifestations, response to therapy, and prognosis.
4. The antisynthetase syndrome is characterized by myositis, interstitial lung disease (ILD), arthritis, mechanic's hands, and Raynaud's phenomenon.
5. Inclusion body myositis should be considered in patients over age 50 with proximal and distal muscle weakness, neuropathic features, and poor response to steroid therapy.

---

1. **How are the idiopathic inflammatory myopathies classified?**
   Although several classification schemes have been devised, the system proposed by Bohan and Peter in 1975 remains the one most commonly referred to:
   1. Adult polymyositis (PM)
   2. Adult dermatomyositis (DM)
   3. PM/DM associated with malignancy (12% of all myositis patients; 50% of myositis patients >age 65 years)
   4. Childhood (juvenile) DM
   5. PM/DM associated with other connective tissue disorders (11% to 40% of all myositis patients)
   6. Sporadic inclusion body myositis (s-IBM) has recently been added to this list of idiopathic inflammatory myopathies and may be one of the most common accounting for 16% to 28% of all inflammatory myopathies.

   Other classification systems add the following to the above list of inflammatory diseases of the muscle:
   - Other forms of inflammatory myopathy
     - Myositis associated with eosinophilia
     - Myositis ossificans
     - Focal myositis
     - Giant cell myositis
   - Myopathies caused by infections
   - Myopathies caused by drugs and toxins

2. **What are some of the epidemiologic features of PM/DM?**
   - Annual incidence of 2 to 10 cases/million
   - Peak age of onset is bimodal in distribution for dermatomyositis: one peak at 5 to 15 years of age, and the other at 45 to 65 years. Polymyositis rarely occurs in patients less than age 15 with mean age of onset 50 to 60 years of age.
   - The female to male ratio is 2–3:1 overall. The female to male ratio in childhood DM is close to 1:1. In PM/DM associated with other connective tissue disorders it is 8–10:1.
   - In the United States, African Americans are affected more commonly than caucasians at a ratio of 3–4:1 in some studies.

3. **What are the major diagnostic criteria for PM/DM? Describe their features.**
   - **Proximal motor weakness**: Weakness occurs earliest and insidiously over 3 to 6 months. It occurs most severely around the shoulder/pelvic girdles and neck flexors. Ocular and facial motor weakness is strikingly unusual and should make one consider another diagnosis. Pain is typically absent or minimal (25%) and if significant should suggest a necrotizing autoimmune myopathy (NAM).
   - Other striated muscle groups that can be involved include pharyngeal muscles causing dysphonia and upper esophageal muscles causing dysphagia (10% to 30%). Nasal regurgitation of fluids can occur. Involvement of these muscles indicates more severe disease.

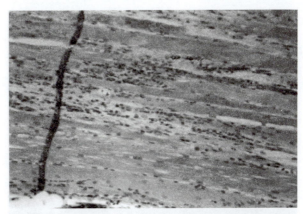

Figure 20-1. Muscle biopsy demonstrating inflammatory infiltrate and muscle fiber necrosis in a patient with polymyositis.

- **Elevated serum muscle enzymes**: Creatine kinase (CK) is elevated in almost all patients at some time during the course of active disease. Other markers of muscle damage include elevated levels of aldolase, myoglobin, aspartate and alanine aminotransferase (AST and ALT), and lactate dehydrogenase (LDH). Myoglobinuria can be seen in active disease.
- **Abnormal neurodiagnostic studies**: The electromyogram (EMG) in PM/DM has a good sensitivity (85%) but low specificity (33%). It shows a typical but not specific pattern consisting of: (1) increased insertional activity with spontaneous fibrillations; (2) myopathic low amplitude and short duration polyphasic motor unit action potentials (MUAPs); (3) complex repetitive discharges. Nerve conduction velocity (NCV) studies are normal in the idiopathic inflammatory myopathies, with the exception of inclusion-body myositis in which neuropathic disease can develop along with the myopathy.
- **Muscle biopsy**: Muscle biopsy should be performed in most cases to confirm the suspected diagnosis. The histologic pattern can be helpful both diagnostically and prognostically (Question 14) (Figure 20-1).
- **Characteristic rash of dermatomyositis**: Skin biopsy shows an interface dermatitis similar to systemic lupus erythematosus (SLE) (Question 4).

4. Describe the dermatologic manifestations of dermatomyositis.

Heliotrope (lilac-colored) **rash**: purple to erythematous rash affecting the eyelids, malar region, forehead, and nasolabial folds. (Eyelids and nasolabial folds are typically spared in the rash of SLE).
Gottron's papules: purple to erythematous flat or raised lesions over the dorsal surface of metacarpals and interphalangeal regions of the fingers (i.e., knuckles). Can also occur over extensor surfaces of wrists, elbows, and knees.
V-sign rash: confluent erythematous rash over the anterior chest and neck.
Shawl-sign rash: erythematous rash over the shoulders and proximal arms.
Holster-sign rash: erythematous rash over lateral aspect of proximal thighs
Mechanic's hands: characterized by cracking and fissuring of the skin of the finger pads, *especially the radial side of the index finger*. Associated with presence of antisynthetase antibodies. More commonly seen in PM than DM.
Nailfold abnormalities: periungual erythema, cuticular overgrowth, dilated capillary loops. (See Chapter 74.)
Subcutaneous calcification: seen nearly exclusively in the juvenile form of DM; can be very extensive.
Dermatomyositis mimics: these can include cutaneous manifestations of trichinosis, allergic contact dermatitis, and drug reactions (hydroxyurea, penicillamine, diclofenac, anti-TNF agents).
PEARL: a patient with proximal muscle weakness, elevated muscle enzymes, and the characteristic rash of DM rarely needs a muscle biopsy to confirm the diagnosis.

5. What measures can be taken to maximize muscle biopsy yield? How can muscle magnetic resonance imaging help?

- Biopsy a muscle that is clearly weak, but not severely so.
- Biopsy the muscle contralateral to one that is abnormal by EMG (i.e., perform neurodiagnostic studies unilaterally, and biopsy the contralateral side based on EMG results). Do not biopsy a muscle that has undergone recent (<2 to 4 weeks) EMG evaluation to avoid spurious results (i.e., EMG artifact).
  - Do not biopsy a muscle within three months of an episode of rhabdomyolysis.
- **Magnetic resonance imaging (MRI) scanning** of the muscle can be helpful to direct muscle biopsy with a sensitivity of 96% to 100%. Areas of inflamed muscle demonstrate increased signal on T2-weighted images with fat suppression (STIR images) but not T1-weighted images, denoting areas of edema/inflammation. In chronic disease, MRI can also show fatty degeneration on T1-weighted images which is unlikely to improve with medications (Figure 20-2).

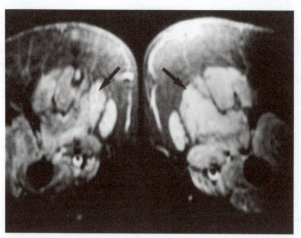

Figure 20-2. MRI scan of a patient with polymyositis. T2-weighted images demonstrate increased signal intensity of affected muscle tissue *(arrows)*.

6. What is amyopathic dermatomyositis?

Occasionally, the cutaneous manifestations of DM occur in the absence of clinically apparent muscle involvement. Such is referred to as **clinically amyopathic dermatomyositis (CADM)**. Perhaps half or more of such patients will develop muscle disease over time, but a significant proportion will manifest skin-limited disease only. This form can be associated with malignancy whereas other patients may develop extramuscular manifestations such as rapidly progressive interstitial lung disease even in the absence of myositis. Over half of these patients have anti-MDA-5 (anti-CADM-140) autoantibodies (Question 12).

7. List some of the extramuscular or extradermatologic manifestations of PM/DM.

Constitutional symptoms: fatigue, low-grade fever, weight loss
Musculoskeletal: arthralgias/arthritis (20% to 70%); associated with antisynthetase antibody syndrome
Pulmonary: interstitial lung disease (70% of patients with antisynthetase antibodies); aspiration pneumonia; respiratory muscle weakness; pulmonary hypertension
Gastrointestinal: esophageal dysmotility (10% to 30%); reflux due to lower esophageal sphincter weakness (15% to 50%); rectal incontinence due to sphincter ani weakness; intestinal perforation due to vasculitis (primarily in juvenile DM)
Cardiac: ECG abnormalities (dysrhythmias, conduction blocks); myocarditis
Vascular: vasculitis (juvenile DM), skin ulcerations (juvenile DM); livedo reticularis, Raynaud's phenomenon (20% to 40%)
Other: manifestations of other connective tissue diseases when PM/DM occurs in "overlap" syndromes or in association with mixed connective tissue disease (MCTD)

8. Is there an association between PM/DM and underlying neoplastic disease?

Associated cancers are present in about 10% to 20% of adult (not juvenile) patients with PM/DM and over 50% of patients who develop PM/DM after age 65 years old. Most have DM (80%) with the remainder having PM (20%). The malignancy is present at onset of myositis or within the first year in 68%. If associated with a malignancy, the cancer almost always occurs within 3 years of myositis onset. Cancers reported in association with PM/DM include, among others, breast, lung, pancreas, stomach, colon, ovary, and Hodgkin's lymphoma. Taiwanese patients also have nasopharyngeal and cervical tumors. This association has long been controversial, but recent studies have shown a 3–6 times increased risk for malignancy in DM and a 1.4–2 times increased risk for PM. Therefore, it is generally advised that patients with PM, and especially those with adult DM, be screened for underlying neoplastic disease. This screen should be age appropriate and include a complete history and exam (including breast, pelvis, prostate), stool occult blood testing, chest x-ray, mammogram, and routine laboratory tests. Recently, the myositis-specific autoantibody, **anti-155/140**, directed against the transcription intermediary factor 1 (TIF-1) family proteins has been reported to be associated with adult cancer-associated DM. Notably, the myositis-specific antisynthetase antibodies (anti-Jo-1 etc.) and anti-Mi-2 have a negative association with malignancy. Some clinicians also recommend an abdominal/pelvic CT scan owing to the high incidence of lymphoma and ovarian cancer, whereas others feel a positron emission tomography (PET) scan is a cost-effective screen. Although controversial some physicians advocate testing for tumor markers associated with common cancers (CEA, CA 125, CA 19-9). If the initial cancer screen is negative, the physician should be alert for future development of cancer over the next 3 to 5 years. A PET scan yearly for 3 to 5 years may be a cost-effective method for screening.
PEARL: Ulcerative skin lesions in an adult DM patient are highly associated with an underlying malignancy.

9. **Which laboratory abnormalities are seen in PM/DM?**
   - Nonspecific abnormalities
     Elevated muscle enzymes: The combination of elevated creatine phosphokinse (CPK), aldolase, AST, and CPK MB >2% to 3% of total CPK is highly characteristic of an inflammatory myopathy. CPK MB is released by regenerating skeletal muscle fibers (not the heart) which occurs in patients with an inflammatory myositis and not in other causes of myopathies. Notably, some PM/DM patients have an elevated aldolase but a normal CPK.
     Erythrocyte sedimentation rate (elevated in 50%)
     C-reactive protein: may be normal; when elevated it can indicate muscle fiber necrosis and resistance to therapy
   - Myositis-associated autoantibodies
     ANA (50% to 80%)
     Anti-RNP antibody (MCTD and "overlap" syndromes)
     Anti-PM-Scl antibody (PM-scleroderma overlap with nucleolar staining ANA)
     Anti-Ku antibody (PM-scleroderma overlap)
   - Myositis-specific autoantibodies (Questions 11 and 12)

10. **Does an elevated serum CPK MB band indicate myocardial involvement?**
    Elevations in CPK MB do not correlate with the presence or extent of myocardial disease, because regenerating skeletal muscle fibers release this isoform of the enzyme. Troponin I is elevated in PM/DM patients with myocardial involvement.

11. **What are some of the more common myositis-specific autoantibodies? (Table 20-1)**

12. **What is the clinical significance of myositis-specific autoantibodies?**
    The presence of myositis-specific autoantibodies (MSAs) helps to predict clinical manifestations and prognosis.
    - **Antisynthetase syndrome:** this syndrome is seen in myositis patients with antibodies directed against amino-acyl t-RNA synthetases which are in charge of facilitating amino acid binding to its cognate t-RNA. The most common is anti-Jo-1 which is directed against histidyl-tRNA synthetase and is present in 15% to 30% of PM patients and 10% of DM patients. The other antisynthetase antibodies are in less than 3% to 5% of PM/DM patients. Patients never have more than one of these MSAs. The antisynthetase syndrome is characterized by:
      - Myositis, interstitial lung disease (40% to 90%), Raynaud's phenomenon (60%), symmetric nonerosive small joint arthritis (60%), mechanic's hands (70%), and occasionally fever. ANA is typically negative since these MSAs stain cytoplasmic antigens.
      - The ILD may be the initial presentation and/or predominant symptom in up to 20% of patients. It may be mild and steroid responsive or severe and resistant to therapy. Lung disease characterized histopathologically as cryptogenic organizing pneumonia is more responsive to therapy than other pathologies. Patients with anti-PL-7 and anti-PL-12 are more likely to have severe ILD and mild or absent myositis.
      - Some patients also have anti-SSA/Ro antibodies. These patients have worse arthritis and their myositis is more resistant to therapy.
      - Up to 5% to 8% of antisynthetase syndrome patients have overlap features of another connective tissue disease (SLE, SS, etc.).
      - Myositis patients with these MSAs rarely if ever have an associated cancer.
    - **Anti-signal recognition particle (SRP) syndrome:** this syndrome typically has a very acute and severe onset of polymyositis with significant muscle pain due to muscle fiber necrosis. Has increased incidence of cardiac involvement. Poor overall response to corticosteroid therapy with 5 year survival 30%. The autoantibody is directed against a 54-kDa protein in an RNA complex involved with intracytoplasmic protein translocation. ANA is negative.

Table 20-1. Myositis-specific Autoantibodies

AUTOANTIBODY	ANTIGEN	PREVALENCE PM/DM	CLINICAL ASSOCIATION	HLA DISSOCIATION
Antisynthetase*	Aminoacyl-tRNA synthetase	20% to 50%	Antisynthetase syndrome	DRw52, DR3
Anti-SRP	Signal recognition particle	5%	Severe, resistant PM	DRw52, DR5
Anti-Mi-2	Helicase components of histone deacetylase complexes	5% to 30%	Classic DM	DRw53, DR7

*Frequency in idiopathic inflammatory myositis: anti Jo-1 (histidyl) (15% to 20%), PL-7 (threonyl) (5% to 10%), PL-12 (alanyl) (<5%), EJ (glycyl) (5% to 10%), OJ (isoleucyl) (<5%), KS (asparaginyl) (<5%), Zo (phenylalanyl) (<1%), Ha-YRS (tyrosyl) (<1%), Mas (serine) (<1%).

- **Anti-Mi-2 syndrome:** syndrome characterized by acute onset of classic skin (V and shawl sign), periungual/cuticle overgrowth, and muscle features of dermatomyositis. It is seen in 5% to 30% of DM patients and occasionally in PM patients. Manifestations respond very well to corticosteroids with 5-year survival over 90%. The autoantibody targets the chromodomain helicase DNA binding protein (CHD4) which is part of the NuRD complex that participates in the remodeling of chromatin by deacetylating histones. Patients have a positive ANA with speckled pattern.
- **Anti-155/140:** this MSA is seen in juvenile DM and adult cancer-associated DM. Patients have heliotrope rash and Gottron's papules. It is present in 23% to 29% of juvenile DM patients and is not associated with cancer. However, in adult DM patients, the sensitivity for diagnosing cancer-associated DM is up to 78% and specificity is 89%. The diagnostic OR is 27 with a positive predictive value of 58% and negative predictive value 95%. The autoantibody targets transcription intermediary factor 1 (TIF-1) family proteins, especially TIF-1gamma. Notably TIF-1 proteins are interferon responsive and have both positive and negative roles in carcinogenesis including p53 (tumor suppressor) regulation. Patients have a low titer positive ANA with a speckled and homogenous pattern.
- **Anti-MDA-5 (anti-CADM-140):** patients with this MSA present with DM with skin ulcerations, palmar papules, and rapidly progressive ILD (70% to 95%). Some patients (20%) have clinically amyopathic DM (hence the name of the autoantibody, anti-CADM). The overall prognosis is poor. This MSA targets the melanoma differentiation-associated gene 5 protein which is a cytoplasmic RNA helicase that has an important role in the innate immune system response during RNA viral infections. ANA is negative.
- **Others:** anti-SSAE (5% DM patients); anti-PMS-1 (7% PM/DM patients), anti-MJ (NXP-2) (25% of juvenile DM especially with calcinosis).

13. What type of myopathy is associated with statin therapy?

The HMG-CoA reductase inhibitors (statins) can cause myalgias and cramps with or without a mildly elevated creatine kinase level in 1 in 10,000 individuals on low doses of statins and up to 1% of individuals on high doses. A small percentage of patients can develop a severe polymyositis that does not resolve with discontinuation of the statin and may require immunosuppressive therapy. These patients are characterized by having **anti-200/100 antibodies** that target HMG-CoA reductase. Notably muscle biopsies characteristically show muscle necrosis *without* inflammation. Patients prone to develop a statin myopathy appear to have a genetic variant (C allele) of the *SLCO1B1* gene on chromosome 12 which codes for a protein involved with the uptake of statins and other compounds into the liver. Up to 2% of the population have two copies of this variant allele which gives them a 15% risk of developing a statin myopathy since more statin is available for uptake by the muscle. Interestingly other lipid-lowering agents can also cause a necrotizing myopathy including fibric acid derivatives (gemfibrozil) and nicotinic acid.

14. Describe the four histologic patterns seen on muscle biopsies in patients with an idiopathic inflammatory myositis.

- **Dermatomyositis:** this is a complement-mediated process with the microvasculature being the primary target. Biopsies show perivascular inflammatory infiltrates that predominate in the perimysium and perifasicular endomysium leading to **perifasicular atrophy of muscle fibers** which is highly characteristic of this pattern. The infiltrate consists of T cells (CD4+ >CD8+), plasmacytoid dendritic cells, and some B cells. Upregulation of MHC Class I antigens on muscle fibers in the perifasicular areas is common. Microvascular changes are prominent. Note that this pattern can be seen in patients who do not have the characteristic rash of dermatomyositis.
- **Polymyositis:** this is a T cell-mediated process with the myocyte being the primary target. It is characterized by focal endomysial infiltrates (CD8+ cytotoxic T cells) that surround and invade non-necrotic muscle fibers. In contrast to DM, the vasculature is spared. MHC Class I antigens are upregulated on the surface of most muscle fibers.
- **Necrotizing autoimmune myopathy (NAM):** presents similar to PM except for more muscle pain. It differs histologically from PM by the presence of marked muscle necrosis with regeneration. There is an invasion of macrophages but a lack of lymphocytic infiltrates and lack of widespread MHC Class I upregulation on muscle fibers. This pattern is associated with anti-SRP syndrome, statin therapy (anti 200/100), malignancy, HIV-associated myositis, and in some patients with the antisynthetase syndrome.
- **Unspecified myositis:** this is the second most common pattern. There is an inflammatory infiltrate without specific localization or upregulation of MHC Class I expression. This is most commonly seen in overlap myositis, especially anti-Ku and anti-PM-Scl.

15. Which conditions should be considered in the differential diagnosis of inflammatory myopathies? (Box 20-1)

16. What is the approach to treatment of PM/DM?

Poor prognostic features in PM/DM patients include severe weakness, dysphagia, respiratory muscle weakness, ILD, myocardial involvement, anti-SRP/anti-MDA-5/anti-155/140 antibodies, necrotizing myopathy on pathology, and malignancy. All patients need corticosteroids and immunosuppressive agents early.

Box 20-1. Differential Diagnosis of Myopathies

Drug and toxin-induced myopathies
(especially statins, IFNα, d-penicillamine, colchicine, amiodarone, antimalarials, AZT, alcohol, cocaine, antifungals, anti-TNF inhibitors)

Neuromuscular disorders
Muscular dystrophies (e.g., Duchenne's)
Neuromuscular junction disorders (e.g., myasthenia gravis, Eaton-Lambert syndrome)
Denervating conditions (e.g., amyotrophic lateral sclerosis)

Endocrine disorders
Hypothyroidism (may see CK as high as 3000)
Hyperthyroidism
Acromegaly
Cushing's disease
Addison's disease

Miscellaneous
Sarcoidosis
Other rheumatic disorders (e.g., polymyalgia rheumatica, fibromyalgia syndrome, inflammatory arthritides, vasculitis)
Carcinomatous neuromyopathy
Acute rhabdomyolysis

Infectious myositis
Bacterial (*Staphylococcus, Streptococcus, Borrelia burgdorferi*)
Viral (e.g., HIV, adenovirus, influenza)
Parasitic (e.g., *Toxoplasma, Trichinella, Taenia*)

Metabolic myopathies
Glycogen storage diseases (e.g., McArdle's or myophosphorylase deficiency, acid maltase deficiency)
Abnormalities of lipid metabolism (e.g., carnitine deficiency, carnitine palmitoyl transferase deficiency)
Mitochondrial myopathies
Nutritional disorders (malabsorption, vitamin D and E deficiencies)
Electrolyte disorders (hypocalcemia and hypercalcemia, hypokalemia, hypophosphatemia)
Organ failure (uremia, liver failure)
Amyloidosis

Corticosteroids (CS) are the mainstay of therapy for PM/DM. Commonly, prednisone is started at a dose of 1 to 1.5 mg/kg/day (up to 80 mg/day) in divided doses, and the dose is maintained until remission is achieved (improved strength and normalization of muscle enzymes). IV pulse methyl-prednisolone is used for life-threatening disease. Subsequently, the dose is slowly tapered while monitoring for recurrence of disease activity. Most experts recommend combining corticosteroids with immunosuppressive agents from the onset of therapy to facilitate the steroid taper since over 50% fail CS alone.

Immunosuppressive agents are used early to help reduce the corticosteroid dose. Methotrexate (up to 25 mg/wk) and azathioprine (2 to 3 mg/kg/day) are used most often but can take up to several months to be maximally effective. Mycophenylate mofetil (MMF) (1 to 1.5 g BID) and leflunomide have also been used. MMF may be more effective for ILD and rash. Cyclophosphamide or combinations of immunosuppressive agents (methotrexate plus azathioprine) are used rarely but have been reported to be of benefit in refractory and life threatening disease and in juvenile DM with vasculitis. Hydroxychloroquine and avoidance of the sun can be helpful adjuncts in treating the cutaneous manifestations of DM.

Tacrolimus (0.1 mg/kg/day; 2 to 5 mg BID) is effective in resistant T cell-mediated PM and lung disease (especially cryptogenic organizing pneumonia). Cyclosporine (3 to 5 mg/kg/day) has also been used with success but tacrolimus seems to be better tolerated.

Intravenous immunoglobulin (IVIG) (2 g/kg over 5 days [0.4 g/kg/day] initially, followed by monthly 3-day courses) has been reported to be effective in severe, refractory DM especially in patients with dysphagia. Although not FDA-approved most clinicians feel it also works in patients with PM.

Rituximab has recently been shown to be effective in DM patients and in PM patients with myositis-specific antibodies. In the future, anti-interferon α (IFNα) therapy may be beneficial in DM patients where IFNα appears to be involved in disease pathogenesis.

Repository corticotropin injection (H.P. Acthar gel): this is derived from pituitary glands obtained from pigs. It contains not only adrenocorticotropic hormone but other melanocortins that are suspected to have immunomodulating properties when they bind to one of five melanocortin receptors. This is FDA approved for treatment of DM/PM. Because of its cost ($28,000/5-mL vial) it is reserved for resistant cases. Each 5-mL vial has a concentration of 80 USP units/mL. The recommended dose is 80 USP units subcutaneously twice a week for 3 months then attempt to decrease the dose.

In the initial stages of disease, when muscle inflammation is most severe and when the patient is most weak, **rehabilitation** is recommended to involve only passive/active assisted range of motion exercises. Later, as strength returns and muscle inflammation subsides, exercise for strengthening can slowly be added to the physical therapy regimen. All patients should receive appropriate vaccinations as well as osteoporosis and pneumocystis prophylaxis.

17. **What is the overall prognosis for these disorders?**

    Clinical subgroups: Similar 5-year survival (5YS) rates are seen in idiopathic PM/DM and in those cases with associated connective tissue diseases (77% to 85%). Old age, ILD, dysphagia, cardiac involvement, and non-white race are associated with a poor prognosis (5YS = 40%). In patients with associated neoplastic disease, a much poorer survival rate is observed.

Table 20-2. IBM vs. Polymyositis

	IBM	POLYMYOSITIS
Demographics	M > F Age >50	F > M All ages
Muscle involvement	Proximal and distal Asymmetric	Proximal Symmetric
Other organ involvement	Neuropathy	Interstitial lung disease, arthritis, heart involvement
Antinuclear antibodies	Sometimes	Sometimes
Myositis-specific antibodies	No	Yes
EMG	Myopathic and neuropathic	Myopathic
Muscle biopsy	CD8+T-cell infiltrate Red-rimmed vacuoles with beta-amyloid	CD8+T-cell infiltrate
Response to immunosuppressive therapy	No	Frequent

Serologic subgroups: Patients with the anti-Mi-2 antibody appear to have a very favorable prognosis, with a 5YS of >90%. Patients who are myositis-specific antibody negative and those with anti-synthetase antibodies have a less favorable prognosis, but still have 5YS rates of >65%. The worst prognosis is seen in patients with an associated anti-SRP antibody, in whom 5YS rates are approximately 30%. Patients with myositis and anti-MDA-5 also do poorly primarily due to their lung disease whereas those with anti-155/140 and malignancy do the worst.

18. What is sporadic inclusion body myositis?

Sporadic inclusion body myositis (s-IBM) predominantly affects white males over the age of 50. The onset of painless weakness is slow and insidious over months to years. Proximal muscles are involved, but distal muscles (forearm finger flexors) are also affected early in the disease course. Weakness is usually bilateral, but asymmetry is common. The legs, especially the anterior thigh muscles, are typically affected more than the arms, and muscle atrophy can be prominent. Dysphagia is common and a late manifestation. At presentation, CPK may be normal (20% to 30%) and if elevated is less than 600 to 800 mg/dL.

Some patients have a mild peripheral neuropathy with loss of deep tendon reflexes. An EMG usually shows both myopathic and neuropathic changes. Extraskeletal muscle involvement of the lungs, joints, and heart rarely occurs in these patients. There may be an association with Sjögren's syndrome but the risk of an associated malignancy is very low. Antinuclear antibodies can be present (<20%), but myositis-specific autoantibodies (e.g., anti-Jo-1) do not occur. Recently an antibody against a 43-kDa muscle autoantigen has been described in 50% of patients. Muscle biopsy shows foci of chronic inflammatory cells (mainly CD8+ T lymphocytes) within the endomysium and no evidence of perifascicular atrophy. MHC Class I antigens are expressed on muscle fibers separating it from hereditary forms of IBM that are due to mutations of a specific isomerase gene involved in aminosugar metabolism. The characteristic findings in s-IBM on muscle biopsy are **red-rimmed vacuoles** containing beta-amyloid seen best on Gomori-Trichrome staining. Patients respond poorly to immunosuppressive therapy, and the course is typically progressive. Rarely a patient will respond to prednisone alone or in combination with methotrexate or azathioprine so patients are typically treated for 3 to 6 months to see if they improve.

19. How does inclusion body myositis differ from polymyositis?

Despite IBM and polymyositis both being inflammatory myopathies, there are several clinical and immunologic differences that distinguish between them (Table 20-2).

PEARL: a patient with PM who fails to respond to prednisone should be reexamined for IBM.

20. How do you separate steroid myopathy from a polymyositis exacerbation?

Polymyositis patients initially responding to prednisone may later complain of weakness while maintained on prednisone, especially when greater than 20 mg/day. Keep in mind that this may represent development of a steroid myopathy. To separate the two, look at the CPK. Steroid myopathy does not cause an elevated CPK or aldolase because it causes type IIb muscle fiber *atrophy*, whereas polymyositis causes inflammation with muscle fiber *necrosis* causing release of muscle enzymes, including CPK. If still not certain, a muscle MRI with STIR images will identify if active inflammation is still present.

BIBLIOGRAPHY

Amato AA, Barohn RJ: Inclusion body myositis: old and new concepts, J Neurol Neurosurg Psychiatry 80:1186–1193, 2009.
Andras C, Ponyi A, Constantin T, et al: Dermatomyositis and polymyositis associated with malignancy: 21 year retrospective study, J Rheumatol 35:438–444, 2008.

Chaisson NF, Paik J, Orbai A-M, et al: A novel dermato-pulmonary syndrome associated with MDA-5 antibodies: report of 2 cases and review of the literature, Medicine 91:220–228, 2012.

Dalakas MC, Illa I, Dambrosia JM, et al: A controlled trial of high-dose intravenous immune globulin infusions as treatment for dermatomyositis, N Engl J Med 329:1993, 1993.

Del Grande F, Carrino JA, Del Grande M, et al: Magnetic resonance imaging of inflammatory myopathies, Top Magn Reson Imaging 22:39–43, 2011.

Fathi M, Lundberg I, Tornling G: Pulmonary complications of polymyositis and dermatomyositis, Semin Respir Critical Care Med 28:451–458, 2007.

Greenberg SA: Inflammatory myopathies: evaluation and management, Semin Neurol 28:241–249, 2008.

Gunawardena H, Betteridge ZE, McHugh NJ: Myositis-specific autoantibodies: their clinical and pathologic significance in disease expression, Rheumatology 48:607–612, 2009.

Lazarou IN, Guerne PA: Classification, diagnosis, and management of idiopathic inflammatory myopathies, J Rheumatol 40:550–564, 2013.

Mammen AL, Chung T, Christopher-Stine L, et al: Autoantibodies against HMG CoA reductase in patients with statin-associated autoimmune myopathy, Arthritis Rheum 63:713–721, 2011.

Mann HF, Vencovsky J: Clinical trials roundup in idiopathic inflammatory myopathies, Curr Opin Rheumatol 23:605–611, 2011.

Oddis C, Reed A, Aggarwal R, et al: Rituximab in the treatment of refractory adult and juvenile dermatomyositis and adult polymyositis: a randomized, placebo-phase trial, Arthritis Rheum 65:314–324, 2013.

Sato S, Kuwana M: Clinically amyopathic dermatomyositis, Curr Opinion Rheumatol 22:639–643, 2010.

Trallero-Araguás E, Rodrigo-Pendás JÁ, Selva-O'Callaghan A, et al: Usefulness of anti-p155 autoantibody for diagnosing cancer-associated dermatomyositis: a systemic review and meta-analysis, Arthritis Rheum 64:523–532, 2012.

Wilkes MR, Sereika SM, Fertig N, et al: Treatment of antisynthetase-associated interstitial lung disease with tacrolimus, Arthritis Rheum 52:2439–2446, 2005.

FURTHER READING

www.myositis.org

CHAPTER 21: MIXED CONNECTIVE TISSUE DISEASE, OVERLAP SYNDROMES, AND UNDIFFERENTIATED CONNECTIVE TISSUE DISEASE

Vance J. Bray, MD

KEY POINTS

1. Mixed connective tissue disease (MCTD) manifests overlap features of systemic sclerosis (SSc), systemic lupus erythematosus (SLE), and polymyositis (PM) associated with high titer anti-U1-RNP antibodies.
2. Severe renal disease, neurologic disease, or the absence of Raynaud's phenomenon should suggest a disease other than MCTD.
3. Pulmonary arterial hypertension (PAH) and/or interstitial lung disease are major causes of mortality in patients with MCTD.
4. Up to half of patients presenting with features of a connective tissue disease (CTD) are undifferentiated and do not fulfill criteria for a defined CTD.
5. One third to half of patients with an undifferentiated CTD evolve into a defined CTD within 3 years from initial diagnosis.

1. **What is the difference between MCTD, overlap syndrome, and undifferentiated connective tissue disease?**
    - **MCTD:** first described by Sharp and co-workers in 1972. It is an overlap syndrome characterized by a combination of manifestations similar to those seen in SLE, SSc, and inflammatory myositis similar to PM. Some patients may develop an erosive arthritis similar to rheumatoid arthritis (RA). The diagnosis requires the presence of high titer anti-U1-RNP antibodies, which causes a high titer, speckled antinuclear antibody (ANA). These patients lack other specific autoantibodies such as anti-Sm, anti-SS-B, anti-double-stranded (ds) DNA, and anticentromere.
    - **Overlap syndrome:** these syndromes occur when patients meet criteria for the diagnosis of more than one of the six classic systemic autoimmune rheumatic diseases (SLE, SSc, PM, dermatomyositis, RA, and Sjögren's syndrome). Although the features of both diseases may occur concurrently, usually one disease predominates clinically. As many as 25% of patients with features of a connective tissue disease have or will develop an overlap syndrome. Some overlap syndromes such as MCTD and certain myositis overlap syndromes have specific autoantibody associations.
    - **Undifferentiated connective tissue disease (UCTD):** typically describes a syndrome in which a patient has some of the clinical features of one of the systemic autoimmune rheumatic diseases and a positive ANA but do not meet criteria for a more specific diagnosis. Most have Raynaud's phenomenon and/or arthralgias/synovitis. Over time, 33% to 50% of patients will develop additional clinical features that will meet criteria for a specific disease diagnosis, whereas the other 50% to 66% will remain undifferentiated.

MIXED CONNECTIVE TISSUE DISEASE

2. **Describe the typical MCTD patient.**
    MCTD is 15 times more common in women than men. The mean age at diagnosis is 37 years, with a range of 4 to 80 years. There is no apparent racial or ethnic predisposition.

3. **What are the early clinical manifestations of MCTD, and how do they change over time?**
    The onset of MCTD is characterized by features of SSc, SLE, PM, and RA that occur simultaneously but usually develop sequentially over time. The most common manifestations at onset are:
    - Raynaud's phenomenon (>90%).
    - Synovitis (>90%).
    - Swollen hands with puffy fingers (>70%).
    - Myositis (>50%).

    Raynaud's phenomenon is present in almost all MCTD patients and if not present should make one question the diagnosis. Joint involvement is common and can result in deformities that resemble Jaccoud's arthropathy.

Table 21-1. Clinical Features of Patients With Mixed Connective Tissue Disease

CLINICAL MANIFESTATION	FREQUENCY (%)
Arthritis/arthralgias	55 to 100
—Jaccoud's arthropathy	30
—Erosions	20
Swollen hands and puffy fingers	66 to 75
Raynaud's phenomenon	90
—Nailfold capillary changes	50
Esophageal dysmotility	43 to 88
Mucocutaneous lesions	
—Sclerodermatous changes	33 to 67
—Skin rash	38 to 50
—Mouth sores	45
Muscle involvement	25 to 63
Lymphadenopathy	39 to 50
Fever	33
Serositis	27 to 30
Hepatosplenomegaly	15 to 25
Trigeminal neuralgia	15
Renal disease (membranous glomerulonephritis)	10
Myocarditis	Rare
Hypertensive crisis	Rare
Aseptic meningitis	Rare

Skin changes seen in the early stages are usually limited to edematous hands; only a minority of patients have more widespread skin changes. Esophageal dysmotility is common. *The absence of severe renal and CNS disease is a hallmark of MCTD and if present should suggest another diagnosis.* The inflammatory symptoms including synovitis, myositis, and serositis generally respond to therapy with corticosteroids. Over time, the manifestations of MCTD tend to become less severe and less frequent. Inflammatory symptoms and signs including arthralgias, arthritis, myositis, serositis, fever, lymphadenopathy, hepatomegaly, and splenomegaly become much less common. Persistent problems are most often those associated with SSc, such as sclerodactyly, Raynaud's phenomenon, and esophageal dysmotility. Pulmonary hypertension is the primary disease-associated cause of death. A few patients develop an erosive, destructive arthritis (Table 21-1).

4. What are the common gastrointestinal manifestations of MCTD?

The most common gastrointestinal (GI) manifestations are similar to those of scleroderma: upper and lower esophageal sphincter hypotension with gastroesophageal reflux heartburn/dyspepsia (60% to 70%), esophageal dysmotility and/or stricture with dysphagia (40%), and pulmonary aspiration. Esophageal function is abnormal in up to 85% of patients, although it may be asymptomatic. Small bowel and colonic disease is less common in MCTD than in scleroderma. Other less common GI complications include intestinal vasculitis, acute pancreatitis, and chronic active hepatitis.

5. What are the pulmonary manifestations of MCTD, and how are they managed?

Involvement of the lungs is common (75%) in MCTD, although most patients are asymptomatic. The typical manifestations and their frequencies are detailed in Table 21-2.

Management involves identifying the specific abnormalities and directing therapy appropriately. Active inflammation, such as pleuritis or nonspecific interstitial pneumonitis (NSIP) may respond to nonsteroidal antiinflammatory drugs (NSAIDs) or corticosteroids, respectively. Other medications such as azathioprine, mycophenolate mofetil, or cyclophosphamide may be used to treat interstitial lung disease. Without therapy

Table 21-2. Pulmonary Manifestations of Mixed Connective Tissue Disease

Symptoms	
—Dyspnea	15% to 20%
—Chest pain and tightness	7%
—Cough	5%
Chest X-ray findings	
—Interstitial changes/NSIP	15% to 30%
—Small pleural effusions	5% to 10%
HRCT scan findings	
—Interstitial lung disease/NSIP	66%
Pulmonary function studies	
—Restrictive pattern	69%
—Decreased carbon monoxide diffusion	66%
Pulmonary hypertension	23% to 30%

HRCT, High-resolution computed tomography; *NSIP,* nonspecific interstitial pneumonitis.

up to 25% will develop severe pulmonary fibrosis. Aspiration secondary to esophageal disease may also contribute to pulmonary disease, so treatment with acid lowering therapies (proton pump inhibitors, antacids), even in the absence of reflux symptoms, is indicated. PAH is a major cause of mortality and morbidity in patients with MCTD. It is usually due to bland intimal proliferation and medial hypertrophy of pulmonary arterioles, which may respond to calcium channel blockers, angiotensin-converting enzyme inhibitors, sildenafil, endothelin receptor antagonists, or prostacyclin infusions depending on severity. Patients with the scleroderma pattern of nailfold capillary abnormalities are most at risk. Other causes of PAH, which are treated differently, include hypoxemia associated with progressive pulmonary fibrosis (oxygen), pulmonary vasculitis (immunosuppressives), and recurrent thromboemboli (anticoagulation). Elevation of N-terminal pro-brain natriuretic factor levels and/or diffusing capacity of carbon monoxide (DLCO) <70% with % forced vital capacity (FVC)/%DLCO >1.6 may identify patients who have PAH.

6. What are the common nervous system manifestations of MCTD?
Severe central nervous system involvement is unusual with MCTD. Trigeminal neuralgia is the most common problem, as it occurs in progressive systemic sclerosis. Sensorineural hearing loss is reported. Headaches consistent with migraines (Raynaud's phenomenon?) are also relatively common, but convulsions and psychosis rarely occur.

7. What are the typical laboratory findings in a patient with MCTD?
The typical findings are detailed in Table 21-3.
Anemia is usually that of chronic disease. Coombs positivity is detected in up to 60% of patients, although overt hemolytic anemia is uncommon. Thrombocytopenia is uncommon. The sedimentation rate is usually elevated due to hypergammaglobulinemia. Hypocomplementemia is not associated with any particular clinical manifestation. Antibodies against other common nuclear antigens are rarely seen.

8. What is U1-RNP?
U1-RNP is a uridine-rich (hence U) small nuclear ribonucleoprotein (snRNP) that consists of U1-RNA and U1-specific polypeptides 70 kDa, A, and C. U1-RNP is one of the spliceosomal snRNP (U1, U2, U4/U6, U5, others) complexes whose function is to assist in splicing premessenger RNA to mature "spliced RNA." Patients with MCTD form high titers of antibodies against U1-RNP, particularly U1-70 kDa and U1-RNA, but also polypeptides A and C, which results in a high titer ANA with a speckled pattern. This antibody can be present in other autoimmune diseases such as SLE and scleroderma but typically in lower titer. Patients with MCTD appear to mount an antigen-driven immune response directed against U1-RNP, especially against an immunodominant epitope on the 70-kDa polypeptide. One hypothesis is that a genetically predisposed (i.e., HLA-DR4) individual mounts a specific immune response against a microbial antigen (cytomegalovirus glycoprotein) that cross-reacts with the U1-70 kDa peptide that has been modified during cellular apoptosis.

9. What is the course and prognosis of MCTD?
Over a 10-year period, 58% of patients are still classified as MCTD. The remainder evolve in to SSc (17%), SLE (9%), or RA (2.5%). There is a low incidence of life-threatening renal disease and neurologic disease

Table 21-3. Laboratory Findings in Patients With Mixed Connective Tissue Disease

ABNORMALITY	FREQUENCY (%)
Anemia	65 to 75
Leukopenia/lymphopenia	57 to 75
Hypergammaglobulinemia	80
Rheumatoid factor	50
Antinuclear antibody (>1:1000)	100
Anti-U1-RNP	100
Hypocomplementemia	25

in MCTD. The major mortality results from progressive pulmonary hypertension and its cardiac sequelae. Patients with abnormal nailfold capillaries and/or anticardiolipin antibodies are predisposed to developing pulmonary hypertension. The general consensus is that patients with MCTD have a better prognosis than those with SLE, but because there is tremendous variability in disease severity and manifestations, it is misleading to tell an individual that he or she has an excellent prognosis. The development of end-organ involvement dictates the morbidity and mortality.

As a general rule, the SLE-like features of arthritis and pleurisy are treated with NSAIDs, antimalarials, low-dose prednisone (<20 mg/day), and occasionally methotrexate. Inflammatory myositis is treated with high doses of prednisone (60 mg/day) and rarely methotrexate or azathioprine. SSc-like features of Raynaud's phenomenon, dysphagia, and reflux esophagitis are treated as described in Chapter 18. Vigorous therapy of myocarditis, NSIP, and/or early pulmonary hypertension with corticosteroids and cyclophosphamide or another immunosuppressive can be beneficial. Symptomatic and progressive pulmonary hypertension is treated as indicated in Question 5. Lung transplantation may be the only option in severe cases, although experience with this procedure in MCTD is limited.

OVERLAP SYNDROMES

10. What is the most common disease in overlap syndromes, and with which other diseases is it associated?

Sjögren's syndrome is the most common overlap and is seen with RA, SLE, SSc, PM, MCTD, primary biliary cirrhosis (PBC), necrotizing vasculitis, autoimmune thyroiditis, chronic active hepatitis, mixed cryoglobulinemia, and hypergammaglobulinemic purpura.

11. What other overlap syndromes are seen?

Other overlap syndromes *not* associated with high titer anti-U1-RNP antibodies are:
- SLE is associated with PM in 4% to 16% of cases.
- SLE can be associated with RA (RUPUS) with positive rheumatoid factor, nodules, and erosive polyarthritis.
- SSc can be associated with myositis. Antibodies to PM-Scl are found in 40% to 50% of patients. The PM-Scl antigen is a complex of 16 polypeptides located at the site of ribosomal assembly in the nucleolus. Thus, patients will have a nucleolar ANA. Anti-PM-Scl antibodies are strongly associated with HLA-DR3. In Japanese patients, who rarely are HLA-DR3 positive, anti-Ku antibodies are more commonly found in patients with this overlap.
- Limited SSc (CREST) can be associated with PBC. CREST antedates PBC by an average of 14 years. Antimitochrondrial antibody can be seen in 18% to 27% of CREST patients. Many also have Sjögren's syndrome.
- SSc and limited SSc can develop antineutrophil cytoplasmic antibody (ANCA) vasculitis (perinuclear ANCA/antimyeloperoxidase).
- Myositis overlap syndromes: antisynthetase antibody syndromes (see Chapter 20).
- RA can overlap with SSc, SLE, MCTD, or Sjögren's syndrome. Patients with anti-RA-33 (hnRNP-A2) are most likely to develop an erosive arthritis.

UNDIFFERENTIATED CONNECTIVE TISSUE DISEASE

12. How common is UCTD?

Up to 50% of patients with early connective tissue disease symptoms may not fulfill criteria for a defined CTD at the time of presentation. However, over time (1 to 3 years) 33% to 50% of these cases will evolve into a

Table 21-4. Clinical and Serologic Manifestations of Undifferentiated Connective Tissue Disease

MANIFESTATION	FREQUENCY (%)
Arthralgias/arthritis	37 to 86
Raynaud's phenomenon	33 to 56
Sicca symptoms	7 to 41
Photosensitivity	10 to 24
Serositis	5 to 16
Oral ulcers	3 to 27
Hematologic	11 to 41

defined connective tissue disease, leaving approximately 15% to 20% of all CTDs remaining UCTD. The majority of patients with UCTD are female (80% to 95%) with disease onset during the fourth decade (30 to 40 years old).

13. What are the clinical and serologic characteristics of UCTD? Do any predict the future development of a defined CTD?

The most frequent manifestations of UCTD are arthralgias/arthritis, Raynaud's phenomenon, mucocutaneous manifestations, and sicca symptoms. Major organ involvement is rare. Most patients (up to 90%) are ANA positive but lack specific autoantibodies against Sm, dsDNA, and centromere. Some patients have anti-SSA antibodies, which correlate with sicca symptoms and mucocutaneous lesions; others have low titer anti-RNP antibodies, which correlate with Raynaud's phenomenon and arthritis. Table 21-4 lists the common manifestations of patients with UCTD.

Certain combinations of features are predictive for development of a defined CTD: UCTD patients with fever, serositis, and/or anti-Sm or anti-dsDNA antibodies are more likely to develop SLE; patients with Raynaud's phenomenon, abnormal nailfold capillaries, and nucleolar ANA develop scleroderma; patients with xerostomia and anti-SSA/SSB antibodies develop Sjögren's syndrome; patients with polyarthritis and high titer anti-U1-RNP develop MCTD; and patients with myositis and antisynthetase antibodies develop myositis–interstitial lung disease overlap. Notably, some patients with UCTD may have severe involvement in only one major organ. This is particularly likely with lung involvement (lung-dominant connective tissue disease).

14. What are suggested classification criteria for UCTD?
- Signs and symptoms of a CTD, but not fulfilling the criteria for any of the defined CTDs for at least 3 years, and
- Presence of ANAs on two different occasions.

BIBLIOGRAPHY

Aringer M, Smolen JS: Mixed connective tissue disease: what is behind the curtain? Best Pract Res Clin Rheumatol 21:1037, 2007.

Burdt MA, Hoffman RW, Deutsher SL, et al: Long-term outcome in mixed connective tissue disease, Arthritis Rheum 42:899–909, 1999.

Cappelli S, Bellando Randone S, Martinovic D, et al: "To be or not to be," ten years after: evidence for mixed connective tissue disease as a distinct entity, Semin Arthritis Rheum 41:589–598, 2012.

Fagundes MN, Caleiro MT, Navarro-Rodriguez T, et al: Esophageal involvement and interstitial lung disease in MCTD, Respir Med 103:854, 2009.

Fischer A, West SG, Swigris JJ, et al: Connective tissue disease-associated interstitial lung disease: a call for clarification, Chest 138:251, 2010.

Furst D, Grossman J: Mixed connective tissue disease, Rheum Dis Clinics North Am 31:411–574, 2005.

Hassoun PM: Pulmonary arterial hypertension complicating connective tissue diseases, Semin Respir Crit Care Med 30:429, 2009.

Hoffman RW, Maldonado ME: Immune pathogenesis of mixed connective tissue disease: a short analytical review, Clin Immunol 128:8, 2008.

Mosca M, Tani C, Talarico R, et al: Undifferentiated connective tissue diseases (UCTD): simplified systemic autoimmune disease, Autoimmun Rev 10:256–258, 2011.

Rodriguez-Reyna TS, Alarcon-Segovia D: Overlap syndromes in the context of shared autoimmunity, Autoimmunity 38:219, 2005.

Sharp GC, Irvin WS, Tan EM, et al: Mixed connective tissue disease—an apparently distinct rheumatic disease syndrome associated with a specific antibody to an extractable nuclear antigen (ENA), Am J Med 52:148–159, 1972.

van der Helm-van Mil AH, le Cessie S, van Dongen H, et al: A prediction rule for disease outcome in patients with recent-onset undifferentiated arthritis: how to guide individual treatment decisions, Arthritis Rheum 56:433, 2007.

SJÖGREN'S SYNDROME

Vance J. Bray, MD

CHAPTER 22

KEY POINTS

1. Sjögren's syndrome is the most common autoimmune disease and should be considered in any patient with unexplained symptoms and a positive antinuclear antibody.
2. The most common symptoms are keratoconjunctivitis sicca, xerostomia, and parotid gland swelling but any organ can be involved.
3. Antibodies against Ro/SS-A and La/SS-B are the serologic hallmarks of primary Sjögren's syndrome.
4. A minor salivary gland lip biopsy showing a chronic lymphocytic infiltrate is the diagnostic gold standard.

1. Who was Sjögren, and what is his syndrome?

Henrich Sjögren was born in 1899 in Stockholm and received his MD from the Karolinska Institutet in 1927. In 1933, he published a monograph associating dry eyes with arthritis. He also introduced Rose Bengal staining to identify corneal lesions and introduced the term **keratoconjunctivitis sicca (KCS)** to describe the ocular manifestations. Sjögren's syndrome (SS) has also been known as Mikulicz's disease, Gougerot's syndrome, sicca syndrome, and autoimmune exocrinopathy.

SS refers to a slowly progressive, inflammatory autoimmune disease that primarily affects exocrine organs (lacrimal, salivary, and parotid glands). Lymphocytic cells infiltrate into these organs causing decreased exocrine secretions both by glandular destruction and effects on neural stimulation.

2. What is the difference between primary and secondary SS?

- **Primary** Sjögren's is diagnosed in a patient with KCS who does not have another underlying rheumatic disease. Primary SS is immunogenetically associated with HLA-DRB1*0301 and DRB1*1501, and serologically associated with antibodies to Ro/SS-A and La/SS-B.
- **Secondary** Sjögren's is diagnosed when there is accompanying evidence of another connective tissue disease, most frequently rheumatoid arthritis (RA). The immunogenetic and serologic findings are usually those of the accompanying disease (e.g., HLA-DR4-positive if associated with RA).

Clinical manifestations such as dry eyes and dry mouth are similar in primary and secondary SS. Extraglandular features including parotid enlargement, lymphadenopathy, and renal involvement are more common in primary SS.

3. Who typically develops SS?

Primary SS is one of the most common autoimmune diseases affecting 1% to 4% of the population depending on criteria used. It typically affects females between ages 30 and 50 years (female/male = 9:1). It has rarely been reported in children. Symptoms progress relatively slowly and there is frequently 8 to 10 years between the onset of symptoms and diagnosis. Secondary SS occurs in up to 15% to 20% of patients with RA or other connective tissue diseases.

4. What are the common initial manifestations of primary SS?

Manifestations can be divided into local sicca symptoms and systemic extraglandular manifestations. The initial clinical manifestations of primary SS are as follows:

- Sicca symptoms
  - Xerophthalmia   47%
  - Xerostomia   42%
  - Parotid gland enlargement   24%
  - Dyspareunia   5%
- Systemic manifestations
  - Arthralgias/arthritis   28%
  - Raynaud's phenomenon   21%
  - Fever/fatigue   10%
  - Lung involvement   2%
  - Kidney involvement   1%

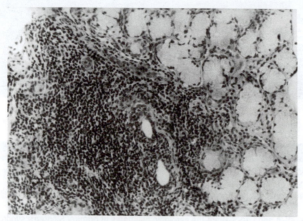

Figure 22-1. Minor salivary gland biopsy demonstrating mononuclear cell infiltration and salivary gland destruction.

5. What is the underlying pathology and pathogenesis of primary SS?

The manifestations of SS result from a predominantly lymphocytic cell infiltration of glandular and nonglandular organs. The cellular infiltration of the lacrimal glands and salivary glands interferes with the production of tears and saliva, respectively. Cellular infiltration of other organs, such as the lungs and gastrointestinal tract, results in a variety of major organ manifestations. Over 90% of the infiltrating cells are CD4+ T lymphocytes with memory phenotype (70%) and B lymphocytes (20%). The remaining 10% are an admixture of plasma cells, CD8+ T lymphocytes, T regulatory cells, natural killer cells, and dendritic cells. Analysis of T cell cytokines from biopsies suggests that this is a predominantly T helper (Th)1-driven response and Th17-driven response (Figure 22-1).

There are two models for the pathogenesis of SS. One postulates that an autoimmune attack on acinar epithelium results in cytotoxic cell death and apoptosis. The other model suggests that glandular function is inhibited by antibodies against the muscarinic receptor type 3 and by cytokine effects resulting in accelerated breakdown of acetylcholine reducing neural stimulation of secretions. Both models are likely to play a role.

6. What are the most common ocular symptoms of SS?

Normal precorneal tears consist of an inner mucin layer produced by conjunctival goblet cells, a middle aqueous layer secreted by lacrimal glands, and an outer lipid layer made by meibomian glands. Patients with SS most often complain of dry and painful eyes, also known as **xerophthalmia** or **KCS**. These symptoms result from a deficient aqueous middle layer of precorneal tear film, which normally comprises 90% of tear volume. These patients may experience a foreign-body or gritty sensation, a burning sensation, itchiness, blurred vision, redness, and/or photophobia. Symptoms worsen as the day progresses, owing to evaporation of ocular moisture during the time that the eyes are open. Notably, some of the eye pain is due to central nervous system (CNS) input because topical anesthetics do not eliminate the pain completely. This pattern contrasts with blepharitis, a low-grade infection of the meibomian glands, in which crusting and discomfort are most pronounced in the morning on awakening. KCS can lead to infections, corneal ulceration, and visual loss.

7. What are other causes of dry eyes besides SS?

Sarcoidosis, chronic hepatitis C, chronic graft-versus-host disease, poorly controlled diabetes, age-related, vitamin A deficiency, pemphigoid, blepharitis, viral infections, contact lens irritation, and medications such as antihistamines, diuretics, tricyclic antidepressants, and benzodiazepines.

8. What tests are used to document dry eyes in a patient with suspected SS?

The most common tests of tear production and adequacy are the **Schirmer's test** and tests using vital dyes that detect disturbances in the normal mucin coating of the conjunctival surface. The **Schirmer's I test** involves placing a piece of filter paper under the inferior eyelid and measuring the amount of wetness over a specified time (Figure 22-2). Normal wetting is >15 mm in 5 minutes, whereas <5 mm is a strong indication of diminished tear production. **Schirmer's II test** involves putting a Q-tip into the nose, which will maximally stimulate output of major and minor lacrimal glands through the nasolacrimal gland reflex. There is a 15% false-positive and false-negative rate with Schirmer's testing. The **Zone-Quick Diagnostic Threads** method of testing for dry eyes is gaining popularity. It uses a sterile cotton thread treated with pH indicator, Phenol Red. The yellow thread turns to red when it comes into contact with tears. The advantages are that the thread does not cause reflex tearing and the test only takes 15 seconds.

Lissamine green or fluorescein dye can be applied topically and the eye examined with a slit lamp. Lissamine green stains epithelial surfaces lacking mucin, whereas fluorescein dye targets areas of cellular disruption, thus

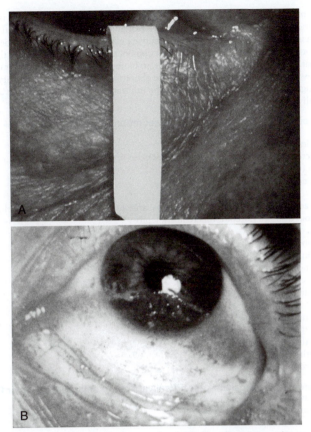

Figure 22-2. **A**, Schirmer's test demonstrating decreased tear production. **B**, Rose Bengal test with increased dye uptake in areas of devitalized epithelium. *(Copyright 2014 American College of Rheumatology. Used with permission.)*

documenting dryness of enough severity to injure corneal tissue. The area of maximum uptake is along the palpebral fissure, where the maximum exposure to the environment and evaporation of tears occur. **Rose Bengal**, which stains dead/dying cells and decreased mucin, is less often used due to its toxic effects on the cornea. There is a 5% false-positive and false negative rate for a score of ≥4 out of 9.

9. **What are the common symptoms of decreased production of saliva?**

   Normal saliva production is 1 to 1.5 L/day. Dry mouth sensation, known as **xerostomia**, occurs when the salivary flow rate decreases to less than 50% of the basal flow rate. It may result in a variety of problems, including:
   - Difficulty swallowing dry food (17%).
   - Inability to speak continuously.
   - Change in taste (metallic, salty, bitter) (33%).
   - Burning sensation (30% to 40%).
   - Increase in dental caries, cracked teeth, loose fillings.
   - Problems wearing dentures.
   - Gastroesophageal reflux symptoms (due to lack of salivary buffering).
   - Disturbed sleep (due to dry mouth and/or nocturia).
   - Predisposition to oral candidiasis (atrophic variant most common).

10. **How can salivary gland involvement be determined?**

    A variety of methods are used to determine salivary function. **Sialometry** (sensitivity 56%, specificity 81%) can be used to quantitate saliva production. An unstimulated whole salivary flow rate of ≤1.5 mL/15 minutes meets criterion for xerostomia. **Sialography** will outline the salivary duct anatomy but may be painful, predispose to infections, or cause obstruction. **Scintigraphy** (sensitivity 75%, specificity 78%) utilizes the uptake and secretion of ^{99m}Tc pertechnetate during a 60-minute period following intravenous injection to quantitate salivary flow rates. **Ultrasonography** (sensitivity 63%, specificity 99%) can detect parenchymal inhomogeneity.

Minor salivary gland (MSG) biopsy (sensitivity 64% to 86%, specificity 90% to 92%) is the gold standard for SS diagnosis. An incisional biopsy through the lower labial mucosa yielding 5 to 10 minor glands is adequate for assessment. An area of >50 lymphocytes around salivary gland acini or ducts is defined as a focus, with ≥1 focus/4 mm² supporting the diagnosis of the salivary component of SS. The findings in the minor salivary glands generally parallel involvement of other organs, so biopsy of the parotid glands or major salivary glands is generally not necessary. The MSG biopsy also may be abnormal before decreased salivary flow can be documented with scintigraphy, because it takes time for the infiltrate to destroy enough salivary gland tissue to cause decreased saliva production.

11. What are some causes of decreased salivary secretion other than SS?
- Temporary
  - Short-term drug use (e.g., antihistamines).
  - Viral and bacterial infections (especially mumps).
  - Dehydration (thermal, trauma, diabetes).
  - Psychogenic causes (fear, depression).
- Chronic
  - Chronically administered drugs (antidepressants, anticholinergics, neuroleptics, clonidine, diuretics).
  - Granulomatous diseases (sarcoid, tuberculosis, leprosy).
  - Amyloidosis.
  - HIV infection.
  - Hepatitis C infection.
  - Chronic graft-versus-host disease.
  - Cystic fibrosis.
  - Diabetes mellitus (uncontrolled).
- Other
  - Therapeutic radiation to the head and neck.
  - Trauma or surgery to the head and neck.
  - Absent or malformed glands (rare).
  - Type V hyperlipidemia.
  - Multiple sclerosis.

12. What is the differential diagnosis of parotid/salivary gland enlargement other than SS?
- **Usually unilateral**
  - Primary salivary gland neoplasms.
  - Lymphoma.
  - Bacterial infection.
  - Chronic sialadenitis.
  - Obstruction.
- **Usually bilateral** (asymmetric)
  - Viral infection (mumps, cytomegalovirus, influenza, coxsackie A).
  - IgG4-related disease.
  - Granulomatous diseases (sarcoid, tuberculosis, leprosy).
  - Recurrent parotitis of childhood.
  - HIV infection (DILS) (see Chapter 42).
- **Bilateral, symmetric** (soft, nontender)
  - Idiopathic   Hepatic cirrhosis   Acromegaly.
  - Diabetes mellitus   Anorexia/bulimia   Gonadal hypofunction.
  - Hyperlipoproteinemia   Chronic pancreatitis   Alcoholism.

13. What other exocrine glands can be involved in SS?
Any exocrine gland can be involved. Patients can have dried nasal mucosa leading to obstruction and bleeding. In addition involvement of the larynx (hoarseness), trachea (cough), vagina (dyspareunia), bowel (constipation), and dry skin (pruritus) can be seen.

14. List the common extraglandular manifestations of primary SS.
Up to 70% to 75% of SS patients can have clinical manifestations of extraglandular disease:
- Fatigue   60% to 70%
- Arthralgias/arthritis   45% to 60%
- Raynaud's phenomenon   13% to 33%
- Esophageal dysfunction   30% to 35%
- Autoimmune thyroiditis   14% to 33%
- Lymphadenopathy   15% to 20%
- Vasculitis   5% to 10%
- Annular skin lesions (subacute cutaneous lupus erythematosus)   5% to 10%
- Lung involvement   10% to 20%

- Kidney involvement   10% to 15%
- Liver involvement   5% to 10%
- Peripheral neuropathy   2% to 5%
- CNS disease   1% to 2%
- Myositis   1% to 2%
- Lymphoma (B cell)   4% to 8%

15. Describe the arthritis of primary SS.
The distribution of Sjögren's arthritis is similar to that of RA. The patient experiences symmetric arthralgias and/or arthritis of the wrists, metacarpophalangeal and proximal interphalangeal joints, frequently associated with morning stiffness and fatigue. In contrast to RA, Sjögren's arthritis is nonerosive and tends to be mild. It usually responds to medications such as nonsteroidal antiinflammatory drugs (NSAIDs), antimalarials (hydroxychloroquine) (controversial), and/or low doses of prednisone (≤5 mg).

16. Describe the clinical characteristics of other extraglandular manifestations of primary SS.
- **Lung manifestations:** all sites of the airways can be involved. Patients can have xerotrachea/xerobronchitis, nonspecific interstitial pneumonitis (NSIP), lymphocytic interstitial pneumonitis (LIP), usual interstitial pneumonitis (UIP), bronchiolitis (constrictive), and lymphoma. Owing to thick secretions and recurrent pneumonia, patients can develop bronchiectasis (8%).
  PEARL: consider SS in any patient with unexplained lung disease and a positive antinuclear antibody (ANA).
- **Renal disease:** characteristic but unusual manifestations include type I renal tubular acidosis (10%) and tubular interstitial nephritis (<5%). Glomerulonephritis and nephrogenic diabetes insipidus have been described.
- **Gastrointestinal:** patients with primary SS may have an increased incidence of **celiac disease** because both diseases share similar genetics of HLA-DRB1*0301 and HLA-DQB1*0201. Suspect in patients with diarrhea and vitamin D deficiency. Primary biliary cirrhosis (3% to 8%), autoimmune hepatitis, and recurrent pancreatitis (<5%) have been described.
- **CNS disease:** CNS vasculopathy causing strokes, multiple sclerosis-like lesions, and cranial nerve (V, VII, VIII) defects has been reported. Patients typically have evidence of skin vasculitis. Recently, a **longitudinal transverse myelitis** (≥4 vertebral segments) and optic neuritis associated with antiaquaporin-4 antibodies (antineuromyelitis optica) has been described. This syndrome is identical to Devic's disease (neuromyelitis optica) and is highly associated with anti-SSA/Ro antibodies. Relapses are frequent. Any patient presenting with transverse myelitis or optic neuritis should have occult SS ruled out. Cyclophosphamide or rituximab with corticosteroids alone or following plasmapheresis can be effective.
- **Peripheral nervous system:** peripheral neuropathy can be motor (mononeuritis multiplex), pure sensory, or sensorimotor. Patients with burning paresthesias and normal nerve conduction velocities may have a **small fiber neuropathy.** These patients have a selective loss of pinprick and temperature sensation (small fibers) while having normal vibratory sensation and deep tendon reflexes (large fibers). Small fiber neuropathy is diagnosed by specially stained skin biopsies taken proximally and distally showing a reduction in intradermal nerve fiber density in the distal specimen. Patients may respond to intravenous immunoglobulin (IVIG) therapy.
- **Vasculitis:** an immune complex mediated small (palpable purpura) or medium (mononeuritis multiplex, bowel infarction) vessel vasculitis can develop. This can be related to macroglobulinemia (Waldenström's) or cryoglobulinemia in the absence of hepatitis C.
- **Pregnancy:** pregnant SS patients with anti-SSA antibodies have an increased risk of delivering a fetus with skin rashes or complete heart block.
  PEARL: often the patient presenting with one of these extraglandular manifestations do not have KCS symptoms or a known diagnosis of SS. Consider primary SS in the differential of any patient presenting with one of these manifestations especially if they are ANA positive.

17. What are the typical laboratory and autoantibody findings in patients with primary SS?
- Erythrocyte sedimentation rate   80% to 90%
- Hypergammaglobulinemia   80%
- Anemia of chronic disease   25%
- Leukopenia   10%
- Thrombocytopenia   Rare
- Autoantibodies
  - —Rheumatoid factor   50% to 60%
  - —ANA   85% to 90%
  - —Anti-SS-A antibody   50% to 70%
  - —Anti-SS-B antibody   33% to 50%

PEARL: it is difficult to make a diagnosis of SS without serologic evidence of autoimmunity (i.e., positive rheumatoid factor or ANA).

18. What is the risk of cancer in SS patients?

SS patients are at a 13-fold to 44-fold greater risk of developing lymphoma than age-matched controls, with an overall frequency of lymphoma of 4% to 8%. Lymphomas are usually non-Hodgkin's B cell lymphomas. Marginal zone B cell lymphoma, particularly the mucosa-associated lymphoid tissue lymphoma subtype, is the predominant type of non-Hodgkin lymphoma associated with SS and occurs at a median time of 8 years after the initial diagnosis of SS. The onset of lymphoma may be preceded by the development of a monoclonal gammopathy (IgMκ most common). Alternatively, concern for lymphoma is raised by the loss of a previously positive rheumatoid factor, the loss of the monoclonal gammopathy, or the development of hypogammaglobulinemia. In primary SS patients, a five times increased risk of developing lymphoma is conferred by the presence of parotid gland enlargement, regional or generalized lymphadenopathy, splenomegaly, leukopenia, cryoglobulinemia (purpura), monoclonal spike, low C4, and/or the presence of germinal centers on the initial MSG biopsy. Patients with a high focus score (≥ 3) on MSG biopsy also had an increased risk (odds ratio = 8×) for subsequent development of lymphoma.

19. What are the new American College of Rheumatology classification criteria for SS?

The classification of SS, which applies to individuals with signs/symptoms that may be suggestive of SS, will be met in patients who have at least two of the following three objective features:
1. Positive serum anti-SSA/Ro and/or anti-SSB/La **or** a positive rheumatoid factor and ANA titer $\geq 1:320$.
2. Labial salivary gland biopsy exhibiting focal lymphocytic sialadenitis with a focus score ≥ 1 focus/4 mm^2.
3. KCS with ocular staining score ≥ 3 (assuming that the individual is not currently using daily eye drops for glaucoma and has not had corneal surgery or cosmetic eyelid surgery in the past 5 years).

Previous diagnosis of any of the following conditions would exclude participation in SS studies or therapeutic trials because of overlapping clinical features or interference with criteria tests:
- History of head and neck radiation treatment.
- Hepatitis C infection.
- Acquired immunodeficiency syndrome.
- Sarcoidosis.
- Amyloidosis.
- Graft-versus-host disease.
- IgG4-related disease.

These criteria have a sensitivity of 73% to 93% and specificity of 90% to 95% for SS. Although not part of these criteria, the addition of parotid ultrasound may increase the sensitivity of these criteria.

20. How is the xerophthalmia of SS treated?

- **Modify the environment**: increase fluid and omega-3 free fatty acid intake. Reduce caffeine intake and smoking. Limit time at computer and turn off ceiling fans. Eliminate offending medications (see Question 7).
- **Eye drops**: many preparations with differing degrees of viscosity are available. Most are cellulose-based (Refresh Tears, Genteal, TearsNaturale) or polyol/glycerine-based (Blink Tears). Artificial tears containing polyvinyl alcohol and/or vasoconstrictors (Visine) should be avoided. Those with a watery consistency may require frequent applications; more viscous preparations (Celluvisc, Systane Ultra) may provide longer benefit but may blur vision in some patients. **Preservative-free artificial tears** (Refresh, TheraTears, Soothe, Systane) are generally less irritating and should be used if patients use topical tears four or more times a day. **Lacriserts** (hydroxypropyl cellulose) are slow-release artificial tears that can be used but require a small amount of residual tear production to be effective and are expensive.
- **Lubricant ointments** (Refresh PM, Lacrilube) are available and may be especially useful during the night.
- **Cyclosporine-A ophthalmic emulsion** 0.05% (Restasis) twice a day should be considered in patients with severe dry eyes (≤ 5 mm wetting at 5 minutes). It can initially sting and takes 4 to 12 weeks to effectively reduce inflammation.
- **Humidifiers** are useful in arid climates and at high altitudes. Evaporation of tears may be slowed by the use of glasses with side shields; swim goggles are an inexpensive means of obtaining occlusive eyewear.
- **Punctal occlusion**, performed by the ophthalmologist, will obstruct the normal lacrimal drainage system, allowing tears to last longer. Temporary plugs (silicone, collagen) are generally inserted before permanent obstruction is considered.
- **Autologous tears**: use for severe ocular surface disease (scleritis, inflammatory nodules, corneal ulcers).
- **Boston scleral lens** with a moisture reservoir can also be used but are expensive ($5000/set).
- Blepharitis is treated with warm compresses, avoid local irritants (mascara), topical azithromycin, and rarely systemic antibiotics (doxycycline).

21. Describe the management for other mucosal dryness and complications in SS.

The complications of xerostomia are best prevented by good dental care, with frequent use of fluoridated toothpaste and mouthwash, daily flossing, as well as regular professional dental attention. Sugars (fructose, sucrose) and potato chips should be reduced. Carbonated beverages should be avoided because they lower oral

pH to <5.5, which is critical to cavity formation. Approaches to relieving symptoms and treating complications include:
- Sugar-free (not just sugarless) gum, mints, or candies may stimulate salivary flow without increasing the risk of dental caries.
- Oral wetting agents: omega 3 fatty acids, olive oil, and flaxseed oil in water. Avoidance of alcohol, frequent water ingestion, and removal of nasal polyps to limit mouth breathing will help oral dryness.
- Commercial products to relieve symptoms of dry mouth include Mouth Kote, Biotene mouthwash, NeutraSal, and saliva substitutes (Salivart, Xero-lube), as well as systemically administered cholinergic drugs (pilocarpine, cevimeline).
- Oral candidiasis is best treated with oral application of nystatin elixir or clotrimazole troches for 10 to 14 days. Topical drugs may be necessary because with significant salivary hypofunction systemically administered antifungal drugs may not reach the mouth in therapeutically adequate amounts. Dentures must be removed while the mouth is being treated and may also need to be treated in order to cure and prevent recurrence of oral candidiasis. Oral fluconazole for 2 weeks can be used in resistant cases.
- Vaginal dryness is treated with topical lubricants. Dry skin usually improves with lotions, creams, and emollients with urea/lactate.

22. How do the cholinergic drugs help dryness?
Patients with significant oral and ocular dryness have been noted to have only 30% of their salivary/lacrimal glands infiltrated with lymphocytes and only 30% to 50% of the glands destroyed. Consequently, the remaining functioning glands can be stimulated to produce more tears and saliva with the use of oral secretaogues. Pilocarpine (Salagen 5 mg QID) and cevimeline (Evoxac 30 mg TID) stimulate the M3 muscarinic receptors on lacrimal and salivary acinar glands. This results in stimulation of ATPase needed for secretion. Cevimeline has a longer half-life (4 hours versus 1.5 hours) and higher specificity of the M3 receptor, thereby lessening cardiac and pulmonary toxicity (heart and lungs have M2 receptors). Patients with some tear production on Schirmer's II testing are more likely to respond to these drugs. Patients with narrow-angle glaucoma, asthma, or on beta blockers should avoid these drugs or be monitored closely. Common side effects are sweating, flushing, and gastrointestinal disturbances.

23. How are the extraglandular manifestations of SS managed?
Fatigue is a common symptom that may be difficult to alleviate (rule out hypothyroidism). If associated with poor sleep, treatment similar to that recommended for fibromyalgia may be of benefit, although tricyclic antidepressants are likely to aggravate dryness of the mucous membranes. The best tricyclic antidepressant is desipramine, owing to low anticholinergic effects. If there are associated inflammatory parameters, such as an elevated sedimentation rate and/or hypergammaglobulinemia, the patient may benefit from treatment with an antimalarial or a low dose of prednisone (controversial).

Arthritis generally responds to NSAIDs, antimalarials, and low doses of prednisone. Severe extraglandular disease may require higher doses of systemic corticosteroids, azathioprine, mycophenolate mofetil, methotrexate, or cyclophosphamide. IVIG may be beneficial for small fiber neuropathy. Rituximab in early trials has shown some benefit for organ threatening disease but does not help sicca symptoms and fatigue. Belimumab and abatacept are being tested in trials. Lymphoma should be treated in consultation with an oncologist and based on the type and stage of disease.

Bibliography
Baimpa E, Dahabreh IJ, Voulgarelis M, et al: Hematologic manifestations and predictors of lymphoma development in primary Sjögren's syndrome: clinical and pathophysiologic aspects, Medicine (Baltimore) 88:284–293, 2009.
Birnbaum J: Peripheral nervous system manifestations of Sjögren's syndrome: clinical patterns, diagnostic paradigms, etiopathogenesis, and therapeutic strategies, Neurologist 16:287–297, 2010.
Brito-Zerón P, Ramos-Casals M, Bove A, et al: Predicting adverse outcomes in primary Sjögren's syndrome: identification of prognostic factors, Rheumatology (Oxford) 46:1359–1362, 2007.
Christodoulou MI, Kapsogeorgu EK, Moutsopoulos HM: Characteristics of the minor salivary gland infiltrates in Sjögren's syndrome, J Autoimmun 34:400–407, 2010.
Cobb BL, Lessard CJ, Harley JB, et al: Genes and Sjögren's syndrome, Rheum Dis Clin N Am 34:847–868, 2008.
Cornec D, Jousse-Joulin S, Pers JO, et al: Contribution of salivary gland ultrasonography to the diagnosis of Sjögren's syndrome: toward new diagnostic criteria? Arthritis Rheum 65:216–225, 2013.
Fauchais A, Ouattara B, Gondran G, et al: Articular manifestations in primary Sjögren's syndrome: clinical significance and prognosis of 188 patients, Rheumatology (Oxford) 49:1164–1172, 2010.
Gottenberg JE, Cinquetti G, Larroche C, et al: Efficacy of rituximab in systemic manifestations of primary Sjögren's syndrome: results in 78 patients of the Autoimmune and Rituximab registry, Ann Rheum Dis 72:1026–1031, 2013.
Guellec D, Cornec D, Jousse-Joulin S, et al: Diagnostic value of the labial minor salivary gland biopsy for Sjögren's syndrome: a systemic review, Autoimmun Rev 12:416–420, 2013.
Ito I, Nagai S, Kitaichi M, et al: Pulmonary manifestations of primary Sjögren's syndrome. A clinical, radiologic, and pathologic study, Am J Respir Crit Care Med 171:632–638, 2005.
Kahlenberg JM: Neuromyelitis optica spectrum disorder as an initial presentation of primary Sjögren's syndrome, Semin Arthritis Rheum 40:343–348, 2011.

Maripuri S, Grande JP, Osborn TG, et al: Renal involvement in primary Sjögren's syndrome: a clinicopathologic study, Clin J Am Soc Nephrol 4:1423–1431, 2009.

Ng WF, Bowman SJ: Primary Sjögren's syndrome: too dry and too tired, Rheumatology (Oxford) 49:844–853, 2010.

Ramos-Casals M, Anaya J, Garciz-Carrasco M, et al: Cutaneous vasculitis in primary Sjögren's syndrome. Classification and clinical significance of 52 patients, Medicine 83:96–106, 2004.

Ramos-Casals M, Brito-Zerón P, Font J: The overlap of Sjögren's syndrome with other systemic autoimmune diseases, Semin Arthritis Rheum 36:246–255, 2007.

Ramos-Casals M, Brito-Zeron P, Siso-Almirall A, et al: Primary Sjögren's syndrome, Br Med J 344:e3821, 2012.

Ramos-Casals M, Solans R, Rosas J, et al: Primary Sjögren's syndrome in Spain. Clinical immunologic expression in 1010 patients, Medicine (Baltimore) 87:210–219, 2008.

Ramos-Casals M, Tzioufas AG, Stone JH, et al: Treatment of primary Sjögren's syndrome: a systematic review, JAMA 304: 452–460, 2010.

Shiboski SC, Shiboski CH, Criswell L, et al: American College of Rheumatology classification criteria for Sjögren's syndrome: a data-driven, expert consensus approach in the Sjögren's International Collaborative Clinical Alliance cohort, Arthritis Care Res 64:475–487, 2012.

St Clair EW, Levesque MC, Prak ET, et al: Rituximab therapy for primary Sjögren's syndrome: an open-label clinical trial and mechanistic analysis, Arthritis Rheum 65:1097–1106, 2013.

Szodoray P, Barta Z, Lakos G, et al: Coeliac disease in Sjögren's syndrome – a study of 111 Hungarian patients, Rheumatol Int 24:278–282, 2004.

Further Reading

http://www.sjogrens.org

CHAPTER 23: ANTIPHOSPHOLIPID ANTIBODY SYNDROME

Sterling G. West, MD and Karen E. Hansen, MD, MS

KEY POINTS

1. One-in-five rule: 20% of deep venous thromboses, 20% of young adult strokes, and 20% of miscarriages are due to antiphospholipid antibody syndrome.
2. Over 50% of patients who have had a clot or miscarriage due to antiphospholipid antibodies will have a recurrence without therapy.
3. Anticoagulation and not immunosuppression is the main therapy to prevent recurrent thrombosis.

1. What are antiphospholipid antibodies?

Antiphospholipid antibodies (aPL abs) are a heterogeneous group of antibodies that bind to plasma proteins with an affinity for phospholipid surfaces. Most of the antigens (e.g., prothrombin and β2-glycoprotein I [β2GPI]) are involved in blood coagulation. These antibodies include the **lupus anticoagulant, anticardiolipin antibodies (aCL abs), anti-β2GPI antibodies**, and antiprothrombin antibodies. In a given patient, one or more of these antibodies may be present.

2. How are aPL abs measured?

  i. To test for the lupus anticoagulant, a phospholipid-dependent screening assay is performed and if prolonged, normal plasma is added in a 1:1 mix. If the lupus anticoagulant is present, addition of platelet-poor normal plasma does not correct the prolonged assay but addition of excess phospholipid does. If a factor deficiency is present, the assay does correct with addition of normal plasma.
  ii. Anticardiolipin antibodies are measured by an enzyme-linked immunosorbent assay (ELISA) test for immunoglobulin G (IgG), IgM, and IgA isotypes.
  iii. Anti-β2GPI antibody is measured by an ELISA test for IgG, IgM, and IgA isotypes.
  iv. Antiprothrombin antibodies are also measured by an ELISA test.

PEARL: unfortunately there is poor agreement among laboratories testing aPL abs with up to a 25% false-positive rate.

3. What is the value of a false-positive Venereal Disease Research Laboratory test?

The Venereal Disease Research Laboratory (VDRL) test measures agglutination (flocculation) of lipid particles that contain cholesterol and the negatively charged phospholipid cardiolipin. aPL abs bind to the cardiolipin in these particles and cause flocculation, indistinguishable from that seen in patients with syphilis. A false-positive VDRL may be a clue to the presence of other aPL abs, but in and of itself, is not a good way to screen for the presence of aPL abs. A false-positive VDRL or rapid plasma reagin (RPR) is seen in, at most, 50% of patients with aCL abs and as such, is not recommended as an additional laboratory test in assessing an individual with suspected aPL abs. Patients with only a false-positive VDRL and no other aPL abs are not at increased risk for clot or fetal loss.

4. What is the clinical significance of a positive aPL ab result? When should a physician suspect a patient has antiphospholipid antibody syndrome?

Low titer (usually IgM and transient) aCL abs are seen in up to 1% to 5% of the normal population. Less than 1% will have a moderate or high titer. aPL abs can occur de novo or be associated with an autoimmune disease, acute and chronic infections, medications, and neoplasms (especially lymphoma). Overall, the positive predictive value of an aPL ab predicting a future stroke, venous thrombosis, or recurrent fetal loss is between 10% and 25% depending on the aPL antibody type and titer.

Antiphospholipid antibody syndrome (APS) should be suspected in any of the following situations:
- Arterial thrombosis before age 50 years.
- Unprovoked venous thrombosis before age 50 years.
- Recurrent thromboses.
- Both arterial and venous thrombotic events.
- Thromboses at unusual sites (renal, hepatic, cerebral sinuses, mesenteric, vena cava, retinal, subclavian, etc.).
- Obstetrical: fetal loss or recurrent miscarriages; early or severe preeclampsia; unexplained intrauterine growth restriction.

5. **What are the updated International Consensus Classification Criteria for definite APS?**
   - At least one of the following clinical criteria:
     - Vascular thrombosis: one or more clinical episodes of arterial, venous, or small vessel thrombosis in any tissue or organ confirmed by imaging studies, Doppler studies, or histopathology and not able to be attributed to another cause.
     - Pregnancy morbidity occurring in a morphologically normal fetus by ultrasound or direct examination:
     - One or more unexplained fetal deaths at more than 10 weeks of gestation.
     - One or more premature births at less than 34 weeks of gestation due to severe preeclampsia, eclampsia, or placental insufficiency.
     - Three or more unexplained consecutive spontaneous abortions at less than 10 weeks of gestation, excluding maternal anatomic or hormonal abnormalities and paternal and maternal chromosomal causes.
   AND
   - At least one of the following laboratory criteria on two or more occasions at least 12 weeks apart and not more than 5 years before the clinical manifestation:
     - IgG and/or IgM aCL abs in moderate or high titer (>40 units of either, or >99th percentile for laboratory tests).
     - IgG and/or IgM antibody to β2GPI at >99th percentile for laboratory tests.
     - Lupus anticoagulant activity according to following guidelines:
     - Prolonged phospholipid-dependent coagulation test (activated partial thromboplastin time [aPTT], Kaolin clotting time, dilute Russell viper venom time [dRVVT], hexagonal phase phospholipid assay [STACLOT-LA test]).
     - Failure to correct the prolonged coagulation time by a mix of platelet-poor normal plasma.
     - Shortening or correction of the prolonged coagulation time with excess phospholipid.
     - Exclusion of other coagulopathies (e.g., factor deficiencies or inhibitors, heparin).

6. **Which clinical and laboratory manifestations that can occur in APS are not included in the updated APS criteria?**
   Clinical: valvular heart disease, certain neurologic manifestations (chorea, seizures), nephropathy, livedo reticularis, pulmonary hypertension, thrombocytopenia, Coombs positive hemolytic anemia.
   Laboratory: IgA aCL abs or IgA anti-β2GPI abs; antibodies against other candidate antigens (prothrombin, phosphatidylserine, others).

7. **Discuss the difference between primary versus secondary APS?**
   Primary APS (PAPS) (Hughes syndrome) occurs in 0.5% of the population. Females outnumber males 3.5:1 and the mean age is 34 years. It is defined as the presence of aPL abs in the setting of thrombosis without another associated disease. Thrombocytopenia, recurrent miscarriage, and/or livedo reticularis may be present. Virtually any venous or arterial site has been affected by thrombosis from these antibodies. In a large group of patients with thrombosis related to aPL abs, approximately two out of three thrombotic events are venous, whereas one out of three are arterial. The site of initial thrombosis often predicts the site of recurrent thrombosis in a given individual. Typical thrombotic events include deep vein thrombosis (DVT), pulmonary embolus, transient ischemic attack, stroke, and myocardial infarction. aPL abs account for approximately 20% of women who experience recurrent miscarriages, 20% of DVTs, and 20% of young patients (<age 50 years) who get strokes (**"One-in-five rule"**). Notably up to 10% of patients with PAPS will evolve into systemic lupus erythematosus (SLE) within 10 years.
   Up to 50% of patients with SLE have aPL abs and the presence of aPL abs has now been added to the list of criteria for the diagnosis of SLE (under the "Immunologic" criterion). In the group with both lupus and aPL abs, up to a half will subsequently develop a thrombotic event (secondary APS). Prospectively, 3% to 7% of SLE patients per year who have aPL abs will experience a new thrombotic event.

8. **How does the lupus anticoagulant affect prothrombin time and aPTT?**
   Prothrombin time (PT) should not be affected by the lupus anticoagulant especially with the newer assays that are insensitive to this antiphospholipid antibody. Over half of patients with the lupus anticoagulant have a prolonged aPTT. However, a normal aPTT does not exclude the presence of a lupus anticoagulant. NOTE: If an APS patient has a prolonged PT they may also have antibodies against factor II (prothrombin), which can lead to hypoprothrombinemia causing an increased chance of hemorrhage when they are anticoagulated (see Question 10).

9. **What are the dRVVT and hexagonal phase II phospholipid assay (STACLOT-LA) tests?**
   These are confirmatory tests for the lupus anticoagulant. Some hematologists recommend doing both tests because in any one individual with a lupus anticoagulant one of these confirmatory tests may be positive, whereas the other is not abnormal owing to the heterogeneity of the lupus anticoagulants. Russell viper venom directly activates factor X and thereby bypasses the factors required in the intrinsic pathway of coagulation. dRVVT is performed similar to the aPTT, except intrinsic coagulation factors proximal to factor X are not required and less phospholipids are present in the reaction. Therefore, the dRVVT test is not affected by factor deficiencies and is more sensitive in the detection of the lupus anticoagulant than

prolongation of the aPTT test. If the dRVVT test is prolonged it is repeated with excess phospholipid added. In patients with the lupus anticoagulant, the excess phospholipid will neutralize the lupus anticoagulant and normalize the dRVVT test. A ratio of dRVVT/dRVVT plus phospholipid of >1.2 is diagnostic of a lupus anticoagulant.

The hexagonal phase phospholipid neutralization assay (STACLOT-LA) is a two part aPTT assay. The plasma being tested is incubated with and without phospholipid and then an aPTT test is performed on the two samples. If the difference between the two aPTT tests are >8 seconds then a lupus anticoagulant is present.

10. What is the significance of a prolonged PT in a patient with the lupus anticoagulant?
A prolonged PT might indicate an extremely high level of lupus anticoagulant, but could also indicate the presence of a prothrombin (factor II) deficiency. This condition can be caused by hereditary factor II deficiency, liver disease, vitamin K deficiency, or anticoagulation with warfarin. In addition, acquired factor II deficiency due to autoantibodies to factor II is rarely associated with autoimmune disorders, including SLE. It is extremely important to detect factor II deficiency, because it is associated with excessive bleeding rather than hypercoagulability. If both the aPTT and PT are prolonged, a prothrombin level should be measured directly to exclude a deficiency.

11. In a patient with thrombosis due to aPL abs, how frequently are the lupus anticoagulant and aCL abs both positive?
- aCL positive and lupus anticoagulant positive 70%.
- aCL positive and lupus anticoagulant negative 15%.
- aCL negative and lupus anticoagulant positive 15%.
- aCL negative and lupus anticoagulant negative <1%.

12. Can a patient with thrombosis due to aPL abs ever have negative aPL abs (seronegative APS)?
Yes. Rarely, patients with large clots will presumably consume the aPL abs into the clot, leading to false-negative results. Consequently, repeating the tests for aPL abs at 12 weeks after the thrombotic event may show they are positive.

Another possibility is that the pathogenic aPL abs are directed against other targets not detected by the aPL ab assays. Such candidate antigens include prothrombin, phosphatidylserine, phosphatidylethanolamine, vimentin–cardiolipin complex, annexin A5, thrombomodulin, protein C, and protein S. Of these, **antiphosphatidylserine-dependent prothrombin antibodies** are the most pathogenic. Furthermore, antibodies directed specifically against β2GPI and not picked up by the aCL ELISA assay have been reported to be associated with clots in some individuals. In addition IgA aPL abs (aCL, anti-β2GPI) should be tested for in patients who are negative for IgG and IgM aPL abs.

Other causes (inherited hypercoagulable states, etc.) for thrombosis should always be assessed in patients with negative lupus anticoagulant and aCL ab tests. The concept of "seronegative" APS is not recognized unless other causes of thrombosis and antibodies against other candidate antigens are rigorously excluded.

13. What is the antigenic determinant for anti-β2GPI antibodies?
β2GPI (apolipoprotein H) is an anionic phospholipid-binding glycoprotein that exists in the blood in a circular conformation. It contains five domains (sushi domains) and belongs to the complement control protein superfamily. It binds through its fifth domain to anionic phospholipid membranes and receptors. After binding, it undergoes a conformational change to an open "hockey stick" conformation. With this change it becomes antigenic by exposing hidden epitopes in the first domain. In addition, the clustering of these molecules provides a high antigenic density. The pathogenic anti-β2GPI antibodies bind to an epitope (D8, D9, R39, G40, R43) in the **first domain** of the β2GPI molecule.

In vivo, β2GPI binds to phosphatidylserine on activated or apoptotic cell membranes (such as those seen in the developing placenta). The anti-β2GPI antibodies then bind to β2GPI dimers on the cell surface. This can lead to complement activation with C5a release leading to recruitment and activation of neutrophils, monocytes, and platelets. Other receptors have been identified that can bind β2GPI or the β2GPI–anti-β2GPI complexes leading to cellular activation, adhesion molecule upregulation, and tissue factor release causing a prothrombotic state. Putative receptors are Toll-like receptors (TLR2, TLR4), important during times of infection, annexin A2, GPIbα, and low-density lipoprotein (LDL) receptors (apoER2, LRP8). Therefore, the inciting prothrombotic stimulus and cells involved may differ between episodes of thrombosis. Notably, a positive aCL ab ELISA test is usually due to binding by anti-β2GPI antibodies.

14. What is the clinical significance of antiprothrombin antibodies?
Antibodies to prothrombin may be responsible for a positive lupus anticoagulant test increasing the risk for thrombosis. Conversely, antibodies to prothrombin may deplete prothrombin leading to hemorrhage.

15. Is the level of aPL abs stable over time?
No. aPL ab levels may fluctuate widely over time spontaneously or in response to clinical events such as a flare of lupus, change in pregnancy status, infection, or thrombosis. aPL ab levels may or may not change with immunosuppressive therapy or anticoagulation for thrombosis.

16. **List the "main" types of diseases associated with increased aPL ab production.**
    Increased aPL ab production is frequently associated with chronic immune stimulation. The primary conditions can be remembered by the mnemonic **MAIN**:
    M—Medications.
    A—Autoimmune diseases.
    I—Infectious diseases.
    N—Neoplasms.

17. **What medications are associated with elevated levels of aPL abs?**
    Although many drugs have been associated with elevated aPL abs, the most common are the phenothiazines and other drugs associated with drug-induced lupus: chlorpromazine (a phenothiazine), procainamide, and quinidine. Hydralazine, phenytoin, α interferon, interleukin-2 therapy, tumor necrosis factor (TNF)-α inhibitors, and a few other drugs have also been a cause of aPL abs. Levamisole-tainted cocaine can also cause these antibodies as well as cold agglutinins.

18. **Which infectious diseases are associated with elevated levels of aPL abs, and what is the clinical significance?**
    Many acute infections, both bacterial and viral (especially herpes), have been associated with transiently or persistently elevated levels of aPL abs. Chronic infections, such as HIV and hepatitis C, are also associated with increased aPL abs; 60% to 80% of patients who are HIV-positive have elevated levels of aPL abs. aPL abs induced by infections are in general not associated with increased thrombotic risk because they are not usually directed against β2GPI. Therefore, patients who have positive aCL abs by ELISA but a negative anti-β2GPI antibody test are usually not at increased risk for clotting.

19. **Which neoplasms are associated with aPL abs?**
    Many neoplasms have been reported, but the most common is lymphoma.

20. **Which clinical syndromes are most commonly associated with elevated levels of aPL abs?**
    Clinical syndromes most commonly associated with aPL abs can be remembered by the mnemonic **CLOT**:
    C—Clot: recurrent arterial and/or venous thromboses (clots).
    L—Livedo reticularis: lace-like rash over the extremities and trunk exaggerated by cold conditions.
    O—Obstetrical loss: recurrent fetal loss.
    T—Thrombocytopenia.

21. **What is the risk of thrombosis in a person with aPL abs?**
    This depends on the clinical setting and the type of aPL ab present. The presence of a lupus anticoagulant increases the risk of thrombosis more than aCL/anti-β2GPI abs with the following odds ratios (OR):
    - Venous thromboembolism (OR 11) in patients <age 50 years.
    - Stroke (OR 8.1) in patients <age 50 years.
    - Fetal loss (OR 7.8).
    - Thrombosis in an SLE patient (OR 5.6).

    PEARL: patients who have all three aPL abs ("triple positives") including lupus anticoagulant, aCL abs, anti-β2GPI abs have the highest risk for thromboses (OR 34.4).

22. **What central nervous system thrombotic manifestations can occur in patients with aPL abs?**
    Stroke is the most common central nervous system (CNS) manifestation. aPL abs have been found in 5% to 10% of unselected patients with stroke and 45% to 50% of patients <50 years old with stroke. This gives a relative risk of 2.3 for aPL abs and stroke for all patients and 8.1 for young stroke patients. Notably, multiple strokes can lead to dementia.

    Thromboses can occur in other areas leading to ischemic optic neuropathy, retinal artery or vein occlusion, sensorineural hearing loss, chorea, transverse myelitis, and cavernous or sagittal sinus thrombosis causing pseudotumor cerebri. Some patients with neurologic symptoms have been misdiagnosed as having multiple sclerosis, based on brain magnetic resonance imaging (MRI) results. However, patients with aPL abs and neurologic symptoms usually have a normal IgG index and negative oligoclonal bands in their cerebrospinal fluid.

23. **What other thrombotic manifestations can occur in patients with aPL abs?**
    Virtually any organ can be involved. Skin thrombosis can cause cutaneous ulceration. Digital gangrene can result from arterial occlusion. Renal artery or vein thrombosis and a thrombotic microangiopathy can cause renal insufficiency. Pulmonary emboli occur in 30% of patients with PAPS and can lead to pulmonary hypertension in 5%. Budd–Chiari syndrome due to venous thrombosis of the liver has been reported. Vena cava syndromes and subclavian vein thromboses can occur. Avascular necrosis is increased in SLE patients with aPL. Retinal artery and vein thrombosis can lead to blindness.

24. **How do elevated levels of aPL abs cause thrombosis in vivo?**
    Because many of the antigens involved in the production of aPL abs are components of the clotting cascade, it is believed that the antibodies directly interfere with normal anticoagulation. The two-hit hypothesis postulates that aPL abs are necessary but not sufficient to cause APS. It proposes that aPL abs *plus* another

prothrombotic factor (infection, pregnancy, etc.) are both necessary to "tip" the clotting cascade toward thrombosis. The prothrombotic factors that coexist in aPL ab patients with and without thrombosis is an area of ongoing research. Recently, β2GPI has been shown to bind to TLR2 and TLR4. It is postulated that bacterial products such as lipopolysaccharide could cause an upregulation of TLR4. The increased number of TLR4 could bind to β2GPI from the plasma inducing a conformational change. Anti-β2GPI antibodies could bind to the TLR4–β2GPI complex causing activation of TLR4 with release of cytokines and other inflammatory mediators, which could increase the risk of thrombosis. This provides an explanation on how infections can trigger a thrombotic event by linking the innate and adaptive immune systems (see also Question 13).

25. **What factors may increase the risk of thrombosis in a patient with aPL abs?**
At the time of thrombosis, over 50% of APS patients will have one or more of the following thrombosis risk factors:
- Antibody characteristics
  - Triple positives (lupus anticoagulant, aCL, anti-β2GPI abs).
  - IgG with anti-β2GPI reactivity especially against the first domain.
  - High titers of antibody (>40 units).
  - Lupus anticoagulant.
- Increased tissue factor release
  - Infection.
  - Surgery.
- Abnormal endothelium
  - Active vasculitis/inflammatory disease (SLE).
  - Atherosclerosis and risk factors (diabetes, hyperlipidemia, high blood pressure [HBP], etc.).
  - Catheterization for arteriography/intravenous (IV) access.
- Prothrombotic risk factors
  - Smoking.
  - Oral contraceptives.
  - Pregnancy.
  - Homocystinemia (MTHFR gene mutation A1298C).
  - Hereditary hypercoagulable disorders.
- Factor V Leiden (APC resistance).
- Protein C or S deficiency.
- Prothrombin gene mutation (G20210A).
- Antithrombotin III deficiency.
- History of previous thrombosis or fetal loss
- Use of cycloxygenase-2 specific inhibitors (controversial).

26. **What other clinical manifestations are associated with aPL abs?**
- Migraine headaches (controversial). Some physicians give a 3- to 4-week trial of low-molecular-weight heparin (LMWH) to see if headaches are improved.
- Seizures (even with normal brain MRI).
- Valve disease—mitral > aortic valve. Occurs in 10% to 50% of patients with aPL abs and SLE. Can cause embolic strokes, and 5% need valve replacement.
- Accelerated atherosclerosis (controversial).
- Hemolytic anemia (Coombs positive): associated with IgM aCL abs.
- Endocrine: adrenal or pituitary infarction.

27. **What is MAPS?**
MAPS refers to microvascular and microangiopathic thromboses that can occur in patients with APS. Patients with classic primary and secondary APS typically have clots predominantly in medium or larger vessels. However, it has become increasingly recognized that small vessels may be involved in visceral organs leading to clinical manifestations resulting from microinfarcts (skin necrosis, cerebral microinfarcts, gastrointestinal and hepatic microinfarcts, alveolar hemorrhage, renal insufficiency, hearing loss, bone marrow infarction, others). In some of these patients profound endothelial injury occurs in these microvessels leading to a microangiopathy with microangiopathic hemolytic anemia, severe thrombocytopenia, and thromboses of multiple small vessels. In patients with the catastrophic antiphospholipid syndrome (CAPS) this microangiopathic and microvascular thrombotic process predominates over the larger vessel thromboses typical of classic APS.

28. **What is CAPS and how does it present?**
CAPS stands for Catastrophic AntiPhospholid Syndrome (Asherson's syndrome), which occurs in less than 1% of patients with APS (both primary and secondary APS). Although rare it is the initial presentation of APS in 50% of patients who develop CAPS. It is a very severe presentation and is defined as having three or more organs involved simultaneously or within 1 week. Small vessel thromboses predominate. The most common presenting manifestations are cardiopulmonary (25%) with acute respiratory failure from hemorrhage (11%), CNS manifestations (22%), abdominal pain (22%), renal insufficiency (14%), and cutaneous disease

Table 23-1. Differential Diagnosis of CAPS

	CAPS	TTP	HUS	HELLP	MALIG HBP	SLE FLARE	ACUTE DIC
Thrombocytopenia	60%	+++ <20,000	++ >20,000	++ >20,000	+	+/− Immune	++/+++
Hemolytic anemia	33%	+++ Schistos >3% to 5%	+++ Schistos >3% to 5%	++ Schist >1% to 2%	+/− Few Schistos	Coombs +	+/++ Few Schistos
Fever	—	30%	—	—	—	+/−	—
Thromboses and/or sxs	Diffuse	CNS 66% Renal 50%	Renal 100%, N/V	Liver 100%, N/V, HA	CNS, renal sxs	Many sxs possible	None
PT/PTT fibrinogen/ FDPs	NI/LA + NI/NI	NI/NI NI/ Inc	NI/NI NI/ Inc	NI/NI NI/Inc	NI/NI NI	NI/LA+ NI	Inc/Inc Dec/Inc
Other	+ aPL abs	Low (5%) AD-AMTS13; very high LDH (>1000)	High C5b-C9; very high LDH (>1000)	High LAEs and LDH (>600); preeclampsia 80%	Severe HBP 100%	Low complements, high anti-dsDNA abs	Low factors V and VIII

aPL abs, Antiphospholipid antibodies; CAPS, catastrophic antiphospholipid syndrome; CNS, central nervous system; Dec, decreased; DIC, disseminated intravascular coagulation; ds, double-stranded; HBP, high blood pressure; FDP, fibrin degradation products; HUS, hemolytic uremic syndrome; Inc, increased; LA, lupus anticoagulant; LAE, liver enzymes; LDH, lactate dehydrogenase; Malig, malignant; NI, normal; N/V, nausea/vomiting; PT, prothrombin time; PTT, partial thromboplastin time; Schistos, schistocytes; SLE, systemic lupus erythematosus; sxs, symptoms; TTP, thrombotic thrombocytopenia purpura.

(10%). As the disease progresses these organs are involved over 60% of the time. Thrombocytopenia occurs in 60% and hemolytic anemia in 33%. In those who develop thrombotic microangiopathy, the thrombocytopenia and hemolysis can be severe and needs to be differentiated from thrombotic thrombocytopenia purpura (TTP), hemolytic uremic syndrome (HUS), malignant hypertension, and disseminated intravascular coagulation (DIC). In pregnant patients it must be separated from HELLP syndrome (Table 23-1). The inciting event for CAPS is unknown in 45% of patients. Infections (20%) and surgery (14%) even when minor are known inciting events. Even with aggressive therapy, mortality is 50%. If they survive the episode of CAPS, 33% of patients get recurrent thromboses over the next 5 years even on adequate anticoagulation.

29. **Based on available evidence, what are the current recommendations for treatment of a patient with aPL abs who has never had a clot or a previous pregnancy complication?**
    - Although controversial, the APLASA study (*Arth Rheum* 56:2382, 2007) showed no benefit from low-dose aspirin (ASA) in otherwise asymptomatic patients with aPL abs. Therefore, low-risk patients should not receive ASA.
    - Asymptomatic patients with aPL abs who are at high risk for clots should receive low-dose ASA (81 mg daily). Patients who have not had a previous clot but are at increased risk for clots in the future include: (i) triple positive aPL abs; (ii) lupus anticoagulant or high titer anti-β2GPI abs; and (iii) SLE patients. SLE patients may also lessen clot risk with hydroxychloroquine therapy. Hydroxychloroquine may prevent aPL abs from binding and disrupting Annexin A5, which is a potent anticoagulant (*Blood* 112:1687, 2008).
    - All patients should have modifiable risk factors treated: smoking, lipids, hypertension, diabetes mellitus, immobilization, birth control pills.

30. **How should a patient with aPL abs and no previous history of thrombosis be treated if they are undergoing a high risk procedure?**
    Asymptomatic patients (particularly those with high-risk profile) should receive prophylactic treatment to prevent clots when undergoing high-risk procedures even if they have no previous history of clot. The following recommendations (*J Rheumatol* 29:843, 2002) should be continued at least 7 days postoperative or postpartum:
    - General surgery: low-dose unfractionated heparin: 5000 units subcutaneous (SC) q8 to q12 hours starting 1 to 2 hours before surgery; or, LMWH such as enoxaparin 30 mg SC q12 hours starting 12 to 24 hours after surgery, or 40 mg SC q24 hours starting 1 to 2 hours before surgery.

- Orthopedic surgery: low-dose unfractionated heparin: 5000 units SC q8 to q12 hours starting 12 to 24 hours after surgery; or, LMWH such as enoxaparin 30 mg SC q12 hours starting 12 to 24 hours after surgery, or 40 mg q24 hours starting 10 to 12 hours before surgery
- Pregnancy: during pregnancy patients should receive ASA (81 to 325 mg daily). Postpartum patients should get LMWH described above for general surgery prophylaxis.

31. **What parenteral anticoagulants are available for treatment of patients with APS?**
    - Unfractionated heparin
        - Prophylactic dose: 5000 units SC twice a day.
        - Treatment of clot dose: 80 units/kg bolus followed by 18 units/kg/h IV maintenance.
        - Monitor PTT, antifactor Xa level (6 hours after dose adjustment), or heparin level.
        - Precautions: heparin-induced thrombocytopenia (HIT), osteoporosis.
    - LMWHs
        - Prophylactic dose.
            - Dalteparin (Fragmin): 5000 international units SC q24 hours.
            - Enoxaparin (Lovenox): 30 mg SC q12 hours (or 40 mg SC q24 hours).
            - Tinzaparin (Innohep): 75 international units/kg SC q24 hours.
        - Treatment of clot dose.
            - Dalteparin (Fragmin): 100 international units/kg SC q12 hours (or 200 international units/kg SC q24 hours).
            - Enoxaparin (Lovenox): 1 mg/kg SC q12 hours (or 1.5 mg/kg SC q24 hours).
            - Tinzaparin (Innohep): 175 international units/kg SC q24 hours.
            - Use cautiously with dose adjustment if creatinine clearance (CrCl) <30 mL/min.
        - Monitor: antifactor Xa level 4 hours after dose.
        - Precautions: less risk of HIT and osteoporosis. Not dialyzable. More expensive than unfractionated heparin.

32. **What parenteral anticoagulants are available to treat a patient with APS who has a history of HIT?**
    - Direct thrombin (IIa) inhibitor.
        - Argatroban.
    - Treatment of clot dose: 2 µg/kg/min IV.
    - Monitor: PTT. Follow chromogenic factor X when transitioning to warfarin.
    - Use cautiously with dose adjustment in liver insufficiency.
    - Synthetic pentasaccharide (inhibits factor Xa via antithrombin similar to heparin).
        - Fondaparinux (Arixtra).
    - Prophylactic dose: 2.5 mg SC q24 hours.
    - Treatment of clot dose: 7.5 mg (if >50 kg weight) or 10 mg (if >100 kg weight) SC q24 hours.
    - Monitor: antifactor Xa level 4 hours after dose.
    - Do not use if CrCl <30 mL/min.

33. **How should heparinization be monitored in patients who already have a prolonged aPTT from the lupus anticoagulant? How about warfarin?**
    In patients who are heparinized, heparin levels can be monitored directly to give an indication of anticoagulant effect. In addition, antifactor Xa level or thrombin time (which measures the clotting system distal to the effects of aPL abs) can be used as good indicators of heparinization. In a patient on warfarin, the PT/international normalized ratio (INR) is not usually affected by the lupus anticoagulant and can be used to monitor the adequacy of anticoagulation.

34. **What is the treatment for a patient who has had a venous thrombosis and elevated levels of aPL abs?**
    Two prospective trials (N Engl J Med 349:1133, 2003; J Thromb Haemost 3:848, 2005) have shown that after initial heparin therapy transitioning to moderate intensity warfarin therapy (INR: 2 to 3) is sufficient to prevent further venous clots. Because the risk of recurrent thrombosis is between 44% and 69%, most individuals will require lifelong anticoagulation. However, patients who had a provoked DVT (without a pulmonary embolus) due to a reversible risk factor (surgery, cast, estrogen therapy, pregnancy, immobilization) may be considered for withdrawal of anticoagulation after 6 months if the proximal venous clot has resolved on ultrasound and D-dimer is normal (controversial). Patients in the high-risk group (triple positive aPL abs, high-titer aPL abs or lupus anticoagulant, previous history of clot, SLE, hereditary thrombophilia) should have lifelong anticoagulation even if the DVT was caused by mitigating factors.

35. **What is the treatment for a patient who had a cerebral arterial clot and elevated levels of aPL abs?**
    There is significant debate over how to manage patients following an arterial thrombosis associated with aPL abs. One area of controversy is the value of antiplatelet agents compared to warfarin as the best therapy. The

one prospective trial (APASS–WARSS study) (JAMA 291:576, 2004) had significant flaws making definitive recommendations difficult. Several retrospective studies and data from stroke studies not specifically including APS patients suggest the following for a patient with a stroke and aPL abs:
- Thrombolytic therapy per expert guidelines.
- Evaluation for other causes of cerebral thrombosis: transthoracic echocardiogram with bubble study to rule out patent foramen ovale and a transesophageal echocardiogram to rule out valvular lesions and an intramural clot.
- Treatment during first 48 hours: low-dose ASA (81 mg daily) and prophylactic dose LMWH. If large stroke, may continue this therapy for 2 weeks to prevent bleeding into damaged area of the brain.
- If the patient's stroke is due to a cardioembolic source (atrial fibrillation, heart valve, intracardiac thrombus), then the patient should be treated with warfarin maintaining an INR between 2 and 3 (some recommend INR 3 to 4).
- If the patient's stroke is not cardioembolic and the patient is medium risk for recurrence, then treatment can be ASA (81 to 325 mg daily) or combination antiplatelet agents (ASA [81 mg daily] plus dipyridamole [200 mg twice a day], clopidogrel [75 mg daily], or ticagrelor [90 mg twice a day]). *Although warfarin (INR 2 to 3) with or without ASA (81 mg daily) has also been used, many experts feel that combination of antiplatelet agents (ASA plus clopidogrel or ticagrelor) is more effective than warfarin-based therapies for **any arterial thrombosis**.*
- If the patient's stroke is not cardioembolic and the patient is high risk for recurrence (triple positive aPL abs, multiple lesions on brain MRI, previous arterial clot, active SLE, smoking), then treatment should be combination antiplatelet agents (ASA plus clopidogrel or ticagrelor), warfarin (INR 2 to 3) plus aspirin (81 mg daily), or high-dose warfarin (INR 3 to 4).

Because the risk of recurrent arterial thrombosis is over 50%, the patient should remain on therapy lifelong. Smoking must be discontinued and hypertension, hyperlipidemia, and diabetes should be controlled. The risk of major bleeding on therapy is <1% on antiplatelet therapy, 2.5% for warfarin therapy (INR 2 to 3), and 4% for combination of the two therapies. Ticagrelor causes more bleeding than clopidogrel. Patients should be assessed for clinical factors and medications that increase bleeding risk before choosing therapy.

36. **What is the treatment for a patient who had a noncerebral arterial thrombosis and elevated levels of aPL abs?**
Recommendations differ depending on whether the arterial thrombosis is cardiac or noncardiac:
- Treatment of noncardiac arterial thrombosis: combination antiplatelet agents (ASA [81 mg daily] plus clopidogrel [75 mg daily] or ASA plus ticagrelor [90 mg twice a day]) or warfarin (INR 2 to 3) plus ASA (81 mg daily). *Many experts feel that combination of antiplatelet agents (ASA plus clopidogrel or ticagrelor) is more effective than warfarin-based therapies for **any arterial thrombosis**.*
- Treatment of cardiac arterial thrombosis:
  - If a patient is at medium risk for recurrence, then treatment should be combination antiplatelet agents (ASA [81 mg daily] plus clopidogrel [75 mg daily] or ASA plus ticagrelor [90 mg twice a day]).
  - If a patient is at high risk for recurrence (triple positive aPL abs, active SLE, smoking), then treatment should be combination antiplatelet agents (ASA plus clopidogrel or ticagrelor), warfarin (INR 2 to 3) plus ASA (81 mg daily), or high-dose warfarin (INR 3 to 4).
  - If a patient is at high risk for recurrence and has a stent, then treatment should be warfarin (INR 2 to 3), ASA (81 mg daily), and clopidogrel (75 mg daily), or ticagrelor (90 mg twice a day) in combination.

Adjunctive therapy should be directed at modifying cardiac risk factors. Notably, statin therapy may decrease clotting risk by decreasing endothelial activation in APS patients.

37. **When do fetal losses typically occur in patients with aPL abs?**
Up to 2% of normal pregnant women have aPL abs, whereas 15% to 20% of women with recurrent pregnancy losses have these antibodies. The pregnancy is usually lost before the 10th week. The proposed pathogenesis is that anti-β2GPI antibodies bind to β2GPI bound to the anionic phospholipid membrane of trophoblasts. This binding leads to complement fixation, complement split product (C5a) release, and influx of inflammatory cells causing a prothrombotic state. Anti-β2GPI antibodies bound to trophoblasts can also alter adhesion molecule expression and downregulates human chorionic gonadotropin, prolactin, and insulin-like growth factor-binding protein-1 secretion leading to inadequate trophoblastic invasion.

Patients with aPL abs are also at risk for later obstetric complications including preeclampsia, fetal death after 10th week, intrauterine growth restriction, and preterm labor. These manifestations are due to placental insufficiency from thromboses causing placental infarcts.

38. **What is the best treatment for the pregnant patient with elevated aPL abs who has had previous fetal loss but no previous history of thrombosis?**
ASA (81 to 100 mg) daily is prescribed before conception. Once conception has occurred, heparin 7500 to 10,000 units SC twice a day or LMWH (such as enoxaparin 40 mg SC daily) is added and continued until at least 34 weeks of gestation. The platelet count should be monitored every 2 to 4 weeks to monitor for HIT. With this combination, the rate of fetal loss is decreased by 54%. Heparin and LMWH at higher

antithrombotic doses do not work any better than prophylactic doses. It is postulated that heparin and LMWH at these low doses have the ability to inhibit complement and this is the major reason they can prevent fetal demise (see Question 37). Heparin or LMWH is stopped before delivery and then reinstituted and continued at prophylactic doses for 1 week postdelivery. Patients at high risk (triple positive aPL, cesarean section, >age 35 years, obesity, severe preeclampsia, twin pregnancy) should continue prophylaxis for 6 weeks postpartum. Coumadin is contraindicated during pregnancy owing to fetal malformations. All patients with aPL abs should have the placenta examined for evidence of infarction even if no problems occurred during pregnancy.

APS patients with a previous history of venous or arterial clot who are on chronic coumadin and become pregnant should be switched to full therapeutic doses of LMWH and low-dose ASA throughout pregnancy. In the postpartum period they can be switched back to warfarin.

39. Outline an approach for treatment of APS patients who have a recurrent clot while receiving anticoagulation.

If an APS patient has a clot while on anticoagulation, it is imperative to establish that the patient was adequately anticoagulated at the time of the recurrent thrombosis. The APS patient on warfarin should have an INR of 2 to 3 and a confirmed chromogenic factor X level of 20% or less. If the patient is adequately anticoagulated and had a venous clot, then the INR should be increased to 3 to 4 or the patient switched to LMWH if the INR is difficult to maintain in a therapeutic range consistently. If the patient has an arterial clot, then the INR can be increased to 3 to 4 and/or low-dose ASA or clopidogrel can be added.

If the APS patient clots while receiving LMWH, an antifactor Xa level should be checked to make sure it is in the therapeutic range. If the patient is therapeutic but has a venous clot and is on once a day enoxaparin, then using twice-a-day dosing may be helpful. If the patient has an arterial clot, then low-dose ASA can be added. If the patient is already on ASA, they can be switched to clopidogrel or use it in combination with ASA.

Use of heparin pumps, intravenous immunoglobulin (IVIG), rituximab, corticosteroids, and/or immunosuppressive medications for patients who have recurrent thromboses while on therapeutic anticoagulation is based on anecdotal reports. Recently, bortezomib (Velcade) has been successfully used in a few patients to kill plasma cells and lower aPL ab levels and clot risk.

There are no data on the effectiveness of the new oral anticoagulants in APS including the direct thrombin inhibitor, dabigatran (Pradaxa), or the direct factor Xa inhibitors, rivaroxaban (Xarelto) and apixaban (Eliquis). Many experts refer to these as "oral LMWH." Trials are planned. The concern is that if the patient misses even one dose they will become subtherapeutic. This is less likely with warfarin.

40. Outline an approach to the treatment of a patient who presents with CAPS.

Owing to the high mortality (50%) in patients who develop CAPS, every effort should be made to prevent its development. APS patients and asymptomatic patients with aPL abs must have infections (including minor infections) treated aggressively and given prophylactic anticoagulation for surgery and in the postpartum period as outlined previously. Patients who develop CAPS can be treated as follows:
- First-line therapy.
  - IV unfractionated heparin (not LMWH).
  - Methylprednisolone 1000 mg daily for 3 to 5 days followed by high-dose oral prednisone.
- Second-line therapy.
  - Plasmapheresis daily for first 3 days. Replacement fluid should be albumin and not fresh frozen plasma unless patient also has TTP/HUS.
  - IVIG after pharesis completed: 0.4 g/kg/day for 5 days.
- Third-line therapy.
  - Cyclophosphamide and/or rituximab, especially if associated with active SLE.

Anticoagulation should be initiated as soon as possible when considered safe. Anticoagulation may need to be delayed if the patient is having life-threatening hemorrhagic complications (pulmonary hemorrhage, intracerebral hemorrhage) as part of their CAPS presentation. The combination of plasmapheresis, corticosteroids, and anticoagulation ("triple therapy") has decreased CAPS mortality by 33% compared to any one therapy alone.

41. How can aPL abs be detected in a patient who is already anticoagulated?

Measurement of aCL abs and anti-β2GPI abs are not affected by anticoagulation and can therefore be used to determine aPL ab levels in a patient on heparin or warfarin. However, coagulation tests to detect the lupus anticoagulant are affected by heparin and warfarin, and care must be taken in determining lupus anticoagulants in this situation. In the patient on heparin, plasma can be treated with heparinase to remove the heparin before the coagulation tests. In a patient on warfarin, it is the PT that is primarily affected, and the aPTT is usually not prolonged. Thus, prolongation of aPTT in a patient on warfarin is still suggestive of the presence of a lupus anticoagulant. Because warfarin depletes vitamin K-dependent factors, a 1:1 mix of the patient's plasma with normal plasma should correct the factor deficiencies induced by warfarin. Thus, if the alterations of clotting parameters are due to warfarin, the PT as well as aPTT will correct. However, as discussed earlier, a prolonged aPTT that does not correct in this situation may be indicative of a lupus anticoagulant.

42. A patient with APS on warfarin comes in with a dangerously high INR. What can be done?
Most patients will not have excessive major bleeding risk unless the INR is 5 or greater. Most of the time you can instruct the patient to hold warfarin until the INR decreases to the desired range. If you must decrease it more quickly, the patient can be given 1 mg of vitamin K orally or intravenously (not subcutaneously). This will decrease the excessive anticoagulation within 12 hours without making them resistant to warfarin for several days, which happens if vitamin K is given subcutaneously. If the patient has a high INR and is severely bleeding, they need to receive fresh frozen plasma to replace coagulation factors acutely. However, this will put them at risk for clotting.

BIBLIOGRAPHY

Asherson RA, Cervera R, Piette JC, et al: Catastrophic antiphospholipid syndrome, Medicine 80:355–377, 2001.
Cohen D, Berger SP, Steup-Beekman GM, et al: Diagnosis and management of the antiphospholipid syndrome, BMJ 340: 1125–1132, 2010.
Crowther MA, Ginsberg JS, Julian J, et al: A comparison of two intensities of warfarin for the prevention of recurrent thrombosis in patients with antiphospholipid antibody syndrome, N Engl J Med 349:1133–1138, 2003.
DeGroot PG, Meijers JCM: β2-Glycoprotein I: evolution, structure, and function, J Thromb Haemost 9:1275–1284, 2011.
Dlott JS, Roubey RA: Drug-induced lupus anticoagulants and antiphospholipid antibodies, Curr Rheumatol Rep 14:71–78, 2012.
Empson M, Lassere M, Craig J, et al: Prevention of recurrent miscarriage for women with antiphospholipid antibody or lupus anticoagulant, Cochrane Database Syst Rev CD002859, 2005.
Erkan D, Harrison MJ, Levy R, et al: Aspirin for primary thrombosis prevention in the antiphospholipid syndrome, Arthritis Rheum 56:2382–2391, 2007.
Erkan D, Leibowitz E, Berman J, et al: Perioperative medical management of antiphospholipid syndrome, J Rheumatol 29:843–849, 2002.
Finazzi G, Marchioli R, Brancaccio V, et al: A randomized clinical trial of high-intensity warfarin vs. conventional antithrombotic therapy for the prevention of recurrent thrombosis in patients with antiphospholipid syndrome (WAPS), J Thromb Haemost 3:848–853, 2005.
Giannakopoulos B, Krilis SA: How I treat the antiphospholipid syndrome, Blood 114:2020–2030, 2009.
Khamashta MA, Cuadrado MJ, Mujie F, et al: The management of thrombosis in the antiphospholipid-antibody syndrome, N Engl J Med 332:993–997, 1995.
Laskin CA, Spitzer KA, Clark CA, et al: Low molecular weight heparin and aspirin for recurrent pregnancy loss: results from the randomized, controlled HepASA Trial, J Rheumatol 36:279–287, 2009.
Levine JS, Branch DW, Rauch J: The antiphospholipid syndrome, N Engl J Med 346:752–763, 2002.
Love PE, Santoro SA: Antiphospholipid antibodies: anticardiolipin antibodies and the lupus anticoagulant in systemic lupus erythematosus (SLE)and in non-SLE disorders, Ann Intern Med 112:682–698, 1990.
Miyakis S, Lockshin MD, Atsumi T, et al: International consensus statement on an update of the classification criteria for definite antiphospholipid syndrome (APS), J Thromb Haemost 4:295–306, 2006.
Ortega-Hernandez OD, Agmon-Levin N, Blank M, et al: The physiopathology of the catastrophic antiphospholipid syndrome: compelling evidence, J Autoimmunity 32:1–6, 2009.
Praprotnik S, Ferluga D, Vizjak A, et al: Microthrombotic/microangiopathic manifestations of the antiphospholipid syndrome, Clin Rev Allerg Immunol 36:109–125, 2009.
Rosborough TK, Jacobsen JM, Shepherd MF: Factor X and factor II activity levels do not always agree with warfarin-treated lupus anticoagulant patients, Blood Coagul Fibrinolysis 21:242–244, 2010.
Ruiz-Irastorza G, Khamashta MA: Stroke and antiphospholipid syndrome: the treatment debate, Rheumatology 44:971–974, 2005.
Tripodi A, deGroot PG, Pengo V: Antiphospholipid syndrome: laboratory detection, mechanism of action and treatment, J Int Med 270:110–122, 2011.

FURTHER READING

http://www.apsfa.org

CHAPTER 24

ADULT-ONSET STILL'S DISEASE

Vance J. Bray, MD

KEY POINTS

1. Systemic illness characterized by quotidian fevers, transient rashes, and an inflammatory polyarthritis.
2. No specific test is diagnostic but a ferritin level >1000 ng/mL is common.
3. Macrophage activation syndrome is a severe, life-threatening complication occurring in 5% to 10% of patients.
4. Nonsteroidal antiinflammatory drugs and corticosteroids control 50% of patients with 33% going into remission.
5. Methotrexate and biologics are required for 50% of patients including the 33% with a chronic disease course.

1. What is Still's disease?

Still's disease is a variant of juvenile idiopathic arthritis that is characterized by seronegative chronic polyarthritis in association with a systemic inflammatory illness. It was initially described in 1897 by George F. Still, a pathologist. The characteristic features of this illness have subsequently been reported in adults, as detailed by Eric Bywaters in 1971.

2. How do patients with adult-onset Still's disease generally present?

Patients are usually young adults (75% before age 35 years) who present with a prolonged course of nonspecific signs and symptoms. The most striking manifestations are severe arthralgias/arthritis, spiking high fevers, and transient rashes. A prodromal sore throat due to perichondritis of the cricothyroid cartilage can occur days to weeks before other symptoms in 70% of cases. These patients appear severely ill and have often received numerous courses of antibiotics for presumed sepsis, although cultures are negative. As many as 5% of patients being evaluated for "fever of unknown origin" may be diagnosed eventually with Still's disease. A few patients may have had similar episodes of illness as children.

3. Describe the characteristic fever of Still's disease.

The fever in Still's disease generally occurs only once a day, usually in the late afternoon or early evening and lasts 2 to 4 hours. The temperature elevation is often marked (>39 °C). Characteristically, the patient's temperature returns to normal or below normal between fever spikes. This pattern is known as a **quotidian** fever. In 20% of cases, the patient may have an additional early morning spike (**double quotidian** fever). The differential of a double quotidian fever is limited to adult-onset Still's disease (AOSD), kala-azar, mixed malarial infections, Kawasaki's disease, right-sided gonococcal or meningococcal endocarditis, and miliary tuberculosis (TB). Note that in up to 20% of cases the patient's temperature may not completely normalize between fever spikes.

Patients with Still's disease generally feel very ill when febrile but feel well when their body temperature is normal. This poses a dilemma for physicians, because hospital rounds and clinic visits may not occur during the times when the patient is febrile. The fever pattern in Still's disease contrasts with the pattern seen in the setting of infection; infections generally cause a baseline elevation in body temperature in addition to episodic fever spikes.

4. What are the common and uncommon signs and symptoms seen in Still's disease?

The common signs and symptoms of Still's disease are shown in Table 24-1. Unusual manifestations include alopecia, mucosal ulcers, subcutaneous nodules, necrotizing lymphadenitis (Kikuchi's disease), amyotrophy, acute liver failure, pulmonary fibrosis, pulmonary hypertension, cardiac tamponade, aseptic meningitis, peripheral neuropathy, interstitial nephritis, amyloidosis, hemolytic anemia, disseminated intravascular coagulation (DIC), thrombotic thrombocytopenic purpura, orbital pseudotumor, uveitis, sensorineural hearing loss, myositis (10%), and reactive hemophagocytic syndrome (macrophage activation syndrome).

5. Describe the rash associated with Still's disease.

Although the rash is said to occur in the vast majority of patients with Still's disease, it is often unappreciated unless specifically sought. The characteristic appearance is that of evanescent, salmon-colored, macular or maculopapular lesions that are nonpruritic. The rash is usually seen on the trunk, arms, legs, or areas of mechanical irritation such as tight clothing (beltline). Often, it is only seen when the patient is febrile. The rash can sometimes be elicited with heat, such as that produced by applying a hot towel or taking a hot bath

Table 24-1. Signs and Symptoms of Adult-Onset Still's Disease

MANIFESTATION	FREQUENCY
Arthralgias	98% to 100%
Fever (>39°C)	83% to 100%
Myalgias	84% to 98%
Arthritis	88% to 94%
Sore throat	50% to 92%
Rash	87% to 90%
Weight loss (>10%)	19% to 76%
Lymphadenopathy	48% to 74%
Splenomegaly	45% to 55%
Pleuritis	23% to 53%
Abdominal pain	9% to 48%
Hepatomegaly	29% to 44%
Pericarditis	24% to 37%
Pneumonitis	9% to 31%

or shower. Koebner phenomenon (i.e., the rash can be induced by rubbing the skin) is reported in approximately 40% of patients. Atypical skin rashes and urticarial lesions have also been reported. Skin biopsies and immunofluorescent studies are nondiagnostic, showing dermal edema and a perivascular mononuclear cell infiltrate.

6. **Describe the arthritis associated with Still's disease.**
The arthritis associated with Still's disease may be overshadowed by the systemic features of the illness. It may not be present at the time of disease onset, may involve only one or a few joints, or be fleeting. With time, the arthritis frequently becomes polyarticular affecting both small and large joints. The joints involved in descending order include: knees, wrists (very common), ankles, elbows, proximal interphalangeals (PIPs), shoulders, metacarpophalangeals (MCPs), metatarsophalangeals (MTPs), hips, distal interphalangeals (DIPs), and temporomandibular joints (TMJs). Neck pain is seen in 50% of cases. Arthrocentesis generally yields class II inflammatory synovial fluid (mean 13,000 cells/μL), and radiographs usually reveal soft-tissue swelling, effusions, and occasionally periarticular osteoporosis. Joint erosions and/or fusion of the carpal bones (40% to 50%), tarsal bones (20%), and cervical spine (10%) may be seen but are more common in children than adults. A destructive arthritis occurs in up to 20% to 25% of cases.

7. **What are the characteristic laboratory features of Still's disease?**
There is no diagnostic test for Still's disease. Rather, the diagnosis is one of exclusion, made in the setting of the proper clinical features and laboratory abnormalities and the absence of another explanation (such as infection or malignancy) (Table 24-2).
PEARL: aldolase is frequently elevated, whereas creatine phosphokinase is normal. Aldolase elevation is due to liver inflammation.

8. **What is the diagnostic significance of an elevated ferritin?**
An extremely elevated serum ferritin (>1000 ng/mL) in the proper clinical setting is suggestive of Still's disease and seen in 70% of cases. Values over 4000 are seen in <50% of cases. In addition to AOSD, the differential diagnosis of fever with hyperferritinemia includes infections (HIV, TB, CMV), malignancies (colon, prostate, breast, lung), lymphomas, hepatic cancer, liver metastasis, and systemic lupus erythematosus. However, unlike these other causes, the elevated ferritin in AOSD is mostly nonglycosylated (H-ferritin) with the glycosylated form (L-ferritin) being <20% of total ferritin. This pattern of ferritin (ferritin >1000 ng/mL, <20% glycosylated) has a 40% to 60% sensitivity and 80% to 90% specificity for AOSD. The etiology of the elevated ferritin is postulated to be from cytokines (tumor necrosis factor [TNF], interleukin-6 [IL-6], IL-18) inducing the heme-degrading enzyme, heme oxygenase-1, on macrophages and endothelial cells causing the release of iron from heme, which stimulates ferritin synthesis. Some experts recommend following ferritin levels for response to therapy.

Table 24-2. Laboratory Findings in Adult-Onset Still's Disease

LABORATORY TEST	FREQUENCY
Elevated erythrocyte sedimentation rate (>50)	96% to 100%
Elevated C-reactive protein (often >10× ULN)	90% to 100%
Leukocytosis (range 12 to 40,000/mm^3)	71% to 97%
Anemia	59% to 92%
Neutrophils (≥80%)	55% to 88%
Hypoalbuminemia	44% to 85%
Elevated hepatic enzymes	35% to 85%
Thrombocytosis	52% to 62%
Positive antinuclear antibodies	0% to 11% (should be)
Positive rheumatoid factor	2% to 8% (negative)

9. **What are the Yamaguchi classification criteria?**
Several criteria have been proposed with the Yamaguchi criteria being most commonly used. Five or more criteria including two or more major criteria yields a 96% sensitivity and 92% specificity to classify a patient as having AOSD.

YAMAGUCHI CLASSIFICATION CRITERIA
- Major criteria
  - Fever >39 °C for >7 days.
  - Arthralgias or arthritis ≥2 weeks.
  - Characteristic rash.
  - Leukocytosis (≥10,000/μL with ≥80% neutrophils).
- Minor criteria
  - Sore throat.
  - Lymphadenopathy.
  - Hepatomegaly or splenomegaly.
  - Abnormal aminotransferases.
  - Negative rheumatoid factor and antinuclear antibody.

Exclusion: malignancy (especially lymphoma), infection (especially Epstein–Barr virus), other connective tissue diseases (especially vasculitis), and drug reactions.

10. **How is Still's disease treated?**
    - **Mild disease:** occurs in 25% of cases with fever, rash, and arthralgias. In these patients, nonsteroidal antiinflammatory drugs (naprosyn 500 mg BID) alone can adequately control Still's disease. If symptoms are not controlled in 2 weeks then they are switched to low-dose prednisone (0.5 mg/kg/day).
    - **Moderate disease:** patients who present with high fever, disabling arthritis, and mild internal organ involvement are started on high-dose prednisone (1.0 mg/kg/day) immediately. If prednisone cannot be tapered to a low dose without disease recurrence, methotrexate is added. There is little experience using any of the other disease-modifying antirheumatic drugs (DMARDs) (antimalarials, azathioprine, mycophenolate mofetil, leflunomide, cyclosporine). Sulfasalazine should be avoided owing to a high rate of side effects.
    - **Severe disease:** patients who present with life-threatening organ manifestations (liver necrosis, cardiac tamponade, macrophage activation syndrome [MAS], DIC) are treated with pulsed methylprednisolone followed by high-dose prednisone and early use of biologic therapy.
    - **Resistant disease:** patients who have life-threatening presentations or patients who continue to require high-dose corticosteroids (>20 mg/day) in spite of 2 months of therapy with methotrexate or another DMARD may benefit from therapy with one of the biologics. Patients with AOSD have high serum levels of TNFα, IL-1, IL-6, and IL-18. Consequently, therapy that blocks one of these cytokines including anti-TNF therapy, IL-1 inhibitors (anakinra), and IL-6 inhibitors (tocilizumab) have induced remission in 72% to 91% of AOSD patients. Anakinra and tocilizumab are more effective than TNF inhibitors especially for systemic manifestations. Patients with prominent joint disease may benefit more from TNF inhibitors (infliximab) and methotrexate. Rituximab, abatacept, intravenous immunoglobulin (IVIG), and stem cell transplant have been used for resistant cases.

11. What is the clinical course and prognosis of Still's disease?

The course of illness generally follows one of three patterns, with approximately one third of patients pursuing each: self-limited illness, intermittent flares of disease activity, or chronic Still's disease. The patients who experience a self-limited course undergo remission within 6 to 9 months. Of those with intermittent flares, two thirds will only have one recurrence, occurring from 10 to 136 months after the original illness. A minority of patients in this group will experience multiple flares, with up to 10 flares being reported at intervals of 3 to 48 months. The recurrent episodes are generally milder than the original illness and respond to lower doses of medications. In the group that experiences a chronic course, arthritis and loss of joint range of motion become the most problematic manifestations and may result in the need for joint arthroplasty, especially of the hip. The systemic manifestations tend to become less severe.

The presence of polyarthritis or large-joint (shoulder, hip) involvement and an elevated ferritin level at onset are poor prognostic signs associated with the development of chronic disease. The 5-year survival rate in AOSD is 90% to 95%. Deaths occurring in Still's disease have been attributed to infections, liver failure, amyloidosis (2% to 4%), adult respiratory distress syndrome, heart failure, status epilepticus, and hematologic manifestations including DIC, thrombotic thrombocytopenic purpura, and reactive hemophagocytic syndrome.

12. What is MAS or reactive hemophagocytic syndrome?

MAS is a life-threatening (20% mortality) secondary (reactive) hemophagocytic syndrome occurring in 5% to 12% of AOSD patients. The pathophysiology involves dysregulation of T lymphocytes and excessive production of cytokines resulting in abnormal proliferation of macrophages and a consumptive coagulopathy. MAS may mimic a flare of AOSD with high fever, hepatosplenomegaly, and an extremely high ferritin (often >10,000) but typically do not manifest arthritis or rash. In addition, unlike AOSD, they have rapidly progressive cytopenias (≥two of three cell lines) due to phagocytosis of hematopoietic cells by macrophages in the bone marrow and reticuloendothelial system. In addition, they develop liver injury (elevated aminotransferases), fasting hypertriglyceridemia (>180 mg/dL), and a consumptive coagulopathy (DIC with elevated prothrombin time/partial thromboplastin time) causing a low fibrinogen level resulting in a low sedimentation rate. Soluble IL-2 receptor (CD25) levels are extremely elevated. Diagnosis is confirmed by a bone marrow aspirate showing hemophagocytosis by macrophages. Hemophagocytosis may also be seen in lymph node, liver, or spleen biopsies. Therapy includes high-dose corticosteroids. Up to 50% may not respond and will require a second-line agent including cyclosporine, etoposide, immunosuppressants (methotrexate, azathioprine, mycophenolate mofetil), and/or IVIG. Biologics (anakinra, TNF inhibitors) may also be useful. All patients should be screened by polymerase chain reaction for an active Epstein-Barr or other viral (CMV, parvo) infection which can initiate MAS.

BIBLIOGRAPHY

Affleck AG, Littlewood SM: Adult-onset Still's disease with atypical cutaneous features, J Eur Acad Dermatol Venereol 19: 360–363, 2005.

Burgi U, Mendez A, Hasler P, et al: Haemophagocytic syndrome in adult-onset Still's disease: a must for biologics? – Case report and brief review of the literature, Rheumatol Int 32:3269–3272, 2012.

Bywaters EGL: Still's disease in the adult, Ann Rheum Dis 30:121–133, 1971.

Chen DY, Lan HH, Hsieh TY, et al: Crico-thyroid perichondritis leading to sore throat in patients with active adult-onset Still's disease, Ann Rheum Dis 66:1264–1266, 2007.

Crispin JC, Martinez-Banos D, Alcocer-Varela J: Adult-onset Still's disease as a cause of fever of unknown origin, Medicine (Baltimore) 84:331–337, 2005.

de Boysson H, Fevrier J, Nicolle A, et al: Tocilizumab in the treatment of the adult-onset Still's disease: current clinical evidence, Clin Rheumatol 32:141–147, 2013.

Fautrel B: Adult-onset Still's disease, Best Pract Res Clin Rheumatol 22:773–792, 2008.

Fautrel B: Tumor necrosis factor alpha blocking agents in refractory adult onset Still's disease: an observational study of 20 cases, Ann Rheum Dis 64:262–266, 2005.

Fautrel B, LeMoël G, Saint-Marcoux B, et al: Diagnostic value of ferritin and glycosylated ferritin in adult onset Still's disease, J Rheumatol 28:322–329, 2001.

Fitzgerald A, Leclercq SA, Yan A, et al: Rapid responses to anakinra in patients with refractory adult-onset Still's disease, Arthritis Rheum 52:1794–1803, 2005.

Franchini S, Dagna L, Salvo F, et al: Efficacy of traditional and biologic agents in different clinical phenotypes of adult-onset Still's disease, Arthritis Rheum 62:2530–2535, 2010.

Fukaya S, Yasuda S, Hashimoto T, et al: Clinical features of haemophagocytic syndrome in patients with systemic inflammatory autoimmune diseases: analysis of 30 cases, Rheumatology (Oxford) 47:1686–1691, 2008.

Giampietro C, Ridene M, Lequerre T, et al: Anakinra in adult onset Still's disease: long term treatment in patients resistant to conventional therapy, Arthritis Care Res (Hoboken) 65:822–826, 2013.

Kong X, Xu D, Zhang W, et al: Clinical features and prognosis in adult-onset Still's disease: a study of 104 cases, Clin Rheumatol 29:1015–1019, 2010.

Yamaguchi M, Ohta A, Tsunematsu T, et al: Preliminary criteria for classification of adult Still's disease, J Rheumatol 19:424–430, 1992.

CHAPTER 25

POLYMYALGIA RHEUMATICA
James D. Singleton, MD

KEY POINTS

1. Polymyalgia rheumatica (PMR) is a common inflammatory disorder in the elderly.
2. Patients present with subacute onset of severe pain and stiffness in proximal limbs and a high erythrocyte sedimentation rate (ESR).
3. PMR may appear synchronously or sequentially in patients with giant cell arteritis.
4. Patients typically respond dramatically to prednisone at 15 to 20 mg/day.
5. PMR treatment often extends for 2 years or more and relapses are frequent.

1. **How does "SECRET" describe the clinical features of PMR?**
   S = Stiffness and pain
   E = Elderly individuals
   C = Constitutional symptoms, Caucasians
   R = Arthritis (rheumatism)
   E = Elevated ESR
   T = Temporal arteritis

2. **Where did the term polymyalgia rheumatica originate?**
   Reports of this syndrome appeared in the medical literature for years under a variety of designations. The name polymyalgia rheumatica was introduced by Barber in 1957 in a report of 12 cases.

3. **Define polymyalgia rheumatica.**
   PMR is an inflammatory syndrome of older individuals that is characterized by pain and stiffness in the shoulder and/or pelvic girdles. Constitutional symptoms are common (33% to 50% of patients). Core criteria include:
   - Patient age ≥50 years
   - Bilateral aching involving the shoulder girdle for ≥2 weeks
   - ESR >40 mm/h and/or elevated C-reactive protein (CRP)
   - Morning stiffness for >45 minutes
   - Bilateral hip pain or a limited range of motion
   - Absence of rheumatoid factor (RF) and antibodies to citrullinated antigens (ACPAs)
   - Rapid response to corticosteroids (prednisone 15 mg daily)
   - Exclusion of other diagnoses except giant cell arteritis (GCA); see Question 16.

   Recently, experts from the ACR and EULAR have established provisional classification criteria using a point system to help in research studies. All patients were required to have the first three criteria (age ≥50 years, bilateral shoulder aching, and abnormal ESR or CRP). The point system applied to morning stiffness (2 points), hip pain (1 point), absence of RF/ACPA (2 points), and absence of other joint pain (1 point). The diagnostic accuracy of the required three criteria plus a score of at least 4 points for the other criteria yielded sensitivity of 68% and specificity of 78%. Addition of shoulder ultrasound increased the diagnostic accuracy marginally.

4. **Who is affected by PMR?**
   PMR is the second most common autoimmune syndrome (after rheumatoid arthritis), with a lifetime risk of 2.4% for women and 1.7% for men. PMR rarely affects those <50 years of age and becomes more common with increasing age. Most patients are >60 years of age, with a mean age of onset of approximately 70 years. Women are affected twice as often as men. PMR, like GCA, largely affects whites and is uncommon in Blacks, Hispanic, Asian, and Native American individuals.

5. **Describe the typical stiffness and pain of PMR.**
   - Stiffness and pain are usually subacute or insidious in onset, symmetric, and profound, and they involve more than one area (neck, shoulders, pelvic girdle). However, at times the onset is abrupt or the initial symptoms are unilateral and then progress to symmetric involvement.

- The shoulder is often (70% to 95% of patients) the first area to be affected. The neck and pelvic girdle are involved in 50% to 70% of cases. A single area may be the predominant source of pain. Symptoms may start unilaterally but usually become bilateral within weeks.
- The magnitude of the pain limits mobility; stiffness and gelling phenomena are dramatic. Pain at night is common and may wake the patient.
- Patients may complain of a sensation of muscle weakness due to the pain and stiffness.

6. Describe the arthritis of PMR.
Approximately 50% of patients can have peripheral joint manifestations. Nonerosive, asymmetric arthritis of the distal joints has been described in up to 30% of cases. Knee effusions, wrist synovitis (often with carpal tunnel syndrome), and sternoclavicular arthritis are detected most frequently. Knee effusions can be large (30 to 150 mL). Ankle and metatarsophalangeal joint (MTP) arthritis are rare and should prompt consideration of another diagnosis. Other peripheral manifestations include remitting seronegative symmetric synovitis with pitting edema (RS3PE syndrome) and tenosynovitis of the extensor tendons of the hands. These may be present initially or occur later during the course of PMR.

7. What are the findings on physical examination of patients with PMR?
Physical findings are less striking than the history would lead the clinician to believe. Up to 33% of patients have constitutional symptoms/signs and appear chronically ill, with weight loss, fatigue, depression, and low-grade fever. High, spiking fevers are unusual unless GCA is present. The neck and shoulders are often tender, and active shoulder motion may be limited by pain. For longer illness duration, capsular contracture of the shoulder (limiting passive motion) and muscle atrophy may occur. Joint movement increases the pain, which is often felt in the proximal extremities, not the joints. Clinical synovitis is most frequently noted in the knees, wrists, and sternoclavicular joints. Carpal tunnel syndrome may be present. Muscle strength testing is often confounded by the presence of pain. However, strength is normal unless disuse atrophy has occurred.

8. What is the etiopathogenesis of PMR?
The cause of PMR is unknown but there is no evidence of an infectious agent or toxin. Clues are presumably provided by the epidemiology of the disease, yet the association of PMR with aging is without clear explanation. The higher prevalence in whites has suggested a genetic predisposition, and an association with human leukocyte antigen DR4 has been reported. The immune system is implicated in the pathogenesis. One model suggests that both PMR and GCA start with activation of dendritic cells at the adventitia–media border, which results in production of IL-1 and IL-6 and causes systemic signs/symptoms and elevated acute-phase reactants. Unlike GCA, patients with PMR do not recruit T cells capable of producing IFN-γ. Without IFN-γ to stimulate macrophages, the arterial inflammation characteristic of GCA does not develop.

9. Explain the source of the symptoms of PMR.
PMR is a systemic inflammatory syndrome, accounting for the frequent constitutional symptoms. Synovitis of the hips and shoulders is difficult to detect clinically but many authors believe it is the cause of the proximal stiffness and pain. This is supported by scintigraphic evidence of axial synovitis, synovial fluid analysis, and synovial biopsy. Some authors have proposed tenosynovitis (biceps) and bursitis (subdeltoid, subacromial, trochanteric, and interspinous muscles) rather than synovitis as the source of symptoms. Magnetic resonance imaging of the shoulders has demonstrated this in some patients. Muscle biopsies are usually normal or show nonspecific changes and no inflammation.

10. What is the most characteristic laboratory finding? Is it always present?
Elevated ESR, often >100 mm/h, is the characteristic laboratory finding. PMR may occasionally (7%) occur with normal or only mildly elevated ESR (<40 mm/h). CRP is usually elevated.

11. Are there other commonly encountered laboratory abnormalities?
Findings reflecting the systemic inflammatory process (normochromic normocytic anemia, thrombocytosis, increased gamma globulins, elevated acute-phase reactants) are common. Liver-associated enzyme abnormalities may be seen in up to one third of patients; an increased alkaline phosphatase level is most common. Renal function, urinalysis, and serum creatine kinase levels are normal. Tests for antinuclear antibodies, RF, and ACPAs are negative.

12. Describe the results of synovial fluid analysis.
Synovial fluid is typically inflammatory with a poor mucin clot. However, leukocyte counts have varied from 1000 to 20,000 cell/uL (mean 2900) with 40% to 50% polymorphonuclear leukocytes. Culture and crystal examinations are negative.

13. How are PMR and GCA related?
PMR and GCA frequently occur synchronously or sequentially in individual patients. PMR has been noted in 40% to 60% of patients with GCA and may be the initial symptom complex in 20% to 40% of cases. Conversely, GCA may occur in 30% of patients with PMR. It is notable that the presence of histologic GCA has been reported in 10% to 15% of patients with PMR who had no clinical evidence of arteritis, and positron emission tomography scans have shown increased uptake in the aorta in 30% of PMR patients, suggesting

subclinical arteritis can occur. The clinical significance and outcome of this occult GCA in patients with PMR are unclear.

14. **When should a temporal artery biopsy be performed on a patient with PMR? (controversial)**
Temporal artery biopsy is usually not necessary unless symptoms or signs suggest the presence of GCA. The patient should be queried regarding current or recent headache, jaw claudication, visual disturbance, scalp tenderness, and other features of GCA. Patients with fever are more likely to have occult GCA. The arteries of the head, neck, torso, and extremities should be examined for tenderness, enlargement, bruits, and decreased pulsation. Constitutional symptoms and laboratory values in PMR and GCA are similar and therefore are not of discriminatory value. However, failure of prednisone (15 to 20 mg/day) to significantly improve symptoms or to normalize ESR/CRP within 1 month should suggest the presence of GCA and prompt temporal artery biopsy.

15. **How is the diagnosis of PMR established?**
The diagnosis of PMR is a clinical one, relying on features in the clinical definition. Several different classification criteria are published (see Question 3).

16. **What other diagnoses should be considered before to diagnosing PMR? How are they differentiated?**
Table 25-1 lists factors to consider in the differential diagnosis of PMR.

Table 25-1. Differential Diagnoses in Polymyalgia Rheumatica/Giant Cell Arteritis

DIAGNOSIS	DISTINGUISHING FEATURES
Fibromyalgia syndrome	Tender points, normal ESR
Hypothyroidism	Elevated thyroid-stimulating hormone, normal ESR
Depression	Normal ESR
Shoulder OA, rotator cuff, frozen shoulder	Physical examination, x-rays, normal ESR
Polymyositis	Weakness predominates; elevated creatine kinase; abnormal electromyography
Malignancy (especially lymphoma, myeloma)	Clinical evidence of neoplasm (except for possibly myelodysplastic syndromes there is no association of cancer with PMR)
Occult infection (TB, HIV, SBE)	Clinical suspicion of infection; cultures, and serologies
Late-onset spondyloarthropathy	Low back pain, abnormal spine x-rays, psoriasis
Rheumatoid arthritis	Positive rheumatoid factor, small joint involvement, especially MTPs

ESR, Erythrocyte sedimentation rate; OA, osteoarthritis; PMR, polymyalgia rheumatics; TB, tuberculosis; HIV, human immunodeficiency virus; SBE, subacute bacterial endocarditis; MTP, metatarsophalangeal joint.

17. **How is PMR distinguished from rheumatoid arthritis?**
It is often difficult to distinguish PMR from the onset of rheumatoid arthritis in older patients, in whom constitutional symptoms and morning stiffness often surpass joint manifestations. Features that support the diagnosis of PMR are as follows:
- Absence of RF and anti-CCP antibodies
- Lack of involvement of small joints (metacarpophalangeal and proximal interphalangeal joints, MTPs) of the hands and feet
- Lack of development of joint damage
- Absence of erosive disease during follow-up

The response to glucocorticoids is not a reliable distinguishing feature.

18. **How are nonsteroidal antiinflammatory drugs used in the treatment of PMR?**
Nonsteroidal antiinflammatory drugs (NSAIDs) are an effective therapy in only 10% to 20% of patients and are best used in those with mild symptoms. As with other diseases, no individual NSAID is necessarily more effective than another, and selection is based on the perception of tolerability and safety for the patient. NSAIDs may be added to glucocorticoid therapy to facilitate steroid tapering. However, the toxicities of NSAIDs need to be kept in mind, particularly given the age of these patients and the duration of therapy.

19. **Describe the use of glucocorticoids in PMR.**
Prednisone at a dose of 15 to 20 mg/day usually evokes a dramatic and rapid response, although up to 25% of patients will not respond dramatically and the treatment will take a few days to be maximally effective.

Prednisone is highly lipophilic, so some investigators recommend a dose of 0.20 mg/kg based on body weight. Using this guideline, lean individuals may be treated with lower doses (10 to 15 mg/day) initially, whereas obese patients will need higher doses. Most patients are significantly better within 1 to 2 days, although others may take longer (1 to 2 weeks) to respond completely. A single daily dose is more effective than alternate-day dosing.

Patients with mild PMR who are at high risk of steroid side effects may be treated more safely with intramuscular methylprednisolone at 120 mg every 4 weeks, which is reduced by 20 mg every 3 months if symptoms and ESR/CRP remain normal.

Tapering of an oral prednisone dose is based on the patient's clinical response. PMR symptoms and ESR/CRP are the most reliable parameters to follow. CRP normalizes more quickly than ESR, which should steadily decline to normal within 1 month. Failure to normalize these acute-phase reactants should prompt a search for occult GCA or an alternative diagnosis. Once ESR and CRP are normalized, the prednisone dose is decreased by 2.5 mg every 2 to 4 weeks until a dose of 10 mg/day is attained. Further tapering is by 1 mg every 1 to 2 months while the patient and ESR or CRP are monitored. During the tapering, an increase in ESR or CRP in an otherwise asymptomatic patient does not justify an increase in prednisone dosage. However, the dose should not be tapered any further until alternative causes of the elevated acute-phase reactant have been investigated.

20. What is the course of PMR?

The course of PMR is longer and recurrences are more frequent than once believed. Possible predictors of a poor clinical course include older age at diagnosis, female sex, and very high ESR/CRP with failure to normalize CRP within 1 week of starting prednisone. Overall, some 75% of patients are able to taper off their prednisone treatment within 2 years. However, between 25% and 35% of patients require low doses of glucocorticoids indefinitely because of a relapse each time the prednisone is tapered off. In those who are able to stop taking glucocorticoids, PMR relapse can occur in 10% to 20% of patients some months or even years later. In these patients, ESR may not be as high as on their original presentation.

21. Given the course of PMR, for how long should prednisone be continued?

Optimally, prednisone administration should be tapered off and discontinued as quickly as possible because side effects are common (65% of patients). However, relapse can result if the tapering off is too rapid. If relapse occurs, control is often regained via only a small increase in dosage. Slow tapering can again be carried out, halting at a dose just above that at which relapse occurred. This is often 5 mg/day or less. Further tapering (1 mg every 2 months) is attempted again after a period of 6 months to 1 year. In patients with steroid-dependent PMR, use of methotrexate can facilitate tapering of steroids. Biologic therapy such as steroid-sparing agents has had mixed results. Reports from uncontrolled studies suggest that etanercept is effective, whereas a controlled trial using infliximab did not show benefit. It was recently reported that tocilizumab is effective, highlighting the prominent role of IL-6 in the pathogenesis of PMR.

22. Other than medication, what should be included in the treatment plan for PMR?

- Reassurance
- Patient education
- Regular physician monitoring
- Range-of-motion exercises, especially where muscle atrophy and/or contracture have occurred
- Attention to glucocorticoid side effects, especially osteoporosis, glucose intolerance, and hyperlipidemia
- Immunizations, including a flu shot, Pneumovax, and zoster vaccine

Bibliography

Barber HS: Myalgic syndrome with constitutional effects: polymyalgia rheumatica, Ann Rheum Dis 16:230–237, 1957.
Blockmans D, DeCeuninck L, Vanderschueren S, et al: Repetitive 18-fluorodeoxyglucose positron emission tomography in isolated polymyalgia rheumatica: a prospective study in 35 patients, Rheumatology 46:672–677, 2007.
Caporali R, Cimmino MA, Ferraccioli G, et al: Prednisone plus methotrexate for polymyalgia rheumatica: a randomized, double-blind, placebo-controlled trial, Ann Intern Med 141:624–628, 2004.
Crowson CS, Matteson EL, Myasoedova E, et al: The lifetime risk of adult-onset rheumatoid arthritis and other inflammatory autoimmune rheumatic diseases, Arthritis Rheum 63:633–639, 2011.
Dasgupta B, Borg FA, Hassan N, et al: BSR and BHPR guidelines for the management of polymyalgia rheumatica, Rheumatology 49:186–190, 2010.
Dasgupta B, Cimmino MA, Kremers HM, et al: 2012 provisional classification criteria for polymyalgia rheumatica, Arthritis Rheum 64:943–954, 2012.
Gabriel SE, Sunku J, Salvarani C, et al: Adverse outcomes of antiinflammatory therapy among patients with polymyalgia rheumatica, Arthritis Rheum 40:1873–1878, 1997.
Gran JT, Myklebust G: The incidence and clinical characteristics of peripheral arthritis in polymyalgia rheumatica and temporal arteritis: a prospective study of 231 cases, Rheumatology 39:283–287, 2000.
Hagihara K, Kawase I, Tanaka T, Kishimoto T: Tocilizumab ameliorates clinical symptoms in polymyalgia rheumatica, J Rheumatol 37:1075–1076, 2010.
Hernandez-Rodriguez J, Cid MC, Lopez-Soto A, et al: Treatment of polymyalgia rheumatica, Arch Intern Med 169:1839–1850, 2009.

Mackie SL, Hensor EM, Haugeberg G, et al: Can the prognosis of polymyalgia rheumatica be predicted at disease onset? Results from a 5-year prospective study, Rheumatology 49:716–722, 2010.
Proven A, Gabriel SE, O'Fallon WM, Hunder GG: Polymyalgia rheumatica with low erythrocyte sedimentation rate at diagnosis, J Rheumatol 26:1333–1337, 1999.
Salvarini C, Cantini F, Consonni D, et al: Acute-phase reactants and risk of relapse/recurrence in polymyalgia rheumatica: a prospective followup study, Arthritis Rheum 53:33–38, 2005.
Salvarani C, Cantini F, Hunder GG: Polymyalgia rheumatica and giant-cell arteritis, Lancet 372:234–245, 2008.
Salvarani C, Cantini F, Olivieri I, et al: Proximal bursitis in active polymyalgia rheumatica, Ann Intern Med 127:270–331, 1997.
Salvarani C, Gabriel S, Hunder GG: Distal extremity swelling with pitting edema in polymyalgia rheumatica. Report on nineteen cases, Arthritis Rheum 39:73–80, 1996.
Salvarani C, Macchioni P, Manzini C, et al: Infliximab plus prednisone or placebo plus prednisone for the initial treatment of polymyalgia rheumatica: a randomized controlled trial, Ann Intern Med 146:631–639, 2007.

IV

THE VASCULITIDES AND RELATED DISORDERS

We are too much accustomed to attribute to a single cause that which is the product of several, and the majority of our controversies come from that.

Baron Justus Von Liegig (1803–1873)
German chemist

APPROACH FOR PATIENTS WITH SUSPECTED VASCULITIS

Marc D. Cohen, MD

CHAPTER 26

> **KEY POINTS**
> 1. There is no single typical presentation of vasculitis.
> 2. Vasculitides are classified by the size of the blood vessel involved: large-, medium-, or small-vessel vasculitis.
> 3. The types of vasculitis differ widely with regard to age, gender, ethnicity, and clinical presentation.
> 4. Appropriate tissue biopsies or angiographic studies are usually necessary for diagnosis.
> 5. The aggressiveness of treatment should be commensurate with the extent of end-organ involvement.

1. **What is the definition of vasculitis? What are the vascular consequences?**
   Vasculitis is inflammation and necrosis of a blood vessel with subsequent impairment of blood flow. The vessel wall destruction leads to perforation and hemorrhage into adjacent tissues. The endothelial injury leads to thrombosis and subsequent impairment of blood flow causing ischemia/infarction of dependent tissues. Long-term consequences include accelerated secondary atherosclerosis of the involved vessel, which contributes to morbidity and mortality.

2. **What are the characteristic histologic features of vasculitis?**
   - Infiltration of the vessel wall by neutrophils, mononuclear cells, and/or giant cells
   - Fibrinoid necrosis (panmural destruction of the vessel wall)
   - Leukocytoclasis (dissolution of leukocytes, yielding "nuclear dust")

   Perivascular infiltration is a nonspecific histologic finding observed in a variety of disease processes and is not considered diagnostic of vasculitis, even though it may coexist in vasculitic tissues.

   Figure 26-1 shows vasculitis in a bowel specimen from a patient with polyarteritis nodosa (PAN).

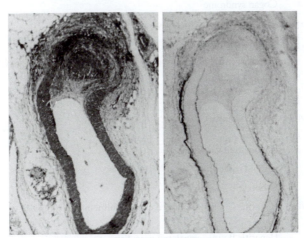

Figure 26-1. Necrotizing vasculitis in a bowel specimen from a patient with polyarteritis nodosa. The arterial lumen is partially occluded by thrombus. The adjacent arterial wall is necrotic, resulting in destruction of the elastic laminae: *(left)* hematoxylin–eosin staining; *(right)* elastic tissue staining; lower power. (Copyright 2014 American College of Rheumatology. Used with permission.)

3. **Via which immune mechanism does vasculitis occur?**
   Cell-mediated, immune-complex-mediated, and **antineutrophil cytoplasmic antibody (ANCA)-associated** mechanisms are involved, depending on the vasculitis. Examples of cell-mediated vasculitis include giant cell arteritis (GCA), Takayasu arteritis, and primary central nervous system (CNS) vasculitis. Examples of

immune-complex-mediated vasculitis include PAN, Henoch–Schönlein purpura, cryoglobulinemic vasculitis, and cutaneous leukocytoclastic angiitis. The ANCA-associated vasculitides, which may involve both cellular and humoral mechanisms, include granulomatosis with polyangiitis (GPA; Wegener granulomatosis), microscopic polyangiitis (MPA), and eosinophilic granulomatosis with polyangiitis (EGPA; Churg–Strauss syndrome). The immune mechanisms of the other types of vasculitis are less certain.

4. **What is the international Chapel Hill consensus conference nomenclature for the vasculitides?**
Table 26-1 describes the vasculitis nomenclature agreed at the Chapel Hill consensus conference.

Table 26-1. Vasculitis Nomenclature Agreed at the International Chapel Hill Consensus Conference

NOMENCLATURE	VASCULITIS
Large-vessel vasculitis	Takayasu arteritis
	Giant cell (temporal) arteritis (GCA)
Medium-vessel vasculitis	Polyarteritis nodosa (PAN)
	Kawasaki disease
Small-vessel vasculitis	Immune-complex-mediated
	Anti-glomerular basement membrane (anti-GBM) disease
	Cryoglobulinemic vasculitis
	IgA vasculitis (Henoch–Schönlein purpura)
	Hypocomplementemic urticarial vasculitis (HUVS, anti-Clq vasculitis)
	Antineutrophil cytoplasmic antibody-associated (pauci-immune)
	Granulomatosis with polyangiitis (GPA)(Wegener's granulomatosis)
	Microscopic polyangiitis (MPA)
	Eosinophilic granulomatosis with polyangiitis (EGPA) (Churg-Strauss)
Variable-vessel vasculitis*	Behçet disease
	Cogan syndrome
Single-organ vasculitis	Cutaneous leukocytoclastic vasculitis
	Cutaneous arteritis
	Primary central nervous system vasculitis (isolated angiitis of CNS)
	Isolated aortitis
	Others
Vasculitis associated with systemic disease	Lupus vasculitis
	Rheumatoid vasculitis
	Sarcoid vasculitis
	Others
Vasculitis associated with probable etiology	Hepatitis C virus-associated cryoglobulinemic vasculitis
	Hepatitis B virus-associated vasculitis
	Syphilis-associated vasculitis
	Drug-associated immune complex vasculitis (hypersensitivity vasculitis)
	Drug-associated ANCA-associated vasculitis
	Cancer-associated vasculitis
	Others

*Thromboangiitis obliterans (Buerger disease) was not classified at this conference but probably best fits as variable-vessel vasculitis.

Note: There are specific American College of Rheumatology classification criteria for many of the major types of vasculitis. These differentiate one vasculitis from another, rather than describing all of the manifestations of a particular form of vasculitis. Thus, these criteria are rarely useful for diagnosis, and appropriate tissue biopsy is generally necessary for confirmation.

5. How should the physician approach the diagnosis of vasculitis?
1. Suspect the disease.
2. Define the extent of the disease.
3. Rule out vasculitis mimics.
4. Confirm the diagnosis.

6. How does vasculitis typically present?
There is no single typical presentation of vasculitis. Vasculitis should be suspected in any constitutionally ill patient who has evidence of multisystem inflammatory disease. The clinical manifestations may suggest the size of vessel involved and the most likely vasculitis. Typical presentations are as follows:
- **Large-vessel vasculitis:** limb claudication, bruits, asymmetric blood pressures, absence of pulses
- **Medium-vessel vasculitis:** cutaneous nodules, ulcers, livedo reticularis, digital gangrene, mononeuritis multiplex, renovascular hypertension
- **Small-vessel vasculitis:** palpable purpura, urticaria, glomerulonephritis, alveolar hemorrhage, scleritis

PEARL: Headache or visual loss in the elderly (GCA), asymmetric pulses with bruits in a patient <30 years of age (Takayasu arteritis), mononeuritis multiplex (PAN), rapidly progressive pulmonary–renal syndrome (ANCA-associated vasculitis), and palpable purpura (immune-complex-mediated vasculitis) are the most common presentations suggesting vasculitis.

7. When should the rheumatologist suspect vasculitis mimics?
Because of its protean manifestations, vasculitis can easily be confused with other diseases. Mimics of vasculitis must be excluded early in the evaluation because treatment varies dramatically and misdiagnosis may result in morbidity and/or mortality. Vasculitis mimics should be suspected when there is:
1. A new heart murmur (subacute bacterial endocarditis, SBE)
2. Necrosis of lower-extremity digits (cholesterol emboli)
3. Splinter hemorrhages (SBE)
4. Prominent liver dysfunction (hepatitis C)
5. Drug abuse (human immunodeficiency virus, HIV; hepatitis B/C; cocaine, etc.)
6. Prior diagnosis of neoplastic disease
7. Unusually high fever (SBE)
8. History of high-risk sexual activity (HIV)

8. What disorders can mimic vasculitis?
The following disorders can mimic vasculitis (common clinical entities in italics):

Large arteries: *Fibromuscular dysplasia*, radiation fibrosis, neurofibromatosis type I, congenital coarctation of aorta, genetic diseases (Marfan syndrome, Loeys–Dietz syndrome), syphilitic aortitis, IgG4 disease

Medium arteries: *Cholesterol emboli syndrome, atrial myxoma, fibromuscular dysplasia*, lymphomatoid granulomatosis, angioblastic T-cell lymphoma, thromboembolic disease, ergotism, type IV Ehlers–Danlos syndrome, segmental arterial mediolysis, Grange syndrome, pseudoxanthoma elasticum

Cerebral arteries: *Reversible cerebral vasoconstrictive syndrome, reversible posterior encephalopathy syndrome, cerebral amyloid angioapthy*, CADASIL syndrome, Susac syndrome, progressive multifocal leukoencephalopathy, Moyamoya disease, intravascular lymphoma, infections

Small arteries: *Infectious endocarditis, mycotic aneurysm with emboli, cholesterol microemboli syndrome, antiphospholipid antibody syndrome, sepsis (gonococcal, meningococcal)*, ecthyma gangrenosum (*Pseudomonas*), thrombotic thrombocytopenia purpura, cocaine, amphetamines, minocycline, hydralazine, HIV, hepatitis C, amyloidosis, systemic rheumatic diseases (*systemic lupus erythematosus*, SLE; *Sjögren's syndrome*), bacteremias (*SBE, Rickettsia*), other systemic viral infections, common variable immunodeficiency, calciphylaxis, livedoid vasculopathy (atrophie blanche), malignant atrophic papulosis (Degos disease)

To rule out vasculitis mimics, consider blood cultures, viral hepatitis studies, HIV testing, urinary toxicology screening, echocardiography, antinuclear antibody (ANA), rheumatoid factor (RF), antiphospholipid antibodies, and/or angiography/magnetic resonance angiography, depending on the clinical situation.

9. What localizing clinical features suggest the different types of vasculitis?
Table 26-2 lists features suggestive of different types of vasculitis. These features occur either before, during, or after the constitutional features and are also relatively nonspecific, with considerable overlap.

Table 26-2. Localized Clinical Features that Suggest Different Types of Vasculitis	
SYMPTOMS	**DIAGNOSIS**
Jaw claudication, visual loss, palpable, thickened, tender temporal artery, or	Giant cell arteritis (GCA)
Diminished temporal artery pulsation	
Absent radial pulses, difficulty obtaining a blood pressure in one arm	Takayasu arteritis or large artery involvement in GCA
Sinus involvement, otitis media, scleritis	GPA (Wegener) or EGPA (Churg–Strauss syndrome)
Hypertension, renal vascular involvement	Polyarteritis nodosa or Takayasu arteritis
Asthma	EGPA (Churg–Strauss syndrome)
Testicular tenderness	Polyarteritis nodosa
Pulmonary–renal syndromes (hemoptysis and glomerulonephritis)	GPA (Wegener) and microscopic polyangiitis

10. **What skin lesions are suggestive of vasculitis?**
    - Medium-vessel vasculitis: subcutaneous nodules, "punched-out" skin ulcers, livedo reticularis, digital gangrene
    - Small-vessel vasculitis: palpable purpura, splinter hemorrhages, hemorrhagic macules, vesiculobullous lesions, and urticaria lasting >24 hours

    Examples are shown in Figure 26-2.

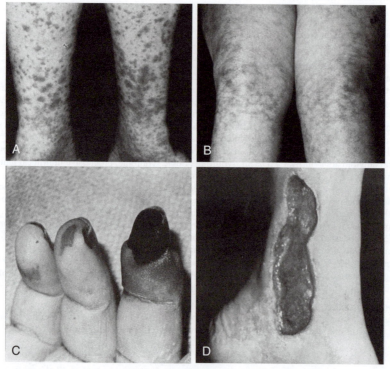

Figure 26-2. A, Palpable purpura. B, Livedo reticularis. C, Digital infarction. D, "Punched out" ulcer. (A, C, D, Copyright 2014 American College of Rheumatology. Used with permission. B, From Colledge N, Walker B, Ralston S: Davidson's principles and practice of medicine, ed 21, Philadelphia, 2010, Churchill Livingstone, Figure 25-37.)

11. **Which laboratory tests are useful in the evaluation of suspected vasculitis?**
    - Tests suggesting systemic inflammation

    Complete blood count: look for anemia of chronic disease and thrombocytosis. White blood cell count and differential to look for neutrophilia or eosinophilia.
    - Primary systemic vasculitis *never* causes pancytopenia (must rule out SLE, B cell lymphoma, myeloma, leukemia)

    Westergren ESR and CRP. ESR >100 mm/h and CRP >10 mg/dL in the absence of bacterial infection and widespread cancer should suggest vasculitis.

    Low albumin: this is a negative acute-phase reactant and decreases with systemic inflammation.
    - Tests suggesting organ involvement

    Creatinine and urinalysis

    Liver-associated enzymes: if extremely elevated, consider hepatitis B/C

    Creatine kinase

    Stool for occult blood

    Chest radiograph

    Brain magnetic resonance imaging or an abdominal computed tomography (CT) scan if symptoms suggest involvement
    - Tests suggesting immune complex formation and/or deposition

    RF and ANA:
    - RF and ANA should not be positive in **primary** systemic vasculitis. If RF is positive, consider cryoglobulinemia and SBE. If ANA is positive, consider SLE or Sjögren's syndrome.

    Cryoglobulins: if positive, rule out hepatitis C.

    Complement levels—C3/C4 are low in cryoglobulinemia, HUVS, and SLE. Other vasculitides usually have normal values except PAN, where they are low in up to 25% of cases, and in some cases of hypersensitivity vasculitides.
    - Tests suggesting ANCA-related vasculitis

    c-ANCA: if against serine proteinase 3, usually GPA; sometimes MPA.

    p-ANCA: if against myeloperoxidase, consider MPA and EGPA; sometimes GPA.

    Cocaine-associated vasculitis can be c-ANCA, p-ANCA, and/or atypical ANCA (anti-human neutrophil elastase [HNE]) positive.
    - Tests suggesting etiology

    Blood cultures: rule out SBE

    Infectious serologies: Hep BsAg (PAN), hepatitis C (cryoglobulinemia), parvovirus IgM (GPA, PAN), herpes (IgM), cytomegalovirus (CMV) (IgM), Epstein–Barr virus (EBV), (IgM), HIV (any vasculitis)

    Serum protein electrophoresis: rule out myeloma

    Cerebrospinal fluid studies: herpes, varicella-zoster virus

    Urinary toxicology screen: rule out cocaine use

    Not all of these tests are ordered for all patients. The physician must choose which test to order according to the clinical situation.

12. **How might ANCAs be helpful in differentiating vasculitis?**
    The c-ANCA directed against serine proteinase 3 is highly specific for GPA with widespread systemic involvement (>90%). Less specific is p-ANCA with anti-myeloperoxidase specificity, which may be found in MPA and EGPA (Churg–Strauss vasculitis). If the p-ANCA is not against myeloperoxidase, inflammatory diseases other than vasculitis should be considered (inflammatory bowel disease, infections). In some patients, ANCAs may have predictive value for relapses and ongoing disease activity. ANCAs may be pathogenic as part of several simultaneous or sequential events.

13. **When are hepatitis serologies helpful when vasculitis is suspected?**
    The presence of hepatitis B surface antigen may be found in some patients (10% to 25%, depending on risk factors) with PAN. Hepatitis C antibodies are often found in patients with essential mixed cryoglobulinemic vasculitis and rarely in PAN.

14. **What other diagnostic studies are commonly used in the evaluation of suspected vasculitis?**
    - Chest x-ray
    - Echocardiography
    - Sinus x-rays or CT scan
    - Angiography (if renal function acceptable)
    - Electromyography and nerve conduction studies
    - Tissue biopsy

15. **What is the role of tissue biopsy in the diagnosis of vasculitis and in what type of vasculitis might tissue biopsy be helpful?**
    Tissue biopsy is unquestionably the procedure of choice in the diagnosis of vasculitis. Some frequently approached biopsy sites are as follows:
    - **Common sites:** Skin, sural nerve (PAN, EGPA; only biopsy if abnormal electromyogram [EMG]/nerve conduction velocity [NCV]), temporal artery (GCA), muscle (PAN), kidney (GPA, MPA; rare to see vasculitis, usually see focal necrotizing glomerulonephritis with or without crescents), lung (GPA, MPA)
    - **Less common sites:** Testicle (PAN), rectum/gut, liver, heart, brain (primary CNS vasculitis), sinus (GPA)

16. **If tissue biopsy is not feasible, what alternative procedures can yield a diagnosis?**
    Angiography at the following sites may be helpful for diagnosis of certain types of vasculitis:
    - Abdomen (celiac trunk, superior mesenteric, and renal arteries) for diagnosis of PAN
    - Aortic arch for diagnosis of Takayasu arteritis and GCA with large-vessel involvement.
    - Extremities for diagnosis of Buerger disease
    - Cerebral sites for diagnosis of primary CNS vasculitis

17. **List two characteristic (but not diagnostic) angiographic features of vasculitis.**
    - Irregular tapering and narrowing (Figure 26-3)

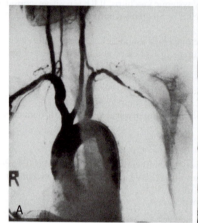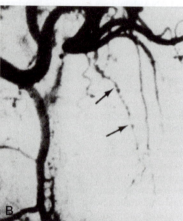

Figure 26-3. Angiography in vasculitis. **A,** Irregular tapering and narrowing of the left subclavian artery in Takayasu arteritis. **B,** Typical "rosary bead" aneurysm formation in a patient with isolated central nervous system.

- Aneurysms ("beading")

18. **What noninvasive tests can be used to determine vessel involvement in patients with vasculitis?**
    - Doppler ultrasound of temporal arteries can localize the area of narrowing in GCA and help determine biopsy sites.
    - Magnetic resonance angiography of the aorta can reveal aortic wall thickening (enhancement with gadolinium indicates inflammation) and areas of stenosis in patients with Takayasu arteritis or GCA with large-artery involvement.
    - Positron emission tomography can reveal enhancement of the aortic and subclavian vessel wall if active inflammation occurs in patients with Takayasu arteritis and GCA.

19. **Describe the general approach to the treatment of a vasculitis.**
    - Identify and remove inciting agents (i.e., medications, infection, etc.).
    - Treat the primary underlying disease associated with the vasculitis (antibiotics for endocarditis, antiviral therapy for hepatitis B or C).
    - Initiate antiinflammatory and/or immunosuppressive therapy commensurate with the extent of the vasculitis. Small-vessel vasculitis confined to the skin usually needs less aggressive treatment than systemic vasculitis involving large and/or medium-sized arteries
    - The combination of cyclophosphamide and prednisone is often regarded as the first choice for induction therapy of generalized and severe types of vasculitis. New targeted biologic agents may replace cyclophosphamide as induction therapy for some forms of vasculitis (e.g., rituximab for ANCA-associated vasculitis).

Maintenance therapies are less well-defined but typically involve the use of azatioprine, methotrexate, or mycophenolate mofetil.
- Prevent complications such as infection (PPD, Pneumovax, and other immunizations; trimethoprim–sulfamethoxazole prophylaxis if on high dose prednisone), osteoporosis, and atherosclerosis (control blood pressure and lipids).

Bibliography

Bacon PA: Endothelial cell dysfunction in systemic vasculitis: new developments and therapeutic prospects, Curr Opin Rheumatol 17:49–55, 2004.
Carlson JA, Ng BT, Chen KR: Cutaneous vasculitis update, Am J Dermatopathol 27:504–528, 2005.
Cohen MD, Conn DL: Approach to the patient with suspected vasculitis, Bull Rheum Dis 48:1–4, 1999.
Gonzalez-Gay MA, Garcia-Porrua C, Pujol RM: Clinical approach to cutaneous vasculitis, Curr Opin Rheumatol 17:56–61, 2005.
Holle JU, Gross WL: ANCA-associated vasculitides: pathogenetic aspects and current evidence-based therapy, J Autoimmun 32:163–171, 2009.
Jennette JC, Falk RJ, Bacon PA, et al: 2012 revised international Chapel Hill consensus conference nomenclature of vasculitides, Arthritis Rheum 65:1–11, 2013.
Langford CA: Vasculitis, J Allergy Clin Immunol 125(Suppl 2):216–225, 2010.
Miller A, Chan M, Wiik A, et al: An approach to the diagnosis and management of systemic vasculitis, Clin Exp Immunol 160:143–160, 2010.
Molloy ES, Langford CA: Vasculitis mimics, Curr Opin Rheumatol 20:29–34, 2008.
Pipitone N, Versari A, Salvarani C: Role of imaging studies in the diagnosis and follow-up of large-vessel vasculitis: an update, Rheumatology 47:403–408, 2008.
Russell JP, Weening RH: Primary cutaneous small vessel vasculitis, Curr Treat Options Cardiovasc Med 6:139–149, 2004.
Rodriguez-Pla A, Stone JH: Vasculitis and systemic infections, Curr Opin Rheumatol 18:39–47, 2006.
Seo P, Stone JH: Large-vessel vasculitis, Arthritis Rheum 51:128–139, 2004.
Seo P, Stone JH: Small-vessel and medium-vessel vasculitis, Arthritis Rheum 57:1552–1559, 2007.
Stone JH, Nousari HC: Essential cutaneous vasculitis: what every rheumatologist should know about vasculitis of the skin, Curr Opin Rheumatol 13:23–34, 2001.
Stone JH: Vasculitis: a collection of pearls and myths, Rheum Dis Clin North Am 33:691–739, 2007.

CHAPTER 27

LARGE-VESSEL VASCULITIS: GIANT CELL ARTERITIS, TAKAYASU ARTERITIS, AND AORTITIS

Puja Chitkara, MD and Gregory J. Dennis, MD

KEY POINTS

1. Giant cell arteritis (GCA) is the most common vasculitis in adults >50 years of age.
2. Jaw claudication is the most specific symptom for GCA.
3. GCA frequently affects the aorta, which can lead to aneurysm formation.
4. Consider Takayasu arteritis (TA) in any young woman with asymmetric blood pressure (BP) and bruits.
5. IgG4-related disease should be ruled out in patients with thoracic aortitis and aneurysm.

1. **List the primary large-vessel vasculitides and the rheumatic diseases associated with large-vessel vasculitis.**
   GCA, TA, and other rheumatic diseases associated with aortitis such as the seronegative spondyloarthropathies, relapsing polychondritis, Behçet disease, Cogan syndrome, and sarcoidosis.

GIANT CELL ARTERITIS

2. **What are other names for GCA?**
   Cranial arteritis, temporal arteritis, and Horton headache.

3. **Discuss the usual demographic characteristics of a patient with GCA.**
   GCA occurs primarily in patients >50 years of age. The incidence increases with age, and GCA is almost 10 times more common among patients in their 80s than in patients aged 50 to 60 years. GCA is two to three times more common among women than men. Siblings of a patient with GCA are at increased risk (tenfold) of getting the disease. GCA has been most commonly reported in whites of Northern European descent. Epidemiological studies suggest that the incidence of GCA in blacks, Hispanics, and Asians is not as rare as once thought, but is still uncommon.

4. **How do patients with GCA present clinically?**
   Most patients will have one of five presentations:
   - Some 20% of patients have cranial symptoms with superficial headache, scalp tenderness, jaw and tongue claudication, and rarely scalp necrosis, diplopia, or blindness. Jaw claudication is the most specific symptom for GCA although amyloid light-chain amyloidosis can also cause this symptom. New-onset diplopia in an elderly patient is also highly suggestive of GCA.
   - Approximately 40% of patients have polymyalgia rheumatica (PMR) with pain and stiffness of proximal muscle groups, such as the neck, shoulders, hips, and thighs. Muscle symptoms are usually symmetric and the shoulders are most commonly involved. Note that 10% to 20% of patients presenting with PMR develop GCA on follow-up.
   - Some 20% of patients have both cranial and PMR symptoms. About 40% to 50% of patients with GCA have PMR symptoms.
   - About 15% of patients have fever and systemic symptoms without any localized symptoms. Patients can present with a fever of unknown origin (FUO). GCA is the cause in 15% of elderly patients with an FUO.
   - Some 5% of patients have other symptoms, such as cough, claudication (upper > lower extremity), or synovitis.

   The onset of symptoms may be acute or insidious. Most patients have fever (40%), weight loss (50%), fatigue, and malaise (40%) as nonspecific symptoms. Tenosynovitis, carpal tunnel syndrome, and relapsing seronegative symmetric synovitis with pitting edema (RS3PE) can occur. When looked for clinically, evidence of large-vessel vasculitis (e.g., subclavian arteries) is found in up to 20% of patients with GCA who present with cranial symptoms and/or PMR.

5. Are there any physical findings that may be helpful in suggesting a diagnosis of GCA?

Several physical abnormalities are highly specific for GCA, but unfortunately most have a low or only moderate degree of sensitivity for the diagnosis. **Scalp tenderness** and **temporal artery abnormalities**, such as a reduction in the pulse in conjunction with palpable tenderness, yield the greatest specificity for diagnosis. The presence of a visual abnormality (diplopia, amaurosis fugax, unilateral loss of vision, optic neuritis, and optic atrophy) may lend additional support for the diagnosis but are relatively less sensitive. Owing to frequent (15% to 30% of cases) involvement of the aorta and its primary branches, BP and pulses should be checked in both arms to look for discrepancies (>10 mmHg difference in systolic BP between arms) and the carotid and subclavian vessels should be auscultated for the presence of bruits.

6. When should GCA be suspected?

There are no pathognomonic clinical features. GCA should be suspected in individuals aged >50 to 60 years with new onset of unexplained pain above the neck (headache, jaw claudication, other areas mimicking sinusitis/ear pain), unexplained fever, or PMR.

7. What is the most dreaded complication of GCA? How commonly does it occur?

Visual loss occurs in 15% of patients, can be an early symptom, and is most commonly caused by ischemic optic neuritis. Anatomic lesions that produce anterior ischemic optic neuritis result from arteritis involving the posterior ciliary branches of the ophthalmic arteries. The blindness is abrupt and painless. Retinal and ophthalmic artery thromboses and occipital strokes are relatively less common causes of blindness. Blindness occurs in less than 10% of patients after corticosteroid treatment is initiated. Visual symptoms in GCA patients on corticosteroids may be caused by cataracts, glaucoma, and central serous retinopathy.

8. The clinical manifestations of GCA might also include what other ocular problems?

Blurring of vision, transient visual loss (amaurosis fugax), iritis, conjunctivitis, scintillating scotomata, photophobia, glaucoma, and ophthalmoplegia from ischemia of extraocular muscles may also occur. Amaurosis fugax is the most predictive factor (relative risk 6.35) for future development of sudden and permanent blindness.

9. Does GCA only involve the cranial circulation?

Although cranial (not intracranial) involvement is the most frequently recognized and characteristic anatomic location for GCA, the process is a generalized vascular disease not limited to the cranial vessels. Extracranial GCA usually involves the aorta and its major branches and is clinically detectable in 15% to 20% of patients. Positron emission tomography (PET) scans suggest that the aorta is frequently involved (50% to 80%) even if not detectable clinically. Involvement of intracranial vessels is rare.

10. Are neurologic complications common in patients with GCA?

Neurologic complications are relatively rare in GCA. The internal carotid and vertebral arteries may be involved, leading to strokes (3%), seizures, acute hearing loss, vertigo, cerebral dysfunction, and depression. Involvement of the intracranial arteries is unusual because these vessels lack an internal elastic lamina.

11. List the resulting manifestations when GCA involves a particular vascular distribution.

Table 27-1 lists the GCA signs for particular vascular distributions.

Note that GCA can involve both large and medium arteries. Pulmonary artery involvement is unusual. Small-artery involvement is much less common, so skin manifestations are rare.

Table 27-1. Complications for Different Vascular Distributions in Giant Cell Arteritis

VASCULATURE	COMPLICATION
Ophthalmic	Blindness
Subclavian	Absent pulses
Renal	Hypertension
Coronary	Angina pectoris
Carotid	Stroke
Vertebral	Dizziness, stroke
Iliac	Claudication
Mesenteric	Abdominal pain

12. What are the possible clinical consequences occurring late in patients with GCA involvement of their aorta?

Aortitis can lead to aortic aneurysms and dissection. GCA patients have a seventeenfold increased relative risk of developing a thoracic aortic aneurysm and a 2.4-fold increased risk of an abdominal aortic aneurysm compared to control individuals. An aortic valve insufficiency murmur, hyperlipidemia, and coronary artery disease are risk factors for development of an aneurysm. Any GCA patient presenting with unexplained midthoracic or low back pain should be evaluated for aortic aneurysm and dissection. Patients with clinical aortic involvement should be followed with magnetic resonance angiography (MRA) or computed tomography angiography (CTA) every 6 to 12 months for the development of new lesions/stenoses or the development of aneurysms. The monitoring appropriate for GCA patients without known clinical aortic involvement is unclear. Bilateral arm BP measurements, listening for an aortic valve insufficiency murmur and vascular bruits, and palpating for an aortic aneurysm during the clinic visit seem prudent. A yearly chest radiograph or echocardiogram and an abdominal ultrasound looking for aortic enlargement have also been recommended.

13. Which tests are most helpful in the diagnosis of GCA?
The erythrocyte sedimentation rate (ESR) is the most useful laboratory test and tends to be higher in GCA than in other vasculitides. It is almost always >50 mm/h, averaging 80 to 100 mm/h by the Westergren method. Although ESR is a sensitive indicator of GCA in the appropriate clinical setting, its specificity is <50%. Other laboratory abnormalities include anemia, thrombocytosis, abnormal liver function tests (especially alkaline phosphatase), and increased C-reactive protein (CRP; frequently to very high levels, >10 mg/dL). Serologies (rheumatoid factor, anti-CCP, ANA) should be negative.

14. Is it possible for patients with GCA to present with "normal" ESR?
Yes but rarely. Although the vast majority (85% to 90%) of GCA patients present with ESR >50 mm/h, there are case series describing the association of biopsy-proven GCA with ESR of 40 to 50 mm/h in 10% and <40 mm/h in 5% of patients. Systemic symptoms are less common in GCA patients with ESR <50 mm/h. When ESR is <40 to 50 mm/h in a patient suspected of having GCA, elevated CRP provides further evidence of an acute-phase response. Temporal artery biopsy is necessary to confirm the diagnosis in all such cases.

15. What test, if any, is used for confirmation of the clinical diagnosis of GCA?
Temporal artery biopsy of the most abnormal segment is the diagnostic test of choice. In the absence of a palpable abnormality of the temporal artery, biopsy of the main trunk on the most symptomatic side is performed first. **Temporal artery duplex ultrasound** showing homogeneous wall thickening (**halo sign**) has 75% sensitivity and 83% specificity in predicting a positive temporal artery biopsy. In the presence of extracranial involvement, **MRA, CTA,** or catheter **angiography** may provide sufficient support for the diagnosis in the absence of a confirmatory biopsy. ^{18}**F-Fluorodeoxyglucose (FDG)-PET** scans demonstrate extracranial artery and/or aortic involvement in 80% of GCA patients with high sensitivity (89%) and specificity (95%). PET scans are more reliable than magnetic resonance imaging (MRI)/MRA for monitoring disease activity during immunosuppressive therapy. Active lesions have uptake of the same or greater intensity than that of the liver. PET scan uptake can predict individuals at risk of later development of aneurysms.

16. What characteristic of the disease process may hamper the ability to demonstrate vasculitis on biopsy?
GCA is characterized by patchy or segmental arterial involvement. Consequently, a 3- to 6-cm segment should be obtained when the physical findings are indeterminate. The arterial biopsy specimen should be sliced through the cross-section at 1- to 2-mm intervals and examined histologically at multiple levels.

17. How often does a properly performed temporal artery biopsy define the need for therapy?
A properly performed biopsy will define the need for therapy in approximately 85% of cases. However, if the biopsy is negative and the clinical suspicion for disease remains high, consideration should be given to biopsy of the opposite side, which will be positive in an additional 3% to 5% of cases. The negative predictive value of **bilateral** negative temporal artery biopsies is 91% for GCA. However, there are notable exceptions. Patients presenting with posterior headaches may have a positive superficial occipital artery biopsy and negative temporal artery biopsy. In addition, GCA patients presenting with aortitis and large-vessel vasculitis (aortic arch syndrome) typically do not have cranial symptoms and have a negative temporal artery biopsy in 40% of cases. These patients are diagnosed on the basis of a characteristic MRA or CTA for vasculitis of the great vessels. Finally, there are other diseases that can mimic GCA and involve the temporal artery such as amyloidosis, which can be diagnosed after staining of specimens with Congo red.

18. Describe the characteristic histologic findings on temporal artery biopsy in GCA.
Histologically, two patterns are seen. In 50% of cases there is the classic granulomatous inflammation of the inner half of the media centered on the internal elastic membrane marked by a mononuclear infiltrate, multinucleate giant cells, and fragmentation of the internal elastic lamina. Giant cells (foreign body and Langhans) occur in 50% to 66% of these cases (Figure 27-1). In the other 50% of cases, granulomas and giant cells are absent, and there is only a nonspecific panarteritis with a mixed inflammatory infiltrate composed largely of lymphocytes and macrophages admixed with a few eosinophils. Neutrophils are rare. Fibrinoid necrosis should not be seen and if present should suggest a different vasculitis.

There are recent reports of a few patients with GCA (<5%) with biopsies showing periadventitial small-vessel vasculitis (SVV) and/or vasculitis of the vasa vasorum (VVV) surrounding an uninflamed temporal artery. Patients with isolated SVV tend to have lower ESR/CRP and less severe clinical manifestations and

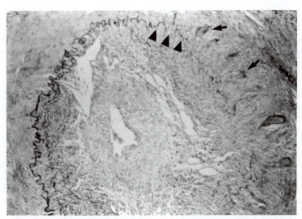

Figure 27-1. Temporal artery biopsy in a patient with giant cell arteritis showing the disrupted internal elastic lamina (*arrowheads*) and giant cells (*arrows*).

disease course than patients with isolated VVV or a classic biopsy for GCA. However, all these patients, regardless of biopsy findings, can develop blindness in up to 15% of untreated cases.

19. **What pitfalls can confuse a pathologist in correctly diagnosing GCA from a temporal artery biopsy?**
    - Up to 50% of positive biopsies show a diffuse lymphocytic infiltrate without evidence of granulomatous inflammation or giant cells.
    - Fragmentation and fraying of the internal elastic lamina are constant features of all aging arteries, and alone are not indicative of active or healed arteritis. There must be an inflammatory cell infiltrate to diagnose GCA.
    - Healed temporal arteritis (because of long-term corticosteroid use) can still be diagnosed because it is characterized by intimal fibrosis, medial scarring, and eccentric destruction of the internal elastic lamina. Corticosteroid therapy does not "normalize" the affected artery; it just gets rid of the inflammatory infiltrate.

20. **Is GCA a genetic disease? How does heredity relate to its pathogenesis?**
    The cause of GCA is unknown and its pathogenesis is poorly understood. The majority of GCA patients express the human leukocyte antigen (HLA)-DRB1*04 haplotype variant (60%), which has a common sequence motif in the second hypervariable region of the B1 molecule. Interestingly, association of GCA with this HLA-DRB1 genotype appears to confer increased susceptibility to the disease, but is not a predictor of disease severity. Other gene polymorphisms have also been reported.

    The environmental trigger is unknown. An attenuated *Burkholderia pseudomallei*-like bacterium was recently isolated from the arterial walls of GCA patients. Early in disease, lymphocytic inflammation is confined to the adventitia and elastic lamina. In the adventitia, antigen-presenting dendritic cells produce IL-18, which recruits T cells to the area and activates Th1 cells to secrete IFNγ and IL-2, and Th17 cells to secrete IL-17. Macrophages that secrete IL-1, IL-6, and TGF-β are also present. IFNγ production activates macrophages in the media to form giant cells and to produce matrix metalloproteinases that destroy the internal elastic lamina. Growth and angiogenic factors (VEGF) support the further influx of T cells and macrophages to the area. Closer to the intima, neovascularization and macrophage-produced cytokines (PDGF, IL-1) cause prominent intimal proliferation that leads to ischemia. Notably, the T-cell cytokine IFNγ is abundantly expressed in GCA but is absent from the arteries of PMR patients without GCA.

21. **Is there a standard treatment for the management of GCA?**
    High-dose corticosteroids (prednisone, 30 mg twice a day) are the cornerstone of therapy. One study suggested that the initial use of pulse therapy (methylprednisolone, 1 g daily for 3 days) was associated with a higher subsequent remission rate. Alternate-day corticosteroid regimens are not effective. It was recently shown that methotrexate is an effective steroid-sparing medication and is recommended to help accelerate tapering off of steroid therapy and to lessen the chance of relapse. One trial did not find that an anti-TNFα inhibitor (infliximab) was effective as a steroid-sparing agent. Recent case reports suggest that an anti-IL-6R biologic (tocilizumab) was effective for steroid-dependent, treatment-resistant GCA. Finally, all GCA patients should be on low-dose aspirin (81 mg/day) to reduce cardiovascular events and blindness.

22. **Should therapy be implemented before a temporal artery biopsy is obtained?**
    The timing for therapy initiation depends on the assessed risk of a serious complication and how soon the biopsy can be obtained. Symptoms for which corticosteroid therapy might be instituted sooner include risk of visual loss, stroke, and angina. In general, there should be a low threshold for starting corticosteroids early in patients who have a clinical syndrome compatible with GCA.

23. **Does treatment with corticosteroids influence the biopsy findings?**
    Although it is possible that corticosteroid therapy may influence temporal artery biopsy findings, recent studies have shown that biopsies may show arteritis after more than 14 days of corticosteroid therapy. In general, the biopsy should be obtained within 7 days of starting corticosteroid therapy whenever possible. Notably, corticosteroid therapy never normalizes all the temporal artery pathology (see Question 19).

24. **Do patients respond rapidly to initiation of appropriate therapy?**
    Corticosteroids usually are dramatically effective in suppressing the systemic symptoms of GCA within 72 hours after initiation of therapy. Localized manifestations of arteritis, such as headaches, scalp tenderness, and jaw or tongue claudication, steadily improve over a longer period of time.

25. **Does initiation of corticosteroid therapy prevent catastrophic events such as blindness and strokes?**
    There have been many instances that support the hypothesis that corticosteroid therapy can prevent catastrophic events in patients with temporal arteritis. Sudden blindness and other stroke-like events have occasionally been reversed in 33% of patients by institution of high-dose corticosteroid therapy (1 g of intravenous methylprednisolone daily for 3 days) if started within 24 hours of the event.

26. **When should the level of corticosteroid medication be reduced?**
    Patients should undergo close periodic observation to identify potential harbingers of complications and for gradual discontinuation of corticosteroid therapy. When clinical evidence of the inflammatory process, including symptoms and laboratory evidence of inflammation, have subsided, the corticosteroid dosage can be lowered safely. A good rule of thumb is to begin tapering off after clinical and laboratory parameters, particularly ESR/CRP, have normalized. If patients do not achieve complete remission or it is not possible to taper off corticosteroid therapy to low doses (<10 to 20 mg of prednisone daily), additional immunosuppressive medications should be considered. Many physicians start low-dose weekly methotrexate (15 mg per week) simultaneously with institution of corticosteroid therapy to allow more rapid tapering off of the latter.

27. **For how long do patients with GCA usually receive corticosteroid therapy?**
    Treatment usually continues for at least 6 months and often for 2 years. Up to 40% of patients need low-dose prednisone indefinitely. It has been well documented that discontinuation of corticosteroid medications too early is associated with worsening of disease activity. Moreover, recurrences are known to occur several years after completion of an appropriate therapeutic regimen. Every effort should be made to treat and limit side effects of corticosteroids such as osteoporosis (calcium and vitamin D therapy, bisphosphonates), diabetes mellitus, hypertension, hyperlipidemia, steroid myopathy, cataracts, infection, and herpes zoster infections.

28. **What is the recommended corticosteroid tapering schedule for a patient with GCA?**
    After normalization of symptoms, ESR, and CRP (usually takes 1 month) on prednisone at 30 mg twice a day, the following tapering schedule can be tried:
    - Taper the dose by 5 mg every 1 to 2 weeks to 30 mg once a day.
    - Decrease the dose by 2.5 mg every 1 to 2 weeks to 15 mg once a day.
    - Further taper the dose by 2.5 mg every 4 weeks to 10 mg daily.
    - Decrease the dose by 1 mg every 4 weeks until the patient is off prednisone.

    Clinical symptoms and CRP should be monitored for every taper in dose. Spontaneous recurrences occur in up to 50% of cases. Up to 40% of patients (especially women) need corticosteroid therapy for years.

29. **Is mortality increased in GCA patients compared with the general elderly population?**
    The risk of death from GCA appears to be increased (threefold) within the first 4 months of starting therapy. Patients typically die of vascular complications, such as stroke or myocardial infarction, supporting the use of low-dose aspirin (81 mg/day) in patients diagnosed with GCA. BP must be controlled and the patient should stop smoking. After 4 months, mortality is similar to that for an aged-matched general population except for increased prevalence (seventeenfold) of thoracic aortic aneurysm and aortic dissection, for which the patient should be monitored. Surgery is considered when the aneurysm enlarges to greater than 5 cm or dissects. Overall, the incidence of malignancy is not increased in GCA patients.

TAKAYASU ARTERITIS

30. **List other names for TA.**
    - Pulseless disease
    - Aortic arch syndrome
    - Occlusive thromboaortopathy

31. **Discuss the typical demographic characteristics of a patient with TA.**
    TA occurs most commonly in young women (female/male ratio 8:1). The median age of onset is 25 years, but 25% of cases occur before age 20 years and 15% occur after age 40 years. TA occurs most commonly in Asian (Japan, China, India, SE Asia) females but has been reported worldwide in all racial groups.

32. **What are the major clinical presentations of TA?**
    A triphasic pattern of progression of disease has been described:
    - **Phase I:** pre-pulseless, inflammatory period characterized by nonspecific systemic complaints such as fever, arthralgias, and weight loss. These patients are often diagnosed as having a prolonged viral syndrome. Patients <20 years of age frequently present with disease in this phase.
    - **Phase II:** vessel inflammation dominated by vessel pain and tenderness.
    - **Phase III:** fibrotic stage, when bruits and ischemia predominate.

    Patients can present in any phase or combination of phases because TA is a chronic, recurrent disease. Up to 10% present with no symptoms, and the incidental finding of unequal pulses/BPs, bruits, or hypertension prompts further evaluation.

33. **List some of the more common clinical features occurring in TA.**
    - Bruits (80%)
    - Claudication (70%)
    - Decreased pulses (60%)
    - Arthralgias (50%)
    - Asymmetric BP (50%)
    - Constitutional symptoms (40%)
    - Headache (40%)
    - Hypertension (30%)
    - Dizziness (30%)
    - Pulmonary involvement (25%)
    - Cardiac involvement (10%)
    - Erythema nodosum (8%)

    Symptoms occur primarily as a result of stenoses of the aorta and its branches. A comprehensive vascular examination (BP, pulse, bruits) in both arms and legs is mandatory. The aortic arch and abdominal aorta are most commonly affected. Upper-extremity and thoracic vessels (subclavian, carotid, vertebral) are more commonly involved than iliac arteries. Pulmonary artery involvement can occur in up to 70% of patients, with <25% having symptoms of pulmonary hypertension. Cardiac involvement with angina, myocardial infarction, heart failure, sudden death, and aortic valvular regurgitation occurs in up to 15% of patients.

34. **Are there any specific laboratory tests useful for the diagnosis of TA?**
    No specific tests are useful. Nonspecific laboratory studies indicate active inflammation such as anemia of chronic disease, thrombocytosis, and elevated ESR and CRP. ESR does not always follow the degree of active, ongoing inflammation and may be normal in 33% to 50% of patients with active disease on arterial biopsy.

35. **How is the diagnosis of TA made?**
    Angiography is the gold standard for detecting arterial involvement in TA. However, MRA and CTA are noninvasive tests that are replacing catheter angiography and can also detect vessel wall thickness. The lesions of TA are most often long-segment stenoses or arterial occlusions of aorta and visceral vessels at their aortic origins. Aneurysms can occur (see Chapter 26). PET scans can also detect vessel wall inflammation with sensitivity/specificity of >90%.

36. **Is the histopathologic description of TA the same as that for GCA?**
    The histologic appearance of TA is a focal panarteritis that can be very similar to GCA. Like GCA, focal "skip lesions" are common. One point that helps in separating TA from GCA is that the cellular infiltrate in TA tends to localize in the adventitia and outer parts of the media including the vasa vasorum, whereas the inflammation of GCA concentrates around the inner half of the media. In addition, lymphocytes in the vessel walls of TA patients are mostly perforin-secreting killer T lymphocytes and NK cells, in contrast to the lymphocyte phenotype (Th1/Th17) seen in GCA patients. Biopsy of a vessel is not necessary to establish a diagnosis of TA if the angiogram and clinical symptoms are characteristic.

37. **Is TA a genetic disease?**
    The etiology and pathogenesis of TA are unknown. Studies linking TA to HLA class I (Bw52, others) and II genes have provided conflicting results and differ between ethnicities. There is no link to HLA-DR4 as seen in GCA.

38. **What is the treatment for TA?**
    High-dose corticosteroids (prednisone, 30 mg twice a day) are the initial therapy for active inflammatory TA. Alternate-day regimens are not successful. Corticosteroids are maintained at high doses until symptoms and laboratory evidence (ESR, CRP) of inflammation normalize. Unfortunately, ESR correlates with the degree of inflammation observed on a biopsied blood vessel in only 50% of cases. With control of inflammation, corticosteroid therapy can be tapered off.

    Relapses do occur, and up to 40% of TA patients will require additional immunosuppressive therapy. Methotrexate is preferred owing to its limited toxicity and its ability to induce remission in 80% of patients. Mycophenolate mofetil, azathioprine, and cyclophosphamide have also been used. However, up to 20% of

TA patients never achieve remission. These patients may benefit from infliximab, tocilizumab, or rituximab therapy.

Other medical therapy includes antihypertensive therapy (vasodilators should be avoided unless the patient has heart failure), antiplatelet therapy to prevent thrombosis, calcium therapy to prevent osteoporosis, and control of hyperlipidemia. Smoking should be stopped and immunization updated. BP should be taken at an extremity without vessel stenosis to obtain an accurate measurement. Surgery is used to bypass stenotic lesions that fail to improve with medical management. Percutaneous transluminal angioplasty has been used in some patients to treat stenotic vessels once inflammation is controlled.

39. If normal ESR does not reflect the degree of ongoing inflammation of the great vessels in TA, are there any other ways to assess disease control?
- MRI with gadolinium: increased gadolinium uptake in the thickened aortic wall suggests ongoing inflammation.
- PET scan: increased uptake (equivalent to liver intensity) of FDG suggests ongoing inflammation.
- Vessel wall biopsy: practical only if the patient is having a vessel bypass as a result of stenosis.

40. What is the prognosis for patients with TA?
Up to 45% of patients develop aortic aneurysms and nearly 40% develop cardiac abnormalities. Echocardiography should be performed to assess for left ventricular hypertrophy, aortic root dilatation, aortic valve insufficiency, and pulmonary hypertension. Sudden death may occur as a result of myocardial infarction, stroke, or aneurysmal rupture or dissection. Cardiac and renal failure can occur. Long-term survival rates are 80% to 90%.

ISOLATED AORTITIS AND CHRONIC PERIAORTITIS

41. What are some infectious causes of aortitis?
Bacterial aortitis due to *Salmonella*, *Staphylococcus*, or *Streptococcus* usually results from bacterial seeding of an atherosclerotic plaque or aneurysmal sac via tha vasa vasorum. Tuberculous aortitis results from direct seeding from adjacent infected tissue or miliary spread. Syphilitic aortitis involves the ascending aorta and is associated with thoracic aortic aneurysm.

42. Describe the classification of idiopathic isolated aortitis.
Inflammation of the aorta is discovered as an incidental histologic finding in 3% to 10% of patients undergoing aortic aneurysm surgery. The classification is based on location:
- Isolated idiopathic thoracic aortitis
  - Giant cell aortitis: inflammation indistinguishable from GCA
  - Lymphoplasmacytic infiltrate: a significant percentage (75%) of these patients have IgG4-related systemic disease
- Chronic periaortitis (abdomen)
  - Idiopathic retroperitoneal fibrosis (Ormond disease)
  - Inflammatory abdominal aortic aneurysm: associated with smoking and family history of aortic aneurysm, and can be associated with retroperitoneal fibrosis; some of these patients have IgG4-related systemic disease
  - Idiopathic isolated abdominal periaortitis: occurs without associated aneurysm or retroperitoneal fibrosis

43. What is Ormond disease?
In 1948, Ormond published histopathologic findings for **idiopathic retroperitoneal fibrosis** (IRPF). Retroperitoneal fibrosis is idiopathic in 70% of cases and is thought to be a subset of **idiopathic multifocal fibrosclerosis**. It is rare, affects men more than women (3:1) of all ethnicities, and occurs at an average age of 40 to 60 years. Patients present (90%) with pain in the lower back, abdomen, flank, and/or scrotum. Some patients have systemic symptoms that include fever, anorexia, and malaise. The physical examination is usually (75%) unremarkable, although hypertension is common. Lower-extremity edema and phlebitis can be seen. Laboratory findings are nonspecific, including elevated ESR/CRP (75% to 90% of cases) and azotemia (50%). Serologies are typically negative. Radiographic CT findings show a homogeneous mass surrounding the aorta that follows the iliac bifurcation. Lymphadenopathy is rare. Medial deviation of the mid part of the ureter and hydronephrosis are common (60% to 75%). Open, laparoscopic, or CT-guided biopsy shows sclerosis and infiltration of mononuclear cells. Small-vessel vasculitis is seen in 50% of cases. Biopsy helps to rule out secondary causes of RPF (drugs, malignant disease, infections, IgG4-related systemic disease). The etiology of IRPF is unknown but may be an exaggerated local inflammatory reaction to oxidized low-density lipoprotein from aortic atherosclerosis. An autoimmune process is also proposed because RPF can occur in patients with other autoimmune diseases. Treatment includes high-dose prednisone for 1 month with tapering off to 10 mg/day by 3 to 6 months. Maintenance prednisone continues for 1 to 3 years. Recurrence of the disease (10% to 30% of cases) or treatment resistance is treated with mycophenolate mofetil, tamoxifen, or methotrexate. Patients are monitored in terms of ESR/CRP, creatinine, and CT scans every 3 months while on therapy and every 6 months when off treatment.

44. When should the rheumatologist suspect that a patient has IgG4-related systemic disease?

IgG4-related systemic disease has recently been described and occurs mostly in older males (60% to 80% of cases are aged >50 years) who frequently (≤40%) have a past or present history of allergic diseases (eczema, asthma). This condition presents with tumor-like lesions in one or more organs, which biopsy reveals as dense lymphoplasmacytic infiltrates enriched in IgG4-positive plasma cells (>30 cells per high-power field and IgG4/IgG positive cell ratio >50%) organized in a **storiform pattern** with fibrosis and obliterative phlebitis. An elevated serum IgG4 level is seen in 60% to 80% of patients. It can involve multiple organs simultaneously (60% to 90% of cases) although one organ is usually most prominently affected. The two most common presentations are type 1 autoimmune pancreatitis (up to 70% of cases associated with IgG4 sclerosing cholangitis) and salivary gland disease including gland enlargement (Mikulicz disease) and sclerosing sialadenitis (Kuttner tumor). Almost any organ can be involved (orbital pseudotumor, lymphadenopathy, lacrimal gland enlargement, interstitial pneumonitis and pulmonary pseudotumors, kidney disease with tubulointerstitial nephritis, pachymeningitis, Reidel thyroiditis). **Chronic lymphoplasmacytic aortitis** involving the thoracic more commonly than the abdominal aorta can lead to aneurysm formation. A subset of patients with idiopathic retroperitoneal fibrosis have this disease, usually in conjunction with other organ involvement. Serologies are negative except for the elevated (>135mg/dL) IgG4 level (60% to 70% of cases). Treatment includes high-dose corticosteroids. Azathioprine, mycophenolate mofetil, or rituximab is used for corticosteroid-dependent or corticosteroid-resistant disease. Of these, rituximab appears to be most effective. Patients may be at increased risk of developing non-Hodgkin lymphoma.

BIBLIOGRAPHY

Agard C, Barrier JH, Dupas B, et al: Aortic involvement in recent-onset giant cell arteritis: a case–control prospective study using helical aortic computed tomodensitometric scan, Arthritis Rheum 59:670–676, 2008.
Alberts MS, Mosen DM: Diagnosing temporal arteritis: duplex vs biopsy, Q J Med 100:785–789, 2007.
Blockmans D, Bley T, Schmidt W: Imaging for large-vessel vasculitis, Curr Opin Rheumatol 21:19–28, 2009.
Cronin C, Lohan D, Blake M, et al: Retroperitoneal fibrosis: a review of clinical features and imaging findings, Am J Roentgenol 191:423–431, 2008.
Gonzalez-Gay MA, Barros S, Lopez-Diaz MJ, et al: Giant cell arteritis: disease patterns of clinical presentation in a series of 240 patients, Medicine 84:269–276, 2005.
Gonzalez-Gay MA, Garcia-Porrua C, Llorca J, et al: Biopsy-negative giant cell arteritis: clinical spectrum and predictive factors for positive temporal artery biopsy, Semin Arthritis Rheum 30:249–256, 2001.
Gonzalez-Gay MA, Lopez-Diaz MJ, Barros S, et al: Giant cell arteritis: laboratory tests at time of diagnosis in a series of 240 patients, Medicine 84:277–290, 2005.
Gornik HL, Creager MA: Aortitis, Circulation 117:3039–3051, 2008.
Hoffman GS, Cid MC, Rendt-Zagar KE, et al: Infliximab for maintenance of glucocorticoid-induced remission of giant cell arteritis, Ann Intern Med 146:621–630, 2007.
Mahr AD, Jover JA, Spiera RF, et al: Adjunctive methotrexate for treatment of giant cell arteritis: an individual patient data meta-analysis, Arthritis Rheum 56:2789–2797, 2007.
Maksimowicz-McKinnon K, Clark T, Hoffman GS: Takayasu and giant cell arteritis: a spectrum within the same disease? Medicine 88:221–226, 2009.
Mason JC: Takayasu's arteritis: advances in diagnosis and management, Nat Rev Rheumatol 6:406–415, 2010.
Mazlumzadeh M, Hunder GG, Easley KA, et al: Treatment of giant cell arteritis using induction therapy with high-dose glucocorticoids: a double-blind, placebo-controlled, randomized prospective clinical trial, Arthritis Rheum 54:3310–3318, 2006.
Molloy ES, Langford CA, Clark TM, et al: Anti-tumour necrosis factor therapy in patients with refractory Takayasu's arteritis: long-term follow-up, Ann Rheum Dis 67:1567–1569, 2008.
Mukhtyar C, Guillevin L, Cid MC, et al: EULAR recommendations for the management of large vessel vasculitis, Ann Rheum Dis 68:318–323, 2009.
Narvaez J, Bernard B, Roig-Vilaseca D, et al: Influence of previous corticosteroid therapy on temporal biopsy yield in giant cell arteritis, Semin Arthritis Rheum 37:13–19, 2007.
Nesher G, Berkun Y, Mates M, et al: Low-dose aspirin and prevention of cranial ischemic complications in giant cell arteritis, Arthritis Rheum 50:1332–1337, 2004.
Nuenninghoff DM, Hunder GG, Christanson TJ, et al: Incidence and predictors of large artery complications in patients with giant cell arteritis: a population-based study over 50 years, Arthritis Rheum 48:3522–3531, 2003.
Restuccia C, Cavazza A, Boiardi L, et al: Small-vessel vasculitis surrounding an uninflammed temporal artery and isolated vasa vasorum vasculitis of the temporal artery: two subsets of giant cell arteritis, Arthritis Rheum 64:549–556, 2012.
Salvarani C, Cantini F, Hunder GG: Polymyalgia rheumatica and giant cell arteritis, Lancet 372:234–245, 2008.
Salvarani C, Hunder GG: Giant cell arteritis with low sedimentation rate: frequency of occurrence in a population-based study, Arthritis Rheum 45:140–145, 2001.
Stone JH, Zen Y, Deshpande V: IgG4-related disease, N Engl J Med 366:539, 2012.
Unizony S, Arias-Urdaneta L, Miloslavsky E, et al: Tocilizumab for treatment of large vessel vasculitis (giant cell arteritis, Takayasu's) and polymyalgia rheumatica, Arthritis Care Res 64:1720–1729, 2012.
Weyend C, Liao Y, Goronzy J: The immunopathology of giant cell arteritis: diagnostic and therapeutic indications, J Neuroophthalmol 32:259–265, 2012.

FURTHER READING

www.rarediseases.org
www.vasculitisfoundation.org

CHAPTER 28: MEDIUM-VESSEL VASCULITIDES: POLYARTERITIS NODOSA, THROMBOANGIITIS OBLITERANS, AND PRIMARY ANGIITIS OF THE CENTRAL NERVOUS SYSTEM

Ramon A. Arroyo, MD

KEY POINTS

1. Polyarteritis nodosa (PAN) should be considered in any noninfected, systemically ill patient who has multiple organ involvement including the peripheral nerves, skin, gut, and/or kidney.
2. PAN does not affect the lungs and sinuses.
3. Hepatitis B virus-associated PAN is treated differently compared to other causes of PAN.
4. Thromboangiitis obliterans occurs in both genders, affects any distal extremity, and is associated with tobacco use.
5. Primary angiitis/vasculitis of the central nervous system (CNS) has an insidious onset of multiple neurologic abnormalities and an abnormal cerebrospinal fluid (CSF) analysis.
6. Reversible cerebral vasoconstriction syndrome has an acute onset of headache, normal CSF, and reversible angiographic findings.

1. What are the medium-vessel vasculitides?
- Polyarteritis nodosa
- Kawasaki disease (see Chapter 71)
- Thromboangiitis obliterans (TO; Buerger disease)
- Primary angiitis of the CNS (PACNS)

2. Are there other sized vessels involved in medium-vessel vasculitides?
Yes, pathologic changes are not restricted to medium vessels alone. Large-vessel and, more frequently, small-vessel changes are often found.

POLYARTERITIS NODOSA

3. What is polyarteritis nodosa?
PAN is a multisystem condition characterized by necrotizing inflammation of small and medium arteries without glomerulonephritis or antineutrophil cytoplasmic antibodies (ANCAs). Patients present with symptoms related to the organs most frequently involved, which include vessels of the peripheral nerves, skin, abdomen, muscle, and kidney in that order. Involvement of other organs such as the lungs and ears/nose/throat (ENT) is unlikely and should prompt another diagnosis.

4. How common is PAN?
PAN is uncommon and has an annual incidence of two to nine cases per 1,000,000. There is no gender difference. PAN affects all racial groups, with average age at diagnosis ranging from the mid-40s to the mid-60s.

5. What are the clinical features of PAN?
The disease presents in a variety of ways. Typically, patients experience constitutional features (>90%) of fever, malaise, and weight loss, along with the manifestations of multisystem involvement listed in Table 28-1.

6. Are any specific laboratory tests helpful in the diagnosis of PAN?
No, most tests are nonspecific and reflect the systemic inflammatory nature of PAN. Elevated erythrocyte sedimentation rate (ESR)/C-reactive protein (CRP), normocytic normochromic anemia, thrombocytosis, and diminished levels of albumin are usually present. Decreased complement levels are unusual. Hepatitis B surface antigen is present in 10% to 50% of cases, depending on the series. Patients with hepatitis B virus (HBV)-associated PAN will also be positive for HBeAg and HBV DNA. Antineutrophil cytoplasmic antibody (ANCA), rheumatoid factor, antinuclear antibody (ANA), and cryoglobulins should be negative in classic primary PAN.

CHAPTER 28 MEDIUM-VESSEL VASCULITIDES

Table 28-1. Prevalence and Manifestations of Polyarteritis Nodosa in Various Organs*

ORGAN	MANIFESTATION	PREVALENCE (%)	COMMENTS
Peripheral nerves	Mononeuritis multiplex	50-70	Motor and sensory deficits
Kidney	Renal artery aneurysms and infarcts	70	Hypertension, occasionally severe
Skin	Palpable purpura, ulcers, livedo, nodules	50	Mainly over the lower extremities
Joint	Arthralgias	50	
	Arthritis	20	
Muscle	Myalgias	50-60	
Gut	Abdominal pain, liver function abnormalities	30-35	Due to mesenteric arteritis
Heart	Congestive heart failure, myocardial infarction	Low	
CNS	Seizures, stroke	Low	
Respiratory	Ear, nose, and throat, lungs	None	
Temporal artery	Jaw claudication	Low	
Testis	Pain	20	More common with hepatitis B
Eye	Retinal hemorrhage, optic ischemia	Low	

*Polyarteritis nodosa (PAN) can be limited to one organ without detectable systemic involvement in up to 10% of cases. This usually presents as cutaneous PAN.

7. How is the diagnosis of PAN made?
Diagnosis of PAN is often difficult. PAN should be suspected in any patient who presents with constitutional symptoms and multisystem involvement. Key **clinical features** suggestive of PAN include skin lesions (e.g., palpable purpura, livedo, necrotic lesions, infarct of the fingertips), peripheral neuropathy (most frequently mononeuritis multiplex), abdominal pain (mesenteric vasculitis), and hypertension with microscopic hematuria/proteinuria. Once PAN is suspected, **biopsy** of accessible tissues should determine the diagnosis. If clinically involved tissues are not amenable to biopsy, a visceral **angiogram** should be performed.

8. What tissue should be sampled to diagnose PAN?
The likelihood of finding arteritis is greatest when symptomatic sites are examined. The most accessible tissues are the skin, sural nerve, skeletal muscle, rectum, and testicle. Biopsy of asymptomatic sites is not recommended. A sural nerve biopsy should never be done in patients with a normal electromyograph.

9. Can a kidney biopsy be diagnostic of PAN?
No, in cases with abnormalities of urinary sediment or proteinuria, renal biopsy will usually reveal coagulative necrosis from renal infarction. This can be seen in other vasculitides, so renal biopsy is not helpful in differentiating medium-vessel vasculitides, but it could be useful if no other tissues are involved or available for diagnosis.

10. Describe the histologic features in PAN.
The pathologic lesion defining classic PAN is **focal and segmental transmural necrotizing vasculitis** of medium and small arteries (Figure 28-1). It less commonly affects arterioles, and involvement of large vessels (i.e., aorta) and veins does not occur. The lesions occur in all parts of the body, but less so in the splenic arteries and not in the pulmonary arteries. The inflammation is characterized by **fibrinoid necrosis** and pleomorphic cellular infiltration of the vessel wall, predominantly polymorphonucleocytes and variable numbers of lymphocytes and eosinophils. The normal architecture of the vessel wall, including the elastic laminae, is disrupted. Coexistence of different stages of inflammation, scarring, and normal vessel walls is common. Thrombosis or aneurysmal dilation may occur at the site of the lesion.

11. When is an angiogram performed for diagnosis of PAN?
An angiogram is performed when clinically involved tissue is not available for biopsy (e.g., a patient who presents with constitutional symptoms and digital ischemia). Angiographic evaluation for PAN usually requires study of the abdominal viscera. The best plan is to study clinically involved organs: the kidney, liver, spleen, stomach, and small/large bowel. In rare cases, hand or foot arteriography is necessary. The sensitivity/specificity

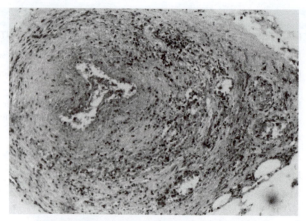

Figure 28-1. Polyarteritis nodosa involving a medium artery.

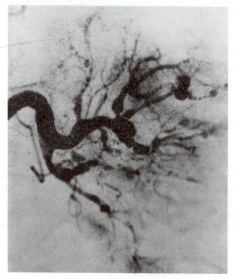

Figure 28-2. Angiogram of a kidney in a patient with polyarteritis nodosa demonstrating multiple aneurysmal dilatations.

of visceral angiography is 90%. MRA and CTA are less sensitive in demonstrating microaneurysms, but are less invasive and may show organ infarcts.

12. **Describe the angiographic findings in PAN.**
    Small saccular aneurysms (microaneurysms), occlusions/cut-offs, luminal irregularities, and stenoses of the small and medium vessels of the viscera (Figure 28-2).

13. **What are some other diseases that can show aneurysms on abdominal visceral angiography?**
    - **Segmental arterial mediolysis (SAM):** nonatherosclerotic, noninflammatory arterial disease that affects mainly muscular arteries and can yield an angiogram that mimics PAN. SAM characteristically involves splanchnic arteries in middle-aged and elderly patients, basilar cerebral arteries in adults, and coronary arteries in children and young adults. The aorta is not involved. Most patients present with life-threatening hemorrhages from aneurysmal rupture. Arterial dissection, stenoses, and thromboses can also occur. Pathologically there is lytic loss of medial muscle causing arterial dilation and aneurysms. The putative cause is vasospasm or a variant of fibromuscular dysplasia. SAM diagnosis is made by clinical presentation, angiographic appearance, and biopsy. Therapy is surgical repair but recurrences are common and the prognosis is poor.
    - **Ehlers–Danlos syndrome (vascular type, formerly type IV):** aneurysms due to vessel wall weakening caused by a defect in the production of type III collagen.
    - Fibromuscular dysplasia.
    - Others: pseudoxanthoma elasticum, neurofibromatosis, and atrial myxoma, among others.

14. What causes PAN?
The cause of PAN is unknown. An immune complex-mediated mechanism is frequently considered, but immune complex deposits or complement components are seldom found in involved vessels. Direct endothelial injury with subsequent release of cytokines and mediators of inflammation is another theory, but the triggering factor or antigen has not been found. Several conditions have been associated with PAN or PAN-like vasculitis, including the following:
- Viral infections such as hepatitis B (HBV) CMV, HTLV-1, human immunodeficiency virus (HIV), parvovirus, EBV, and hepatitis C (rare)
- Autoimmune disorders such as systemic lupus erythematosus (SLE), rheumatoid arthritis, dermatomyositis, and Cogan syndrome
- Medications such as allopurinol and sulfa drugs
- Hairy cell leukemia
- Adenosine deaminase 2 loss of function mutation: cause of autosomal recessive familial PAN

15. How is PAN treated?
Decisions regarding the initial management of PAN without HBV infection depend on the extent of disease, rate of disease progression, and organs involved. Treatment of this systemic vasculitis should include high doses of corticosteroids. If severe, intravenous pulse methylprednisolone (1 g/day for 3 days or 10 mg/kg every 2 weeks three times and then every 3 weeks three times) is frequently used combined with prednisone at a dose of 1 to 2 mg/kg per day in divided doses. Corticosteroid therapy is gradually changed to a single daily dose and slowly tapered off. Cytotoxic medications such as cyclophosphamide (2 mg/kg daily oral or 15 mg/kg IV monthly with dose adjusted for age and renal disease, or 500 to 1000 mg/m^2 IV monthly with dose adjusted according to white blood cell count) are added to the corticosteroid regimen in cases with major organ involvement (CNS, mononeuritis multiplex, gastrointestinal tract, kidney, or heart) or inability to taper off steroid therapy. After 6 to 12 months of therapy the cyclophosphamide can usually be switched to azathioprine (or leflunomide, methotrexate, or mycophenolate mofetil). Patients who fail to respond to cyclophosphamide may benefit from infliximab therapy (3 to 5 mg/kg monthly).

16. How does the therapy for HBV-associated PAN differ from that for PAN not associated with HBV?
Owing to HBV vaccination, HBV-associated PAN now only accounts for <10% of cases of PAN. PAN usually occurs within 6 months of HBV acquisition. HBV-associated PAN has more orchitis, hypertension, and renal infarcts. In HBV-associated PAN, the traditional treatment with corticosteroids and cyclophosphamide jeopardizes the patient's outcome by allowing the virus to persist and cause further liver damage and ongoing antigenemia. Consequently, patients who are HBsAg- and HBeAg-positive are treated with the following combination:
- Prednisone 60 mg/day for 1 week to control systemic symptoms, then the dose is tapered off by 50% daily until it has been decreased to zero by the end of the second week.
- Plasmapheresis to remove circulating immune complexes (thrice weekly for 3 weeks, twice weekly for 2 weeks, then once weekly until the patient is negative for HBeAg).
- Antiviral agents (lamivudine or alternative) to eliminate the virus. The antiviral agent should be **given on plasmapheresis days after the procedure** to maintain blood levels.

Successful therapy will be accompanied by seroconversion from HBeAg to anti-HBe antibodies, which can be achieved in 50% of patients. Patients who are negative for hepatitis C, HIV, and delta virus do best, with an 81% remission rate and a 10% risk of relapse.

17. What is the prognosis for PAN?
The outcome of PAN depends on the presence and extent of visceral and CNS involvement. Most deaths occur within the first year, usually as a result of uncontrolled vasculitis (60% to 70%), a delay in diagnosis, or complications of treatment. Deaths occurring after the first year are usually due to complications of treatment, infections, or a vascular event such as myocardial infarction or stroke due to accelerated atherosclerosis. The overall 5-year survival rate is 65% to 75% with aggressive treatment. The **five factor score** assessed at the time of diagnosis can be used to predict prognosis. It assigns one point each for proteinuria, elevated creatinine (>1.58 mg/dL), and gastrointestinal tract, CNS, and heart involvement. The 6-year survival rate is 86% for patients with no points, 69% for those with 1 point, and 47% for those with ≥2 points.

18. Can PAN affect only one organ?
Localized PAN is uncommon but has been reported as an isolated finding in the skin, gallbladder, uterus, breast, appendix, and peripheral nerves. Cutaneous PAN is the most common presentation. Patients present with multiple, tender nodular skin lesions (0.5 to 2 cm in diameter) usually located on the legs and feet but sometimes on the arms and trunk. Livedo is found in 60% and mild polyneuropathy in 33% of cases. Internal organ involvement is absent, but fever, myalgias, and arthralgias can be seen during the acute phase. Only 10% of cases progress to systemic PAN during follow-up. Owing to the benign prognosis, patients can be treated with prednisone at 20 to 40 mg/day with subsequent tapering off. Low-dose methotrexate, azathioprine, dapsone, and colchicine have been successfully used as steroid-sparing agents. Cyclophosphamide is not needed, unlike in systemic PAN. In patients who develop cutaneous PAN after a streptococcal infection, antibiotic therapy is effective.

THROMBOANGIITIS OBLITERANS

19. Is TO a true vasculitis?
TO, also known as **Buerger disease**, is an inflammatory, obliterative, nonatheromatous vascular disease that most commonly affects the small and medium arteries, veins, and nerves. In the acute phase of TO, a highly inflammatory thrombus forms, and although there is some inflammation in the blood vessel wall itself, the inflammatory changes are not nearly as prominent as in other forms of vasculitis. However, because of the associated mild inflammatory changes within the blood vessel, TO is pathologically considered as vasculitis.

20. What is the etiology of TO?
Although it is clear that tobacco use plays a major role in the initiation and continuation of this disease, TO pathogenesis remains unknown. Other etiologic factors may be important as well, such as genetic predisposition and possibly autoimmune mechanisms (antiendothelial antibodies).

21. Who is affected by TO?
Typically young smokers aged 18 to 50 years, and rarely in older individuals. The average age at diagnosis is the mid-30s. Most reports describe heavy smokers, but TO has been reported for smokers who have smoked three to six cigarettes a day for a few years. The disease has also been reported for pipe smokers, marijuana users, and tobacco chewers.

TO is predominantly a disease of males but is seen in women as well. The disease is more prevalent in the Middle East and Far East than in North America and Western Europe.

22. What are the clinical features of TO?
Usually, the initial manifestation of TO is ischemia or claudication of both legs, and sometimes the hands, which begins distally and progresses cephalad. Two or more limbs are commonly involved. Superficial thrombophlebitis and the Raynaud phenomenon are described in 40% of cases.

23. What are some of the presenting symptoms that prompt the TO patient to seek medical attention?
1. Claudication, pain at rest, and digital ulceration are the primary manifestations. Because the disease starts distally, dysesthesia, sensitivity to cold, rubor, or cyanosis prompts the patient to seek medical attention in one third of cases.
2. Pedal (instep) claudication is characteristic of TO, and patients often seek special shoes or orthopedic or podiatry care before the process is fully appreciated.
3. Gangrene/ulceration or pain at rest is the presenting complaint in one third of patients. This occurs predominantly in the toes and fingers. It may occur spontaneously but more often follows trauma, such as nail trimming or pressure from tight shoes.
4. Superficial migratory thrombophlebitis may be the first manifestation of TO.

24. How is TO diagnosed?
To confirm a clinical diagnosis, conditions that mimic TO must be excluded. The most important and common of these are atherosclerosis, emboli, autoimmune diseases, a hypercoagulable state, and diabetes. There are no specific tests to aid in the diagnosis. Complete blood count, liver function tests, urinalysis, fasting blood glucose, acute-phase reactants (ESR/CRP), and serologic tests (ANA, RF) are usually normal or negative. All patients suspected of having TO should undergo an echocardiogram to rule out cardiac thrombi and an arteriogram to rule out atherosclerosis. The arteriogram will also help to confirm a clinical diagnosis of TO because arteriographic findings are suggestive (although not pathognomonic) of the disease.

25. Describe the arteriographic findings in TO.
Although no single arteriographic feature is specific for TO, the radiographic constellation in conjunction with the clinical picture *is* diagnostic. On arteriograms, there is involvement of the small and medium blood vessels, most commonly the digital arteries of the fingers and toes, as well as the palmar, plantar, tibial, peroneal, radial, and ulnar arteries (Figure 28-3). The angiographic appearance comprises bilateral focal segments of stenosis or occlusion with normal proximal or intervening vessels. An increase in collateral vessels often occurs around areas of occlusion, giving a tree-root, spider-web, or corkscrew appearance. Note that in the arteriographic description, the affected arteries may have normal segments, but the most important characteristic is that the proximal arteries are normal, without evidence of atherosclerosis or emboli.

26. Is a biopsy needed to make a TO diagnosis?
Pathologic specimens are not commonly obtained during the acute phase of TO. Reluctance to obtain biopsy specimens of these vessels is because the distal extremity is usually ischemic and biopsy may lead to new ulceration. Therefore, most pathologic specimens come from amputated limbs. In the acute phase, panvasculitis with a **highly cellular thrombus including microabscesses** in the thrombus and vessel wall are seen. In the subacute phase, the thrombus is less cellular and recanalization of the thrombus is apparent. There may be perivascular fibrosis during this phase. In the late phase, there is often organized and recanalized thrombus and perivascular fibrosis. Unlike other medium-vessel vasculitides, the internal elastic membrane is preserved and venulitis is frequently found.

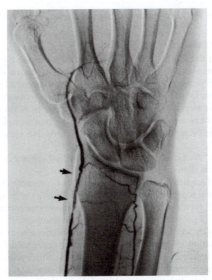

Figure 28-3. Angiogram of hand in thromboangiitis obliterans. Note the irregularity of the radial artery (*arrows*) and the cut-off of the palmar arch vessels with no digital vessels.

27. **What conditions should be included in the differential diagnosis of TO?**
    - Systemic lupus erythematosus
    - Various blood dyscrasias (hyperviscosity syndrome)
    - Rheumatoid arthritis
    - Occupational hazards
    - Systemic sclerosis
    - Hypothenar hammer syndrome and thoracic outlet syndrome
    - PAN
    - Antiphospholipid antibody syndrome
    - Embolic disease (cholesterol emboli, atrial myxoma, thoracic outlet)
    - Giant cell or Takayasu arteritis
    - Small-vessel vasculitides
    - Ergot toxicity
    - Premature atherosclerosis

28. **How is TO treated?**
    1. **Complete discontinuation** of smoking or tobacco use in any form including nicotine replacements (many patients continue to smoke despite disease severe enough to result in amputation)
    2. Treatment of local ischemic ulceration
    3. Foot care (lubricate skin with lanolin-based cream, place lamb's wool between toes, avoid trauma)
    4. Trial of calcium channel blockers and/or pentoxifylline
    5. Iloprost (helps patients with critical limb ischemia get through the period when they first discontinue smoking)
    6. Sympathectomy
    7. Treatment of cellulitis with antibiotics
    8. Treatment of superficial phlebitis with nonsteroidal antiinflammatory drugs
    9. Amputate the limb when all else fails (more than 50% of patients who continue to smoke require amputations)

29. **Is surgical recanalization an option in the treatment of TO?**
    Surgical recanalization is usually not an option. Because vascular involvement is distal, appropriate sites for bypass graft insertion are generally not present. In the few patients who have undergone arterial bypass, long-term results are poor.

PRIMARY ANGIITIS/VASCULITIS OF THE CNS

30. **How common is PACNS and who gets it?**
    PACNS is rare and males are affected more than females (2:1). The median age of onset is 50 years but PACNS can affect any age. Note that in the 2012 International Chapel Hill Consensus Conference, PACNS

was reclassified as single-organ vasculitis (instead of medium-vessel vasculitis) and renamed primary CNS vasculitis (PCNSV).

31. **What are the clinical subsets of PACNS/PCNSV?**
    - **Granulomatous angiitis of the CNS (GACNS)** (50% to 60% of cases): patients typically present with chronic insidious headaches along with focal or diffuse deficits involving the brain, meninges, or spinal cord. Symptoms are usually present or recurring for more than 3 months before a diagnosis is made. Brain magnetic resonance imaging (MRI) is abnormal, showing bilateral infarcts in subcortical white and deep gray matter, and CSF shows aseptic meningitis. Angiograms may be normal. Biopsy demonstrates granulomatous vasculitis. Treatment is with corticosteroids and cyclophosphamide. The prognosis is poor.
    - **Atypical PACNS:** multiple presentations are distinct from GACNS either clinically or pathologically but treatments are the same.
        - Mass-like presentation (5% of cases): patients present with a solitary cerebral mass that is diagnosed by biopsy. An infectious or malignant process must be ruled out.
        - Amyloid β (Aβ)-related angiitis (ABRA) (20% to 25% of patients): Aβ peptide deposition in arteries is seen in sporadic cerebral amyloid angiopathy (CAA). Patients with sporadic CAA are older (age >65 years) than patients with typical PACNS/PCNSV. The most common manifestation is intracerebral hemorrhage. In a subset of patients with CAA, vascular inflammation is also present. This inflammation can be transmural granulomatous vasculitis (40%), nongranulomatous vasculitis (20%), or perivascular nondestructive inflammation (30% to 40%). Patients with vascular inflammation are diagnosed as having ABRA. Patients with ABRA are more prone to present with subacute cognitive decline, hallucinations, mental status changes, seizures, and **cerebral hemorrhage** than patients with typical GACNS. Patients with ABRA frequently have increased gadolinium leptomeningeal enhancement and can respond to immunosuppressive therapy, whereas patients with CAA without inflammation do not.
        - Spinal cord presentations (rare): the lesion is limited to the spinal cord and is diagnosed by biopsy.
        - Nongranulomatous PACNS (20% of patients): pathology shows lymphocytic infiltration or fibrinoid necrosis and no granulomatous findings on biopsy. The clinical presentation, treatment, and prognosis are similar to GACNS. Infection and lymphoproliferative diseases with similar presentation must be ruled out.

32. **What are the typical presenting manifestations of PACNS/PCNSV?**
    The onset is most often insidious (over 1 to 3 months). Patients almost always have a headache. Common presentations are as follows:
    - Chronic meningitis (headaches)
    - Recurrent focal neurologic symptoms
    - Unexplained, diffuse neurologic dysfunction (subacute encephalopathy, behavioral changes, seizures, cerebral hemorrhage), which is most common in older patients with ABRA
    - Unexplained spinal cord dysfunction (myelopathy, radiculopathy)

33. **How is the clinical diagnosis of PACNS/PCNSV confirmed?**
    - Laboratory tests: elevated ESR/CRP, anemia of chronic disease, and thrombocytosis may or may not be present. If results are abnormal, another systemic or infectious disease should also be considered.
    - CSF: lymphocytic pleocytosis (median 20 cells/μL) and elevated protein (median 120 mg/dL) in 80% to 90% of patients. High IgG index and oligoclonal bands can occasionally be seen. If CSF is normal, another condition such as reversible cerebral vasoconstrictive syndrome (RCVS) should be considered (see Question 34).
    - Angiogram: alternating areas of stenosis and ectasia in multiple vessels in more than a single vascular bed. Sensitivity is 56% to 90% and the predictive value is 30% to 50%. Vessels of <500 μm in diameter cannot be visualized. CTA and MRA are less sensitive than a catheter angiogram.
    - Brain MRI: almost always abnormal but is nonspecific, with predictive value of 40% to 70%. Cortical/subcortical infarcts (50%), white matter hyperintensities, and gadolinium-enhanced intracranial lesions (33%) are seen most commonly. Gadolinium-enhanced leptomeninges is common in ABRA.
    - Brain biopsy (gold standard): granulomatous vasculitis is more diagnostic than lymphocytic vasculitis. The highest yield is from a lesion. Tissue cannot be obtained via needle biopsy. If there is no lesion, then leptomeninges and cortex from the nondominant temporal lobe should be biopsied. The sensitivity is 75% and the specificity is 90% to 100%. Note that patients with an abnormal cerebral angiogram frequently have normal leptomeningeal MRI and biopsy, whereas patients with leptomeningeal enhancement on MRI and a normal cerebral angiogram are more likely to have an abnormal leptomeningeal biopsy because of the size of the vessel involved.

34. **Describe how RCVS differs from PACNS/PCNSV.**
    RCVS is more common in women and comprises a group of related disorders characterized by **acute** onset of recurrent headache associated with reversible vasoconstriction of cerebral arteries. These disorders include benign angiitis of CNS (BACNS), Call–Fleming syndrome, postpartum angiopathy, drug-induced angiopathy (serotonergic, sympathomimetic, and illicit drugs), exertional/sex-associated headaches, and

migraine-associated angiopathy. All patients present with an acute thunderclap headache that can be associated with seizures (40%), brain edema (40%), lobar or convexity subarachnoid hemorrhage (20% to 35%), or generalized seizures (15% to 20% of cases). Some patients present with reversible posterior leukoencephalopathy syndrome (RPLS). Laboratory and CSF analyses are typically normal. Angiograms show narrowing of the intracerebral arteries of both hemispheres. Repeat angiograms in 4 to 12 weeks show resolution of such angiographic abnormalities. Failure to reverse angiographic abnormalities within this time period suggests a diagnosis other than RCVS. Treatment includes calcium channel blockers (nimodipine 60 mg every 6 hours, verapamil 80 mg twice daily, or verapamil sustained release 180 to 240 mg daily). Some physicians also give a short course of high-dose prednisone. RCVS can be distinguished from PACNS by the **acuteness** of the onset, a normal CSF examination, and the reversibility of angiographic abnormalities within 1 to 3 months.

35. **What other diseases can mimic CNS vasculitis and must be excluded before giving a patient the diagnosis of PACNS/PCNSV?**
    - Infections: herpes, HIV, varicella zoster virus, syphilis, and progressive multifocal leukoencephalopathy (PML), among others
    - Malignancy-associated vasculitis: CNS lymphoma, lymphomatoid granulomatosis, angiocentric lymphoma
    - Drug use: amphetamines, cocaine, heroin, ephedrine, phenylpropanolamine (may cause vasospasm and not vasculitis)
    - Connective tissue diseases: SLE, Sjögren's syndrome, Behçet disease, PAN, Churg–Strauss syndrome, ANCA-associated vasculitis, antiphospholipid antibody syndrome
    - **Susac syndrome**: endotheliopathy presenting with sensorineural hearing loss, encephalopathy, and retinal artery occlusion
    - Others: sarcoidosis, CADASIL syndrome, fibromuscular dysplasia, dissection, moyamoya disease

36. **Is a cerebral angiogram specific for PACNS/PCNSV?**
    No, several other diseases can have angiographic features similar to those of PACNS/PCNSV, including RCVS, severe hypertension, vasospasm around aneurysmal bleed, cerebral amyloid angiopathy, drug-induced vasospasm, syphilis, CNS lymphoma, and thrombotic disorders.

37. **How is PACNS/PCNSV treated? What is the prognosis?**
    There are no controlled trials. Patients are typically treated with high-dose prednisone and cyclophosphamide for 3 to 6 months, during which time prednisone is tapered to the lowest effective dose. If remission is achieved (no new symptoms or MRI lesions), patients are switched to maintenance therapy (azathioprine, mycophenolate) for at least another year or longer. The mortality rate is 10% to 17% and some 20% of patients experience moderate to severe disability.

BIBLIOGRAPHY

Abgrall S, Mouthon L, Cohen P, et al: Localized neurological necrotizing vasculitides. Three cases with isolated mononeuritis multiplex, J Rheumatol 28:631–633, 2001.
Birnbaum J, Hellmann DB: Primary angiitis of the central nervous system, Arch Neurol 66:704–709, 2009.
Guillevin L, Mahr A, Callard P, et al: Hepatitis B virus-associated polyarteritis nodosa: clinical characteristics, outcome, and impact of treatment in 115 patients, Medicine (Baltimore) 84:313–322, 2005.
Hewins P, Jayne D: Medium vessel vasculitis, Medicine 38:93–96, 2009.
Jannette, et al: 2012 Revised International Chapel Hill Consensus Conference Nomenclature of Vasculitides, Arthrits & Rheumatism, 65(1):1–11, 2013.
Mahr M: Treating PAN current state of the art, Clin Exp Rheum 20(64):110–116, 2011.
Morgan AJ, Schwartz RA: Cutaneous polyarteritis nodosa: a comprehensive review, Int J Dermatol 49:750–756, 2010.
Mukhtyar C, Guillevin L, Cid MC, et al: EULAR recommendations for management of primary small and medium vessel vasculitis, Ann Rheum Dis 68:310–317, 2009.
Olin JW: Thromboangiits obliterans, Curr Opin Rheumatol 18:18–24, 2006.
Pagnoux C, Seror R, Henegar C, et al: Clinical features and outcomes in 348 patients with polyarteritis nodosa: a systemic retrospective study of patients diagnosed between 1963 and 2005 and entered into the French Vasculitis Study Group Database, Arthritis Rheum 62:616–626, 2010.
Rennebohm R, Susac JO, Egan RA, Daroff RB: Susac's syndrome—update, J Neurol Sci 299:86–91, 2010.
Salvarani C, Hunder G, Morris J, et al: Aβ-related angiitis, Neurology 81:1–8, 2013.
Singhal AB, Hajj-Ali RA, Topcuoglu MA, et al: Reversible cerebral vasoconstriction syndromes: analysis of 139 cases, Arch Neurol 68:1005–1012, 2011.
Slavin RE: Segmental arterial mediolysis: course, sequelae, prognosis, and pathologic–radiologic correlation, Cardiovasc Pathol 18:352–360, 2009.
Villa-Forte: EULAR/European Vasculitis Study Group recommendations for the management of vasculitis, Curr Opin Rheumatol 22:49–53, 2010.

FURTHER READING

www.cnsvfing.org
www.nlm.nih.gov/medlineplus/vasculitis.html
www.vasculitisfoundation.org

CHAPTER 29: ANTINEUTROPHIL CYTOPLASMIC ANTIBODY-ASSOCIATED VASCULITIS

Mark Malyak, MD

KEY POINTS

1. Granulomatosis with polyangiitis (GPA) predominantly affects the upper and lower respiratory tracts and kidneys and is associated with proteinase 3 antineutrophil cytoplasmic antibody (PR3-ANCA).
2. Microscopic polyangiitis (MPA) should be considered in all patients presenting with a pulmonary–renal syndrome and is associated with myeloperoxidase (MPO)-ANCA.
3. Eosinophilic granulomatosis with polyangiitis (EGPA) presents as pulmonary infiltrates and eosinophilia in a patient with adult-onset asthma.
4. ANCA is both diagnostic and pathogenic in patients with ANCA-associated vasculitis (AAV).
5. Cyclophosphamide and rituximab (RTX) are important steroid-sparing therapies in patients with life- or organ-threatening AAV.

1. What are the primary ANCA-associated vasculitides?
The AAVs primarily affect small and medium arteries and include:
- Granulomatosis with polyangiitis (GPA, formerly Wegener granulomatosis)
- Microscopic polyangiitis (MPA)
- Eosinophilic granulomatosis with polyangiitis (EGPA) (formerly Churg Strauss syndrome)
- Renal-limited vasculitis with pauci-immune necrotizing/crescentic glomerulonephritis (RLV)

2. List the major autoantigens that ANCAs associated with vasculitis are directed against within neutrophils and monocytes.
- Proteinase-3 (PR3)
- Myeloperoxidase (MPO)
- Lysosome-associated membrane protein 2 (LAMP2)

3. What tests are used to detect ANCAs?
ANCAs are antibodies directed against specific proteins in granules in the cytoplasm of neutrophils and lysosomal proteins in monocytes and are present in the sera of patients with several underlying diseases. When alcohol-fixed neutrophils are used as an antigen source in indirect immunofluorescence tests, three ANCA categories may be detected according to the resulting pattern (Figure 29-1):
- **Cytoplasmic (c)-ANCA** is characterized by diffuse staining of the neutrophil cytoplasm. The protein recognized by c-ANCA is nearly always PR3, a serine proteinase present in primary azurophilic granules of neutrophils.
- **Perinuclear (p)-ANCA** results in perinuclear cytoplasmic staining. The protein recognized by p-ANCA is often MPO and less commonly is elastase or other proteins (lactoferrin, cathepsin G, bactericidal/permeability-increasing protein [BPI], catalase, lysozyme, and others) within primary azurophilic or specific granules of neutrophils. Patients with p-ANCA with MPO specificity are those most likely to have AAV.
- **Atypical ANCA** is the term for patterns not clearly c-ANCA or p-ANCA. The protein target of atypical ANCA is usually unclear, but in many cases is common to p-ANCA. Patients with this pattern or specificity to proteins other than PR3 or MPO are unlikely to have an AAV.

In addition to indirect immunofluorescence ANCAs, specific ELISAs for PR3 and MPO antibodies are now universally available. **Owing to better sensitivity and specificity, all three ANCA, anti-PR3, and anti-MPO tests should be requested when evaluating a patient for suspected AAV.** Note that antibodies against LAMP2 are not usually tested for until pathogenicity is confirmed. However, AAV patients negative for ANCA by standard methods may have antibodies directed against LAMP2 or may have IgA antibodies directed against PR3 or MPO.

4. How does ANCA contribute to the development of AAV? (Controversial)
It is not known how ANCA contributes to the development of AAV. Under certain conditions such as infections and other environmental triggers, release of cytokines (IL-1, TNFα) can cause neutrophils and monocytes to transport PR3 or MPO to their cell surface. Patients with c-ANCA can react with PR3, whereas

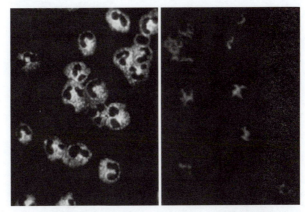

Figure 29-1. c-ANCA (*left*) and p-ANCA (*right*) immunofluorescence patterns using alcohol-fixed neutrophils as an antigen source.

patients with p-ANCA react with MPO, causing activation of neutrophils and monocytes. Cytokines (IL-1, TNFα) also upregulate adhesion molecules on endothelial cells, which the activated neutrophils can bind to and transmigrate into the vessel wall, causing vasculitis. The circulating activated neutrophils and monocytes can degranulate and release reactive oxygen species and lysosomal enzymes, leading to endothelial injury. Other products (e.g., PR3, MPO) released from these degranulating cells may bind to the endothelial cells and serve as target antigens for circulating ANCAs, contributing to the vasculitic response.

5. **What factors predispose some patients to ANCA and AAV?**
   Predisposing factors are unknown. There are geographic and population differences in the relative incidence and clinical expression of the various AAVs. This suggests that both genetic and environmental factors contribute to an individual's risk of developing ANCA and AAV. Several candidate genes (HLA class II, CTLA4, and PTPN22) have been described. Silica and nasal carriage of *Staphylococcus aureus* are environmental factors associated with GPA.

GRANULOMATOSIS WITH POLYANGIITIS

6. **Define GPA.**
   GPA is a primary vasculitis characterized by:
   - **Upper and lower respiratory tract** involvement with granulomatous vasculitis of mostly small vessels, extravascular granulomatous inflammation, and necrosis
   - **Glomerulonephritis** that is pauci-immune, focal and segmental, necrotizing, and often crescentic
   - Strong association with c-ANCA and **anti-proteinase 3 (PR3) antibodies**

   Generalized GPA implies involvement of all three major anatomic sites (upper respiratory tract, lungs, kidneys). **Limited GPA** is defined as the absence of renal involvement. Notably, limited GPA tends to present as a granulomatous disorder without vasculitic features. Only 10% of cases evolve to generalized GPA.
   Although GPA is considered a primary vasculitis syndrome, the inflammatory changes, including granulomas, often occur in parenchymal sites **outside** vessel walls (**extravascular** granulomatous infiltration). Interestingly, granulomas are rarely seen in the kidneys.

7. **How is the upper respiratory tract affected clinically by GPA?**
   Chronic inflammation of the mucosa of the upper respiratory tract characterized by granulomatous inflammation, vasculitis, and necrosis may lead to clinical manifestations in the following locations:
   - **Paranasal sinuses:** Chronic sinusitis is a common presenting manifestation (50%) that ultimately affects 80% of patients. Patients commonly carry *S. aureus* that can lead to infection and is associated with GPA relapses.
   - **Nasal mucosa:** chronic inflammation occurs in approximately 70% of patients, resulting in a chronic purulent nasal discharge, epistaxis, mucosal ulcerations, and, less commonly, perforation of the nasal septum and disruption of the supporting cartilage of the nose (**saddle-nose deformity**).
   - **Oral mucosa:** chronic inflammation may lead to oral ulcers that may or may not be painful.
   - **Pharyngeal mucosa:** chronic inflammation may lead to obstruction of the auditory canal, resulting in acute suppurative otitis media or chronic serous otitis media. New-onset otitis media in an adult should prompt consideration of GPA.
   - **Laryngeal and tracheal mucosa:** chronic inflammation may lead to hoarseness and subglottic stenosis, which in severe cases may result in stridor and respiratory insufficiency.

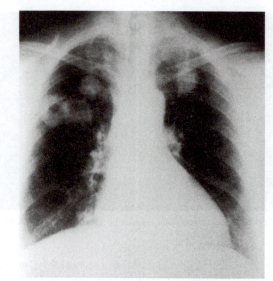

Figure 29-2. Chest radiograph demonstrating nodules (some cavitating) in a patient with WG. (*Copyright 2014 American College of Rheumatology. Used with permission.*)

8. **How does lower respiratory tract involvement manifest clinically and radiographically in GPA? What is the pathology?**
    - Clinical evidence of pulmonary disease is common on presentation (50% of cases) in GPA, ultimately affecting 85% to 90% of patients. Approximately one third of these patients, despite having radiographically evident pulmonary disease, do not have lower respiratory tract symptoms. Patients with relatively normal chest radiographs (CXR) may have abnormal computed tomography scans showing lesions not visible on CXR. The clinical manifestations of pulmonary involvement are highly variable, and can be explained by the underlying pathologic process.
    - **Chronic inflammation** results in the characteristic lesion of GPA, the granuloma, typically occurring in the extravascular interstitium of the alveolar septa, but also within vessel and airway walls. This may lead to the formation of nodules and/or fixed infiltrates on CXR (Figure 29-2). The nodules may cavitate centrally. If this process is extensive, subacute or chronic respiratory insufficiency may result.
    - **Acute inflammation** results in infiltration of neutrophils and other inflammatory cells in vessel walls, the extravascular interstitium, and alveolar spaces. A clinically important manifestation of acute inflammation is capillaritis, characterized by acute neutrophilic infiltration and fibrinoid necrosis within alveolar septa, which may result in life-threatening alveolar hemorrhage.
    - **Fibrosis** may result from healing of acute or chronic inflammation. If fibrosis is diffuse, the patient may experience chronic respiratory insufficiency.

9. **Besides direct involvement, how else may the upper and lower respiratory tracts be affected in GPA?**
    - Bacterial sinusitis, most often due to *Staphylococcus aureus*, commonly occurs as a result of obstruction of the paranasal sinus ostia by the inflammatory process. Similarly, obstruction of bronchi by nodules or intrabronchial lesions may lead to postobstructive bacterial pneumonia.
    - Infections may also result as a complication of treatment-induced immunosuppression. Glucocorticoids (GCs) and cyclophosphamide can suppress both humoral and cellular immunity. Thus, patients are predisposed to pulmonary infections with opportunistic organisms such as *Pneumocystis jiroveci*, herpesviruses, mycobacteria, fungi, and *Legionella*, as well as common suppurative bacteria such as *Streptococcus pneumoniae*.
    - Medications may have direct toxic effects on the lungs. Cyclophosphamide, even at the relatively low doses used to treat GPA, may rarely lead to pulmonary fibrosis. Methotrexate can also be associated with acute pneumotoxicity.

10. **How does involvement of the kidney manifest clinically and pathologically in GPA?**
    Clinical evidence of renal disease occurs in approximately 15% to 30% of patients with GPA on presentation, ultimately affecting 50% to 80%. The pathologic renal lesion is a **pauci-immune, focal and segmental, necrotizing glomerulonephritis**. In more severe cases, crescentic glomerulonephritis may occur. Immunofluorescence studies reveal little or no deposition of immunoglobulin, immune complexes, or complement, which is the reason for the pauci-immune designation. Renal vasculitis of larger vessels and granulomas are uncommon.

Most patients with glomerulonephritis have asymptomatic renal disease, manifesting as an "active" urinary sediment (hematuria, pyuria, proteinuria, and cellular casts) with variable degrees of disturbance of renal function (elevated serum creatinine). Patients with more severe renal involvement may develop progressive renal disease leading to acute or chronic renal failure.

11. Besides the upper and lower respiratory tracts and kidney, what other organ systems may be affected by GPA?

All organ systems may be affected to variable degrees by GPA. In addition, constitutional symptoms such as anorexia, weight loss, fatigue, malaise, and fever are common.

- The **eye** is commonly involved, affecting 30% to 60% of patients. Proptosis due to inflammatory and fibrotic infiltration of the retroorbital space (retroorbital pseudotumor) affects 15% of patients. This process may result in loss of visual acuity due to impingement on the optic nerve and loss of conjugate gaze due to infiltration of the extraocular muscles. Other less specific ocular abnormalities include scleritis, episcleritis, uveitis, conjunctivitis, optic neuritis, nasolacrimal duct obstruction, and retinal artery thrombosis. Eye involvement may be the initial presentation of GPA before other manifestations occur.
- The **skin** is eventually involved in 40% to 50% of patients. Lesions include palpable purpura, ulcers, subcutaneous nodules, and vesicles. Pathologic examination may reveal necrotizing vasculitis with or without granulomatous infiltration of the vessel walls, in addition to extravascular granulomatous infiltration and necrosis. Children with GPA may present with palpable purpura and be misdiagnosed as having IgA vasculitis (Henoch–Schönlein purpura).
- Involvement of the **musculoskeletal system** commonly manifests as arthralgia and myalgia, eventually affecting 67% of patients. Synovitis is less common and, when present, does not result in erosive disease, articular destruction, or joint deformity.
- Involvement of the **peripheral and central nervous systems** (CNS) occurs in 15% and 8% to 10% of patients, respectively. The most common peripheral neuropathy is mononeuritis multiplex; symmetric polyneuropathy is less common. Sural nerve biopsy may show vasculitis. CNS syndromes include chronic pachymeningitis, cranial neuropathies, ocular palsies, cerebrovascular events, seizures, pituitary involvement, brain stem and spinal cord lesions, and brain hemorrhage (cerebral, subarachnoid, subdural).
- **Cardiac** involvement is less common; up to 5% of patients develop pericarditis, which rarely results in interference with ventricular filling. Involvement of the myocardium, endocardium, and coronary vasculature is unusual, but may result in significant morbidity and, rarely, mortality.

Involvement of other organ systems, including the gastrointestinal (intestinal perforations) and genitourinary tracts (bladder/urethral vasculitis, orchitis, epididymitis, prostatitis), salivary gland (mass), pancreas (mass), and liver (granulomatous infiltration) occurs less frequently but may occasionally result in life-threatening complications.

12. Discuss the epidemiology of GPA.

The true prevalence and incidence of GPA are unknown, but it is a rare disorder. It is much less common than other rheumatologic disorders such as rheumatoid arthritis, systemic lupus erythematosus (SLE), polymyalgia rheumatica, and giant cell arteritis. The mean age at diagnosis is 41 years. Although the age range is 5 to 78 years, only 16% of patients are <18 years of age. Males and females are equally affected. Whites are affected seven times more often than blacks.

13. What is the clinical association between ANCA and GPA?

The following statements can be made about the clinical association between ANCA and GPA:

Sensitivity and specificity: Patients with active, generalized GPA have a 90% likelihood of being ANCA-positive, whereas only 60% of limited forms of GPA are ANCA-positive, giving an overall sensitivity of 73% for ANCA positivity. Among GPA patients with positive ANCA, 80% to 90% are c-ANCA-positive with PR3 specificity, whereas 10% to 20% are p-ANCA-positive with MPO specificity. The overall specificity of PR3-ANCA for active generalized GPA is 98%. Consequently, a patient with a characteristic clinical presentation and PR3-ANCA may not need a biopsy for tissue confirmation (controversial).

ANCA titers and disease flares: Overall, ANCA titers correlate with GPA disease activity in 60% of cases. A recent metaanalysis suggests that a rise in ANCA titer (two- to fourfold or a transition from negative to positive) in patients with clinically inactive GPA heralds exacerbation of disease. However, at least 40% of clinically inactive GPA patients who have a rise in ANCA titer will not have a flare of their disease. Therefore, prophylactic increases in immunosuppressive medications in a patient with a rising ANCA titer should not be instituted unless the patient exhibits clinical signs of disease exacerbation. Notably, ANCA titers do not tend to rise during an acute infection, which may aid in distinguishing exacerbation of GPA from an infectious process in patients with previously quiescent disease.

ANCA and relapse risk: Patients on maintenance therapy who have persistently positive ANCA are at increased risk of flares if the therapy is stopped. Therefore, such patients should remain on maintenance therapy indefinitely.

14. In patients with AAV, what is the sensitivity of anti-PR3 and anti-MPO antibodies?

Table 29-1 outlines the sensitivity of anti-PR3 and anti-MPO antibodies in AAV.

Table 29-1. Sensitivity of Anti-PR3 and Anti-MPO antibodies

DISEASE ENTITY	ANTIBODY SENSITIVITY (%)		
	ANTI-PR3	ANTI-MPO	NEGATIVE ANCA
Granulomatosis and polyangiitis (GPA)	66	24	10 (generalized GPA)
Microscopic polyangiitis	26	58	10-15
Renal-limited vasculitis, pauci-immune glomerulonephritis	20	64	15-20
Eosinophilic granulomatosis with polyangiitis	10	50	35-50

ANCA, Antineutrophil cytoplasmic antibody; MPO, myeloperoxidase; PRS, proteinase 3.

Although the presence of c-ANCA associated with anti-PR3 antibodies is quite specific (98%) for GPA, there are other AAV associations, particularly MPA and renal-limited vasculitis with pauci-immune necrotizing/crescentic glomerulonephritis. Interestingly, the glomerular lesions of these three disorders (GPA, MPA, RLV) are indistinguishable and are characterized by scant or no deposition of immunoglobulin (pauci-immune). Thus, these c-ANCA-associated pauci-immune disorders are a distinct category of autoimmune disease and can be distinguished from immune complex disease (e.g., SLE) and anti-basement membrane antibody disease (Goodpasture disease), which can also affect the kidneys (and lungs).

15. **Besides PR3-ANCA, what other tests can be abnormal in GPA?**
The systemic inflammatory nature of GPA often results in anemia of chronic inflammation, leukocytosis, thrombocytosis, and elevation of the erythrocyte sedimentation rate (ESR) and C-reactive protein (CRP). Low serum albumin and elevated globulin levels may also be present. Importantly, leukopenia and thrombocytopenia are unusual, often helping to distinguish GPA from other autoimmune or neoplastic disorders.

Evidence of glomerulonephritis is suggested by the presence of hematuria, pyuria, cellular casts, and proteinuria. If renal function is compromised by the inflammatory process, elevated serum creatinine is expected. Other laboratory tests may be helpful in the investigation of specific end-organ damage, such as electrocardiography and echocardiography for pericarditis, nerve conduction velocity for mononeuritis multiplex, and magnetic resonance imaging for retroorbital infiltration.

16. **The prototypic pulmonary–renal syndromes are GPA/MPA, Goodpasture disease, and SLE. Routine hematoxylin and eosin staining of kidney biopsies in such cases is nonspecific, so what other studies performed on renal tissue may aid in distinguishing these three disorders?**
Immunofluorescence studies can help in this differentiation. **Goodpasture disease (anti-GBM antibody disease)** results from the presence of **anti-basement membrane antibodies**, which bind to epitopes (noncollagen domain 1 of alpha 3 chain of type IV collagen) in the basement membranes of glomeruli and alveoli. The resultant antibody–antigen interaction leads to fixation of complement and initiation of the inflammatory process, causing glomerulonephritis and alveolar hemorrhage. Immunofluorescence staining with Ig antibodies reveals **linear** deposition of Ig in the glomerular basement membranes.

Glomerulonephritis due to **SLE** results from immune complex deposition in the glomerulus. Immunofluorescence studies reveal **granular** (lumpy) deposition of Ig, characteristic of immune complex deposition, within the glomerulus.

The pathophysiology of glomerulonephritis in **GPA/MPA** is unclear, but the disease does not appear to be due to immune complexes or detectable direct antibody binding to epitopes within the glomerular tissue. Thus, immunofluorescence studies are usually negative or reveal only scant Ig deposition, usually in areas of necrosis.

17. **Discuss the differential diagnosis of GPA.**
Table 29-2 lists the distinguishing features of various syndromes that may mimic GPA.

18. **What is the natural history of GPA?**
The presentation and natural history of GPA are highly variable. The spectrum of clinical presentation may range from relatively mild disease limited to the upper respiratory tract to fulminant life-threatening involvement of the upper and lower respiratory tract, kidneys, and other end organs. The disease progression is also variable and protean, including protracted mild disease remaining in the upper respiratory tract despite absence of treatment, widespread but relatively mild and slowly progressive disease, and rapidly progressive pulmonary and renal disease manifesting as alveolar hemorrhage syndrome and rapidly progressive renal failure on presentation. A further caveat is the observation that relatively mild and limited disease may rapidly progress to more diffuse and active disease at any time during the course in at least 10% of cases. The natural history of untreated generalized GPA is well understood. It is a uniformly fatal disorder with a mean survival time of <1 year. Death may result from respiratory failure, renal failure, infection, other end-organ involvement, or as a complication of treatment.

Table 29-2. Distinguishing Features of Syndromes that May Mimic GPA

SYNDROME	EXAMPLE	DISTINGUISHING FEATURES
Primary vasculitis syndromes	EGPA	Atopic history
		Marked eosinophilia
	Microscopic polyangiitis	Destructive upper airway disease unusual
		Cavitary pulmonary nodules unusual
		Absence of granuloma
Angiocentric immunoproliferative lesions	Lymphomatoid granulomatosis	Glomerulonephritis unusual
Pulmonary renal syndromes	Goodpasture disease	Anti-basement membrane antibodies
		Immunofluorescence: linear deposition
	Immune complex disease (e.g., SLE)	ANA, anti-dsDNA and Sm antibodies
		Immunofluorescence: granular deposition
Granulomatous infections	Mycobacterium	Proper stains and cultures
	Fungi	
	Actinomycosis	
	Syphilis	
Intranasal drug abuse	Cocaine	**Antineutrophil elastase antibodies**
		Predominantly nasal septal pathology (CIMDL)
Pseudovasculitis syndromes	Atrial myxoma	Echocardiography
	Subacute bacterial endocarditis	Blood cultures
	Cholesterol emboli syndrome	Echocardiography (transesophageal)
		Angiography
		Skin biopsy
Neoplastic	Lethal midline granuloma	Nose/palate destruction
		NK T cell lymphoma

CIMDL, Cocaine-induced midline destructive lesion, which is usually associated with p-ANCA directed against human neutrophil elastase.

19. How is GPA treated? How are relapses prevented?

INDUCTION THERAPY

- Life-threatening (rapidly progressive glomerulonephritis, diffuse alveolar hemorrhage): IV pulse of methylprednisolone (15 mg/kg ideal body weight or 1 g) daily for 3 to 5 days plus plasmapheresis. This is combined with cyclophosphamide or RTX as outlined below.
- Organ-threatening disease: Oral prednisone (1 mg/kg per day in divided doses) plus:
  - Cyclophosphamide: Monthly IV pulse (0.5 to 1 g/m^2) is as effective (except for more relapse risk) and more safe than a daily oral dose (2 mg/kg per day). Titrate to effect while keeping the total white blood cell count >3500 /μL and the absolute neutrophil count >1000 to 1500 /μL to lessen the risk of infection.

OR
  - RTX: Two doses of 1 g given 2 weeks apart is as effective as four doses of 375 mg/m^2 given at weekly intervals. RTX is as effective as cyclophosphamide and is particularly effective in patients who have only partially responded or relapsed while on cyclophosphamide. Note that RTX is removed by plasmapheresis but not by hemodialysis.

- Non-organ-threatening disease (limited GPA): Prednisone plus weekly methotrexate (15-25mg). Only use if creatinine less than 1.5mg/dL. Patients with subglottic stenosis can also be treated with bronchoscopy, intralesional steroid injections with or without topical mitomycin C, followed by dilation of the airway.
- Notably patients with generalized GPA (vasculitis presentation) may respond better to therapy (cyclophosphamide or RTX) than patients with limited GPA presenting as a granulomatous mass (retroorbital pseudotumor, etc.). These treatment-resistant patients may need a second course of RTX 4-6 months after the first course. However, RTX should not be given sooner than 4 months after a previous dose.
- Prednisone should be tapered after response achieved; however, it should not be tapered to less than 15 mg a day within the first month.

REMISSION THERAPY

Once patients with generalized GPA have been brought into remission using cyclophosphamide in combination with prednisone, they should be switched to another less toxic immunosuppressive medication. This usually can occur within 6 months after starting cyclophosphamide. Several medications frequently used in combination with low-dose prednisone to maintain remission include azathioprine, methotrexate, mycophenolate mofetil, and leflunomide. Clinical trials and experience suggest that azathioprine (2 mg/kg per day) is more effective than the other medications in maintaining remission in patients who have had generalized GPA. Methotrexate may be effective in maintaining remission in patients with limited GPA and those without renal insufficiency.

Patients brought into remission using RTX in combination with prednisone may or may not be put on azathioprine to maintain remission. A recent study (MAINRITSAN trial) definitively showed that RTX 500 mg (one dose) every 6 months was superior to azathioprine in maintaining remission and preventing relapses.

The duration of maintenance therapy for GPA patients is unclear. Patients who have been in complete remission for 12 to 18 months on standard maintenance therapy have a 50% risk of relapse once that therapy is stopped. A recent study suggests that maintenance therapy for more than 36 months is associated with less chance of relapse. However, many rheumatologists feel that GPA patients with persistent ANCA positivity are at increased risk of relapse and should be kept on maintenance therapy indefinitely even if in clinical remission. The 5-year survival is 85% to 90%.

PROPHYLACTIC THERAPY

- Oral trimethoprim/sulfamethoxazole (one double-strength tablet three times a week) provides prophylaxis against *Pneumocystis jiroveci* in patients with vasculitis who are receiving high-dose GC therapy (>15 to 20 mg prednisone per day). This antibiotic therapy also limits recurrent sinus infections, which can exacerbate GPA. Patients allergic to sulfa drugs can receive dapsone, atovaquone, or inhaled pentamidine.
- Nasal irrigation with a suspension of 2% mupuricin (Bactroban) in 1 L of saline (keep refrigerated) can prevent sinus infections. Irrigate the sinuses with nasosinus lavage until clear return of fluid occurs. Apply 2% mupurican ointment with a cotton bud inserted half way into the nasal vestibule between irrigations to diminish carriage of *S. aureus*.
- Therapy to prevent osteoporosis should also be instituted according to guidelines.
- Cardiovascular risk factors (HBP, diabetes, lipids) should be screened for and treated because the incidence of ischemic CV disease is twofold higher in GPA.
- Malignancy screening is recommended for patients who have received cyclophosphamide. Rates of malignancy (skin and bladder cancers and acute myeloid leukemia) are increased, particularly in patients receiving a total dose of >36 g.
- Patients who receive multiple courses of RTX may be at risk of hypogammaglobulinemia. IgG levels <300 mg/dL (or <500 mg/dL with infections) should be treated with replacement doses of IV IgG (0.4 g/kg monthly).
- Ovarian and sperm protection should be discussed if patient is to receive cyclophosphamide. The risk of ovarian failure is up to 50% in patients >20 years of age who receive a total dose of >20 g, those >30 years who receive a total dose of >10 g, and those >40 years who receive a total dose of 5 g. Leuprolide (3.75 g monthly) has been used for ovarian protection. The risk of azospermia occurs with a total dose of 6 to 10 g. Banking of sperm is the only reliable method to assure future fertility. Some centers give testosterone 200 mg IM every 2 weeks in an attempt to preserve testicular function.

SALVAGE THERAPY

- Plasma exchange (PLEX) is used early in life-threatening disease (RPGN, DAH) with good short-term efficacy, and is used as salvage therapy. Note that PLEX removes 25% of an RTX dose if performed within 24 hours of dose administration and removes 50% of the dose if PLEX is performed daily for 3 days after RTX administration.
- Intravenous gammaglobulin (2 g/kg divided over 5 days) provides some short-term benefit.
- Autologous stem cell transplantation, anti-thymocyte globulin, or Campath (alemtuzumab; monoclonal antibody against CD52 on lymphocytes).
- Infliximab (and probably all TNF inhibitors) are not effective.

20. **Can GPA patients who go into renal failure receive a kidney transplant?**
    Yes, a kidney transplant is possible in such patients. However, the GPA should be under control and the ANCA titer low or absent before transplantation. The use of mycophenolate and cyclosporine after transplantation to prevent rejection should help to prevent GPA recurrence.

MICROSCOPIC POLYANGIITIS

21. **What is MPA? How does it differ from classic polyarteritis nodosa (PAN)?**
    MPA is defined as a systemic necrotizing vasculitis that clinically and histologically affects small vessels (i.e., capillaries, venules, or arterioles) with few or no immune deposits. MPA is frequently associated with focal segmental necrotizing glomerulonephritis and pulmonary capillaritis. It can be distinguished from classic PAN primarily because it does not cause microaneurysm formation in abdominal or renal vessels. MPA can be differentiated from GPA because it does not cause granuloma formation or granulomatous vasculitis (Table 29-3). Treatment of MPA is based on the same principles as those outlined for GPA (see Question 19).

22. **Who gets MPA?**
    MPA affects males and females with a peak age 30 to 50 years. However, it can occur at any age.

23. **What is the usual presentation of MPA?**
    Patients typically present with acute onset of rapidly progressive glomerulonephritis (100%) and up to 50% have pulmonary infiltrates and/or effusions. Up to 30% of cases have diffuse alveolar hemorrhage with hemoptysis. Other manifestations include fever (50% to 70%), arthralgias (30% to 65%), gastrointestinal tract involvement (50%), purpura (40%), ears/nose/throat involvement (30%), and peripheral or CNS disease (25% to 30%). Although uncommon, insidious onset of these symptoms occurs in some patients.

24. **What is the characteristic histopathology of MPA?**
    The renal pathology is a focal, segmental necrotizing glomerulonephritis, frequently with crescents. Immunofluorescence and electron microscopy show no immune deposits (i.e., pauci-immune glomerulonephritis). Lung biopsy shows pulmonary capillaritis with negative immunofluorescence. Skin biopsy shows leukocytoclastic vasculitis.

25. **How is the diagnosis of MPA made?**
    MPA diagnosis is made on the basis of a characteristic clinical presentation and a renal biopsy showing necrotizing glomerulonephritis without immune deposits. p-ANCA directed against MPO is found in up to 60% of patients and is supportive of the diagnosis. Notably, some patients (15% to 30%) may have c-ANCA (directed against PR3) but MPA patients are less likely to have upper respiratory tract involvement (i.e., sinusitis), which distinguishes MPA from GPA.

Table 29-3. Clinical Features of Polyarteritis Nodosa (PAN), Microscopic Polyangiitis (MPA), and Granulomatosis With Polyangiitis (GPA)

CLINICAL FEATURES	PAN	MPA	GPA
Kidney involvement			
Renal vasculitis with infarcts and microaneurysms	Yes	No	No
Rapidly progressive glomerulonephritis with crescents	No	Yes	Yes
Lung involvement			
Alveolar hemorrhage	No	Yes	Uncommon
Laboratory data			
Hepatitis B virus infection	Yes (10%)	No	No
Perinuclear antineutrophil cytoplasmic antibody	<10%	50%-80%	10%-20%
Abnormal angiogram with microaneurysms	Yes	No	No
Histology	Necrotizing vasculitis	Necrotizing vasculitis (no granulomas)	Granulomatous vasculitis
Relapses	Rare	Common	Common

26. **What other pulmonary–renal syndromes must be distinguished from MPA?**

    SLE and Goodpasture syndrome can present with rapidly progressive renal dysfunction and pulmonary hemorrhage (see Question 16).

27. **Describe the recommended therapy for MPA and its prognosis.**

    Owing to the serious presentation of this disease, most investigators recommend combined therapy with high-dose GCs and cyclophosphamide or RTX (see Question 19). Plasmapharesis and intravenous gammaglobulins have been used in a few patients with progressive renal failure or pulmonary hemorrhage. Maintenance therapy is similar to that for GPA.

    The prognosis is guarded. Relapses are common (33%). At least 20% of patients end up on dialysis. Pulmonary hemorrhage can be life-threatening. Overall, the 5-year survival rate is 70% to 75%. This may be improved with newer protocols for therapy.

EOSINOPHILIC GRANULOMATOSIS WITH POLYANGIITIS (CHURG–STRAUSS SYNDROME)

28. **What is EGPA?**

    EGPA (formerly Churg-Strauss syndrome, allergic angiitis and granulomatosis) is a granulomatous vasculitis of small- and medium-sized vessels, frequently involving the skin, peripheral nerves, and lungs, and is associated with peripheral eosinophilia. EGPA occurs primarily in patients with a previous history of allergic manifestations, such as rhinitis (often with nasal polyps) (70%) and adult-onset asthma (>95%). Cytokines that affect eosinophils (IL-5) and eosinophil granule proteins (major basic protein, cationic protein) appear to be important in the pathogenesis of this disease.

29. **Describe the three clinical phases of EGPA.**

    The phases may appear simultaneously and do not have to follow one another in the order presented here.
    1. The **prodromal phase** averages 28 months but may persist for years (2 to 7 years). It consists of allergic manifestations of rhinitis, polyposis, and most commonly asthma (80% to 90%). Recurrent fevers occur in 50% of cases during this stage. Asthma frequently worsens before entering the second phase.
    2. **Peripheral blood and tissue eosinophilia** develop, frequently causing a picture resembling Löffler syndrome (shifting pulmonary infiltrates and eosinophilia), chronic eosinophilic pneumonia, or eosinophilic gastroenteritis. Myocarditis can develop. This second phase may remit or recur over years before the third phase. Fever is always present during the flares.
    3. **Life-threatening systemic vasculitis** occurs on average 3 years after the onset of the prodromal phase. Asthma can abruptly abate as the patient moves into this phase. Patients can develop myocarditis, valvular insufficiency, neurologic symptoms (most commonly vasculitic peripheral neuropathy), eosinophilic gastroenteritis, purpura, and testicular pain.

30. **What are the major clinical features of EGPA?**

    Table 29-4 lists the major clinical features of EGPA.

Table 29-4. Major Clinical Features of Eosinophilic Granulomatosis With Polyangiitis

ORGAN	CLINICAL MANIFESTATIONS
Paranasal sinus	Acute or chronic paranasal sinus pain or tenderness, rhinitis (70%), polyposis, opacification of paranasal sinuses on radiographs
Lungs	Asthma (usually adult onset), patchy and shifting pulmonary infiltrates (70%), nodular infiltrates without cavitations, pleural effusions and diffuse interstitial lung disease seen on chest radiograph. Pulmonary hemorrhage can occur.
Nervous system (60-70%)	Mononeuritis multiplex or asymmetric sensorimotor polyneuropathy; rarely CNS or cranial nerve involvement
Skin (50%)	Subcutaneous nodules, petechiae, purpura, skin infarction (occur mainly during the vasculitic phase)
Joints (50%)	Arthralgias and arthritis (rare)
Gastrointestinal tract	Eosinophilic gastroenteritis (abdominal pain, bloody diarrhea), abdominal masses
Miscellaneous	Renal failure (uncommon), congestive heart failure, corneal ulcerations, panuveitis, prostatitis

31. What laboratory abnormalities are seen in EGPA?
The characteristic laboratory abnormality is **eosinophilia** (>1500 cells/μL). Anemia, elevated ESR/CRP, elevated IgE (70%), and positive rheumatoid factor (70%) may be found. ANCAs are present in 50% to 65% of patients. These are directed primarily against MPO and give a p-ANCA pattern. Patients who are ANCA-positive are more likely to develop renal disease, alveolar hemorrhage, mononeuritis multiplex, and purpura. There is no direct correlation between the degree of eosinophilia and disease activity.

32. How is EGPA diagnosed?
EGPA is diagnosed on the basis of its clinical and pathologic features. The diagnosis should be suspected in a patient with a previous history of allergy or asthma who presents with eosinophilia (>1500 cells/μL) and systemic vasculitis involving two or more organs. The diagnosis is corroborated by biopsy of involved tissue. The major differential diagnosis is idiopathic hypereosinophilic syndrome.

33. Describe the histopathologic findings in EGPA.
The characteristic pathologic changes in EGPA include **small necrotizing granulomas** and **necrotizing vasculitis of small arteries and veins**. Granulomas are usually extravascular near small arteries and veins. They are highly specific and composed of a central eosinophilic core surrounded radially by macrophages and giant cells (in contrast to granulomas with a basophilic core seen in other diseases). Inflammatory cells are also present: eosinophils predominate, with smaller numbers of neutrophils and lymphocytes.

34. What drugs have been reported to cause EGPA? (Controversial)
The cysteinyl leukotriene type I receptor antagonists zafirlukast (Accolate), montelukast (Singulair), and pranlukast have been associated with EGPA. Whether they are a direct cause of EGPA is controversial. Some clinicians believe that EGPA is unmasked when patients use these drugs and taper off their GC dose. Others feel that these drugs can directly contribute to the development of EGPA because several patients have developed the disease when these drugs were instituted even when GC doses were not tapered. Consequently, leukotriene inhibitors should not be used in patients with EGPA.

35. How is EGPA differentiated from GPA?
Table 29-5 compares organ involvement in EGPA and GPA.

Table 29-5. Organ Involvement in Eosinophilic Granulomatosis With Polyangiitis (EGPA) and Granulomatosis With Polyangiitis (GPA)

ORGAN	EGPA	GPA
ENT	Rhinitis, polyposis	Necrotizing lesions
Allergy, bronchial asthma	Frequent	No more frequent than in the general population
Renal involvement	Uncommon	Common
Eosinophilia	10% of peripheral leukocytes	Minimally elevated
Histology	Eosinophilic necrotizing granuloma	Necrotizing epithelioid granuloma
Prognosis (major cause of death)	Cardiac	Pulmonary and renal
Antineutrophil cytoplasmic antibodies	p-ANCA 50-65%	c-ANCA 90%

36. What is the Five Factor Score (FFS)?
The FFS describes five features associated with poor prognosis in EGPA:
- Creatinine >1.58 mg/dL
- Proteinuria >1 g/day
- CNS involvement
- Gastrointestinal involvement
- Myocardial involvement

The FFS has recently been applied to GPA and MPA but proteinuria has been excluded as a prognostic marker. Using the four remaining FFS indicators, the 5-year survival for patients with any AAV was 91% for FFS of 0, 79% for FFS of 1, and 60% for FFS ≥2.

37. How is EGPA treated? What is its prognosis?
The treatment of choice is GC therapy. Patients with FFS of 0 may be managed with GCs alone. However, flares occur in 35% of cases when GC doses are tapered off. Patients with poor prognostic factors (FFS ≥1) need GCs (60 to 80 mg/day in divided doses) and cyclophosphamide (monthly pulse). Those with severe presentations may benefit from 3 days of pulsed methylprednisolone (1 g/day) with or without plasmapharesis.

Up to 10% of patients are resistant to conventional therapy. These patients may benefit from RTX or mepolizumab, an anti-IL-5 monoclonal antibody.

The 5-year survival rate for EGPA is 97% for FFS of 0 and 90% for FFS ≥1. The major cause of death is cardiac involvement with myocardial infarction and congestive heart failure.

DRUG-INDUCED ANCA-ASSOCIATED VASCULITIS

38. What drugs have been implicated in causing AAV?

Drug-induced AAV has been reported for **propylthiouracil, methimazole, hydralazine, minocycline,** and **levamisole-cut cocaine**. Other drugs have been implicated. The vasculitis is typically associated with MPO-ANCA. In addition to MPO, most patients also have antibodies against elastase and lactoferrin. A few will have PR3-ANCA. Patients with levamisole-induced AAV may have antibodies against PR3 (50%), MPO (100%), and human neutrophil elastase (HNE). Patients with drug-induced AAV present with constitutional symptoms, arthralgias with occasional synovitis, and cutaneous vasculitis. Minocycline-induced AAV frequently has elevated liver enzymes. Levamisole-induced AAV patients may have leukopenia (28%) due to bone marrow suppression and can also have cold agglutinins causing ear necrosis. Serious end-organ manifestations, including necrotizing glomerulonephritis and alveolar hemorrhage, occur less frequently. Treatment involves withholding the offending drug. More serious cases require systemic GC and cytotoxic agents.

ANCA AND OTHER DISEASES

39. What other disorders are associated with p-ANCA and atypical ANCA?

Whereas c-ANCA represents the presence of anti-PR3 antibodies and is associated with a small number of diseases, p-ANCA and atypical ANCA may be due to a variety of different antibodies and may be present in a wide range of diseases. Specific antibodies that may result in positive p-ANCA or atypical ANCA include antibodies directed against MPO, elastase, cathepsin G, lactoferrin, and β-glucuronidase. p-ANCA in the setting of GPA, MPA, EGPA, or RLV is usually due to anti-MPO antibodies (p-ANCA should be against MPO if the patient has vasculitis). p-ANCA present in other disorders is less well characterized but is usually not due to antibodies directed against MPO:
- Goodpasture (anti-GBM antibody) disease: between 10% and 40% will have positive ANCA, usually against MPO. These patients tend to have worse kidney disease prognosis.
- Most rheumatic disorders (rheumatoid arthritis, SLE, Sjögren's syndrome, systemic sclerosis, polymyositis, Buerger disease, relapsing polychondritis) have had positive ANCAs reported with varying but low frequency (<20%). ANCA is usually p-ANCA directed against proteins other than MPO. The clinical significance is unknown. Several cases of p-ANCA-associated vasculitis have been reported in patients with limited and diffuse systemic sclerosis.
- Inflammatory bowel disease: between 60% and 80% of ulcerative colitis patients and up to 25% of Crohn disease patients have positive ANCA. It is usually p-ANCA directed against a nuclear envelope or a neutrophil granule protein but not MPO.
- Autoimmune liver disease: p-ANCA (not MPO) or atypical ANCA is seen in primary sclerosing cholangitis (70%), chronic active hepatitis, and primary biliary cirrhosis.
- Cystic fibrosis: up to 80% to 90% of patients have positive p-ANCA, most commonly against BPI protein in the primary azurophilic granules of neutrophils. It is notable that patients with cystic fibrosis frequently have gram-negative infections of their airways.
- Infections: human immunodeficiency virus, subacute bacterial endocarditis, leprosy, malaria, acute parvovirus B19, and acute infectious mononucleosis. **Note that all three ANCA patterns have been reported for patients with *Mycobacterium tuberculosis* infections.**

BIBLIOGRAPHY

Bibby S, Healy B, Steele R, et al: Association between leukotriene receptor antagonist therapy and Churg–Strauss syndrome: an analysis of the FDA AERS data-base, Thorax 65:132–138, 2010.

Cohen P, Pagnoux C, Mahr A, et al: Churg–Strauss syndrome with poor-prognosis factors: a prospective multicenter trial comparing glucocorticoids and six or twelve cyclophosphamide pulses in forty-eight patients, Arthritis Rheum 57:686–693, 2007.

Comarmond C, Pagnoux C, Khellaf M, et al: Eosinophilic granulomatosis with polyangiitis (Churg–Strauss): clinical characteristics and long-term followup of the 383 patients enrolled in the French Vasculitis Study Group cohort, Arthritis Rheum 65:270–281, 2013.

de Groot K, Harper L, Jayne DR, et al: Pulse versus daily oral cyclophosphamide for induction of remission in antineutrophil cytoplasmic antibody-associated vasculitis: a randomized trial, Ann Intern Med 150:670–680, 2009.

Faurschou M, Mellemkjaer L, Sorensen IJ, et al: Increased morbidity from ischemic heart disease in patients with Wegener's granulomatosis, Arthritis Rheum 60:1187–1192, 2009.

Ferraro A, Hassan B, Savage COS: Pathogenic mechanisms of anti-neutrophil cytoplasm antibody-associated vasculitis, Expert Rev Clin Immunol 3:543–555, 2007.

Flossmann O, Berden AE, de Groot K, et al: Long-term patient survival in ANCA-associated vasculitis, Ann Rheum Dis 70:488–494, 2011.

Hiemstra TF, Walsh M, Mahr A, et al: Mycophenolate mofetil vs azathioprine for remission maintenance in antineutrophil cytoplasmic antibody-associated vasculitis: a randomized controlled trial, JAMA 304:2381–2388, 2010.

Hogan SL, Falk RJ, Chin H, et al: Predictors of relapse and treatment resistance in antineutrophil cytoplasmic antibody-associated small-vessel vasculitis, Ann Intern Med 143:621–631, 2005.

Holle JU, Gross WL: Treatment of ANCA-associated vasculitis, Autoimmun Rev 12:483–486, 2013.

Holle JU, Gross WL, Holl-Ulrich K, et al: Prospective long-term follow-up of patients with localised Wegener's granulomatosis: does it occur as persistent disease stage? Ann Rheum Dis 69:1934–1939, 2010.

Jayne DR, Chapel H, Adu D, et al: Intravenous gammaglobulin for ANCA-associated systemic vasculitis with persistent disease activity, Q J Med 93:433–439, 2000.

Jayne DRW, Rasmussen N, Andrassy K, et al: A randomized trial of maintenance therapy for vasculitis associated with antineutrophil cytoplasmic autoantibodies, N Engl J Med 349:36–44, 2003.

Jayne JR, Gaskin G, Rasmussen N, et al: Randomized trial of plasma exchange or high dosage methylprednisolone as adjunctive therapy for severe renal vasculitis, J Am Soc Nephrol 18:2180–2188, 2007.

Jones RB, Tervaert JW, Hauser T, et al: Rituximab versus cyclophosphamide in ANCA-associated renal vasculitis, N Engl J Med 363:211–220, 2010.

Klemmer PJ, Chalermskulrat W, Reif MS, et al: Plasmapheresis therapy for diffuse alveolar hemorrhage in patients with small-vessel vasculitis, Am J Kidney Dis 42:1149–1153, 2003.

Martinez V, Cohen P, Pagnoux C, et al: Intravenous immunoglobulin for relapses of systemic vasculitides associated with antineutrophil cytoplasmic autoantibodies: results of a multicenter, prospective, open-label study of twenty-two patients, Arthritis Rheum 58:308–317, 2008.

Mukhtyar C, Guillevin L, Cid MC, et al: EULAR recommendations for the management of primary small and medium vessel vasculitis, Ann Rheum Dis 68:310–317, 2009.

Mukhtyar C, Hellmich B, Bacon P, et al: Outcomes from studies of antineutrophil cytoplasm antibody associated vasculitis: a systematic review by the European League Against Rheumatism systemic vasculitis task force, Ann Rheum Dis 67:1004–1010, 2008.

Ntatsaki E, Watts RA, Scott DG: Epidemiology of ANCA-associated vasculitis, Rheum Dis Clin North Am 36:447–461, 2010.

Pagnoux C, Mahr A, Hamidou MA, et al: Azathioprine or methotrexate maintenance for ANCA-associated vasculitis, N Engl J Med 359:2790–2803, 2008.

Ribi C, Cohen P, Pagnoux C, et al: Treatment of Churg–Strauss syndrome without poor-prognosis factors: a multicenter, prospective, randomized, open-label study of seventy-two patients, Arthritis Rheum 58:586–594, 2008.

Smith R, Jones RB, Guerry MJ, et al: Rituximab for remission maintenance in relapsing antineutrophil cytoplasmic antibody-associated vasculitis, Arthritis Rheum 64:3760–3769, 2012.

Stone JH, Merkel PA, Spiera R, et al: Rituximab versus cyclophosphamide for ANCA-associated vasculitis, N Engl J Med 363:211–232, 2010.

Tomasson G, Grayson PC, Mahr AD, et al: Value of ANCA measurements during remission to predict a relapse of ANCA-associated vasculitis—a meta-analysis, Rheumatology (Oxford) 51:100–109, 2012.

FURTHER READING

www.cssassociation.org
www.vasculitisfoundation.org

CHAPTER 30

IMMUNE-COMPLEX–MEDIATED SMALL-VESSEL VASCULITIDES

Ramon A. Arroyo, MD

KEY POINTS

1. Hypersensitivity vasculitis is most commonly idiopathic or due to a drug or infection.
2. Henoch–Schönlein purpura (HSP) presents with palpable purpura, arthritis, abdominal colic, and renal disease.
3. Skin biopsy in HSP shows leukocytoclastic vasculitis with IgA deposition in vessel walls on direct immunofluorescence.
4. Urticarial lesions lasting longer than 24 to 48 hours and resolving with hyperpigmentation are likely vasculitic.
5. Obstructive pulmonary disease commonly occurs in patients with hypocomplementemic urticarial vasculitis syndrome.

1. What are the small-vessel vasculitides due to immune complex deposition?

Small-vessel vasculitis includes a variety of conditions that are grouped together because of the involvement of small blood vessels (<50 μm in diameter) of the skin, especially arterioles and postcapillary venules. **Leukocytoclastic vasculitis (LCV)** and **necrotizing vasculitis** are terms used to describe the usual histopathology, in which small blood vessels are infiltrated with polymorphonuclear neutrophils (PMNs) and/or mononuclear cells. As the process evolves, **fibrinoid necrosis** of the vessel wall with leukocyte fragments (leukocytoclasis) and destruction of the blood vessel wall is seen. Conditions associated with small-vessel vasculitis due to immune complex deposition include those listed in Table 30-1.

2. What causes this group of small-vessel vasculitides?

The cause of cutaneous vasculitis is not a single factor and depends on underlying associated condition(s). All patients should be asked about **new medications, recent infections, and risk factors for hepatitis C**. Between 30% and 50% of cases have no identifiable cause. **Hypersensitivity vasculitis** is the diagnosis given to these patients when the cause cannot be identified. Regardless of the etiology, the vascular injury is believed to be triggered by the deposition of **immune complexes** in the vessel wall with activation of complement, leading to migration of PMNs to the area, release of lysosomal enzymes, and damage to the vessel wall.

Table 30-1. Conditions Associated With Small-Vessel Vasculitis Due to Immune Complex Deposition

CONDITION	COMMENTS
Hypersensitivity vasculitis	Drug reactions or idiopathic
Urticarial vasculitis	If hypocomplementemic consider HUVS and SLE
IgA vasculitis (Henoch–Schönlein purpura)	Renal and gastrointestinal involvement, IgA in vessel walls
Cryoglobulinemic vasculitis	Hepatitis B and C, rarely HIV, and cancer
Rheumatic disorders	RA, SLE, Sjögren's syndrome, Crohn disease
Infections	SBE, *Neisseria*, influenza, mononucleosis, HIV, hepatitis B and C
Malignancy	Leukemia, lymphoma, myeloma, solid tumors, myelodysplastic syndromes, hairy cell leukemia
Anti-glomerular basement membrane disease	Pulmonary–renal syndrome (Goodpasture syndrome)
Erythema elevatum diutinum	Occurs over the extensor surfaces of joints (hands, knees) and buttocks; responds to dapsone

HIV, Human immunodeficiency virus; *HUVS*, hypocomplementemic urticarial vasculitis syndrome; *RA*, rheumatoid arthritis; *SBE*, subacute bacterial endocarditis; *SLE*, systemic lupus erythematosus.

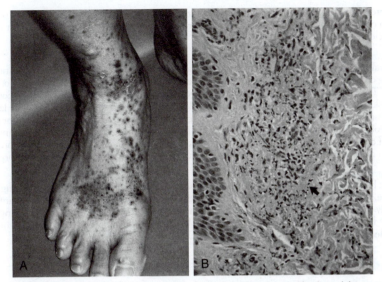

Figure 30-1. Small-vessel vasculitis. **A,** Palpable purpura. **B,** Histopathology of a cutaneous blood vessel demonstrating leukocytoclastic vasculitis with nuclear dust (*arrow*).

3. What is the major clinical manifestation in small-vessel vasculitis?

Palpable purpura is the most common primary lesion in cutaneous vasculitis. Typically, hundreds of discrete, subtly palpable, purpuric spots suddenly appear on the feet and lower extremities (Figure 30-1). The hands, arms, and other body sites also may be affected. In addition to palpability, the presence of a central necrotic punctum is helpful in distinguishing a purpura of vasculitis from purpuras of other causes. These lesions are dynamic, often beginning as asymptomatic, nonpalpable, purpuric macules that eventually become palpable. Some may become nodular, bullous, infarctive, and ulcerative. **Urticarial lesions** are the second most common cutaneous presentation. Other cutaneous manifestations include livedo reticularis and erythema-multiforme–like lesions.

4. Can small-vessel vasculitis only involve the skin? Can patients have systemic manifestations?

The answer to both questions is yes. **Cutaneous leukocytoclastic angiitis** is classified as **single-organ vasculitis** when confined to the skin. When a small-vessel vasculitis is not confined to the skin it can be associated with systemic symptoms. Constitutional symptoms, including fever, arthralgias, and malaise, frequently accompany the appearance of the skin lesions. Frank arthritis is uncommon. Proteinuria, hematuria, and occasional renal insufficiency can occur. Gastrointestinal (GI) manifestations include abdominal pain and GI bleeding, which can be severe and life-threatening. Other organ involvement is less common.

5. What diseases can mimic small-vessel vasculitis?

- Pigmented purpuric dermatoses
- Antiphospholipid syndrome
- Livedoid vasculitis (atrophie blanche)
- Cholesterol emboli
- Low platelet count: Immune thrombocytopenia purpura (ITP), thrombotic thrombocytopenic purpura (TTP), disseminated intravascular coagulation (DIC)
- Meningococcemia
- Calcipylaxis
- Infective endocarditis
- Atrial myxoma
- Scurvy
- Amyloidosis

6. List the laboratory and radiographic tests recommended for a patient presenting with a small-vessel vasculitis.

Most patients presenting with LCV of unknown cause should have the following laboratory tests to look for an etiology: **complete blood count, erythrocyte sedimentation rate (ESR)/C-reactive protein, chemistries, liver-associated enzymes, urinalysis, antinuclear antibody (ANA)/rheumatoid factor (RF), C3/C4 complement, antineutrophil cytoplasmic antibody (ANCA), cryoglobulins, hepatitis serologies, human immunodeficiency virus** (if risk factors), **serum protein electrophoresis,** and **chest x-ray (CXR)**. Unfortunately, the laboratory abnormalities are frequently unrevealing and nonspecific. Notably, malignancy is the cause of LCV in only 1% of patients. Myelodysplastic syndrome and hairy cell leukemia are the most common malignancies.

7. How is small-vessel vasculitis diagnosed?
Patient evaluation requires a full medical evaluation and appropriate laboratory tests (see Question 6), depending on the clinical situation. Diagnosis is made by **skin biopsy** identifying the presence of cutaneous vasculitis. The presence of eosinophils on biopsy suggests drug-induced LCV. Direct immunofluorescence studies of the skin are helpful in differentiating systemic diseases such as IgA vasculitis (HSP). The lack of immune deposits distinguishes microscopic polyangiitis from IgA vasculitis/HSP and mixed cryoglobulinemia, in which immunoglobulins are deposited in the vascular walls. However, except for HSP, skin biopsy cannot discern the etiology of cutaneous vasculitis (infections, drugs, cryoglobulinemia, malignancy, etc.). Therefore, a complete evaluation must be undertaken comprising history, physical examination, and selected laboratory tests.

8. How is small-vessel vasculitis treated?
Treatment has to be determined individually. If the associated disorder can be identified, treating that problem may suffice. Any potential drug or antigen should be discontinued or removed. An underlying infection should be properly treated. Mild cases without internal organ involvement may be self-limited, requiring no specific treatment. If systemic symptoms are present and skin lesions are diffuse, or if internal organ involvement is present, glucocorticoids are usually the treatment of choice.

IGA VASCULITIS (HENOCH–SCHÖNLEIN PURPURA)

9. What are the histopathologic features of IgA vasculitis (IgAV)?
The histopathologic features of IgAV (Henoch–Schönlein purpura) are leukocytoclastic vasculitis or necrotizing small-vessel vasculitis. The characteristic direct immunofluorescence finding is predominantly **IgA deposition** in affected blood vessels. IgA can also be found in the glomerular mesangium. The skin biopsy finding of IgA deposition is what makes this syndrome pathologically different from other forms of small-vessel vasculitis.

10. What is the role of IgA in the pathogenesis of IgAV/HSP?
Many cases of IgAV occur following a respiratory infection, for which IgA is important for mucosal immunity. IgA plays a pivotal role in the pathogenesis of IgAV. There are two subclasses of IgA: IgA1 and IgA2. IgA1 accounts for 80% to 90% of serum IgA, but only 50% of secretory IgA. IgAV is associated with deposition of only IgA1 and not IgA2. Notably, renal-limited IgA nephropathy (Berger disease) involves IgA1 exclusively. For both IgAV and Berger disease, investigators have found that the hinge-region O-linked glycans of IgA1 are deficient in galactose and end with N-acetylgalactosamine (GalNAc). Antiglycan antibodies may recognize the GalNAc moiety on aberrant IgA1 molecules, leading to immune complex formation that is deposited in tissues and activates the alternative complement pathway. In addition, IgA can bind to mesangial cells in the kidney, leading to proliferation and release of proinflammatory cytokines. This kidney receptor binds IgA1 at its hinge region more readily when IgA1 is deficient in galactose.

11. Describe the clinical manifestations of IgA vasculitis.
The classic tetrad of palpable purpura, arthritis, abdominal pain, and renal disease occurs in up to 80% of cases. The rash may begin as macular erythema and urticarial lesions, but may progress rapidly to purpura. The lower extremities and buttocks are the most common sites for the rash. Scrotal and scalp edema can be seen, particularly in children. The joints are involved in 60% to 84% of patients. The involvement is symmetrical and most commonly involves the ankles and knees, which are usually swollen, warm, and tender. GI lesions may cause severe cramping, abdominal pain, intussusception, hemorrhage, and, rarely, ileal perforation. Renal involvement is seen in 50% of patients and is usually manifest as asymptomatic proteinuria and hematuria. However, more marked findings may occur, including nephrotic syndrome and acute renal failure.

IgAV is often acute in onset, and resolution is rapid and complete in 97% of cases, except in a minority of patients (3% to 5%) with chronic renal disease. Persons of any age can be affected, but IgAV occurs primarily in children between the ages of 2 and 10 years. Adults have more severe disease with a higher frequency of renal involvement. Patients of any age (especially adults) suspected of having IgAV for whom a skin biopsy is negative for IgA should be evaluated for ANCA-associated vasculitis, anti-C1q disease, or IgA paraproteinemia.

12. How is IgAV/HSP treated?
The disease is generally self-limited, lasting from 6 to 16 weeks. For mild cases, supportive treatment alone may be adequate. Arthritis responds to nonsteroidal antiinflammatory drugs (NSAIDs). Systemic glucocorticoids (prednisone 1 mg/kg/d × 2 weeks with tapering off over 2 weeks) may be used in patients with GI involvement or bleeding. Progressive renal disease is difficult to treat and usually does not respond to glucocorticoids. Aggressive treatment with high-dose glucocorticoid pulses and cytotoxics should be considered in patients with poor prognostic factors of proteinuria >1 g/day, nephrotic syndrome, and crescentic glomerulonephritis >50% crescents. ANCA-associated vasculitis, which is more likely to respond to rituximab, should be ruled out.

URTICARIAL VASCULITIS

13. What is urticarial vasculitis?
Urticarial vasculitis (UV) is a small-vessel vasculitis presenting with urticarial lesions instead of the more typical palpable purpura. Because of this unusual presentation, UV was separated from the other types of necrotizing small-vessel vasculitis. There are three different syndromes:
- **Normocomplementemic UV** is a self-limited subset of hypersensitivity vasculitis. It is usually idiopathic.
- **Hypocomplementemic UV** comprises two types:
  - The primary type is usually idioathic and not associated with systemic manifestations except occasionally neuropathy.
  - The secondary type is a chronic disorder with features of systemic lupus erythematosus (SLE) including autoantibodies, low complement, and interface dermatitis with a positive lupus band test.
- **Hypocomplementemic UV syndrome (HUVS)** is a severe form of disease with UV and extracutaneous manifestations including obstructive pulmonary disease/emphysema (50%) especially in smokers, uveitis (30%), episcleritis, fever, angioedema (50%), peripheral neuropathy, cardiac valvular lesions, pericarditis (15% to 20%), transient migratory large joint arthritis (50%), recurrent abdominal pain (30%), glomerulonephritis (50%), and seizures. Laboratory abnormalities include **anti-C1q antibodies (C1q precipitins)** (100%), low C3/C4 complement, elevated ESR (67%), positive ANA (65%), and positive RF (<10%). For ANA-positive patients, SLE and Sjögren's syndrome shuld be ruled out. A baseline CXR and pulmonary function tests should be obtained for all patients with HUVS.

14. How is UV differentiated from typical urticaria?
- UV tends to involve the trunk and proximal extremities more than the distal lower extremities, like other causes of LCV.
- UV lesions typically last for more than 24 to 48 hours and often resolve with residual hyperpigmentation. True urticaria lesions (hives) last for <24 hours (usually 8 to 12 hours) and leave no trace.
- UV lesions are often characterized by pain and burning rather than pruritus, the sensory hallmark of true urticaria.
- UV lesions are typically 0.5 to 5 cm in diameter, whereas true urticaria may coalesce into large lesions of >10 cm.
- Symptoms or signs of systemic disease, such as fever, arthralgias, abdominal pain, lymphadenopathy, or abnormal urine sediment, tend to occur in HUVS and rarely in true allergic urticaria.
- The histology is LCV for UV, in contrast to edema of the upper dermis for true urticaria.

15. What are some of the conditions associated with UV? What is the proposed pathogenesis?
UV has been described in association with SLE, Sjögren's syndrome, lymphoma, hepatitis B and C antigenemia, drug reactions, and IgM paraproteinemia (Schnitzler syndrome). The etiology is thought to be related to immune complex deposition. In patients with HUVS, the proposed pathogenesis is that IgG2 anti-C1q antibodies (C1q precipitins) bind to collagen-like regions of the C1q molecule, forming an immune complex that deposits in blood vessels causing activation of complement and other mediators and leading to vasculitic lesions. It has been proposed that the obstructive lung disease observed is a result of binding of anti-C1q antibodies to collagen-like regions of surfactant proteins in pulmonary alveoli. This, in combination with vasculitic lesions in pulmonary capillaries, causes lung injury, possibly due to influx of neutrophils and release of neutrophil elastase. There is controversy over whether or not HUVS is an atypical subset of SLE.

16. How is UV treated?
Therapy consists of supportive measures and treatment of any associated or underlying disorder. Assuming that there is no internal organ involvement, conservative treatment is reasonable. Both H_1 (fexofenadine) and H_2 (ranitidine) antihistamines are used. NSAIDs help with arthralgias and arthritis. In addition, prednisone in doses from 10 to 60 mg may be required. **Dapsone** and hydroxychloroquine benefit some patients with HUVS. For patients with severe disease and major organ involvement, cyclophosphamide, azathioprine, and mycophenolate mofetil are used in combination with prednisone, similar to SLE therapy. Cyclosporine may be beneficial for patients with HUVS who develop progressive airway obstruction. Rituximab and plasmapharesis followed by IV Ig are alternatives for treatment-refractory disease.

ERYTHEMA ELEVATUM DIUTINUM

17. What is erythema elevatum diutinum (EED)?
EED is a form of LCV limited to the skin. The lesions have a characteristic distribution in that they involve the skin over the extensor surface of joints (especially knuckles, knees, and buttocks) symmetrically. They start as pink/yellow papules or plaques and later become red/purple nodules. Biopsy shows LCV with fibrinoid necrosis. Direct immunofluoresence is nonspecific. EED has been associated with connective tissue diseases, infections, and paraproteinemias, especially IgA. Patients respond dramatically to dapsone or sulfapyridine but lesions recur on discontinuation.

BIBLIOGRAPHY

Buck A, Christensen J, McCarty M: Hypocomplementemic urticarial vasculitis syndrome, J Clin Aesthet Dermatol 5:36–46, 2012.
Davis MD, Brewer JD: Urticarial vasculitis and hypocomplementemic urticarial vasculitis syndrome, Immunol Allergy Clin North Am 24:183–213, 2004.
Eustace JA, Nadasdy T, Choi M: Disease of the month: the Churg-Strauss syndrome, J Am Soc Nephrol 10:2048–2055, 1999.
Lau KK, Suzuki H, Novak J, Wyatt RJ: Pathogenesis of Henoch–Schönlein purpura nephritis, Pediatr Nephrol 25:19–26, 2010.
Mukhtyar C, Guillevin L, Cid MC, et al: EULAR recommendations for management of primary small and medium vessel vasculitis, Ann Rheum Dis 68:310–317, 2009.
Park H: Neoplastic and Paraneoplastic Vasculitis, Vasculopathy and Hypercoagulability, Rheum Dis Clin North Am 37:4, 2011.
Ronkainen J, Koskimies O, Ala-Houhala M, et al: Early prednisone therapy in Henoch–Schönlein purpura: a randomized, double-blind, placebo-controlled trial, J Pediatr 149:241–247, 2006.
Saulsbury FT: Henoch–Schönlein purpura, Curr Opin Rheumatol 22:598–602, 2010.
Stone JA: Vasculitis: a collection of pearls and myths, Rheum Dis Clin North Am 33:691–739, 2007.
Ting TV: Diagnosis and management of cutaneous vasculitis in children, Pediatr Clin North Am 61:2, 2014.
Wahl CE, Bouldin MB, Gibson LE: Erythema elevatum diutinum: clinical, histopathologic, and immunohistochemical characteristics of six patients, Am J Dermatopathol 27:397–400, 2005.
Zuberbier T: Urticarial vasculitis and Schnitzier syndrome, Immunol Allergy Clin North Am 34:1, 2014.

FURTHER READING

www.nlm.nih.gov/medlineplus/vasculitis.html

CRYOGLOBULINEMIA
Korey R. Ullrich, MD

> **KEY POINTS**
> 1. Mixed cryoglobulinemia is an immune-complex mediated small-vessel vasculitis commonly associated with chronic hepatitis C virus infection, systemic autoimmune diseases (especially Sjögren's syndrome), and lymphoproliferative disorders.
> 2. Palpable purpura, weakness, and arthralgias are the most common manifestations of mixed cryoglobulinemia, but renal involvement is most closely associated with a poor prognosis.
> 3. Rituximab has recently emerged as an effective treatment option for HCV-associated cryoglobulinemic vasculitis, particularly when used in combination with antiviral agents, and has demonstrated superiority when compared to traditional immunosuppressive regimens.

1. What are cryoglobulins?
Cryoglobulins are immunoglobulins or immunoglobulin-containing complexes that spontaneously precipitate from serum and plasma at low temperatures and become soluble again with rewarming. Cryoprecipitation of human serum components was first described by Wintrobe and Buell in 1933. The term "cryoglobulin" was introduced by Lerner et al in 1947.

2. How are cryoglobulins classified?
Brouet et al studied 86 patients with cryoglobulinemia and, based on those observations, published a classification system in 1974 that is still in use today.
- **Type I:** composed of a single monoclonal immunoglobulin (Ig), with IgM being the most common. Serum levels of the cryoglobulin are typically very high (5 to 30 mg/mL, cryocrit >5%) and precipitation occurs rapidly with cooling (usually <24 hours).
- **Type II:** "mixed" cryoglobulins (MC) composed of a *monoclonal* Ig (typically IgM) that acts as an antibody (e.g., *rheumatoid factor*) against *polyclonal* Ig (typically IgG). Serum levels are usually intermediate (1 to 10 mg/mL, cryocrit 1% to 5%), therefore precipitation may take a few days.
- **Type III:** mixed cryoglobulins similar to Type II, but with *polyclonal* Ig with *rheumatoid factor* activity directed against *polyclonal* Ig. They are usually present in small quantities (0.1 to 1 mg/mL, cryocrit <1%) and precipitate slowly (up to 7 days), so are more difficult to detect.
- **Type II–III:** an unusual variant composed of *oligoclonal* IgM and faint polyclonal immunoglobulins. It is thought to represent a transition from polyclonal (type III) to monoclonal (type II) mixed cryoglobulinemia as clonal expansion of B cells progresses (see Question 10).

3. What is the overall incidence of each cryoglobulin type?
Type I: 10% to 15%, type II: 50% to 60%, type III: 25% to 30%, type II–III: 10%. "Mixed" account for 85% to 90% of all cases.

4. Describe the requirements for collection and processing of blood specimens for cryoglobulin testing.
- Blood is collected into prewarmed tubes. The sample is then allowed to clot for 1 hour, followed by centrifugation and separation of the serum. All of these steps, including transportation of the sample after collection, must be performed at 37 °C. Premature cooling may decrease the cryoglobulin concentration and result in false-negative results.
- The remaining serum is incubated at 4 °C (refrigerator temperature) for 3 to 7 days. A 7-day incubation is ideal because many mixed cryoglobulins will not be identified otherwise due to slow precipitation.
- Centrifugation at 4 °C is performed. Visual inspection of the cryoprecipitate allows for determination of the cryocrit (quantitative measure). Many laboratories only report the cryocrit and no further testing is performed beyond this point.
- If further testing is done (qualitative analysis), the sample is washed so only the precipitate remains. The precipitate is then rewarmed and the quantity and contents of the cryoglobulin (e.g., immunoglobulin type, complement, etc.) are determined by immunodiffusion and immunofixation.

5. **What underlying disorders are associated with type I cryoglobulinemia?**
   Lymphoproliferative disorders that are associated with monoclonal immunoglobulin production such as multiple myeloma, Waldenstrom's macroglobulinemia, chronic lymphocytic leukemia, and B cell lymphomas.

6. **What conditions are associated with the mixed cryoglobulinemias?**
   Hepatitis C (HCV) infection is the most common, followed by autoimmune/autoinflammatory diseases and lymphoproliferative processes. Only a small fraction of cases (<5%) are truly "essential" cryoglobulinemia (i.e., those with no definable underlying illness).

7. **Describe the relationship between hepatitis C infection and mixed cryoglobulinemia.**
   Hepatitis C accounts for up to 90% of type II and up to 70% of type III cases. Overall 30% to 50% of patients with HCV infection have detectable cryoglobulins, but less than 10% of these patients (or <5% of all patients with HCV infection) develop symptomatic vasculitis. The prevalence is highest in the Mediterranean area and lower in Northern Europe, the United States, and the rest of the world. Development of cryoglobulinemic vasculitis is associated with the duration of infection and generally occurs after 10 years.

8. **What other infections are associated with mixed cryoglobulinemia?**
   After HCV, HIV is the most common. Other infectious agents are less frequently seen and the association is not as clearly established in the majority. Many of these cases are associated with the transient appearance of type III cryoglobulins without associated disease. These include hepatitis B, Epstein–Barr virus, cytomegalovirus, hepatitis A, *Coxiella burnetii* (Q fever), Parvovirus B19, poststreptococcal nephritis, subacute bacterial endocarditis, tuberculosis, leprosy, brucellosis, coccidioidomycosis, parasitic infections, and others.
   PEARL: a patient with fever, valvular heart disease, and negative cultures in the setting of MC must be evaluated for Q fever.

9. **Describe the relationship between systemic autoimmune disease and mixed cryoglobulinemia.**
   Autoimmune disorders are the second most commonly associated diagnoses with MC (usually type III) after hepatitis C. Sjögren's syndrome is the most common, followed by systemic lupus erythematosus and rheumatoid arthritis. Cryoglobulins may be seen in up to 15% to 20% of cases, but associated vasculitis is seen in only a small fraction of cases. Levels of circulating cryoglobulins are typically much lower than that seen in HCV cases. The presence of cryoglobulins is associated with extraglandular manifestations, lymphoma, and mortality in Sjögren's syndrome. Cutaneous vasculitis, peripheral neuropathy, elevated rheumatoid factor (RF), and low complement may also be associated with cryoglobulins. Many of these patients are also infected with HCV, so testing for HCV should be conducted in patients with autoimmune disease presenting with cutaneous vasculitis if not already done. Less common associations include systemic sclerosis, polyarteritis nodosa, autoimmune thyroiditis, Henoch–Schönlein purpura, giant cell arteritis, antiphospholipid antibody syndrome, sarcoidosis, Behçet's disease, inflammatory myopathies, antineutrophil cytoplasmic antibody (ANCA)-associated vasculitides, and inflammatory bowel disease.

10. **What are the mechanisms underlying tissue injury in cryoglobulinemic vasculitis?**
    - Cryoglobulin precipitation and vascular occlusion in the microcirculation is the predominant cause of injury in type I cryoglobulinemia and reflects the large concentration and cold-inducible characteristics of the immunoglobulins. Cold-inducible injury is not thought to play a major role in type II and type III MC given the fact that in vitro cold precipitation is much slower.
    - Immune-complex mediated vasculitis is the primary cause in types II and III MC. The small vessels are most commonly affected, but medium vessel involvement may occur. Associated complement fixation, in part, explains the low level of complement in this condition. The higher the thermal range that the cryoglobulin will still precipitate, the more likely it is to activate complement.

11. **Describe the steps involved in mixed cryoglobulin formation and their pathogenicity.**
    This process has been most extensively studied in HCV-associated MC. Expansion of B lymphocytes is the hallmark and is thought to result from chronic immune stimulation. HCV has a membrane protein, E2, that binds to CD81 on B cells and is thought to be directly involved in B cell stimulation. These cells produce immunoglobulins with RF activity, especially a particular variant designated the WA cross-idiotype. Complexes of HCV particles, immunoglobulins, RF, complement, and other particles (e.g., very-low-density lipoprotein) comprise the cryoglobulin. Cryoglobulins may persist despite viral clearance following treatment (and may no longer contain viral particles), suggesting that cryoglobulin formation may initially be a virus-dependent phenomenon that eventually becomes autonomous. Tissue deposition, complement fixation, and the following inflammatory cascade result in vasculitis. The fact that a particular B cell activating factor (BAFF) promoter polymorphism and elevated levels of BAFF are found in patients with MC suggests that it may have a pathogenic role by promoting B cell proliferation and survival.

12. **Summarize the major clinical and laboratory features of cryoglobulinemia.**
    The major clinical and laboratory features of cryoglobulinemia are shown in Figure 31-1.

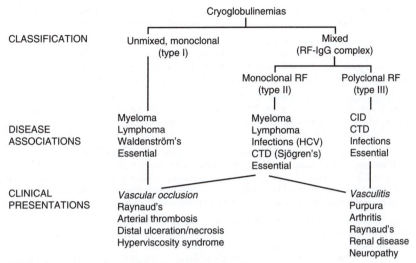

Figure 31-1. The major clinical and laboratory features of cryoglobulinemia.

13. What are the common clinical manifestations?

Hyperviscosity syndrome (bleeding, vision changes, neurologic symptoms, etc.) is the most common manifestation in type I. In MC, cutaneous manifestations are the most common, with arthralgias and neuropathy being other frequent findings. The frequency of manifestations varies between studies, reflecting the characteristics of the patient populations (Table 31-1).

Table 31-1. Common Clinical Manifestations			
Purpura	55% to 100%	Raynaud's phenomenon	5% to 35%
Arthralgias	45% to 100%	Renal	10% to 40%
Weakness	70% to 100%	Sicca	30% to 50%
Meltzer's triad*	40% to 80%	Gastrointestinal	2% to 6%
Neuropathy	20% to 80%	Pulmonary	<5%
Ulcers	10%	Malignancy	10% to 15%
Arthritis	<10%	Endocrine (diabetes mellitus, hypothyroid, erectile dysfunction)	

*Meltzer's triad = purpura + arthralgias + weakness/myalgias.

14. What are the common cutaneous manifestations in MC?

Palpable purpura is the most common manifestation, being seen in up to 100% of cases during the course of disease. Urticarial vasculitis can also occur. Lesions typically affect the lower extremities, but can involve the trunk and upper extremities. They usually resolve spontaneously, but tend to be recurrent. Because cryoglobulinemic vasculitis can involve both small and medium vessels, more severe cutaneous lesions can be seen. For example, large skin ulcers can occur (10%) and generally are above the malleoli (separating them from venous stasis ulcers). Digital necrosis, bullae, and livedo racemosa may also be seen.

15. What is the most common renal finding?

Type 1 membranoproliferative glomerulonephritis is the most common histologic pattern (80% of cases). Frank nephrotic or nephritic syndrome can occur, but patients typically present with less substantial microscopic hematuria or proteinuria. Hypertension and elevated creatinine are common, and renal failure may be mild or severe at presentation.

16. What are the common neurologic manifestations?

A painful sensory polyneuropathy is the most common finding. It can be symmetrical or asymmetrical, and insidious or abrupt in onset. Motor involvement can also occur, typically months to years after the sensory neuropathy. Mononeuritis multiplex may also be seen. Neuropathy is thought to result from vasculitis of the vasa nervorum and is always painful. Central nervous system involvement is exceedingly rare and other causes (e.g., atherosclerotic) should be explored if central nervous system symptoms occur.

17. Describe the typical articular manifestations.
Polyarticular arthralgias are seen in the majority of patients during the course of the disease. Patients may describe profound joint pain, but inflammatory features are lacking on examination. A nonerosive arthritis is much less commonly encountered. Immune-complex deposition is thought to be the cause of joint symptoms.

18. How is malignancy associated with MC?
Symptomatic lymphoma develops in 5% to 20% of patients within 10 years of diagnosis. B cell lymphomas are the most common, whereas hepatocellular carcinoma and papillary thyroid cancer occur less frequently. Treatment of HCV or cryoglobulinemia (e.g., with antivirals and rituximab) may result in resolution or prevention of lymphoma.

19. What are the common laboratory abnormalities in mixed cryoglobulinemic vasculitis?
Elevated RF and hypocomplementemia are seen in almost all patients with MC. Notably, C4 is reduced out of proportion to C3. A polyclonal hypergammaglobulinemia or monoclonal gammopathy are also frequently seen. Autoantibodies (other than RF) are seen in more than half of patients and include antinuclear, anti-smooth muscle, antineutrophil cytoplasmic, antithyroid, antimitochondrial, and antiphospholipid antibodies.

20. How is the diagnosis of mixed cryoglobulinemic vasculitis established?
Detection of cryoglobulins in the right clinical setting is diagnostic. Given the fact that false-negative results are common due to sample mishandling, the absence of cryoglobulins does not exclude the diagnosis. A high level of suspicion should be maintained if characteristic clinical and laboratory features are present. Elevated RF, low complement, and the presence of a monoclonal gammopathy (especially when found together) may serve as a surrogate marker of cryoglobulinemia. Biopsy of affected tissue (typically skin) demonstrates leukocytoclastic vasculitis, and intravascular hyaline thrombi may also be seen. Immunofluorescence typically demonstrates immunoglobulin and C3 deposition. Biopsies of liver or bone marrow may demonstrate clonal expansions of B cells.

21. What is the prognosis of mixed cryoglobulinemic vasculitis?
Approximately 65% have a slow, relatively benign course, and 35% have a moderate-to-severe course. Survival over 10 years is 56% in mixed cryoglobulinemic vasculitis versus 93% in controls. Renal involvement most strongly confers a worse prognosis (62% survival without versus 33% survival with renal involvement), and male gender, age ≥60 years, type II cryoglobulinemia, gastrointestinal involvement, chronic HCV infection, and diffuse vasculitis may also be risk factors. Cryoglobulin levels, complement values, and RF titers have no prognostic significance. Renal failure is the most common cause of death, whereas cirrhosis, widespread vasculitis, malignancy, and infection are less frequent causes.

22. Discuss the treatment options for mixed cryoglobulinemic vasculitis.
Removal of the antigenic stimulus is the primary goal. In HCV-associated mixed cryoglobulinemic vasculitis this involves use of standard antiviral regimens, whereas in malignancy, other infections, and autoimmune diseases, appropriate treatment of these conditions is warranted. Immunosuppression is used to directly control the vasculitis and associated tissue damage. Most data regarding treatment are derived from studies of HCV-associated mixed cryoglobulinemic vasculitis:
- *Glucocorticoids*: high-dose steroids should be used in patients with severe manifestations (e.g., neurologic, renal, or diffuse vasculitis), and short courses of low to intermediate doses can be used during flares. Steroids should be tapered off quickly, and there is no role for chronic therapy.
- *Plasma exchange*: although there is no controlled data supporting its use, expert opinion suggests a role in severe, life-threatening disease. It is the treatment of choice for hyperviscosity syndrome and diffuse alveolar hemorrhage.
- *Cyclophosphamide*: is frequently employed in combination with plasma exchange to treat severe disease, and it can be considered in this setting. It is not recommended for use as monotherapy.
- *Other immunosuppressants*: use of azathioprine, methotrexate, cyclosporine, and other immunosuppressive agents is anecdotal, and no consensus recommendations can be made.
- *Colchicine*: may have favorable effects on pain, weakness, purpura, and leg ulcers. The standard dose is 1 mg/day, and it can be used as long as needed (may be years).
- *Low antigen diet*: can result in substantial improvement of purpura and pain within 4 to 8 weeks. It also has a favorable effect on laboratory abnormalities. It should be considered in all patients.
- *Intravenous immunoglobulin*: there are some reports of its use with plasma exchange to treat cutaneous ulcers. However, several cases of worsening vasculitis associated with its use have been described, so it should be avoided if possible.
- *Antivirals and rituximab (see below)*.

23. Discuss the use of antiviral agents and rituximab in the treatment of mixed cryoglobulinemic vasculitis.
Antiviral (AV) agents should be considered in all patients with hepatitis C associated MC. They have demonstrated response rates of 30% to 80% in MC, but their use may be limited due to contraindications, side effects (interferon-α may exacerbate vasculitis manifestations), and slow onset of action.

Rituximab (RTX) has shown great promise in treating mixed cryoglobulinemic vasculitis and should be considered in all patients with moderate-to-severe disease. Its use in combination with AV has demonstrated superiority over either agent used alone. RTX monotherapy has also been shown to be more efficacious than standard-of-care immunosuppression (high-dose steroids, azathioprine, cyclophosphamide, plasma exchange, or a combination of these). However, either RTX or AV alone is effective, so a contraindication to one should not affect the decision to use the other. Typical response rates with combination therapy are 70% to 80%, with most being complete clinical responders. Addition of RTX to AV seems to particularly predict a more rapid clinical response and better renal response than AV alone. Improvement may be seen as early as 1 month, but typically occurs within 3 to 6 months. Clinical response rates occur more commonly than immunologic and virologic response rates, indicating that viral and immunologic responses are not necessary. Many patients treated with combination therapy were re-treated with AV despite having failed previous AV monotherapy and demonstrated a better response than treatment with RTX alone; therefore, it is reasonable to re-treat these patients with AV regardless of their initial response. The presence of monoclonal B cell expansions, type 1 genotype, initial viral load, and extent of liver disease seem to predict treatment response, but the decision to treat should not be based on these parameters.

There is no consensus regarding how RTX and AV should be administered. The studies using combination therapy have used sequential treatment with AV followed by RTX several weeks later rather than concurrent administration, given the concern for possible adverse events, so this may be a reasonable option. Studies have evaluated dosing RTX 1 g every 2 weeks (2 doses) and 375 mg/m^2 weekly for 4 weeks, and both are effective.

24. Is relapse common after treatment with RTX?
Treatment effect is usually durable and has been demonstrated for >2 years after a single treatment course. Relapse occurs in ~20% of cases and seems to be less frequent with combination therapy versus either RTX or AV monotherapy. Immunologic relapse always precedes clinical relapse, B cell recovery precedes relapse in the majority of cases, and most patients with a clinical relapse have viral recurrence or an initial lack of viral response. However, not all patients with immunologic relapse (decreased C4, increased cryoglobulins, return of B cells) have a clinical relapse, so it is difficult to predict who should be re-treated and when. Re-treatment with RTX after relapse is highly effective and thus should be considered in this setting.

25. Discuss the safety of RTX when used to treat mixed cryoglobulinemic vasculitis?
Overall, safety is similar when compared to other treatments. Serum sickness occurs in ~1% of cases and is usually mild. One study suggested that the administration of RTX 1 g every 2 weeks is more commonly associated with severe systemic reactions (e.g., vasculitis flares) than the weekly dosing schedule. The mechanism is thought to involve cryoglobulins forming immune complexes with RTX by binding to it in an RF-dependent manner, resulting in accelerated immune-complex mediated vasculitis. This was dependent on the level of cryoglobulins (high cryoglobulin concentration, low C4) and dose of RTX, thus the recommendation was to use the lower dose regimen and to perform plasma exchange before administration in patients with high cryoglobulin concentrations (>3%) and/or significant renal insufficiency. One approach is to do plasma exchange every other day for five to seven treatments plus high-dose glucocorticoids followed by RTX (375 mg/m^2 weekly × 4 doses). Notably, HCV viral loads are generally not affected by RTX and worsening liver disease has not been demonstrated.

26. Summarize the general treatment principles of HCV-associated cryoglobulinemia.
The general treatment principles of HCV-associated cryoglobulinemia are shown in Figure 31-2.

27. Define cryofibrinogenemia and describe its diagnosis and clinical manifestations.
Cryofibrinogens are insoluble complexes of fibrin, fibrinogen, fibrin split products, plasma proteins, and immunoglobulins that precipitate with cold exposure. They do not precipitate in serum (plasma only) because the proteins consumed in the clotting process during cooling are the necessary substrates for cryofibrinogens. It is typically associated with malignancy, diabetes mellitus, connective tissue diseases, and infection.

Cutaneous manifestations are the most common and are the result of vascular occlusion and tissue ischemia. They tend to occur in cold-exposed areas and include purpura, livedo, ulcers, and gangrene. Leukocytoclastic vasculitis and necrosis are seen more commonly than isolated microthrombi in biopsy specimens, but they may occur together. Thromboses in larger vessels (strokes, myocardial infarction, etc.) are seen less frequently. Paradoxical bleeding may occur due to depletion of clotting factors. There is an association with cryoglobulins: cryofibrinogens are seen in 70% of patients with cryoglobulins, whereas 60% of cryofibrinogens occur in isolation.

28. Discuss the appropriate collection and processing of specimens being tested for cryofibrinogens.
Blood is collected in nonheparinized tubes (use EDTA or citrate) that does not allow coagulation and is stored at 37 °C until centrifugation. After centrifugation, the remaining plasma is stored at 4 °C for 72 hours and cryofibrinogens, if present, will form during this period. Cryofibrinogens are absorbed by red blood cells (RBCs), so a delay in centrifugation or allowing the sample to cool may result in false-negative results because the RBCs are eventually discarded. Heparin tubes should not be used for collection because heparin may form

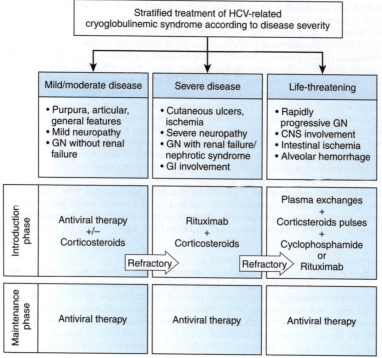

Figure 31-2. The general treatment principles of HCV-associated cryoglobulinemia. CNS, Central nervous system; GI, gastrointestinal; GN, glomerulonephritis.

a cryoprecipitate with plasma factors and lead to false-positive results. It is also recommended that a separate serum sample be obtained by collecting blood in a prewarmed tube that does allow coagulation. The serum sample should be tested for the presence of a cryoglobulins as outlined in Question 4.

PEARL: cryofibrinogens will precipitate in the cold only from the plasma sample, whereas cryoglobulins precipitate in the cold from both the plasma and serum samples.

29. **Discuss the treatment of cryofibrinogenemia.**
    Avoiding cold exposure and keeping the patient at 37 degrees is reasonable. Cutaneous lesions should be treated according to standard gangrene or burn protocols. Streptokinase and stanozolol have been shown to be effective. Steroids alone have not been shown to be beneficial, but may be helpful when combined with other immunosuppressants (azathioprine, chlorambucil). Immunosuppression should be reserved for cases associated with systemic autoimmune disease. There are limited data to support the use of plasma exchange. Heparin is not useful and patients may actually worsen. Warfarin is potentially beneficial, but studies have had mixed results. Aspirin and colchicine have been studied, but have not demonstrated a benefit.

30. **What is cold agglutinin disease?**
    Cold agglutinins are typically IgM antibodies directed against I/i antigens on erythrocytes leading to hemolytic anemia due to complement-mediated RBC destruction in the reticuloendothelial system (typically the liver). Slowing of blood flow with occlusion of superficial vessels by agglutinated RBCs in exposed cooler peripheral tissues can lead to acrocyanosis, Raynaud's-like symptoms, and skin ulcers on ears, nose, and digits. Most cases with chronic manifestations are idiopathic or related to lymphoproliferative diseases. Treatment includes warmth, glucocorticoids, RTX, and rarely plasmapheresis. Alkylating agents are limited to those patients requiring them to treat their lymphomas. Cold agglutinin disease due to infections (mycoplasma pneumoniae, infectious mononucleosis, other viruses) typically are asymptomatic or cause transient clinical manifestations that usually do not require therapy other than warmth. Recently, cold agglutinin disease has been described in patients with ANCA vasculitis related to levamisole-tainted cocaine.

BIBLIOGRAPHY

Agnello V, Elfahal M: Cryoglobulin types and rheumatoid factors associated with clinical manifestations in patients with hepatitis C virus infection, Dig Liver Dis 39(Suppl 1):S25–S31, 2007.

Amdo TD, Welker JA: An approach to the diagnosis and treatment of cryofibrinogenemia, Am J Med 116:332–337, 2004.

Berentsen S: How I manage cold agglutinin disease, Br J Hematol 153:309–317, 2011.

Charles ED, Dustin LB: Hepatitis C virus-induced cryoglobulinemia, Kidney Int 76:818–824, 2009.

Dammacco F, Tucci FA, Lauletta G, et al: PEGylated interferon-α, ribavirin, and rituximab combined therapy of hepatitis C virus-related mixed cryoglobulinemia: a long-term study, Blood 116:343–353, 2010.

De Vita S, Quartuccio L, Isola M, et al: A randomized controlled trial of rituximab for the treatment of severe cryoglobulinemic vasculitis, Arthritis Rheum 64:843–853, 2012.

Ferri C, Antonelli A, Mascia MT, et al: B-cells and mixed cryoglobulinemia, Autoimmun Rev 7:114–120, 2007.

Ferri C, Mascia MT: Cryoglobulinemic vasculitis, Curr Opin Rheumatol 18:54–63, 2006.

Ferri C, Sebastiani M, Giuggioli D, et al: Mixed cryoglobulinemia: demographic, clinical, and serologic features and survival in 231 patients, Semin Arthritis Rheum 33:355–374, 2004.

Gragnani L, Piluso A, Giannini C, et al: Genetic determinants in hepatitis C virus-associated mixed cryoglobulinemia: role of polymorphic variants of BAFF promoter and Fcγ receptors, Arthritis Rheum 63:1446–1451, 2011.

Lamprecht P, Gause A, Gross WL: Cryoglobulinemic vasculitis, Arthritis Rheum 42:2507–2516, 1999.

Motyckova G, Murali M: Laboratory testing for cryoglobulins, Am J Hematol 86:500–502, 2011.

Pietrogrande M, De Vita S, Zignego AL, et al: Recommendations for the management of mixed cryoglobulinemia syndrome in hepatitis C virus-infected patients, Autoimmun Rev 10:444–454, 2011.

Ramos-Casals M, Stone JH, Cid MC, et al: The cryoglobulinemias, *Lancet* 379:348–360, 2012.

Saadoun D, Landau DA, Calabrese LH, et al: Hepatitis C-associated mixed cryoglobulinaemia: a crossroad between autoimmunity and lymphoproliferation, Rheumatology 46:1234–1242, 2007.

Saadoun D, Rigon MR, Sene D, et al: Rituximab plus PEG-interferon-α/ribavirin compared with PEG-interferon-α/ribavirin in hepatitis C-related mixed cryoglobulinemia, Blood 116:326–334, 2010.

Sene D, Ghillani-Dalbin P, Amoura Z, et al: Rituximab may form a complex with IgMκ mixed cryoglobulin and induce severe systemic reactions in patients with hepatitis C virus-induced vasculitis, Arthritis Rheum 60:3848–3855, 2009.

Sneller M, Hu Z, Langford C: A randomized controlled trial of rituximab following failure of antiviral therapy for hepatitis C virus-associated cryoglobulinemic vasculitis, Arthritis Rheum 64:835–842, 2012.

Tedeschi A, Barate C, Minola E, et al: Cryoglobulinemia, Blood Rev 21:183–200, 2007.

Terrier B, Saadoun D, Sene D, et al: Efficacy and tolerability of rituximab with or without PEGylated interferon α-2b plus ribavirin in severe hepatitis C virus-related vasculitis, Arthritis Rheum 60:2531–2540, 2009.

CHAPTER 32

BEHÇET'S DISEASE AND COGAN'S SYNDROME

Sterling G. West, MD

TOP SECRETS

1. Behçet's disease should be considered in any patient with a systemic inflammatory disease characterized by recurrent orogenital ulcers and uveitis.
2. Behçet's disease is the only vasculitis to cause pulmonary aneurysms.
3. Pathergy at the site of needle sticks is characteristic of Behçet's disease.
4. Cogan's syndrome is characterized by ocular interstitial keratitis and audiovestibular disease.

1. **What are the variable vessel vasculitides?**
   The International Chapel Hill Consensus Conference recognized two vasculitides that can affect any size and type (arteries, veins, capillaries) of blood vessel: Behçet's disease and Cogan's syndrome.

BEHÇET'S DISEASE

2. **What are the Revised International Criteria for Adamantiades–Behçet's disease?**
   - **Recurrent oral ulceration** (1 point): recurrent and multiple minor aphthous, major aphthous, or herpetiform ulcerations.
   - **Recurrent genital ulceration** (2 points): aphthous ulceration or scarring.
   - **Eye lesions** (2 points): anterior uveitis, posterior uveitis, or cells in vitreous on slit lamp examination; or retinal vasculitis.
   - **Skin lesions** (1 point): pseudofolliculitis, papulopustular lesions, erythema nodosum-like lesions, pyoderma gangrenosum-like lesions.
   - **Vascular lesions** (1 point): phlebitis, large vein thrombosis, aneurysm, arterial thrombosis.
   - **Positive pathergy test** (1 point): 2 mm erythema 24 to 48 hours after a #20- to 21-gauge needle prick to a depth of 5 mm.

   The diagnosis is confirmed in a patient with three or more points. Note that pulmonary aneurysms, major venous thrombosis, genital ulcers that scar, hypopyon, and pathergy are highly characteristic of Behçet's disease in a patient presenting with recurrent oral ulcers. Note that histopathologic analysis of involved tissues reveals a *neutrophilic vascular reaction* to leukocytoclastic vasculitis.

3. **Behçet's disease is a clinical diagnosis. What other diseases must be considered and ruled out in a patient presenting with possible Behçet's disease?**
   Virtually all the features of Behçet's disease can be seen in Crohn's colitis. Inflammatory bowel disease must be considered particularly in patients with iron deficiency, markedly elevated erythrocyte sedimentation rate (ESR, >100 mm/h), or even minor bowel complaints. Other collagen vascular diseases with oral ulcers, ocular disease, and arthritis need to be considered, including systemic lupus erythematosus, reactive arthritis, herpetic infection, systemic vasculitis, and Sweet's syndrome.

4. **Describe "pathergy."**
   Pathergy is the hyperreactivity of the skin to any intracutaneous injection or needle stick (pathergy test). It frequently occurs at sites of blood draw. Originally described in 1935, this reaction is believed by some to be pathognomonic for Behçet's disease. The mechanism of pathergy in Behçet's disease is unknown, but it is thought to be related to increased neutrophil chemotaxis. The rate of a positive reaction varies in different populations, being more common in Japan and Turkey and less common in England and the United States.

5. **Who gets Behçet's disease?**
   The disease occurs in both males and females equally, with the mean age of patients being approximately 30 years. It is rare to occur in childhood and after the age of 50 years. The highest prevalence is in Turkey and Japan.

6. **What is the relationship between this disease and the old Silk Route of Marco Polo?**
   Although Behçet's disease occurs worldwide, it is much more prevalent in individuals living along the old Silk Route (trade trail of Marco Polo), extending from the Orient (Japan) through Turkey and into the

Mediterranean basin. Japanese and Eastern Mediterranean individuals have a three to six times increased incidence of HLA-B51 in patients with Behçet's disease compared with controls. The presence of HLA-B51 appears to be associated with a more complete expression of manifestations and a more severe clinical course of disease. HLA-B51 is not increased in frequency in patients with Behçet's disease in the United States. Although first described 25 years ago, we still do not know whether the HLA-B51 or a gene in linkage disequilibrium with HLA-B51 is the predisposing locus for Behçet's disease. Genome-wide scans have identified up to 16 additional loci that may contribute to the risk of developing Behçet's disease. Familial clustering has been reported.

7. Describe the aphthous ulcers associated with Behçet's disease.
Aphthous-like stomatitis is the initial manifestation in 25% to 75% of patients with Behçet's disease. Preferential sites of ulceration are the mucous membranes of the lips, gingiva, cheeks (buccal mucosa), and tongue. The palate, tonsils, and pharynx are rarely involved (unlike reactive arthritis or Stevens–Johnson syndrome). Most oral ulcers occur in crops (3 to >10 lesions), are less than 1 cm in diameter, heal without scarring within 1 to 3 weeks, and are recurrent.

8. List a differential diagnosis of aphthous stomatitis.
Underlying conditions may be identified in as many as 30% of patients with severe aphthous stomatitis. Most cases remain idiopathic, however (Table 32-1).

Table 32-1. Differential Diagnosis of Aphthous Stomatitis

CONDITION	AFFECTED POPULATION
Idiopathic	70%
B_{12}/folate/iron deficiency	22%
Gluten-sensitive enteropathy	2%
Menstrually related	2%
Complex aphthosis	2%
Inflammatory bowel disease	1%
Behçet's disease	1%

9. What is complex aphthosis?
This recently described entity describes patients without systemic manifestations of Behçet's disease who have recurrent oral and genital aphthous ulcers or almost constant multiple (>3) oral aphthae. Differentiation from complex aphthosis may be difficult because the initial clinical presentation of Behçet's disease is often confined to oral and genital ulceration.

10. How frequently do the various clinical symptoms of Behçet's disease occur?

Oral aphthous ulcers	97% to 100%
Genital ulcers	80% to 90%
Ocular symptoms	50% to 79%
Arthritis	40% to 50%
Skin lesions	35% to 85%
Central nervous system disease (CNS)	5% to 10%
Major vessel occlusion/aneurysm	5% to 10%
Gastrointestinal involvement	0% to 25%

11. Describe the genital ulcers of Behçet's disease.
Aphthous ulcers similar to those in the mouth also occur on the genitalia, most frequently the scrotum and vulva. The penis and the perianal and vaginal mucosa are less often involved. Lesions in men tend to be more painful than those in women. Genital ulcers are usually deeper than oral lesions and may leave scars after healing (66%). Vulvar ulcers often develop during the premenstrual stage of the cycle.

12. Are nonvenereal genital ulcers commonly due to Behçet's disease?
No. Although genital ulcers are virtually universal in Behçet's disease, Behçet's disease is a rare cause of genital ulceration. Venereal ulcers are the most common type of genital ulceration and include herpes simplex, syphilis, chancroid, lymphogranuloma venereum, and granuloma inguinale (donovanosis). These infections need to be ruled out in patients with suspected Behçet's disease. Nonvenereal causes of genital ulceration include trauma (mechanical, chemical), adverse drug reactions, nonvenereal infections (nonsyphylitic spirochetes, pyogenic, yeast), vesiculobullous skin diseases, and various neoplasms such as precarcinoma (Bowen's

disease) and carcinoma (basal cell carcinoma and squamous cell carcinoma). More common rheumatic causes of genital ulceration include reactive arthritis and Crohn's disease.

13. **What are the ophthalmologic manifestations of Behçet's disease?**
Anterior/posterior uveitis, conjunctivitis, corneal ulceration, papillitis, and retinal vasculitis. Ocular lesions occur in 90% of men and 70% of women. Blindness is limited mostly to patients with posterior uveitis, and occurs on average 4 years after onset of Behçet's disease. All patients with Behçet's disease need ophthalmologic screening.

14. **What is a hypopyon?**
The presence of inflammatory cells in the anterior chamber of the eye. It occurs in up to 20% of patients with Behçet's disease and is a poor prognostic sign because it is frequently associated with retinal involvement. Although initially believed to be pathognomonic of ocular Behçet's disease, hypopyon is more commonly seen with severe B27-associated uveitis (see Chapter 75).

15. **Describe the arthritis associated with Behçet's disease.**
Approximately 50% of patients will develop signs or symptoms of joint involvement. The arthritis is usually migratory, monoarticular or oligoarticular, and asymmetric, principally affecting the knees, ankles, elbows, and wrists. Arthritic flares typically last for several weeks. Enthesopathy is common especially in patients with acneiform lesions. Shoulders, spine, sacroiliac joints, hips, and small joints of the hands and feet are infrequently involved and should suggest another disease (e.g., HLA-B27-associated arthropathy). The arthritis may be polyarticular and occasionally resembles rheumatoid arthritis. Erosive changes are rare. Synovial fluid cell counts average 5000 to 10,000/mm^3, and neutrophils predominate. Note that **arthralgia** is more common in Behçet's disease but lacks diagnostic value.

16. **What are the cutaneous manifestations of Behçet's disease?**
    - Erythema nodosum (50%).
    - Superficial thrombophlebitis (25%).
    - Acneiform skin eruption or pseudofolliculitis (65%): with evidence of vessel-based histology.
    - Pyoderma gangrenosum-like lesions.
    - Sweet's syndrome-like lesions.
    - Cutaneous small vessel vasculitis and pustular vasculitic lesions.
    - Hyperirritability of skin (pathergy)—common in Turkey/Japan. Rare in the United States.

17. **Describe the vascular involvement in Behçet's disease.**
Thrombosis of the large veins and arteries may occur, as can arterial aneurysms. Vascular thrombosis may be seen in a quarter of all patients and include *thrombosis of the superior or inferior vena cava*, portal or hepatic veins, and pulmonary arteries. Emboli from the thromboses are rare. Behçet's disease patients with thrombosis may have the factor V Leiden mutation. Behçet's disease is virtually alone among the vasculitides as a frequent cause of fatal *aneurysms of the pulmonary arterial tree*. **Hughes–Stovin syndrome** is a forme fruste of Behçet's disease characterized by deep venous thrombosis and pulmonary artery aneurysms.

18. **How often do neurologic manifestations occur in Behçet's disease?**

Headaches (52%)	Cerebellar ataxia
Meningoencephalitis (28%)	Hemiplegia/paraparesis
Cranial nerve palsies (16%)	Pseudobulbar palsy
Seizures (13%)	Extrapyramidal signs

Neurologic symptoms occur in 5% to 10% of patients and tend to recur during flares of oral, genital, and joint lesions. CNS involvement, which may be life-threatening, is usually a late manifestation occurring from 1 to 7 years after the initial onset of disease. The most commonly involved region is the brainstem. Intracranial hypertension, mostly resulting from dural sinus thrombosis, is seen in 20% of patients with neurologic disease. Mortality of CNS Behçet's disease is high (40%).

19. **What other organ involvement can be seen in Behçet's disease?**
    - Gastrointestinal involvement is more common in Japan (25% to 30%) and is characterized by mucosal ulcerations in the ileum and the right side of the colon. Ileocecal lesions may perforate.
    - Apart from sporadic reports of valvular lesions, myocarditis, and pericarditis, cardiac involvement in Behçet's disease is uncommon.
    - Epididymitis occurs in 10% of men with Behçet's disease.
    - Renal manifestations including glomerulonephritis are uncommon.
    - Amyloid AA can cause nephrotic syndrome.

20. **What are the common laboratory findings in Behçet's disease?**
Laboratory parameters are nonspecific in Behçet's disease. Some of the common findings include elevated ESR, increased C-reactive protein (CRP), leukocytosis, increased serum levels of immunoglobulin G (IgG),

IgA, and IgM; increased α_2-globulin; elevated cerebrospinal fluid protein and cell count (in patients with neurologic involvement). These findings most often occur during disease exacerbation and often return to normal during remission.

21. **What are the major causes of mortality in Behçet's disease?**
    - CNS involvement.
    - Vascular disease (ruptured pulmonary and peripheral aneurysms).
    - Bowel disease (perforation).

    Men and younger age at onset have the worse prognosis. Mortality may be 15% to 20% in the first 5 years. However, disease exacerbations and mortality decrease over time.

22. **Which drugs are reported to be successful in treating the mucocutaneous lesions of Behçet's syndrome?**
    - Local corticosteroid creams, dexamethasone elixir (0.5 mg/5 mL) swish for 5 to 10 minutes and spit (but do not rinse) three times daily.
    - Topical tacrolimus in combination with topical corticosteroids.
    - Topical tetracycline solutions.
    - Oral colchicine, 0.6 mg two to three times daily. Especially useful for erythema nodosum.
    - Dapsone, 50 to 150 mg/day alone or in combination.
    - Thalidomide, 50 to 150 mg/day but can cause a neuropathy with prolonged use.
    - Azathioprine, 2.5 mg/kg/day or methotrexate, 5 to 20 mg weekly.
    - Interferon-α, 9×10^6 units three times a week for 3 months followed by 3×10^6 units three times a week.
    - Tumor necrosis factor (TNF)-α antagonists.
    - Apremilast: recent trial showed both oral and genital ulcers responded very well to this medication.

23. **Which immunosuppressive agents are reported to be successful in treating severe ocular Behçet's disease?**
    - Systemic corticosteroids and azathiprine, 2.5 mg/kg/day (or mycophenolate mofetil), should be tried first.
    - Cyclosporine, 3 to 5 mg/kg/day, can be added to azathioprine or used alone if azathioprine fails. Cyclosporine should not be used in patients with CNS Behçet's disease because it can worsen CNS symptoms. Tacrolimus, 0.1 mg/kg/day, can be an alternative to cyclosporine.
    - Infliximab, 5 mg/kg monthly intravenous, has been successful if less expensive therapies fail.
    - Interferon-α is a good alternative but should not be used with azathioprine due to additive myelotoxicity.
    - Chlorambucil, 0.1 to 0.2 mg/kg/day and cyclophosphamide are salvage therapies.
    - Rituximab has been successfully used in severe eye disease.

24. **What other therapies can be useful in Behçet's disease?**
    - Arthritis: colchicine. If refractory use sulfasalazine, corticosteroids, azathioprine, methotrexate, TNF-α antagonists.
    - CNS: corticosteroids, azathioprine, interferon-α cyclophosphamide, chlorambucil, TNF-α antagonists. Do not use cyclosporine.
    - Gastrointestinal: corticosteroids, sulfasalazine, azathioprine, TNF-α antagonists.
    - Vascular thromboses: corticosteroids and other immunosuppressives. Do not anticoagulate because patients can have silent aneurysms that may rupture causing a life-threatening hemorrhage.
    - Aneurysms/vasculitis: corticosteroids and cyclophosphamide. Endovascular embolization or surgery for hemorrhage.

25. **Who was Behçet?**

    Hulusi Behçet, a Turkish dermatologist, in 1937 described a chronic relapsing syndrome of oral ulceration, genital ulceration, and uveitis that now bears his name.

26. **Describe the MAGIC syndrome.**

    Although chondritis has been noted in association with many other rheumatic diseases, the relationship between idiopathic relapsing polychondritis and Behçet's disease is particularly close. In 1985, Firestein and colleagues proposed the name "**M**outh **A**nd **G**enital ulceration with **I**nflamed **C**artilage" (MAGIC) syndrome in an attempt to encompass both clinical entities.

27. **Describe the pathogenesis of Behçet's disease.**

    The pathogenesis of Behçet's disease remains unclear. It might not have a primary autoimmune basis. No specific antibodies or clear-cut abnormalities in B cells have been demonstrated. An infectious trigger in a genetically predisposed host is postulated. Heat shock protein release interacting with Toll-like receptors causing release of cytokines such as interleukin (IL)-1, IL-8, IL-12, and IL-17, which leads to neutrophil and T helper 1 cell hyperactivity, has been reported in patients with Behçet's disease. Some investigators think Behçet's may be an autoinflammatory disorder but the rarity of fever during flares, the lack of a defined genetic locus, and the older age of onset makes this less likely.

COGAN'S SYNDROME

28. What is Cogan's syndrome?

Cogan's syndrome has a median age of onset of 25 years. It has the following manifestations:
- Major manifestations: occur concurrently or within 4 months in 75% of patients.
  - Ocular disease (red, painful, photophobic eyes): typical lesion is nonsyphilitis interstitial keratitis. Can have scleritis, episcleritis, uveitis, or chorioretinitis.
  - Audiovestibular symptoms: rapid onset sensorineural hearing loss (often bilateral) and vestibular dysfunction (vertigo and ataxia).
- Other manifestations: tend to occur in patients who are at risk for widespread vasculitis.
  - Constitutional symptoms (50%): fever, weight loss, adenopathy, hepatosplenomegaly.
  - Vasculitis: aortitis with aortic insufficiency/aneurysm (12%), aortic/mitral valvulitis, purpura, gangrene.
  - Laboratory abnormalities: anemia, leukocytosis, thrombocytosis, elevated ESR and CRP. Rarely antimyeloperoxidase.

29. How is Cogan's syndrome treated?

Treatment includes topical steroids for ocular manifestations and high-dose glucocorticoids for audiovestibular and systemic disease. Failure to taper prednisone and treatment-resistant disease is treated with immunosuppressives (methotrexate, azathioprine) and/or cyclosporine. Some patients recover after a single episode. Most patients have exacerbations with over 50% sustaining permanent hearing loss. Cochlear implants can be beneficial for these patients. Aortitis is treated with aggressive immunosuppressive therapy (prednisone, cyclophosphamide, and/or cyclosporine). Vascular surgery may be necessary for aortic valve replacement or aneurysm repair.

Acknowledgement

The author wishes to thank Dr. Raymond Enzenauer for his contributions to this chapter in the previous edition.

BIBLIOGRAPHY

Borhani Haghighi A, Pourmand R, Nikseresht A: Neuro-Behçet disease, Neurologist 11:80–89, 2005.
Calamia KT, Schiirmer M, Melikoglu M: Major vessel involvement in Behçet's disease: an update, Curr Opin Rheumatol 23:24–31, 2011.
Cogan DS: Syndrome of nonsyphilitic interstitial keratitis and vestibuloauditory symptoms, Arch Ophthalmol 33:144, 1945.
Hatemi G, Silman A, Bang D, et al: EULAR recommendations for the management of Behçet disease, Ann Rheum Dis 67:1656–1662, 2008.
Imai H, Motegi M, Mizuki N, et al: Mouth and genital ulcers with inflamed cartilage (MAGIC syndrome): a case report and literature review, Am J Med Sci 314:330, 1997.
International Team for the Revision of International Criteria for Behçet's Disease: Clinical manifestations of Behçet's disease. The ITR-ICBD report, Clin Exp Rheumatol 26(Suppl 50):S1–S18, 2008.
Keogan MT: An approach to the patient with recurrent orogenital ulceration, including Behçet's syndrome, Clin Exp Immunol 156:1–11, 2009.
Kotter I, Hamuryudan V, Oztürk ZE, et al: Interferon therapy in rheumatic diseases: state of the art 2010, Curr Opin Rheumatol 22:278–283, 2010.
Mazlumzadeh M, Matteson EL: Cogan's syndrome: an audiovestibular, ocular, and systemic autoimmune disease, Rheum Dis Clin North Am 33:855, 2007.
Sfikakis PP, Markomichelakis N, Alpsoy E, et al: Anti-TNF therapy in the management of Behçet's disease – review and basis for recommendations, Rheumatology 46:736–741, 2007.
Uzun O, Erkan L, Akpolat J, et al: Pulmonary involvement in Behçet's disease, Respiration 75:310–321, 2008.
Yurdakul S, Yazici H: Behçet's syndrome, Best Pract Res Clin Rheumatol 22:793–809, 2008.

FURTHER READING

http://www.niams.nih.gov/Health_Info/Behcets_Disease/
http://www.behcets.com

CHAPTER 33

RELAPSING POLYCHONDRITIS
Marc D. Cohen, MD

KEY POINTS

1. The diagnosis requires three of the following: recurrent auricular, nasal, tracheolaryngeal chondritis, nonerosive inflammatory polyarthritis, cochlear and/or vestibular damage, and inflammatory eye disease.
2. Auricular chondritis can be separated from cellulitis because it does not affect the earlobe.
3. Many diseases, especially vasculitis and myelodysplasia, are associated with relapsing polychondritis.
4. Corticosteroids are the mainstay of therapy but additional immunosuppressives may be helpful.

1. **Define relapsing polychondritis.**
   Relapsing polychondritis (RPC) is an uncommon episodic systemic disease characterized by recurrent inflammation and destruction of cartilaginous tissues.

2. **Who gets RPC?**
   Patients are predominantly white with a slight female predominance. Persons of all ages can develop RPC with a peak in the fifth decade (40 to 60 years old). There is an association with HLA-DR4 (2× increased risk).

3. **Briefly discuss the etiopathogenetic hypothesis of RPC.**
   The etiology of RPC is unknown but thought to be an autoimmune process. RPC patients and animal models of RPC have demonstrated cellular and humoral immunity against a variety of cartilage components including collagen (types II, IX, XI), matrilin-1, and proteoglycans. In RPC patients, the degree of immune response correlates with clinical disease activity.

   An inciting agent (infectious, toxic, immunologic) has not yet been identified. However, once stimulated, activated lymphocytes and macrophages are thought to secrete mediators that induce the release of lysosomal enzymes, especially proteases. The resulting inflammatory destruction of cartilage generates an attempt at repair by local fibroblasts and chondrocytes, leading to the formation of granulation tissue and fibrosis.

4. **Describe the histopathology of RPC.**
   The histopathology of involved cartilage, regardless of location, is similar and highly characteristic. The cartilage matrix, which is normally basophilic (blue), becomes acidophilic (pink) when examined by routine hematoxylin and eosin staining. Inflammatory cell infiltrates (initially polymorphonuclear cells and later lymphocytes and plasma cells) are seen invading the cartilage from the periphery inward. Granulation tissue and fibrosis develop adjacent to inflammatory infiltrates, occasionally resulting in sequestration of cartilage segments. Increased lipids and lysosomes in chondrocytes are demonstrated by electron microscopy. Immunofluorescence may demonstrate immunoglobulin and complement components in the tissue.

5. **Define the diagnostic criteria for RPC (set forth by Michet et al, 1986).**
   - Major criteria
     - Proven inflammatory episodes involving articular cartilage.
     - Proven inflammatory episodes involving nasal cartilage.
     - Proven inflammatory episodes involving laryngotracheal cartilage.
   - Minor criteria
     - Ocular inflammation (conjunctivitis, keratitis, episcleritis, uveitis).
     - Hearing loss.
     - Vestibular dysfunction.
     - Seronegative inflammatory arthritis.

   The presence of two major criteria or one major and two minor criteria is considered diagnostic of RPC. Histologic examination of cartilage is not required except in atypical cases.

6. **Which target organs are most commonly involved in the clinical presentation and eventual course of RPC?**
   The clinical features of RPC are outlined in Table 33-1.

Table 33-1. Clinical Features of Relapsing Polychondritis

FEATURE	PRESENTING %	CUMULATIVE %
Auricular chondritis	43	89
Arthritis	32	72
Nasal chondritis	21	61
Ocular inflammation	18	59
Laryngotracheal symptoms	23	55
Reduced hearing	7	40
Vestibular dysfunction	4	28
Microhematuria	15	26
Saddle nose	11	25
Cutaneous	4	25
Laryngotracheal stricture	15	23
Vasculitis	2	14
Elevated creatinine	7	13

From Kent PD, Michet CJ, Luthra HS: Relapsing polychondritis, *Curr Opin Rheumatol* 16:56-61, 2004.

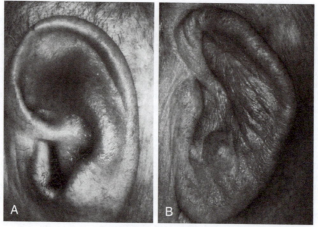

Figure 33-1. A, The ear in early inflammatory relapsing polychondritis. B, Chronic collapse of the cartilaginous pinna in a patient with relapsing polychondritis. (*Copyright 2014 American College of Rheumatology. Used with permission.*)

7. **Discuss the clinical features and potential complications of the auricular and nasal chondritis of RPC.**

   Auricular chondritis is the most frequent and characteristic clinical feature of RPC. It typically presents as the sudden onset of burning pain, warmth, swelling, and purplish-red discoloration of the helix, antihelix, and sometimes tragus of one or both ears (Figure 33-1, A). Because only the cartilaginous portion is affected, the inferior soft lobules are always spared, separating it from cellulitis. Attacks may last from a few days to several weeks. After one or more attacks, the external ear may lose its structural integrity owing to inflammatory dissolution of cartilage. This results in a drooping, floppy ear that has been termed "cauliflower ear" (Figure 33-1, B).

   Nasal chondritis develops suddenly as a painful fullness of the nasal bridge. Epistaxis occasionally accompanies the inflammation. It is less recurrent than auricular chondritis; however, even in the absence of clinical inflammation, cartilage collapse may occur, resulting in a "saddle nose" deformity (Figure 33-2).

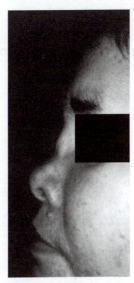

Figure 33-2. Saddle nose deformity due to nasal septal collapse. *(Copyright 2014 American College of Rheumatology. Used with permission.)*

8. **Discuss the distribution of disease, clinical symptoms, and potential complications of the respiratory tract in RPC.**
   Cartilage inflammation may occur early in the larynx and trachea, and later in the first-order and second-order bronchi. Patients with antibodies against matrilin-1 are most likely to develop laryngotracheal disease because matrilin-1 is predominantly located in the trachea. In mild cases, symptoms might consist of throat tenderness, hoarseness, and a nonproductive cough. In severe cases, laryngeal and epiglottal edema may cause choking, stridor, dyspnea, or respiratory failure requiring emergency tracheostomy. Repeated or persistent inflammation of the airways can lead to either tracheal stenosis or dynamic airway collapse caused by dissolution of the tracheal and bronchial cartilaginous rings. Costochondritis can cause respiratory splinting and when severe can cause depression of the anterior chest wall. In addition, respiratory tract infections may complicate the clinical course of these patients.

9. **Describe the arthritis of RPC.**
   The arthritis of RPC is usually an oligoarticular or polyarticular, asymmetric, nonerosive inflammatory arthritis with a predilection for the ankles, wrists, hands, and feet, as well as the sternoclavicular, costochondral, and sternomanubrial joints. Tenosynovitis is common. The arthritis is typically acute, migratory, and episodic resolving spontaneously over days to weeks. Rarely, it can become chronic. When the small joints of the hands and feet are affected, the disease may mimic seronegative rheumatoid arthritis. Flail chest has been described secondary to inflammatory lysis of the costosternal cartilage. Cervical, lumbar, and sacroiliac inflammation can occur. The arthritis activity does not correlate with other disease manifestations of RPC.

10. **Describe the ocular involvement of RPC.**
    Virtually every structure of the eye and surrounding tissues may be affected. Episcleritis, conjunctivitis, and uveitis are most common. Complications may include cataracts, optic neuritis, keratitis, proptosis, corneal ulcerations and thinning, and extraocular muscle palsies. Retinal vasculitis, optic neuritis, and necrotizing scleritis can cause loss of visual acuity and even blindness.

11. **Discuss audiovestibular damage in RPC.**
    Audiovestibular involvement presents as hearing loss, tinnitus, vertigo, and fullness in the ear (due to serous otitis media). Conductive hearing loss results from inflammatory edema or cartilage collapse of the auricle, external auditory canal, and/or eustachian tubes. Sensorineural hearing loss can be caused by inflammation of the internal auditory artery.

12. **Describe the cardiac manifestations of RPC.**
    Aortic insufficiency is the most common cardiac manifestation and, after respiratory involvement, is the most serious complication of RPC. It is usually due to progressive dilatation of the aortic root, which usually distinguishes it from the aortic insufficiency of other common rheumatic diseases (Table 33-2). Less frequent cardiac complications include pericarditis, myocarditis, arrhythmias, coronary aneurysms, valvulitis, and conduction defects.

Table 33-2. Aortic Insufficiency: Patterns of Disease Association

PATHOLOGY	UNDERLYING CONDITION
Valvulitis	Rheumatic fever Rheumatoid arthritis Ankylosing spondylitis* Endocarditis Reactive arthritis Behçet's syndrome
Congenital	Bicuspid aortic valve
Dilatation of valve ring	Marfan's syndrome Syphilis Relapsing polychondritis Dissecting aneurysm Idiopathic

*Ankylosing spondylitis and reactive arthritis can also cause dilatation of the valve ring.

13. What other clinical manifestations occur in RPC?

Vasculitis may occur in up to 30% of cases and indicates a poor prognosis. Involved vessels range in size from capillaries (leukocytoclastic vasculitis) to large arteries (aortitis). Ascending thoracic aortic aneurysms may be a late manifestation.

Neurologic manifestations (5% of patients) may include cranial neuropathies (second, sixth, seventh, eighth), headaches, and more rarely seizures, aseptic meningitis, encephalopathy, hemiplegia, and ataxia.

Renal disease manifested by an abnormal urinalysis can be seen in up to 25% of patients. Renal pathology usually shows a focal glomerulonephritis, but a wide variety of renal lesions have been reported. Renal disease usually indicates a worse prognosis.

Dermatologic manifestations occur in 35% of patients and are most common in patients with RPC and myelodysplasia. Oral aphthosis and leukocytoclastic vasculitis are most common. The aphthosis may resemble Behçet's syndrome and has the acronym **MAGIC syndrome** (mouth and genital ulcers with inflamed cartilage). Multiple other skin lesions can occur including nodules resembling erythema nodosum (15%), alopecia, abnormal nail growth, superficial thrombophlebitis, as well as others.

14. What laboratory data support the diagnosis of RPC?

Laboratory abnormalities are nonspecific and generally reflective of an inflammatory state: elevated erythrocyte sedimentation rate/C-reactive protein (ESR/CRP), leukocytosis, thrombocytosis, chronic anemia, and increased alpha and gamma globulins. Low titers of rheumatoid factor, antinuclear antibody, and antineutrophil cytoplasmic antibodies (ANCAs) may be seen. Antibodies to type II collagen have been found in approximately 20% of patients but are not diagnostic or prognostic of disease activity.

15. Describe the radiographic abnormalities of RPC.

Soft-tissue radiographs of the neck may demonstrate narrowing of the tracheal air column, suggestive of tracheal stenosis. Spiral computerized axial tomography (noncontrast) and/or magnetic resonance imaging (MRI) can more accurately define the degree of tracheal narrowing and inflammation. Repeated inflammation may lead to cartilaginous calcification of the pinnas, which may be seen in other conditions, such as frostbite. Radiographs of the joints may occasionally demonstrate periarticular osteopenia. Erosions are not seen unless the patient has an associated rheumatoid arthritis.

16. What is the differential diagnosis of RPC?

Auricular chondritis due to RPC must be separated from cellulitis (*Pseudomonas*, *Staphylococcus*), infectious perichondritis, frostbite, recurrent trauma (wrestlers), and cocaine-induced vasculitis. Similar to RPC, granulomatosis with polyangiitis (Wegener's), syphilis, cocaine use, and lethal midline granuloma (natural killer/T cell lymphoma) can also cause saddle nose deformities. In children, rare genetic defects can cause nasal chondritis and saddle nose deformity and/or myxoid degeneration of thyroid and cricoid cartilage with laryngeal stenosis. Syphilitic aortitis and Marfan's syndrome can cause dilatation of the aortic root. Cogan's syndrome can cause keratitis and vestibuloauditory dysfunction.

17. Which diseases commonly coexist in patients with RPC?

Up to 33% of RPC patients have or develop an associated disease with vasculitis and myelodysplastic syndromes most commonly identified. Most rheumatologic diseases have been reported in association with RPC, including systemic vasculitis (most common), systemic lupus erythematosus, rheumatoid arthritis, Sjögren's syndrome, and spondyloarthropathy, as well as others. Usually the inflammatory rheumatologic disease precedes the onset of RPC. Hypothyroidism from autoimmune thyroid disease has also been associated with RPC. Myelodysplastic syndromes occur before or simultaneously with RPC. This is more common in men with late-onset RPC. Other malignancies (lymphoma, acute lymphoblastic leukemia) have also occurred in association with RPC.

18. **Which diagnostic modalities are useful in detecting and following disease activity and cartilage damage in patients with RPC?**

ESR and CRP are accurate predictors of disease activity in most patients. Pulmonary complications may be demonstrated by radiographic imaging as outlined previously and by the use of pulmonary function testing with flow volume loops. If compromised, computed tomography or MRI of the tracheobronchial tree should be performed and followed. Echocardiography is useful in the diagnosis and follow-up of valvular heart disease and aortic root dilatation. MR angiograms should be followed in patients with large artery involvement.

19. **What medications are used in the treatment of RPC?**

Nonsteroidal antiinflammatory drugs, colchicine, and low-dose prednisone may be used to control minor inflammatory episodes. However, with more active disease, prednisone doses of 20 to 60 mg/day are usually used until control is attained. Methylprednisolone pulses (1 g/day ×3 days) are used for acute respiratory flares, neurosensory hearing loss, and systemic vasculitis. Continued inflammation or an inability to taper glucocorticoids to safe maintenance doses warrants the addition of a steroid-sparing agent. Dapsone (50 to 200 mg/day) has been useful in this regard in patients without major organ involvement. In patients with ocular, pulmonary, cardiovascular involvement, or systemic vasculitis, other immunosuppressives such as cyclophosphamide, methotrexate (0.3 mg/kg/week), azathioprine, mycophenolate mofetil, and cyclosporine (when cytopenias present) are used. A recommended approach in patients with severe disease is to control manifestations with corticosteroids and cyclophosphamide and later switch to a less toxic medication such as methotrexate. Patients who fail to respond may be candidates for biologic therapies (infliximab [5 mg/kg/month], tocilizumab [8 mg/kg/month]). Anakinra, abatacept, and rituximab have had variable results. Plasmapheresis, intravenous immunoglobulin (2 g/kg/month), or stem cell transplantation have been used as salvage therapies.

20. **When does surgery play a role in the management of RPC?**

Tracheostomy may be required in patients with airway collapse unresponsive to nighttime positive pressure ventilation. Airway obstruction caused by tracheal stenosis or tracheomalacia may require surgical resection. Intrabronchial stent placement has been reported as a potential remedy for dynamic airway collapse. Aortic insufficiency may require valve replacement, and aortic aneurysm formation may necessitate surgical grafting but the risk of dehiscence is high (12%).

Surgical reconstruction of nasal septal collapse is *not* recommended because further collapse and deformity frequently occur postoperatively. Cochlear implants are used for patients with sensorineural hearing loss.

21. **What is the prognosis in patients with RPC?**

In 1976, McAdam et al reported that the 5- and 10-year survival of 112 patients with RPC was 74% and 55%, respectively. Infection and systemic vasculitis were the major causes of death. Fifteen percent died as a direct consequence of cardiovascular or respiratory tract RPC. Poor prognostic indicators included coexistent vasculitis and early saddle nose deformity in younger patients (<age 51 years), and the presence of anemia due to myelodysplasia in older patients. In the 1998 study by Trentham et al, the average disease duration was 8 years and the survival rate was significantly improved at 94%. The most common cause of death is pulmonary infection due to altered anatomy and immunosuppressive therapy. Vasculitis decreases the 5-year survival to 45%.

BIBLIOGRAPHY

Buckner JH, Van Landeghen M, Kwok WW, et al: Identification of type II collagen peptide 261-273 specific T cell clones in a patient with relapsing polychondritis, Arthritis Rheum 46:238–244, 2002.
Del Rosso A, Petix NR, Pratesi M, et al: Cardiovascular involvement in relapsing polychondritis, Semin Arthritis Rheum 26:840–844, 1997.
Frances C, el Rassi R, Laporte JL, et al: Dermatologic manifestations of relapsing polychondritis: a study of 200 cases at a single center, Medicine(Baltimore) 80:173–179, 2001.
Imai H, Motegi M, Mizuki N, et al: Mouth and genital ulcers with inflamed cartilage (MAGIC syndrome): a case report and literature review, Am J Med Sci 314:330–332, 1997.
Lahmer T, Trieber M, von Werder A, et al: Relapsing polychondritis: and autoimmune disease with many faces, Autoimmunity Rev 9:540–546, 2010.
McAdam LP, O'Hanlan MA, Bluestone R, et al: Relapsing polychondritis: prospective study of 23 patients and a review of the literature, Medicine (Baltimore) 55:193–215, 1976.
McCarthy EM, Cunnane G: Treatment of relapsing polychondritis in the era of biologic agents, Rheumatol Int 30:827–828, 2010.
Rafeq S, Trentham D, Ernst A: Pulmonary manifestations of relapsing polychondritis, Clin Chest Med 31:513, 2010.
Trentham DE, Le CH: Relapsing polychondritis, Ann Intern Med 129:114–122, 1998.
Wallace ZS, Stone JH: Refractory relapsing polychondritis treated with serial success with interleukin 6 receptor blockade, J Rheumatol 40:100–101, 2013.
Yoo JH, Chodosh J, Dana R: Relapsing polychondritis: systemic and ocular manifestations, differential diagnosis, management, and prognosis, Semin Ophthalmol 26:261, 2011.

V

SERONEGATIVE SPONDYLOARTHROPATHIES

Which of your hips has the most profound sciatica?

William Shakespeare (1564–1616)
Measure for Measure, I

ANKYLOSING SPONDYLITIS

Robert W. Janson, MD

CHAPTER 34

KEY POINTS

1. Sacroiliitis and enthesitis are the hallmarks of ankylosing spondylitis (AS).
2. Rheumatoid factor (RF) and antinuclear antibody (ANA) are negative (seronegative spondyloarthropathy).
3. Human leukocyte antigen (HLA)-B27 increases the risk of developing AS 50 to 100 times.
4. Only 2% (1 out of 50) of HLA-B27-positive individuals develop AS during their lifetime.
5. Tumor necrosis factor (TNF)-α blocking agents are very effective in AS for both spinal and peripheral joints.

1. What is AS? How was the term derived?

AS is a chronic systemic inflammatory disease affecting the sacroiliac joints, spine, and, not infrequently, peripheral joints. The name is derived from the Greek roots *ankylos*, meaning "bent" (*ankylosis* means joint fusion), and *spondylos*, meaning "vertebra." The diagnosis is "primary AS" if no associated disorder is present and "secondary AS" if associated with reactive arthritis, psoriasis, ulcerative colitis, or Crohn's disease.

Radiographic sacroiliitis is the hallmark of AS. However, it takes an average of 4 to 9 years from onset of inflammatory back pain to the development of definite radiographic sacroiliitis. Patients without sacroiliitis on plain radiograph usually have inflammation detected on magnetic resonance imaging (MRI). These patients are said to have a preradiographic (nonradiographic) axial spondyloarthritis (SpA), which may or may not progress over time to definite radiographic sacroiliitis. Because the majority (70%) of patients in early disease will not have definite radiographic changes at the time of diagnosis, the ASAS (Assessment of SpondyloArthritis International Society) classification criteria were developed for patients with back pain greater than 3 months and age of onset less than 45 years. These criteria have a sensitivity of 83% and specificity of 84% for a patient having an axial SpA (Box 34-1).

Box 34-1. ASAS Classification Criteria for Axial SpA

Sacroiliitis on imaging
plus
≥1 SpA feature

OR

HLA-B27
plus
≥2 other SpA features

- **SpA features:** inflammatory back pain, arthritis, enthesitis (heel), uveitis, dactylitis, psoriasis, Crohn's disease/ulcerative colitis, good response to nonsteroidal antiinflammatory drugs (NSAIDs), family history for SpA, HLA-B27, elevated C-reactive protein (CRP).
- **Sacroiliitis on imaging:** active (acute) inflammation on MRI showing sacroiliitis *or* definite radiographic sacroiliitis.

SpA, Spondyloarthritis.

---

2. AS is also known by what eponyms?

Marie-Strümpell's or von Bechterew's disease, after physicians who contributed to the clinical description of the disease in the late 19th century.

3. Describe the clinical characteristics of AS. How do men and women differ in their presentations?

The clinical manifestations of AS usually begin in late adolescence or early adulthood, with onset after age 45 years being uncommon. It occurs more commonly in males than females (2 to 3:1). AS patients most commonly present with complaints of low back pain with prolonged morning and, often, nocturnal stiffness. This stiffness improves with movement and exercise. Buttock pain may initially alternate from side to side before becoming persistent. Physical examination reveals sacroiliac joint tenderness, decreased spinal mobility, and sometimes reduced chest expansion due to costovertebral joint involvement. AS is often more difficult to diagnose early in females as a result of less pronounced clinical features, atypical presentations (peripheral arthritis, cervical spine disease), and possibly slower development of radiographic changes.

Table 34-1. Differentiation of Low Back Pain

	INFLAMMATORY LBP	MECHANICAL LBP
Age of onset	<40 years of age	Any age
Type of onset	Insidious	Acute
Symptom duration	>3 months	<4 weeks
Morning stiffness	>60 min	<30 min
Nocturnal pain	Frequent	Absent
Effect of exercise	Improvement	Exacerbation
Sacroiliac joint tenderness	Frequent	Absent
Back mobility	Loss in all planes	Abnormal flexion
Chest expansion	Often decreased	Normal
Neurologic deficits	Unusual	Possible

LBP, Low back pain.

4. **What features in the history and physical examination are helpful in differentiating inflammatory low back pain in AS from mechanical low back pain?**
Differentiation of low back pain (LBP) is presented in Table 34-1.
PEARL: a patient less than 40 to 50 years old with three out of four of the following criteria has a high likelihood of having inflammatory back pain: (1) morning stiffness of at least 30 minutes; (2) improvement of back pain with exercise but not rest; (3) awakening because of back pain during the second half of the night only; (4) alternating buttock pain.

5. **Describe six physical examination tests used to assess sacroiliac joint tenderness or progression of spinal disease in AS.**
   - **Occiput-to-wall test.** Assesses loss of cervical range of motion. Normally with the heels and scapulae touching the wall, the occiput should also touch the wall. Any distance from the occiput to the wall represents a forward stoop of the neck secondary to cervical spine involvement with AS. The tragus-to-wall test could also be used.
   - **Chest expansion.** Detects limited chest mobility. Measured at the fourth intercostal space in men and just below the breasts in women, normal chest expansion is approximately 5 cm. Chest expansion less than 2.5 cm is abnormal.
   - **Schober test (modified).** Detects limitation of forward flexion of the lumbar spine. Place a mark at the level of the posterior superior iliac spine (dimples of Venus) and another 10 cm above in the midline. With maximal forward spinal flexion with locked knees, the measured distance should increase from 10 cm to at least 15 cm (Figure 34-1). Other spinal mobility tests will show that lateral flexion and spinal rotation are also diminished, establishing that the patient has a *global* loss of spinal mobility. Lateral flexion is measured by placing a mark at the lateral iliac crest and another 20 cm above in the midaxillary line. The patient bends away laterally and the distance should increase from 20 cm to at least 25 cm.
   - **Pelvic compression.** With the patient lying on one side, compression of the pelvis should elicit sacroiliac joint pain.
   - **Gaenslen's test.** With the patient supine, a leg is allowed to drop over the side of the examination table while the patient draws the other leg toward the chest. This test should elicit sacroiliac joint pain on the side of the dropped leg (Figure 34-2).
   - **Patrick's test.** With the patient's heel placed on the opposite knee, downward pressure on the flexed knee with the hip now in *flexion*, *abduction*, and external *rotation* (FABER) should elicit contralateral sacroiliac joint tenderness (Figure 34-2).

6. **What is an enthesis? How does it relate to the disease process in AS?**
An **enthesis** is a site of insertion of a ligament, tendon, or articular capsule into bone. In AS, the initial inflammatory process involves the enthesis, followed by a process that results in new bone formation or fibrosis. Sites of enthesopathy in AS include the sacroiliac joints; ligamentous structures of the intervertebral discs, manubriosternal joints, and symphysis pubis; ligamentous attachments in the spinous processes, the iliac crests (whiskering), trochanters, patellae, clavicles, and calcanei (Achilles enthesitis or plantar fasciitis); and capsules and intracapsular ligaments of large synovial joints.

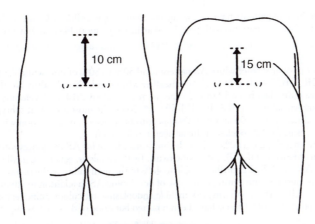

Figure 34-1. Schober test.

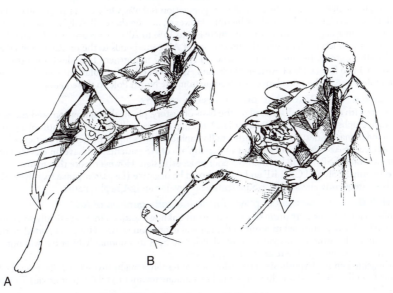

Figure 34-2. A, Gaenslen's test; **B**, Patrick's test.

7. Which peripheral joints are most commonly involved in AS?
Approximately 30% of patients with AS develop a peripheral arthritis. The hips and shoulders (girdle joints) are most commonly involved. Notably, hip involvement in AS is associated with a poor prognosis. Rarely, arthritis of the sternoclavicular, temporomandibular, cricoarytenoid, or symphysis pubis occurs. Involvement of the thoracic costovertebral, sternocostal, and manubriosternal joints may cause chest pain worsened by coughing or sneezing.

8. What are the extraskeletal manifestations of AS?
Remembering the first few letters of the disease's name will help in recalling these.

A—aortic insufficiency (3% to 10%), ascending aortitis, and other cardiac manifestations, such as conduction abnormalities (3% to 9%), diastolic dysfunction, pericarditis, and ischemic heart disease.
N—neurologic: atlantoaxial (C1 to C2) subluxation (2%), cauda equina syndrome from spinal arachnoiditis, traumatic spinal fractures with myelopathy (C5 to C6, C6 to C7 most commonly), ossification of the posterior longitudinal ligament with spinal stenosis.
K—kidney: secondary amyloidosis, immunoglobulin A (IgA) nephropathy, chronic prostatitis.
S—spine: cervical fracture, spinal stenosis, significant spinal osteoporosis.
P—pulmonary: upper lobe fibrosis, restrictive changes.
O—ocular: acute anterior uveitis (25% to 30% of patients).
N—nephropathy (IgA), nephrolithiasis
D—discitis or spondylodiscitis (Andersson lesions).

In addition, 30% to 60% of patients have asymptomatic microscopic colitis or Crohn's-like lesions in their terminal ileum and colon. AS patients with peripheral arthritis are more likely to have colitis lesions.

9. Which HLA shows a strong association with AS? Does this association vary among different racial groups?

HLA-B27 is present in over 90% of white AS patients and 50% to 80% of non-white AS patients. Because the prevalence of the HLA-B27 allele is 6% to 9% in healthy whites and 3% in healthy North American blacks, a HLA-B27-positive individual has a 50 to 100 times increased relative risk of developing AS. Currently, there are over 59 known subtypes (HLA-B*2701-59). B*2705 is the most prevalent subtype. No one subtype predisposes to AS, although B*2706 and B*2709 appear to have less of an association with AS, possibly due to amino acid differences in the "B" pocket of the antigen binding cleft.

Twin studies show that there is a 60% to 75% disease concordance for AS in monozygotic twins and a 12% to 27% disease concordance in HLA-B27 dizygotic twins. By this analysis, genetics contributes 90% to the total risk for developing AS. HLA-B27 contributes 30% to 40% to the heritability of the disease. This suggests that other genetic factors must be contributing to the risk of developing AS in addition to environmental factors. Two genes other than HLA-B27 conferring risk include endoplasmic reticulum aminopeptidase 1 (ERAP-1) and interleukin-23 receptor (IL-23R). Others have been reported but none of these are as important as HLA-B27.

10. How prevalent is AS among individuals who are HLA-B27-positive? Among individuals who are HLA-B27-positive with a relative with AS? Among different ethnic groups?

The overall prevalence of AS in the general U.S. population is 0.5%. Only 2% (1 out of 50) of HLA-B27-positive individuals develop AS during their lifetime. However, among those HLA-B27-positive individuals with an affected first-degree relative, the rate increases to 15% to 20%. AS is associated with HLA-B27 in all ethnic groups, which explains why the prevalence of AS corresponds to the prevalence of HLA-B27 in a particular ethnic group. Because the prevalence of HLA-B27 in northern latitudes is high (up to 15% of Scandinavians) and low (<1% of African blacks and Asians) in ethnic populations near the equator, there is an apparent decrease in the prevalence of AS going from the North Pole to the equator.

11. When should a HLA-B27 test and other tests be ordered?

Most patients with AS can be diagnosed on the basis of history, physical examination, and the finding of sacroiliitis on radiographs, obviating the need for HLA testing. Knowing the HLA-B27 status of a patient with back pain of an inflammatory nature with negative radiographic findings might be helpful, particularly in non-white individuals (see ASAS criteria in Question 1). Up to 75% of AS patients will have an elevated erythrocyte sedimentation rate (ESR) or CRP, which is a poor prognostic sign. However, note that many patients with AS will have a normal ESR and CRP. RF and ANA should be negative (i.e., *seronegative* spondyloarthropathy). IgA levels are frequently elevated in AS patients who develop an IgA nephropathy.

12. How is HLA-B27 hypothesized to play a role in the pathogenesis of AS?

Infection with an unknown organism or exposure to an unknown antigen in a genetically susceptible individual (HLA-B27+) is hypothesized to result in the clinical expression of AS. This is supported by the HLA-B27 transgenic rat model, which will spontaneously develop an SpA in a normal habitat but will not when raised in a germ-free environment. There are four hypotheses:

- **Arthritogenic peptide hypothesis.** The arthritogenic response might involve specific microbial peptides that bind to HLA-B27 and are then presented in a unique manner to CD8+ (cytotoxic) T cells resulting in disease.
- **Molecular mimicry.** The induction of autoreactivity to self-antigens might develop as a result of "molecular mimicry" between sequences or epitopes on the infecting organism or antigen and a portion of the HLA-B27 molecule or other self-peptides.
- **Free heavy chain hypothesis.** HLA-B27 heavy chains can form stable homodimers with no associated β-2 microglobulin on the cell surface. These homodimers can trigger direct activation of natural killer cells through recognition via immunoglobulin receptor (KIR)-like receptors causing cytokine (IL-17, TNF) release.
- **Unfolded protein hypothesis.** HLA-B27 has a propensity to misfold in the endoplasmic reticulum causing an unfolded protein stress response. This results in the release of inflammatory cytokines such as IL-23, which can activate proinflammatory T helper 17 (Th17) cells. Notably, ERAP-1 is involved in the trimming of peptides for loading in MHC (major histocompatibility complex) molecules (i.e., HLA-B27) in the endoplasmic reticulum. Abnormal loading may contribute to misfolding of HLA-B27 resulting in an unfolded protein stress response and IL-23 production. ERAP-1 and IL-23R polymorphisms both contribute to the genetic risk of developing AS.

13. Describe the typical radiographic features of AS.

The radiographic changes of AS are predominantly seen in the axial skeleton (sacroiliac, apophyseal, discovertebral, and costovertebral) as well as at sites of enthesopathy ("whiskering" of the iliac crest, greater tuberosities of the humerus, ischial tuberosities, femoral trochanters, calcaneus, and vertebral spinous processes). Sacroiliitis is usually bilateral and symmetric. Initially it involves the synovial-lined lower two thirds of the sacroiliac joint (Figure 34-3). The earliest radiographic change is erosion of the iliac side of the sacroiliac joint, where the cartilage is thinner and has clefts. Progression of the erosive process results in an initial

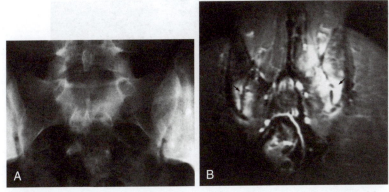

Figure 34-3. A, Radiograph of the pelvis demonstrating bilateral sacroiliitis. B, Magnetic resonance image of the sacroiliac joints demonstrating edema (*arrows*) due to inflammation of these joints.

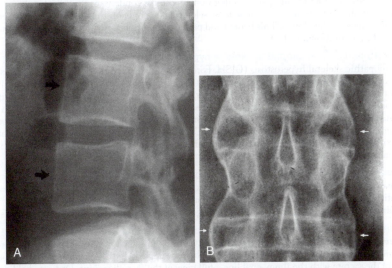

Figure 34-4. A, Lateral radiograph of the lumbar spine demonstrating anterior squaring of vertebrae (*arrows*). B, Anteroposterior radiograph of the spine demonstrating bilateral, thin, marginal syndesmophytes (*arrows*).

"pseudo-widening" of the sacroiliac joint space with bony sclerosis eventually followed by complete bony ankylosis or fusion of the joint (grade 4). In cases of early sacroiliitis where plain radiographs may be normal, a noncontrast MRI will demonstrate inflammation and edema in the majority of cases.

Inflammatory disease of the spine involves the insertion of the annulus fibrosis to the corners of the vertebral bodies, resulting in initial "shiny corners" (Romanus lesion) followed by "squaring" of the vertebral bodies (Figure 34-4). Gradual ossification of the outer layers of the annulus fibrosis (Sharpey's fibers) forms intervertebral bony bridges called **syndesmophytes**. Fusion of the apophyseal joints and calcification of the spinal ligaments along with bilateral syndesmophyte formation can result in complete fusion of the vertebral column, giving the appearance of a "bamboo" spine. Calcification of the supraspinous ligament can end caudally in a tapering point (dagger sign). Some patients develop an inflammatory destructive spondylodiscitis (Andersson lesion) that can mimic infection.

14. **What is the pathophysiology behind the radiographic features seen in AS?**

Unknown. Experimental data from mouse models support that inflammation and bone remodeling are two independent processes. The model shows:
- Bone morphogenic proteins (BMPs) and the WNT family of proteins may contribute to the development of calcification at sites of entheses and the sacroiliac joints. TNF-α has a yin–yang effect on this process. It stimulates BMP production but downregulates WNT signaling through upregulation of DKK1.
- The presence of enthesis-resident T cells (CD3+CD4−CD8−IL-23R+) that respond to IL-23 with resultant release of IL-17 (causing local inflammation) and IL-22 (inducing osteoblast-mediated bone formation).

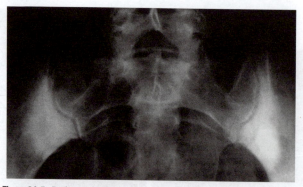

Figure 34-5. Radiograph of the pelvis demonstrating osteitis condensans ilii.

15. What is osteitis condensans ilii?

An asymptomatic disorder of multiparous young women, osteitis condensans ilii (OCI) is characterized by radiographic findings of a triangular area of dense sclerotic bone only on the iliac side and adjacent to the lower half of the sacroiliac joints. This benign and painless condition is not a form of AS and is not associated with HLA-B27 status (Figure 34-5).

16. How are AS and diffuse idiopathic skeletal hyperostosis different?

Diffuse idiopathic skeletal hyperostosis (DISH, Forestier's disease) is a noninflammatory disease occurring most commonly in obese, diabetic males aged greater than 50 years. It is characterized by flowing hyperostosis (bone formation), calcification of the anterior longitudinal ligament of at least four contiguous vertebral bodies, and nonerosive enthesopathies (whiskerings). The disease is not associated with sacroiliitis, apophyseal joint ankylosis, or HLA-B27. The flowing osteophytes in DISH typically occur on the right side of the spine, contralateral to the heart and aorta. On a lateral spine radiograph, a linear area of radiolucency exists between the calcified anterior longitudinal ligament and the anterior surface of the vertebra. (See Chapter 51.)

17. What are other causes of radiographic sacroiliac joint abnormalities?

Inflammatory: spondyloarthropathies, infection (bacterial, fungal, mycobacterial).
Traumatic: fracture, osteoarthritis, osteitis condensans ilii.
Generalized disease: gout, hyperparathyroidism, Paget's disease, paraplegia, neoplastic metastases.

18. Name the radiographic view used to specifically visualize the sacroiliac joints.

An **anteroposterior** projection of the pelvis (AP pelvis) is often sufficient to evaluate the inferior aspects of the sacroiliac joints. The **Ferguson** view (AP with the tube angled 25 to 30 degrees cephalad) counteracts the overlap of the sacrum with the ilium, enabling a full view of the sacroiliac joint. Dedicated **oblique views** of each SI joint can also be done.

19. Describe the natural course of AS.

Although the course is variable, the first 10 years predicts the subsequent course of the disease. The Bath Ankylosing Spondylitis Disease Activity Index (BASDAI, disease activity), Bath Ankylosing Spondylitis Metrology Index (BASMI, spinal mobility), and Bath Ankylosing Spondylitis Functional Index (BASFI) are standardized instruments used by some clinicians to measure disease progression and response to therapy. Early factors that predict a poor prognosis include early hip joint involvement, ESR >30 mm/h or persistently high CRP, poor response to NSAID therapy, and early development of syndesmophytes. Extraarticular manifestations such as uveitis, cardiovascular involvement, and pulmonary fibrosis portend a poor outcome. It is likely that patients with mild AS have a normal life expectancy and will maintain their ability to work. However, patients with poor prognostic signs have a three times increased risk of withdrawing from the workforce and a 1.5 times increased risk of dying. Causes of death include cardiovascular disease, gastrointestinal disease, and spinal fractures.

20. Which medications are helpful in the management of AS?

Although there is no cure for AS, most patients can be managed by controlling inflammatory symptoms and participating in an exercise program to minimize deformity and disability. The following modalities are helpful:

NSAIDs. Indomethacin is the most widely used NSAID for AS. Other NSAIDs may also be beneficial, and the choice is balanced by tolerance and effectiveness. Continuous use of NSAIDs has been associated with a decrease in radiographic progression. Simple analgesics can be added for additional pain relief but should not be used as primary therapy.

Second-line treatment. Sulfasalazine (1500 mg twice a day) may be beneficial in patients with NSAID-resistant peripheral arthritis but does not help sacroiliitis, spondylitis, or enthesitis. Although not well studied, low-dose weekly methotrexate therapy may benefit patients with prominent peripheral joint involvement. Limited data suggest that leflunomide is not beneficial.

Anti-TNF therapy. These agents are highly effective in reducing the inflammatory component of AS including spinal mobility, function, peripheral synovitis, enthesitis, and uveitis while improving quality of life. The highest response rates (ASAS-40 in 50% of patients) have been observed in younger patients with shorter disease duration and elevated CRP but patients with advanced disease may also benefit from this therapy. Concomitant therapy with methotrexate is not required. The 2010 ASAS guidelines recommend the use of anti-TNF agents in patients with AS with predominant axial manifestations who have high disease activity defined as a BASDAI ≥4 (0 to 10) despite adequate trials of two NSAIDs over a 4-week period, and in patients with symptomatic peripheral arthritis despite NSAIDs, disease-modifying antirheumatic drugs (preferably sulfasalazine), and local steroid injection therapies. The effect of anti-TNF agents on radiographic progression is controversial. Recent data suggest that early and prolonged use does decrease syndesmophyte formation.

Other biologics. Abatacept, tocilizumab, and rituximab are not effective for AS. Anti-IL-17 therapies and ustekinumab hold promise.

Corticosteroids. Oral corticosteroids have *no* value in the treatment of the musculoskeletal aspects of AS. Local corticosteroid injections are useful in the treatment of enthesopathies, peripheral synovitis, and recalcitrant sacroiliitis.

Other treatments. Bisphosphonates and calcium/vitamin D replacement should be considered in AS patients with osteoporosis secondary to their inflammatory disease. Anterior uveitis can usually be managed with dilation of the pupil and corticosteroid eye drops. In resistant cases, an anti-TNF-α agent (other than etanercept) can be used to control the uveitis. Cardiovascular risk factors should be treated.

21. **How is physiotherapy used in AS?**
Daily home exercises need to be performed to maintain good posture and chest expansion and to minimize deformities. Hydrotherapy (swimming) provides the best environment to maximize the exercise program. Patients should sleep on a firm mattress fully supine with a small neck-support pillow to prevent progressive deformity. Lying prone for 15 to 30 minutes daily or sleeping prone at night helps prevent kyphosis. Cigarette smoking should be avoided as smoking diminishes response to therapy and accelerates radiographic progression.

22. **When is surgery indicated in AS?**
Total hip replacement is indicated in the setting of severe pain and limitation of motion. Bisphosphonates and NSAIDs may be used for 3 months after surgery to prevent postoperative calcifications around the prosthesis. Vertebral wedge osteotomy to correct severe kyphotic deformities in some patients may be warranted, but it carries the risk of operative neurologic damage. Cardiac manifestations of AS may require aortic valve replacement or pacemaker insertion.

BIBLIOGRAPHY

Amrami KK: Imaging of the seronegative spondyloarthropathies, Radiol Clin N Am 50:841–854, 2012.
Haroon N, Inman RD, Learch TJ, et al: The impact of TNF-inhibitors on radiographic progression in ankylosing spondylitis, Arthritis Rheum 65:2645–2654, 2013.
Lee W, Reveille JD, Weisman MH: Women with ankylosing spondylitis: a review, Arthritis Rheum 59:449–454, 2008.
Lories RJ, Schett G: Pathophysiology of new bone formation and ankylosis in spondyloarthropathies, Rheum Dis Clin N Am 38:555–567, 2012.
Poddubnyy D, Rudwaleit M: Early spondyloarthritis, Rheum Dis Clin N Am 38:387–403, 2012.
Reveille JD: Genetics of spondyloarthritis – beyond the MHC, Nat Rev Rheumatol 8:296–304, 2012.
Robinson PC, Brown MA: The genetics of ankylosing spondylitis and axial spondyloarthritis, Rheum Dis Clin N Am 38:539–553, 2012.
Rudwaleit M, Metter A, Listing J, et al: Inflammatory back pain in ankylosing spondylitis: a reassessment of the clinical history for application as classification and diagnostic criteria, Arthritis Rheum 65:569–578, 2006.
Sieper J, Rudwaleit M, Baraliakos X, et al: The Assessment of SpondyloArthritis International Society (ASAS) handbook: a guide to assess spondyloarthritis, Ann Rheum Dis 68:ii1–ii44, 2009.
van der Heijde D, Sieper J, Maksymowych WP, et al: 2010 update of the international ASAS recommendations for the use of anti-TNF agents in patients with axial spondyloarthritis, Ann Rheum Dis 70:905–908, 2010.
van der Linden SM, Baeten D, Maksymowych WP: Ankylosing spondylitis. In Firestein GS, Budd RC, Gabriel SE, et al: Kelley's textbook of rheumatology, ed 9, Philadelphia, 2013, Elsevier Saunders.
Weber U, Lambert RGW, Ostergaard M, et al: The diagnostic utility of magnetic resonance imaging in spondylarthritis: an international multicenter evaluation of one hundred eighty-seven subjects, Arthritis Rheum 62:3048–3058, 2010.
Yu D, Lories R, Inman RD: Pathogenesis of ankylosing spondylitis and reactive arthritis. In Firestein GS, Budd RC, Gabriel SE, et al: Kelley's textbook of rheumatology, ed 9, Philadelphia, 2013, Elsevier Saunders.

FURTHER READING

http://www.spondylitis.org
http://www.asas-group.org

CHAPTER 35: RHEUMATIC MANIFESTATIONS OF GASTROINTESTINAL AND HEPATOBILIARY DISEASES

Sterling G. West, MD

KEY POINTS

1. Inflammatory arthritis is most likely to occur in inflammatory bowel disease (IBD) patients with extensive colonic involvement.
2. Consider bowel disease in any patient with an intermittent, inflammatory arthritis regardless of presence or absence of gastrointestinal symptoms.
3. Episodes of peripheral arthritis coincide with flares of bowel disease, whereas spinal arthritis occurs independent of bowel disease severity.
4. Type I autoimmune hepatitis (AIH) presenting with polyarthritis and a positive antinuclear antibody (ANA) can mimic systemic lupus erythematosus (SLE).
5. Pancreatic cancer can release enzymes, which cause fat necrosis resulting in a triad of lower extremity arthritis, tender nodules, and eosinophilia (Schmidt's triad).

ENTEROPATHIC ARTHRITIDES

1. **What bowel diseases are associated with inflammatory arthritis?**
   - Idiopathic, inflammatory bowel disease (ulcerative colitis [UC], Crohn's disease) and pouchitis.
   - Microscopic colitis (lymphocytic colitis and collagenous colitis).
   - Infectious gastroenteritis and pseudomembranous colitis.
   - Whipple's disease.
   - Gluten-sensitive enteropathy (celiac disease).
   - Intestinal bypass arthritis.

2. **How often does an inflammatory peripheral and/or spinal arthritis occur in patients with idiopathic IBD?**
   The occurrence of inflammatory peripheral and/or spinal arthritis in patients with idiopathic IBD is shown in Table 35-1.

3. **What are the most common joints involved in UC and Crohn's disease?**
   The most common joints involved in UC and Crohn's disease are shown in Figure 35-1.
   Upper extremity and small joint involvement are more common in UC than in Crohn's disease. Both UC and Crohn's-related arthritis affect the knee and ankle predominantly.

4. **Describe the clinical characteristics of inflammatory peripheral arthritis associated with idiopathic IBD.**
   - **Type 1** (arthritis often parallels IBD activity): occurs in 4% to 6% of IBD patients, affecting males and females equally. Children are affected as commonly as adults. The arthritis is typically acute in onset (80%), asymmetric (80%), and pauciarticular (usually involves less than five joints with the knee and ankle most common). It occurs before (30% of cases) or early in the course of the bowel disease and is strongly associated (80%) with flares of IBD and other extraarticular manifestations (erythema nodosum, uveitis). Synovial fluid analysis reveals an inflammatory fluid [normally 5000 to 12,000 but can be up to 50,000 white blood cells/mm^3 (predominantly neutrophils)] and negative crystal examination and cultures. Most arthritic episodes are self-limited with 80% resolving within 3 months. This type of arthritis does not result in radiographic changes or deformities. There is an increased prevalence of *HLA-B27*, *HLA-B35*, and *HLA-DRB1*0103* in patients with this type of arthritis.
   - **Type 2** (arthritis is independent of IBD activity): is less common occurring in 3% to 4% of IBD patients. The arthritis tends to be symmetric (80%), polyarticular (metacarpophalangeal [MCP] joints > knees and ankles > other joints), runs a course independent of the activity of the inflammatory bowel disease,

Table 35-1. The Occurrence of Inflammatory Peripheral and/or Spinal Arthritis in Patients With Idiopathic Inflammatory Bowel Disease

	ULCERATIVE COLITIS	CROHN'S DISEASE
Peripheral arthritis	5% to 10%	10% to 15%
Sacroiliitis*	15%	15%
Sacroiliitis/spondylitis†	5%	10%

*Many of these patients have asymptomatic radiographic sacroiliitis and is not strongly correlated with HLA-B27.
†Overall, 10% of Crohn's disease and 5% of ulcerative colitis patients develop ankylosing spondylitis, which is correlated with HLA-B27.

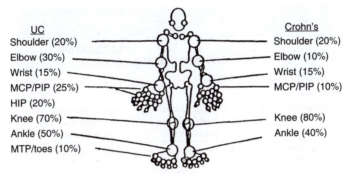

Figure 35-1. The most common joints involved in ulcerative colitis and Crohn's disease. MCP, Metacarpophalangeal; MTP, metatarsophalangeal; PIP, proximal interphalangeal.

and does not correlate with extraarticular manifestations (except uveitis). Active arthritis is chronic (90%) and episodes of exacerbations and remissions may continue for years. Owing to its chronicity, this type of arthritis can cause erosions and deformities. There is an association with *HLA-B44* but not with HLA-B27.

5. **What other extraintestinal manifestations commonly occur with idiopathic IBD and inflammatory peripheral arthritis?**
Approximately 25% of IBD patients have a combination of extraintestinal manifestations, frequently multiple in an individual patient.
P—pyoderma gangrenosum (<2% to 5%).
A—aphthous stomatitis (<10%): more common in UC.
I—inflammatory eye disease (acute anterior uveitis) (5% to 15%): more common in Crohn's disease.
N—nodosum (erythema) (<10% to 15%).

6. **Do the extent and activity of IBD and the activity of peripheral inflammatory arthritis show any correlation?**
UC and Crohn's disease patients are more likely to develop a peripheral arthritis if the colon is extensively involved. In patients with type 1 arthritis, most arthritic attacks occur during the first few years following onset of bowel disease but late occurrences also occur. The episodes of arthritis coincide with flares of bowel disease in 60% to 80% of patients. The arthritis may precede symptoms of IBD in up to 30% of cases, especially in children with Crohn's disease. Consequently, lack of gastrointestinal symptoms or a negative stool guaiac test does not exclude the possibility of occult Crohn's disease in a patient who presents with a characteristic arthritis.

7. **What are the clinical and radiographic characteristics of inflammatory spinal arthritis occurring in idiopathic IBD?**
The clinical and radiographic characteristics and course of spinal arthritis in IBD are similar to those for ankylosing spondylitis.
- Inflammatory spinal arthritis occurs more commonly in males than females (3:1).
- Patients complain of back pain and prolonged stiffness, particularly at night and upon awakening. This improves with exercise and movement.

- Physical examination reveals sacroiliac joint tenderness, global loss of spinal motion, and sometimes reduced chest expansion.
- Bilateral symmetric sacroiliitis with or without thin marginal syndesmophytes similar to idiopathic ankylosing spondylitis (see Chapter 34).

8. Does the activity of inflammatory spinal arthritis correlate with the activity of IBD?

No. The onset of sacroiliitis/spondylitis can precede by years, occur concurrently, or follow by years the onset of IBD. Furthermore, the course of spinal arthritis is completely independent of the course of IBD.

9. What human leukocyte antigen occurs more commonly than expected with inflammatory arthritis secondary to IBD?

Human leukocyte antigen-B27 (HLA-B27): 8% of a normal healthy white population has the HLA-B27 gene, but a patient with IBD who possesses the HLA-B27 gene has a seven to ten times increased risk of developing an inflammatory sacroiliitis/spondylitis compared with IBD patients who are HLA-B27-negative. It should be noted that the mutation of the NOD2(CARD15) gene on chromosome 16 that has been associated with the development of Crohn's disease has not been associated with an increased prevalence of axial or peripheral inflammatory arthritis in patients with IBD (Table 35-2).

Table 35-2. Frequency of HLA-B27 in Inflammatory Bowel Disease

	CROHN'S DISEASE	ULCERATIVE COLITIS
Sacroiliitis/spondylitis	55%	70%
Peripheral arthritis*	Same as normal healthy control population	Same as normal healthy control population

*Some studies report an increase in HLA-B27 in patients with type I arthropathy (26% vs 8% in controls).

10. What other rheumatic problems occur with increased frequency in IBD patients?

- Achilles enthesitis/plantar fasciitis (enthesopathy).
- Granulomatous lesions of bones and joints.
- Hypertrophic osteoarthropathy (periostitis) with clubbing (5%) – more common in Crohn's disease.
- Psoas abscess or septic hip from fistula formation (Crohn's disease).
- Osteoporosis and avascular necrosis secondary to medications (i.e., prednisone).
- Vasculitis.
- Amyloidosis.

11. What serologic abnormalities are seen in patients with IBD?

- Erythrocyte sedimentation rate is elevated, whereas rheumatoid factor and ANA are negative.
- Antineutrophil cytoplasmic antibody (ANCA)–perinuclear ANCA (pANCA) is seen in 55% to 70% of UC patients and <20% of colon-predominant Crohn's disease patients. It is directed against lactoferrin and less commonly bactericidal permeability increasing protein, cathepsin G, lysozyme, or elastase. It is never directed against myeloperoxidase.
- Anti-*Saccharomyces cerevisiae*—present in 40% to 70% of Crohn's disease patients and rarely (<15%) in UC patients.

12. Which treatments are effective for alleviating symptoms of inflammatory peripheral arthritis and/or sacroiliitis/spondylitis in IBD patients?

Treatments that are effective for alleviating symptoms of inflammatory peripheral arthritis and/or sacroiliitis/spondylitis in IBD patients are presented in Table 35-3.

13. What rheumatic disorders have been associated with pouchitis, lymphocytic colitis, and collagenous colitis?

Pouchitis is inflammation of the ileal pouch created following colectomy for UC. It occurs in up to 40% to 60% of patients having this surgery. Patients present with watery or bloody diarrhea. Some will develop arthritic manifestations. Treatment includes metronidazole and ciprofloxacin. Surgical revision may be necessary in treatment-resistant cases.

Microscopic colitis includes both lymphocytic colitis (LC) and collagenous colitis (CC). Patients present with watery diarrhea and may develop arthritic manifestations (10% to 20%) or autoimmune thyroiditis. Patients over 65 years old (80%) and females (60%) are most commonly affected. The diagnosis can only be made by tissue histology obtained by colonoscopy. Budesonide is effective for inducing and maintaining clinical and

Table 35-3. Treatment of Inflammatory Bowel Disease-Related Inflammatory Peripheral or Spinal Arthritis

	PERIPHERAL ARTHRITIS	SACROILIITIS/ SPONDYLITIS
NSAIDS*	Yes	Yes
Intraarticular corticosteroids	Yes	Yes (sacroiliitis)
—Sulfasalazine†	Yes	No
—Mesalamine	No	No
Immunosuppressive medication	Yes	No
Anti-TNF-α‡	Yes	Yes
Bowel resection		
—Ulcerative colitis	Yes	No
—Crohn's disease	No	No

*Nonsteroidal antiinflammatory drugs (NSAIDs) may exacerbate inflammatory bowel disease. Cox-2 selective NSAIDs may be safer.
†Sulfasalazine helps peripheral arthritis in ulcerative colitis patients more than Crohn's disease patients.
‡Antitumor necrosis factor-α (anti-TNF-α) approved and effective include infliximab, adalimumab, golimumab, and certolizumab pegol.

histologic remission for CC and LC, and loperamide may ameliorate diarrhea. Evidence for benefit of bismuth subsalicylate and mesalamine with or without cholestyramine for treatment of CC or LC is weak (Table 35-4).

14. **Why are patients with IBD prone to develop an inflammatory arthritis?**
    The pathogenesis of gut–joint enteropathy is unknown. However, inflammation of the gut and joints appear to be tightly linked. When ileocolonoscopies are done on spondyloarthropathy (ankylosing spondylitis, reactive arthritis) patients without gastrointestinal symptoms, up to 25% have macroscopic lesions and up to 60% have microscopic evidence of asymptomatic Crohn's disease. Over time, 6% to 10% of these patients develop overt symptomatic Crohn's disease. Alternatively, up to 10% of IBD patients without evidence of a spondyloarthropathy at onset of their gastrointestinal symptoms will develop overt arthritis on follow-up.
    Environmental antigens capable of inciting rheumatic disorders enter the body's circulation by traversing the respiratory mucosa, skin, or gastrointestinal mucosa. The human gastrointestinal tract has an estimated surface area of 400 m^2 (200× the body's skin surface area) and functions not only to absorb nutrients but also to exclude potentially harmful antigens. The gut-associated lymphoid tissue, which includes Peyer's patches, the lamina propria, and intraepithelial T cells, constitutes 25% of the gastrointestinal mucosa and helps to exclude entry of bacteria and other foreign antigens. Whereas the upper gastrointestinal tract is normally exposed to 10^3 mucosa-adhering bacteria, the lower gastrointestinal tract is constantly in contact with millions of bacteria (up to 10^{12}/g of feces). The total number of bacterial cells called the *human microbiota* that we are exposed to is 10 times that of the number of cells of the body.
    Inflammation, whether from idiopathic IBD or from infection with pathogenic microorganisms, can disrupt the normal integrity and function of the bowel, leading to increased gut permeability. This increased permeability may allow nonviable bacterial antigens in the gut lumen to enter the circulation more easily. These microbial antigens could either deposit directly in the joint synovia, leading to a local inflammatory reaction, or cause a systemic immune response, resulting in immune complexes that then deposit in joints and other tissues. Genetic susceptibility is required to develop the immunologic response in the gut and joint, which results in persistent inflammation and tissue injury.

15. **What rheumatic manifestations have been described in patients with celiac disease (gluten-sensitive enteropathy)?**
    - Arthritis (4% to 26%)—symmetric, nonerosive polyarthritis involving predominantly large joints (knees and ankles > hips and shoulders). May precede enteropathic symptoms in 50% of cases. Notably, oligoarthritis and sacroiliitis have also been reported. The arthritis responds to a **gluten-free diet** in 40% to 60% of cases.
    - Osteomalacia due to steatorrhea from severe enteropathy causing vitamin D deficiency. Some of these patients are mistakenly diagnosed as fibromyalgia with irritable bowel syndrome.
    - Dermatitis herpetiformis.

Table 35-4. Rheumatic Disorders That are Associated With Pouchitis, Lymphocytic Colitis, and Collagenous Colitis

	POUCHITIS	LC	CC
IBD-like peripheral inflammatory arthritis	Yes	Yes	Yes (10%)
Rheumatoid arthritis	No	Yes	Yes
Ankylosing spondylitis	No	Yes*	No
Thyroiditis/other autoimmune disease	No	Yes	Yes

CC, Collagenous colitis; IBD, inflammatory bowel disease; LC, lymphocytic colitis.
*Up to 60% of patients with idiopathic ankylosing spondylitis have asymptomatic microscopic colitis/Crohn's-like lesions on right-sided colon biopsies. However, only 6% to 10% will evolve into overt IBD.

16. **What HLA is found in patients with celiac disease and how does it contribute to the development of the disease?**
Celiac disease is an enteropathy resulting from an autoimmune reaction to wheat gluten/gliadin by T lymphocytes in the gut in genetically predisposed individuals. It is a relatively common disease (1:300) in white individuals and can occur at any age. HLA-DQ2 and/or HLA-DQ8 (usually in linkage with HLA-DR3) are seen in 99% of celiac disease patients compared with 40% of the normal population. Dietary gluten is partly digested by gastric enzymes to form a 33-amino acid peptide that is deaminated by tissue transglutaminase increasing its immunogenicity. The immunogenic gliadin peptide is then presented in the context of HLA-DQ2 or HLA-DQ8 to CD4+ T cells, resulting in interferon-γ release and inflammation, altered gut permeability, and villous atrophy. Only 66% have characteristic bowel symptoms, whereas others will present with arthritis, vitamin D or vitamin B_{12} deficiency, iron deficiency anemia, cerebellar disease, infertility, or peripheral neuropathy. It is more likely to occur in patients with other HLA-DR3-associated autoimmune diseases such as Sjögren's syndrome, type I diabetes mellitus, autoimmune thyroid disease, or autoimmune liver disease.

17. **How is the diagnosis of celiac disease made?**
The gold standard is jejunal biopsy showing villous atrophy. However, autoantibody testing is very helpful in screening individuals before biopsy. On a gluten-rich diet in people who are not immunoglobulin A (IgA)-deficient, IgA antibodies against **tissue transglutaminase** have a high sensitivity (95%) and specificity (90%) for celiac disease. Owing to poor specificity, antigliadin antibodies are no longer used to screen for celiac disease.

18. **What is the intestinal bypass arthritis–dermatitis syndrome?**
In the past, this syndrome occurred in 20% to 80% of patients who have undergone intestinal bypass (jejunoileal or jejunocolic) surgery for morbid obesity. Owing to the frequency of this complication, this type of obesity surgery has been abandoned. Today it can occur as a rare consequence of bacterial overgrowth in patients with poor intestinal peristalsis (systemic sclerosis, colorectal surgery) or diverticular disease. The arthritis is intensely painful, inflammatory, oligoarticular, and frequently migratory, affecting both upper and lower extremity small and large joints. Radiographs usually remain normal despite 25% of patients having chronic recurring episodes of arthritis. Up to 80% develop dermatologic abnormalities, the most characteristic of which is a maculopapular or vesiculopustular rash. The pathogenesis involves bacterial overgrowth in a blind loop resulting in antigenic stimulation causing immune complex formation (frequently cryoprecipitates containing bacterial antigens, secretory IgA, and complement) in the serum that deposit in the joints and skin. Treatment includes nonsteroidal antiinflammatory drugs (NSAIDs), corticosteroids, and oral antibiotics, which usually improve symptoms. Only surgical reanastomosis of the blind loop can result in complete elimination of symptoms.

RHEUMATIC SYNDROMES AND PANCREATIC DISEASE

19. **What pancreatic diseases have been associated with rheumatic syndromes?**
Pancreatitis, pancreatic carcinoma, and pancreatic insufficiency.

20. **What are the clinical features of the pancreatic, panniculitis, and polyarthritis syndrome?**
    Pancreatic, panniculitis, and polyarthritis syndrome (PPP) is a systemic syndrome occurring in some patients with pancreatitis or pancreatic acinar cell carcinoma due to release of trypsin, lipase, and amylase from the diseased pancreas causing fat necrosis. A good way to remember the clinical manifestations is the mnemonic PANCREAS:
    P—Pancreatitis.
    A—Arthritis (60%) and arthralgias, usually of the ankles and knees. Synovial fluid is typically noninflammatory and creamy in color due to lipid droplets that stain with Sudan black or oil red O.
    N—Nodules that are tender, red, and usually on the extremities. These are frequently misdiagnosed as erythema nodosum but are areas of lobular (not septal) panniculitis with fat necrosis. Fasciitis due to subcutaneous fat necrosis can also be seen.
    C—Cancer of the pancreas more commonly causes this syndrome than does pancreatitis.
    R—Radiographic abnormalities due to osteolytic bone lesions from bone marrow necrosis (10%).
    E—Eosinophilia. The triad of arthritis, nodules, and eosinophilia is called Schmidt's triad.
    A—Amylase, lipase, and trypsin are elevated due to release by a diseased pancreas and cause the fat necrosis in skin, synovium, and bone marrow.
    S—Serositis, including pleuropericarditis frequently with fever.

21. **What other musculoskeletal problem can occur with pancreatic insufficiency?**
    Osteomalacia due to fat-soluble vitamin D malabsorption.

RHEUMATIC SYNDROMES AND HEPATOBILIARY DISEASE

22. **What is lupoid hepatitis?**
    Lupoid hepatitis is now called type I (classic) AIH. It can occur in all age groups (bimodal peak: 10 to 20 years, 45 to 70 years), but most patients are young and predominantly female (70%). Many patients have clinical (arthralgias 50%) and laboratory manifestations that resemble SLE. Patients commonly have positive ANAs, antibodies against smooth muscle antigen characteristically with specificity against F1 actin, hypergammaglobulinemia, and occasionally LE cells. They usually do not have antibodies against double-stranded DNA (dsDNA). Type I AIH has been described in patients with Sjögren's syndrome, SLE, mixed connective tissue disease, and limited systemic sclerosis (CREST syndrome). Patients with type I AIH can have other autoantibodies such as atypical pANCAs (65%) and antibodies against soluble liver antigen (10% to 50%).

23. **To what degree is type I AIH similar to SLE?**
    A comparison of type I AIH and SLE is given in Table 35-5.

Table 35-5. Comparison of Type I Autoimmune Hepatitis and Systemic Lupus Erythematosus

	SLE	TYPE I AIH
Young women	+	+
Polyarthritis	+	+
Fever	+	+
Rash	+	+
Nephritis	+	−
Central nervous system disease	+	−
Photosensitivity	+	−
Oral ulcers	+	−
ANA	99%	70%
LE cells	70%	Uncommon
Polyclonal gammopathy	+	+
Anti-Smith (Sm) antibodies	25%	0
+ anti-ds DNA	70%	Rare
+ anti-Fl actin (Anti-SM)	Rare	80%

AIH, Autoimmune hepatitis; ANA, antinuclear antibodies; ds, double-stranded; SLE, systemic lupus erythematosus.

24. **What is the difference between anti-Sm and anti-SM antibodies?**
Anti-Sm antibodies are antibodies against the Smith antigen, which is an epitope on small nuclear ribonuclear proteins. It is highly diagnostic of SLE. The anti-SM antibody is an antibody against the smooth muscle antigen (FI actin). It is highly diagnostic of AIH. They are frequently confused with one another.

25. **List the common autoimmune diseases associated with primary biliary cirrhosis.**
Primary biliary cirrhosis (PBC) is an autoimmune disease of the liver marked by slow progressive destruction of the small bile ducts. Bile cholestasis leads to tissue damage with fibrosis and cirrhosis. It is more common in females (9:1). Up to 80% have antimitochondrial antibodies. The most specific antimitochondrial antibody is the M2 antibody directed against the E2 subunit of the pyruvate dehydrogenase complex on the inner mitochondrial membrane. Up to 50% of patients with PBC have one or more additional autoimmune disorders:
- Keratoconjunctivitis sicca (secondary Sjögren's syndrome) 25% to 30%.
- Autoimmune thyroiditis (Hashimoto's disease) 20%.
- Raynaud's disease 20%.
- Rheumatoid arthritis 8% to 10%.
- Limited scleroderma (CREST variant) occurs in 4% to 8% of PBC patients and antedates PBC by 14 years. Most have anticentromere antibodies.
- Others: pernicious anemia (4%), celiac disease, SLE (1.5%), polymyositis.

26. **Compare and contrast the arthritis that may occur with PBC and rheumatoid arthritis.**
A comparison of PBC arthritis and rheumatoid arthritis is given in Table 35-6.

Table 35-6. Primary Biliary Cirrhosis Arthritis versus Rheumatoid Arthritis

	PBC ARTHRITIS	RHEUMATOID ARTHRITIS
Frequency in patients with PBC	10% develop RA	1% to 10% develop PBC
Number of joints*	Polyarticular	Polyarticular
Symmetry	Symmetric	Symmetric
Inflammatory	Yes	Yes
Rheumatoid factor	Sometimes	Yes (85%)
Erosions on radiograph	Rare	Common

DIP, Distal interphalangeal; PBC, primary biliary cirrhosis; RA, rheumatoid arthritis.
*PBC can involve DIP joints, whereas RA does not.

27. **What other musculoskeletal manifestations may occur in patients with PBC?**
- Osteomalacia due to fat-soluble vitamin D malabsorption.
- Osteoporosis due to renal tubular acidosis.
- Hypertrophic osteoarthropathy.

28. **What dose adjustments need to be made for antirheumatic medications in patients with severe hepatobiliary disease?**
Severe liver disease can be defined as a combination of one or more of the following factors: elevated bilirubin >3 mg/dL, albumin <3 g/dL with ascites, elevated protime not fully corrected by vitamin K, and/or cirrhosis on liver biopsy. Elevated transaminases greater than three times the upper limit of normal should also be a concern. Also, note that because creatine is synthesized in the liver, serum creatinine may be an overestimate of renal function.
Hepatobiliary disease may substantially impair the elimination or activation of drugs that the liver metabolizes or excretes. Although glucuronidation is spared, oxidation and acetylation are slowed. In addition, decreased synthesis of albumin may lead to increased free fraction of the active drug. Decreased synthesis of vitamin K-dependent clotting factors may lead to increased risk of bleeding if a medication affects platelet function or number.
The following are guidelines for antirheumatic drug therapy in severe liver disease:
- **Prodrug metabolism**—azathioprine, leflunomide, cyclophosphamide, prednisone, and sulindac need to be converted to active moiety by the liver. This is impaired in patients with severe hepatic insufficiency. Consequently, these drugs should be avoided or replaced with active forms (i.e., 6-mercaptopurine, prednisolone).
- **Biliary excretion**—methotrexate, cyclosporine, colchicine, leflunomide, indomethacin, and sulindac are excreted in the bile and undergo enterohepatic circulation. These should be avoided in patients with impaired biliary function.

- **Change in drug dosage for severe liver disease:**
  - Acetaminophen: use up to a maximum dose of 2 g/day.
  - Antimalarials: use with caution and at lower doses. American College of Rheumatology (ACR) guidelines recommend avoid in patients with Child-Pugh C liver disease.
  - Antitumor necrosis factor-α (anti-TNF-α): probably safe.
  - Allopurinol: little data. Use with caution. Can cause severe hepatitis.
  - Azathioprine: use 6-mercaptopurine instead but use at low dose with caution because toxicity can occur quickly.
  - Bisphosphonates: probably safe.
  - Biologics (other): little data. Would avoid or use tocilizumab and tofacitinib with caution because they can have liver toxicity.
  - Colchicine: avoid.
  - Cyclophosphamide: may not be converted to active form.
  - Cyclosporine and tacrolimus: eliminated by liver, so avoid.
  - Febuxostat: metabolized by the liver. Can cause liver toxicity. Avoid or use with caution at lower doses.
  - Leflunomide: avoid.
  - Methotrexate: avoid.
  - Mycophenylate mofetil: no dosage change, but do not exceed 2 g/day.
  - Narcotics: most metabolized by liver. Fentanyl and hydromorphone are the safest. Need to lower dose or extend interval. Avoid meperidine.
  - NSAIDs: lower dose 50%. Avoid diclofenac, sulindac, and indomethacin. Note that NSAIDs even at low doses increase risk of bleeding and renal failure.
  - Prednisone: use prednisolone or methylprednisolone instead.
  - Sulfasalazine: use with caution and at lower doses. Can cause hepatic failure rarely. ACR guidelines recommend avoid in Child-Pugh C liver disease.
  - Tramadol: double dosing interval from 6 to 12 hours. Start at dose of 25 mg.

BIBLIOGRAPHY

Balbir-Gurman A, Schapira D, Nahir M: Arthritis related to ileal pouchitis following total proctocolectomy for ulcerative colitis, Semin Arthritis Rheum 30:242–248, 2001.
Cho JH: The genetics and immunopathogenesis of inflammatory bowel disease, Nature Rev Immunol 8:458, 2008.
Delco F, Tchambaz L, Schlienger R, et al: Dose adjustment in patients with liver disease, Drug Safety 28:529–545, 2005.
Green PHR, Cellier C: Celiac sprue, N Engl J Med 357:1731–1743, 2007.
Holden W, Orchard T, Wordsworth P: Enteropathic arthritis, Rheum Dis Clin N Am 29:513–530, 2003.
Krawitt EL: Autoimmune hepatitis, N Engl J Med 354:54–66, 2006.
Lubrano E, Cicacci C, Amers PR, et al: The arthritis of coeliac disease: prevalence and pattern in 200 adult patients, Br J Rheumatol 35:1314–1318, 1996.
Manns MP, Cjaza AJ, Gorham JD, et al: Diagnosis and management of autoimmune hepatitis, Hepatology 51:2193–2213, 2010.
Marx WJ, O'Connell DJ: Arthritis of primary biliary cirrhosis, Arch Intern Med 139:213–216, 1979.
Narvaez J, Bianchi MM, Santo P, et al: Pancreatitis, panniculitis, and polyarthritis, Semin Arthritis Rheum 39:417–423, 2010.
Rodriguez-Reyna TS, Martinez-Reyes C, Yamamoto-Furusho JK: Rheumatic manifestations of inflammatory bowel disease, World J Gastroenterol 15:5517–5524, 2009.
Tysk C, Bohr J, Nyhlin N, et al: Diagnosis and management of microscopic colitis, World J Gastroenterol 14:7280–7288, 2008.
Watt FE, James OFW, Jones DEJ: Patterns of autoimmunity in primary biliary cirrhosis patients and their families: a population-based cohort study, Q J Med 97:397–406, 2004.
Wollheim FA: Collagenous colitis and rheumatology, Curr Rheumatol Rep 2:183–184, 2000.
Zholudev A, Zurakowski D, Young W, et al: Serologic testing with ANCA, ASCA, and anti-OmpC in children and young adults with Crohn's disease and ulcerative colitis: diagnostic value and correlation with disease phenotypes, Am J Gastroenterol 99:2235–2241, 2004.

FURTHER READING

http://www.celiac.org
http://www.ccfa.org
http://www.niddk.nih.gov
http://www.aasld.org

CHAPTER 36
REACTIVE ARTHRITIS
Richard T. Meehan, MD

KEY POINTS

1. Reactive arthritis (ReA) is a sterile, inflammatory arthritis that is typically preceded by a gastrointestinal or genitourinary infection occurring 1 to 4 weeks previously.
2. Similar to other spondyloarthropathies, patients with ReA are more likely to be human leukocyte antigen-B27 (HLA-B27) positive, which portends a worse prognosis and more joint and extraarticular manifestations.
3. Long-term (3 to 6 months) antibiotics may help *Chlamydia*-induced ReA but does not affect the course of ReA associated with enteric pathogens.
4. Over 50% of patients have a self-limited course lasting 2 to 6 months, 30% have recurrent episodes, and 10% to 20% have a chronic course requiring immunosuppressive therapy.

1. What is Reiter's syndrome?
As originally described in 1916, Reiter's syndrome is the clinical triad of conjunctivitis, nongonococcal urethritis, and arthritis following an infectious dysentery. Reiter's syndrome, a term no longer used, is now considered to be a form of ReA because two thirds of patients do not have all three features of this triad.

2. Define ReA.
ReA is a sterile, inflammatory synovitis occurring within 4 weeks of an infection by organisms that infect mucosal surfaces, especially urogenital or enteric infections. The arthritis is typically an asymmetric oligoarthritis that predominantly involves lower extremity large joints. ReA patients are frequently HLA-B27 positive and commonly exhibit systemic symptoms with unique extraarticular manifestations including skin, eye, and enthesopathy features.

3. How is ReA acquired? What is the influence of HLA-B27?
Susceptibility to ReA may be conferred by the specific class I major histocompatibility antigens, HLA-B27. However, its acquisition is strictly dependent on infection with certain gastrointestinal (enterogenic) or genitourinary (urogenital) pathogens. The most common organisms associated with disease among HLA-B27 patients include *Salmonella, Shigella, Yersinia, Chlamydia*, and *Campylobacter*. Many studies using electron microscopy, polymerase chain reaction (PCR), immunofluorescence, and/or gas chromatography-mass spectrometry techniques have identified microbacterial products including bacterial nucleic acids (*Chlamydia*) and cell wall components within the synovium of some of these patients. In hospital-based reports, HLA-B27 is present in 60% to 80% of patients with ReA. These patients tend to have more severe arthritis, more extraarticular manifestations (uveitis, rash), a higher prevalence of sacroiliitis, and a more prolonged course. Notably, in population-based studies, patients with ReA are less likely to be HLA-B27 positive and have a milder oligoarthritis without systemic symptoms or extraarticular manifestations.

4. What infectious agents "cause" ReA?

Urogenital	***Chlamydia*** *trachomatis, Ureaplasma urealyticum*
Enterogenic	***Salmonella*** *typhimurium, Salmonella enteritidis, Salmonella Heidelberg, Salmonella choleraesuis*
	Shigella *flexneri, Shigella dysenteriae, Shigella sonnei*
	Yersinia *enterocolitica, Yersinia pseudotuberculosis*
	Campylobacter jejuni
Others	*Clostridium difficile*
	Chlamydia pneumoniae
	Vibrio parahaemolyticus
	Borrelia burgdorferi
	Neisseria gonorrhoeae
	Streptococcus (post-Streptococcal ReA)
	Hepatitis C
	Giardia lamblia
	Mycoplasma

Note: In 40% of ReA patients an infectious agent cannot be identified. Urine PCR for *Chlamydia* and stool cultures may be helpful in patients with urethritis or diarrhea, respectively. Serologic tests for *Chlamydia*, *Salmonella*, and *Yersinia* can be done depending on the suspected inciting agent.

5. Who gets ReA?
Primarily young adults, ages 20 to 40 years. Patients with enterogenic ReA exhibit equal sex distribution, whereas those with the urogenital form are predominantly male. ReA is rare in children and uncommon in African Americans. ReA is the most common type of inflammatory arthritis affecting young adult males.

6. After the initial infection, when do symptoms of ReA first appear?
Although the initial infection may be mild or inapparent (10% to 30%), most patients will develop systemic symptoms within 1 to 4 weeks.

7. List the extraarticular manifestations associated with ReA.

Constitutional	**Genitourinary**
Low-grade fever	Infectious urethritis
Weight loss (rare)	Sterile urethritis
	Prostatitis (80%)
Ocular	Hemorrhagic cystitis
Sterile conjunctivitis (60%)	Salpingitis, vulvovaginitis
Anterior uveitis (20%) (acute unilateral, HLA-B27 positive)	**Mucocutaneous**
	Circinate balanitis (30%)
Gastrointestinal	Keratoderma blennorrhagicum (15%)
Infectious ileitis/colitis	Hyperkeratotic nails (10%)
Sterile ileitis/colitis (60%)	Painless oral ulcers (25%)
Cardiac (rare in acute disease)	**Other**
Heart block (1%)	Neuropathy (cranial or peripheral nerve)
Aortic regurgitation	Immunoglobulin A nephropathy
Aortitis (1%)	Renal amyloidosis
Pericarditis	Thrombophlebitis, livedo reticularis
	Erythema nodosum (*Yersinia*)

Note: The frequency of the various extraarticular manifestations depends on both the inciting infectious agent and if the patient is HLA-B27 positive.

8. What two cutaneous lesions are characteristic of ReA?
Circinate balanitis and **keratoderma blennorrhagicum** are relatively specific for ReA. Circinate balanitis is a **painless**, serpiginous ulceration of the glans penis. Similarly, keratoderma blennorrhagicum refers to psoriasiform lesions occurring primarily on the plantar surface of the heel and metatarsal heads. Both lesions are predominantly associated with urogenital ReA (*Chlamydia*) and resolve spontaneously.

9. Describe the musculoskeletal manifestations of ReA.
Arthritis. In ReA, the joints tend to be moderately inflamed and characterized by prolonged stiffness. Joint involvement is typically asymmetric, oligoarticular (less than five joints), and confined to the knees, ankles, and/or feet. Hip involvement is rare. Upper limb arthritis (e.g., wrist and digits) may also occur (50%). Uncommonly it can be a polyarthritis. The arthritis always lasts over 1 month and usually longer. Joint erosions may result from chronic disease.

Enthesitis is an inflammation of the ligament, tendon, joint capsule, or fascia insertion site into bone (enthesis). In ReA, enthesitis commonly causes heel pain (Achilles tendon and plantar fascia), metatarsalgia (plantar fascia), and iliac spine/crest pain.

Dactylitis ("sausage" digits) of fingers and toes are due to a combination of arthritis, enthesitis, and tendinitis.

Spondylitis. Forty percent of patients with ReA may have axial skeleton symptoms, and 25% develop radiographic changes. The risk of developing sacroiliitis and/or spondylitis is related to disease chronicity and HLA-B27.

10. What is the differential diagnosis for ReA?

Most Likely	Less Likely
Gonococcal arthritis	Ankylosing spondylitis
Acute septic arthritis	Rheumatic fever
Psoriatic arthritis	Gout/pseudogout
Inflammatory bowel disease arthritis	Lyme disease
Rheumatoid arthritis	Behçet's syndrome

In addition, ReA must always be considered as a possible complication of hepatitis C and HIV infection.

11. Compare the clinical features of ReA with gonococcal arthritis.
A comparison of the clinical features of ReA with gonococcal arthritis is given in Table 36-1.

Table 36-1. A Comparison of the Clinical Features of Reactive Arthritis With Gonococcal Arthritis

FEATURE	REACTIVE	GONOCOCCAL
Sex ratio	Male > female	Female > male
Age	20 to 40 years	All ages, most 20 to 40 years
Migratory arthralgias	No	Yes
Arthritis	Lower limbs	Upper limbs, knees
Enthesitis	Yes	No
Spondylitis	Yes	No
Tenosynovitis	Yes	Yes
Dactylitis	Yes	No
Urethritis	Yes	Yes
Uveitis	Yes	No
Oral ulcers	Yes	No
Cutaneous lesions	Keratoderma, balanitis	Pustules
Culture positive	No	Yes (<50%)
HLA-B27 positive	Yes (80%)	Same as general population
Penicillin responsive	No	Yes

Table 36-2. A Comparison of the Clinical Features of Reactive Arthritis With Rheumatoid Arthritis

FEATURE	REACTIVE ARTHRITIS	RHEUMATOID ARTHRITIS
Sex ratio	Male > female	Female > male
Age	20 to 40 years	All ages
Arthritis	Oligoarticular	Polyarticular
	Large joints (asymmetric)	MCP, PIP wrist, MTP (symmetric)
Enthesitis	Yes	No
Spondylitis	Yes	No
Ocular disease	Conjunctivitis, uveitis	Keratitis, scleromalacia, sicca, scleritis
Lung disease	No	Yes
Urethritis	Yes	No
Cutaneous lesions	Keratoderma, balanitis	Subcutaneous nodules, vasculitis
Rheumatoid factor positive	No	Yes (85%)
HLA association	HLA-B27 (80% of white males)	HLA-DR4 (70%)

HLA, Human leukocyte antigen; *MCP*, metacarpophalangeal; *MTP*, metatarsophalangeal; *PIP*, proximal interphalangeal.

12. **Compare the clinical features of ReA with rheumatoid arthritis.**
    A comparison of the clinical features of ReA with rheumatoid arthritis is given in Table 36-2.

13. **Which laboratory investigations are useful in confirming the diagnosis of ReA?**
    The diagnosis of ReA is clinical, and no laboratory investigation can substitute for a proper history and physical examination. However, they can be used in confirming the clinical diagnosis. Arthrocentesis is the most valuable test, because it excludes septic and crystalline arthritis (Table 36-3).

14. **What are the usual synovial fluid findings from a patient with ReA?**
    The synovial fluid typically reveals a predominance of leukocytes, ranging from 5000 to 50,000 cells/mm³. In acute ReA, most of these cells are neutrophils, but in chronic disease, either lymphocytes or monocytes may be prevalent.

Table 36-3. Laboratory Investigations That Are Useful in Confirming the Diagnosis of Reactive Arthritis

	EXPECTED RESULT
Primary (essential)	
ESR and or CRP	Elevation
Complete blood count and differential	Polymorphonuclear leukocytosis
	Thrombocytosis and anemia
Rheumatoid factor	Negative
Urinalysis	Pyuria, +/− bacteria
Synovial fluid analysis	Moderate leukocytosis
	Negative Gram stain and no crystals
Cultures and/or PCR	
—Throat	(+/−) (*Chlamydia*)
—Urine	(+/−) (*Chlamydia*)
—Stool	(+/−) (*Yersinia* and *Salmonella* can persist for weeks)
—Synovial fluid	Negative cultures
—Urethra/cervix	(+/−) (*Chlamydia*)
—Sputum	(+/−) (*Chlamydia pneumonia*)
Secondary (optional)	
Antinuclear antibody	Negative
Antibody serology	Positive (e.g., *Yersinia*, *Shigella*, and *Chlamydia*)
Blood cultures	Negative, unless septic
Radiographs	
• Peripheral joints	Arthritis, enthesitis
• Axial joints	Spondylitis, enthesitis
• Anteroposterior pelvis	Sacroiliitis
Electrocardiogram	Heart block
Colonoscopy	Ileitis/colitis

CRP, C-Reactive protein; *ESR*, erythrocyte sedimentation rate; *PCR*, polymerase chain reaction.

Other synovial fluid characteristics include decreased viscosity, normal glucose level, and increased protein. Large, vacuolar macrophages (Reiter's cells), containing intact lymphocytes or fragmented nuclei, are occasionally seen but are not specific for ReA. Synovial fluid PCR for *Chlamydia* can be done but has not been validated.

15. **Describe the radiographic features seen in patients with ReA.**
    Remember your **ABCDE'S**. These radiographic features are typical of all seronegative spondyloarthropathies.
        A—**Ankylosis** of the spine occurs in up to 20% of patients. There are large, nonmarginal syndesmophytes, called "jug-handle" syndesmophytes, which usually occur in an asymmetric distribution. These syndesmophytes can also occur in psoriatic spondylitis but differ from the thin, marginal, bilateral syndesmophytes seen in ankylosing spondylitis (Figure 36-1).
        B—**Bony reactivity** and proliferation at enthesis sites (Achilles tendon and plantar fascia insertions) and periostitis are common. Ossification of tendons may occur. **Bone demineralization** (periarticular osteopenia) may be observed in a periarticular distribution compatible with an inflammatory arthritis.
        C—**Cartilage**-space narrowing occurs uniformly across the joint space of weight-bearing joints compatible with an inflammatory arthritis. No abnormal cartilage or soft tissue **calcifications** are seen.

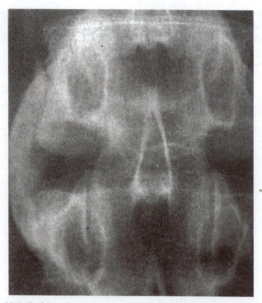

Figure 36-1. Radiograph of spine showing a large "jug-handle" syndesmophyte.

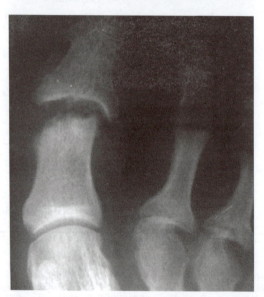

Figure 36-2. Radiograph of foot in a patient with reactive arthritis showing erosions of the interphalangeal joint of the great toe and second and third metatarsophalangeal joints.

  D—Distribution of arthritis is primarily in the lower extremity, whereas psoriatic arthritis usually affects the upper extremity. The sentinel joint involved may be the *interphalangeal joint of the great toe*.
  E—Erosions are common in the metatarsophalangeal joints (Figure 36-2). Sacroiliac joint erosions tend to involve one sacroiliac joint more than the other (asymmetric), which contrasts to the symmetric involvement of ankylosing spondylitis (Figure 36-3).
  S—Soft tissue swelling and dactylitis (diffuse swelling of toes). Psoriatic arthritis causes dactylitis of the fingers more than toes.

16. How do the radiographic features of sacroiliac and spine involvement in ReA compare with those in ankylosing spondylitis?

Note that 100% of patients with ankylosing spondylitis develop radiographic changes in the sacroiliac joints, compared with only 25% of ReA patients (Table 36-4). Patients with inflammatory bowel disease also develop

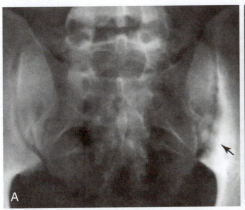
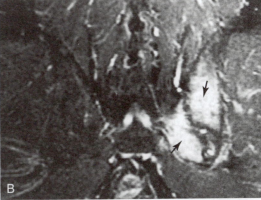

Figure 36-3. **A,** Radiograph of pelvis showing left sacroiliitis (*arrows*). **B,** Magnetic resonance image of pelvis showing left sacroiliitis (*arrows*).

Table 36-4. Radiographic Features of Sacroiliac and Spine Involvement in Reactive Arthritis in Comparison With Those in Ankylosing Spondylitis

	ANKYLOSING SPONDYLITIS	REACTIVE ARTHRITIS
Sacroiliitis	Bilateral, symmetric	Unilateral or asymmetric
Spondylitis	Bilateral, thin, marginal syndesmophytes	Asymmetric, nonmarginal, "jug-handle" syndesmophytes

radiographic changes of their spine similar in appearance to those of ankylosing spondylitis, whereas psoriatic arthritis produces changes similar to ReA.
Note: unilateral sacroiliitis without peripheral arthritis does not occur in ReA and should suggest another diagnosis (e.g., infection).

17. Is HLA-B27 determination useful?

A sufficient number of patients with ReA will not be HLA-B27 positive, thus rendering HLA-B27 determination a poor diagnostic test in screening patients with low back pain, especially because 7% of the normal white population will be positive. Patients with ReA can usually be successfully diagnosed and managed without HLA-B27 determination. However, this test may be of value if the clinical picture is incomplete, such as in the absence of an antecedent infection or lack of extraarticular features. Many rheumatologists find it useful, however, to classify patients as having either "HLA-B27 associated" or "nonassociated" forms of ReA. HLA-B27 status may have prognostic value, as positivity correlates with an increase in disease severity, chronicity, and frequency of exacerbations, as well as development of aortitis, uveitis, and spondylitis.

18. Describe the nonpharmacologic management of ReA.

Initial management begins with bed rest and splinting of the affected joints. Transient relief of joint inflammation may be obtained by use of ice packs and/or warm compresses. Once inflammation subsides (1 to 2 weeks), **passive** strengthening and range of motion exercises should be initiated. Progression to **active** exercises reduces the likelihood of muscle atrophy. Avoidance of behavior promoting reinfection is critical.

19. Describe the pharmacologic management of ReA.

Infectious disease. Elimination of the "triggering" infection with appropriate antibiotics is the first therapeutic goal in ReA. This is especially true for *Chlamydia* infections (azithromycin 1 g single dose or doxycycline 100 mg twice a day for 7 days, both patient and partner).

Extraarticular disease. The mucocutaneous features of ReA are usually self-limited and may require no specific therapy. Topical corticosteroids and keratolytic agents may help keratoderma blennorrhagicum. Symptoms of uveitis should be referred for ophthalmologic evaluation.

Articular disease. In most patients, reduction of inflammation and restoration of function can be achieved with nonsteroidal antiinflammatory drugs (NSAIDs) alone. Indomethacin (150 mg/day in divided doses) is the prototypic NSAID for treatment of ReA but other NSAIDs can be used depending on patient tolerance. Aspirin and propionic acid derivatives (e.g., ibuprofen) seem less effective and are not recommended for initial therapy.

Some patients with recurrent or chronic symptoms may require additional therapeutic measures for disease control. Intraarticular corticosteroids may be used judiciously to alleviate NSAID-resistant synovitis and sacroiliitis. Obviously, joint sepsis must be excluded before corticosteroid injection. Systemic corticosteroids in low or moderate doses (5 to 10 mg/day) are usually ineffective in ReA, but a therapeutic trial of 30 to 60 mg/day may be warranted in patients having resistant disease and disorders (e.g., AIDS) in which cytotoxic therapy is contraindicated.

20. How do you treat refractory ReA?

In most patients (>50%), remission of symptoms usually occurs within 2 to 6 months after disease onset but may take as long as 1 year. Patients experiencing recurrent flares (30% to 35%) or persistence of symptoms (15% to 20%) despite adequate NSAID therapy may require a disease-modifying agent. Sulfasalazine (2 g/day to 3 g/day) is the drug of choice for refractory ReA and may also be safely used in patients with HIV infection. Patients started on sulfasalazine within the first 3 months do best. Other disease-modifying agents, such as methotrexate and leflunomide, have also been used with variable success. Tumor necrosis factor-α blocking agents have been reported to be successful in many patients.

21. Should antibiotics be used in ReA? If so, for how long? (Controversial)

Once an antecedent infection has triggered ReA, it is unlikely that antibiotics will affect the course of illness with the possible exception of *Chlamydia*-triggered ReA. All patients and their sexual partners should be treated for *Chlamydia*-positive urethritis associated ReA (see Question 19). However, because chlamydial organisms have been demonstrated in a metabolically active state in the synovial tissue, some rheumatologists advocate a 3-month trial of doxycycline or minocycline 100 mg twice a day for *Chlamydia*-confirmed or suspected ReA. Recently, the combination of either doxycycline (100 mg twice a day) plus rifampin (300 mg daily) or azithromycin (500 mg daily for 5 days, then twice a week) plus rifampin for 6 months was shown to be effective therapy in some patients with long-standing chronic *Chlamydia*-induced ReA.

Antibiotic therapy for postenteric-associated ReA has not been demonstrated in trials to reduce severity of arthritis. The demonstration of bacterial cell wall antigens but not nucleic acid in synovial tissue suggests that bacterial antigens alone, *not* viable microorganisms, may perpetuate this type of ReA and therefore antibiotics are not effective.

Prophylactic antibiotics should be considered in patients with a previous episode of ReA who later develop urethritis after unprotected sex or traveler's diarrhea. Azithromycin (1 g) as a single dose for urethritis or azithromycin (1 g) as a single dose (*Campylobacter*) plus ciprofloxacin (750 mg) as a single dose (*Salmonella, Shigella,* and *Yersinia*) at onset of diarrhea has anecdotally prevented the subsequent redevelopment of ReA.

22. When should you suspect that ReA may be a complication of HIV infection?

ReA may be the first manifestation of HIV infection. Therefore, HIV antibody status and hepatitis serologies should be determined when the appropriate risk factors and/or clinical features are present. Furthermore, patients with refractory ReA and risk factors for HIV should have antibody determination before the use of immunosuppressive agents.

23. What is the prognosis for patients with ReA?

Although the prognosis of ReA is variable, most patients fully recover from their initial illness. However, a significant number (15% to 50%) will have one or more recurrences of ocular disease, mucocutaneous lesions, and/or arthritis. Up to 20% of patients will manifest some form of chronic peripheral arthritis and/or axial skeleton disease. The spondylitis of ReA is common (15% to 30%) but typically mild. Blindness occurs in 5% who develop uveitis. Factors such as reinfection, male gender, hip arthritis, erythrocyte sedimentation rate (ESR) >30 mm/h, sausage digits, poor response to NSAIDs, genetic susceptibility (HLA-B27), and heel pain are associated with a poorer prognosis. In general, disability due to articular disease is related to responsiveness to medication in the absence of spontaneous remission. Overall, the long-term prognosis for postdysenteric ReA is better than post-*Chlamydia* ReA.

24. What is an undifferentiated peripheral spondyloarthropathy?

An undifferentiated spondyloarthropathy does not meet criteria for ReA or psoriatic arthritis. As many as 40% of patients may be undifferentiated upon presentation with the majority of patients developing additional manifestations later in their disease course enabling a more definitive diagnosis. The Assessment of Spondylo-Arthritis International Society (ASAS) classification criteria for peripheral spondyloarthritis has a sensitivity of 78% and specificity of 83% for detecting a patient who has a peripheral spondyloarthropathy. They are:
- Peripheral arthritis (asymmetric lower extremity) or enthesitis or dactylitis plus one of the following (HLA-B27; genitourinary/gastrointestinal infection; psoriasis; inflammatory bowel disease; or magnetic resonance imaging showing sacroiliitis).

OR

- Peripheral arthritis (asymmetric lower extremity) or enthesitis or dactylitis plus two of the following (arthritis; enthesitis; dactylitis; inflammatory back pain; family history of a spondyloarthropathy).

Bibliography

Carter JD, Espinoza LR, Inman RD, et al: Combination antibiotics as a treatment for chronic Chlamydia-induced reactive arthritis, Arthritis Rheum 62:1298–1307, 2010.
Carter JD, Hudson AP: The evolving story of Chlamydia-induced reactive arthritis, Curr Opin Rheumatol 22:424–430, 2010.
Clegg DO, Redo DJ, Abdellatif M: Comparison of sulfasalazine and placebo for the treatment of axial and peripheral articular manifestations of the seronegative spondyloarthropathies, Arthritis Rheum 42:2325, 1999.
Colmegna I, Cuchacovich R, Espinoza LR: HLA-B27-associated reactive arthritis: pathogenetic and clinical considerations, Clin Microbiol Rev 17:348–369, 2004.
Hannu T, Mattila L, Siitonen A, et al: Reactive arthritis attributable to Shigella infection: a clinical and epidemiological nationwide study, Ann Rheum Dis 64:594–598, 2005.
Jacobs A, Barnard K, Fishel R, et al: Extracolonic manifestations of *Clostridium difficile* infections. Presentation of 2 cases and review of the literature, Medicine 80:88–101, 2001.
Leirisalo-Repo M: Reactive arthritis, Scand J Rheumatol 34:251–259, 2005.
Meyer A, Chatelus E, Wendling D, et al: Safety and efficacy of anti-tumor necrosis factor α therapy in ten patients with recent-onset refractory reactive arthritis, Arthritis Rheum 63:1274–1280, 2011.
Rihl M, Kohler L, Klos A, et al: Persistent infection of Chlamydia in reactive arthritis, Ann Rheum Dis 65:281–284, 2006.
Rohekar S, Tsui FWL, Tsui HW, et al: Symptomatic acute reactive arthritis after an outbreak of Salmonella, J Rheumatol 35:1599–1602, 2008.
Saxena S, Aggarwal A, Misra R: Outer membrane protein of salmonella is the major antigenic target in patients with salmonella induced reactive arthritis, J Rheumatol 32:86–92, 2005.
Schiellerup P, Krogfelt KA, Locht H: A comparison of self-reported joint symptoms following infection with different enteric pathogens: effect of HLA-B27, J Rheumatol 35:480–487, 2008.
Sieper J, Fendler C, Laitko S, et al: No benefit of long-term ciprofloxacin treatment in patients with reactive arthritis and undifferentiated oligoarthritis, Arthritis Rheum 42:1386, 1999.
Sieper J, Rudwaleit M, Braun J, et al: Diagnosing reactive arthritis: role of clinical setting in the value of serologic and microbiologic assays, Arthritis Rheum 46:319–327, 2002.

Further Reading

http://www.spondylitis.org

CHAPTER 37

ARTHRITIS ASSOCIATED WITH PSORIASIS AND OTHER SKIN DISEASES

William R. Gilliland, MD, MHPE

KEY POINTS

1. Inflammatory joint disease occurs on average in 26% of patients with psoriasis.
2. There are five clinical and overlapping subsets of psoriatic arthritis. Distal interphalangeal (DIP) involvement is the most characteristic pattern.
3. Dactylitis, enthesitis, and tenosynovitis are common musculoskeletal features accompanying psoriatic arthritis.
4. Antitumor necrosis factor-α (anti-TNF-α) agents are effective for peripheral and axial arthritis as well as skin disease.
5. Psoriatic patients have a higher mortality rate due to an increased incidence of the metabolic syndrome and premature atherosclerosis.

---

1. **How prevalent is psoriasis and psoriatic arthritis in the general population?**
   Epidemiologic studies suggest that the prevalence of psoriasis is approximately 2% to 3%. Whites are affected (two times) more often than other ethnic groups. The estimates of inflammatory arthritis accompanying psoriasis range from 7% to 42% (average 26%).

2. **Do genetic and environmental factors play a role in psoriatic arthritis?**
   Yes. Twin studies, family studies, and genome-wide association studies (GWAS) suggest a genetic predisposition to psoriatic arthritis. Concordance among monozygotic twins ranges from 35% to 70%, compared to 12% to 20% for dizygotic twins. Epidemiologic studies have found that first-degree relatives of psoriatic arthritis patients are 27 to 50 times more likely to develop arthritis. Up to 40% of patients with psoriatic arthritis have a family history of psoriasis.

   Psoriatic arthritis is a polygenic disorder. GWAS have identified a number of possible genes. *HLA-Cw6* is associated with severe, early-onset skin psoriasis. *HLA-B38* and *HLA-B39* are associated with psoriatic arthritis and *HLA-B27* is associated with sacroiliitis and spondylitis. Notably, only 50% of patients with psoriatic sacroiliitis/spondylitis are HLA-B27 positive. Recently *MICA* and other genes in linkage disequilibrium with other susceptibility genes have been found to be associated with peripheral psoriatic arthritis. *HLA-DR*04* is associated with worse radiographic progression.

   Evidence suggests that trauma and infection play a role in psoriatic arthritis. Trauma to a joint (*deep Koebner phenomenon*) is reported in 25% of patients before the onset of a patient's psoriatic arthritis. Subclinical trauma may explain DIP involvement. Bacterial agents such as streptococcal pharyngitis have been reported before the onset of guttate psoriasis. Notably, there is an association of psoriasis with obesity.

3. **Does gender play a role in its prevalence? How old is the typical patient?**
   Unlike the classic connective tissue disorders such as systemic lupus erythematosus or rheumatoid arthritis, the overall prevalence of arthritis is relatively equal between the sexes. However, in patients with spinal involvement, the male to female ratio is almost 3:1. Men also tend to have a higher prevalence of DIP-only involvement, whereas women tend to have a higher prevalence of symmetric polyarthritis.

   Most patients present between the ages of 35 and 50 years. However, juvenile psoriatic arthritis is also well recognized and usually presents between ages 9 and 12 years.

4. **Is there a relationship between the onset of psoriasis and the onset of arthritis?**
   - Psoriasis precedes arthritis by an average of 8 to 10 years in 67% of patients.
   - Arthritis precedes psoriasis or occurs simultaneously in 33% of patients, particularly in childhood and in older patients (>age 50 years).

5. **If psoriasis is not obvious, what areas should be closely examined?**
   Umbilicus, scalp, anus, and behind ears.

6. **Is there a relationship between the extent of skin involvement and arthritis?**
   No particular pattern (plaque, pustular, guttate) or extent of psoriasis is associated with arthritis. However, some suggest that arthritis is more deforming and widespread with extensive skin involvement as indicated by a Psoriasis Assessment Severity Index (PASI) greater than 10 (range of PASI score is 0 to 72). Up to 35% report that their skin and joint disease flare at the same time. Notably CD8+ T cells appear to be involved in the skin and entheseal lesions.

7. **What are the current classification criteria for psoriatic arthritis?**
   The **CASPAR** (Classification of Psoriatic Arthritis) criteria are:
   1. Evidence of psoriasis (current, past, family): two points if current history of psoriasis, one point others.
   2. Psoriatic nail dystrophy: one point
   3. Negative rheumatoid factor: one point.
   4. Dactylitis (current, past history): one point.
   5. Radiographic evidence of juxtaarticular new bone formation: one point.
   Three or more points have 99% specificity and 92% sensitivity for diagnosis of psoriatic arthritis.

8. **What are the characteristic patterns of joint involvement in psoriatic arthritis?**
   Approximately 95% of patients with psoriatic arthritis have peripheral joint disease [synovitis, tenosynovitis (dactylitis), enthesitis]. Another 5% have axial spine involvement exclusively. In 1973, Moll and Wright divided psoriatic arthritis into five broad categories. In reality, they overlap, creating a heterogeneous combination of joint disease. For instance, only 2% to 5% of psoriatic arthritis patients have predominantly DIP involvement, whereas over 50% of patients have DIP involvement in association with another pattern. As mentioned above, 5% of patients have only axial spine involvement but up to 40% of patients with one of the other patterns of psoriatic arthritis will also have coexistent axial involvement (Table 37-1). *Importantly, these patterns are not mutually exclusive.*

Table 37-1. Classification of Joint Involvement in Psoriatic Arthritis

SUBTYPE	PERCENTAGE	TYPICAL JOINTS
1. Asymmetric oligoarticular disease	15 to 20	DIP joints and PIP joints of hands and feet. MCP joints, MTP joints, knees, hips, and ankles
2. Predominant DIP involvement	2 to 5	DIP joints
3. Arthritis mutilans	5	DIP joints, PIP joints
4. Polyarthritis "rheumatoid-like"	50 to 60	MCP joints, PIP joints, and wrists
5. Axial involvement (isolated)	2 to 5	Sacroiliac, vertebral

DIP, Distal interphalangeal; *MCP,* metacarpophalangeal; *MTP,* metatarsophalangeal; *PIP,* proximal interphalangeal.

9. **What other features are associated with certain subtypes?**
   - Asymmetric oligoarthritis—dactylitis.
   - Predominant DIP involvement—nail changes.
   - Arthritis mutilans—osteolysis of involved joints, "telescoping" of digits.
   - "Rheumatoid-like" disease—fusion of wrists.
   - Axial involvement—asymmetric sacroiliitis and "jug handle"-like syndesmophytes.

10. **Which is the most "classic" pattern of psoriatic arthritis?**
    Predominant DIP involvement, but note it is one of the least common patterns. However, very few inflammatory arthritides involve the DIP joints. When a patient has DIP inflammatory arthritis, psoriatic arthritis should be high on the differential.

11. **How does the axial involvement in psoriatic arthritis differ from that in other seronegative spondyloarthropathies?**
    Asymmetric sacroiliac involvement is typical of psoriatic arthritis and reactive arthritis. The other major seronegative spondyloarthropathies, ankylosing spondylitis and inflammatory bowel disease, tend to be more **symmetric**. Additionally, syndesmophytes are characteristically large, nonmarginal ("jug handle"-like), as opposed to the thin, marginal, symmetric syndesmophytes that occur in ankylosing spondylitis (see Chapter 34).

12. **What clinical features suggest psoriatic arthritis rather than other polyarticular arthritic diseases such as rheumatoid arthritis?**
    - Asymmetric joint involvement.
    - Absence of rheumatoid factor.
    - Significant nail pits (>60 total pits is pathognomonic) or nail dystrophy.
    - Involvement of DIP joints in the absence of osteoarthritis.
    - "Sausage digits" (dactylitis): seen in 30% to 50%. Due to synovitis and flexor tenosynovitis.
    - Enthesitis: seen in 35% to 40%. Most common Achilles and plantar fascia insertion.
    - Family history of psoriasis or psoriatic arthritis.
    - Axial radiographic evidence of sacroiliitis, paravertebral ossification, and syndesmophytes.
    - Peripheral radiographic evidence of erosive arthritis with relative lack of periarticular osteopenia.
    - Synovial biopsies show increased vascularity and the presence of macrophages (CD163+), lymphocytes, and neutrophils.

13. Are there any extraarticular features associated with psoriatic arthritis?

Unlike rheumatoid arthritis, psoriatic arthritis is associated with only a few extraarticular features. **Nail changes** are seen in 80% of patients with arthritis, as opposed to only 30% with psoriasis only. These changes include pitting, transverse ridging, onycholysis, hyperkeratosis, and yellowing. **Eye disease** includes conjunctivitis in 20% and acute iritis in over 7% of cases. Iritis can be bilateral and is more commonly associated with axial involvement. Other less common features include oral ulcers, urethritis, nonspecific colitis, and rarely dilatation of base of aortic arch causing aortic insufficiency.

14. Discuss the association between flares of skin and nail disease and flares of psoriatic arthritis?

The relationship between skin and joint disease activity is variable. Patients with the simultaneous onset of psoriasis and psoriatic arthritis have reported that when one manifestation flares the other is likely to flare. However, for most patients the skin and arthritis run separate courses. Patients with DIP involvement are more likely to have worse nail involvement. This is partly because the extensor tendon enthesis inserts in an area adjacent to the nail root. When the enthesis becomes inflamed nail growth is affected adversely.

15. Are there additional concerns when someone presents acutely with severe psoriasis or psoriatic arthritis?

Especially in young or middle-aged men, one needs to consider concurrent HIV infection. Clinically, psoriasis or psoriatic arthritis associated with HIV infection is more aggressive and difficult to control with traditional medical therapy. As you might suspect, the detection of HIV is also important therapeutically, because drugs such as methotrexate have been associated with worsening immunodeficiency and death. Although it was initially thought that immunosuppressive drugs such as methotrexate were contraindicated in HIV-positive patients, with close monitoring many patients have been successfully treated with agents such as methotrexate.

16. Can laboratory tests help in diagnosing psoriatic arthritis?

By definition, psoriatic arthritis is classified as a "seronegative" arthritis, meaning that the rheumatoid factor is typically negative. However, low titer rheumatoid factor can be detected in 5% to 9% and anticitrullinated peptide antibodies in 5% of psoriatic arthritis patients. This can make it difficult to separate from coexistent rheumatoid arthritis. However, the presence of DIP involvement, enthesitis, and dactylitis supports a diagnosis of psoriatic arthritis regardless of the serologies. Antinuclear antibodies are reported in 10% to 15%. As in other inflammatory diseases, erythrocyte sedimentation rates (ESR), C-reactive protein (CRP), and anemia may vary with disease activity. Patients with an elevated ESR and CRP are more likely to have polyarticular disease and a worse prognosis. Hyperuricemia is seen in 20% and is not due to the extent of skin involvement but related to the increased incidence of the metabolic syndrome seen in patients with psoriatic disease. Analysis of synovial fluid reveals inflammatory fluid with a neutrophilic predominance.

17. What radiographic features help to differentiate psoriatic arthritis from other inflammatory diseases?

Overall, 45% to 50% of patients will develop erosions within the first 2 years of their disease and eventually 67% will develop radiographic changes:
- Asymmetric involvement.
- Relative absence of juxtaarticular osteopenia.
- Involvement of DIP joints.
- Erosion of the terminal tufts (acroosteolysis).
- Whittling of the phalanges.
- Cupping of the proximal portion of the phalanges (pencil-in-cup deformity).
- Bony ankylosis distal to metacarpophalangeal (MCP) joints.
- Osteolysis of bones (arthritis mutilans).
- Polyarticular unidigit—MCP, proximal interphalangeal (PIP), and DIP of same finger involved.
- Sacroiliac and spondylitic changes (usually asymmetric).
- Musculoskeletal ultrasound showing enthesitis and dactylitis.
- Magnetic resonance imaging showing enthesitis and bone marrow edema at insertion sites of entheses. Sacroiliitis before X-ray changes.

Psoriatic arthritis, showing erosions and ankylosis of DIP and PIP joints, is shown in Figure 37-1.

18. What principles should be used to guide treatment of psoriatic arthritis? How should the arthritis be treated?

Patients should be treated similar to other inflammatory arthritides. Polyarticular disease and an elevated ESR/CRP indicate a worse prognosis. Some patients can be managed with nonsteroidal antiinflammatory drugs (NSAIDs) alone. Intraarticular steroid injections are also helpful in joints that are resistant to NSAIDs and proven not to be infected. When NSAIDs fail to control the inflammation with three or more joints involved or the PASI is greater than 10, disease-modifying agents should be considered.

Methotrexate, sulfasalazine, leflunomide, and cyclosporine have all been reported to have a small effect on skin involvement, peripheral arthritis, enthesitis, and dactylitis. However, none of these medications have been shown to halt radiographic progression and none are effective for axial disease or nail disease.

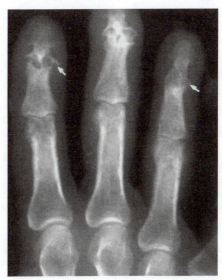

Figure 37-1. Psoriatic arthritis, showing erosions and ankylosis of DIP *(arrows)* and PIP joints. *DIP,* Distal interphalangeal; *PIP,* proximal interphalangeal. *(From Perlman SG, Barth WF: Psoriatic arthritis: diagnosis and management, Compr Ther 5:60-66, 1979.)*

Owing to large amounts of TNF-α found in psoriatic arthritis synovium, anti-TNF-α agents with or without methotrexate have been shown to be effective therapy for arthritis, dactylitis, enthesitis, spondylitis, and skin disease. Obesity appears to lessen the effectiveness of anti-TNF agents. Additionally, T helper 17 (Th17) cells have been shown to play a role in psoriasis and less so in psoriatic arthritis. Interleukin-23 (IL-23) is a cytokine involved in the differentiation of naïve T cells to Th17 cells. Ustekinumab (Stelara) is a monoclonal antibody that binds to the p40 subunit common to both IL-12 and IL-23 preventing their binding to a common receptor. Owing to successful trials, ustekinumab has been approved for the treatment of both psoriasis and peripheral psoriatic arthritis. Abatacept, alefacept, and rituximab have been used to treat psoriatic arthritis with limited or no success.

The role of antimalarials (hydroxychloroquine) is controversial. Exacerbation of psoriasis and erythroderma can occur with antimalarials, and consequently some consider them to be contraindicated. Systemic glucocorticoids should also be used cautiously because of the risk of inducing a flare of skin disease if tapered too rapidly.

19. **How does the prognosis of psoriatic arthritis compare with that of rheumatoid arthritis?**
    Psoriatic arthritis and rheumatoid arthritis have a similar prognosis and effect on quality of life. Overall, 60% have erosive arthritis in five or more joints, 40% have joint deformities and/or spine involvement, and up to 19% experience arthritis mutilans in at least one joint. Up to 20% will develop ACR (American College of Rheumatology) class III or class IV functional impairment with disability. A younger age of onset, female gender, acute onset of arthritis, polyarticular disease, and elevated ESR/CRP predicted a poor prognosis. In addition, mortality is increased with a standardized mortality ratio of 1.36. Recent studies show a link among psoriasis, obesity, the metabolic syndrome, hyperuricemia, and premature atherosclerosis.

20. **Are there any other medications that may be available now or in the future to treat psoriatic arthritis?**
    Apremilast is an oral small molecule that inhibits phosphodiesterase 4 (PDE4). By inhibiting PDE4 the hydrolysis of intracellular cyclic adenosine monophosphate (cAMP) is abrogated. This causes a buildup of cAMP intracellularly which triggers the protein kinase A pathway, which decreases production of TNF-α, IL-12, IL-23, and others by lymphocytes and macrophages resulting in modulation of the immune response. Apremilast trials using 30 mg twice a day show modest efficacy in psoriatic arthritis, enthesitis, and dactylitis. Its major side effect is nausea and diarrhea.
    Monoclonal antibodies that block IL-17A (secukinumab, ixekizumab) or the IL-17 receptor A (brodalumab) are promising biologics that are currently in trials for psoriasis and psoriatic arthritis.

21. **What other dermatologic conditions have been associated with arthritis?**
    Palmoplantar pustulosis, acne conglobata, acne fulminans, psoriatic onychopachydermoperiostitis, and hidradenitis suppurativa. Note that acne vulgaris is not included.

22. **What musculoskeletal symptoms are associated with these cutaneous pustular lesions?**
    - Anterior chest wall—pain and swelling in the sternoclavicular, manubriosternal, and sternocostal joints (probably SAPHO variant).

- Axial skeleton—chronic cervical or lumbar pain. Symphysis pubis is common.
- Peripheral arthritis—least common type; usually involves less than three joints (wrist, PIP, elbow, acromio-clavicular, and metatarsophalangeal [MTP] joints are the most common).

23. What is SAPHO syndrome?

S—Synovitis (90% of patients): oligo asymmetric (large > small joints), axial (sternal), and sacroiliac joints (unilateral).
A—Acne (18%): cystic acne conglobata, acne fulminans.
P—Pustulosis (66%): pustular psoriasis, palmoplantar pustulosis, or hidradenitis suppurativa.
H—Hyperostosis: especially of anterior chest wall with sternocostoclavicular hyperostosis.
O—Osteitis: symphysis pubis, sacroiliitis (33%), spondylodiscitis, anterior chest wall, vertebral sclerosis more than long bones.

The name was proposed in 1987 by Chamot et al because they were impressed by the association of a sterile arthritis (frequently involving the anterior chest) and various skin conditions. Etiology is unclear, although *Propionibacterium acnes* as a causative agent has been implicated. HLA-B27 is positive in 13% of cases. Therapy includes NSAIDs, intraarticular and systemic corticosteroids, sulfasalazine, doxycycline, intravenous bisphosphonates, methotrexate, and anti-TNF agents. Note that anti-TNF agents (especially infliximab) can exacerbate pustular psoriasis.

24. What is chronic recurrent multifocal osteitis and how does it relate to SAPHO?

Chronic recurrent multifocal osteitis (CRMO) is a chronic sterile inflammatory and multifocal disease of bone that preferentially affects children, females (F > M 2:1), but with no racial predilection. Bone sites involved differ according to age of the patient. The metaphysis of the long bones is preferentially affected in children and adolescents, whereas anterior thoracic, vertebral, and/or unilateral sacroiliac lesions predominate in adults. Bone biopsies are necessary to rule out bacterial osteomyelitis, tumor, and eosinophilic granuloma. Many patients with CRMO have Crohn's disease or psoriasis or skin lesions associated with SAPHO. Over time, most patients with CRMO evolve to satisfy criteria for a spondyloarthropathy, although they usually are HLA-B27 negative. Treatments used have been similar to those used in SAPHO.

BIBLIOGRAPHY

Bogliolo L, Alpini C, Caporali R, et al: Antibodies to cyclic citrullinated peptides in psoriatic arthritis, J Rheumatol 32:511, 2005.
Bruce IN, Schentag C, Gladman DD: Hyperuricemia in psoriatic arthritis does not reflect extent of skin involvement, J Clin Rheumatol 6:6, 2000.
Chandran V, Schentag CT, Gladman DD: Reappraisal of the effectiveness of methotrexate in psoriatic arthritis: results from a longitudinal observational cohort, J Rheumatol 35:469, 2008.
Clegg DO, Reda DJ, Mejias E, et al: Comparison of sulfasalazine and placebo in the treatment of psoriatic arthritis, Arthritis Rheum 39:2013–2020, 1996.
Coates LC, Tillett W, Chandler D, et al: The 2012 BSR and BHPR guideline for the treatment of psoriatic arthritis with biologics, Rheumatology 52:1754–1757, 2013.
Colina M, Govoni M, Orzincolo C, et al: Clinical and radiologic evolution of synovitis, acne, pustulosis, hyperostosis, and osteitis syndrome: a single center study of a cohort of 71 subjects, Arthritis Rheum 61:813, 2009.
Duffin KC, Chandran V, Gladmann DD, et al: Genetics of psoriasis and psoriatic arthritis: update and future direction, J Rheumatol 35:1449, 2008.
Gelfand JM, Gladman DD, Mease PJ, et al: Epidemiology of psoriatic arthritis in the population of the United States, J Am Acad Dermatol 53:573, 2005.
Gladman DD, Ang M, Su L, et al: Cardiovascular morbidity in psoriatic arthritis, Ann Rheum Dis 68:1131, 2009.
Jurik AG: Chronic recurrent multifocal osteomyelitis, Semin Musculoskel Radiol 8:243, 2004.
Kaltwasser JP, Nash P, Gladman D, et al: Efficacy and safety of leflunomide in the treatment of psoriatic arthritis: a multinational, double-blind, randomized, placebo-controlled clinical trial, Arthritis Rheum 50:2004, 1939.
McDonagle D, Lories RJ, Tan AL, et al: The concept of a "synovio-entheseal complex" and its implications for understanding joint inflammation and damage in psoriatic arthritis and beyond, Arthritis Rheum 56:2482, 2007.
Nestle FO, Kaplan DH, Barker J: Psoriasis, N Engl J Med 361:496, 2009.
Ritchlin CT: Pathogenesis of psoriatic arthritis, Curr Opin Rheumatol 17:406, 2005.
Ritchlin CT, Kavanaugh A, Gladman DD, et al: Treatment recommendations for psoriatic arthritis, Ann Rheum Dis 68:1387, 2009.
Saad AA, Symmons DP, Noyce PR, et al: Risks and benefits of tumor necrosis factor-alpha inhibitors in the management of psoriatic arthritis: systemic review and metaanalysis of randomized controlled trials, J Rheumatol 35:883, 2008.
Scarpa R, Cosentini E, Manguso F, et al: Clinical and genetic aspects of psoriatic arthritis "sine psoriasis," J Rheumatol 30:2638, 2003.
Siannis F, Farewell VT, Cook RJ, et al: Clinical and radiological damage in psoriatic arthritis, Ann Rheum Dis 65:478, 2006.
Taylor W, Gladman D, Helliwell P, et al: Classification criteria for psoriatic arthritis: development of new criteria from a large international study, Arthritis Rheum 54:2665, 2006.
Turkiewicz AM, Moreland LW: Psoriatic arthritis: current concepts on pathogenesis-oriented therapeutic options, Arthritis Rheum 56:1051, 2007.

FURTHER READING

http://www.psoriasis.org

VI
ARTHRITIS ASSOCIATED WITH INFECTIOUS AGENTS

As it takes two to make a quarrel, so it takes two to make a disease, the microbe and its host.

Charles V. Chapin
(1856–1941)

IV.
ARTHRITIS ASSOCIATED WITH INFECTIOUS AGENTS

BACTERIAL SEPTIC ARTHRITIS, BURSITIS, AND OSTEOMYELITIS

William R. Gilliland, MD, MHPE

CHAPTER 38

KEY POINTS

1. *Staphylococcus aureus* is the most common cause of septic arthritis and osteomyelitis.
2. Large weight-bearing joints, particularly the knee, are the most prone to developing septic arthritis.
3. The initial choice of antibiotic therapy is based on the Gram stain and clinical situation.
4. More than 50% of women who develop disseminated gonococcal infections (DGIs) do so within 1 week of onset of menses.
5. Any patient with fever, arthralgias, and tenosynovitis should be evaluated for a DGI.

---

1. **How do gonococcal and nongonococcal septic arthritis differ? (Table 38-1)**

2. **What clinical manifestations are typical of nongonococcal septic arthritis?**
   An abrupt onset of swelling, warmth, and pain involving one joint is the classic presentation, the exception being an infected joint prosthesis where the presentation may be more indolent (delayed-onset type). Many patients have serious underlying illnesses and may be febrile or have rigors. However, depending on the patient, the presence of fevers over 38° C ranges from 40% to 90% of cases and the percentage of cases with rigors ranges from 20% to 60%. Large joints (knee, hip) are most commonly involved. Patients keep the knee flexed or hip flexed, abducted, and externally rotated to maximize intracapsular volume. Both passive and active range of motion are very painful. Children and most adults refuse to use the involved extremity.

3. **How do organisms reach the synovium to cause septic arthritis?**
   - Hematogenously from a remote infection (70%)
   - Dissemination from adjacent osteomyelitis (especially in children)
   - Lymphatic spread from a soft tissue infection near the joint
   - Iatrogenic infections from arthrocentesis or arthroscopy (20%)
   - Penetrating trauma from plant thorns or other contaminated objects

4. **What factors predispose an individual to develop septic arthritis?**
   Impaired host defense (50%)
   - Neoplastic disease
   - Elderly (>80 years old) or children (<5 years old)
   - Chronic, severe illness (i.e., alcoholism, diabetes, cirrhosis, chronic renal disease, human immunodeficiency virus [HIV])
   - Cutaneous ulcers and skin infections
   - Sickle cell disease (susceptibility to encapsulated organisms owing to splenic dysfunction)
   - Hypogammaglobulinemia (susceptibility to *Mycoplasma* infections)
   - Immunosuppressive agents (i.e., glucocorticoids, chemotherapy, biologics)

   Direct penetration
   - Intravenous drug abuse; puncture wounds; invasive procedures

   Joint damage
   - Prosthetic joints (over 50% occur in patients over 70 years old)
   - Chronic arthritis [i.e., rheumatoid arthritis (RA), hemarthrosis, osteoarthritis]

   Host phagocytic defects
   - Late complement-component deficiencies (susceptibility to *Neisseria*); impaired chemotaxis

5. **Which joints are most commonly involved in nongonococcal septic arthritis in adults?**

Knee	55%
Hip	11%
Ankle	8%
Shoulder	8%
Wrist	7%
Elbow	6%
Others	5%
Polyarticular	10% to 19% (usually only two to three joints)

Table 38-1. Differentiating Gonococcal from Nongonococcal Arthritis

	GONOCOCCAL	NONGONOCOCCAL
Host	Young, healthy adults	Small children, elderly, immunocompromised
Pattern	Migratory polyarthralgias/arthritis	Monoarthritis
Tenosynovitis	Common	Rare
Dermatitis	Common	Rare
Positive joint cultures	<25%	>95%
Positive blood cultures	Rare	40-50%
Outcome	Good in >95%	Poor in 30-50%

6. **Which bacteria are usually responsible for nongonococcal septic arthritis in adults?**
   Overall, a causative pathogen is documented by culture in approximately 70% to 90% of septic arthritis patients and include:

S. aureus	44% to 66% (most penicillin-resistant, up to 50% methicillin-resistant [MRSA])
Group A/B streptococci	18% to 28% (group B more common in the elderly)
Gram-negative bacilli	9% to 19%
Streptococcus pneumoniae	3%
Polymicrobial	4%

7. **Why does S. aureus cause most cases of septic arthritis?**
   S. aureus preferentially localizes to joints owing to the presence of microbial surface components recognizing adhesive matrix molecules (MSCRAMMs) that are embedded in the cell wall peptidoglycan. MSCRAMMs bind to host proteins including collagen, fibrinogen, fibronectin, and others. A collagen-binding protein, under the influence of a *cna* gene, has been found to be the most important virulence factor contributing to joint localization. Clumping factors (A and B) binds to fibrinogen and fibronectin-binding protein (A and B) binds to fibronectin. Exotoxins produced by the bacteria contribute to the inflammatory response and bacteria survival.

8. **Which organisms are commonly involved in septic arthritis in children?**
   Considerable institutional variation exists, but the most common organisms in various age groups are as follows:

Neonates (<2 months)	Age 2 months to 5 years	Age 5 to 15 years
S. aureus (hospital-acquired)	Kingella kingae	S. aureus
Streptococci (Group B)	S. aureus	Streptococcus pyogenes
Gram-negative bacilli	S. pyogenes	
	S. pneumoniae	
	Haemophilus influenza (less common due to vaccination)	

9. **Name the organisms that are associated with underlying disorders in septic arthritis.**

RA	S. aureus (frequently polyarticular)
Alcoholism/cirrhosis	Gram-negative bacilli
	S. pneumoniae
Malignancies	Gram-negative bacilli
Diabetes mellitus	Gram-negative bacilli
	Gram-positive cocci
Drug abuse	Pseudomonas aeruginosa
	Serratia marcescens
	S. aureus
Dog/cat bites	Pasteurella multocida
Hemoglobinopathies	S. pneumoniae
	Salmonella spp. (osteomyelitis)
Hemochromatosis	Vibrio vulnificus (oyster-eating)
	Yersinia species (especially in the prosthetic joints)
Raw milk/dairy products	Brucella spp.
Systemic lupus erythematosus (SLE)	Encapsulated organisms (Neisseria, Salmonella, Proteus)

10. **How helpful are synovial fluid analysis and culture in nongonococcal septic arthritis?**
    Arthrocentesis with demonstration of the bacteria on Gram stain or culture establishes the diagnosis of septic arthritis. Of the tests that can be run on the synovial fluid, culture, Gram stain, and leukocyte (white blood cell, WBC) counts are the most useful (Table 38-2).

Table 38-2. Laboratory Tests in Nongonococcal Septic Arthritis		
PROCEDURE YIELD	**TECHNICAL ASPECTS**	**DIAGNOSTIC**
Culture	Plate or inoculate culture bottles immediately	70-90% positive in nongonococcal arthritis
Gram stain	May increase yield by centrifuging synovial fluid	75% in gram-positive cocci, 50% in gram-negative bacilli
WBC count	Usually 50,000 cells/mm^3 with 40% having >100,000 cells/mm^3 (>85% PMNs)	Counts often overlap other inflammatory diseases (gout, RA, reactive arthritis)
Glucose	<50% of serum glucose	Helpful if present
Cell wall antigens	CIE or PCR	Only helpful in *Haemophilus influenza*, *Streptococcus pneumonia*, and *Kingella kingae*

CIE, Counterimmunoelectrophoresis; *PCR*, polymerase chain reaction; *PMN*, polymorphonuclear leukocyte; *RA*, rheumatoid arthritis; *WBC*, white blood cell.

PEARL: Only 40% to 50% of all patients with septic arthritis have synovial fluid WBC counts over 100,000 cells/mm^3. So even if the synovial fluid WBC is not "classic" for septic arthritis, there can still be an infection even with WBC counts less than 50,000 cells/mm^3. Notably, crystal-induced arthritis (gout, pseudogout) can coexist with septic arthritis.

11. **Are any blood tests useful in septic arthritis?**
    Blood cultures are probably the most useful because approximately 50% (24% to 76%) of patients with nongonococcal septic arthritis have positive cultures. Blood cultures may be positive whereas synovial fluid cultures are negative in up to 10% of cases. **Leukocytosis, elevated sedimentation rate,** and **elevated C-reactive proteins (CRP)** are seen in most individuals (60% to 90%) but are not discriminative owing to overlap with other inflammatory arthritic diseases. Over 90% of patients with septic arthritis have an elevated CRP greater than 2 mg/dL (20 mg/L) therefore values lower than this are helpful in excluding septic arthritis. An elevated serum **procalcitonin** level may be supportive of the diagnosis but nondiagnostic by itself.

12. **Do plain radiographs play a role in diagnosing septic arthritis?**
    Initial radiographs should be obtained to rule out adjacent osteomyelitis and to establish a baseline. Early radiographic changes occurring within a few days include periarticular osteopenia, joint effusion, and soft tissue swelling. However, definitive changes of septic arthritis may take up to 2 to 3 weeks to develop and include periosteal reaction, joint space loss, erosions, and subchondral bone destruction.

13. **How can I remember the radiologic and/or pathologic changes in septic arthritis?**
    Remember **A-B-C-D-E-S** (Table 38-3).

Table 38-3. Nongonococcal Septic Arthritis: Radiographic and Pathologic Correlates		
	RADIOGRAPHIC SIGN	**PATHOLOGIC CORRELATE**
A	Bony **ankylosis**	Fibrous or bony ankylosis (endstage)
B	**Bone** mineralization decreased	Osteopenia from increased flow, inflammatory cytokines
C	**Cartilage** space loss	Pannus with cartilage destruction
D	Joint **deformity**	End stage of arthritic destruction
E	**Erosions**	Pannus with bony destruction
S	Joint effusion (the first sign), soft-tissue **swelling**	Edema of synovium with fluid production

14. **Can any other radiographic studies be helpful in septic arthritis?**
    Other radiographic tests are especially helpful in visualizing joints that are deep or difficult to palpate (i.e., hip, sacroiliac, and sternoclavicular joints). They are also helpful early on in a septic process, when plain films do not yet demonstrate any abnormalities (Table 38-4).

Table 38-4. Specialized Radiographic Studies in Septic Arthritis

PROCEDURE	UTILITY
Technetium-99m bone scan	Often positive in 24-48 h, but not specific for septic synovitis
Indium-111 scan	Less sensitive than bone scan but more specific because it relies on direct labeling of WBCs that migrate to the area of infection; especially helpful in evaluation of prosthetic joints
CT	Visualizes bony changes, such as erosions, before the use of plain films
MRI with contrast	Provides early detection of soft-tissue changes, such as edema and effusions with 100% sensitivity; also demonstrates osteomyelitis

CT, Computed tomography; MRI, magnetic resonance imaging; WBC, white blood cell.

15. **How do you treat nongonococcal septic arthritis?**
    - Choose an effective antibiotic based on patient age, clinical situation, and Gram stain findings.
    - Prompt and adequate drainage of the joint on a frequent basis (sometimes several times a day if using needle drainage) is essential. Always send synovial fluid for cell count, Gram stain, and culture to make sure therapy is succeeding as evidenced by decreasing cell count and cultures becoming negative. Although controversial, many clinicians feel that surgical (open, arthroscopic) drainage should be done instead of needle drainage (see Question 17).
    - Analgesics are useful as adjunctive therapy.
    - Physical therapy is important.
      - Passive range of motion after pain has improved.
      - Active range of motion when inflammation has substantially improved.
      - Weight-bearing when inflammation has resolved.

16. **Which antibiotic should you choose? How long do you treat nongonococcal septic arthritis?**
    Antibiotics should be started after cultures are obtained, with the choice of antibiotics determined by the suspected organism based on the initial Gram stain and the clinical situation (note that doses listed are for adults):
    - **Gram-positive cocci on Gram stain:** start vancomycin 30 mg/kg/day IV in two divided doses, but do not exceed 2 g/day. If allergic to vancomycin, one can use daptomycin (6 mg/kg/day IV), linezolid (600 mg IV BID), or clindamycin (900 mg IV TID).
    - **Gram-positive rod:** usually *Listeria* in an immunocompromised host. Treated with ampicillin (2 g IV every 4 hours) plus gentamycin (3 mg/kg IV in three divided doses). If allergic to penicillin, one can use trimethoprim-sulfamethoxazole, meropenem, or linezolid.
    - **Gram-negative diplococci:** usually *Neisseria gonorrhoeae* or *Neisseria meningitidis*. Treated with a third-generation cephalosporin such as ceftriaxone (1 g IV daily) or cefotaxime (1 g IV every 8 hours).
    - **Gram-negative rod:** start a third-generation cephalosporin such as ceftriaxone (2 g IV daily) or cefotaxime (2 g IV every 8 hours). If allergic to cephalosporin, one can use ciprofloxacin (400 mg IV every 12 hours).
    - **Negative Gram stain** (immunocompetent patient): start vancomycin.
    - **Negative Gram stain** (immunosuppressed patient, IV drug abuser, or trauma-related septic arthritis): start vancomycin plus third-generation cephalosporin (e.g. ceftriaxone).

    Once the organism has been identified, the antibiotic regimen (Table 38-5) can be tailored as follows: parental therapy should be initiated for at least 2 weeks, followed by 2 to 4 weeks of oral therapy. Intraarticular antibiotics should not be used. The total duration of therapy is variable and depends on the patient's clinical response.

17. **When is surgical drainage absolutely indicated for a septic joint?**
    - Infected hip joints and probably shoulder joints
    - Vertebral osteomyelitis with cord compression
    - Anatomically difficult-to-drain joints (i.e., sternoclavicular joint)
    - Inability to remove purulent fluid by needle drainage because fluid is too thick or loculated
    - Joints failing to respond to needle drainage (i.e., persistent positive cultures of synovial fluid or failure of synovial WBC to decrease)
    - Prosthetic joints
    - Associated osteomyelitis requiring surgical drainage
    - Arthritis associated with a foreign body
    - Delayed onset of therapy (>7 days)—irreversible cartilage damage starts within 1 week

18. **What is the prognosis in patients with nongonococcal septic arthritis?**
    Despite better drainage and antibiotics, this remains a serious disease with 2% to 10% mortality. Most of these patients (25% to 60%) have a chronic debilitating underlying disease (i.e., RA, polyarticular sepsis, cirrhosis, hemodialysis, and renal transplant) that contributes to the mortality. Of the surviving patients, between 30% and 50% have residual abnormalities (pain or limited motion of the joint).

Table 38-5. Nongonococcal Septic Arthritis: Antibiotic Choice for Specific Organisms

ORGANISM	ANTIBIOTIC OF CHOICE	ALTERNATIVES
Staphylococcus aureus	Nafcillin	Cefazolin Vancomycin Clindamycin
Methicillin-resistant *S. aureus* (MRSA)	Vancomycin	Deptomycin Linezolid Clindamycin
Streptococcus pyogenes or *Streptococcus pneumonia*	Penicillin or nafcillin	Cefazolin Vancomycin Clindamycin
Enterococcus	Ampicillin plus gentamicin	Vancomycin plus aminoglycoside
Haemophilus influenzae	Ampicillin	Third-generation cephalosporin Cefuroxime Chloramphenicol
Enterobacteriaceae	Third-generation cephalosporin or levofloxacin	Imipenem Aztreonam Ampicillin Aminoglycoside (not alone)
Pseudomonas	Aminoglycoside plus antipseudomonal penicillin	Aminoglycoside plus ceftazidime, imipenem, or aztreonam

19. **What factors suggest a poor outcome in nongonococcal septic arthritis?**
    RA, delayed diagnosis, polyarticular sepsis, immunosuppressive therapy, positive blood cultures, Gram-negative organisms, elderly age, renal transplant/dialysis or cirrhosis.

20. **How does septic arthritis differ in children?**
    - The age of the patient is very helpful in determining the likely organism (see question 8).
    - Arthritis is often secondary to adjacent osteomyelitis.
    - Children have a higher incidence of hip involvement.
    - Dislocation of the femoral head is unique to hip infections in neonates.

21. **Discuss the important aspects in the association of RA and septic joints.**
    Previously damaged joints and the use of **immunosuppressive agents** are probably responsible for the increased risk (≤3%) of septic arthritis in patients with RA. The incidence may be increasing with the use of biologic therapy such as anti-tumor necrosis factor (TNF) agents. The patients are usually those with longstanding seropositive disease, marked disability, and a history of corticosteroid use. Unfortunately, the steroids may blunt the typical symptoms of septic arthritis, causing it to be mistaken for a "flare" of RA. Gram-positive organisms, especially *S. aureus*, account for 75% to 90% of infections. Rare organisms and polymicrobial infections have also been reported. The most important feature is the poor prognosis. The mortality is 25%, with only half of those surviving attaining their preinfection level of functioning.

22. **Are there any peculiarities about septic arthritis in intravenous drug abusers?**
    1. Higher incidence of gram-negative organisms, especially *Pseudomonas* and *Serratia*. However, *S. aureus* is the most common organism.
    2. More insidious course with longer duration of symptoms.
    3. Increased propensity to affect the axial skeleton (especially the lumbar vertebrae, sacroiliac joint, symphysis pubis, ischium, and sternocostal articulations).
    4. In general, if given proper therapy, have a very low risk of death and high likelihood of preserved joint function unless they have HIV.

23. **What is the incidence of prosthetic joint infections? What are the risk factors?**
    The overall infection rate in primary total joint replacement is approximately 1% to 2%. Risk factors include distant site of infection, impaired host defense, RA, diabetes mellitus, revision arthroplasty (5 to 10 times increased risk), increased operative time, and superficial joint replacements (i.e., knee, elbow, ankle).

24. **What are the most common organisms causing prosthetic joint infection?**
    Early infections (<3 months post total joint arthroplasty) are caused by *S. aureus*, *Streptococcus*, or gram-negative bacilli. Usually due to surgical contamination. These patients present with fever and local signs of wound infection typical of septic arthritis.

Delayed infections (3 to 24 months) are usually caused by coagulase-negative staphylococci (*Staphylococcus epidermidis*). These organisms can get into the polysaccharide mucoid biofilm (glycocalyx) that forms on the prosthetic joint and provides a protective environment for bacterial growth. Patients present with progressive joint pain but frequently do not have other symptoms typical of septic arthritis. Fever occurs in less than 50% and leukocytosis in 10%. Elevated erythrocyte sedimentation rate (ESR) and CRP are common.

Late infections (>24 months) are the result of hematogenous seeding from a distant site of infection such as the skin, mouth, or urinary tract. Patients have acute onset of joint pain, swelling, and fever typical of septic arthritis.

25. How can a prosthetic infection be separated from aseptic loosening?
Infection should be suspected in any patient with progressive pain in a prosthetic joint. Fever may or may not be present but ESR and CRP are frequently elevated (75% and 88%, respectively). The synovial fluid will be inflammatory. Radiographs may show greater than 2 mm lucency between bone and cement but this does not separate infection from aseptic loosening. Magnetic resonance imaging (MRI), computed tomography (CT) scan, and positron emission tomography-18F-fluorodeoxyglucose (PET-FDG) scans are of limited value owing to the artifact of the prosthesis. The procedure of choice is combined bone marrow scan/indium scan showing increased uptake around the prosthesis (the bone scan should normally be negative 8 months after surgery). This imaging has an overall accuracy of 88% to 98%. However, positive cultures of synovial fluid or tissue are needed to confirm the diagnosis. The presence of granulocytes in biopsies of periprosthetic tissue is supportive diagnostically.

26. How are prosthetic joint infections treated? What measures can be done to prevent them?
Prolonged antibiotics and surgical intervention. Occasionally (<10% of large joint prosthesis infections) patients who have had symptoms for less than 1 week, negative preoperative synovial fluid cultures, no sinus tract, and a stable implant can be treated with debridement and antibiotics without removal of the prosthesis. However, most surgeons favor a three-stage procedure: (1) prosthesis and cement removal with stabilization of the joint using an antibiotic-impregnated spacer; (2) prolonged (6 weeks) systemic antibiotics; and (3) delayed implantation with antibiotic-impregnated cement. Rifampin use in conjunction with other antibiotics has been an effective additive therapy. The success rate is 80% to 90% using the three-stage approach. Mortality rates are 5% to 20%.

Steps to prevent prosthetic joint infections include: (1) preoperative evaluation to rule out occult infections (dental, bacteriuria, skin) and MRSA carrier status; (2) perioperative antibiotic prophylaxis; (3) timing of surgery and administration of biologic therapy; (4) some advocate prophylactic antibiotics for dental procedures in patients who have had large joint arthroplasties within the previous 2 years (controversial).

27. What is "pseudoseptic" arthritis?
Pseudoseptic arthritis is seen in the setting of poorly controlled RA in which the patient presents with one or more inflamed joints with very high synovial fluid WBC counts (>100,000 cells/mm^3). The cultures are negative, and patients respond to increased corticosteroids rather than antibiotics. *However, infection always needs to be ruled out first!* This presentation may also be seen in the crystal-induced arthritides, seronegative spondyloarthropathies, and viscosupplementation for osteoarthritis especially in a patient with calcium pyrophosphate dihydrate deposition disease (CPPD) who receives Synvisc.

28. Who is at risk for a DGI?
Unlike nongonococcal septic arthritis, the typical patient who develops gonococcal arthritis is a young, healthy person. Women are more commonly affected than men, and are more prone to develop a DGI around menstruation, pregnancy, and postpartum. Other risk factors include urban residence, non-white race, low socioeconomic status, low educational status, prostitution, and previous gonococcal infection. Septic arthritis as a result of a DGI used to be the most common cause of septic arthritis in adults less than 30 years of age. Today, the incidence has declined to about 1% of all septic arthritides due to effective sexually transmitted disease (STD) control programs.

29. How soon after infection do arthritic symptoms develop in DGI?
Arthritis complicates 1% to 3% of patients with gonorrhea. Typically, symptoms develop 1 day to several weeks after the sexual encounter and commonly (in 50% of female patients) occur during the week of the menstrual period in women.

30. What bacterial characteristics increase the potential for *N. gonorrhoeae* to disseminate?
1. Small, sharply bordered colonies with **surface pili (serotype Por.IA)** are more virulent than large colonies.
2. The presence of **outer membrane opacity-associated protein** increases its virulence and also its ability to disseminate.
3. **Nutritional requirements**, in that organisms requiring arginine, hypoxanthine, proline, and uracil (AHPU) are more likely to disseminate.
4. Some strains have **resistance to the bactericidal effects** of human serum.
5. **Antibiotic resistance** may be mediated by plasmids or chromosomal-mediated mutations.

31. What host factors enhance susceptibility?
1. High-risk sexual practices (i.e., multiple partners and prostitutes).
2. Local environment of the cervix (i.e., changes in pH that occur during menstruation).

3. Congenital or acquired complement deficiencies, especially of C6–C8, predispose to recurrent *Neisseria* infections. The interaction between the neisserial organism and the complement system is critical to eradicating it from the blood stream.
PEARL: Always measure the serum 50% hemolytic complement (CH50) level in a patient with recurrent neisserial infections. If it is 0, work up the patient for complement deficiency.
4. Asplenia or reticuloendothelial dysfunction such as may occur in SLE and sickle cell anemia patients.

32. What patterns of arthritis are associated with gonorrhea?

Migratory polyarthralgia	70%
Tenosynovitis	67%
Purulent arthritis	42%
Monoarthritis	32%
Polyarthritis	10%

An important diagnostic clue is **tenosynovitis**. It most commonly affects the dorsum of the wrists, fingers, toes, and ankles. The pain is often out of proportion to what is seen on physical examination. Patients should also be examined for meningitis and endocarditis.

33. Apart from articular complaints, what other symptoms are associated with DGI?
The clinical manifestations have been classified into two stages:
- **Bacteremic stage:** polyarthralgias (migratory or additive), tenosynovitis, fever (60%), and **dermatitis** (75%) (Figure 38-1). Classically, the dermatitis is maculopapular or vesicular. The lesions may or may not be symptomatic and occur on the trunk and extremities. However pustules, hemorrhagic bullae, vasculitis, and erythema multiforme may be seen. At this stage, blood cultures may be positive but synovial fluid cultures are negative. This stage lasts 48 to 72 hours.
- **Suppurative stage:** About 50% of patients will develop a septic arthritis. It is usually monoarticular but can involve more than one joint. The knee is most commonly involved followed by the wrist, ankle, and elbow. Unlike other causes of septic arthritis, the small joints of the hand are frequently involved. At this stage, synovial fluid cultures can be positive but blood cultures are negative. Notably, patients can present with this septic arthritis without having previous symptoms of the bacteremic stage.

It is important to note that only 25% of patients with a DGI have **genitourinary symptoms** (i.e., pelvic inflammatory disease [PID]) consistent with a localized gonorrhea infection. Therefore, lack of symptoms of PID either in the past or present does not rule out a DGI.

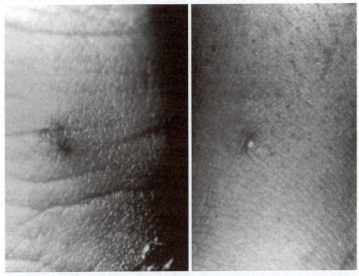

Figure 38-1. The vesicle and pustular rash of disseminated gonococcal infection (DGI). *(Copyright 2014 American College of Rheumatology. Used with permission.)*

34. How useful are cultures and Gram stains in diagnosing gonococcal septic arthritis?
Unlike nongonococcal arthritis, in gonococcal arthritis the Gram stains of synovial fluid are positive in less than 25% of cases. Cultures improve the diagnostic yield. Because urethritis is often asymptomatic, appropriate smears and urethral cultures should always be obtained. Urethral smears and cultures are more useful in men (>90% sensitivity) than in women (Table 38-6).

Table 38-6. Culture Positivity in Disseminated Gonococcal Infection (DGI)

SITE	ISOLATION RATE
Genitourinary	80%
Synovial fluid	25-70%
Rectum	20%
Pharynx	10%
Blood	5-10%
Skin	Rare

PEARL: Specimens should be collected with dacron or rayon swabs because calcium alginate is toxic to gonococci. Additionally, specimens obtained from contaminated sites (genitourinary tract, pharynx, and rectum) should be cultured on Thayer–Martin media. Specimens from noncontaminated areas (synovial fluid and blood) should be cultured on chocolate agar. Always use culture plates that have been warmed to body temperature and plate specimens immediately, often at the bedside. This is because the neisserial organism causing DGI can be killed by vancomycin in Thayer–Martin media and cold temperatures.

35. Are other laboratory tests helpful in DGI?

Much like nongonococcal septic arthritis, in DGI leukocytosis and elevated sedimentation rates are common but nonspecific. Synovial fluid WBC counts range from 34,000 to 68,000 cells/mm^3 with a mean of 50,000/mm^3. Nucleic acid hybridization/amplification tests (NAATs) can detect *N. gonorrhoeae* DNA in culture-negative synovial fluid as well as other sites (urine, endocervical, vaginal, urethra in men).

36. How are DGIs treated?

In the past, a dramatic improvement on administration of penicillin was believed to be diagnostic of a DGI. However, with the emergence of antibiotic-resistant strains (penicillin and quinolones), the initial drug of choice for gonorrhea has changed:

Local (cervicitis)   **Ceftriaxone**, 250 mg IM × 1 dose (or cefixime 400 mg orally × 1 dose), followed by **doxycycline**, 100 mg orally twice daily for 7 days (or azithromycin 1 g × 1 dose).

DGI   **Ceftriaxone**, 1 g IM or IV per day until signs and symptoms have become much improved, which may take 7 to 10 days, followed by daily outpatient therapy with **cefixime** 400 mg orally two times daily for an additional week.

Alternative antibiotics can be used depending on sensitivities and local policy.

If the patient is allergic to cephalosporins, spectinomycin (2 g IM every 12 hours) can be used if available. If not available, consult your infectious disease specialist. Skin testing for cephalosporin allergy may be indicated. If the strain is not resistant to penicillin, parental penicillin or amoxicillin (1 g IV every 8 hours) may be used. Repeated joint aspirations are necessary until the synovial fluid WBC count decreases to a low level.

Patients and their partners should also receive empiric treatment for coexistent and/or silent *Chlamydia* infections (doxycycline, 100 mg orally twice daily for 7 days or azithromycin 1 g × 1 dose, especially if the patient is pregnant). Patients should also be tested for syphilis (using the Venereal Disease Research Laboratory [VDRL] test) and HIV.

37. Can *N. meningitidis* cause a septic arthritis?

Acute meningococcemia can cause arthralgias in up to 40% of cases. An acute purulent arthritis can later follow in a minority of cases (2% to 10%). It usually involves the knee. Only 25% of patients have an associated meningitis. Many will have an associated maculopapular rash. Synovial fluid cultures are positive in 20% and should be kept for 7 days instead of the usual 3 days. Polymerase chain reaction (PCR) testing of synovial fluid may be useful if cultures are negative and suspicion is high. Most patients respond well to antibiotics (third-generation cephalosporin) and joint drainage.

38. Can syphilis cause arthritis?

Secondary syphilis due to *Treponema pallidum* can cause a polyarthritis that can be confused with multiple other connective tissue diseases such as SLE, RA, vasculitis, sarcoidosis, and spondyloarthropathies. One should suspect syphilis in patients with polyarthritis who have a maculopapular rash on their palms and soles (75% to 100%), generalized lymphadenopathy (75%), headache (50%), fever (50%), sore throat (33%), mucosal ulcers, and condyloma lata. The arthritis is symmetric and involves the knees and ankles more than the small joints of the hands. Tenosynovitis may be present. Synovial fluid cell counts range from 4000 to 13,000/mm^3. Spirochetes cannot be seen in the fluid on dark field exam or cultured. Diagnosis is made by syphilis serologies (fluorescent treponemal antibody-absorption, FTA-ABS) and clinical presentation. The treatment is penicillin. Concomitant HIV infection should be ruled out.

39. Can bursae become infected?

The olecranon (adults) and prepatellar (children) bursae are the most common sites of septic bursitis. Most septic bursitis occurs in patients who constantly traumatize the skin in these areas (carpenters, laborers). Alcoholism, diabetes, and preexisting bursal disease are also risk factors. More than 50% also have a surrounding cellulitis and a few patients may get a noninflammatory sympathetic joint effusion of the underlying joint. Over 80% of septic bursitis is due to *S. aureus*. Blood cultures are rarely positive because the organisms get into the bursa by transcutaneous spread through skin abrasions. Patients usually have abrupt onset of pain, swelling, and erythema. Diagnosis is made by aspiration, Gram stain, and culture of bursal fluid. Bursal fluid cell counts are elevated but not as much as in septic joints. Antibiotics should be administered intravenously initially and the bursa aspirated repeatedly or incised and drained. This is especially important for febrile patients or those who are immunocompromised. After control of the infection, oral antibiotics are taken for an additional 2 to 3 weeks. Failure to respond is an indication for bursectomy.

40. What is the difference between acute and chronic osteomyelitis?

Acute osteomyelitis occurs predominantly in children. Over half occur in children less than age 5 years. It is usually due to *S. aureus* (90%), which seeds the metaphysis of long bones by hematogenous spread. Patients typically present within a few days with fever, pain, and decreased range of motion of the involved bone/joint. Laboratory tests show leukocytosis and elevations of ESR/CRP. Blood cultures are positive in 50%. Radiographs are frequently normal for the first 2 to 3 weeks. Focal osteopenia and a periosteal reaction is seen in 90% by 1 month. Indium-111-labeled leukocyte scan (90%) or MRI (100%) are abnormal at an early stage. Bone scans may be difficult to interpret as a result of growth plate activity in children. Treatment is with appropriate antibiotics for 4 to 6 weeks.

Chronic osteomyelitis usually occurs in adults secondary to an open wound or fracture. Vertebral osteomyelitis as a result of hematogenous spread and spine surgery is also seen. Localized bone pain, erythema, and draining sinus tract are typically present. Radiographic changes are seen 2 to 3 weeks after the onset of infection and reveal osteolysis, periosteal reaction, and sequestra. Bone scan, indium scan, CT scan, MRI, and PET scans are abnormal. A specific bacterial diagnosis is made by bone biopsy, which is essential. Culture of the sinus tract is not reliable. *S. aureus* is the most common organism, but gram-negative bacteria are also isolated, especially if the chronic osteomyelitis occurs as a result of trauma. Therapy includes antibiotics for 6 weeks and debridement of bone.

41. What is the difference between a sequestra and Brodie's abscess?

- Sequestra—segments of necrotic bone that are separated from living bone by granulation tissue; must be removed by debridement, owing to the inability of antibiotics to sterilize them.
- Brodie's abscess—a bone abscess found during the chronic stage of hematogenous osteomyelitis; it usually has a sclerotic margin on radiography.

BIBLIOGRAPHY

Chihara S, Segreti J: Osteomyelitis, Dis Mon 56:5–31, 2010.
Del Pozo JL, Patel R: Infection associated with prosthetic joints, N Engl J Med 361:787–794, 2009.
Gutierrez K: Bone and joint infections in children, Pediatr Clin North Am 52:779–794, 2005.
Hanrahan JA: Recent developments in septic bursitis, Curr Infect Dis Rep 15:421–425, 2013.
Hariharan P, Kabrhel C: Sensitivity of erythrocyte sedimentation rate and C-reactive protein for the exclusion of septic arthritis in emergency department patients, J Emerg Med 40:428, 2011.
Manadan AM, Block JA: Daily needle aspiration versus surgical lavage for the treatment of bacterial septic arthritis in adults, Am J Ther 11:412–415, 2004.
Margaretten ME, Knowles J, Moore D, et al: Does this adult patient have septic arthritis ? JAMA 297:1478–1488, 2007.
Mathews CJ, Kingsley G, Field M, et al: Management of septic arthritis: a systematic review, Ann Rheum Dis 66:440–445, 2007.
Mathews CJ, Weston VC, Jones A, et al: Bacterial septic arthritis in adults, Lancet 375:846–855, 2010.
Palestro CJ, Love C, Miller TT: Diagnostic imaging tests and microbial infections, Cell Microbiol 9:2323–2333, 2007.
Ravindran V, Logan I, Bourke BE: Medical vs surgical treatment for native joint in septic arthritis: a 6-year, single UK academic centre experience, Rheumatology 48:1320–1322, 2009.
Rice PA: Gonococcal arthritis, Infect Dis Clin North Am 19:853–861, 2005.
Ross JJ, Shamsuddin H: Sternoclavicular septic arthritis: review of 180 cases, Medicine (Baltimore) 83:139, 2004.
Singleton JD, West SG, Nordstrom DM: "Pseudoseptic" arthritis complicating rheumatoid arthritis: a report of 6 cases, J Rheumatol 18:1319, 1991.
Zimmerli W: Clinical practice: vertebral osteomyelitis, N Engl J Med 362:1022–1029, 2010.
Zimmerli W: Infection and musculoskeletal conditions: prosthetic-joint-associated infections, Best Pract Res Clin Rheumatol 20:1045–1063, 2006.

FURTHER READING

www.cdc.gov/std/treatment/2010/gonococcal-infections.htm

CHAPTER 39

LYME DISEASE
John K. Jenkins, MD

KEY POINTS

1. Lyme disease is the most common vector-borne disease with peak onset during spring and summer months.
2. Erythema chronicum migrans (ECM) is the diagnostic skin lesion that occurs at the site of the tick bite.
3. Disseminated infection can affect the heart, nervous system, and joints.
4. Diagnosis is confirmed by a positive immunoglobulin G (IgG) Western blot for *Borrelia burgdorferi* in the serum of a patient with appropriate clinical findings.
5. Oral antibiotics are effective for prevention and early disease but intravenous antibiotics are necessary for disseminated disease.
6. Coinfection with *Babesia* or *Anaplasma* in any patient with hemolysis, neutropenia, and/or thromboctopenia should be considered.

1. How was Lyme disease recognized as a distinct clinical entity?
Lyme disease was first recognized as a distinct entity in Old Lyme, Connecticut, in 1975. A neighborhood outbreak of juvenile rheumatoid (idiopathic) arthritis (JIA) was reported to the state public health department by the mothers of the affected children because they believed the neighborhood clustering to be more than coincidence. The outbreak in this rural community was consistent with an infectious etiology transmitted by an arthropod vector. To put things in perspective, Lyme disease is the most common vector-borne disease in the United States and Europe and the second most common in the world (malaria being the most common).

2. What is the etiology of Lyme disease?
Lyme disease in the United States is caused by an infection with the tick-borne spirochete, *B. burgdorferi*, which was discovered in 1982. Only three species within the genus *B. burgdorferi sensu lato* cause infection in humans. Only one of these three pathogenic species (*B. burgdorferi sensu stricto*) occurs in North America, whereas the other two occur in Asia (*Borrelia garinii*, *Borrelia afzelii*) and all three occur in Europe. There are many similarities to syphilis; it is a multisystem disease that occurs in stages that can mimic other diseases. *Borrelia* can only rarely be cultured from the blood or other infected tissues, and the incubation period is 3 to 32 days. Because *Borrelia* is rarely found in tissues, the pathogenesis of Lyme disease manifestations is felt to be the result of the host's inflammatory response to the spirochete.

3. What is the geographic distribution and seasonal occurrence of Lyme disease in the United States? In what other countries has it been reported?
Lyme disease is tick-borne and is most prevalent from April or May to November in the endemic areas. The peak incidence is in late spring and the early summer months of June and July. Lyme disease has been reported in many of the 48 contiguous states, but most cases occur in three regions:
- The northeast coast, between Maine and Maryland
- The midwest, in Wisconsin and Minnesota
- Along the western coast of northern California and Oregon

The disease also occurs in Europe (highest in Slovenia, Austria), Scandinavia (Sweden), China, Asia, Japan, and Australia.

4. Name the arthropod vector of *B. burgdorferi* and its animal hosts. Describe how Lyme disease is transmitted.
Ixodes scapularis (previously called *Ixodes dammini*) was the tick first described to carry the causative organism and is the vector in the northeast and midwest United States. Up to 50% of adult ticks are infected in endemic areas. *Ixodes pacificus* is the vector on the west coast, and its preferential host is the lizard, which is not a very good reservoir for *Borrelia*. Other *Ixodid* species are the vectors in other parts of the world: *Ixodes ricinus* in Europe, where Lyme disease is common, and *Ixodes persculatus* in the former Soviet Union and Asia. Small and large mammals are generally the preferred hosts.

The *I. scapularis* egg mass is laid in the leaf clutter at the bottom of the forest (consequently, this tick does not exist in dry climates). Larvae emerge in the summer and fall. They require a blood meal that they get from the white-footed mouse, which is an asymptomatic reservoir for *Borrelia*. The tick larvae acquire *Borrelia* with their blood meal, fall off the mouse, and molt to nymphs that lay dormant until late spring and summer of the following year. At that time the nymphs emerge again to get a blood meal (and *Borrelia*) from the white-footed mouse. Infected nymphs can pass *Borrelia* on to other mice and humans when they take a blood meal. Later the nymphs become adults and the females feed on white-tailed deer (in the region of their shoulder, hence *I. scapularis*) to get blood nutrients to make eggs. The eggs are laid in leaf clutter. The eggs are not infected with *Borrelia* even if the female tick is. The deer does not remain infected with *Borrelia*. After the eggs are laid, the 2-year life cycle starts over again.

Borrelia infection occurs through the bite of the *Ixodid* tick, an event remembered by only half of patients with Lyme disease—a key point to remember when taking a history. The tick is also very small (the size of a freckle) and often simply overlooked. The intestinal tract of the tick is the reservoir for *Borrelia*. The tick has a slow, extended feeding cycle, and hours after feeding it regurgitates transmitting *Borrelia* to the animal host. Other ticks have been shown to harbor *Borrelia*, including the Lone Star tick (*Amblyomma americanum*) and the American dog tick (*Dermacentor variabilis*). In the southern United States, an ECM-like rash and flu-like symptoms, called Southern tick-associated rash illness (STARI), are caused by the bite of the Lone Star tick infected with *Borrelia lonestari*.

5. **What organ systems are involved in Lyme disease?**
The disease is frequently thought of as a "rash-arthritis" complex, even though the arthritis may be a late manifestation. Not all patients have rash or arthritis. In addition, the nervous system (both central and peripheral) and cardiac system may be involved. In the United States, a patient infected with *B. burgdorferi* who develops the typical skin rash, ECM, and who is *not treated* with antibiotics has a 1% to 5% chance of developing cardiac manifestations, a 15% chance of developing neurologic manifestations, and a 70% chance of developing arthritis (60% migratory polyarthritis, 10% chronic monoarthritis). In Europe, where all three strains of *Borrelia* can cause infection, arthritis is less common (15%) but meningoradiculoneuritis as a result of *B. garinii* is more common.

6. **Describe the typical rash of Lyme disease.**
In 80% to 90% of patients with Lyme borreliosis in the United States (60% in Europe), the disease begins with ECM, which usually occurs at the site of the tick bite. The ticks are attracted to warm, carbon dioxide-exhaling animals. The ticks prefer warm and moist areas to dine. Consequently, ECM is frequently found behind the knee or in the groin, beltline, or axilla. ECM begins as a red macule or papule that expands to form **a large annular lesion** 20 cm or more in diameter with **partial central clearing** and a bright red outer border (Figure 39-1). Atypical skin lesions can be seen and include diffuse erythema, urticaria, evanescent rashes, and a malar rash.

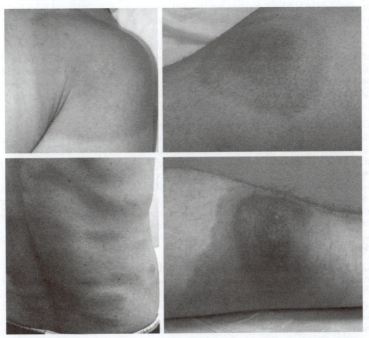

Figure 39-1. The lesions of erythema chronicum migrans (ECM). (*Courtesy Juan Salazar, MD, University of Connecticut Health Center.*)

7. **What are the stages of Lyme disease, their temporal relation, and which organ systems are involved in each stage?**
   Lyme disease has three stages:
   - Early localized ECM—skin (ECM), regional lymphadenopathy, flu-like symptoms
   - Disseminated infection—nervous and cardiac systems, skin and musculoskeletal (but potentially any organ) system
   - Persistent infection (late disease)—musculoskeletal and nervous systems

   After the incubation period (mean 7 to 10 days), the first stage of Lyme disease or ECM occurs. Regional lymphadenopathy (25%) may occur, leading to confusion with tularemia. "Flu-like" symptoms such as headache, fatigue, arthralgias, and fever (15%) may occur, but ECM usually fades in several days to a few weeks. The second stage, or disseminated infection, may begin within days to 10 months after ECM occurs and is the result of hematogenous spread. The third stage occurs an average of 6 months after disease onset but may occur as soon as 2 weeks or as late as 2 years after disease onset.

8. **What clinical manifestations occur in the second stage (disseminated infection) of Lyme disease?**
   Characteristically, the central nervous system (CNS) is involved. Approximately 10% develop neurologic symptoms 1 to 2 weeks into the disease. Cranial nerve palsy (especially unilateral or bilateral Bell's palsy) and meningitis are most common. A motor or sensory radiculoneuritis, subtle encephalitis with cognitive dysfunction, mononeuritis multiplex, myelitis, chorea, and cerebellar ataxia can also occur. Cardiac manifestations occur in less than 3% of untreated patients during the second stage and include varying degrees of atrioventricular (AV) block (usually temporary) and myo- or pancarditis. The heart valves are not involved, distinguishing it from acute rheumatic fever. Secondary (satellite) skin lesions are common (50%) and indicate spirochetal dissemination. Lymphadenopathy, splenomegaly, mild hepatitis, sensorineural hearing loss, iritis/keratitis, and severe fatigue can occur. Migratory arthralgias, bursitis, and tendon involvement are common and transient. Frank arthritis is usually not prevalent until the third stage.

9. **Describe the clinical manifestations of the third stage (late disease) of Lyme disease.**
   The third stage of Lyme disease occurs in 10% of untreated patients and represents persistent infection as a result of *B. burgdorferi*, which has mechanisms that enable it to evade the immune system. This stage usually involves episodic attacks of an asymmetric oligoarticular arthritis affecting the large joints (the knee 80% of the time). Other large joints can be involved whereas small joints are rarely affected. Over time, the arthritic attacks typically resolve. In less than 10% of patients, the arthritis becomes more persistent and chronic, usually affecting the knee. Fatigue frequently accompanies the arthritis episodes, but in general fever and other systemic symptoms do not. Serologies (rheumatoid factor [RF], antinuclear antibody [ANA], anticyclic citrullinated peptides [anti-CCP], human leukocyte antigen-B27 [HLA-B27]) are typically negative. Synovial fluid is inflammatory (average WBC 25,000/mm^3 with neutrophil predominance).

   Chronic nervous system involvement may occur in the third stage but is rare. Manifestations include an encephalomyelitis (in Europe, usually owing to *B. garinii*), a mild sensorimotor neuropathy in a "stocking and glove" distribution, or an encephalopathy (affecting memory, mood, and sleep). Finally, a late skin lesion, *acrodermatitis chronica atrophicans*, can occur. It is most commonly seen in Europe and is the result of *B. afzelii* infection. It manifests as a blue/red area of the skin with swelling that may lead to skin atrophy, wrinkling, and protruding veins. Thickened patches of skin called morphea may also rarely occur in this stage.

10. **How is ECM treated in adults and children over 8 years old?**
    When treating ECM, the physician needs to make sure that no other systemic manifestations suggesting disseminated infection are present (i.e., neurologic or cardiac). If none are present, oral antibiotics are adequate when given for 14 to 21 days for early Lyme disease. In general, *Borrelia* species are less sensitive to penicillin by in vitro testing than to amoxicillin, doxycycline, and second- and third-generation cephalosporins. The drugs of choice are doxycycline (100 mg bid in adults; 4 mg/kg/day in two divided doses [max 100 mg/dose] in children > 8 years) or amoxicillin (500 mg tid in adults; 50 mg/kg/day in three divided doses [max 500 mg/dose] in children > 8 years). In the case of penicillin allergy, cefuroxime (500 mg bid in adults; 30 mg/kg/day in two divided doses [max 500 mg/dose] in children > 8 years) or erythromycin (500 mg qid in adults; 12.5 mg/kg qid [max 500 mg/dose] in children > 8 years) may be used. Erythromycin may be less effective clinically. Overall, antibiotics cure more than 90% of patients with ECM.

11. **How is ECM treated in young children and pregnant women?**
    Doxycycline should be avoided in children less than 8 years old and pregnant women, owing to its effect on developing teeth. For children less than 8 years old, amoxicillin, 50 mg/kg/day in three divided doses (up to 250 mg tid), and for pregnant women, amoxicillin 500 mg tid for 14 to 21 days, are recommended. If allergic to penicillin, cefuroxime 30 mg/kg/day in two divided doses (up to 125 mg bid) or erythromycin 30 mg/kg/day in three divided doses (up to 250 mg tid) for children less than age 8 years and cefuroxime (500 mg bid) or erythromycin (500 mg qid) for pregnant women for 14 to 21 days is used. Maternal–fetal transmission of *B. burgdorferi* is very rare and does not harm the fetus.

12. **What diagnostic tests are available for Lyme disease?**
In addition to clinical diagnosis (tick bite in an endemic area followed by ECM and arthritis), serologic testing by enzyme-linked immunosorbent assay (ELISA) is commonly used. Detection of diagnostic levels of antibodies to B. burgdorferi is done by a two-tiered approach of ELISA/indirect immunofluorescence assay for screening followed by Western blot testing for confirmation in a reference laboratory and interpreted according to Centers for Disease Control (CDC) criteria.

Serodiagnostic tests are unreliable within the first month of disease onset. Therefore, patients with obvious ECM should be treated without serologic testing. Within 2 to 4 weeks, 70% to 80% of patients are IgM-positive by ELISA. IgM antibodies peak at 6 to 8 weeks. IgG antibodies by ELISA are positive after 4 weeks and peak at 4 to 6 months after infection. Therefore, in a person with acute disease (without classic ECM lesions) of less than 1 month's duration, IgM and IgG antibody responses should be measured in both acute and convalescent sera. The height of the titer does not indicate more severe disease activity. Both IgM and especially IgG antibodies can remain positive for years after successful therapy with antibiotics. Therefore, persistent IgM antibodies do not indicate active or inadequately treated infection. In addition, many individuals (7%) in an endemic area who have never had clinical disease or treatment can be positive for these antibodies, presumably indicating they had subclinical infections that their own immune system eradicated without the help of antibiotics.

The second test of the two-tiered approach is Western blot analysis, which can be used to detect antibodies to the various specific *Borrelia* proteins in a patient's serum and may discriminate between cross-reacting antibodies from other sources and those directed toward *Borrelia* proteins. Western blot analysis is more specific but not more sensitive than ELISA for diagnosing Lyme disease. Therefore, it is not used for screening owing to its cost. It is used to confirm all indeterminate or positive ELISA results. A positive result in the right clinical setting is strong evidence for infection whereas a negative result is strong evidence against an infection. Both IgM and IgG Western blots are performed. Within the first month of symptoms, the IgM Western blot may be the only positive one. *After the first month of infection, only the IgG Western blot is used to support the diagnosis. If after the first month of infection only the IgM Western blot is positive and not the IgG blot, then the IgM blot is likely to be a false-positive result.* Western blot positivity is interpreted as follows:
- the IgM Western blot is positive if at least two of the following three bands are present (first month of infection): 23 (OspC), 39 (BmpA), or 41 (Fla) kDa.
- the IgG Western blot is positive if five of the following 10 bands are positive (after the first month of infection): 18, 21, 28, 30, 39, 41, 45, 58, 66, or 93 kDa.

The sensitivity of two-tiered testing is 30% to 40% in ECM during the acute phase, up to 78% in ECM during the convalescent phase, and 95% in patients with later stages of disease. Recently, an ELISA that uses a highly conserved region of the variable protein-like sequence expressed (VlsE) protein has been developed. This is called a C6 peptide ELISA and has high sensitivity and specificity for Lyme disease in all stages but should also be confirmed with Western blot analysis. Finally, in cases of neuroborreliosis, the ratio of cerebrospinal fluid (CSF) to serum IgG antibodies to *Borrelia* can prove intrathecal antibody production.

The gold standard is culture of B. burgdorferi in Barbour–Stoenner–Kelly medium from ECM lesions in early disease. Tissue cultures are uniformly negative late in disease and polymerase chain reaction (PCR) analysis of bodily fluids and tissue is a better (although not Food and Drug Administration [FDA]-approved) test. PCR can detect B. burgdorferi DNA in skin, spinal (40% sensitivity) and synovial fluid (85% sensitivity), and synovial tissue. However, a positive PCR result from any bodily fluid is always a false positive in a patient with a negative serodiagnostic test (ELISA/Western blot). The Lyme urine antigen test is of no value.

13. **Name the most common explanations for a false-negative Lyme test.**
Specific antibodies to *Borrelia* may not be present early (within the first month of infection), leading to a false-negative result. Therefore, it is helpful to draw acute and convalescent sera in this case. Additionally, antibiotics, either complete and adequate therapy or partial therapy with residual infection, may halt the immune response and subsequent development of measurable levels of specific antibody if given early in the first stage of Lyme disease.

14. **Why might a false-positive serologic test for Lyme disease occur?**
- In endemic areas, a large percentage (7%) of the population may have had a subclinical infection and be seropositive without acute or chronic illness.
- Adequately treated patients may remain seropositive long after an infection is eradicated.
- Antibodies directed toward other spirochetes may cross-react to the *Borrelia* antigen(s) used in the ELISA. This is particularly likely in a patient with over 1 month of nonspecific symptoms and a positive IgM ELISA but a negative IgG ELISA (patients with true Lyme disease should develop an IgG response). For example, patients with antibodies to syphilis (*Treponema pallidum*) or Rocky Mountain spotted fever or those who recently had a dental procedure that exposed them to spirochetes in the oral cavity (*Treponema denticola*) may have IgM antibodies to these organisms that react positive in the Lyme ELISA. In addition, certain acute viral infections (Epstein–Barr virus [EBV], cytomegalovirus [CMV], parvovirus) and human granulocytic anaplasmosis can give false-positive IgM seroreactivity to B. burgdorferi. Not recognizing a

false-positive result will lead to a patient being treated for Lyme disease while his or her underlying disease goes untreated.
- Interlaboratory variability and lack of standardization of the test may result in both false-positives and false-negatives.

The quality and nonspecificity of Lyme titers suggest that Lyme testing should only be used in a confirmatory manner in patients suspected of having clinical Lyme disease—not in screening patients with multiple vague complaints.

15. **Describe laboratory abnormalities that may be seen in Lyme disease.**
The neurologic manifestations of Lyme disease that occur during the second stage often involve symptoms of meningeal irritation. As one would expect, there may be a mild cellular pleocytosis and elevated protein in the CSF upon spinal tap. This may also occur in late stages of disease with chronic CNS symptoms that are not as suggestive of meningeal involvement. In these patients, a high IgG index and oligoclonal bands may be seen in the CSF. Intrathecal antibodies against *Borrelia* may be positive but PCR testing of CSF has low sensitivity (40%). Cranial magnetic resonance images (MRIs) show focal nodular or patchy white matter lesions consistent with inflammation that resolve with therapy.

During episodes of arthritis, synovial fluid cell counts range from 1000 to 100,000/mm^3 and are predominantly polymorphonuclear leukocytes. PCR can detect *B. burgdorferi* DNA in synovial fluid and synovial tissue. It is more sensitive (85%) than culture and more specific than ELISA but difficult to perform. ANAs and RF are no more prevalent than in the general population.

16. **How should the second (disseminated disease) and third (late disease) stages of Lyme disease be treated?**
In stages 2 and 3, intravenous antibiotics are generally indicated. For neurologic manifestations or a high degree of AV block, ceftriaxone (2 g IV daily for 2 to 4 weeks) or cefotaxime (2 g IV every 8 hours for 2 to 4 weeks) is commonly used. In children, ceftriaxone (50 to 75 mg/kg/day IV with max of 2 g/day) or cefotaxime (150 mg/kg/day IV in three to four divided doses with max 6 g/day) is used. Mild neurologic (Bell's palsy alone) or cardiac (first-degree AV block with a PR interval of less than 0.3 seconds) disease may be treated with oral antibiotics as outlined in the treatment for ECM above, but therapy should be for 3 to 4 weeks.

For stage 3 with chronic arthritis, oral antibiotics may be used for 30 to 60 days if there is arthritis *without neurologic manifestations*: doxycycline (100 mg PO bid) or amoxicillin (500 mg PO tid). Some physicians prefer the IV regimens for chronic Lyme arthritis. Other IV regimens include penicillin G (20 million U, six divided doses) for 2 to 4 weeks. Late neurologic manifestations, which may occur after adequate treatment of arthritis with oral agents, definitely require IV antibiotics as outlined above for stage 2. Some consider ceftriaxone the drug of choice for any form of late Lyme disease, although oral doxycycline or amoxicillin for 1 month has been shown to work very well in arthritis. Note that 15% of patients may experience a Jarisch–Herxheimer reaction within 24 to 48 hours of starting antibiotics.

17. **Why does chronic Lyme arthritis not respond well to antibiotic treatment? What other therapy is available?**
Up to 10% of chronic Lyme arthritis is antibiotic refractory. This may be the result of persistent infection or a chronic immune process resulting from the infection rather than persistent infection itself. Supportive evidence for this hypothesis is that there appears to be a genetic predisposition to the development of chronic arthritis in patients with particular class II major histocompatibility complex (MHC) genes (human leucocyte antigen [HLA]-DR4 and -DR2 alleles). The HLA-DRB molecules that comprise these alleles can bind an epitope of *B. burgdorferi* outer surface protein A (OSPA$_{163-175}$). Patients with antibiotic-refractory arthritis have T cell recognition of this epitope.

A rational approach is to treat chronic Lyme arthritis with 1 month of oral antibiotics. If there is some response and the arthritis is mildly persistent at the end of that month, then retreatment for an additional month of oral antibiotics is recommended. If the persistent arthritis is more severe, then the second month of treatment should be with IV antibiotics. If the arthritis persists after 2 months of antibiotics, then the synovial fluid should be analyzed by PCR for *B. burgdorferi* DNA. If the PCR is positive, the patient should receive a third month of IV antibiotics. If the PCR is negative, the patient should be treated with nonsteroidal antiinflammatory drugs (NSAIDs). Intraarticular corticosteroids are rarely used. In the uncommon patient who fails to respond to the above therapy, hydroxychloroquine (200 mg BID) or methotrexate should be tried. Most patients will resolve their arthritis within 4 to 5 years. If the arthritis fails to resolve, then the patient should be offered arthroscopic synovectomy, which is usually curative in 50%. Patients who refuse or are not candidates for synovectomy have been treated with infliximab therapy.

18. **How can Lyme disease be prevented?**
Good tick bite prevention is, of course, necessary in endemic areas. Clothing that completely covers the body, for example, shirts and pants legs tucked in, should be worn. Light-colored clothing allows detection and removal of ticks. Tick repellent should be used. There are no published recommendations on the use of antibiotics for tick bites once they occur, but a physician should use antimicrobial agents judiciously in this setting. Oral antibiotics (one dose of doxycycline 200 mg) are commonly used in endemic areas although one study in

an endemic area suggested that the chance of developing an adverse reaction to oral antibiotics for tick bites was as high as the likelihood of developing Lyme disease from the untreated bite. In nonendemic areas where most of the ticks probably do not harbor *Borrelia*, the prudent thing to do is remove ticks promptly (it takes several hours to engorge and then regurgitate *Borrelia*), have an appropriate index of suspicion, and recognize and treat disease in its early stages with appropriate antimicrobials.

DIFFICULT CLINICAL SITUATIONS

19. **A patient reports that she has had diffuse arthralgias/myalgias for many months and has a diagnosis of fibromyalgia. She reports that she used to visit New York, although never went camping or hiking. Her physician ordered a Lyme test, and the IgM ELISA returned positive. Should she get antibiotics?**
No. The ELISA tests give many false positives. The IgM Western immunoblots can also give false-positive results and are useful only in the first few weeks of an infection. Patients with symptoms for greater than 1 to 2 months who have a negative IgG ELISA and/or IgG Western blot do not have Lyme disease. In other words, IgG seropositivity is virtually universal in late Lyme disease.

20. **A patient with a history of definite Lyme disease in the past has been treated with two courses of appropriate IV antibiotics for 1 month each time. She has persistent myalgias and has been diagnosed with fibromyalgia. Should she receive another course of therapy with a different antibiotic?**
No. Posttreatment Lyme disease syndrome (PLDS) occurs in 15% to 25% of patients (especially those with a history of neurologic involvement) but does not respond to antibiotics. Patient symptoms resemble fibromyalgia/chronic fatigue syndrome with subjective cognitive and memory difficulty, widespread pain, sleep disturbance, and fatigue. The symptoms start within 6 months of Lyme disease onset and persist for over 6 months. The pathophysiology of these symptoms is unclear but has been reported in other postinfectious illnesses such as West Nile encephalitis. They usually have normal cranial MRIs, brain positron emission tomography (PET) scans, and functional MRIs, although up to 50% have nonspecific abnormalities. In these patients, there is little evidence to support a persistent CNS infection with *Borrelia* following adequate antibiotic treatment as evidenced by normal CSF studies including cell count, protein, PCR for *Borrelia* DNA, negative antibodies against B. burgdorferi, normal IgG index, and negative oligoclonal bands. Additionally, it should be noted that both IgM and IgG antibodies to *Borrelia* may persist in the serum for years after therapy and do not indicate persistent infection. Therefore, the patient with PLDS should not be treated with prolonged IV antibiotics but rather receive standard treatment for fibromyalgia. Over time most patients improve.

21. **A mother brings her child for examination and reports that he was bitten by a tick the previous day. The tick was not engorged. Should the child receive antibiotics prophylactically?**
Controversial. The risk of contracting Lyme disease is 1% to 3% if the tick has not been attached for 48 hours or not engorged. The bite site should be observed for the development of ECM and the child treated if ECM develops. A patient claiming a bite within 72 hours by an engorged tick in an endemic area should receive prophylactic antibiotics (doxycycline 200 mg, one dose) because the risk of infection is 25% and can be prevented (87% efficacy) with prophylactic antibiotics.

22. **An adult is referred to you for a positive IgG ELISA and Western blot test for exposure to *B. burgdorferi*. The test was obtained by his primary care physician as part of an annual physical examination because the patient frequently hikes and camps in an area with known Lyme disease. He has never had symptoms of Lyme disease and is asymptomatic. Do you treat him with antibiotics?**
Controversial. Treatment of seropositive asymptomatic patients is debated. Some argue that a 1-month course of oral antibiotics (doxycycline or amoxicillin) is indicated to assure eradication of the spirochete, much like what would be done in an asymptomatic patient found to have a positive fluorescent treponemal antibody-absorption (FTA-ABS) for syphilis. Others argue that the patient had a subclinical infection and the patient's immune system has already eradicated the *Borrelia*.

23. **How can you tell if a patient has been infected with other *Ixodes*-transmitted pathogens in addition to *B. burgdorferi*?**
I. scapularis can transmit other parasites at the time it transmits B. burgdorferi. The two most common are *Babesia microti* (babesiosis) and *Anaplasma phagocytophilum* (human granulocytic anaplasmosis). **Any patients with suspected Lyme disease who have leukopenia or thrombocytopenia should be investigated for coinfection with one of these pathogens.**
Babesiosis causes hemolysis, thrombocytopenia, and elevated liver-associated enzymes. Intraerythrocytic organisms may be seen on peripheral blood smear. Treatment requires therapy with atovaquone (Mepron) plus azithromycin or IV clindamycin plus oral quinine for 7 to 10 days. *Human granulocytic anaplasmosis* causes fever, headache, arthralgias, leukopenia, and thrombocytopenia. If it is misdiagnosed as Lyme disease, it still responds to doxycycline but not to amoxicillin therapy. Treatment includes doxycycline (100 mg bid) for 10 days. Patients allergic to or unable to take doxycycline (pregnant women, children < 8 years old) should be treated with rifampin (300 mg bid for adults; 10 mg/kg twice a day for children) for 10 days.

Bibliography

American College of Physicians: Guidelines for laboratory evaluation in the diagnosis of Lyme disease, Ann Int Med 127:1106–1108, 1997.
Cerar D, Cerar T, Ruzic-Sabljic E, et al: Subjective symptoms after treatment of early Lyme disease, Am J Med 123:79–86, 2010.
Costello CM, Steere AC, Pinkerton RE, et al: Prospective study of tick bites in an endemic area for Lyme disease, J Infect Dis 159:136–139, 1989.
Ginsberg HS: Transmission of risk of Lyme disease and implications for tick management, Am J Epidemiol 138:65–73, 1993.
Girschick HJ, Morbach H, Tappe D: Treatment of lyme borrellosis, Arth Res Ther 11:258, 2009.
Hu LT: In the clinic. Lyme disease, Ann Int Med 157, 2012. ITC-2-ITC2-16.
Klempner MS, Hu LT, Evans J, et al: Two controlled trials of antibiotic treatment in patients with persistent symptoms and a history of Lyme disease, N Engl J Med 345:85–92, 2001.
Lightfoot RW, Luft BJ, Rahn DW, et al: Empiric parental antibiotic treatment of patients with fibromyalgia and fatigue and a positive serologic result for Lyme disease: a cost effective analysis, Ann Intern Med 119:503–509, 1993.
Magid D, Schwartz B, Craft J, et al: Prevention of Lyme disease after tick bite: a cost-effective analysis, N Engl J Med 327:534, 1992.
Mitchell P, Reed KD, Hofkes JM: Immunoserologic evidence of coinfection with Borrelia burgdorferi, Babesia microtic, and human granulocytic *Ehrlichia* species in residents of Wisconsin and Minnesota, J Clin Microbiol 34:724, 1996.
Nadelman RB, Nowakowski J, Fish D, et al: Prophylaxis with single-dose doxycycline for the prevention of Lyme disease after an *Ixodes scapularis* tick bite, N Engl J Med 345:79–84, 2001.
Nocton JJ, Dressler F, Rutledge BJ, et al: Detection of *Borrelia burgdorferi* DNA by polymerase chain reaction in synovial fluid from patients with Lyme arthritis, N Engl J Med 330:229–234, 1994.
O'Connell S: Lyme borreliosis: current issues in diagnosis and management, Curr Opin Infect Dis 23:231–235, 2010.
Sigal LH: The Lyme disease controversy: the social and financial costs of the mismanagement of Lyme disease, Arch Intern Med 156:1493, 1996.
Sood SK, Salzman MB, Johnson BJB, et al: Duration of tick attachment as a predictor of the risk of Lyme disease in an area in which Lyme disease is endemic, J Infect Dis 175:996–999, 1997.
Steere AC, Angelis SM: Therapy for Lyme arthritis: strategies for the treatment of antibiotic-refractory arthritis, Arthritis Rheum 54:3079–3086, 2006.
Steere AC, Dwyer E, Winchester R: Association of chronic Lyme arthritis with HLA-DR4 and HLA-DR2 alleles, N Engl J Med 323:219–223, 1990.
Steere AC, Malawista SE, Snydman DR, et al: An epidemic of oligoarticular arthritis in children and adults in three Connecticut communities, Arthritis Rheum 20:7–17, 1977.
Warshafsky S, Nowakowsky J, Nadelman RB, et al: Efficacy of antibiotic prophylaxis for prevention of Lyme disease, J Gen Intern Med 11:329, 1996.
Wormser GP, Dattwyler R, Shapiro ED, et al: The clinical assessment, treatment, and prevention of Lyme disease, human granulocytic anaplasmosis, and babesiosis: clinical practice guidelines by the Infectious Disease Society of America, Clin Infect Dis 43:1089–1134, 2006.

Further Reading

www.cdc.gov/Lyme
www.lyme.org

MYCOBACTERIAL AND FUNGAL JOINT AND BONE DISEASES

William R. Gilliland, MD, MHPE

KEY POINTS

1. Osteoarticular tuberculosis accounts for 10% of all cases of extrapulmonary disease.
2. Tuberculous and fungal arthritis typically presents insidiously as a chronic monoarthritis affecting the knee.
3. Nontuberculous mycobacterial musculoskeletal infections most commonly present as hand tenosynovitis.
4. Brucellosis caused by ingestion of unpasteurized dairy products usually presents with sacroiliitis and fever.

1. **What percentage of patients with tuberculosis (TB) have bone or joint involvement?**
   The number of cases of *Mycobacterium tuberculosis* (MTB) infection has risen because of its association with human immunodeficiency virus (HIV) infections and the use of immunosuppressant medications. Extrapulmonary disease accounts for 35% of all cases of TB. Approximately **1% to 3%** of all presentations of TB and 10% of all cases of extrapulmonary TB have osteoarticular involvement.

2. **How is TB disseminated to the bones and joints?**
   - Hematogenous spread
   - Lymphatic spread from distant focus
   - Contiguous spread from infected areas

   Although joint involvement may be secondary to hematogenous spread, it usually is secondary to an adjacent osteomyelitis. Therefore, tuberculous arthritis usually comprises a combination of bone and joint involvement.

3. **Who is at risk of osteoarticular TB?**
   - Alcoholics
   - Drug abusers
   - HIV-positive patients
   - Elderly nursing home patients
   - Immigrants from countries where TB is endemic
   - Immunosuppressed patients
   - Patients treated with immunosuppressive therapy including biologics (the risk is greater for TNF antagonists than for other drugs)

   Glucocorticoids at a prednisone dose of ≥10 mg/day significantly increase the risk for all of these patients.

4. **What bones and joints are commonly affected by osteoarticular TB?**
   Spine involvement (Pott disease) accounts for 50% of cases, with the thoracolumbar spine most frequently involved. The disease usually involves the anterior vertebral border and disc, ultimately progressing to disc narrowing, vertebral collapse, and kyphosis (Gibbus deformity). Although TB may affect only the vertebral body, it usually crosses the disc and involves adjacent vertebrae. Complications include paravertebral cold abscesses, spread beneath the anterior longitudinal ligament causing scalloping of anterior vertebral bodies, psoas abscesses, sinus tract formation, and neurologic compromise. Sacroiliac joint involvement accounts for 10% of osteoarticular TB; it is usually unilateral when it occurs and may be misdiagnosed as a spondyloarthropathy.

   Peripheral joint involvement typically occurs in weight-bearing joints, usually the hip, knee, and ankle, and is monoarticular. Subchondral bone involvement may precede cartilage destruction, so joint space narrowing is often a late finding. Adjacent osteomyelitis is very common. It accounts for approximately 30% of all cases of osteoarticular TB.

   Osteomyelitis and **dactylitis** account for 2% to 3% of all osteoarticular TB and may only involve the appendicular skeleton; peripheral involvement depends on the age of the patient. In adults, metaphyseal regions of the long bones, most commonly the femur and tibia, are affected. Ribs and other bones may be involved. In children, the metacarpals and phalanges are more likely to be affected and their involvement resembles dactylitis.

   Tenosynovitis and bursitis occur more commonly in atypical mycobacterial infections.

5. **What are the typical signs and symptoms of osteoarticular TB?**
   Constitutional symptoms (fever, weight loss, malaise) may or may not be present.
   - **Spinal tuberculosis**: Back pain (especially with movement), spasm, local tenderness, kyphosis, cord compression, mycotic aneurysm of aorta

- **Peripheral joints:** Slow-onset chronic monoarthritis
  - Hip: pain in the thigh and groin with a limited range of motion
  - Knee: insidious pain with swelling and a limp (especially in children)
  - Hand/wrist: carpal tunnel syndrome, swelling, pain
- **Osteomyelitis:** Pain and lytic lesions on radiographs without a periosteal reaction
  - Dactylitis (85% of cases occur in children of <6 years of age)

6. What is Poncet disease?
In patients with visceral (usually lymph nodes) or pulmonary TB, an acute polyarthritis (presumably reactive) may develop, accompanied by fever. Tuberculous organisms are not cultured from the involved joints but a purified protein derivative (PPD) test is positive. Although any joint may be involved, the knees, ankles, and elbows are most commonly affected.

7. How is osteoarticular TB diagnosed?
Diagnosis may be difficult and is often delayed by up to 12 to 18 months because of the insidious onset of nonspecific symptoms. In addition, the chest radiograph may be normal in 50% of patients with osteoarticular TB. A PPD skin test will be positive unless the patient is anergic, which occurs in 10% to 30% of cases. An interferon-γ release assay (IGRA; QuantiFERON-TB Gold and T-SPOT.TB) is more sensitive than a PPD test and is not affected by previous BCG vaccination.

A definitive diagnosis is established by demonstrating MTB presence in tissue or synovial fluid. The yield for several common procedures is as follows:

Synovial fluid smear for TB	20%
Synovial fluid adenosine deaminase (>31 U/L)	80%
Synovial fluid culture for TB	80%
Synovial biopsy and culture	>90%

Nucleic acid amplification tests (NAATs) on synovial fluid and tissue may help to confirm TB within 1 to 2 days instead of the 3 to 6 weeks for conventional culture. However, NAATs do not have 100% sensitivity and therefore culture remains the gold standard. Cultures are mandatory to determine mycobacterial drug sensitivities.

8. What are the characteristics of synovial fluid and tissue biopsies in osteoarticular TB?
Synovial fluid analysis reveals elevated protein in virtually all patients with arthritis, and low glucose is seen in 60% of cases. Cell counts are highly variable and range from 1000 to 100,000 cells/mm^3, but in most cases fall in the range from 10,000 to 20,000 cells/mm^3. Polymorphonuclear cells predominate. Synovial membrane biopsies typically show caseating granulomas in 80% of cases. Osteomyelitis is diagnosed by needle biopsy, which usually reveals a granulomata that may or may not be associated with caseating necrosis.

9. What are the characteristic radiographic features of osteoarticular TB?
No pathognomonic radiographic signs of tuberculosis exist. However, several signs may be helpful.
- Spine
  - Narrowing of joint spaces with vertebral collapse (vertebra plana)
  - Anterior vertebral scalloping and soft-tissue swelling (paravertebral abscess)
  - Extensive vertebral destruction with relative preservation of disc spaces (Figure 40-1)
- Peripheral joints
  - Soft-tissue swelling with effusion
- Phemister triad:
  - Juxtaarticular osteoporosis
  - Peripheral subchondral osseous erosions
  - Articular destructive lesions with little periosteal reaction
  - Narrowing of joint spaces occurs as a late finding
- Osteomyelitis
  - Lytic lesion with a lack of periosteal reaction
- Dactylitis (mainly in children)
  - Short bones of the hand exhibit a ballooned-out lytic appearance with a lack of periosteal reaction (spina ventosa)

10. How is osteoarticular TB treated?
The current guidelines of the CDC, American Thoracic Society, and Infectious Disease Society of America recommend 6 to 9 months of therapy. If rifampin cannot be used, the patient should be treated for at least 9 months. Most patients are started on four drugs initially (IREZ therapy): **isoniazid** (5 mg/kg, up to 300 mg daily), **rifampin** (10 mg/kg, up to 600 mg daily), **ethambutol** (15 mg/kg daily, up to 1600 mg daily), and **pyrazinamide** (15 to 30 mg/kg, up to 2 g daily). Directly observed therapy is highly recommended. Once MTB sensitivity to isoniazid is confirmed, the ethambutol can be stopped. Pyrazinamide is continued for the first 2 months and then stopped. For the remainder of the treatment time, isoniazid plus rifampin 5 days

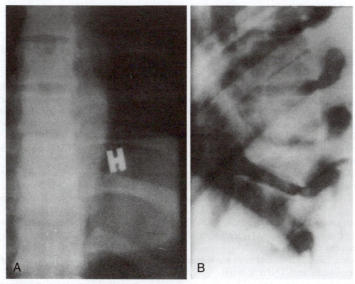

Figure 40-1. A, Abscess formation on an anterior view of the thoracic spine. B, Vertebral collapse with angulation (Pott disease) on a lateral view. *(Copyright 2014 American College of Rheumatology. Used with permission.)*

a week is adequate. Pyridoxine (25 to 50 mg daily) should be used with isoniazid. Patients with mutidrug-resistant TB (1% of all U.S. cases) should be treated with other drug regimens prescribed by an expert in TB therapy for 18 to 24 months or longer.

For those with arthritis or minimal osteomyelitis, antituberculous therapy is often the only therapy needed. However, if bone involvement is extensive, spinal kyphosis is greater than 40 degrees, multidrug-resistant TB is present, or there is neurologic compromise, surgery is often necessary to debride the abscess and hasten recovery.

11. What musculoskeletal problems can be caused by atypical mycobacteria?

Unlike MTB, nontuberculous (atypical) mycobacteria (NTM) are not spread from human to human and have a propensity to involve the tendons and joints of the hands. In fact, 50% of infections affect the hands, whereas only 20% affect the knees. Polyarticular disease and spinal involvement are much less common.
- *Mycobacterium avium–intracellulare* (M. avium complex, MAC)
    - Most common systemic mycobacterial infection in patients with HIV (25% of AIDS patients)
    - Tenosynovitis, bursitis, and osteomyelitis are all well described
- *Mycobacterium kansasii*
    - Found primarily in the southwestern United States
    - May cause all of the syndromes listed for MAC plus reactivation after total hip replacement
- *Mycobacterium marinum*
    - Aquatic organism that is an occupational hazard of oyster shuckers, aquarium enthusiasts, and others
    - Tenosynovitis of the hands or wrist is the classic presentation, although synovitis and osteomyelitis have been reported
- Other atypical mycobacterial species include M. *simiae*, M. *szulgai*, and M. *ulcerans*

12. What conditions predispose patients to NTM infection?
- Prior surgery or trauma
- Direct inoculation and/or environmental exposure (soil, water, animals)
- Intraarticular steroid injections and preexisting joint disease
- Open wounds on the hands or fingers
- Immunosuppression and biologic therapy

13. How are atypical mycobacterial osteoarticular infections treated? What is the prognosis?
- These infections require multiple drugs (consult a specialist).
- Surgical debridement plays an important role in debulking the infection.
- Prolonged therapy is necessary.
- Relapses are common, even with the best therapy.

14. **List the guidelines for mycobacterial infection prevention in patients who are to receive biologic agents (especially anti-TNFα agents).**
    - All patients who are to receive biologic agents should have MTB (latent and active) and NTM screening.
      - A risk factor assessment, physical examination, and chest radiograph should be performed for all patients.
      - The tuberculin skin test (TST, also known as PPD) only has sensitivity and specificity of 70%. PPD >5 mm at 48 hours should be considered positive even if the patient has a history of BCG vaccination.
      - Many patients with immune-mediated inflammatory diseases are on prednisone and other immunosuppressants, which can make TST/PPD tests unreliable. Therefore, IGRA screening is often recommended. Notably, up to 10% of IGRA tests may be indeterminate in patients on immunosuppressive medications and their risk of latent MTB should be assessed clinically.
      - Screening procedures decrease reactivation of MTB by 80%. Notably, NTM (especially MAC) infections are becoming more common than MTB.
    - Monoclonal antibodies (especially infliximab) against TNFα have the highest risk and abatacept and rituximab have the lowest risk for MTB and NTM infection. Reactivation of MTB tends to occur within 6 months of starting anti-TNFα therapy and usually presents as extrapulmonary disease, especially lymphadenitis.
    - Patients with latent MTB and a normal chest radiograph should start biologics (especially anti-TNFα agents) after 1 month of therapy. Patients should receive a complete course for latent MTB (9 months of INH or 4 months of rifampin).
    - Patients with active MTB should have a complete course of anti-tuberculous (IREZ) therapy before starting a biologic (especially anti-TNFα agents).
    - Patients with a history of treated NTM infection should be evaluated by a specialist before a biologic is used. Some NTM infections such as pulmonary MAC are hard to cure and anti-TNFα agents should be avoided. Rituximab or abatacept may be safer agents.

15. **Are any musculoskeletal conditions associated with *Mycobacterium leprae* (leprosy)?**
    Erythema nodosum leprosum is seen in lepromatous leprosy and probably represents a reactive arthritis. Clinical manifestations include fever, subcutaneous nodules, arthralgias, and frank arthritis.
    Symmetric polyarthritis is usually insidious and involves the wrist, small joints of the hands and feet, and the knees. The onset is months to years after the initial infection. It is most often seen in tuberculoid or borderline leprosy. Patients may be positive for rheumatoid factor.
    Bony abnormalities secondary to neuropathy include resorption of the distal metatarsals, aseptic necrosis, claw hands, and Charcot joints.
    Direct infection of the bone typically affects the distal phalanges.
    Lucio phenomenon is necrotizing vasculitis of the skin due to lepromatous leprosy.

16. **How do fungal infections of the bones and joints present clinically? What are the risk factors?**
    Osteomyelitis is the most common fungal musculoskeletal syndrome. **Septic arthritis** may arise via direct extension from bone or, less frequently, inoculation or hematogenous spread. In general, monarthritis is indolent, with delays in diagnosis of months to years. Acute arthritis is unusual except in *Candida* and *Blastomyces* infections. Risk factors are similar to those for osteoarticular TB: environmental exposure, HIV and other immunodeficiencies, and immunosuppressive medications including biologic therapy such as anti-TNFα agents (especially infliximab).

17. **How helpful are synovial fluid analyses and cultures in fungal septic arthritis?**
    As in TB, **cell counts** are highly variable. Typically, white blood cell counts range from 10,000 to 60,000 cell/mm^3, with either polymorphonuclear or mononuclear cells predominating.
    Culture of synovial fluid is critical in establishing the diagnosis, but colony counts are often low. Laboratory personnel must be alerted to the possibility of fungal disease so that they do not use inhibitory media. Amplification techniques based on polymerase chain reaction have recently been developed for many species of mycobacteria and fungi and these may be useful diagnostic techniques in the future.

18. **Describe the epidemiology of some of the fungi that cause septic arthritis.**
    Table 40-1 lists the mode of infection for fungal species that cause septic arthritis and the and geographic areas where they occur.

19. **How frequently is bone or articular involvement seen with these fungi and at what locations does it occur?**
    Histoplasma capsulatum: In the acute setting, large joint polyarthritis with or without erythema nodosum can be seen and can resemble acute sarcoid arthritis. In the chronic setting, arthritis is very rare. Disseminated histoplasmosis is seen in immunosuppressed patients. Serologic tests, serum and urine antigen screening, and biopsy and cultures can confirm the diagnosis.
    Cryptococcus neoformans: Osteomyelitis occurs in 5% to 10% of infections. Arthritis is very rare and almost always involves the knee. Serum antigen screening and tissue biopsy and culture can confirm the diagnosis.

Table 40-1. Epidemiology of Fungi Causing Septic Arthritis

FUNGUS	MODE OF INFECTION	GEOGRAPHIC AREA
Histoplasma capsulatum	Inhalation; aerosolized from soil rich in bird (especially chicken) and bat feces	Worldwide, but highest in Ohio and Mississippi River valleys
Cryptococcus neoformans	Inhalation; aerosolized from pigeon droppings; also seen in immunosuppressed	Worldwide
Coccidioides immitis	Inhalation; especially in dry months; also seen in immunosuppressed and AIDS patients	Southwestern U.S., Central and South America (especially in arid and semiarid regions)
Blastomyces dermatitidis	Usually inhalation, but rare case of dog-to-human, human-to-human, and inoculation reported; male/female ratio of 9:1	Mississippi and Ohio River basins, Middle Atlantic states, Canada, Europe, Africa, and northern South America
Sporothrix schenckii	Cutaneous disease from scratch or thorn prick; systemic disease is due to inhalation; also seen in immunosuppressed, alcohol abusers, and gardeners	Worldwide
Candida species	Endogenous; common in premature infants and other compromised hosts (malignancies, indwelling catheters, immunosuppression, broad-spectrum antibiotic use)	Worldwide
Aspergillus fumigatus	Inhalation of decaying matter or hospital air; also seen in surgical or trauma patients and immunocompromised	Worldwide
Madurella species	Implantation of aerobic bacteria or true fungi into uncovered feet	Worldwide, but typically in tropical climates where no shoes are worn (rare in U.S.)

Coccidioides immitis: Bone and joint involvement is seen in 10% to 50% of infections with extrathoracic disease. Osseous involvement may involve multiple sites. Monarthritis of the knee is the most common arthritis. Serologic testing, urine antigen screening, and tissue biopsies with stains and cultures are necessary to confirm the diagnosis. Synovial fluid cultures are rarely positive.

Blastomyces dermatitidis: Bone and joint involvement is seen in 20% to 60% of patients with disseminated disease. Osseous involvement typically affects the **vertebrae**, ribs, tibia, skull, and feet. Arthritis is usually monoarticular, occurring in 3% to 5% of cases. Synovial fluid is often purulent. Serum and urine antigen screening, synovial fluid cultures, and tissue biopsy and cultures can confirm the diagnosis.

Sporothrix schenckii: Bone and joint involvement is seen in 80% of systemic cases. Arthritis is mono- or pauciarticular. The knee and all the upper extremity joints are most commonly involved. **Hand and wrist involvement distinguishes this from other fungal arthritides**. Infection occurs via entry through the lungs with dissemination and uncommonly through skin inoculation. Most patients are immunosuppressed. Serologic testing is unreliable. Synovial fluid and tissue biopsy and culture confirm the diagnosis.

Candida species: This type of infection is rare but is increasing with greater use of broad-spectrum antibiotics and indwelling catheters in immunosuppressed patients. Osteomyelitis and monoarticular arthritis are both uncommon. The arthritis may have an acute presentation with positive cultures.

Aspergillus fumigatus: Osteomyelitis and arthritis are both rare but can occur via direct spread from the lung. Serum biomarker antigen detection and tissue biopsy with culture confirm the diagnosis.

Madurella species: Bone and joint involvement is common, with spread of soft-tissue infection to bones, fasciae, and joints.

Scedosporium species: These species have a predilection for bone and cartilage after cutaneous inoculation and dissemination.

20. **How is fungal septic arthritis treated?**
    Amphotericin B has historically been the most effective therapy for most fungi but is limited by its renal toxicity. To limit this toxicity, liposomal and other formulations of amphotericin and, more recently, caspofungin have been introduced. One of these drugs is indicated for all severe fungal infections or for fungi that are resistant or do not respond to one of the oral antifungal agents. One of these agents is typically used first until antifungal sensitivity has returned, especially in seriously ill or immunocompromised patients.

Oral antifungal agents may be used for treatment of osteoarticular mycotic infections, depending on the fungus and the severity of the infection. These include itraconazole (coccidioidomycosis, blastomycosis, sporotrichosis, histoplasmosis) and fluconazole (*Cryptococcus*, candidiasis), and newer antifungals such as voriconazole (aspergillosis, scedosporiosis), posaconazole, and micafungin. The length of treatment is 6 to 12 months. In immunocompromised patients (i.e., HIV), oral antifungal agent use may be lifelong owing to the high frequency of recurrence. Therapeutic debridement is needed in many cases.

21. **List some other organisms that might cause osteoarticular problems in other areas of the world although rarely within the United States.**
    - **Brucellosis:** Gram-negative, intracellular coccobacillus transmitted to humans mainly through ingestion of unpasteurized dairy products (cheese). The febrile illness can have an acute or insidious onset, with 33% of patients developing musculoskeletal manifestations. Sacroiliitis (50%) is the most common presentation, followed by peripheral arthritis (35%), spondylitis (25%), and osteomyelitis (5%). Peripheral joint involvement is usually a monarthritis typically involving the hip or knee. Treatment is a combination of doxycycline and rifampin for 6 weeks.
    - **Parasitic infection:** Protozoan, cestode, nematode, or trematode infection should be considered in patients who present with oligoarthritis, myositis, or vasculitis after visiting an area in which such infections are endemic. Eosinophilia and a lack of response to antirheumatic treatment should prompt consideration of a parasitic infection causing the musculoskeletal problems.

BIBLIOGRAPHY

American Thoracic Society: CDC, Infectious Diseases Society of America: Treatment of tuberculosis, MMWR Recomm Rep 52(RR11):1–77, 2003.
Cuellar ML, Silveira LH, Citera G, et al: Other fungal arthritides, Rheum Dis Clin North Am 19:439–455, 1993.
DeVuyst D, Vanhoenacker F, Gielen J, et al: Imaging features of musculoskeletal tuberculosis, Eur Radiol 13:1809–1819, 2003.
Foocharoen C, Sarntipipattana C, Foocharoen T, et al: Synovial fluid adenosine deaminase activity to diagnose tuberculous septic arthritis, Southeast Asian J Trop Med Public Health 42:331–337, 2011.
Griffith DE, Aksamit T, Brown-Elliot BA, et al: An official ATS/IDSA statement: Diagnosis, treatment, and prevention of non-tuberculous mycobacterial diseases, Am J Resp Crit Care Med 175:367–416, 2007.
Hirsch R, Miller SM, Kazi S, et al: Human immunodeficiency virus-associated atypical mycobacterial skeletal infections, Semin Arthritis Rheum 26: 3470–356, 1996.
Huang TY, Wu TS, Yang CC, et al: Tuberculous arthritis: a fourteen-year experience at a tertiary teaching hospital in Taiwan, J Microbiol Immunol Infect 40:493–499, 2007.
Kroot EJ, Hazes JM, Colin EM, Dolhain RJ: Poncet's disease: reactive arthritis accompanying tuberculosis, Rheumatology 46:484–489, 2007.
Malaviya AN, Kotwal PP: Arthritis associated with tuberculosis, Best Pract Res Clin Rheumatol 17:319–343, 2003.
Marquez J, Espinoza LR: Mycobacterial, brucellar, fungal, and parasitic arthritis. In Hochberg MC, Silman AJ, Smolen JS, et al: Rheumatology, ed 5, Philadelphia, 2011, Mosby.
Mertz LE, Blair JE: Coccidiodomycosis in rheumatology patients, Ann NY Acad Sci 1111:343–357, 2007.
Pai M, O'Brien R: New diagnostics for latent and active tuberculosis: state of the art and future prospects, Semin Respir Crit Care 29:560–568, 2008.
Pereira HL, Ribeiro SL, Pennini SN, Sato EI: Leprosy-related joint involvement, Clin Rheumatol 28:407–414, 2009.
Priest JR, Low D, Wang C, Bush T: Brucellosis and sacroiliitis: a common presentation of an uncommon pathogen, J Am Board Fam Med 21:158–161, 2008.
Saiz P, Gitelis S, Virkus W, et al: Blastomycosis of long bones, Clin Orthop 421:255–259, 2004.

FURTHER READING

www.cdc.gov/Tb/

VIRAL ARTHRITIDES

Carolyn Anne Coyle, MD

CHAPTER 41

> **KEY POINTS**
> 1. Hepatitis B virus infection presents as an arthritis–urticaria syndrome.
> 2. Hepatitis C virus infection can cause autoantibodies and polyarthritis.
> 3. Hepatitis C virus can cause cryoglobulinemuic vasculitis syndrome.
> 4. Parvovirus is the most common viral arthritis in the United States.
> 5. Viral arthritis should be considered in any patient presenting with polyarthritis, fever, and rash.

1. **List three general characteristics of viral arthritis.**
    - Viral arthritis often occurs during the viral prodrome, at the time of the characteristic rash.
    - The most common viral arthritides in the United States generally present with symmetrical small-joint involvement, although different patterns of joint and soft-tissue involvement occur with each virus.
    - In all instances, the arthritis associated with viral infections is nondestructive and does not lead to any currently recognized form of chronic joint disease.

HEPATITIS A AND B

2. **Is hepatitis A virus infection associated with any rheumatic manifestations?**
    Hepatitis A virus infections are not commonly associated with extrahepatic manifestations. Arthralgias and rash are observed in 10% to 14% of patients and usually occur early during the acute phase of the disease.

3. **Arthritis is frequently observed with hepatitis B. Describe the general clinical course of hepatitis B virus (HBV) infection.**
    HBV is a partially double-stranded DNA virus consisting of a nucleocapsid core with two antigenically distinct constituents, hepatitis B core antigen (HBcAg) and hepatitis Be antigen (HBeAg). The core is surrounded by a nucleocapsid coat, or surface antigen (HBsAg).
    HBV is primarily transmitted parenterally and much less commonly through sexual contact. Most individuals exposed to HBV experience a clinically silent, self-limited infection resulting in an antibody response to HBsAg. Acute icteric infection occurs 40 to 120 days after exposure to the virus, although approximately 20% of cases remain anicteric. IgM antibodies against HBcAg indicate an acute HBV infection. Infection resolves in 90% to 95% of cases, with the remainder developing chronic infections. In approximately 5% to 10% of cases, HBV infection proceeds to a chronic phase characterized serologically by HBeAg, anti-HBcAg (IgG), and HBsAg. Of these patients, 30% proceed to chronic active hepatitis. Risk factors for chronicity include male sex, immunocompromised state, and infection at birth.

4. **What arthritic symptoms are associated with HBV infection?**
    Arthralgias are estimated to occur in 20% of patients. Frank arthritis is less common, occurring in approximately 10% of cases. Joint symptoms are typically present during the prodromal phase of acute HBV infection and may precede clinical jaundice by days to weeks. Articular symptoms usually have a rapid onset, occur in a symmetrical additive or migratory fashion, and primarily involve small joints of the hands and the knees. **Urticaria** frequently accompanies the acute arthritis. These symptoms persist for 1 to 3 weeks and subside quickly after the onset of jaundice. In patients with acute hepatitis, joint symptoms are self-limited and have not been associated with chronic joint disease or permanent damage. In patients with chronic active hepatitis, arthralgias and arthritis may be present or recur over long periods of time. Treatment involves joint rest and nonsteroidal antiinflammatory drugs. The joint manifestations may occur in the setting of nonicteric hepatitis, so only a high incidence of suspicion can lead to the diagnosis of HBV.

5. **How does HBV infection produce these arthritic symptoms?**
    It is believed that arthritic manifestations are due to deposition of HBsAg-anti-HBsAg immune complexes in synovial tissue, leading to a secondary nonspecific inflammatory response. This antibody response to HBsAg occurs earlier in the disease course in patients with arthritic symptoms compared to those without arthritic symptoms.

6. **Describe other rheumatologic manifestations of HBV.**
   A variety of extrahepatic manifestations occur in addition to arthralgias/arthritis, including an arthritis–dermatitis syndrome, nephropathy (typically membranous), and systemic necrotizing vasculitis, in particular polyarteritis nodosa (PAN).

7. **Is there any association between the duration of articular symptoms and the development of systemic vasculitis?**
   Prolonged articular symptoms may be a harbinger of systemic necrotizing vasculitis. The latter usually occurs within the first 6 to 12 months of HBV infection, but occasionally can occur in late, chronic disease. Systemic necrotizing vasculitis implies HBV antigenemia and persistent circulating immune complexes. Originally thought to be responsible for as many as 40% of PAN cases, HBsAg positivity is now found in only 5% to 10% of cases. In HBsAg-positive PAN patients, there appears to be a higher prevalence of malignant hypertension, bowel ischemia, and orchitis, whereas glomerulonephritis is uncommon and the antineutrophil cytoplasmic antibody status is usually negative.

8. **What serum antibodies and other laboratory findings are commonly seen with HBV infection and arthritic symptoms?**
   The diagnosis of HBV infection is made by confirming the presence of one or more HBV antigens or antibodies to these antigens in the sera of patients with HBV infection. Typically, during the period of joint involvement, free HBsAg, viral DNA, and IgM anti-HBcAg are present in serum. In general, liver-associated enzymes are abnormal. Synovial fluid is inflammatory. With the onset of jaundice and resolution of arthritic symptoms, the HBsAg titer falls and IgG anti-HBsAg and anti-HBcAg titers increase. Other laboratory tests that are occasionally abnormal include low rheumatoid factor (RF) titers and complement levels (10% to 25% of patients).

9. **What rheumatic symptoms are associated with hepatitis B vaccination?**
   Although unusual and controversial, several rheumatic syndromes have been reported following recombinant hepatitis B vaccination: rheumatoid arthritis (RA), erythema nodosum, uveitis, systemic lupus erythematosus (SLE), and others.

HEPATITIS C

10. **Discuss the epidemiology of hepatitis C virus infection.**
    Hepatitis C virus (HCV) was discovered in 1988 and is a linear, single-stranded RNA (ssRNA) virus with extensive genomic variability. There are six different HCV subtypes. HCV is the most common blood-borne infection in the United States, with a prevalence of 1% to 2% in the general population. Nationwide, HCV affects approximately 2.7 million people, with 19,000 new lives affected each year. It is estimated that 8000 to 13,000 new deaths per year are related to HCV. Like HBV, HCV is primarily transmitted parenterally via blood products or contact with contaminated needles, although the mode of transmission remains obscure in up to 50% of cases. Although HCV is found in saliva in up to 50% of infected patients, oral transmission has not been clearly demonstrated.

11. **Describe the clinical course of hepatitis in HCV infection.**
    The incubation period for HCV is approximately 6 weeks. The initial infection is usually less clinically severe than for HBV, with only 25% of adult patients ever developing jaundice (compared to 80% for HBV infection). HCV causes more modest elevations in liver function tests than HBV does; however, more than 60% of acute infections lead to chronicity. Some 20% to 50% of HCV infections ultimately lead to cirrhosis and consequent increased prevalence of hepatocellular carcinoma.

12. **Describe the diagnostic studies used in the diagnosis of HCV.**
    Diagnostic testing for HCV infection usually begins with identification of anti-HCV antibodies in the sera of infected patients using enzyme immunoassay (EIA) and recombinant immunoblot assay (RIBA) methodology. The sensitivity of EIA studies is 80% to 90% but they may be fairly nonspecific. False positives may occur in the setting of hypergammaglobulinemia, RF positivity, or recent influenza vaccination. The RIBA method is highly specific and sensitive, and it is believed that in the presence of elevated transaminases it is diagnostic of HCV infection. Among high-risk populations and EIA-positive patients, confirmation of HCV infection by RIBA approaches 95%. The gold standard of HCV detection remains the HCV RNA PCR test, which should be ordered in atypical cases of HCV and in situations that may influence therapeutic decisions.

13. **Discuss the autoantibodies that may be present in HCV infection.**
    Some 40% to 65% of chronically infected HCV patients have a low antinuclear antibody (ANA) titer, antithyroid antibodies, anticardiolipin antibodies, anti–smooth-muscle antibodies, and/or positive RF frequently associated with hypocomplementemia due to an associated cryogloulinemia. Antibodies against cyclic citrullinated peptide are usually negative. These associations with HCV infection justify its consideration in the differential diagnosis of rheumatic disease. In fact, any patient suspected of having seropositive RA who has elevated liver-associated enzymes must be screened for HCV infection.

14. **Describe the rheumatologic manifestations of HCV.**
    - Cryoglobulins (types II and III) can be detected in up to 35% to 55% of patients with chronic HCV infection. However, only 3% to 5% develop cryoglobulinemic vasculitis. This syndrome name has been applied to patients with type II or III cryoglobulins associated with a variety of distinctive features including palpable purpura, arthralgia, and multiple organ involvement such as glomerulonephritis (33%), mesenteric vasculitis (20%), and peripheral neuropathy (50% to 86%). RF positivity and low complement levels (especially C4) are frequently present owing to immune complex formation. In recent years it has been established that HCV infection is found in 80% to 90% of patients with cryoglobulinemic vasculitis and that it is directly involved in the pathogenesis, as evidenced by the presence of HCV RNA in the majority of the cryoprecipitates.
    - Two arthritic syndromes are observed in 2% to 20% of patients with HCV: (1) nonerosive polyarthritis of small joints similar to RA, and (2) intermittent oligoarthritis associated with the cryoglobulinemia. In addition, Sjögren's syndrome has been described in a number of HCV patients. These patients differ from patients with primary Sjögren's syndrome in that there is a lower female predominance, ANA and anti-SSA/SSB antibodies are absent, and milder histology is observed on salivary gland biopsy. The clinical symptoms are also less significant, with only 30% of patients having xerostomia and virtually no xerophthalmia.
    - Several recent reports describe a possible association between fibromyalgia and HCV, and many believe the association is greater than would be expected by chance alone. In one study, 10% of HCV patients fulfilled the fibromyalgia diagnostic criteria, compared to 2% of control patients. No relationship between the severity of HCV-associated liver disease and other immunological alterations was seen. HCV infection should be considered in selected patients with fibromyalgia, especially those with atypical features and particularly in the presence of elevated transaminases (even modest elevations) or risk factors for infection with blood-borne pathogens.
    - Osteosclerosis of all bones except the cranium has been observed in rare cases. Patients have limb pain, high bone turnover markers, and elevated bone density. It has been postulated that abnormal functions of IGF-1 and IGF-2 cause this manifestation. Bone lymphoma must be excluded.

15. **Discuss the treatment of HCV hepatitis and its extrahepatic manifestations.**
    The FDA-approved treatment for HCV infection includes once weekly Peg-IFN-α2a (180 µg) or Peg-IFN-α2b (1.5 µg/kg) combined with ribavirin (1000 to 1200 mg/day) subcutaneously for 24 weeks (genotypes 2 and 3) or 48 weeks (genotypes 1 and 4). IFN doses and the use of ribavirin are determined according to renal function. Approximately 50% (genotypes 1 and 4) and 75% (genotypes 2 and 3) of patients have a virologic response, but relapses are common. In the past few years, three protease inhibitors (boceprevir, telaprevir, simeprevir) and one nucleotide analog inhibitor (sofosbuvir) have been FDA-approved as additional therapies for hepatitis C which has markedly decreased relapses or lead to a cure. See Chapter 31 for a discussion of the treatment of HCV-associated cryoblobulinemic vasculitis.

RUBELLA

16. **Natural rubella infection or rubella vaccination is frequently associated with arthritic syndromes. When in the clinical course of natural rubella infection do arthritic symptoms appear?**
    Rubella virus infection is symptomatic in 50% to 75% of individuals and is characterized by an acute mild to severe viral exanthem consisting of a maculopapular rash and significant lymphadenopathy. The incubation period is approximately 18 days. The rash appears first on the face as a light pink maculopapular eruption and then spreads centrifugally to involve the trunk and extremities, sparing the palms and soles. The onset of joint symptoms occurs rapidly and within several days either before or after the skin rash. Rubella infection associated with joint symptoms is seen most commonly in women who are 20 to 40 years old. Approximately 30% of female patients and 6% of male patients with rubella have joint symptoms.

17. **What are the typical joint manifestations associated with natural rubella virus infection and how are they treated?**
    Joint involvement is usually symmetrical and affects the small joints of the hands, followed by the knees, wrists, ankles, and elbows. Periarthritis leading to tenosynovitis and carpal tunnel syndrome is a well-recognized complication of rubella infection. Joint symptoms are usually self-limited; however, there are case reports of chronic arthritis, without joint destruction, lasting months to years. As with all virus-associated arthritides, no specific therapy is available. Restriction of activity and antiinflammatory therapy are effective in most patients. Hydroxychloroquine can be tried in patients with chronic arthritis.

18. **Discuss the pathogenesis of the arthritic manifestations associated with rubella infection.**
    Wild-type rubella and some vaccine strains replicate in synovial organ cultures. A number of case reports of rubella-associated arthritis have also demonstrated persistent rubella virus infection of synovial tissue. These data and others support the belief that active viral replication in synovial tissues may be responsible for the joint symptoms. However, immune complexes have also been isolated from involved joints. More recently, rubella virus has been isolated from lymphocytes of patients who had experienced rubella-associated arthritis years earlier. Virus in these lymphocytes would serve as a source for later direct viral seeding of the joint or for antigen release and subsequent immune complex formation.

19. **Are any important laboratory abnormalities seen in rubella-associated arthritis?**
Diagnosis of rubella infection may be confirmed by direct viral isolation from nasopharyngeal cultures or antirubella antiIgM antibodies. There are no other distinctive laboratory abnormalities in patients with rubella-associated arthritis. Synovial fluid has occasionally yielded rubella virus, with mildly elevated protein levels and leukocyte counts (predominately mononuclear cells).

20. **What are the arthritic symptoms associated with rubella vaccine?**
Arthritic symptoms occur approximately 2 weeks after rubella vaccination, a time coincident with seroconversion and the ability to isolate rubella virus from the pharynx of inoculated individuals. Joint symptoms are similar to those in natural infection, and involve the knees more frequently than the small joints of the hands. The rate of arthralgia or arthritis following vaccination (RA 27/3 strain) is approximately 15% to 25% in seronegative adult women, with far fewer women reporting more prolonged joint symptoms for up to 1 year. In children, the frequency of joint manifestations is approximately 1% to 5%. Joint symptoms are usually self-limited, lasting 1 to 5 days, and most studies have failed to demonstrate the development of any form of chronic arthritis.

21. **What are the rheumatic syndromes caused by rubella infections or the rubella vaccine in children?**
Two syndromes are seen in children 1 to 2 months after infection or vaccination. (1) Catcher's crouch syndrome is a lumbar radiculopathy causing popliteal fossa pain on arising in the morning. Pain is exacerbated by knee extension, causing the child to assume a baseball catcher's crouch. (2) Arm syndrome is a brachial neuropathy causing arm and hand dysesthesias that are worse at night. Both these syndromes can last for up to 2 months but may recur for up to 1 year. There are no chronic sequelae.

PARVOVIRUS

22. **What diseases are associated with human parvovirus (HPV) B19 infection?**
Parvovirus B19 is a small, single-stranded, species-specific DNA virus that replicates in dividing cells and has a remarkable tropism for human erythroid progenitor cells. It is a pathogen responsible for several diseases, including erythema infectiosum (fifth disease); transient aplastic crisis, especially in patients with underlying hematologic conditions such as sickle cell disease, thalassemia, and other bone marrow disorders; anemia in HIV disease; fetal hydrops in infected mothers; and polyarthritis/rash syndrome in adults. Parvovirus B19 is the most common viral arthritis in the United States. Rarely, patients can develop a mild myocarditis, peripheral neuropathy, and/or hepatitis.

23. **How is parvovirus B19 transmitted and what is the clinical course?**
It is presumed that parvovirus B19 is transmitted via respiratory secretions. The secondary attack rate among susceptible household contacts is approximately 50%. Some individuals develop a flu-like syndrome, whereas most (70%) remain asymptomatic. In children, rash is common and appears as bright red "slapped cheeks." In adults, the rash is on the trunk and extremities but the "slapped cheeks" appearance is not seen. In rare cases adults can develop "socks and gloves" acral erythema. Joint symptoms are rare in children but common in adults.

24. **Describe the arthritic symptoms in HPV infection.**
The arthropathy associated with HPV infection is similar to that seen after natural rubella or vaccine-associated infection. There is rapid onset of symmetrical polyarthritis in peripheral small joints, primarily of the hands and wrists. Joint symptoms are more common in adults (60%) than in children (5% to 10%) and in women than in men. In general, the symptoms are self-limited (several weeks), but they may persist for months or even years in certain individuals. As with other viral arthropathies, no long-term joint damage or significant functional disability has been reported after HPV infection. The pathogenesis of acute joint symptoms appears to be secondary to immune-complex deposition and a nonspecific inflammatory response. Patients with chronic joint symptoms have B19 DNA in their synovium and bone marrow. Nonstructural proteins (NS1) on the surface of B19 virions can upregulate IL-6 and lead to low-grade inflammation and apoptosis of host cells.

25. **How is the serologic diagnosis of HPV B19 infection made?**
The definitive diagnosis of B19 infection relies on detection of B19 IgM antibodies or viral B19 DNA. IgM antibodies occur early, increasing at approximately 1 month, but are often undetectable by 2 to 3 months. Detection of viral B19 DNA by PCR may persist even after IgM antibodies disappear. IgG persists for years and perhaps for life. Thus, the finding of IgG antiB19 antibodies without IgM antibodies has little diagnostic significance and in fact is found in approximately 60% of the healthy adult population.

26. **Why is it important to make a diagnosis of HPV B19 infection?**
The clinical presentation of HPV B19 infection may resemble adult RA or juvenile idiopathic arthritis, especially in patients who do not present with the typical HPV exanthem and who have a clinical course of greater than 2 months in duration. Many chronic B19 patients meet American College of Rheumatology criteria for the diagnosis of RA, and some even have low to moderate serum RF titers. In addition, B19 infection

may mimic SLE. Both may present with rash, fever, myalgia, arthropathy, cytopenias, hypocomplementemia, antiphospholipid antibodies, and positive ANA. The symptoms and signs in B19 patients tend to be short-lived, although prolonged symptoms have been reported. The possibility of B19 infection should be considered in these patients, because diagnosis of HPV would avoid inappropriate treatment for other rheumatic conditions.

27. **How are patients with chronic joint symptoms arising from HPV 19 infection treated?**
Treatment is symptomatic with antiinflammatory medications. Hydroxychloroquine has been used successfully in some patients. It has recently been found that patients with chronic B19 arthropathy are unable to develop IgG antibodies to the minor capsid protein VP1, which encodes neutralizing epitopes. This may account for their inability to clear viral B19 DNA. In these patients with chronic joint pain and persistent B19 IgM antibodies and/or viral B19 DNA, IVIG may be an effective treatment although it appears to be more effective in immunocompromised patients. The IVIG may contain antibody against VP1 from donors who have mounted a successful immune response against HPV B19 enabling the patient receiving the IVIG to better clear the virus.

OTHER VIRUS INFECTIONS

28. **What six alphavirus infections have rheumatic complaints as a major feature?**
With worldwide travel being more common, physicians may have patients who become infected with one of the alphaviruses listed in Table 41-1.

Table 41-1. Geographic Distribution of Various Alphaviruses

ALPHAVIRUS	GEOGRAPHIC DISTRIBUTION
Chikungunya	East Africa, India, Southeast Asia, the Philippines, Caribbean, Central/South America
O'nyong-nyong	East Africa
Ross River	Australia, New Zealand, South Pacific islands
Mayaro	South America (Bolivia, Brazil, Peru)
Barmah Forest	Australia
Sindbis (Karelian fever)	Sweden, Finland, Isthmus of Russia

29. **Describe the clinical syndromes associated with alphavirus infection. How does it differ from dengue infection?**
The mosquito-transmitted illnesses arising from infection by the six alphaviruses (ssRNA) listed in Table 41-1 share a number of clinical features, of which fever, arthritis, and rash are the most constant and characteristic. Arthritis may be severe. The joints most frequently affected are the small joints of the hands, and the wrists, elbows, knees, and ankles. The arthritis is generally symmetrical and polyarticular. In the majority of alphavirus infections, joint symptoms resolve over 3 to 7 days. Joint symptoms persisting for longer than 1 year have been reported, although there is no evidence of permanent joint damage.
Dengue fever is caused by a Flaviviridae virus transmitted by a mosquito. The illness has been described in over 100 countries, many of which also harbor the alphaviruses. Dengue infection presents with fever, headache, a measles-like rash, and severe myalgias and arthralgias (60% to 80% of cases), earning it the name "break bone fever." It differs from the alphavirus diseases in that patients with dengue infection can have leukopenia, thrombocytopenia, and elevated liver enzymes. A small percentage of patients have a severe illness with dengue hemorrhagic fever and shock.

30. **Describe the clinical features and course of mumps virus infection**
Mumps virus is a member of the Paramyxoviridae family. It is an ssRNA virus surrounded by a lipoprotein envelope. Subclinical infections with mumps virus are seen in 20% to 40% of patients. Some of the features of clinical infection include low-grade fever, anorexia, malaise, headache, myalgia, and parotitis. Epididymoorchitis is the most common extrasalivary gland manifestation of mumps infections and is observed in 20% to 30% of postpubertal males. Central nervous system involvement occurs in approximately 1 in 6000 cases. Myocarditis is also not an uncommon finding.

31. **When do the rheumatologic manifestations occur in patients with mumps viral infection?**
Although rare, arthritis has been associated with mumps viral infection. Patients most commonly present at 1 to 3 weeks after the clinical viral infection with a migratory polyarthritis that principally involves the large more than the small joints. The duration of symptoms is variable, and symptoms usually resolve in approximately 2 weeks without residual joint damage.

32. Are any rheumatic symptoms associated with enterovirus or adenovirus infection?

Coxsackieviruses and echoviruses are among the enteroviruses that cause a wide spectrum of clinical disease. Self-limited arthritis in both large and small joints has been observed in a limited number of patients with coxsackievirus or echovirus infection. Cocksackievirus can cause rash, pleuritis, and myocarditis as extraarticular manifestations. **Echovirus can cause myositis in patients with agammaglobulinemia**. Adenovirus rarely causes a self-limited syndrome of low-grade fever, arthralgias/arthritis, and rash.

33. Is arthritis frequently associated with clinical infections by the herpetoviruses?

Arthritis is rarely reported as a complication of herpetovirus infections. The Herpetoviridae family includes herpes simplex virus, varicella-zoster virus, Epstein–Barr virus, and cytomegalovirus (bone marrow transplant patients). Herpes hominis may cause knee arthritis in wrestlers (herpes gladiatorum).

BIBLIOGRAPHY

Cacoub P, Renou C, Rosenthal E, et al: Extrahepatic manifestations associated with hepatitis c virus infection. A prospective multicenter study of 321 patients. The GERMIVIC, Medicine 79:47, 2000.

Ganem D, Prince AM: Hepatitis B virus infection—natural history and clinical consequences, N Engl J Med 350:1118, 2004.

Iannuzzella F, Vaglio A, Garini G: Management of hepatitis C virus-related mixed cryoglobulinemia, Am J Med 123:400–408, 2010.

Maillefert JF, Sibilia J, Toussirot E, et al: Rheumatic disorders developed after hepatitis B vaccination, Rheumatology (Oxford) 38:978–983, 1999.

Naides SJ: Rheumatologic manifestations of human parvovirus B19 infection in adults, Rheum Clin North Am 24:375–401, 1998.

Ramos-Casals M, Loustaud-Ratti V, DeVita S, et al: Sjögren's syndrome associated with hepatitis C virus: a multicenter analysis of 137 cases, Medicine 84:81, 2005.

Ramos-Casals M, Munoz S, Medina F, et al: Systemic autoimmune disease in patients with hepatitis C virus infection: characterization of 1020 cases (the HISPAMES Registry), J Rheumatol 36:1442, 2009.

Rivera J, de Diego A, Trinchet M: García Monforte A: Fibromyalgia-associated hepatitis C virus infection, Br J Rheumatol 36:981–985, 1997.

Rosner I, Rosenbaum M, Toubi E, et al: The case for hepatitis C arthritis, Semin Arthritis Rheum 33:375, 2004.

Schmidt AC: Response to dengue fever—the good, the bad, and the ugly? N Engl J Med 363:484, 2010.

Sene D, Ghillani-Dalbin P, Amoura Z, et al: Rituximab may form a complex with IgMκ mixed cryoglobulin and induce severe systemic reactions in patients with hepatitis C virus-induced vasculitis, Arthritis Rheum 60:3848–3855, 2009.

Simon F, Parola P, Grandadam M, et al: Chikungunya infection: an emerging rheumatism among travelers returned from India Ocean islands. Report of 47 cases, Medicine 86:123, 2007.

Toivanen A: Alphaviruses: an emerging cause of arthritis? Curr Opin Rheumatol 20:486, 2008.

Young N, Brown NE: Parvovirus B19, N Engl J Med 350:586, 2004.

CHAPTER 42: HIV-ASSOCIATED RHEUMATIC SYNDROMES

Daniel F. Battafarano, DO

KEY POINTS

1. Screen for a human immunodeficiency virus (HIV) infection in any patient with reactive arthritis, psoriatic arthritis, or psoriasis that is unresponsive to conventional therapy.
2. Bone and joint infections from bacteria do not occur any more frequently in HIV-infected individuals compared to other patients.
3. Highly active retroviral therapy (HAART) has resulted in increased prevalence of osteonecrosis and immune reconstitution inflammatory syndrome (IRIS) in HIV-infected patients, whereas diffuse infiltrative lymphocytosis syndrome (DILS), spondyloarthropathies, and the painful articular syndrome occur less commonly.

1. How common are rheumatic manifestations in HIV patients? Has HAART affected this?

It is estimated that 35 million people are infected with HIV worldwide. The overall prevalence of rheumatic manifestations associated with HIV is approximately 9%. With the use of HAART the overall prevalence of spondyloarthropathies, DILS, and painful articular syndrome has decreased, whereas complications of HIV and its therapy (osteopenia, avascular necrosis, immune reconstitution inflammatory syndrome) have increased.

2. What are the rheumatic manifestations associated with HIV?

Box 42-1 describes rheumatic manifestations associated with HIV.

Box 42-1. Rheumatic Manifestations Associated With Human Immunodeficiency Virus (HIV) Before and After Highly Active Antiretroviral Therapy (HAART)

Pre-HAART	HAART
Articular	**IRIS**
Arthralgias (5%)	Sarcoidosis
HIV-associated arthritis (1%)	Rheumatoid arthritis
Reactive arthritis	Systemic lupus erythematosus
Psoriatic arthritis	Reactive arthritis
Undifferentiated spondyloarthropathy	Sjögren's syndrome
Painful articular syndrome (10%)	Subacute cutaneous lupus
Muscular	Graves' disease
Myalgias/fibromyalgia (30%)	**Drug-induced conditions**
Polymyositis (2%)	Zidovudine myopathy
Nemaline rod myopathy	Mitochondrial myopathies from newer NRTIs
Inclusion body myositis	Rhabdomyolysis
HIV wasting syndrome	Gout/hyperuricemia
Diffuse infiltrative lymphocytosis syndrome (3%)	Lipodystrophy
Vasculitis	**Osseous conditions**
Infection	Osteopenia/osteoporosis
Septic arthritis	Osteomalacia
Pyomyositis	Osteonecrosis
Gout/hyperuricemia	Osteomyelitis

Adapted from Patel N, Patel N, Espinoza, LR: HIV infection and rheumatic diseases: the changing spectrum of clinical enigma, Rheum Dis Clin North Am 35:139-161, 2009.

IRIS, Immune reconstitution inflammatory syndromes; *NRTIs*, nucleoside reverse transcriptase inhibitors.

3. **Does HIV infection have a direct role in the pathogenesis of rheumatic syndromes?**
   A wide spectrum of rheumatic syndromes/diseases in HIV-positive individuals has been described. Many of the rheumatic disorders are encountered in nonHIV populations, but some are unique to patients with HIV infection, including the following:
   - HIV-associated arthritis
   - Painful articular syndrome
   - DILS

   A direct role of HIV infection in rheumatic syndromes has not been well established. Although the specific mechanism is unclear, many of the rheumatic syndromes (polymyositis, vasculitis, HIV-associated arthritis, and DILS) occur in the presence of profound immunodeficiency. Decreasing frequencies of some rheumatic syndromes/diseases in HIV-infected individuals treated with HAART suggest at least an indirect role of HIV infection. In addition, with CD4⁺ T-cell depletion, diseases in which CD8⁺ T cells are predominant, such as psoriasis, reactive arthritis, and DILS, are more commonly seen. T regulatory cells, a subset of CD4⁺ T cells whose main function is to maintain self-tolerance and avoid the development of autoimmunity, are depleted in patients with HIV infection. It is believed that depletion of these regulatory cells and the production of various cytokines play an important role in the pathogenesis of HIV and may contribute to the development of autoantibodies and autoimmune complications. As CD4⁺ T-cell numbers decline (<300 cells/μL), the risk of opportunistic infections rises.

4. **What role do autoantibodies have in HIV-associated rheumatic syndromes?**
   In untreated HIV-positive patients, the most common laboratory abnormalities are a polyclonal gammopathy in up to 45%, low-titer rheumatoid factor and antinuclear antibodies in up to 20%, and IgG anticardiolipin antibodies in over 90% of patients. Anticardiolipin antibodies are rarely of clinical significance because they are not associated with anti-β2 glycoprotein I antibodies. Cryoglobulins can occur in HIV patients with coexisting hepatitis C infection. Both cytoplasmic and perinuclear antineutrophil cytoplasmic antibodies have been described, although without characteristic vasculitis. Therefore, although autoantibodies are common, there is no clinical correlation with the development of a particular rheumatic syndrome. However, patients presenting with arthralgias and one of these autoantibodies may be initially misdiagnosed as having a particular rheumatic disease and not HIV infection.

5. **What is HIV-associated arthritis? How does it differ from the painful articular syndrome?**
   HIV-associated arthritis is typically seronegative and oligoarticular, involving joints of the lower extremities (knees and ankles). The synovial fluid is noninflammatory, with negative cultures and normal radiographs. The symptoms tend to be self-limited, lasting 1 to 6 weeks, and respond to rest, physical therapy, nonsteroidal antiinflammatory drugs (NSAIDs), and low-dose corticosteroids. Unlike reactive arthritis and undifferentiated spondyloarthropathies, there is no enthesopathy, mucocutaneous involvement, or HLA-B27 association, and symptoms do not recur. Once the clinical disorder resolves, the medications can be successfully discontinued. Rarely, a more prolonged arthritis can occur that results in narrowing of joint spaces. These patients may respond to hydroxychloroquine and/or sulfasalazine.

   The **painful articular syndrome** is acute in onset, involves the knees, shoulders, and elbows, and lasts for <24 hours. It occurs in late stages of HIV infection. It is speculated that this may represent transient bone ischemia, because there is no evidence of synovitis. Narcotics are often necessary to relieve symptoms.

6. **How does reactive (Reiter-like) arthritis typically present in a HIV patient?**
   The incidence of reactive arthritis/Reiter syndrome associated with HIV infection is 0.5% to 3% but has declined significantly since HAART was introduced. The onset may precede the diagnosis of AIDS by up to 2 years, occur concomitantly, or most commonly present with severe immunodeficiency. Seronegative oligoarthritis of the lower extremities and urethritis are common, but conjunctivitis is rare. Enthesopathy, plantar fasciitis, dactylitis, stomatitis, and skin and nail changes are common, and balanitis may be seen. Axial skeletal involvement and uveitis are unusual. Synovial fluid is inflammatory (2000 to 10,000 cells/μL) and cultures are negative. The clinical course is typically one of mild arthritis with remissions and recurrences. Severe erosive arthritis does occur and can be very debilitating. The frequency of HLA-B27 in HIV-positive reactive arthritis patients is the same (70% to 90% of patients) as that found in HIV-negative reactive arthritis patients of the same race.

7. **What is the conventional treatment for reactive arthritis in HIV-infected patients?**
   NSAIDs are generally effective, along with physical therapy modalities. It has even been shown that indomethacin inhibits HIV replication in vitro. Intraarticular and soft-tissue cortisone injections are especially therapeutic for localized involvement. Low-dose corticosteroids (<10 mg/day) and sulfasalazine (1.5 g/day) may be effective agents for severe enthesopathy/arthritis. Hydroxychloroquine (up to 600 mg/day) and etretinate (0.5 to 1 mg/kg per day) have been useful as additional second-line agents for refractory arthritis or cutaneous lesions. Methotrexate (<20 mg/week) and other immunosuppressive or biologic agents (TNFα antagonists) should be used with caution and only in patients with CD4⁺ T-cell counts >200 cells/μL and a HIV viral load <60,000 copies/mm³. Patients must be monitored closely because use of these agents may precipitate fulminant AIDS, Kaposi sarcoma, or opportunistic infections.

8. **What is the association between psoriasis and HIV infection?**
Psoriasis and psoriatic arthritis tend to occur late in the course of HIV infection. The full spectrum of psoriaform skin manifestations can be observed in the same patient. Psoriatic arthritis is treated similarly to reactive arthritis. Antiretroviral treatment is very effective for both psoriasis and psoriatic arthritis. Methotrexate, biologics, and phototherapy are reserved for refractory skin or joint involvement because they can precipitate worsening immunosuppression or the onset of Kaposi sarcoma (see Question 7). Lastly, any patient with a severe unexplainable flare of psoriasis or the onset of psoriasis that is unresponsive to conventional therapy should be evaluated for HIV infection.

9. **Why are many HIV patients with arthritis categorized as having undifferentiated spondyloarthropathy?**
Many patients develop oligoarthritis, enthesitis, dactylitis, onycholysis, balanitis, uveitis, or spondylitis without sufficient criteria to be classified as having reactive arthritis/Reiter syndrome or psoriatic arthritis. These patients are ultimately given a diagnosis of undifferentiated spondyloarthropathy. Local treatment, NSAIDs, intraarticular cortisone injections, and sulfasalazine are the conventional approaches for treatment. Other immunosuppressives or biologics such as anti-TNFα agents are used with caution (see Question 7).

10. **What are the HIV-associated muscle diseases?**
Muscle involvement in HIV-infected patients is common, can occur at any stage of disease, and can be inflammatory or noninflammatory. A **noninflammatory necrotizing myopathy** and **HIV-related wasting syndrome** (slim disease) has been described in over 40% of HIV patients diagnosed with myopathy. Muscle biopsies show atrophy and necrosis without inflammation. It has been speculated that the pathogenesis is immune-mediated or may be related to metabolic or nutritional factors. Patients infected with HIV in the pre-HAART era more commonly develop polymyositis, nemaline rod myopathy, and HIV wasting syndrome. Patients treated with HAART tend to develop drug-induced conditions such as mitochondrial myopathy, rhabdomyolysis, and lipodystrophy. Rhabdomyolysis is of particular concern when protease inhibitors are used concurrently with statins.

11. **How can HIV-associated polymyositis and zidovudine (AZT) myopathy be clinically distinguished?**
HIV-associated polymyositis is clinically identical to idiopathic polymyositis with proximal muscle weakness, creatine kinase (CK) elevation, myopathic electromyography (EMG), abnormal muscle magnetic resonance imaging (MRI), and an inflammatory muscle biopsy with CD8+ infiltrates and viral antigen. Autoantibodies such as anti Jo-1 and Mi-2 are absent. *Toxoplasma gondii* must be excluded. Most patients respond well to corticosteroid therapy (0.5 mg/kg per day) for 6 to 12 weeks, with the dose adjusted according to the clinical course. Corticosteroids and HAART may be useful in combination. Methotrexate may benefit selected patients with persistent myositis as a second-line agent but close monitoring is required.

Myopathy induced by AZT (>600 mg/day) occurs after a mean therapy duration of 11 months. This syndrome is clinically indistinguishable from polymyositis. It is associated with mild elevation of muscle enzymes, myopathic EMG, and inflammatory muscle biopsy. The muscle biopsy may reveal AZT-induced toxic mitochondrial myopathy with the appearance of so-called ragged red fibers, which is indicative of abnormal mitochondrial and paracrystalline inclusions. In general, EMG and muscle biopsy are not necessary. The clinical recommendation for evaluating muscle weakness in a patient on AZT is to hold the drug for 4 weeks and reassess the patient via examination and CK measurement. AZT-induced myopathy symptoms and laboratory test results will improve within 4 weeks, and muscle strength will return 8 weeks after discontinuing AZT. High-dose AZT has rarely been used since the advent of HAART, and this myopathy is therefore much less common. Other nucleoside reverse transcriptase inhibitors such as didanosine may also cause this myopathy.

12. **Describe DILS in a patient with HIV infection.**
Diffuse idiopathic lymphocytic syndrome (DILS) is diagnosed according to (1) HIV-positive infection, (2) presence of bilateral, painless salivary gland enlargement or xerostomia persisting for more than 6 months, and (3) histologic confirmation of salivary or lacrimal gland lymphocytic infiltration with predominantly CD8+,CD29- T cells in the absence of granulomatous or neoplastic enlargement or confirmatory ^{67}Ga scintigraphy. There is a much higher prevalence of DILS in Africa compared to the United States. The onset of symptoms usually presents at a mean period of 3 years before diagnosis of HIV infection. DILS is characterized by xerophthalmia, xerostomia, parotid gland enlargement, parotid cysts, persistent circulating CD8 T-cell lymphocytosis, and diffuse visceral lymphocytic infiltration. Pulmonary involvement as a result of lymphocytic interstitial pneumonitis is the most serious complication of DILS and has decreased significantly with HAART. Cranial nerve palsies (VII due to parotid compression), aseptic meningitis, and symmetrical peripheral motor neuropathy may occur. Lymphocytic hepatitis, interstitial nephritis, type IV renal tubular acidosis, polymyositis, and lymphoma have also been observed. Low to moderate doses of corticosteroids are beneficial for glandular enlargement and sicca symptoms. Topical treatment is usually satisfactory, but pilocarpine (5 to 10 mg three times per day) may be necessary for severe sicca symptoms. High-dose corticosteroids and HAART are used for severe extraglandular involvement.

Table 42-1. Comparison of Sjögren's Syndrome and Diffuse Infiltrative Lymphocytosis Syndrome (DILS)

	SJÖGREN'S SYNDROME	DILS
Parotid swelling	Uncommon	Common
Sicca symptoms	Common	Common
Extraglandular manifestations	Uncommon	Common
Infiltrative lymphocytic phenotype	CD4 T cell	CD8 T cell
Autoantibodies (RF, ANA, anti-SS-A/SS-B)	Common	Rare
HLA association	DRB1*0301	DRB1*1102, 1301, 1302
Corticosteroids for glandular symptoms	Rarely helpful	Beneficial

ANA, Antinuclear antibody; RF, rheumatoid factor.

13. **Compare DILS to Sjögren's syndrome.**
    Table 42-1 compares features of Sjögren's syndrome and DILS.

14. **List the forms of vasculitis that have been described for HIV infection and/or following institution of HAART.**
    - Polyarteritis nodosa; usually presents as a sensorimotor neuropathy
    - Large artery/aorta vasculitis; more common in Africa
    - Hypersensitivity angiitis due to AZT and didanosine
    - Henoch–Schönlein purpura
    - Granulomatosis with polyangiitis (Wegener granulomatosis)
    - Primary vasculitis of the central nervous system
    - Behçet syndrome
    - Kawasaki disease in both children and adults
    - Eosinophilic granulomatosis with polyangiitis (Churg–Strauss vasculitis)

15. **Is septic arthritis and/or bone infection more common in HIV-infected patients?**
    No, bone and joint infections from bacteria do not occur any more frequently in HIV-positive compared with HIV-negative individuals. Intravenous drug abusers and hemophiliacs are clearly at increased risk of septic arthritis. The most common bacterial organism is *Staphylococcus aureus*, especially in IV drug abusers, whereas *Salmonella* is most common in hemophiliacs. *Mycobacterium tuberculosis* arthritis and/or osteomyelitis can occur at any time in the course of HIV infection and may be multifocal (30%). Atypical mycobacterial and fungal musculoskeletal infections typically occur with severe immunosuppression (<100 cells/μL). Overall, bacterial joint infections are most common when the $CD4^+$ count is greater than 250 cells/μL, and opportunistic infections occur in patients with lower $CD4^+$ counts. Osteomyelitis may occur independently at any bony site or may coexist with septic arthritis.

16. **How does pyomyositis present clinically?**
    Pyomyositis is rarely observed in developed countries but is still commonly diagnosed in Africa and India. Patients are usually in late-stage disease with $CD4^+$ counts <200 cells/μL. Pyomyositis presents with fever, local muscle pain, erythema, swelling, and leukocytosis. This uncommon infection typically involves the quadriceps muscle, and a single abscess is present in 75% of cases. *S. aureus* is identified in the vast majority of these cases, but opportunistic infections may occur. Patients are diagnosed using ultrasound, computed tomography scanning, MRI, and cultures, and respond to conventional surgical drainage and antibiotics.

17. **Name the rheumatic diseases that have a negative association with AIDS.**
    Systemic lupus erythematosus (SLE) and rheumatoid arthritis (RA) are both mediated via a process involving interaction between MHC class II gene products and CD4 T lymphocytes. Therefore, SLE and RA may become quiescent with progressive HIV infection and decreasing $CD4^+$ T cell counts. Notably, however, some RA patients may not go into remission. When a HIV-infected patient with previously diagnosed SLE or RA is being treated with HAART, the resultant immune reconstitution can cause recurrence of their previously inactive SLE or RA.

18. **What is the immune reconstitution inflammatory syndrome (IRIS)?**
    After initiation of HAART in a HIV-infected individual, cellular immunity improves. There is an increase in $CD4^+$ cells, the $CD4^+/CD8^+$ ratio, and cytokines such as IL-6 and IFN-γ, along with an imbalance in Th1/Th2 cells and expression of CCR-3 and CCR-5 on monocytes and granulocytes. As a result, some patients (up to 13%) develop a very profound inflammatory systemic response known as IRIS within 3 to 27 months

(mean 9 months) after starting HAART. This syndrome is less likely to occur if the CD4+ count is >200 to 350 cell/μL when HAART is initiated. AIDS patients can be diagnosed with IRIS if they develop severe systemic inflammatory symptoms on HAART associated with increasing CD4+ counts and decreasing HIV-1 viral load, and the symptoms cannot be explained by a new etiology or infection. The first phase of IRIS occurs within 8 to 12 weeks after initiation of HAART and results from an increase in memory CD4+ cells. It can be associated with exacerbation of preexisting RA, SLE, or sarcoidosis. The second phase occurs after 6 months of HAART and results from naïve CD4+ cells and their cytokines. This can be associated with the onset of a new systemic or organ-specific autoimmune disease such as RA, SLE, Still disease, polymyositis, reactive arthritis, autoimmune thyroid disease, subacute cutaneous lupus, or Guillain–Barré syndrome. In addition, opportunistic infections under treatment can worsen during this phase. IRIS tends to be a self-limited syndrome and in general HAART is continued. If the inflammatory response is severe and threatens irreversible damage to the eyes or central nervous system, then HAART may need to be discontinued and the patient treated with corticosteroids.

19. **Can a patient with severe RA or a spondyloarthropathy and a coexisting HIV infection be treated with anti-TNFα therapy?**
    Guidelines for the use of immunosuppressives and/or TNF inhibitors in a HIV-infected individual with a severe rheumatic disease include restricting use to patients who have:
    - CD4 T-cell count of >200 cells/μL
    - HIV viral load of <60,000 copies/μL

20. **What other miscellaneous rheumatic syndromes are described in patients with HIV?**
    Fibromyalgia has been observed in 10% to 30% of HIV-infected patients. Tendinitis, bursitis, carpal tunnel syndrome, adhesive capsulitis, and Dupuytren contracture may occur, particularly in patients treated with protease inhibitors (indinavir). Hyperuricemia is common in HIV patients and gout can occur. There may be an association with ritonavir and indinavir.

21. **What bone diseases occur more commonly in HIV patients?**
    - **Osteoporosis** risk is three times greater in patients with HIV. The cause is multifactorial. Vitamin D deficiency is common. Therapy includes calcium, vitamin D, and bisphosphonate therapy according to current recommendations.
    - **Osteonecrosis (avascular necrosis)** can occur in any joint, with the hip being most common. The prevalence is 4% to 5%. Risk factors include dyslipidemia associated with protease inhibitors, corticosteroid use, and the HIV infection itself when the patient has a very low CD4 count (<60 cells/μL).
    - **Hypertrophic osteoarthropathy (HO)** can develop in patients with *Pneumocystis jiroveci* pneumonia. Treatment of the pneumonia improves the HO.

22. **Do any other retroviruses cause rheumatic diseases?**
    Human T lymphotropic virus type I (HTLV-I) is a complex type C RNA retrovirus. It infects millions worldwide, particularly in the Caribbean, southern Japan, South Africa, and South America, especially Brazil. It is transmitted via breast milk, sexual intercourse, and blood products. The virus causes two types of disease: (1) adult T-cell leukemia/non-Hodgkin lymphoma (5% lifetime risk), frequently with hypercalcemia and skin involvement; and (2) a variety of chronic inflammatory syndromes (lifetime risk 2%). These inflammatory syndromes include seronegative oligo- or polyarthritis with tenosynovitis and nodules with fibrinoid necrosis. Other syndromes include polymyositis-like disease, dermatitis, uveitis, and transverse myelitis, also known as HTLV-1-associated myelopathy/tropical spastic paraparesis (HAM/TSP). Diagnosis is made by ELISA detection of antibodies with confirmation by Western blotting and the observation of so-called **flower cells** on a peripheral smear. Treatment options are poor. Cases of this viral infection are being seen more frequently in the United States as a result of immigration and screening of donated blood.

BIBLIOGRAPHY

Authier FJ, Chariot P, Gherardi RK: Skeletal muscle involvement in human immunodeficiency virus (HIV)-infected patients in the era of highly active antiretroviral therapy (HAART), Muscle Nerve 32(3):247–260, 2005.
Calabrese L, Kircher E, Shrestha E: Rheumatic complications of human immunodeficiency virus (HIV) infection in the era of highly active antiretroviral therapy (HAART): emergence of a new syndrome of immune reconstitution and changing pattern of pattern of disease, Semin Arthritis Rheum 35:166–174, 2005.
Foulon G, Wislez M, Maccache JM, et al: Sarcoidosis in HIV-infected patients in the era of highly active antiretroviral therapy, Clin Infect Dis 38:418–425, 2004.
Guillevin L: Vasculitides in the context of HIV infection, AIDS 22(Suppl 3):S27–S33, 2008.
Maganti RM, Reveille JD, Williams FM: Therapy insight: the changing spectrum of rheumatic disease in HIV infection, Nat Clin Pract Rheumatol 4(8):428–438, 2008.
Marquez J, Restrepo CS, Candia L, et al: Human immunodeficiency virus-associated rheumatic disorders in the HAART era, J Rheumatol 31:741–746, 2004.
Medina F, Pérez-Saleme L, Moreno J: Rheumatic manifestations of human immunodeficiency virus infection, Infect Dis Clin North Am 20(4):891–912, 2006.

Muller M, Wandel S, Colebunders R, et al: Immune reconstitution inflammatory syndrome in patients starting antiretroviral therapy for HIV infection: a systemic review and meta-analysis, Lancet Infect Dis 10:251–261, 2010.

Paccou J, Viget N, Legrout-Gerot I, et al: Bone loss in patients with HIV infection, J Bone Spine 76:637–641, 2009.

Patel N, Patel N, Espinoza LR: HIV infection and rheumatic diseases: the changing spectrum of clinical enigma, Rheum Dis Clin North Am 35:139–161, 2009.

Further Reading

http://www.rheumatology.org/public/factsheets/diseases.../HIV.asp

WHIPPLE'S DISEASE
Carolyn Anne Coyle, MD

KEY POINTS

1. Whipple's disease is a rare, systemic, infectious disorder caused by the actinomycete *Tropheryma whipplei*.
2. Joint manifestations of Whipple's disease often antedate the gastrointestinal symptoms by years and typically affect large joints in a migratory, intermittent pattern resembling palindromic rheumatism.
3. The diagnosis is established by demonstrating the organism on biopsy of the small bowel or other affected organ using immunohistochemical staining and quantitative PCR analysis.
4. Treatment consists of prolonged antibiotic therapy.

1. What is Whipple's disease?
Whipple's disease is an uncommon chronic systemic disorder caused by the gram-positive bacillus *Tropheryma whipplei* (from the Greek *trophe* meaning nourishment and *eryma* meaning barrier, which refers to the malabsorption seen in this disease). It can present with polyarthritis, fever, malabsorption, and central nervous system (CNS) manifestations. Because of its nonspecific presentation, the condition is usually diagnosed when it is in an advanced stage. The typical patient is a middle-aged white man presenting with abdominal pain, diarrhea, weight loss, and arthritis.

2. When did Dr. Whipple first describe the disease and bacillus that now bear his name?
In 1907, Dr. George Hoyt Whipple reported a "hitherto undescribed disease" in a 36-year-old medical missionary with migratory arthritis, cough, fever, diarrhea, malabsorption, weight loss, skin hyperpigmentation, and abdominal swelling with mesenteric lymphadenopathy. In Whipple's original case report, the patient's "first symptoms were attacks of arthritis coming on in several joints." At autopsy, Whipple noted "great numbers of rod-shaped organisms" in silver-stained sections of a mesenteric lymph node and speculated that this organism might be the causative agent of the disease.

3. Describe the clinical presentation of patients with Whipple's disease.
Whipple's disease is a systemic illness affecting primarily white men (86%) over age 40 years (mean 49 years). Over 66% have had occupational exposure to soil (farmers), sewage water, or animals. Patients usually present with a history of intermittent arthralgias/arthritis (60% to 80%) involving multiple joints over a period of years. Later, they gradually develop diarrhea (80%), steatorrhea, weight loss (93%), and other organ involvement, including cardiac, CNS, and renal involvement. Hyperpigmentation of the skin is found in 50% of patients; low-grade fever (35% to 40%) and lymphadenopathy (50%) are common.

The multisystem manifestations of Whipple's disease can be remembered using the following mnemonic:

Wasting/weight loss	Diarrhea
Hyperpigmentation (skin)	Interstitial nephritis
Intestinal pain	Skin rashes
Pleurisy	Eye inflammation
Pneumonitis	Arthritis
Lymphadenopathy	Subcutaneous nodules
Encephalopathy	Endocarditis
Steatorrhea	

4. Describe the arthritis associated with Whipple's disease.
Seronegative migratory oligo- or polyarthritis/arthralgia primarily involving large joints (knees) characterized by brief episodic attacks lasting a few days in a pattern akin to palindromic rheumatism is associated with Whipple's disease. Arthritis/arthralgia is the presenting symptom in 60% of 70% of reported cases and is present in 90% of all patients. It does not correlate with intestinal symptoms and can precede the intestinal manifestations in 75% of patients by a mean interval of 6 years. Sacroiliitis is present in 7% and spondylitis in 4% of cases. Joint fluid examination may reveal periodic acid–Shiff (PAS)-positive material; however, joint fluid cultures are negative. Radiographs usually remain unremarkable.

5. **Describe the synovial fluid and microscopic results from arthrocentesis and synovial biopsies for patients with Whipple's disease.**

   Arthrocentesis for patients with Whipple's disease and arthritis usually reveals an inflammatory fluid with white blood cell (WBC) counts between 2000 and 30,000 cells/mm^3 with greater than 50% polymorphonuclear cells. Repeat arthrocentesis after antibiotic therapy shows resolution of inflammation, with WBC counts between 100 and 300 cells/mm^3 and less than 50% polymorphonuclear cells. Synovial biopsy also demonstrates an inflammatory picture, with focal synovial lining cell hyperplasia and moderate perivascular lymphocytosis. Importantly, there are also PAS-positive granules in macrophages (foamy macrophages) within the synovial membrane, most likely representing degenerated bacterial forms.

6. **What is the etiology of Whipple's disease?**

   Multiple tissues from patients with Whipple's disease show PAS staining deposits. These deposits contain non–acid-fast, PAS-positive, rod-shaped bacilli that on electron microscopy have an unusual trilamellar plasma membrane surrounded by a cell wall. PCR identification of the DNA sequence encoding 16S rRNA revealed that the bacterium causing Whipple's disease (*T. whipplei*) is closely related to other soil-borne, gram-positive actinomycetes. Modifications of this PCR technique are currently used as one of the standard methods for establishing a diagnosis of Whipple's disease and are more sensitive than histopathologic analysis.

7. **What are some of the immunologic defects in patients who develop Whipple's disease?**

   T. whipplei is an ubiquitous organism and its DNA has been detected by PCR in the saliva and stool of 1% of individuals without evidence of Whipple's disease. Why some people develop clinical Whipple's disease is unclear. It is postulated that these patients have genetic or acquired defects in the mucosal and peripheral immune system that may predispose them to symptomatic infection with this bacillus. Defects in the cell-mediated immune response with reduced TH1 cytokines (IL-12 and IFN-γ), accompanied by increased secretion of TH2 cytokines (IL-4), have been described for affected individuals. It is unclear if these defects are primary and predispose a person to the infection or are the result of the bacillus growing within macrophages.

8. **How is the diagnosis of Whipple's disease most commonly made?**

   Before the PCR technique was developed, a definitive diagnosis was established only when microscopic examination of a jejunal biopsy of small intestinal mucosa showed infiltration of the lamina propria by large macrophages that contained diastase-resistant, PAS-positive inclusions. In 1961, electron microscopy demonstrated that the PAS-positive materials were rod-shaped bacilli. These bacilli can be found in multiple other tissues (lymph nodes, pericardium, myocardium, liver, spleen, kidney, synovium, and brain) and are located both intra- and extracellularly. Since the advent of the PCR technique in the 1990s, diagnosis can now be made without biopsy, in cases who present with extraintestinal disease, or when biopsy results are inconclusive. However, the best evidence of infection is demonstration of the organism in tissue with immunohistochemical staining with antisera specific for *T. whipplei*. Quantitative PCR for *T. whipplei* DNA is used as a confirmatory test performed on tissue (small bowel, endocardium, synovium, lymph node, brain) and body fluid (blood, vitreous fluid, synovial fluid, and cerebrospinal fluid [CSF]). PCR testing of saliva and stool as a screening tool has a 95% positive predictive value if both are positive and a 98% negative predictive value if both are negative. Notably, some (<5%) normal individuals without Whipple's disease can be PCR-positive. PCR of whole blood is useful if positive, but a negative test does not rule out the disease. The organism can be grown in culture but takes an average of 30 days, requires special culture techniques that are not generally available, and remains a research tool.

9. **In addition to arthritis and intestinal manifestations, how else can Whipple's disease present?**

   - Up to 10% of Whipple's disease patients present with neurologic manifestations, and up to 40% will eventually develop CNS symptoms. Even in Whipple's patients without neurologic symptoms, 50% can have PCR-positive CSF and therefore all patients should have CSF tested before therapy, regardless of symptoms. In patients who develop neurologic symptoms, dementia is the most frequent symptom (70%). Psychiatric symptoms (50%), supranuclear vertical gaze palsy (50%), hypothalamic involvement (33%), and myoclonus (25%) are also common. Progressive supranuclear palsy with oculomasticatory and/or oculofacioskeletal myorhythmias is pathognomonic for CNS Whipple's disease but occurs in only 20% of cases. Brain biopsy and positive PCR of CSF are diagnostic in 90% of cases.
   - *T. whipplei* has been a rare cause of culture-negative endocarditis. Cardiac involvement of the pericardium, myocardium, and endocardium including valves is found at autopsy in all patients with classic Whipple's disease. However, only 17% to 55% of cases are symptomatic.
   - Panuveitis diagnosis is made by PCR testing of the vitreous humor.
   - Other manifestations typically accompany a classic Whipple's presentation. These include pulmonary involvement (30%), mesenteric more than peripheral adenopathy with noncaseating granulomas (9%), and rarely genitourinary involvement.

10. **What is the therapy currently recommended for Whipple's disease?**

    Before the use of antibiotics, Whipple's disease was uniformly fatal. There is no general consensus on the best antibiotic regimen for treatment of Whipple's disease. Current recommendations include a 2-week course of parenteral therapy (ceftriaxone 2 g/day) followed by long-term therapy with double-strength trimethoprim/sulfamethoxazole (TMP/sulfa; 160 mg/800 mg twice per day for 1 to 2 years). It is critical that an antibiotic that penetrates the CNS is used to lessen the chance of treatment failures and relapses. Tetracycline is recommended for those who are allergic to TMP/sulfa.

11. **How frequently do patients experience clinical relapses of disease following 1 year of treatment?**
Because Whipple's disease is uncommon, formal prospective studies of therapeutic regimens have not been carried out. It is estimated that up to 35% of patients with Whipple's disease who had long-term treatment relapsed after an average of 5 years. Neurologic relapses are most common and are particularly hard to treat. More long-term data are needed regarding the choice and duration of antibiotic therapy. Recommendations for treating disease relapses include ceftriaxone (2 g IV twice per day) or meropenem for 4 weeks followed by doxycycline (100 mg twice per day) plus hydroxychloroquine (200 mg three times per day) or TMP/sulfa (twice per day) for a year. PCR may have a role in monitoring the eradication or persistence of infection and in providing physicians with information regarding treatment decisions such as choice, duration, and alteration of antibiotic therapy. Recent PCR studies show a correlation between persistent PCR positivity and the relapse rate.

12. **Describe the Jarisch–Herxheimer reaction and immune reconstitution inflammatory syndrome (IRIS) that can occur during antibiotic therapy for Whipple's disease.**
    - The Jarisch–Herxheimer reaction was initially described as a systemic reaction that occurs 1 to 2 hours after initial treatment of syphilis with effective antibiotics, especially penicillin. It consists of abrupt onset of fever, chills, myalgias, headache, tachycardia, hyperventilation, vasodilatation with flushing, and mild hypotension. It has been well correlated with the release of heat-stable pyrogens from spirochetes. The reaction is self-limited; however, it can be prevented by administration of oral prednisone. The Jarisch–Herxheimer reaction has been reported after initial treatment of a number of infectious diseases besides syphilis, including leptospirosis, Lyme disease, relapsing fever, rat-bite fever, and Whipple's disease.
    - IRIS occurs within the first few weeks following initiation of antibiotic therapy and is manifest by progression of disease symptoms and high fever. It is most common in patients who have received prior immunosuppressive therapy or who have CNS involvement. Corticosteroids can be beneficial in the control of these symptoms.

Bibliography

Dobbin WO: Whipple's disease: an historical perspective, Q J Med 56:523, 1985.
Fenollar F, Puechal X, Raoult D: Whipple's disease, N Engl J Med 356:55–66, 2007.
Feurle GE, Junga NS, Marth T: Efficacy of ceftriazone or meropenem as initial therapies in Whipple's disease, Gastroenterology 138:478, 2010.
Gerard A, Sarrot-Reynauld F, Liozon E, et al: Neurologic presentation of Whipple's disease: report of 12 cases and review of the literature, Medicine (Baltimore) 81:443, 2002.
Lagier JC, Lepidi H, Raoult D, Fenollar F: Systemic *Tropheryma whipplei*: clinical presentation of 142 patients with infection diagnosed and confirmed in a reference center, Medicine (Baltimore) 89:337, 2010.
Louis ED, Lynch T, Kaufmann P, et al: Diagnostic guidelines in central nervous system Whipple's disease, Ann Neurol 40:561–568, 1996.
Moos V, Schmidt C, Geelhaar A, et al: Impaired immune functions of monocytes and macrophages in Whipple's disease, Gastroenterology 138:210, 2010.
O'Duffy JD, Griffing WL: Whipple's arthritis: direct detection of *Tropheryma whippelii* in synovial fluid and tissue, Arth Rheum 42:812–817, 1999.
Ramzan NN, Loftus Jr E, Burgart LJ, et al: Diagnosis and monitoring of Whipple disease by polymerase chain reaction, Ann Int Med 126:520–527, 1997.
Relman DA, Schmidt TM, MacDermott RP, Falkow S: Identification of the uncultured bacillus of Whipple's disease, N Engl J Med 327:293–301, 1992.
Schneider T, Moos V, Loddenkemper C, et al: Whipple's disease: new aspects of pathogenesis and treatment, Lancet Infect Dis 8:179, 2008.
Whipple GH: A hitherto undescribed disease characterized anatomically by deposits of fat and fatty acids in the intestinal and mesenteric tissues, Bull Johns Hopkins Hosp 18:382, 1907.

CHAPTER 44

ACUTE RHEUMATIC FEVER AND POSTSTREPTOCOCCAL ARTHRITIS

Carolyn Anne Coyle, MD

KEY POINTS

1. Acute rheumatic fever (ARF) occurs in 1% to 6% of patients with streptococcal pharyngitis.
2. The arthritis of ARF is a self-limited migratory polyarthritis of large joints that develops 2 to 3 weeks after streptococcal pharyngitis and resolves within 1 month.
3. Rheumatic fever causes 25% to 40% of all cardiovascular disease in the world.
4. Prompt antibiotic treatment of streptococcal pharyngitis decreases the subsequent development of ARF by 80%.

1. **What is acute rheumatic fever?**
   ARF is a systemic inflammatory disease that occurs as a delayed complication of pharyngeal infection with group A streptococci (GAS). It involves multiple organ systems including the heart, joints, central nervous system, skin, and subcutaneous tissues. The most common clinical manifestations include migratory polyarthritis, fever, carditis, and, less often, chorea, subcutaneous nodules, and erythema marginatum. Although joint manifestations may be prominent enough to group ARF among the rheumatic diseases, its greatest significance relates to its adverse effects on the heart, both acutely and chronically leading to rheumatic heart disease, a chronic condition caused by scarring and deformity of the heart valves. As concisely stated by Lasegue many years ago, rheumatic fever "licks the joints and bites the heart."

2. **When were the first studies on ARF published? When was the association with GAS made?**
   The classic works in the field of ARF were published in 1836 by Jean-Baptiste Bouillard and in 1889 by Walter B. Cheadle. They included extensive studies on "rheumatic arthritis" and carditis. The specific rheumatic lesion in the myocardium was described by Ludwig Aschoff in 1904. The introduction of Rebecca Lancefield's grouping system for β-hemolytic streptococci in 1933 allowed clarification of the epidemiology of the disease by a number of investigators.

3. **How is the diagnosis of ARF established?**
   The Jones criteria for guidance in the diagnosis of ARF were first published by T. Duckett Jones in 1944 and have been revised over the years by the American Heart Association. The current revised Jones criteria for the diagnosis of ARF are listed in Box 44-1.
   All patients should have evidence of a preceding GAS infection (with few exceptions) **and** the presence of two major manifestations **or** one major and two minor manifestations. Fulfillment of these criteria indicates a high probability of ARF. Note that a minor criterion should not be counted if the patient exhibits that manifestation as a major criterion (e.g., a patient with polyarthritis cannot also be counted as having the minor criterion of arthralgia).

4. **Is there an easier way to remember the major manifestations of the Jones criteria for ARF? (Submitted by Christopher T. Parker)**
   Yes, simply use the word "Jones" and replace the "o" with a heart-shaped symbol.
   J = joints (75%)
   O = carditis (40% to 50%)
   N = nodules (<10%)
   E = erythema marginatum (<10%)
   S = Sydenham chorea (15%)
   Percentages listed in parentheses denote the incidence of a particular symptom during a child's initial attack.

5. **In what situations can a diagnosis of ARF be made without strict adherence to the Jones criteria?**
   There are three circumstances in which a diagnosis of rheumatic fever can be made without strictly adhering to the Jones criteria:
   1. Chorea may occur as the only manifestation of ARF many months after the streptococcal pharyngitis and serologic evidence of an antecedent infection may be lacking. **Antideoxyribonuclease-B (antiDNase-B)** is the antibody most likely to be positive in a patient with chorea because it is the longest lasting.

Box 44-1. Revised Jones Criteria for Acute Rheumatic Fever

Major Manifestations	Supporting Evidence of GAS Infection	Minor Manifestations
Carditis	Positive throat culture or rapid streptococcal antigen test	Clinical findings
Polyarthritis		Arthralgia
Chorea	Elevated or rising antibody titers	Fever
Subcutaneous nodules	Recent scarlet fever	Previous ARF or rheumatic heart disease
Erythema marginatum		Laboratory findings
		Elevated acute phase reactants
		Erythrocyte sedimentation rate
		C-reactive protein
		Prolonged P–R interval

ARF, Acute rheumatic fever.

2. Indolent carditis and/or typical chronic valve lesions (mitral, aortic) may also present as the only manifestation of ARF. Again, the prolonged latent period between clinical infection and the patient coming to medical attention may make documentation of antecedent streptococcal infection difficult.
3. In patients with a history of ARF or rheumatic heart disease, a new episode of ARF may be difficult to diagnose. Although most patients fulfill the Jones criteria, a different heart lesion would need to be present to distinguish between old and new cardiac pathology.

6. **Describe the natural history of ARF and its relationship to the clinical and laboratory criteria necessary to establish a diagnosis.**
   There is usually a latent period of approximately 18 days between the onset of streptococcal pharyngitis and ARF. This period is rarely less than 1 week or longer than 5 weeks. Overall only 70% of older children/adults and 20% of younger children remember having had pharyngitis. In addition, a positive throat culture for *Streptococcus* is found in only approximately 25% of patients with ARF and may be negative owing to the latent period. Several rapid GAS antigen detection tests are commercially available. These tests are generally very specific (97%) but less sensitive (89%). Neither a throat culture nor an antigen test for GAS distinguishes between a carrier state and infection. As many as one third of patients with ARF do not remember having any illness in the month preceding the onset of rheumatic fever.
   Streptococcal antibodies may be more useful because (1) they reach a peak titer at about the time of onset of rheumatic fever, (2) they indicate true infection rather than transient carriage, and (3) any significant recent streptococcal infection can be detected by performing several tests for different antibodies.

7. **What specific antibodies are used to help confirm a diagnosis of ARF?**
   The specific antibody tests that have been used are directed against extracellular products found in the supernatant broth of streptococcal cultures. They include antistreptolysin-O (ASO), antiDNase-B, antistreptokinase, antihyaluronidase, and antiNADase (antiDPNase). The normal ranges for all of these antibody titers depend on several factors, including the patient's age, geographic location, epidemiologic circumstances, and time of the year. The most commonly used tests are ASO, antiDNase-B, and antistreptokinase. The antibody levels peak at 4 to 5 weeks after the pharyngeal infection. Failure to demonstrate evidence of recent infection by a battery of these three serologic tests makes diagnosis of ARF doubtful.
   As a general reference, an ASO titer is considered to be elevated at 240 Todd units in adults and 320 Todd units in children. AntiDNase-B titers of >120 Todd units in adults and >240 Todd units in children are also considered to be elevated. Samples should be drawn at 2- to 4-week intervals and all samples processed simultaneously. The ASO test is the most widely used serological test for detection of GAS infections. Elevated ASO titers are found in approximately 80% of patients with clinical manifestations of ARF. The sensitivity can be increased even further to 90% using two serological tests and up to 95% using three serological tests. Elevated ASO titers should be interpreted with caution, however, because they are not very specific and other streptococcal groups (including groups C and G) and other species of bacteria produce ASO-like products that result in an elevated ASO titer but have no association with ARF. Therefore, when streptococcal infection is suspected, it is advisable to measure not only ASO but also a second type of more specific streptococcal antibody such as the antiDNase-B titer.
   Clinicians should be aware that high titers for ASO or other antistreptococcal antibodies can also be found in patients (particularly children) with other known rheumatic diseases and no associated ARF. This is usually a result of nonspecific immune stimulation resulting in a polyclonal gammopathy demonstrating past streptococcal exposure.

8. **How useful is the Streptozyme test for diagnosis of ARF?**
   The Streptozyme test is a slide hemagglutination test that detects antibodies to five or more extracellular streptococcal antigens. However, the nature of the antibodies assayed and the antigens they are directed against are not well characterized. There is also considerable lot-to-lot variability in the standardization of the reagent. Consequently, this is not a good test for confirming a diagnosis of ARF.

9. What is known about the biology of GAS in relation to ARF?

Streptococcus pyogenes (group A streptococcus) is a ubiquitous human pathogen that causes a wide array of infections. Streptococcal infections at other sites, such as skin and wounds and in puerperal sepsis or pneumonia, have not been associated with rheumatic fever. An exception to this may occur in Aboriginal communities of Australia, where ARF is associated with pyoderma caused by GAS. Notably, the so-called nephritogenic GAS has very rarely if ever been shown to cause ARF in well-defined epidemics of nephritis, that is, the coexistence of ARF and acute glomerulonephritis in the same patient is quite unusual. It has become clear that changes in the biologic properties and clinical virulence of prevalent streptococcal strains influence the rheumatogenic potential of GAS. The M protein is the chief virulence factor of GAS, and antigenic differences are used to divide GAS into serotypes. Only streptococcal strains with certain M serotypes are known to be highly virulent and strongly associated with ARF. The degree of encapsulation varies greatly among GAS strains, and strains that are both rich in M protein and heavily encapsulated are readily transmitted from person to person and tend to produce severe infections.

10. How does GAS cause ARF?

Many hypotheses have been advanced to explain the occurrence of ARF and the exact genesis of rheumatic carditis and other clinical manifestations of the disease. The most acceptable has been that the disease represents a damaging immune response on the part of the host to an antecedent GAS infection involving microbial antigens crossreacting with target organs (**molecular mimicry**). The GAS cytoplasmic membrane is surrounded by an outer peptidoglycan layer. This layer is covered by a surface layer containing carbohydrates (group A specific), proteins (M proteins), and glycoproteins. Antigens in the GAS membrane and layers can cross react with heart antigens. For example, GAS cytoplasmic membrane antigens can crossreact with sarcolemmal antigens. Streptococcal M protein peptides can crossreact with cardiac myosin and articular cartilage/synovium and are contained in some "rheumatogenic" M protein serotypes. The group A carbohydrate rhamnose-N-acetylglucosamine can crossreact with the glycosides of heart valves. So-called heart-reactive antibodies (HRAs) are found in higher titers in 33% to 85% of patients with rheumatic heart disease compared to those without the disease. Immunoglobulin and complement have been found bound to the myocardium of children dying of rheumatic carditis, which suggests that circulating HRAs may have pathogenetic significance. Another hypothesis postulates that M protein and streptococcal pyrogenic exotoxin may function as "superantigens" capable of strongly activating a broad range of T lymphocytes, which may also contribute to the pathogenesis of ARF, although evidence of this is lacking.

11. What host factors contribute to the pathogenesis of ARF?

ARF is most frequent among children in the 4- to 15-year-old group. Some observers have questioned whether repeated "primary" infections might be a prerequisite for the development of ARF. It is very rare in children less than 4 years of age. There is no clear-cut sex predilection overall, although host factors including sex and age at the time of GAS infection undoubtedly play some role. The incidence of chorea is equal among prepubescent boys and girls, but is very rare in sexually mature men and is exaggerated during pregnancy. Other examples of sex predilection include a higher frequency of tight mitral stenosis in females and aortic stenosis in males. The attack rate of ARF after untreated streptococcal exudative tonsillitis ranges from 1% to 6% (average 3%), and the disease may cluster in families, especially twins. Interestingly, a B lymphocyte alloantigen (designated **D8/17**) has been found in 66% to 100% of ethnically diverse ARF patients and in only 10% of control individuals. The presence of this antigen may be useful in diagnosis. Associations between ARF susceptibility and certain HLA class II antigens have been conflicting.

12. Describe the arthritis associated with ARF.

The arthritis of ARF usually involves the large joints, particularly the knees (75%), ankles (50%), and elbows/wrists/hips (15%), and occurs in 75% of patients. The shoulder (8%), spine (2%), and smaller joints of the hands and feet are less commonly involved. In a classic attack, several joints are involved in quick succession and each for a brief period of time, resulting in the typical picture of a migratory polyarthritis accompanied by signs and symptoms of an acute febrile illness. Acute polyarthritis involving 6 to 16 joints occurs early in the course of ARF and can be exceptionally painful with only mild signs of inflammation. The onset of arthritis is almost always associated with a rising or peak titer of streptococcal antibodies. Patients are usually symptomatic for 1 to 2 weeks, and only rarely do symptoms exceed a 4-week course. ARF never causes permanent joint deformities, with the rare exception of Jaccoud-type deformity, which can occur in individuals who have had multiple attacks of ARF.

The pathologic changes in the joints in ARF include a serous effusion, with a thickened, erythematous synovial membrane covered by a fibrinous exudate. Microscopically, there is a diffuse cellular infiltrate of polymorphonuclear leukocytes and lymphocytes. Focal fibrinoid lesions and histiocytic granulomas may be late findings. Synovial fluid is sterile and inflammatory.

13. Is there a poststreptococcal reactive arthritis (PSRA) distinct from ARF?

Several investigators have described the inverse relationship between the incidence and severity of carditis and the severity of joint involvement in ARF. Some investigators have described patients with a poststreptococcal "reactive" arthritis that occurs after a brief latent period (1 to 2 weeks), persists longer than the typical 4-week period that is typical of ARF, and responds poorly to salicylates/nonsteroidal antiinflammatory drugs (NSAIDs). It appears that this so-called PSRA is more common in females than males and that PSRA patients tend to be older (frequently young adults) than those who develop ARF. The arthritis has been described as predominantly nonmigratory as opposed to the classic migratory arthritis described in ARF. Some have described PSRA as a *forme fruste* of ARF and hypothesize that it may be caused by different strains of GAS and have a more benign prognosis. However, because no clear data exist to distinguish PSRA from ARF, it is generally recommended that all episodes of poststreptococcal arthritis that fulfill the revised Jones criteria be assumed to represent ARF and be treated as such.

14. Describe the characteristics of some of the other manifestations occurring in ARF.
- **Carditis** occurs in 50% to 65% of patients; the younger a person is, the greater is the likelihood of carditis. All three layers of the heart are affected (pericardium, myocardium, and valves). The mitral valve is most often involved, followed by the aortic valve. Echocardiograms show more valve involvement (90% of patients) than appreciated clinically. The significance of valvulitis on echocardiogram when no murmur is heard is unclear and the condition may heal without sequelae. Congestive heart failure due to myocarditis occurs in 5% to 10% of patients, never occurs without valve involvement, and occurs more commonly during recurrences of ARF. All degrees of heart block can occur.
- **Subcutaneous nodules** (<10%) are similar to those found in rheumatoid arthritis and in systemic lupus erythematosus, and are usually associated with severe carditis and not arthritis. The nodules (average of three to four) are firm and painless, range from a few millimeters to 2 cm, and can resolve within days.
- **Erythema marginatum** (<10%) is an irregular, serpiginous, nonpruritic rash that spreads centrifugally on the arms and trunk (never on the face). The condition only in patients with carditis.
- **Fever** can be high, especially in first week. However, in up to 30% of patients the body temperature does not exceed 38° C. Fever does not last for longer than 4 weeks.

15. What is St. Vitus' dance?
St. Vitus' dance is **Sydenham chorea**. It is a neurologic disorder characterized by emotional lability and rapid, uncoordinated, involuntary purposeless movements most notable in the face, hands, and feet. Movements are more marked on one side than the other. The "milking" sign is characteristic. Sensation is not affected, but weakness can occur. The choreiform movements disappear during sleep. The latent interval between streptococcal pharyngitis and chorea onset may be prolonged, and is frequently greater than 6 to 8 weeks. Consequently, ASO titers may be normal although antiDNase-B may still be elevated. Brain MRI shows inflammation in the basal ganglia. Therapy is symptomatic. Symptoms can last 2 to 4 months and may be the only manifestation of ARF. Up to 33% of patients will develop rheumatic heart disease, particularly if a murmur is noted at time chorea presents. Patients are at higher risk of developing obsessive compulsive disorder in the future.

16. Describe the treatment of ARF.
When a diagnosis of ARF is established, treatment with antibiotics sufficient to eradicate pharyngeal carriage of GAS is indicated, even in patients with no symptoms of pharyngitis (Table 44-1).

The other objectives of ARF therapy are to quiet inflammation, decrease fever and toxicity, and control cardiac failure. Analgesics without antiinflammatory properties are recommended for patients with mild disease. This allows complete expression of the clinical manifestations to aid in diagnosis and avoids posttherapeutic rebounds. Most patients, however, require salicylates. Salicylate levels of 20 to 30 mg/dL are required to control the inflammatory response. Controlled trials with other NSAIDs are not available but naproxen has been used successfully in children. Corticosteroids may be indicated to control the joint and systemic symptoms in more severe cases, with special consideration of dose tapering to prevent rebound symptoms. Most patients with severe myocarditis causing heart failure are treated with corticosteroids; however, it is not clear if this therapy alters the course of their disease.

17. What is the major sequela of ARF?
Most of the manifestations of ARF are transient without long-term sequelae, with cardiac involvement being the exception. Damage to heart valves may occur and may be chronic and progressive. Severe cardiac failure, total disability, and death may ensue years after the acute attack. In fact, the earliest structural change of rheumatic inflammation—fibrinoid degeneration—is found in the collagen of the connective tissues of the heart. The characteristic Aschoff nodule is now believed to be derived from connective tissue elements. Rheumatic carditis is characteristically a pancarditis involving the pericardium, myocardium, and free borders of valve cusps. **Pediatric autoimmune neuropsychiatric disorders associated with streptococci (PANDAS)** have recently been described. Patients with preceding streptococcal infections may have an increased risk of developing Tourette syndrome or obsessive–compulsive disorder following a streptococcal infection. There is high association with a B cell alloantigen (D8/17).

18. What is the recommended therapy for prevention of ARF?
Prevention of ARF in patients who present with GAS pharyngitis and do not have a prior history of ARF (**primary prevention**) involves antimicrobial therapy consisting of a single injection of 600,000 units for children <60 lb (27 kg) or 1.2 million units for larger individuals >60 lb (27 kg) of benzathine penicillin G, or oral therapy with penicillin V, 250 mg two to three times a day for patients <60 lb (27 kg) and 500 mg two

Table 44-1. Current Recommendations for Treatment of Acute Rheumatic Fever*

ANTIBIOTIC	DOSE
Benzathine penicillin G	600,000 units for patients <60 lb, IM, one dose
Penicillin V	1,200,000 units for patients >60 lb, IM, one dose **or**
	250 mg three times daily by mouth for 10 days for children **or**
	500 mg twice daily for 10 days for adolescents and adults **or**
Amoxicillin	750 mg once daily for 10 days
For individuals allergic to penicillin	
Erythromycin estolate	20–40 mg/kg per day in divided doses (maximum 1 g/day) given by mouth for 10 days **or**
Erythromycin ethylsuccinate or stearate	40 mg/kg per day in divided doses (maximum 1 g/day) given by mouth for 10 days

*Massive antibiotic therapy will not alter the course of acute rheumatic fever or the frequency or severity of cardiac involvement. Clarithromycin and azithromycin can also be used in penicillin-allergic patients but are more expensive. Cephalosporins (cefuroxime) have been effective in shorter courses (4 to 6 days) and should be considered for a penicillin-allergic patient in areas where group A streptococcal strains are resistant to macrolides (erythromyicn, azithromycin, etc.).

Table 44-2. Acute Rheumatic Fever Prophylaxis (Secondary Prevention)

ANTIBIOTIC	DOSE
Benzathine penicillin G	600,000 units for patients <60 lb, IM, every 4 wks
	1,200,000 units for patients >60 lb, IM, every 4 wks **or** *
Penicillin V	250 mg twice daily **or**
Sulfadiazine	0.5 g once daily for patients <60 lb
	1.0 g once daily for patients >60 lb
For individuals allergic to penicillin and sulfadiazine	
Erythromycin stearate	250 mg twice daily

*In high-risk situations, administration every 3 weeks is justified and recommended.

to three times a day in adolescents and adults for 10 days. In penicillin-allergic patients, the dosage is erythromycin estolate, 20 to 40 mg/kg per day (maximum 1 g/day), or erythromycin ethylsuccinate, 40 mg/kg per day (maximum 1 g/day), administered in two to four equally divided daily doses for 10 days. Antibiotic therapy for suspected streptococcal pharyngitis reduces the risk of developing ARF by 80%. Unfortunately, many patients fail to continue oral treatment for the full 10 days needed to eradicate the infecting organism because they are asymptomatic after the first few days of treatment.

Patients with a prior history of ARF (**secondary prevention**) are at progressively increased risk of developing recurrent ARF with each streptococcal infection and require continuous prophylaxis to prevent intercurrent streptococcal infections. The recurrence rate per infection may be as high as 50% in the first year and decreases sharply until 4 to 5 years after the attack, when it levels off to 10% per year. The recommended regimens are listed in Table 44-2.

Note that sulfa medications can be used for prophylaxis but not for primary treatment of streptococcal infections. Patients with a history of ARF with mild cardiac involvement should receive treatment for 10 years or until the age of 25, whichever is longer. Patients with a history of severe carditis or valve surgery should receive lifelong antibiotic prophylaxis. Patients with a history of ARF without cardiac involvement should receive antibiotic prophylaxis for 5 years or until the age of 18, whichever is longer. ARF patients without cardiac involvement who have frequent exposure to children (mothers, daycare workers) should receive prophylaxis for as long as this exposure continues.

It is hoped that as more is learned about the virulence factors of various GAS strains, an effective vaccine can be developed for eradication of ARF.

19. **What is a reasonable differential diagnosis when confronted with a patient with migratory polyarthritis?**
Gonococcal polyarthritis, subacute bacterial endocarditis, persistent viremias, rubella, hepatitis B, sarcoid arthritis, and Whipple's disease.

It is important to bear in mind that ARF does not cause urticaria, angioneurotic edema, or clinically overt glomerulonephritis. In addition, serum complement levels are increased and antinuclear and other autoantibodies do not appear in the course of ARF, no matter how persistent the disease.

20. **What is the worldwide impact of ARF?**
    The frequency and severity of ARF have been declining rapidly in North America, Europe, and Japan (although a series of unexpected outbreaks in the United States occurred in the mid-1980s). These declining trends were beginning even before the widespread use of antibiotics, and changes in social conditions and improved access to health care have undoubtedly contributed to the decline. ARF is, however, rampant in the Middle East, the Indian subcontinent, and areas in Africa and South America. It has been estimated that there are 20 million new cases of ARF each year, and rheumatic heart disease accounts for 25% to 40% of all cardiovascular disease in many developing countries.

Bibliography

Altamimi S, Khalil A, Khalaiwi KA, et al: Short versus standard duration antibiotic therapy for acute streptococcal pharyngitis in children, Cochrane Database Syst Rev CD004872, 2012.

Bryant PA, Robins-Browne R, Carapetis JR, Curtis N: Some of the people, some of the time: susceptibility to acute rheumatic fever, Circulation 119:742–753, 2009.

Carapetis JR, McDonald M, Wilson NJ: Acute rheumatic fever, Lancet 366:155–168, 2005.

Dajani A, Taubert K: Treatment of acute streptococcal pharyngitis and prevention of rheumatic fever: a statement for health professionals, Pediatrics 96:758–764, 1995.

Dajani AS, Ayoub EM, Bierman FZ, et al: Guidelines for the diagnosis of rheumatic fever, JAMA 268:2069–2073, 1992.

Dajani AS, Ayoub EM, Bierman FZ, et al: Guidelines for the diagnosis of rheumatic fever: Jones criteria, updated 1992, Circulation 87:302, 1993.

Ellis NM, Kurahara DK, Vohra H, et al: Priming the immune system for heart disease: a perspective on group A streptococci, J Infect Dis 202:1059–1067, 2010.

Jansen TL, Jansen M, van Riel PL: Acute rheumatic fever or post-streptococcal reactive arthritis: a clinical problem revisited, Br J Rheumatol 37:335–340, 1998.

Kasitanon N, Sukitawut W, Louthrenoo W: Acute rheumatic fever in adults: case report together with analysis of 25 patients with acute rheumatic fever, Rheumatol Int 29:1041–1045, 2009.

Mackie SL, Keat A: Poststreptococcal reactive arthritis: what is it and how do we know? Rheumatology (Oxford) 43:949, 2004.

Shulman ST: Pediatric autoimmune neuropsychiatric disorders associated with streptococci (PANDAS): update, Curr Opin Pediatr 21:127, 2009.

Valtonen JM, Koskimies S, Miettinen A, Valtonen VV: Various rheumatic syndromes in adult patients associated with high antistreptolysin O titres and their differential diagnosis with rheumatic fever, Ann Rheum Dis 52:527–530, 1993.

World Health Organization: Rheumatic fever and rheumatic heart disease: report of a WHO Expert Consultation, Geneva, 2004, WHO.

Zabriskie J, Lavenchy D, Williams RC, et al: Rheumatic fever–associated B cell alloantigens as identified by monoclonal antibodies, Arthritis Rheum 28:1947, 1985.

VII
RHEUMATIC DISORDERS ASSOCIATED WITH METABOLIC, ENDOCRINE, AND HEMATOLOGIC DISEASES

Screw up the vise as tightly as possible—you have rheumatism; give it another turn, and that is gout.

Anonymous

GOUT
Robert W. Janson, MD

CHAPTER 45

KEY POINTS

1. Gout is the most common cause of inflammatory arthritis in men over 40 years of age.
2. Gout should not occur in a premenopausal woman.
3. Hyperuricemia and gout are strongly associated with obesity and the metabolic syndrome.
4. Dietary and lifestyle modifications are recommended for the management of gout.
5. The rheumatologist should always look for gout in all undiagnosed joint conditions even if the serum uric acid level is normal, the involved joint is atypical, and the flare is chronic and polyarticular.
6. The patient's comorbid medical conditions should be assessed, including renal and hepatic function, to guide the safest treatment options for acute gout and chronic symptomatic hyperuricemia, with a serum uric acid goal of <6.0 mg/dL.

1. What is gout? How was the term derived?
Gout is a disease in which tissue deposition of monosodium urate (MSU) crystals occurs as a result of hyperuricemia (MSU supersaturation of extracellular fluids), resulting in one or more of the following manifestations:
- Gouty arthritis
- Tophi (aggregated deposits of MSU occurring in articular, osseous, cartilaginous, or soft tissue areas)
- Gouty nephropathy
- Uric acid nephrolithiasis

The term *gout* is derived from the Latin *gutta*, which means a drop. In the 13th century, it was thought that gout resulted from a drop of evil humor affecting a vulnerable joint.

2. Hyperuricemia is defined as a serum uric acid concentration above what levels in males and in females? What are the most common factors associated with hyperuricemia and gout?
Serum uric acid concentrations are both age- and sex-dependent. Uric acid concentrations rise in association with the onset of puberty in males and menopause in females. Gout is rare in males under age 30 and in premenopausal females. The onset of gout in men under the age of 25 is usually associated with an inherited defect in the purine degradation pathway, alcoholism, and/or renal insufficiency including familial juvenile hyperuricemic nephropathy and medullary cystic kidney disease. The peak age for onset of gout is 40 to 50 years in males and after 60 years in females. Hyperuricemia is defined as a serum uric acid concentration >7.0 mg/dL in males and >6.0 mg/dL in females. Body mass index and alcohol intake are the most important predictors of hyperuricemia and gout in the majority of individuals.

3. How prevalent is gout? Discuss the epidemiology of gout.
Overall, the prevalence of gout increases with age and serum urate concentrations. The prevalence of gout according to the third National Health and Nutrition Examination Survey (NHANES-III) is >2% in men over 30 years of age and women over 50 years of age. Over 80 years of age, the prevalence of gout is 9% in men and 6% in women. Therefore, gout is the most common cause of inflammatory arthritis in men over 40 years of age. Recent data suggest that the prevalence of gout has further increased over the past two decades secondary to diet, obesity, metabolic syndrome, and medication use such as low-dose aspirin and diuretics. The male to female ratio is 2:1 to 7:1. Although only 15% of all patients with hyperuricemia develop gout, the risk increases to 30% to 50% if their serum uric acid concentration is >10 mg/dL. Overall, 25% of gouty patients have a positive family history of gout.

4. Uric acid is a product of the metabolism of which group of nucleotides?
Uric acid is the end product of the degradation of **purines**. Humans lack the enzyme *uricase*, which in other species oxidizes uric acid (sparingly soluble) to the highly soluble compound allantoin. The lack of this enzyme subjects humans to the potential risk of tissue deposition of uric acid crystals. Although humans possess the uricase gene, it is inactive. It is postulated that humans have acquired the propensity to become hyperuricemic because uric acid may have powerful antioxidant and free radical scavenger properties.

5. **What pathogenic processes are responsible for the development of hyperuricemia?**
   - Overproduction of urate (endogenous or exogenous dietary purine precursors)
   - Underexcretion of urate (abnormal renal handling of urate)
   - A combination of both processes

   Most patients with hyperuricemia and primary gout are underexcreters of uric acid (90%).

6. **What test determines if a patient with gout is an overproducer or underexcreter of uric acid?**
   A 24-hour urine collection is obtained for determination of uric acid and creatinine excretion (to ensure adequate 24-hour collection). On a regular purine diet, a urate value >800 mg per 24 hours suggests overproduction of uric acid. A 24-hour urate value <800 mg suggests underexcretion.

7. **Name the two inherited enzyme abnormalities in the urate biosynthesis pathway that can cause urate overproduction.**
   - Overactivity of phosphoribosylpyrophosphate (PRPP) synthetase
   - Partial deficiency of hypoxanthine–guanine phosphoribosyltransferase (HGPRT) (Kelley–Seegmiller syndrome)

   These enzyme abnormalities, which cause uric acid overproduction, are inherited as X-linked traits. Patients with these abnormalities often present with early adult-onset gout (male <25 years of age) and a high incidence of uric acid nephrolithiasis. Complete deficiency of HGPRT results in the **Lesch–Nyhan syndrome** (mental retardation, spasticity, choreoathetosis, and self-mutilation). In addition, patients with **glucose-6-phosphatase deficiency** (von Gierke glycogen storage disease) also exhibit urate overproduction due to accelerated breakdown of ATP during hypoglycemia-induced glycogen degradation. Inhibition of renal tubular urate secretion can also occur in this disease as a result of competitive anions from lactic acidosis. Finally, patients with hereditary fructose intolerance caused by **fructose-1-phosphate aldolase deficiency** can develop hyperuricemia in part because of accelerated ATP catabolism.

   Figure 45-1 shows the urate biosynthesis pathway.

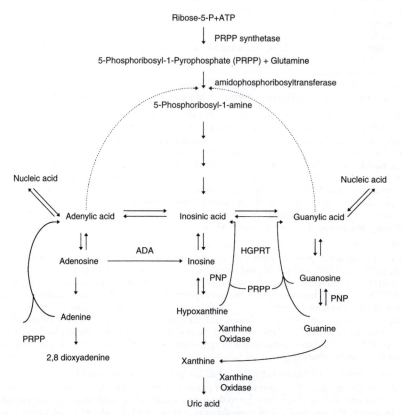

Figure 45-1. Urate biosynthesis. Dotted arrows represent feedback inhibition. *ADA*, Adenosine deaminase; *HGPRT*, hypoxanthine–guanine phosphoribosyltransferase; *PNP*, purine nucleloside phosphorylase.

8. **What are the acquired causes of hyperuricemia?**
   Urate overproduction: excess dietary purine consumption, accelerated hepatic ATP degradation in alcohol abuse or fructose ingestion, and increased nucleotide turnover in myeloproliferative and lymphoproliferative disorders
   Urate underexcretion: renal disease, lead nephropathy (saturnine gout), inhibition of tubular urate secretion (keto- and lactic acidosis), and miscellaneous causes such as hyperparathyroidism, hypothyroidism, and respiratory acidosis

9. **Name the drugs that cause hyperuricemia due to decreased renal excretion of urate.**
   The mnemonic **CAN'T LEAP** can be used to remember these drugs:

Cyclosporine	Lasix (furosemide) (and other loop diuretics)
Alcohol	Ethambutol
Nicotinic acid	Aspirin (low dose)
Thiazides	Pyrazinamide

   Other drugs that can cause hyperuricemia by unknown mechanisms include levodopa, theophylline, and didanosine. By contrast, the commonly used drugs losartan, amlodipine, and fenofibrate have mild uricosuric effects that can help lower uric acid.

10. **Why does excessive alcohol consumption often lead to hyperuricemia and gout?**
    The quantity of alcohol consumed strongly correlates with the risk of developing gout. Consumption of more than 30 to 50 g of alcohol a day (three to four beers, glasses of wine, or liquor shots) increases the relative risk of developing gout by a factor of 2 to 2.5 compared to zero alcohol consumption. Alcohol consumption increases the synthesis of urate by accelerating the degradation of hepatic ATP. Alcohol consumption is also associated with the production of lactic acid, which reduces renal excretion of urate. Beer, which contains a substantial amount of the purine guanosine, confers a more than twofold greater risk of gout over liquor. Moderate wine drinking (14 g or 5 oz per day) does not increase the risk of gout or serum uric acid levels.

11. **What are the four stages of gouty arthritis?**
    - **Asymptomatic hyperuricemia**: elevated serum uric acid level without gouty arthritis, tophi, or uric acid nephrolithiasis. Up to 15% of these patients will eventually develop gout. In those who develop gout, most patients will have had 20 years of asymptomatic hyperuricemia before their first gout attack.
    - **Acute gouty arthritis**: a single joint is involved in 85% to 90% of patients, whereas up to 15% will have polyarticular involvement with their first attack.
    - **Intercritical gout**: the asymptomatic intervals between acute attacks of gout. Over 60% of patients will have a second attack within 1 to 2 years, whereas 5% to 10% may never have another attack.
    - **Chronic tophaceous gout**: development of subcutaneous, synovial, or subchondral bone deposits of MSU crystals.

12. **Describe the characteristics of an acute attack of gout.**
    Early episodes of acute gouty arthritis are typically **monoarticular** (85%), begin abruptly, and reach maximal intensity within hours. The onset of attacks often occurs during the **night** or **early morning** when the joint is coolest. The affected joint becomes exquisitely painful, warm, red, and swollen. A low-grade fever may be present. The **periarticular erythema and swelling** may progress to resemble a noninfectious cellulitis termed gouty cellulitis. Acute gout may also occur in nonarticular sites, such as the olecranon bursa, prepatellar bursa, and Achilles tendon. Early attacks often spontaneously resolve over 3 to 10 days. **Desquamation of the skin** overlying the affected joint can occur with resolution of the inflammation. Subsequent attacks of gout can occur more frequently, become polyarticular, and persist for longer.

13. **What joints are most commonly involved in gout?**
    The joints of the lower limbs are typically involved more often than those of the upper limbs. The **first metatarsophalangeal (MTP) joint of the great toe** is involved in >50% of initial attacks and over time is affected in >90% of patients. Acute gout of the first MTP is termed **podagra**. In order of frequency of involvement after the MTP joints are the instep, ankle, heel, knee, wrist, fingers, and elbow. Attacks of gout at more axial sites (spine) are rare. Gout and tophi have a predilection for cooler, acral sites, where the solubility of MSU crystals may be diminished as a result of the cooler temperature. In addition, joints that have undergone degenerative changes provide a nidus that facilitates crystal formation.

14. **What events may trigger an acute attack of gout?**
    - Alcohol ingestion
    - Hemorrhage
    - Dietary excess of purines
    - Acute medical illness including infections
    - Exercise
    - Drugs

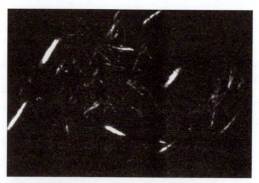

Figure 45-2. Polarized light microscopy showing needle-shaped uric acid crystals in synovial fluid.

- Trauma
- Radiation therapy
- Fructose drink ingestion
- Surgery (postoperative days 3 to 5)

15. Can symptomatic hyperuricemia (gout) be managed by diet alone?
Unfortunately, it is often difficult to manage gout by diet alone because the purine content of the diet typically contributes only 1.0 mg/dL to the total serum uric acid concentration. Patients should be advised to limit their consumption of the following purine-rich foods:
- Meats, particularly organ meats (liver, kidney, etc.)
- Seafood, particularly shellfish, sardines, and anchovies

Excessive fructose consumption (sodas, fruit juices, energy drinks) is also associated with higher incidence of gout. Fructose is metabolized in the liver to ATP, which contributes to the urate load. By contrast, moderate intake of purine-rich vegetables (asparagus, cauliflower, spinach, and mushrooms), nuts, legumes (beans and peas), and vegetable protein is not associated with increased risk of gout. Coffee intake through a noncaffeine mechanism, vitamin C (500 mg/day), reduced-fat dairy intake (milk, yogurt), and tart cherries can reduce the risk of gout.

16. How is a diagnosis of gout established?
Fresh synovial fluid or a tophus aspirate must be evaluated for the presence of MSU crystals. The intra- or extracellular crystals are typically needle-shaped and negatively birefringent (yellow when parallel to the axis of a red compensator) on polarized microscopy (Figure 45-2) (see Chapter 7). Intracellular crystals are diagnostic of an acute gout attack. Extracellular crystals may be found in previously affected joints during the intercritical phases of gout.

The synovial fluid is inflammatory (typically 20,000 to 100,000 leukocytes/mm^3) with a predominance of neutrophils. Septic synovial fluids may contain urate crystals so it is important to obtain a synovial fluid Gram stain and culture if clinical suspicion of a septic joint exists.

Serum uric acid levels will be elevated at some time in almost all patients with gout, but the level can be normal at the time of an acute gouty attack in as many as 30% of patients. This appears to be caused by IL-6 generation via the acute inflammatory response, which facilitates renal uric acid excretion. Finally, hematologic evaluation may show an elevated erythrocyte sedimentation rate (ESR), mild neutrophil leukocytosis, and possibly reactive thrombocytosis.

17. What are the typical radiographic features of gout?
Soft tissue swelling around the affected joint can be seen in early acute attacks of gout. In chronic gout, **tophi** and **bony erosions** can be seen (Figure 45-3). Articular tophi produce irregular soft-tissue densities that occasionally are calcified. Bony erosions in gout appear "punched out" with sclerotic margins and **overhanging edges**, sometimes termed **rat bite erosions**. The joint space is typically preserved until late in the disease and juxtaarticular osteopenia is absent.

18. What roles do ultrasonography and dual-energy computerized tomography have in the diagnosis of gout?
- **Ultrasonagraphy**: musculoskeletal ultrasound can show a superficial, hyperechoic band (deposition of urate crystals) on the surface of articular cartilage ("double contour sign") in gouty patients (Figure 45-4). Tophi appear as nonhomogeneous material surrounded by an anechoic rim.
- **Dual-energy computerized tomography (DECT)**: this is a CT scanning technique in which two x-ray tubes with different voltages are aligned at 90 degrees to one another. This allows identification of urate crystal deposits because the chemical composition of uric acid causes lower attenuation of x-ray photons tracking through it in comparison to bone calcium. The urate deposits can be easily separated from surrounding tissues with a high degree of sensitivity and specificity, which aids in the diagnosis of difficult cases.

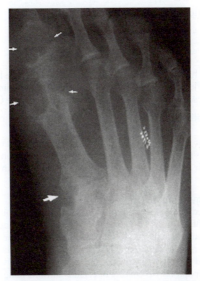

Figure 45-3. Radiograph of a foot showing erosive changes (*arrows*) of chronic tophaceous gout.

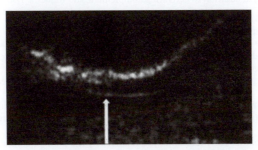

Figure 45-4. Ultrasound of a metatarsophalangeal joint showing the "double contour" sign (*arrow*).

19. How long is the interval from an initial attack of gout until the appearance of tophi? Where do tophi commonly occur?

In patients with untreated gout, tophi develop on average 10 years after the initial attack of gout. Tophi may occur at any site; common locations are the synovium, subchondral bone, digits of the hands and feet, olecranon bursa, extensor surface of the forearm, Achilles tendon, and, less commonly, the antihelix of the ear. Tophi can ulcerate through the skin and extrude a white, chalky material consisting of a dense concentration of MSU crystals. Although rare, an ulcerated tophus can become infected.

20. What medical conditions associated with hyperuricemia and gout must be excluded as part of the evaluation of a gouty patient?

The two most common medical conditions associated with hyperuricemia and gout are:
- Obesity; weight loss can improve hyperuricemia
- Alcohol abuse

Other medical conditions and causes of hyperuricemia are:
- Drugs (see Question 9)
- Renal insufficiency
- Hypothyroidism
- Myeloproliferative disease, lymphoproliferative diseases, hemolytic anemias, polycythemia vera
- Hyperparathyroidism, diabetic ketoacidosis, diabetes insipidus, Bartter syndrome
- Autosomal dominant medullary cystic kidney disease, lead nephropathy, familial juvenile hyperuricemic nephropathy
- Sarcoidosis, psoriasis
- Dehydration

Other common medical conditions frequently seen in gouty patients are:
- Hypertension
- Dyslipidemia
- Atherosclerosis
- Glucose intolerance and the metabolic syndrome

Therefore, in addition to a good history and physical examination, appropriate laboratory evaluation of a patient with gouty arthritis should include a complete blood count; chemistries including creatinine and blood urea nitrogen, calcium, liver enzymes, and serum uric acid; thyroid-stimulating hormone (TSH); a lipid profile; and urinalysis.

21. How do women with gout differ from male patients with regard to disease onset and clinical features?
Female patients develop gout at an older age (typically after menopause). Polyarticular acute gouty attacks are more common. Female patients frequently have osteoarthritis, hypertension, and mild chronic renal insufficiency or are being treated with diuretics. Tophi are particularly common in previously damaged joints including Heberden nodes, and in the finger pads.

22. Discuss the pathophysiology of acute gouty arthritis.
Acute gouty arthritis is triggered by precipitation of MSU crystals in the joint. Initial recognition of naked MSU crystals by Toll-like receptors 2 and 4 on chondrocytes and macrophage lineage cells appears to be critical to the expression of proinflammatory cytokines and initiation of the inflammatory response. It is also thought that the inflammatory nature of the crystals is determined by a balance of certain proteins that can coat the crystals; crystals coated with IgG react with Fc receptors on responding cells and promote an inflammatory response, whereas apolipoprotein-B coating of crystals inhibits phagocytosis and a cellular response. Urate crystals stimulate the production of chemotactic factors, cytokines (IL-1β via activation of the NLRP3 inflammasome, IL-6, IL-8, and TNF), prostaglandins, leukotrienes, and oxygen radicals by neutrophils, monocytes, and synovial cells, in addition to activating complement and inducing lysosomal enzyme release.

23. Why are early attacks of acute gouty arthritis often self-limited?
The following mechanisms have been postulated:
- The cellular response may be modulated by different proteins coating the crystals. Inflammation allows more apolipoprotein-B to leak from the blood to the synovial fluid, which can coat the urate crystals and make them less phlogistic.
- Phagocytosis and clearance of crystals by neutrophils decrease the crystal concentration; neutrophil apoptosis occurs.
- The heat associated with the inflammation results in increased urate crystal solubility.
- Enhanced adrenocorticotropic hormone secretion in response to pain/stress may suppress the inflammatory response.
- Proinflammatory cytokines (IL-1 and TNF) are balanced by the production of cytokine inhibitors and regulatory cytokines such as TGF-β.

24. Name the types of renal disease associated with hyperuricemia.
- **Urate nephropathy**: deposition of MSU crystals in renal interstitial tissue with a surrounding giant-cell reaction. This may cause mild and intermittent proteinuria and rarely causes renal dysfunction (associated hypertension is more often the cause).
- **Uric acid nephropathy**: precipitation of uric acid crystals in the collecting ducts and ureters results in acute renal failure, as in the acute tumor lysis syndrome. This condition is most likely to occur following chemotherapy for lymphoma, leukemia, and medulloblastoma.
- **Uric acid nephrolithiasis**: Occurs in up to 10% to 25% of primary gout patients. The frequency parallels increases in serum and urinary concentrations of uric acid and in urine acidity. Uric acid stones are radiolucent. The incidence of calcium stones is also higher in patients with gout, particularly those with hyperuricosuria. Uric acid serves as a nidus for calcium stone formation. Between 10% and 40% of gouty patients have one or more attacks of renal colic before their first gout attack.
- **Others**: autosomal dominant medullary cystic kidney disease (one third of patients have gout), lead intoxication (saturnine gout), and familial juvenile hyperuricemic nephropathy.

25. Discuss the renal transport of uric acid and how this can contribute to hyperuricemia and gout.
Renal urate transport consists of glomerular filtration followed by near-complete reabsorption of filtered urate, subsequent secretion back into the tubule, and reabsorption in the distal proximal tubule, with net renal excretion of 10% of the filtered uric acid (see Figure 86-1). **URAT1** is an important renal urate-anion exchanger on the apical surface of proximal tubular epithelial cells responsible for reabsorption of filtered urate. Inhibition of URAT1 results in enhanced renal excretion of uric acid (uricosuria) and lower uric acid levels. Drugs that inhibit URAT1 include probenecid, sulfinpyrazone, benzbromarone, metabolites of losartan, and high-dose aspirin. Specific URAT1 inhibitors (lesinurad) are in development. URAT1 is stimulated by the following drugs and results in decreased renal urate excretion with resultant hyperuricemia: lactate, nicotinate,

pyrazinoate, low-dose aspirin, and possibly diuretics. Other less important renal apical surface urate transporters are OAT4 and OAT10.

GLUT9A is the major transporter on the basolateral surface of proximal tubular epithelial cells responsible for transporting urate from tubular cells into the renal interstitium. Mutations of GLUT9A cause less reabsorption of uric acid, leading to lower uric acid levels and less risk of developing gout.

There are other transport proteins in renal proximal tubular epithelial cells that regulate uric acid secretion. OAT1 and OAT3 on the basolateral surface transport urate from the renal interstitium into epithelial cells. **ABCG2** and MRP4 are the two major proteins on the apical surface that extrude urate from epithelial cells into tubular urine. Polymorphisms of ABCG2 are associated with decreased renal secretion of uric acid resulting in hyperuricemia and gout.

26. When should treatment of asymptomatic hyperuricemia be considered?

Asymptomatic hyperuricemia characterized by no prior history of gouty arthritis, tophaceous deposits, or nephrolithiasis should only be treated in situations in which there may be acute overproduction (e.g., chemotherapy, radiation) of uric acid, as in the acute tumor lysis syndrome. Some recommend treatment if urinary uric acid excretion is greater than 1100 mg/d because of 50% risk of nephrolithiasis. Otherwise, there are currently no widely accepted indications for treatment of asymptomatic hyperuricemia other than nonpharmacologic interventions (weight loss, dietary modification, and decrease alcohol intake).

27. Discuss the treatment options for acute gouty arthritis.

The 2012 American College of Rheumatology (ACR) guidelines for the management of gout recommend the following medications to treat acute gout: **nonsteroidal antiinflammatory drugs (NSAIDs; full dose), oral colchicine, or corticosteroids** (Table 45-1). Patients with a severe gouty attack may require a combination of two of these agents (the combination of NSAIDs and oral corticosteroids is less desirable because of the potential for gastrointestinal toxicity). Topical ice can also be used. Most NSAIDs appear to be efficacious provided they are dosed at full antiinflammatory levels. In patients with permissive renal and hepatic function, oral colchicine is dosed at 1.2 mg followed by 0.6 mg 1 hour later; this can be followed by prophylaxis dosing of 0.6 mg once or twice daily. Corticosteroids can be administered by oral, IV, intramuscular, or intraarticular routes. The role of an IL-1 inhibitor in treating acute gout is uncertain because of an undefined risk/benefit ratio. Urate-lowering therapy (ULT) should never be started until after complete resolution of the acute gouty attack, nor should it be stopped if an acute gouty attack occurs while the patient is on ULT.

Table 45-1. Treatment Options for Acute Gout

TREATMENT OPTIONS	DOSAGE	COMMENTS
NSAIDs (indomethacin)	Oral 50 mg four times per day for 24-48 h, then 50 mg three times per day for 48 h; taper and discontinue after the attack subsides	Indomethacin is the drug of choice; other NSAIDs with a short half-life are probably as effective
Oral colchicine	1.2 mg followed by 0.6 mg 1 h later	Most effective within the first 36 h of an attack. Contraindicated in the elderly or significant renal or hepatic insufficiency. Avoid use with concomitant P450 3A4 and P-glycoprotein inhibitors including cyclosporine, clarithromycin, erythromycin, ketoconazole, itraconazole, disulfiram, HIV protease inhibitors, diltiazem, verapamil, and grapefruit juice
Intraarticular steroids (triamcinolone or methylprednisolone)	40 mg for large joints, 10-20 mg for small joints or bursae	Useful in the treatment of 1 or 2 involved joints or bursae. Effective within the first 24 h of an attack in 90% of patients
Systemic corticosteroids	Prednisone 0.5 mg/kg per day for 5-10 days or for 2-5 days then taper for 7-10 days or triamcinolone acetonide 60 mg IM, can repeat once	Rebound arthropathy may occur; may be used in patients with CKD
Adrenocorticotropic hormone	25-40 IU subcutaneously every 12 h as needed (1-3 doses typical)	Much more costly than alternative therapies

CKD, Chronic kidney disease; *HIV*, human immunodeficiency virus; *NSAID*, nonsteroidal antiinflammatory drug.

28. What are the indications for chronic treatment of symptomatic hyperuricemia?
Lifelong therapy with an antihyperuricemic drug is indicated in the following situations:
- More than two or three acute attacks of gout within 1 to 2 years
- Renal stones (urate or calcium)
- Tophaceous gout
- Established gout with chronic kidney disease stage 2 or worse

The indications for xanthine oxidase inhibitors versus probenecid therapy, along with their dosing and side-effect profiles, are discussed in Chapter 86. A xanthine oxidase inhibitor, such as **allopurinol** or **febuxostat**, is first-line therapy. The starting dose of allopurinol is 100 mg/day (50 mg/day in stage 4 chronic kidney disease, CKD) with gradual upward titration (often >300 mg/day) to a serum uric acid goal of <6 mg/dL, even in patients with renal impairment provided regular monitoring is in place. Patients at increased risk of severe allopurinol hypersensitivity reaction (e.g., Koreans with stage 3 or worse CKD; patients of Han Chinese or Thai descent) should undergo HLA-B*5801 screening before initiation of allopurinol therapy. Febuxostat is dosed at 40 to 80 mg per day as needed and may be used in patients with stage 3 CKD. Probenecid is contraindicated in patients who are overproducers of uric acid (see Question 6), have a history of nephrolithiasis, or have a glomerular filtration rate (GFR) <50 mL/min.

29. Acute gouty attacks can be precipitated by initiation of antihyperuricemic therapy. How can this risk be minimized?
According to the ACR guidelines for management of gout, the ULT dose should be gradually increased and combined with use of either a low-dose NSAID (e.g., naproxen 250 mg twice daily) or colchicine 0.6 mg orally once or twice daily as prophylaxis. If the patient is elderly or has a GFR of 30 to 50 mL/min, colchicine should be dosed at 0.6 mg/day or every other day. Acute or prophylactic colchicine should be avoided if the GFR is <30 mL/min.
Prophylaxis should be continued for the greater of:
- at least 6 months

OR
- 3 months after achieving the serum uric acid goal in patients without tophi
- 6 months after achieving the serum uric acid goal in patients with one or more tophi

Low-dose prednisone (≤10 mg/day) can be used as prophylaxis in patients with contraindications to NSAIDs or colchicine. Patients with continued acute gouty activity should remain on prophylaxis for gout for a more prolonged period of time.

30. What is the treatment for tophaceous gout?
The treatment goal is to substantially lower serum uric acid (goal <5 mg/dL) to permit urate resorption from the tophi. In rare cases, probenecid is added to allopurinol to help the kidney to excrete the uric acid load mobilized from resolving tophi. Chronic prophylaxis with oral colchicine or NSAIDs is often helpful in these patients to reduce the frequency of acute gouty attacks. **Pegloticase** is considered in patients with a severe gout burden who are intolerant of oral ULT or have refractory disease despite ULT (see Chapter 86).

31. Why is gout relatively common in organ transplant recipients?
Therapy with cyclosporine or tacrolimus, which reduces urinary urate excretion, is probably the most significant factor. Polyarticular attacks of gout and early development of tophi can be observed. Treatment of acute attacks and normalization of the hyperuricemia are often problematic. NSAIDs are relatively contraindicated in the setting of cyclosporine or tacrolimus therapy or renal insufficiency, and allopurinol therapy with concomitant azathioprine may result in significant neutropenia. Intraarticular or systemic corticosteroids may be the safest treatment options for acute gouty attacks. Synovial fluid cultures should be performed routinely. Uricosurics are often ineffective in these patients as a result of a GFR <50 mL/min. Allopurinol can be used if the patient is not on azathioprine (see Chapter 86). Even if the dose of azathioprine is reduced by 50% to 75% while the patient is on allopurinol, this is a dangerous combination that may result in severe leukopenia or bone marrow failure. **Finally, colchicine should never be used in patients taking cyclosporine or tacrolimus because rare, severe cases of neuromyopathy have been reported, even for patients on low doses for <1 week.**

32. Who was Podagra?
In mythology, Podagra was the foot-torturer born of the seduction of Venus by Bacchus. This terrible-tempered virgin goddess even inspired fear in Jove.

BIBLIOGRAPHY

Burns CM, Wortmann RL: Clinical features and treatment of gout. In Firestein GS, Budd RC, Gabriel SE, et al: Kelley's textbook of rheumatology, ed 9, Philadelphia, 2012, Elsevier Saunders.
Choi HK: A prescription for lifestyle change in patients with hyperuricemia and gout, Curr Opin Rheumatol 22:165–172, 2010.
Choi HK, Mount DB, Reginato AM: Pathogenesis of gout, Ann Intern Med 143:499–516, 2005.
George RL, Keenan RT: Genetics of hyperuricemia and gout: implications for the present and future, Curr Rheumatol Rep 15:309–320, 2013.
Keenan RT: Safety of urate-lowering therapies. Managing the risks to gain the benefits, Rheum Dis Clin North Am 38:663–680, 2012.

Keenan RT, Nowatzky J, Pillinger MH: Etiology and pathogenesis of hyperuricemia and gout. In Firestein GS, Budd RC, Gabriel SE, et al: Kelley's textbook of rheumatology, ed 9, Philadelphia, 2012, Elsevier Saunders.
Khanna D, Fitzgerald JD, Khanna PP, et al: 2012 American College of Rheumatology guidelines for management of gout. Part 1. Systematic nonpharmacologic and pharmacologic therapeutic approaches to hyperuricemia, Arthritis Care Res 64:1431–1446, 2012.
Khanna D, Khanna PP, Fitzgerald JD, et al: 2012 American College of Rheumatology guidelines for management of gout. Part 2. Therapy and anti-inflammatory prophylaxis of acute gouty arthritis, Arthritis Care Res 64:1447–1461, 2012.
Neogi T: Gout: N Engl J Med 364:443–452, 2011.
Terkeltaub RA: Colchicine update: 2008, Semin Arthritis Rheum 38:411–419, 2009.
Terkeltaub RA, Furst DE, Bennett K, et al: High versus low dosing of oral colchicine for early acute gout, Arthritis Rheum 62:1060–1068, 2010.
Zhu T, Pandya BJ, Choi HK: Prevalence of gout and hyperuricemia in the US population, Arthritis Rheum 63:3136–3141, 2011.

FURTHER READING

http://www.niams.nih.gov/Health_Info/Gout/
http:/www.gouteducation.org

CHAPTER 46: CALCIUM PYROPHOSPHATE DEPOSITION DISEASE

Frederick T. Murphy, DO

KEY POINTS

1. Calcium pyrophosphate deposition disease (CPPD) is a disease of the elderly, with onset and increasing frequency after the age of 50 years.
2. Patients younger than 55 years with chondrocalcinosis (CC) should be evaluated for a familial form or metabolic diseases associated with CPPD.
3. Chronic CPPD should be considered in any elderly patient with symptoms suggesting seronegative rheumatoid arthritis or polymyalgia rheumatica.
4. Chronic CPPD should be considered in any patient with diffuse osteoarthritis (OA) in atypical joints such as the metacarpophalangeal joints (MCPs), wrists, elbows, and shoulders.
5. The mnemonic ABC (**A**lignment **B**lue **C**alcium) is useful for remembering the color of a CPPD crystal parallel to the first-order red compensator when viewing synovial fluid by polarized light microscopy.

1. **What is calcium pyrophosphate dihydrate?**
   Calcium pyrophosphate dihydrate is a calcium salt ($Ca_2P_2O_7 \cdot 2H_2O$) that in crystalline form (called CPP crystals) is deposited in cartilage and other articular tissues, leading to a variety of clinical manifestations. CPPD is the preferred umbrella term for all presentations related to CPP crystal deposition. Other terms such as CPPDD/CPDD (calcium pyrophosphate dihydrate deposition disease) are the same as CPPD.

2. **List the clinical presentations associated with CPPD.**
   CPPD-associated arthritis is the third most common cause of inflammatory arthritis, occurring in 3.4% of adult patients. However, it can present in a number of different ways. It should be considered in the diagnosis of any acute or chronic mono-, oligo-, or polyarticular inflammatory or noninflammatory arthritis occurring in patients over the age of 55 years. If it occurs in a patient aged <55 years, then familial forms, certain metabolic diseases (hyperparathyroidism, hemochromatosis, hypomagnesemia, dialysis-dependent renal failure, others), and/or a history of joint trauma/meniscectomy need to be considered. Clinical presentations that can overlap CPPD include the following:
   - **Asymptomatic CPPD** (lanthanic): this is radiographic CC without clinical manifestations and usually involves the knee.
   - **Acute CPP crystal arthritis** (pseudogout): a mono- or oligoarticular arthritis is the most common (89%) presentation when it presents as an inflammatory arthritis. The knee and wrist are the most commonly involved joints.
   - **Chronic CPP crystal inflammatory arthritis** (pseudorheumatoid pattern): a polyarticular arthritis is the less common (11%) presentation of CPPD-associated inflammatory arthritis. This should be considered in any elderly patient with seronegative rheumatoid arthritis or polymyalgia rheumatica.
   - **Pyrophosphate arthropathy** (pseudoOA): OA changes associated with CPPD. Patients may (50%) or may not have superimposed attacks of acute CPP crystal arthritis (pseudogout). CPPD causes OA in joints that are not usually involved by OA, such as the MCPs and radiocarpal and elbow joints.
   - **Other presentations**
     - Tumoral (pseudotophaceous pattern) CPP crystal deposition in periarticular and bony structures
     - Tendon deposits, most commonly in the Achilles, triceps, and obturator tendons
     - Pseudoneuropathic pattern: the radiographic appearance is Charcot-like but the patient has normal pain perception
     - Cervical stenosis: from CPPD in the ligamentum flavum and/or transverse ligament of the atlas
     - Crowned dens: CPPD above the odontoid process can lead to acute neck pain and meningismus with crystal shedding
     - Axial involvement: intervertebral disc calcifications and sacroiliac joint involvement are more common in familial forms

3. **What factors predispose patients to CPPD development?**
   - Idiopathic (sporadic): the greatest risk factors are advancing age (odds ratio [OR] 2.25 for each decade over age 40) and primary OA (OR 2.66). Note that sex and obesity are not risk factors.
   - Consequence of mechanical joint trauma or meniscectomy (OR 5.0)

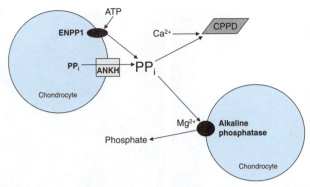

Figure 46-1. Factors contributing to calcium pyrophosphate crystal deposition.

- Familial predisposition: in young-onset CPPD. Mutations of the *ANKH* gene (gain of function) on chromosome 5p (CCAL2) and unknown genes on chromosome 8q (CCAL1). Patients tend to present in their 20s and 30s and are more likely to have spinal involvement.
- Specific disease associations: primary hyperparathyroidism (OR 3.0), long-standing hypomagnesemia (OR 13.5), hypophosphatasia, and hemochromatosis. Other diseases have been associated with CPPD but evidence is not as strong as for the diseases listed. Rheumatoid arthritis has a negative association (OR 0.18).

4. **Discuss the pathogenesis of CPPD.**
   Figure 46-1 shows factors that contribute to CPP deposition.
   - A high level of inorganic pyrophosphate (PPi) in cartilage is an important contributor to CPP crystal formation:
     - ANKH mutations: transport of more pyrophosphate from chondrocytes into cartilage
     - Ectonucleotide pyrrophospatase/phosphodiesterase 1 (ENPP1) and ENPP3 overactivity: generates more intracellular and extracellular pyrophosphate via hydrolysis of ATP.
     - Tissue-nonspecific lack of alkaline phosphatase (ALP) or underactivity (hypophosphatasia): magnesium is a cofactor for ALP so hypomagnesemia lessens its activity. In addition, calcium (hyperparathyroidism), iron (hemochromatosis), and copper (Wilson disease) inhibit ALP. The normal function of ALP is to break down PPi. When ALP function is abnormal, PPi levels increase.
   - Enhanced nucleation of CPP crystals in cartilage is an important contributor to CPP crystal formation:
     - Increased calcium concentrations (hyperparathyroidism) enhance crystal formation
     - Enhanced nucleation of CPP crystals due to increased iron (hemochromatosis) and copper (Wilson disease)
     - Lack of inhibitors of nucleation: magnesium inhibits nucleation so low levels contribute to crystal formation
     - Multiple changes in osteoarthritic cartilage composition (CILP, osteopontin) facilitate CPP crystal formation/deposition

5. **How common is CC?**
   Cross-sectional studies show that 8% of community-dwelling individuals have CC on knee radiographs (Figure 46-2). However, CC is rare before age 50 and increases with age, with up to 30% of the population having CC on roentgenograms by the ninth decade of life. Asymptomatic CC is the most common clinical presentation of CPPD. In patients with CPPD, the most common sites for finding radiographic CC are the knees and triangular fibrocartilage of the wrists (>90%). Calcifications should be bilateral.

6. **Is all CC caused by CPP crystal deposition?**
   Calcium salts other than CPP, such as basic calcium phosphate (BCP), can appear as CC. For example, the calcification of intervertebral disc cartilage seen in ochronosis largely consists of calcium hydroxyapatite. Clinicians usually assume that certain radiographic patterns of CC, such as the triangular fibrocartilage complex in the wrist or the hyaline cartilage and menisci in the knees, are due to CPP deposition. However, this is not always the case and dystrophic calcifications comprising BCP deposition due to trauma can be seen in these areas, particularly if only found unilaterally.

7. **Do all patients with CPPD have CC?**
   CPPD can cause arthritis without being seen as CC on roentgenograms. This can occur in up to 20% of patients with symptomatic CPPD. This is one reason why an acutely inflamed joint must be aspirated to identify the cause. An elderly patient who presents with an acutely inflamed knee could have gout or pseudogout as a cause of the arthritis, even if a roentgenogram is normal. The only way to tell is to aspirate the joint. The phrase **pyrophosphate arthropathy** has been used to describe structural damage to a joint associated with CPPD, with or without radiographic CC.

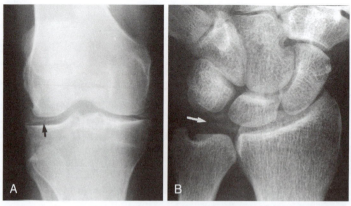

Figure 46-2. A, Chondrocalcinosis of the knee. B, Triangular fibrocartilage complex of the wrist.

8. **What is acute CPP crystal arthritis? How does it present?**

   Acute CPP crystal arthritis (pseudogout) is an acute arthritis caused by release of CPP crystals from the cartilage or synovium into the joint space. CPP crystals can interact with cell membranes, causing nonspecific activation of signal transduction pathways and inducing the release of prostaglandins, leukotrienes, and cytokines. The CPP crystals also interact with Toll-like receptor 2 on cells, which engulfs the CPP crystals. The crystals interact with the intracellular NLRP3 (cryopyrin) inflammasome, resulting in caspase-1 activation and IL-1 and IL-18 release, which causes intense inflammation of the joint. CXCL8 stimulates ingress of neutrophils into the joint, which is critical in triggering crystal-induced inflammation and the resultant synovitis. Symptoms of acute pseudogout are the same as for any acute arthritis, with rapid onset of pain and swelling. Physical examination reveals warmth, swelling with effusion, tenderness, and limited motion of the involved joint(s). Overlying erythema may simulate cellulitis. Occasionally systemic symptoms such as malaise and fever will also raise suspicion of infection (**pseudoseptic arthritis**).

   The presentation of pseudogout can mimic gout, but the causative crystal is CPP dihydrate rather than monosodium urate. Attacks of pseudogout tend to be less painful and take longer to reach peak intensity in comparison to gout. Usually, only a single joint is affected, although oligo- and polyarticular pseudogout have been described. Large joints are affected more commonly than small joints are, with the knee and wrist being the joints most frequently involved. Notably, the first MTP is rarely involved by pseudogout. Untreated pseudogout is self-limited, resolving within 7 to 10 days or longer. Patients are typically asymptomatic between attacks.

9. **How is acute CPP crystal arthritis diagnosed?**

   When a patient presents with an acute mono- or oligoarthritis, the critical and immediate diagnostic procedure is aspiration of the joint(s). The fluid obtained may appear yellow and cloudy or even opaque and chalky white because of suspended crystals. Synovial fluid is sent to the laboratory for a cell count and differential, as well as a Gram stain and bacterial culture. Synovial fluid leukocytosis with a predominance of polymorphonuclear leukocytes (PMNs) is present. A specimen of synovial fluid is also promptly analyzed for crystals by **polarized light microscopy**. The presence of **intracellular** CPP crystals confirms the diagnosis of pseudogout. Rarely, a definitive diagnosis requires special methods of crystal identification such as x-ray diffraction.

10. **How is polarized light microscopy performed to definitively diagnose CPPD?**

    A drop of synovial fluid is placed on a clean microscope slide and covered with a cover slip. The slide is first examined under an ordinary light microscope but the crystals are rarely visible. Therefore, a polarizer is typically needed to find CPP crystals, which appear as bright rhomboid or rectangular crystals with blunt or squared ends (see Chapter 7). For a definitive diagnosis a first-order red compensator is applied. CPP crystals are referred to as **weakly positively birefringent**. This means that CPP crystals appear blue when viewed under polarized light, with the long axis of the crystal parallel to the *direction of slow vibration of light in the first-order red compensator*. The mnemonic **ABC** (**A**ligned **B**lue **C**alcium) is useful: if the crystal is aligned with the red compensator and is blue, then it is CPP. CPP crystals lying with their long axes at right angles to the direction of slow vibration will appear yellow rather than blue. Observation of crystals inside a PMN instead of floating free helps to confirm that the CPP crystals are causing the arthritis.

11. **What are the pitfalls to be wary of when diagnosing acute CPP crystal arthritis?**

    1. **Septic arthritis** can coexist (in up to 1% of cases) with any acute crystalline arthritis, including CPPD. Enzymes that degrade cartilage can be released into the joint either from the infecting bacteria or the PMNs. These enzymes are able to strip crystals from the structures in and around the joint, and an unwary clinician might miss a septic joint. This is why joint fluid is sent for a Gram stain and culture on all arthrocenteses of acute arthritis.

2. It is possible for a patient to have simultaneous gout and pseudogout. Although rare, this condition is easily diagnosed via careful polarized light microscopy.
3. Acute pseudogout in the wrist of an elderly person may cause a carpal tunnel syndrome. Any patient with carpal tunnel syndrome requires a careful history and physical examination. Similarly, CPP deposition can cause cubital tunnel syndrome.
4. Acute pseudogout is frequently precipitated by an urgent medical illness, such as myocardial infarction, or by a surgical procedure. Fluid shifts with fluctuations in serum calcium levels are thought to play a role in such attacks. An elderly hospitalized patient who complains of new joint pain should be investigated for pseudogout. Note that most patients with idiopathic pseudogout are older than 55 to 60 years. There are recent reports of pseudogout after administration of intraarticular hyaluronate containing high concentrations of phosphate (Synvisc). Intravenous bisphosphonates have also been implicated in attacks when hypercalcemia is rapidly normalized. Parenteral granulocyte colony-stimulating factor may cause attacks by stimulating neutrophils.
5. Up to 20% of patients with pseudogout may not have CC on radiography. The synovial fluid **must** be examined for crystals.

12. How is acute CPP crystal arthritis treated?

The principles for treating acute pseudogout are the same as those for treating acute gout, although the disease is not as well studied.
1. In some cases, ice packs, temporary rest, and thorough aspiration of the affected joint with removal of the offending CPP crystals may halt the attack. Most rheumatologists offer other therapy in addition to these steps.
2. **Nonsteroidal antiinflammatory drugs (NSAIDs)** prescribed at full antiinflammatory doses may be effective but should be used with caution in elderly patients with multiple chronic illnesses, such as renal insufficiency and peptic ulcer disease.
3. In the patient at risk of side effects from NSAIDs, an option is **joint injection** with a long-acting corticosteroid preparation, such as **triamcinolone hexacetonide**. Triamcinolone hexacetonide at a dose of 40 mg is injected into large joints, such as the knee and shoulder. Smaller joints, such as the wrist, may be treated with 10 to 20 mg. Local injection is the best method to provide prompt, complete relief of the attack with little risk of systemic adverse effects.
4. One or two intramuscular injections of 60 mg **triamcinolone acetonide** is as effective as indomethacin. This approach has been useful in hospitalized patients with contraindications to NSAIDs who decline an intraarticular injection. In rare cases adrenocorticotropic hormone can be considered but is very expensive.
5. Oral **prednisone** can be used but has not been formally studied in pseudogout. This approach could be considered if an intraarticular or intramuscular injection is not desirable, as in a patient with a bleeding diathesis. The patient is started on 40 mg of oral prednisone daily, which is tapered to zero in 10 to 14 days. Of course the side effects of any steroid preparation must be kept in mind, including the potential for temporary worsening of diabetic glucose control or exacerbation of an infection.
6. Oral **colchicine** is known to interrupt acute pseudogout attacks. To lessen the side effects, a loading dose of 1.2 mg followed by 0.6 mg 1 hour later is recommended in patients with a glomerular filtration rate of >50 mL/min. Colchicine is not favored by rheumatologists for pseudogout because it has significant potential toxicity in the elderly population.
7. IL-1 inhibitors such as **anakinra** (100 mg subcutaneously daily for 3 to 5 days) are effective, but are not FDA-approved and are expensive; they could be considered in the rare circumstance of treatment-resistant disease.
8. Polyarticular attacks of pseudogout may be managed using NSAIDs, any of the systemic steroid regimens noted, colchicine, or anakinra.

13. Can any therapy prevent attacks of acute CPP arthritis from occurring?

Fortunately, most patients only have a few attacks that are widely separated in time, and thus require no prophylaxis against pseudogout. For patients with frequent attacks, colchicine at 0.6 mg twice a day prevents recurrences. Some rheumatologists use daily low doses of an NSAID or low-dose prednisone for the same purpose, although there are no reported studies of this approach.

14. Can CPPD disease be confused with rheumatoid arthritis?

Differentiating CPPD disease and RA can be difficult. Up to 5% of patients with CPPD arthritis have involvement of multiple joints, particularly the knees, wrists, and elbows, with chronic low-grade inflammation persisting for weeks or months. In the past this was called the pseudorheumatoid pattern of CPPD disease. Joint involvement may be symmetric, and systemic symptoms such as fatigue or morning stiffness are present. Physical examination reveals synovial thickening, loss of joint motion, and flexion contractures.

Serologically, the erythrocyte sedimentation rate and C-reactive protein can be elevated. Up to 10% of patients with CPPD will test positive for rheumatoid factor (RF) because of their age. If present, RF is usually a low titer. Higher RF titers, antibodies against cyclic citrullinated peptide, more widespread synovitis, involvement of the hands and feet, and characteristic erosions distinguish true RA from pseudoRA.

Before making a diagnosis of seronegative RA in an elderly patient, or RA with only a low positive RF, it is prudent to consider the possibility of CPPD by reviewing roentgenograms and clinical features and by aspirating a joint to examine synovial fluid for crystals if necessary. Notably, if NSAIDs are ineffective in controlling symptoms, hydroxychloroquine and methotrexate may be useful for patients with this CPPD presentation.

15. **What features suggest that a patient has pyrophosphate arthropathy rather than typical OA?**
Pyrophosphate arthropathy (pseudoOA) is seen in approximately half of patients diagnosed with symptomatic chronic CPPD. The pattern of joint involvement is different from that seen in primary OA. Patients with CPPD presenting as pyrophosphate arthropathy commonly have severe degenerative changes in the MCPs, radiocarpal joints, elbows, and shoulders, as well as the knees. Of these joints, only the knees are typically involved in primary OA. Therefore, any patient with OA in atypical joints should be evaluated for CPPD. Patients with pyrophosphate arthropathy are treated with NSAIDs, analgesics, physical therapy, and joint surgery, similar to the therapy for primary OA.

16. **What radiographic features in the knee suggest CPPD rather than typical primary OA?**
The knee is the most common joint involved in CPPD. Certain radiographic features help in separating pyrophosphate arthropathy from OA. In primary OA the medial compartment of the knee is more commonly involved, resulting in varus changes or so-called bow legs. Pyrophosphate arthropathy from CPPD is more likely to affect the lateral compartment, causing bi- or unilateral valgus changes or so-called knock knees. Isolated patellofemoral OA, bilateral involvement, **exuberant osteophytosis**, and flexion contractures are also more common in pyrophosphate arthropathy than in primary OA.

Radiographs typically show CC, but not always. Recent studies have shown that ultrasonography of the knee (and wrist and shoulder) is useful in detecting calcifications in cartilage with high sensitivity (0.87) and specificity (0.96) compared to plain radiographs. This will be a useful radiographic tool in the future.

17. **Describe the appropriate laboratory workup in a patient with newly diagnosed CPPD.**
Most cases of CPPD are sporadic or associated with normal aging. If the CPPD is severe or affects many joints, or the patient is younger than 50 years, it is reasonable to search for a metabolic cause. Evaluations must be individualized for persons older than 55 years, with hyperparathyroidism a primary consideration. Recommended laboratory studies include:
- Calcium (rule out hyperparathyroidism)
- Phosphorus
- Magnesium (rule out hypomagnesemia, usually from renal wasting)
- ALP (rule out hypophosphatasia)
- Ferritin, iron, total iron-binding capacity (rule out hemochromatosis)
- Renal function

There is a general consensus that hypothyroidism does not cause CPP crystal deposition. However, initiation of thyroxine therapy in a hypothyroid patient who has CPPD may precipitate a pseudogout attack, so many clinicians order measurement of thyroid-stimulating hormone.

18. **Does any treatment retard or reverse deposition of CPP crystals causing the arthritis?**
Unfortunately there is no therapy to prevent deposition of CPP crystals or remove CPP deposits already present. Patients with an underlying disease such as primary hyperparathyroidism should have the disease treated. This may retard further CPP crystal deposition but will not resolve the crystals already deposited. Some patients have been treated with the following:
- **Magnesium**: may be useful in patients with low magnesium levels. Has also been used in patients with normal levels because *in vitro* studies showed that magnesium has inhibitory effects on CPP crystal nucleation and growth. Note that loop and thiazide diuretics, proton pump inhibitors, and calcineurin inhibitors (cyclosporine, tacrolimus) can cause hypomagnesemia.
- **Probenecid**: it is postulated that probenecid lowers high PPi levels by blocking the ANKH anion channel.
- **Phosphocitrate**: lowers PPi levels but needs to be given intravenously because of poor oral absorption.

BIBLIOGRAPHY

Chollet-Janin A, Finckh A, Dudler J, Guerne P-A: Methotrexate as an alternative therapy for chronic pyrophosphate deposition disease: an exploratory analysis, Arthritis Rheum 56:688–692, 2007.

Doherty M, Abhishek A: Calcium pyrophosphate crystal-associated arthropathy. In Hochberg MC, Silman AJ, Smolen JS, et al: Rheumatology, ed 5, Philadelphia, 2011, Mosby Elsevier.

Martinez Sanchis A, Pascual E: Intracellular and extracellular CPPD crystals are a regular feature in synovial fluid from uninflamed joints of patients with CPPD related arthropathy, Ann Rheum Dis 64:1769–1772, 2005.

McGonagle D, Tan AL, Madden J, et al: Successful treatment of resistant pseudogout with anakinra, Arthritis Rheum 58:631–633, 2008.

Richette P, Bardin T, Doherty M: An update on the epidemiology of calcium pyrophosphate dihydrate crystal deposition disease, Rheumatology 48:711–715, 2009.

Roane DW, Harris MD, Carpenter MT, et al: Prospective use of intramuscular triamcinolone acetonide in pseudogout, J Rheumatol 24:1168–1170, 1997.

Rothschild B, Yakubov LE: Prospective 6-month double blind trial of hydroxychloroquine treatment of CPDD, Compr Ther 23:327, 1997.
Shah K, Spear J, Nathanson LA, et al: Does the presence of crystal arthritis rule out septic arthritis? J Emerg Med 32:23–26, 2007.
Wu DW, Reginato AJ, Torriani M, et al: The crowned dens syndrome as a cause of neck pain: report of two new cases and review of the literature, Arthritis Rheum 53:133–137, 2005.
Zhang W, Doherty M, Bardin T, et al: European League Against Rheumatism recommendations for calcium pyrophosphate deposition. Part I: terminology and diagnosis, Ann Rheum Dis 70:563–570, 2011.
Zhang W, Doherty M, Pascual E, et al: EULAR recommendations for calcium pyrophosphate deposition. Part II: management, Ann Rheum Dis 70:571–575, 2011.

Chapter 47: BASIC CALCIUM PHOSPHATE AND OTHER CRYSTALLINE DISEASES

Frederick T. Murphy, DO

KEY POINTS

1. Basic calcium phosphate (BCP) crystals deposit most commonly in the shoulder tendons/bursa but can occur in other periarticular areas.
2. BCP crystal deposits can remain asymptomatic or shed, causing acute calcific periarthritis.
3. BCP crystals are involved in the pathogenesis of a large joint destructive arthritis such as Milwaukee shoulder syndrome and may contribute to osteoarthritis (OA) in other joints.

1. **Are the crystals that cause gout and pseudogout the only crystals seen in synovial fluid?**
   Although monosodium urate crystals, which cause gout, and calcium pyrophosphate dihydrate (CPPD) crystals, which cause pseudogout, are the most commonly identified crystals in synovial fluid, many other crystals or particles may be encountered during polarized light microscopy. Some of these crystals cause disease and some are just interesting incidental findings (Box 47-1).

Box 47-1. Crystals and Particles Seen in Synovial Fluid

- Monosodium urate crystals
- Calcium pyrophosphate dihydrate crystals
- Calcium hydroxyapatite crystals (and other basic calcium phosphate crystals)
- Calcium oxalate crystals
- Injectable corticosteroid crystals
- Starch from examination gloves
- Cholesterol crystals
- Lipid droplets
- Foreign organic matter (e.g., plant thorns)
- Metallic fragments from prosthetic joints
- Immunoglobulin crystals in cryoglobulinemia
- Hemoglobin
- Aluminum
- Cystine
- Xanthine
- Charcot–Leyden crystals
- Amyloid

2. **What is the relationship between calcium hydroxyapatite and BCP crystals?**
   Calcium hydroxyapatite ($Ca_5(PO_4)_3 \cdot 2H_2O$) is a calcium-containing mineral found in bone. Partially carbonate-substituted hydroxyapatite and two other calcium-containing minerals (octacalcium phosphate and tricalcium phosphate) may be found in soft tissue and tendon calcifications and in some forms of arthritis. Collectively, these calcium-containing minerals are referred to as **basic calcium phosphate**.

3. **What diseases are associated with BCP crystals?**
   - Calcific periarthritis
     - Calcific deposits in tendons, bursae, joint capsules
     - Acute calcific periarthritis
   - BCP arthropathy
     - Acute synovitis
     - Destructive arthropathy
   - Subcutaneous/soft tissue calcifications
     - Connective tissue diseases: systemic lupus erythematosus, systemic sclerosis, mixed connective tissue disease, dermatomyositis
     - Metastatic calcifications: chronic renal failure with high calcium–phosphorus product (>70)
     - Tumoral calcinosis

4. **Where are periarticular calcium deposits most often seen?**
   BCP deposition is common in the shoulder. Up to 5% of shoulder roentgenograms in adults have periarticular calcium deposits, usually in the supraspinatus tendon. These deposits can be asymptomatic or cause pain and impingement. Tendons around other joints may also be affected, including the hand, wrist, hip, knee, foot, and neck (longissimus colli muscle at its insertion into the anterior tubercle of the atlas). Radiographically the calcific deposits can be dense and globular when asymptomatic or fragmented and fluffy due to the effects of inflammation.

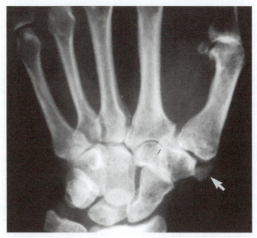

Figure 47-1. Amorphous homogeneous deposits of basic calcium phosphate near the first carpometacarpal joint *(arrow)*.

5. Why do the calcifications occur most commonly in the shoulder?

The supraspinatus tendon is prone to impingement. The tendon is poorly vascularized a few millimeters from its insertion into the humeral head. Therefore its ability to recover from the repetitive trauma of impingement is poor, resulting in ischemia and necrosis. This "critical zone" is prone to accumulating calcium salts (BCPs) causing calcific deposits in the tendon and bursa. Notably, other tendons that develop calcifications have a similar pathogenesis, with deposition at relatively avascular and traumatized sites in the tendon. Therefore the calcification may be the *result* of chronic tendinitis rather than the cause.

6. How is calcific tendinitis treated?

Asymptomatic BCP deposits require no therapy. Patients with symptoms of bursitis or tendinitis are managed conservatively, with physical therapy and nonsteroidal antiinflammatory drugs (NSAIDs). Local injection with a short-acting corticosteroid such as betamethasone should be used sparingly because steroids may promote calcification in the long term. Occasionally, use of a needle to disrupt the calcification causes more rapid dissolution of the deposit by stimulating phagocytosis of the BCP. Surgical or arthroscopic debridement of very large or severely symptomatic calcific deposits may be necessary. Pulsed ultrasound therapy has shown recent promise for dissolving BCP crystals.

7. What is acute calcific periarthritis?

When BCP crystals are shed from a calcific deposit, there is an intense local inflammatory reaction to the crystals, similar to other crystalline arthritides. If this reaction occurs around a joint, the clinical picture is an acute arthritis with pain, warmth, loss of motion, and swelling. Roentgenograms reveal the BCP deposit and thus identify the crystal causing the problem. Acute calcific periarthritis most commonly occurs in the shoulder from calcifications in the supraspinatus tendon. Attacks of calcific periarthritis can occur in other joint areas either spontaneously or after minor trauma.

8. What is hydroxyapatite pseudopodagra? What is the crowned dens syndrome?

Hydroxyapatite pseudopodagra is acute calcific periarthritis occurring near the first metatarsophalangeal (MTP) joint, causing podagra identical to that seen in gout. This presentation is more common in young women who excessively pronate their feet; walking or running causes repetitive trauma to this area. The condition may be distinguished from gout according to the premenopausal status of the patient, the absence of monosodium urate crystals in synovial fluid, and characteristic calcifications around the joint on roentgenography. Symptoms subside over several weeks, either spontaneously or with treatment. Interestingly, the calcific deposit may dissolve during the acute inflammatory episode, leading to disappearance of the calcification on follow-up roentgenograms. This can also occur in other joint areas (Figure 47-1).

Crowned dens syndrome can cause acute neck pain due to calcifications surrounding the odontoid process. These calcifications are frequently a combination of BCP and CPPD crystals. This condition occurs most commonly in the elderly and can cause fever and associated neurologic symptoms including headache, confusion, and aseptic meningitis. Calcifications are seen best on an open-mouth view of the odontoid process or a computed tomography scan of the area.

9. Describe the treatment for acute calcific periarthritis?

Attacks of calcific periarthritis may be managed similarly to other crystalline arthritides. NSAIDs given in full doses are the mainstay of therapy. For acute crystalline arthritis, indomethacin 50 mg orally three times daily for 1 to 2 days and then tapered off is the classic approach. Other NSAIDs are probably just as effective. The patient's age, underlying renal disease, and history of peptic ulcer disease are factors in the decision on whether to use NSAIDs. It has been reported that colchicine therapy is successful for acute calcific periarthritis. Aspiration of the joint and injection of a corticosteroid is often the most expedient way to provide relief.

10. **Can BCP crystals cause an inflammatory synovitis?**
Acute attacks of arthritis due to BCP crystals in the knee and other joints have been described. The attacks resemble gout. A more chronic arthritis leading to erosive OA changes in the fingers has also been linked to BCP crystals. Unfortunately both these presentations are difficult to prove because of the difficulty in identifying BCP crystals in synovial fluid.

11. **How are BCP crystals identified if they are suspected of causing a joint problem?**
Identification of BCP crystals is difficult. If characteristic calcifications are observed on roentgenograms, it is often presumed that BCP is the cause of the symptoms. Aspiration of a calcific deposit may yield material that looks like toothpaste. Individual BCP crystals are so small that they cannot be seen. Plain and polarized light microscopy may reveal aggregated BCP crystals with an appearance described as "shiny coins" (Figure 47-2). BCP crystals are not birefringent and so are not seen on polarized light microscopy. Special stains, such as alizarin red, can confirm the presence of calcium in the aspirated material but are not widely available to clinicians and are not specific for BCP. Precise crystal identification requires techniques such as transmission electron microscopy, which is available only in large referral hospitals and is not practical for the clinician.

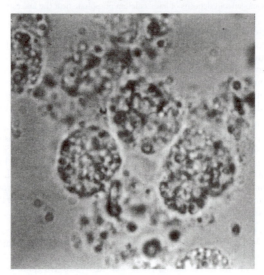

Figure 47-2. Aggregates of basic calcium phosphate crystals seen in neutrophils under light microscopy.

12. **How does Milwaukee shoulder syndrome (apatite-associated arthropathy or rotator cuff tear arthropathy) present?**
Milwaukee shoulder syndrome is characterized by severe degenerative arthritis of the glenohumeral joint with loss of the rotator cuff associated with the presence of BCP crystals (Figure 47-3). Often, large joint effusions are present on physical examination. Patients with Milwaukee shoulder syndrome are usually women in their 70s. Bilateral shoulder involvement is common, with the dominant side more severely affected. Many of these patients have had shoulder impingement with calcific tendonitis in the past. It is postulated that BCP crystals shed from the tendon/bursa deposit calcium into the joint. These BCP crystals localize to the synovium, where they act as mitogens, causing cytokine and matrix metalloproteinase (MMP, e.g., collagenase) production by synovial macrophages and fibroblasts. In turn, the collagenase and other MMPs contribute to the rotator cuff disruption and accelerated degenerative changes in the shoulder.

Symptoms vary from minimally symptomatic with shoulder motion to severe pain at rest. Physical examination reveals reduced active and passive ranges of motion with glenohumeral crepitus. Effusions can be large. Synovial fluid, which often has streaks of blood, is noninflammatory with few white blood cells that are predominantly mononuclear. Roentgenograms show severe OA of the glenohumeral joint associated with upward migration of the head of the humerus, indicating a defect in the rotator cuff. Notably, there is a relative paucity of osteophytes (atrophic degenerative arthritis) compared to CPPD disease and primary OA. Soft tissue calcifications may also be present.

BCP arthropathy can affect other joints as well, particularly the knees and hips. A loss of joint space in the lateral compartment in the knees distinguishes this from primary OA, similar to CPPD-associated arthropathy. Rapidly destructive arthritis of the finger due to BCP has been called **Philadelphia finger**.

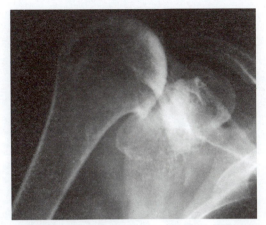
Figure 47-3. Milwaukee shoulder. Note the upward migration of the humeral head indicating a rotator cuff tear.

13. **How is Milwaukee shoulder syndrome treated?**
    Treatment can be unsatisfactory. Some patients do well with a daily low dose of NSAIDs and/or analgesics. Local heat is frequently beneficial. If large effusions are present, repeated arthrocenteses sometimes relieve symptoms. Intraarticular steroids should be used sparingly. Joint usage needs to be reduced for severe symptoms. At the same time, physical therapy is vital to maintain the range of motion and strengthen the surrounding muscles. Surgical intervention may be considered for advanced degenerative changes.

14. **Do BCP crystals contribute to OA?**
    BCP crystals are frequently found in OA joints. It is not believed that they come from bone underlying denuded cartilage. Instead it is postulated that low levels of extracellular inorganic pyrophosphate in degenerative cartilage of some patients with OA allows the formation of hydroxyapatite crystals in extracellular matrix vesicles. These are shed from the cartilage into the synovial fluid and deposit in the synovium. The calcium-containing crystals are mitogenic, causing synovial proliferation with production of MMPs and prostaglandins. This may result in more rapid progression of OA. Patients with OA in whom BCP crystals have been demonstrated in noninflammatory synovial fluid seem to have larger effusions and more destructive OA compared to OA patients without BCP crystals. This association remains controversial.

15. **Describe the appearance and clinical presentation of other crystals in synovial fluid.**
    - **Calcium oxalate crystals** are characteristically bipyramidal in appearance. They occur in effusions from patients with primary oxalosis or end-stage renal disease. Ascorbic acid is metabolized to oxalate, so dialysis patients taking Vitamin C supplements are prone to this condition. So-called oxalate gout may cause both intra- and extraarticular manifestations.
    - **Cholesterol crystals** are found in synovial fluid from *chronic* joint effusions, usually rheumatoid arthritis. The crystals are square and plate-like with a single notched corner. Cholesterol crystals are beautifully birefringent, both positively and negatively. They do not cause inflammation. They are a sign of a chronic inflammatory effusion and form from the cholesterol in the cell membranes of neutrophils after they break down in the joint.
    - **Steroid crystals** in synovial fluid may be confused with CPPD crystals because they are often small, irregularly shaped or rectangular, and weakly birefringent. Intracellular steroid crystals in synovial fluid are not uncommon. Careful polarized microscopy is necessary because steroid crystals may be positively or negatively birefringent (both types are often seen in the same field), whereas CPPD crystals are always weakly positively birefringent. The patient will also have a history of joint injection with corticosteroid, possibly weeks earlier. Patients sometimes do not volunteer this information, so a specific question about previous joint injection must be asked.
    - **Talc (or starch) particles** from examination gloves are an artifact occurring during preparation of synovial fluid slides. They resemble small beach balls when viewed under polarized light microscopy.
    - **Lipid droplets** have a "Maltese cross" appearance under polarized light microscopy. Lipid droplets in synovial fluid may represent a subchondral fracture or may be seen occasionally in medical conditions, including pancreatitis. Lipid droplets look like starch particles, although the size of starch particles is more variable.

    There are many other types of particles or contaminants that can appear in synovial fluid, such as glass fragments from cover slips and specks of cartilage, so all synovial fluids must be examined carefully (Figure 47-4).

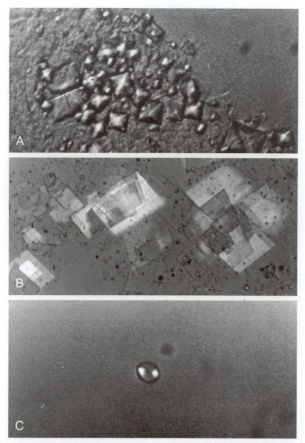

Figure 47-4. Other synovial fluid crystals. **A,** Calcium oxalate crystals have a characteristic bipyramidal shape under ordinary light microscopy. **B,** Plane-shaped cholesterol crystals are strongly birefringent when viewed under polarized light microscopy. These crystals were obtained from an aspirate of a knee effusion in a patient with rheumatoid arthritis. **C,** Starch (talc) from examination gloves is a common artifact during slide preparation. (**A,** *Courtesy The Upjohn Company.* **B,** *Linda Sakai, MD.* **C,** *Courtesy The Upjohn Company.*)

Bibliography

Ea HK, Liote F: Advances in understanding calcium-containing crystal disease, Curr Opin Rheumatol 21:150–157, 2009.
Ecklund KJ, Lee TQ, Tibone J, Gupta R: Rotator cuff tear arthropathy, J Am Acad Orthop Surg 15:340–349, 2007.
Fam AG, Stein J: Hydroxyapatite pseudopodagra in young women, J Rheumatol 19:662–664, 1992.
Halverson PB, Carrera GF, McCarty DJ: Milwaukee shoulder syndrome: fifteen additional cases and a description of contributing factors, Arch Intern Med 150:677–682, 1990.
MacMullan P, McMahon G, McCarthy G: Detection of basic calcium phosphate crystals in osteoarthritis, Joint Bone Spine 78:358–363, 2011.
Rosenthal AK: Crystals, inflammation, and osteoarthritis, Curr Opin Rheumatol 23:170–173, 2011.
Schumacher HR, Chen LX: Other crystal-related arthropathies. In Hochberg MC, Silman AJ, Smolen JS, et al: Rheumatology, ed 5, Philadelphia, 2011, Mosby.
Schumacher HR, Reginato AJ: Atlas of synovial fluid analysis and crystal identification, Philadelphia, 1991, Lea & Febiger.
Terkeltaub R: Calcium crystal diseases: calcium pyrophosphate dihydrate and basic calcium phosphate. In Firestein GS, Budd RC, Gabriel SE, et al: Kelley's textbook of rheumatology, ed 9, Philadelphia, 2013, Elsevier Saunders.
Whelan LC, Morgan MP, McCarthy GM: Basic calcium phosphate crystals as a unique therapeutic target in osteoarthritis, Front Biosci 10:530–541, 2005.
Wu DW, Reginato AJ, Torriani M, et al: The crowned dens syndrome as a cause of neck pain: report of two new cases and review of the literature, Arthritis Rheum 53:133–137, 2005.

ENDOCRINE-ASSOCIATED ARTHROPATHIES

Edmund H. Hornstein, DO

CHAPTER 48

KEY POINTS

1. The diabetic stiff hand syndrome is related to disease duration and therapy and predicts microvascular complications of diabetes.
2. Frozen shoulder is a common and often overlooked diagnosis in patients with diabetes.
3. Carpal tunnel syndrome can be the initial manifestation of hypothyroidism, diabetes mellitus, and acromegaly.
4. Hypothyroidism should be ruled out in patients with muscle symptoms and an elevated creatine kinase.
5. Osteoporosis with fractures can be the presentation of hyperparathyroidism, Cushing's syndrome, and hyperthyroidism.

1. **What signs or symptoms should prompt a search for an occult endocrinopathy?**
   - Entrapment neuropathy, particularly carpal tunnel syndrome.
   - Calcium pyrophosphate dihydrate (CPPD) arthropathy.
   - Diffuse myalgia with or without muscle weakness.
   - Raynaud's phenomenon.

2. **Which endocrine diseases have well-described rheumatologic manifestations associated with them?**

Diabetes mellitus	Hyperparathyroidism
Hypothyroidism	Acromegaly
Hyperthyroidism	Cushing's syndrome
Hypoparathyroidism	Hyperlipoproteinemia

DIABETES MELLITUS

3. **What rheumatologic syndromes are more common in patients with diabetes mellitus?**
   - Intrinsic complications of diabetes mellitus.
     - Diabetic stiff hand syndrome (limited joint mobility syndrome, diabetic cheiroarthropathy).
     - Neuropathic arthropathy (Charcot joint) and diabetic osteolysis.
     - Diabetic amyotrophy.
       - Diabetic muscle infarction.
   - Conditions with increased incidence in diabetes mellitus.
     - Adhesive capsulitis of the shoulder (frozen shoulder).
       - Calcific shoulder periarthritis (tendinitis).
       - Complex regional pain syndrome (shoulder–hand syndrome).
     - Flexor tenosynovitis of the hands (trigger fingers).
     - Dupuytren's contractures.
     - Carpal tunnel syndrome.
     - Diffuse idiopathic skeletal hyperostosis (DISH).
     - Septic joint/osteomyelitis.

4. **How does the diabetic stiff hand syndrome present?**
   This syndrome, also known as limited joint mobility syndrome and diabetic cheiroarthropathy, presents with the insidious development of flexion contractures involving the small joints of the hands, starting with the distal interphalangeal joints (DIPs) and proximal interphalangeal joints (PIPs) and moving proximally over time. This condition occurs in both type 1 diabetics (8% to 50%) and type 2 diabetics (increased) and correlates with disease duration, glucose control, and renal/retinal microvascular disease.
   The "prayer sign" observed on physical examination reflects the inability to fully extend the joints of the fingers (Figure 48-1). These finger contractures are attributed to excessive glycosylation of dermal and periarticular collagen, decreased collagen degradation, and increased dermal hydration resulting in indurated and thickened skin around the joints. This condition can be confused with scleroderma. Laboratory serologies

357

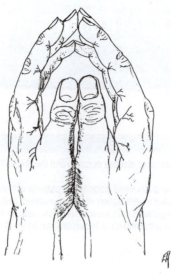

Figure 48-1. Prayer sign in a patient with limited joint mobility due to diabetes mellitus.

and hand radiographs are unremarkable. Treatment is physical therapy and control of the underlying diabetes. Contractures usually progress slowly but rarely limit function significantly.

5. **Discuss the relationship between Charcot joint and diabetes mellitus.**
   Charcot joint occurs in <1% of all diabetics (both type 1 and type 2). It occurs in both males and females with equal frequency. Most patients (>66%) are over age 40 years and have had long-standing (>10 years), poorly controlled diabetes complicated by a diabetic peripheral neuropathy. Patients present with relatively painless swelling and deformity usually of the foot (most commonly tarsometatarsal joints) and ankle, although knee, hip, and spine can be involved. Occasionally it can be of sudden onset mimicking an infection. With progression of disease, the patient can develop "rocker bottom" feet owing to midtarsal collapse. Skin over bony prominences can ulcerate and become infected without the patient's knowledge owing to abnormal sensation resulting from the neuropathy. Radiographs frequently show severe abnormalities characterized by the **5 Ds**: destruction, density (increased), debris, disorganization, and dislocation (Figure 48-2). The *increased* density and sharp margins of the bony debris help separate a Charcot joint from infection. The etiology is a combination of repetitive microtrauma to a desensate foot and autonomic dysfunction leading to increased blood flow, hyperemia, and osteoclastic resorption of bone. Treatment includes protected weight-bearing, soft casts, good shoes, and aggressive treatment and prevention of skin ulcerations. Charcot joints, however, usually progress. There is no role for surgery (fusion, arthroplasty) other than amputation for severe cases. Diabetes mellitus has replaced neurosyphilis as the most common cause of a Charcot joint today.

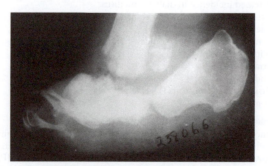

Figure 48-2. Charcot joints of foot and ankle.

6. **What is diabetic osteolysis?**
   Diabetic osteolysis is a condition specifically occurring in diabetics. The osteolysis is characterized by osteoporosis and variable degrees of resorption of distal metatarsal bones and proximal phalanges in the feet. Pain

is variable. Radiographs have a characteristic "licked candy" appearance. The pathogenesis is unclear, as this syndrome can occur at any time during the course of diabetes. The primary consideration in the differential diagnosis is osteomyelitis. Treatment is conservative and includes protected weight-bearing. The process may terminate at any stage and in some cases may completely resolve.

7. **How does diabetic amyotrophy present? How is it different from diabetic muscle infarction?**
Diabetic amyotrophy presents with severe pain and dysesthesia involving most commonly the proximal muscles of the pelvis and thigh. The perispinal and shoulder girdle muscles can also be involved. The condition may be bilateral in 50% of cases. Anorexia, weight loss, and unsteady gait owing to muscle wasting and weakness may be seen. The typical patient is a 50-year-old to 60-year-old man with well-controlled, mild noninsulin-dependent diabetes mellitus of several years' duration, although it can be the presenting sign of diabetes. Usually the patient has no evidence of diabetic retinopathy or nephropathy but may have a distal symmetric sensory neuropathy.

Laboratory evaluation is usually unremarkable except for an elevated cerebrospinal fluid protein. Electromyography/nerve conduction velocity (EMG/NCV) testing demonstrates changes compatible with a neuropathy, and muscle biopsy shows muscle fiber atrophy without an inflammatory infiltrate. The etiology is unclear but may be as a result of an immune-mediated vasculopathy affecting the lumbosacral plexus or femoral nerve. Treatment includes pain control and physical therapy. Increasingly, immunomodulating agents (intravenous immunoglobulin, intravenous methylprednisolone) are being used. Over 50% recover within 3 to 18 months, although recovery is often incomplete. Some patients have recurrent episodes.

Diabetic muscle infarction is the spontaneous infarction of muscle. It occurs in long-standing insulin-dependent diabetics with multiple other microvascular complications. Patients present with acute onset of pain and swelling over days to weeks of thigh or calf. Creatine kinase may be elevated. Clinical presentation, laboratory findings, and muscle magnetic resonance imaging help to rule out infection/abscess or malignancy, although an excisional biopsy may be necessary.

8. **What is diabetic periarthritis of the shoulder?**
Diabetic periarthritis of the shoulder is also known as **frozen shoulder** or **adhesive capsulitis**. It occurs in 10% to 33% of diabetics and is five times more common in diabetics than in nondiabetics. The typical patient is female with type 2 diabetes of long duration who presents with diffuse soreness and global loss of motion of the shoulder. Up to 50% of patients have bilateral involvement, although the nondominant shoulder is frequently more severely involved. Laboratory studies and radiographs are unremarkable. Some patients have **calcific (hydroxyapatite) periarthritis/tendinitis**, which is three times more common in diabetics than in patients without diabetes and may increase the risk of developing frozen shoulder. Treatment includes nonsteroidal antiinflammatory drugs (NSAIDs), rarely intraarticular steroids, and vigorous physical therapy to improve range of motion. For unclear reasons, this syndrome may spontaneously remit after weeks to months.

9. **The shoulder–hand syndrome can be a complication of frozen shoulder. What is it?**
When a frozen shoulder (with or without calcific periarthritis) is accompanied by vasomotor changes of reflex sympathetic dystrophy/chronic regional pain syndrome, it is known as shoulder–hand syndrome (see Chapter 65).

10. **How commonly does flexor tenosynovitis or Dupuytren's contractures occur in patients with diabetes mellitus?**
Flexor tenosynovitis occurs in 5% to 33% of diabetic patients. Females with long-standing diabetes are more commonly affected than males. Patients complain of aching and stiffness in the palmar aspect of the hand. Symptoms are worse in the morning. A "trigger" finger may occur as a result of an inflammatory nodule getting caught in the proximal pulley at the base of the finger. The thumb of the dominant hand is most commonly involved (75%), although multiple fingers on both hands can be affected. Laboratory findings and radiographs are unremarkable. Treatment includes NSAIDs, local steroid injections, and surgery.

Dupuytren's contractures occur in 30% to 60% of patients with type 1 diabetes. Patients present with nodular thickening of the palmar fascia, leading to flexion contractures usually of the fourth and fifth digits. Patients usually have long-standing diabetes, although there is no association with control of the diabetes. The pathogenesis is thought to be a result of contractile myofibroblasts producing increased collagen secondary to microvascular ischemia. Treatment includes NSAIDs, physical therapy, local steroid injections, local collagenase injections, and rarely surgery.

11. **What is the relationship between diabetes mellitus and carpal tunnel syndrome?**
Carpal tunnel syndrome commonly (20%) occurs in diabetic patients. Patients present with numbness in the median nerve distribution. Nocturnal paresthesias, hand pain, and pain radiating to the elbow or shoulder (Valleix phenomenon) can also occur. Tinel's and Phalen's signs may be positive. Thenar atrophy is a late sign and indicates muscle denervation. The neuropathy may be from extrinsic compression or owing to microvascular disease causing vasa nervorum ischemia. Treatment includes splints, NSAIDs, diuretics, local steroid injections into the carpal tunnel, and surgical decompression (see Chapter 62).

12. **What is DISH? How commonly does it occur in diabetes mellitus?**
    DISH is diffuse idiopathic skeletal hyperostosis, also known as Forestier's disease. It occurs in up to 20% of type 2 diabetic patients who are typically obese and over age 50 years. Patients present with neck and back stiffness associated with loss of motion. *Pain is not prominent.* Radiographs are diagnostic and consist of at least four vertebrae fused together as a result of ossification of the anterior longitudinal ligament. Disc spaces, apophyseal joints, and sacroiliac joints are normal, helping to separate it from osteoarthritis and ankylosing spondylitis. Treatment is usually NSAIDs and physical therapy (see Chapter 51).

13. **What diabetes-associated rheumatologic syndromes have features in common with scleroderma?**
    The syndrome of limited joint mobility in which findings in the fingers are reminiscent of the sclerodactyly seen in the CREST syndrome.
    Scleredema diabeticorum occurs primarily in type 2 diabetics and is characterized by thickened, edematous areas of skin most commonly on the upper back and neck. This has also been called scleredema adultorum of Buschke, type 3.

THYROID DISEASE

14. **Describe the arthropathy associated with severe hypothyroidism.**
    Myxedematous arthropathy usually affects large joints such as the knees. The patient presents with swelling and stiffness. Synovial thickening, ligamentous laxity, and knee effusions with a characteristic slow fluid wave (bulge sign) are common. The synovial fluid is noninflammatory with an increased viscosity owing to high hyaluronic acid levels giving a string sign of 1 foot to 2 feet instead of the normal 1 inch to 2 inches. Radiographs are typically normal.
    Osteonecrosis can also occur (controversial). In adults, it typically involves the hip or tibial plateau. In children, abnormal epiphyseal ossification may occur, which can be confused with epiphyseal dysplasia or juvenile avascular necrosis (Legg–Calvé–Perthes disease) of the hip.

15. **What other common rheumatologic syndromes are associated with hypothyroidism?**
    Think of **TRAP**:
    T—Tunnel (carpal) syndrome (15% of hypothyroid patients).
    R—Raynaud's phenomenon.
    A—Aching muscles with findings indistinguishable from those of fibromyalgia (up to 30% of hypothyroid patients).
    P—Proximal muscle weakness and stiffness with an elevated creatine kinase. Thyroid-stimulating hormone (TSH) always very high (>20) and thyroxine (T4) low.
    Although chondrocalcinosis has also been ascribed to hypothyroidism, it probably does not occur more commonly than in age-matched controls.

16. **What is the relationship between Hashimoto's thyroiditis and other collagen vascular diseases?**
    Hashimoto's thyroiditis occurs with increased frequency in several collagen vascular diseases. It has been described in systemic lupus erythematosus (SLE), Sjögren's syndrome, and rheumatoid arthritis, as well as mixed connective tissue disease, scleroderma, and polymyositis. The increased prevalence of human leukocyte antigen-B8 (HLA-B8), DR3, DR5 in patients with Hashimoto's thyroiditis accounts for it occurring with diseases that have similar HLA associations. Any patient with a collagen vascular disease should be followed closely for development of hypothyroid symptoms.

17. **Which rheumatic problems occur in patients with hyperthyroidism?**
    - Thyroid acropachy.
    - Painless proximal muscle weakness (70% of hyperthyroid patients)—more common in elderly patients with apathetic hyperthyroidism.
    - Osteoporosis—most common musculoskeletal manifestation.
    - Adhesive capsulitis of the shoulders (controversial)—especially in patients with proximal muscle weakness.

18. **Describe thyroid acropachy.**
    Thyroid acropachy is a rare (1%) complication of Graves' disease consisting of soft tissue swelling of the hands, digital clubbing, and periostitis particularly involving the metacarpal and phalangeal bones. Radiographs are characteristic (Figure 48-3). It is strongly associated with ophthalmopathy and pretibial myxedema. The symptoms usually occur after the patient becomes euthyroid. Pain is variable but usually mild. There is no effective therapy.

19. **How do you differentiate hyperthyroid myopathy from the myopathies of hypothyroidism and idiopathic inflammatory myopathy (polymyositis)?**
    The differences among hyperthyroid myopathy, myopathies of hypothyroidism, and idiopathic inflammatory myopathy (polymyositis) are presented in Table 48-1.

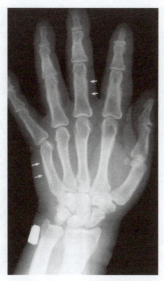

Figure 48-3. Thyroid acropachy. Note the periosteal reaction along shafts of the metacarpals and phalanges (*arrows*).

Table 48-1. Differences Among Hyperthyroid Myopathy, Myopathies of Hypothyroidism, and Idiopathic Inflammatory Myopathy (Polymyositis)

	TSH	T4	CK	WEAKNESS	BIOPSY
Inflammatory myopathy	Normal	Normal	Increased	Mild to severe	Inflammation
Hypothyroidism	Increased	Decreased	Increased	Usually mild	Normal
Hyperthyroidism	Decreased	Increased	Normal	Usually mild	Normal

CK, Creatine kinase; *T4*, thyroxine; *TSH*, thyroid-stimulating hormone.

20. What medications used to treat hyperthyroidism can cause rheumatic syndromes?
- Propylthiouracil—can cause a systemic vasculitis (perinuclear antineutrophil cytoplasmic antibody positive).
- Methimidazole—lupus-like syndrome and a syndrome of diabetes mellitus owing to antiinsulin antibodies.

PARATHYROID DISEASE

21. List the rheumatic syndromes associated with primary hyperparathyroidism.
- Painless proximal muscle weakness with normal muscle enzymes but a neuropathic EMG.
- Chondrocalcinosis with pseudogout attacks usually owing to CPPD crystals.
- Osteogenic synovitis owing to subchondral bony collapse from thinning of bone (leading to osteoarthritis).
- Osteoporosis.
- Ectopic soft tissue calcifications.
- Tendon ruptures.

22. What are the skeletal ramifications of primary hyperparathyroidism?
Osteitis fibrosa cystica represents the classic sequela of prolonged hyperparathyroidism from any cause. It most commonly occurs in patients with hyperparathyroidism associated with end stage renal disease and is diagnosed by X-ray findings that are most prominent in the hands. Subperiosteal resorption with a blurring of the cortical margins on the radial side of the phalanges is seen, accompanied by a decrease in bone diameter and resorption of the tufts of the distal phalanges (Figure 48-4). Diffuse osteopenia is common, and erosions may be seen in the joints of the hands, axial skeleton, and at the ends of the clavicles. Discrete lytic lesions owing to focal aggregates of osteoclastic giant cells and fibrous tissue with decomposing blood may occur and are known as **brown tumors**. Spinal compression fractures are common.

23. What is the relationship between chondrocalcinosis and primary hyperparathyroidism?
Up to 15% of patients with chondrocalcinosis will be found to have primary hyperparathyroidism. Conversely, over 50% of patients with long-standing primary hyperparathyroidism will have radiographic evidence of chondrocalcinosis.

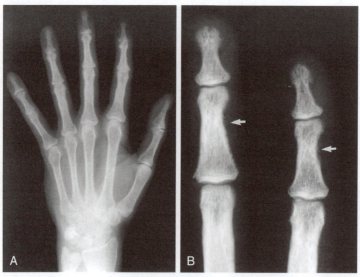

Figure 48-4. A, Radiograph of hand of a patient with hyperparathyroidism. B, Close-up of phalanges demonstrating subperiosteal resorption (*arrows*).

24. What is the knuckle, knuckle, dimple, knuckle sign?
Patients with type Ia pseudohypoparathyroidism (autosomal dominant Albright's hereditary osteodystrophy) may have a skeletal deformity with a short fourth metacarpal. When they clench their hand to form a fist, a dimple appears where the fourth knuckle should be, emphasizing the short fourth metacarpal bone. These patients will also have parathyroid hormone resistance (low calcium, high phosphorous, high parathyroid hormone [PTH]), short stature, ectopic calcifications around weight-bearing joints and perispinal ligaments, and may have mental retardation. It is as a result of a defect in *GNAS1* resulting in PTH resistance. Patients with pseudopseudohypoparathyroidism have a short fourth metacarpal (and metatarsal) bone but none of the other clinical or biochemical manifestations.

ACROMEGALY

25. How often does arthropathy occur in acromegaly?
It is common and may be seen in up to 74% of affected patients. Degenerative disease is the most common manifestation and crepitus on examination is the most common finding. The knees, shoulders, hips, lumbosacral spine, and cervical spine are the most frequently symptomatic areas, but the hands reveal the most characteristic radiographic changes. Clinical and radiographic changes occur due to excess growth hormone-stimulating hepatocytes to produce somatomedin C (insulin-like growth factor), which affects osteocytes, chondrocytes, and fibroblasts.

26. List the radiographic findings in the hands of patients with acromegaly.
- Soft tissue thickening.
- Deformation of epiphyses with squaring of enlarged terminal phalanx/phalanges (spade-like).
- Chondrocalcinosis (rare).
- Increased joint/disc space.
- Periosteal apposition of tubular bones (Figure 48-5).

27. What other rheumatologic syndromes may accompany acromegaly?
- Carpal tunnel syndrome (up to 50% of patients).
- Proximal muscle weakness with normal EMG and normal muscle enzymes.
- Raynaud's phenomenon (up to 33% of patients).
- Chondrocalcinosis (rare).

CUSHING'S SYNDROME

28. List the rheumatic syndromes associated with excessive glucocorticoids.
- Proximal muscle weakness.
- Osteoporosis (all doses).
- Osteonecrosis.
- Steroid withdrawal syndrome.

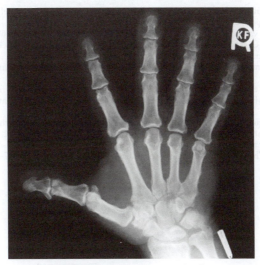

Figure 48-5. Acromegaly of the hand.

29. **Describe the myopathy seen with excessive glucocorticoids.**
    Proximal muscle weakness without muscle enzyme elevations can be seen in patients with Cushing's syndrome or in patients receiving >10 mg of prednisone a day. EMG findings are usually normal or nonspecific. Muscle biopsy can show type 2b muscle fiber atrophy, which is nonspecific and can be seen with disuse atrophy. Patients should be treated with physical therapy, as muscle-strengthening exercises may delay the onset or improve this myopathy.

30. **Which is more likely to cause osteonecrosis: endogenous Cushing's syndrome or iatrogenic Cushing's syndrome?**
    Iatrogenic Cushing's syndrome (i.e., prednisone therapy) is much more likely than Cushing's syndrome to cause osteonecrosis.

31. **What is the steroid withdrawal syndrome?**
    This syndrome, sometimes called Slocumb's syndrome, is characterized by myalgias, arthralgias, and lethargy following too rapid a taper of corticosteroids. Sometimes patients can develop noninflammatory joint effusions, particularly in the knees. Low-grade fevers occasionally occur. This withdrawal syndrome can be confused with reactivation of the primary disease for which the corticosteroids were used. Increasing the corticosteroids, tapering the steroids more slowly, and using NSAIDs can all help the symptoms.

FAMILIAL HYPERLIPOPROTEINEMIA

32. **Describe the musculoskeletal disorders that have been associated with familial hyperlipoproteinemia.**
    - Types I, IV, V—gout is associated with the hypertriglyceridemia seen in these hyperlipidemias. Type IV patients can have chronic arthralgias.
    - Types II, III—tendinous xanthomas on digital extensor tendons and Achilles tendon. Achilles tendinitis can occur. Tuberous xanthomas on extensor surfaces (elbows, knees, hands) can mimic gouty tophi or rheumatoid nodules.
    - Type II—episodic, acute, migratory inflammatory arthritis resembling acute rheumatic fever can occur in up to 50% of patients. Arthritis resolves in 2 weeks but frequently recurs. Cholesterol crystals are *not* found in the synovial fluid.
    - Type III—osseous xanthomas in long bones can lead to pathologic fractures.

BIBLIOGRAPHY

Anwar S, Gibofsky A: Musculoskeletal manifestations of thyroid disease, Rheum Dis Clin North Am 36:665–680, 2010.
Arkkila PE, Kantola IM, Viikari JS, et al: Shoulder capsulitis in type I and type II diabetic patients: association with diabetic complications and related diseases, Ann Rheum Dis 55:907, 1996.
Bauer DC, Ettinger B, Nevitt MC, Stone KL: Risk of fracture in women with low serum levels of thyroid-stimulating hormone, Ann Int Med 134:561–568, 2001.
Chammas M, Bousquet P, Renard E, et al: Dupuytren's disease, carpal tunnel syndrome, trigger finger, and diabetes mellitus, J Hand Surg Am 20:109, 1995.

Cutolo M: Endocrine diseases and the musculoskeletal system. In Firestein GS, Budd RC, Gabriel SE, et al: Kelley's textbook of rheumatology, ed 9, Philadelphia, 2013, Elsevier Saunders.
Dixon RB, Christy NP: On the various forms of corticosteroid withdrawal syndrome, Am J Med 68:224–230, 1980.
Hartl E, Finsterer J, Grossegger C, et al: Relationship between thyroid function and skeletal muscle involvement in subclinical and overt hypothyroidism, Endocrinologist 11:217, 2001.
Kapoor A, Sibbitt WL Jr: Contractures in diabetes mellitus: the syndrome of limited joint mobility, Semin Arthritis Rheum 18:168, 1989.
Killinger Z, Payer J, Lazurova I, et al: Arthropathy in acromegaly, Rheum Dis Clin North Am 36:713–720, 2010.
Klemp P, Halland AM, Majoos FL, et al: Musculoskeletal manifestations of hyperlipidemia: a controlled study, Ann Rheum Dis 52:44–48, 1993.
Lebiedz-odrobina D, Kay J: Rheumatic manifestations of diabetes mellitus, Rheum Dis Clin North Am 36:681–699, 2010.
Markenson JA: Rheumatic manifestations of endocrine diseases, Curr Opin Rheumatol 22:64–71, 2010.
Ormseth MJ, Sergent JS: Adrenal disorders in rheumatology, Rheum Dis Clin North Am 36:701–712, 2010.
Wen HY, Schumacher HR Jr, Zhang LY: Parathyroid disease, Rheum Dis Clin North Am 36:647–664, 2010.

ARTHROPATHIES ASSOCIATED WITH HEMATOLOGIC DISEASES

Kevin D. Deane, MD, PhD

KEY POINTS

1. If a fracture is suspected as a cause of hemarthrosis, evaluate the synovial fluid for fat droplets, which indicates release of bone marrow elements through bony disruption.
2. Joint aspiration is generally safe up to an international normalized ratio (INR) of 4.5. However, if septic arthritis is possible, the joint should be aspirated regardless of the INR.
3. If a symptomatic joint in a patient with hemophilia does not improve with factor replacement, consider infection.
4. *Salmonella* accounts for 50% of osteomyelitis infections in patients with sickle cell disease.
5. Up to 40% of sickle cell patients will experience osteonecrosis of the femoral or humeral head.

1. What is a hemarthrosis?

Hemarthrosis is defined as extravasation of blood into a joint's synovial cavity. The diagnosis may be readily apparent in the setting of hemophilia, but in other circumstances it is less clear. Streaks of blood, as opposed to the uniformly bloody fluid of a hemarthrosis, may be seen in the synovial fluid during routine arthrocentesis because of needle trauma to skin or other periarticular structures. Blood that appears in the synovial fluid at the end of an arthrocentesis is also because of trauma, particularly if the initial synovial fluid was not bloody. During an arthrocentesis, if frankly bloody fluid is seen initially on entering the joint, hemarthrosis must be suspected. The best option is to withdraw the needle and re-enter the joint at another site. If the original arthrocentesis was traumatic, synovial fluid obtained from the new site should become clear or be only blood-tinged. If diffusely bloody synovial fluid is seen again, hemarthrosis is likely. If you are still uncertain, check a hematocrit on the bloody synovial fluid. A hematocrit similar to peripheral blood is more likely from a traumatic arthrocentesis, whereas fluid from a hemarthrosis has a hematocrit less than peripheral blood. A synovial fluid hematocrit >10% will make the fluid appear grossly bloody.

2. Why is it important to accurately identify hemarthrosis?

A major concern with hemarthrosis is long-term joint damage owing to inflammation resulting from recurrent bleeding. This is of particular concern with syndromes such as hemophilia. In addition, fracture can cause hemarthrosis. As such, accurately identifying hemarthrosis and instituting appropriate treatment can reduce long-term joint-related disability.

3. What are the causes of hemarthrosis?

The causes of hemarthrosis are listed in Box 49-1.

4. What finding in the bloody synovial fluid may indicate a fracture has caused the hemarthrosis?

A fracture may release blood and bone marrow elements including lipids into the synovial fluid. These fat globules may be seen floating at the top of the synovial fluid by bedside visualization of the fluid in the syringe or collection tube. If there are fat globules present in the synovial fluid identified by oil red O staining, a fracture should be suspected. Subtle fractures through bony endplates adjacent to joints may be difficult to see on plain radiography, and computed tomography or magnetic resonance imaging (MRI) may be necessary to identify the fracture.

5. Is it safe to perform arthrocentesis when a patient has a prolonged prothrombin time from warfarin therapy?

If a patient on warfarin develops an acute monoarthritis, diagnostic aspiration is warranted, even if the prothrombin time is excessively prolonged. It is suggested that joint aspiration is safe if the INR is <4.5. In addition, some authorities report that reversal of anticoagulation is not necessary if the proper technique is carefully observed and an appropriately small gauge needle is used. However, bleeding into the joint may occur following such arthrocentesis. Caution should be observed, particularly in large joints where it is difficult to apply direct pressure, such as the shoulder or knee. There are no specific published guidelines for reversal of anticoagulation before arthrocentesis; however, fresh frozen plasma or small doses of vitamin K (0.5 mg to 2 mg) given intravenously have been noted to rapidly reverse the effects of warfarin to allow surgical interventions where significant bleeding is not expected; however, this has not been studied for arthrocentesis. Vitamin K should never be given subcutaneously as it may cause prolonged reversal of anticoagulation from warfarin.

> **Box 49-1. Causes of Hemarthrosis**
>
> **Trauma**
> Injury with or without fracture
> Postsurgical
> Postarthrocentesis
> **Bleeding disorders**
> Hemophilia
> von Willebrand disease
> Thrombocytopenia
> Excessive anticoagulation
> Thrombolytic therapy for myocardial infarction
> **Disorder of connective tissue**
> Ehlers–Danlos syndrome
> Pseudoxanthoma elasticum
> **Tumors**
> Pigmented villonodular synovitis
> Tumors metastatic to joints
> Secondary tumors of synovium
> Hemangiomas
>
> **Miscellaneous**
> Scurvy
> Sickle cell disease and other hemoglobinopathies
> Myeloproliferative diseases with thrombocytosis
> Munchausen's syndrome
> Acute septic arthritis
> Lyme disease
> Arteriovenous fistula
> Ruptured aneurysm
> Charcot arthropathy
> Gaucher's disease
> Amyloid arthropathy
> Acute crystalline arthritis
> Postdialysis
>
> From Gatter RA, Schumacher HR: A practical handbook of joint fluid analysis, Philadelphia, 1991, Lea & Febiger.
> NOTE: Any condition causing intense inflammation will cause synovial vessels to be congested and friable, predisposing patients to hemarthrosis after seemingly insignificant trauma.

6. **What can be done for hemarthrosis in the setting of warfarin therapy?**
    Spontaneous hemarthrosis in the setting of warfarin therapy is uncommon and almost always occurs with an INR prolonged >2.5 times control and underlying joint damage from diseases such as *osteoarthritis* and rheumatoid arthritis being present in the majority of cases. The knee is the most commonly affected joint. In the absence of underlying arthritis, spontaneous hemarthrosis is rare unless the INR is >5. For treatment, the affected joint is drained (for pain relief) and then rested. A mild compression bandage and ice may be applied and analgesia provided with acetaminophen or narcotics. Symptoms usually spontaneously subside if the prothrombin time is reduced from supratherapeutic to simply therapeutic. If the patient's underlying condition permits, complete reversal of anticoagulation will hasten recovery. Occasionally, an intraarticular injection of corticosteroids such as triamcinolone hexacetonide will be needed to control symptoms. Destructive arthritis from a single episode of hemarthrosis is rare; however, chronic joint destruction resulting from recurrent bleeding from warfarin therapy has been reported.

7. **What rheumatologic problems can occur in patients with hemophilia?**
    - Acute hemarthrosis.
    - Subacute or chronic arthropathy.
    - End stage arthropathy.
    - Intramuscular or soft tissue hemorrhage (may cause pseudotumor or compartment syndrome).
    - Subperiosteal hemorrhage (may cause bone pseudotumor).
    - Septic arthritis.

8. **How does acute hemarthrosis present in a patient with hemophilia?**
    Hemophilia A (factor VIII deficiency) and hemophilia B (factor IX deficiency) are associated with hemarthrosis. Prodromal symptoms of stiffness or warmth occur in the affected joint. As the joint capsule distends, severe pain follows with swelling from effusion and decreased range of motion. The swelling will eventually tamponade the bleeding and the hemarthrosis will gradually resolve over a matter of days to weeks. Almost all patients with severe hemophilia (<1% of normal factor activity) and half of patients with moderate disease (1% to 5% factor activity) will have recurrent hemarthroses spontaneously or following minor trauma. Large joints (knees, elbows, ankles) are most commonly involved. If factor levels are >5% of normal, hemarthroses tend to be less frequent or occur following more significant trauma. Hemarthroses first begin to occur in weight-bearing joints when a child is just learning to walk.

9. **How do you treat an acute hemarthrosis in a patient with hemophilia?**
    The mainstay of therapy for acute hemarthrosis in hemophilia is rapid replacement of deficient factor to achieve a level of ≥30%. A useful rule of thumb is that each international unit of virally inactivated

plasma-derived or recombinant factor VIII (or IX) concentrate infused per kilogram of body weight causes a rise in factor levels by 2% or two international units per deciliter. In appropriate patients, factor replacement therapy can be promptly instituted by the family at the first symptoms of hemarthrosis to decrease the risks of sequelae. Transmission of HIV is no longer a risk and transmission of hepatitis is significantly reduced with factor replacement currently given. Patient education and involvement are critical for the success of any treatment program. Other initial treatment consists of placing the joint at rest in as much extension as can be tolerated (to prevent contractures), with applications of ice packs and other local measures. Analgesics are given for pain. Mild compression bandaging may be useful. Some authors have advocated intraarticular glucocorticoids. Arthrocentesis, after appropriate factor replacement, may help relieve symptoms. Once acute bleeding and pain are controlled, graded physical therapy to prevent muscle atrophy and contractures should be instituted.

10. **When should septic arthritis be suspected if a hemophiliac develops acute monoarthritis?**
    The presence of blood in the joint can act as a culture medium. The presence of fever and/or if the pain of a suspected hemarthrosis fails to improve after factor replacement, concomitant septic arthritis must be suspected and aspiration of the joint becomes mandatory. Of note, HIV infection in the setting of hemophilia is the most significant risk factor for septic arthritis. Any synovial fluid obtained on routine aspiration of a hemarthrosis should be submitted for Gram stain and culture. *Staphylococcus aureus* and *Streptococcus pneumoniae* are most common organisms identified (Box 49-2).

> **Box 49-2. Diagnostic Clues for Septic Arthritis Coexisting With Hemarthrosis**
>
> Failure of joint pain to resolve with factor replacement
> Fever >38 C
> Peripheral leukocytosis
> HIV infection
> Previous arthrocentesis in the same joint
> Presence of arthroplasties
> Underlying joint damage (chronic arthropathy)
> Intravenous drug use

From Ellison RT, Reller LB: Differentiating pyogenic arthritis from spontaneous hemarthrosis in patients with hemophilia, West J Med 144:42-45, 1986.

11. **Do recurrent hemarthroses have any long-term consequences in patients with hemophilia?**
    As the patient approaches adulthood, acute hemarthroses become less frequent but chronic joint symptoms supervene. Recurrent hemarthroses lead to accumulation of hemosiderin in the joint lining tissues. Proliferative synovitis develops and the joint cartilage is degraded. The end result is a chronically swollen joint, less painful than seen in acute hemarthroses, with decreased range of motion. Surrounding muscles become atrophic and joint contracture is a frequent complication. Examination reveals bony enlargement, coarse crepitus, and deformity. Patients may be significantly disabled by chronic hemophilic arthropathy. The regular administration of factor replacement prophylactically has reduced the risk of developing subsequent chronic arthropathy.

12. **Are there any characteristic radiographic findings?**
    Radiographs in acute hemarthrosis will be remarkable for soft tissue swelling, increased synovial density (iron deposition), and effusion. Chronic arthropathy of hemophilia may have both inflammatory (erosive) and degenerative features. Specific findings include proximal radial head enlargement, widening of the femoral and humeral intercondylar notches, talar flattening, and squaring of the inferior patella (Figure 49-1).

13. **What is the treatment of chronic hemophilic arthropathy?**
    The treatment principles for chronic hemophilic arthropathy are outlined in Box 49-3.
    Treatment programs must be individualized for each patient. Difficult patients are frequently referred to specialized treatment centers.

14. **Does sickle cell anemia have any rheumatologic manifestations?**
    - Hand–foot syndrome
    - Bone infarction
    - Osteonecrosis of bone
    - Noninflammatory joint effusions adjacent to areas of bony crisis
    - Chronic inflammation of joints
    - Hyperuricemia and gout
    - Hemarthrosis
    - Septic arthritis
    - Osteomyelitis
    - Focal muscle necrosis
    - Rhabdomyolysis

15. **How does hand–foot syndrome present in a patient with sickle cell disease?**
    Hand–foot syndrome, or sickle cell dactylitis, is a problem in infants with sickle cell disease. Children present with acute pain and swelling diffusely in the fingers or toes, usually as a first manifestation of sickle cell

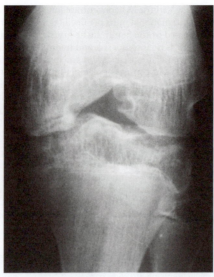

Figure 49-1. Knee of young patient with hemophilia. Note degenerative and erosive changes of both femoral condyles and the tibial plateau.

Box 49-3. Treatment Principles for Chronic Hemophilic Arthropathy

Prophylactic infusions of factor VIII to prevent recurrences of hemarthrosis (factor goal >5%)
Nonweight-bearing rest periods to allow synovitis to regress
Physical therapy to improve joint stability and maintain muscle strength
Intraarticular glucocorticoids to reduce symptoms and recurrent hemarthroses
Nonacetylated salicylates or cox-2 specific inhibitors (celecoxib) for pain and swelling
Arthroscopic synovectomy for chronic synovitis unresponsive to conservative therapy
Total joint arthroplasty for end stage joint disease. Arthrodesis for ankles
Consider rifampicin chemical synoviorthesis (particularly small joints)
Consider radioisotope synovectomy (particularly if factor inhibitor present) with P32 or 90-yttrium

From York JR: Musculoskeletal disorders in the haemophilias, Baillière's Clin Rheumatol 5:197-220, 1991.

---

disease. Fever and leukocytosis may accompany the dactylitis. The etiology is thought to be local bone marrow ischemia. Subperiosteal new bone formation may be seen on radiographs of the metacarpal or metatarsal bones 2 weeks after the acute episode. Symptoms generally spontaneously subside in a few weeks.

16. What causes joint pain in patients with sickle cell disease?

Patients with sickle cell (S-S) disease or the heterozygous state (sickle-β thalassemia, S-C, S-D disease) frequently experience polyarthralgias. Local sickling of cells leads to obstruction of the microcirculation and to bone infarctions. During painful crises, patients may experience chest, abdominal, back, muscle, and joint pain caused by microinfarctions. Treatment of painful crises includes hydration, oxygen, and analgesics. Hydroxyurea can reduce the frequency of painful crises. Other musculoskeletal manifestations including painful large joint arthritis (usually the knees) often with noninflammatory synovial effusions lasting a few days to 3 weeks can also occur. These effusions are attributable to bone infarctions causing a "sympathetic" transudative effusion, which is unresponsive to intraarticular corticosteroids. Alternatively, some patients during an acute painful crisis will develop a monoarticular or oligoarticular inflammatory arthritis that resolves within a week. Cultures and crystal examinations are negative. Finally, osteonecrosis of larger bones (frequently multifocal) such as the femoral or humeral head is seen in up to 40% of patients with sickle cell disease. Initially, radiographs may be normal. MRI is the most sensitive method to detect early osteonecrosis of the bone.

17. **Name two characteristic radiographic findings that can be seen in the spine in patients with sickle cell disease.**
    Vertebral bodies can have a characteristic "Lincoln log" or H-shaped appearance owing to epiphyseal infarction from sickled cells causing endplate collapse. A second radiographic abnormality that may be observed is a central cup-like indentation ("codfish vertebrae") owing to osteoporotic weakness of the vertebrae caused by marrow expansion.

18. **Can osteonecrosis of the femoral head be treated in the setting of sickle cell disease?**
    Treatment is very unsatisfactory. The patient may be put on nonweight-bearing status in an attempt to allow revascularization and prevent collapse of the affected bone, although this is rarely effective. An orthopedic surgeon should be consulted promptly. Core decompression of the femoral head may be attempted in early cases. Prosthetic joint replacement is often the treatment used when joint damage is advanced, although results are suboptimal. In one series, 19% of total hip replacements for avascular necrosis of the femoral head in sickle cell disease required revision within 5 years. Perioperative worsening of sickle cell disease is common.

19. **Is gout seen frequently in sickle cell disease?**
    In children with sickle cell disease, hyperuricosuria without hyperuricemia occurs, probably as a result of increased red cell turnover associated with crises. Up to 40% of adult sickle cell patients will have hyperuricemia, caused by renal tubular damage with decreased uric acid excretion. However, gout is surprisingly uncommon. Occasionally, gout may be seen, so crystals should be looked for in joint effusions seen during sickle cell crisis.

20. **What is the most common musculoskeletal infectious problem seen in sickle cell disease?**
    Osteomyelitis is seen more than 100 times more frequently in sickle cell disease than in normal individuals. It is frequently multifocal. Because of functional asplenia, *Salmonella* infections account for 50% of osteomyelitis especially in children with sickle cell disease. Fortunately, septic arthritis is infrequent but is usually caused by *Staphylococcus aureus* or a gram-negative organism other than *Salmonella* when it occurs. The large proportion of gram-negative infections may be as a result of bacterial translocation across bowel mucosa that has been compromised by microinfarcts from sickling cells (Box 49-4).

> **Box 49-4. Factors Predisposing Sickle Cell Patients to Infection**
>
> Functional asplenia with decreased clearance of bacteria
> Tissue damaged by crisis
> Decreased neutrophil function at lower oxygen tensions
> Decreased opsonization
> Decreased interferon-γ production
> Increased risk of nosocomial infection

21. **How does osteomyelitis present in sickle cell disease?**
    Presentation of osteomyelitis may be subtle, mimicking sickle crisis or affecting multiple areas. Both sickle crisis and osteomyelitis may present with bone pain, fever, and leukocytosis, and radiographs may be identical although patients with osteomyelitis have more severe symptoms. An absolute **band** neutrophil count of >1000/mm³ is more suggestive of osteomyelitis than infarction or crisis. Contrast-enhanced MRI can help differentiate between infection and infarction.

22. **What is the management of suspected osteomyelitis in sickle cell disease?**
    The management of suspected osteomyelitis in sickle cell disease is outlined in Box 49-5.

23. **Do the other hemoglobinopathies have any rheumatologic manifestations?**
    Hemoglobin SC disease and sickle-β thalassemia may develop similar manifestations to sickle cell disease, including hand–foot syndrome and gout. Osteonecrosis of bone has been reported in both conditions. Generally, rheumatologic manifestations are less common in these other hemoglobinopathies. There are case reports of osteonecrosis occurring in patients with sickle cell trait, but the incidence is the same as in age-matched controls with normal hemoglobin. Patients with β thalassemia major (Cooley's anemia) may develop arthropathy from marrow expansion, microfractures from osteoporosis, and scoliosis in patients surviving two decades. They do not get osteonecrosis. Chelation therapy with deferiprone (to reduce iron overload from transfusions) can cause arthralgias in 20% of patients.

24. **What are some rheumatic disease mimics associated with use of hydroxyurea?**
    Hydroxyurea is used in sickle cell to increase levels of fetal hemoglobin which does not readily sickle; in addition, hydroxyurea is used for other hematologic conditions such as myelofibrosis and thrombocytosis. There are several rheumatic disease mimics associated with hydroxyurea. These include skin ulcers that are typically seen in the lower extremities and can mimic systemic vasculitis. Hydroxyurea has also been associated with development of a painful discoloration of the hands and feet (palmar-plantar erythrodysethesia) that is also occasionally associated with blisters. It has also been associated with alopecia, and dermatomyositis-like and scleroderma-like syndromes. Treatment is typically withdrawal of hydroxyurea.

Box 49-5. Management of Suspected Osteomyelitis in Sickle Cell Disease

1. Admit patient to hospital for thorough evaluation.
2. Immobilize affected bones to avoid pathologic fracture.
3. Check baseline complete blood count, erythrocyte sedimentation rate, and C-reactive protein.*
4. Consult hematology and infectious disease services.
5. Obtain blood cultures.
6. Order febrile agglutinins and stool cultures for *Salmonella*.
7. Obtain plain radiographs of all involved bones; repeat these in 10 to 14 days if the originals are normal.
8. Consider magnetic resonance imaging of affected area. Obtain a radionuclide bone or gallium scan.†
9. Aspirate for culture any bones that are suspected for infection.
10. After a diagnosis is established, preoperative measures are instituted to decrease the risk of surgical complications (transfusions to achieve hemoglobin A level 60% of total hemoglobin, maintenance of adequate oxygenation and hydration).
11. All abscesses in bones should be promptly decompressed to restore blood supply.
12. Avoid tourniquets for intraoperative hemostasis.
13. Do not start antibiotics until adequate specimens of blood, bone, and pus are obtained for culture and Gram stain.
14. Initiate antibiotics based on Gram stain results, considering the possibility of *Salmonella*.
15. Parenteral antibiotics are continued for 6 to 8 weeks.‡

*C-Reactive protein is more useful than erythrocyte sedimentation rate to follow response to treatment and for differentiating osteomyelitis from sickle cell crisis. Note that sickle cell disease is associated with an abnormally low erythrocyte sedimentation rate because the sickled cells cannot form good rouleaux.
†Radionuclide scans are not as useful for differentiating bony infarction and osteomyelitis but will identify affected areas in the spine or pelvis, or unsuspected multifocal involvement.
‡Prolonged therapy is necessary because both infection and sickle cell crisis impair blood flow to the affected bone.
From Epps CH Jr, Bryant DD, Coles MJM, Castro O: Osteomyelitis in patients who have sickle cell disease, Bone Joint Surg 73-A:1281-1294, 1991.

BIBLIOGRAPHY

Anand AJ, Glatt AE: *Salmonella* osteomyelitis and arthritis in sickle cell disease, Semin Arthritis Rheum 24:211–221, 1994.
Angastiniotis M, Eleftheriou A: Thalassaemic bone disease, Pediatr Endocrinol Rev 6(Suppl 1):73–80, 2008.
Best PJ, et al:Hydroxyurea-induced leg ulcers in 14 patients, Ann Int Med 128(1):29–32, 1998.
Ellison RT, Reller LB: Differentiating pyogenic arthritis from spontaneous hemarthrosis in patients with hemophilia, West J Med 144:42–45, 1986.
Epps Jr CH, Bryant DD, Coles MJM, Castro O: Osteomyelitis in patients who have sickle-cell disease, J Bone Joint Surg 73-A:1281–1294, 1991.
Jean-Baptiste G, De Ceulaer K: Osteoarticular disorders of haematologic origin, Best Pract Res Clin Rheumatol 14:307–323, 2000.
Luck JV, Silva M, Rodriguez-Merchan EC, et al: Hemophilic arthropathy, J Am Acad Orthop Surg 12:234–245, 2004.
Manco-Johnson MJ, Abshire TC, Shapiro AD, et al: Prophylactic versus episodic treatment to prevent joint disease in boys with severe hemophilia, N Engl J Med 357:535–544, 2007.
Marti-Carvajal A, Dunlop R, Agreda-Perez L: Treatment for avascular necrosis of bone in people with sickle cell disease, Cochrane Database Syst Rev 4:CD004344, 2004.
Prabhakar H, Haywood C Jr, Molokie R: Sickle cell disease in the United States: looking back and forward at 100 years of progress in management and survival, Am J Hematol 85:346–353, 2010.
Shupak R, Teital J, Garvey MB, et al: Intra-articular methylprednisolone in hemophilic arthropathy, Am J Hematol 27:26–29, 1988.
Thumboo J, O'Duffy JD: A prospective study of the safety of joint and soft tissue aspirations and injections in patients taking warfarin sodium, Arthritis Rheum 41:736–739, 1998.
Wild JH, Zvaifler NJ: Hemarthrosis associated with sodium warfarin therapy, Arthritis Rheum 19:98–102, 1976.
Wong AL, Sakamoto KM, Johnson EE: Differentiating osteomyelitis from bone infarction in sickle cell disease, Pediatr Emerg Care 17:60–63, 2001.
York JR: Musculoskeletal disorders in the haemophilias, Baillière's Clin Rheumatol 5:197–220, 1991.

FURTHER READING

www.hemophilia.org
www.sicklecelldisease.org

MALIGNANCY-ASSOCIATED RHEUMATIC DISORDERS

Daniel F. Battafarano, DO

CHAPTER 50

> **KEY POINTS**
>
> 1. Lymphoma and common solid tumors may be associated with connective tissue disease.
> 2. When palmar fasciitis presents in a woman, think ovarian carcinoma.
> 3. Rheumatoid arthritis, systemic lupus erythematosus, and Sjögren's syndrome are all associated with an increased risk for lymphoma.
> 4. Leukocytoclastic vasculitis is the most common paraneoplastic vasculitis presentation.

1. Is there a causal relationship between malignancies and rheumatic disorders?
It is uncommon for a rheumatic disease to mimic malignancy. However, rheumatic syndromes have been associated with various malignancies, and patients with preexisting connective tissue disease have developed malignancies. Approximately 10% to 15% of patients hospitalized with advanced malignancy will manifest a paraneoplastic syndrome. Endocrine syndromes secondary to ectopic hormone production account for one third of all paraneoplastic syndromes followed by connective tissue, hematologic, and neuromuscular syndromes. The majority of rheumatic syndromes associated with malignancies do not demonstrate significant causal relationships. Therefore, it is not recommended or cost effective to have an extensive search for occult malignancy with common rheumatic syndromes.

2. What are the mechanisms that malignancy can cause musculoskeletal symptoms?
- Direct tumor invasion of bones and joints.
- Paraneoplastic rheumatic syndromes.
- Malignancy developing in a preexisting connective tissue disease as a result of the disease or its therapy.
- Rheumatic syndromes attributable to chemotherapy used to treat malignancy.

3. What are the accepted direct associations between musculoskeletal syndromes and malignancy?
Metastatic disease, leukemia, lymphoma, and primary synovial and bone tumors are directly associated with the pathologic mechanisms of the underlying tumor. Bone metastases typically involve the long bones, spine, or pelvis and generally arise from breast, lung, and prostate more than kidney and thyroid neoplasms. The majority of skeletal metastases do not produce pain. Metastases or carcinomatous invasion of the synovium may rarely be the initial manifestation of a malignancy. Lung neoplasms are the most common primary tumor. Large joints are most likely to be involved with monoarthritis of the knee the most common presentation. Metastases to joints distal to the elbows and knees are very rare and are usually attributable to lung cancer. Severe joint pain especially at night with a noninflammatory (monoarticular predominance) or hemorrhagic joint effusion that rapidly reaccumulates after aspiration should suggest carcinomatous invasion of the synovium. Synovial fluid cytology and/or synovial biopsy will be diagnostic.

4. What are the musculoskeletal features of leukemia and lymphoma?
Leukemia can present as a symmetric, asymmetric, or migratory polyarthritis or as bone pain. It can be the presenting manifestation in 5% to 6% of patients with leukemia. Overall, articular manifestations in acute leukemia occur in approximately 14% to 50% of children (acute lymphoblastic leukemia being the most common) and 4% to 16% of adults. Joint pain usually involves the ankle, shoulder, or knee and has been attributed to leukemic synovial infiltration. Bone pain occurs in up to 50% of patients and is attributable to subperiosteal infiltration. Long bone pain is more common in children and back pain is more common in adults. The joint and bone pain are more severe than the clinical findings and may be nocturnal. Synovial effusions are uncommon, mildly inflammatory, and leukemic cells are rare. Hemorrhage into the joint can occur. The white blood cell count may be normal, but lactate dehydrogenase is always elevated. Plain radiographs may be normal at the onset of the bone pain in 50% of cases, but bone scintigraphy will detect involvement early. Metaphyseal rarefaction and osteolytic lesions are characteristic radiographic findings. The diagnosis is confirmed by bone marrow and/or synovial biopsy. The joint or bone pain is optimally treated with systemic chemotherapy.

Up to 25% of patients with non-Hodgkin's **lymphoma** can have musculoskeletal symptoms with bone pain most common. Lymphomatous arthritis is rare but should be suspected in patients with constitutional symptoms out of proportion to the severity of the arthritis especially if periarticular osteolytic lesions are present on radiographs. Patients are seronegative. The diagnosis is confirmed by bone or synovial biopsy.
Notably, both patients with leukemia and lymphoma can develop secondary gout especially on initiation of chemotherapy.

5. What musculoskeletal paraneoplastic syndromes are associated with malignancy?
   Musculoskeletal paraneoplastic syndromes that are associated with malignancy are outlined in Table 50-1.

Table 50-1. Musculoskeletal Paraneoplastic Syndromes Associated With Malignancy

PARANEOPLASTIC SYNDROME	MALIGNANCY	CLINICAL ASSOCIATION
Myopathy		
Dermatomyositis	Adenocarcinoma, nasopharyngeal cancer (Southeast Asians)	Cancer may precede, coincide, or follow diagnosis of myositis
Polymyositis	Adenocarcinoma	Lower risk than dermatomyositis (9% of PM versus 15% of patients with DM)
Arthropathy		
Hypertrophic osteoarthropathy	Various types	Lung cancer (nonsmall cell) is most common
Amyloidosis	Multiple myeloma	25% of primary (AL) amyloidosis is associated with multiple myeloma
Secondary gout	Myeloproliferative disorders	Tumor lysis syndrome
Carcinomatous polyarthritis	Solid tumor or hematologic disorders	80% of women have breast cancer
Atypical polymyalgia rheumatica	Renal, lung, colon, myeloma	Age < 50, not responsive to prednisone
RS3PE*	Several tumors	Rapid onset wrist, hand, and ankle arthritis with edema. May have fever. Poor response to prednisone
Vascular		
Necrotizing vasculitis	Lymphoproliferative, various types	Chronic unexplained necrotizing vasculitis
Polyarteritis nodosa	Hairy cell leukemia	Polyarteritis-like clinically and by arteriography
Digital necrosis	Gastrointestinal and lung cancer	Severe Raynaud's phenomenon after age 50 years
Cryoglobulinemia	Plasma cell dyscrasias, non-Hodgkin's lymphoma	Refractory Raynaud's phenomenon
Cutaneous		
Sweet's syndrome	Leukemia (AML), others	Associated with malignancy in 15%
Palmar fasciitis and polyarthritis	Ovarian is most common	Also seen in breast, gastric, endometrial, lung, and hepatocellular cancers
Scleroderma	Adenocarcinoma	Women > men; anti-RNAP III
Panniculitis	Pancreatic > breast, prostate, hematologic cancer	Subcutaneous nodules and arthritis, eosinophilia
Erythromelalgia	Myeloproliferative disorders	Severe burning pain, erythema, and warmth primarily in feet

Table 50-1. Musculoskeletal Paraneoplastic Syndromes Associated With Malignancy *(Continued)*

PARANEOPLASTIC SYNDROME	MALIGNANCY	CLINICAL ASSOCIATION
Multicentric reticulohistiocytosis	Adenocarcinoma, ovarian, lung, and others	Associated with malignancy in 30%
Miscellaneous		
Pyogenic arthritis	Colon cancer, multiple myeloma	Intestinal flora cultured Rare cause of primary septic arthritis
Lupus-like syndrome	Hairy cell leukemia Ovary, breast, lymphoma	Polyarthritis, serositis, rash, Raynaud's phenomenon, positive ANA
Antiphospholipid antibodies	Solid tumors Lymphoproliferative	Association with thrombosis is unclear
Oncogenic osteomalacia	Solid tumors; tumors of mesenchymal origin	Bone pain, muscle weakness low phosphorous, elevated FGF23 Octreotide scan to localize tumor
Sarcoidosis	Solid tumors, lymphoma	Draining lymph nodes show noncaseating granuloma
Lymphomatoid granulomatosis	Lymphoma	Angiodestructive lesions, EBV-associated

AML, Acute myeloid leukemia; ANA, antinuclear antibodies; DM, dermatomyositis; EBV, Epstein–Barr virus; PM, polymyositis.
*RS3PE, Remitting seronegative symmetric synovitis with pitting edema; RNAP III, RNA polymerase III.

6. **Discuss the occurrence of cancer in patients with dermatomyositis and polymyositis.**
   Dermatomyositis (DM) and polymyositis (PM) without an associated connective tissue disease have an increased risk (3 to 7 times for DM and 1.4 to 2 times for PM) for malignancy, primarily with solid tumors. The risk of malignancy is also increased in patients with amyotrophic DM. The onset of DM or PM may precede (1 to 2 years), coincide, or occur up to 5 years after the malignancy is diagnosed. The most common malignancies are ovarian, lung, stomach, pancreas, bladder, and cervix, which accounts for 70% of cases in Western populations, whereas nasopharyngeal malignancies are most common in Asian populations. Patients with myositis-specific autoantibodies (antisynthetase antibodies) and children with DM rarely have an associated malignancy. Creatine kinase levels and muscle biopsy findings are not useful for distinguishing DM and PM in patients with or without malignancy. However, it has been noted that patients with DM or PM who have a normal creatine kinase but elevated aldolase are more likely to have a malignancy. All adult patients with new onset DM or PM should undergo an age-specific examination for occult malignancy. In addition, a chest/abdominal/pelvic computed tomography scan or positron emission tomography/computed tomography scan should be done because of the high incidence of lymphoma and ovarian cancer. Many experts recommend testing for tumor antigens CA125, CA19-9, and CEA. A malignancy should be highly suspected in patients over age 65 years, patients with treatment-resistant myositis, patients with pharyngeal and diaphragmatic involvement, and in patients with DM who have ulcerative skin lesions especially on the trunk. Recently, anti-p155/p140 antibodies have been described and are highly predictive of cancer-associated DM. If the initial cancer screen is negative, annual screening for cancer for the next 3 to 5 years is indicated particularly for high-risk patients.

7. **What is hypertrophic osteoarthropathy?**
   Hypertrophic osteoarthropathy (HOA) is a syndrome that includes (1) clubbing of fingers (Hippocratic fingers) and toes, (2) periostitis of tubular bones, and (3) arthritis with a noninflammatory synovial fluid. Primary HOA (pachydermoperiostosis) is autosomal dominant, appears during childhood mostly in males (male/female, 9:1), and is characterized by clubbing, skin hypertrophy (pachyderma), coarse facial features, seborrhea, and hyperhidrosis. The secondary form can be divided into generalized or localized forms. The generalized form is most often associated with intrathoracic malignant neoplasms (nonsmall cell lung cancer, mesothelioma, and others) in 90% of cases. It also occurs in patients with other malignancies (hepatic, gastrointestinal, POEMS), chronic infections (lung, subacute bacterial endocarditis, HIV, and others), cystic fibrosis, congenital cyanotic heart disease, inflammatory bowel disease, cirrhosis, Graves' disease, or on certain drugs (voriconazole). The localized form of HOA has been associated with hemiplegia, aneurysms, infective arteritis, and patent ductus arteriosus. The clinical course of secondary HOA is determined by the underlying primary disease. Platelet/endothelial cell activation with release of vascular endothelial growth factor and platelet-derived growth factor appears to play a key role in the etiology of HOA (Figure 50-1).

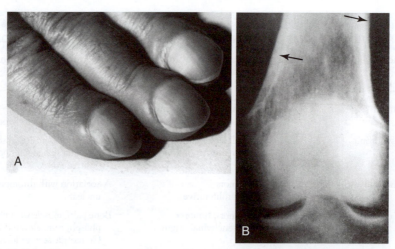

Figure 50-1. **A,** Clubbing of fingers. Soft tissue proliferation of the nailbed and distal tissues of the digits is seen. Usually the nail makes an angle of 20 degrees or more with the projected line of the digit. When clubbing occurs, subungual proliferation causes diminution of the angle. **B,** Roentgenogram of the knee shows subperiosteal new bone formation of the lower femoral shafts (*arrows*). New bone is separated from the old cortex by a t radiolucent line (*right*); a later subperiosteal lesion is seen (*left*). (Copyright 2014 American College of Rheumatology. Used with permission.)

8. **What is carcinomatous polyarthritis?**
   Polyarthritis can rarely (<2%) be the presenting manifestation of an occult malignancy. The association of polyarthritis and malignancy is suggested by:
   1. A close temporal relationship (average 10 months) between the onset of a seronegative arthritis and the diagnosis of malignancy.
   2. Improvement of the arthritis with treatment of the underlying cancer.
   3. Recurrence of the arthritis with tumor recurrence.

   Carcinomatous polyarthritis should be strongly suspected in a patient with the following features: explosive onset of an asymmetric oligoarthritis or polyarthritis, late age of onset, predominant lower extremity involvement, spares the wrists and small hand joints, and absence of rheumatoid factor, erosions, or rheumatoid nodules. Radiographs show no periosteal reaction. Note that polymyalgia rheumatica-like symptoms unresponsive to prednisone have also been described as a presentation of various malignancies.

9. **Vasculitis occurs as a paraneoplastic syndrome with which malignancies?**
   Vasculitis is more common with myelodysplastic disorders, leukemia, and lymphomas but may occur with common solid tumors. Leukocytoclastic vasculitis is the most frequent paraneoplastic presentation. Henoch–Schönlein purpura, medium vessel vasculitis, and granulomatous vasculitis have been described. A polyarteritis nodosa-like vasculitis has been described most commonly in patients with hairy cell leukemia and less commonly in other malignancies. Vasculitis may precede (by up to 2 years), coincide, or follow the malignancy diagnosis. Proposed mechanisms for vasculitis as a paraneoplastic syndrome include immune complex formation, direct vascular injury by antibodies to endothelial cells, and a direct effect of leukemic cells (i.e., hairy cells) on the endothelium.

10. **What is Sweet's syndrome?**
    Sweet's syndrome is also known as acute febrile neutrophilic dermatosis and mimics vasculitis. It is associated with malignancy in 10% to 15% of patients. Sweet's syndrome is most commonly seen with acute myelogenous leukemia, but has been described with many malignancies. It has been associated with acute, self-limited polyarthritis in 20% of cases. It can be treated effectively with nonsteroidal antiinflammatory drugs (NSAIDs) or corticosteroids, although malignancy associated Sweet's syndrome may be treatment-resistant.
    The cardinal features are:
    - abrupt onset of raised, often painful papules and plaques on the extremities (dorsum of hands), face, neck, or trunk;
    - fever;
    - peripheral neutrophilic leukocytosis; and
    - dense dermal neutrophilic infiltrates without vasculitis on biopsy.

11. Which rheumatic syndromes or signs have been described with ovarian carcinoma?

Dermatomyositis/polymyositis	Carpal tunnel syndrome
Palmar fasciitis	Adhesive capsulitis
Shoulder–hand syndrome	Fibromyalgia
Lupus-like syndrome	Positive antinuclear antibody

Acute febrile neutrophilic dermatosis (Sweet's syndrome)

12. Describe the features of palmar fasciitis syndrome?

Palmar fasciitis syndrome (also known as palmar fibromatosis) is most commonly associated with ovarian carcinoma, although it can be seen with other malignancies (breast, stomach, pancreas, lung, and colon). Palmar fasciitis has features of pain, swelling, flexion deformities of the fingers, and vasomotor instability similar to complex regional pain syndrome. A symmetric polyarthritis can accompany the fibrosis. Progressive changes lead to a "woody hands" texture and appearance. The presence of palmar fasciitis portends a poor prognosis because it typically manifests after tumor metastasis. Plantar fasciitis with lower extremity involvement can occur in some cases.

Histologic examination of the involved tissues reveals extensive fibrosis with increased fibroblast and mononuclear cell infiltration. There is no evidence of collagen deposition similar to that seen in scleroderma, and the nailfold capillary examination is normal. Deposits of immunoglobulin G in the palmar fascia and the presence of low-titer antinuclear antibodies in some patients suggest an immunopathologic mechanism. Treatment response with NSAIDs, corticosteroids, ganglionic blockade, and/or physical therapy is usually poor. Successful removal of the underlying tumor may result in dramatic clinical improvement of the palmar fasciitis syndrome.

13. What is the shoulder–hand syndrome?

The **shoulder–hand syndrome** is much milder than the palmar fasciitis syndrome. This syndrome is most often described with ovarian carcinoma or with lung cancer localized to the superior sulcus (Pancoast tumor). Pain in the shoulder with loss of motion may result in adhesive capsulitis, and the hand of the involved side becomes puffy and stiff with vasomotor instability. Conventional treatment for complex regional pain syndrome provides variable relief.

14. Which malignancies are associated with preexisting connective tissue disease?

Malignancies that are associated with preexisting connective tissue disease are outlined in Table 50-2.

Table 50-2. Preexisting Connective Tissue Disease Associated With Malignancy

DISEASE	MALIGNANCY	CLINICAL RISKS
Rheumatoid arthritis	Lymphoproliferative disorders (2 to 3 times increased risk) Lung cancer (2 times risk) Melanoma and other skin cancers	Longer disease duration, immunosuppression, Felty's syndrome, paraproteinemia
Systemic lupus erythematosus	Lymphoproliferative disorders (2 to 4 times increased risk) Cervical cancer	Adenopathy, splenomegaly
Discoid lupus	Squamous cell epithelioma	HPV-related, in plaques > 20 years
Sjögren's syndrome	Lymphoproliferative disorders, hematologic malignancies (4% to 10% lifetime risk)	Palpable purpura, cutaneous ulcers, cryoglobulinemia, adenopathy, splenomegaly, MALT lymphoma
Systemic sclerosis	Alveolar cell carcinoma, nonmelanoma skin cancer, adenocarcinoma of esophagus lymphoproliferative disorders	Pulmonary fibrosis, areas of skin fibrosis, Barrett's metaplasia
Dermatomyositis	Adenocarcinoma, melanoma, lymphoproliferative disorders, nasopharyngeal tumors (Asians)	Older age, ulcerative skin lesions, anti-p155/p140
Polymyositis	Adenocarcinoma	Polymyositis < dermatomyositis
Paget's disease	Osteogenic sarcoma	Occurs in 1% of lesions
Eosinophilic fasciitis	Lymphoproliferative disorders	Aplastic anemia, thrombocytopenia

HPV, Human papillomavirus; MSG, minor salivary gland biopsy.

15. **What malignancies are associated with tumor necrosis factor inhibitors in pediatric and adult patients?**

    Long-term observations since 1998 have indicated that there have been 48 cases of malignancies in children and adolescents treated with tumor necrosis factor (TNF) blockers for juvenile idiopathic arthritis, rheumatoid arthritis, psoriatic arthritis, plaque psoriasis, Crohn's disease, and ankylosing spondylitis. Half of the pediatric cases have been lymphomas (Hodgkin's and non-Hodgkin's) and other malignancies reported are leukemia, melanoma, and solid tumors. Most (88%) of the pediatric patients were on other immunosuppressive medications such as azathioprine and methotrexate. These determinations are primarily from infliximab and etanercept data because there has been minimal use of other TNF inhibitors in pediatric patients. In adults, there is an increased risk for developing nonmelanoma skin cancer but conflicting or little evidence that other malignancies are increased. TNF inhibitors appear to worsen melanomas.

16. **List the immunosuppressive drugs/agents used to treat connective tissue disease and their potential malignancies?**

    A list of the immunosuppressive drugs/agents used in the treatment of connective tissue disease and their potential malignancies are presented in Table 50-3.

Table 50-3. Immunosuppressive Drugs/Agents Used in the Treatment of Connective Tissue Diseases and Their Potential Malignancies

TREATMENT	MALIGNANCIES
Hydroxychloroquine	None
Sulfasalazine	None
Methotrexate	Minimal risk for EBV-induced lymphoma
Leflunomide	None
Azathioprine	Possible risk for non-Hodgkin's lymphoma
Cyclosporine	EBV-induced lymphoma
TNF blocker(s)	Nonmelanoma skin cancers
Mycophenolate mofetil	Possible risk for lymphoma
Cyclophosphamide (IV) cancer	Minimal risk for lymphoma or bladder
Cyclophosphamide (oral)	Bladder carcinoma (2 to 4 times), non-Hodgkin's lymphoma, leukemia, skin cancer
Other biologics	Insufficient data but no definite increase

EBV, Epstein–Barr virus; IV, intravenous; TNF, tumor necrosis factor.

17. **Can chemotherapy for malignancy cause "rheumatism"?**
    - **Postchemotherapy rheumatism**—myalgias and migratory arthralgias can occur in some patients 1 to 3 months after therapy for carcinoma of breast, ovary, or non-Hodgkin's lymphoma. Usually resolves within a year.
    - **Aromatase inhibitors**—arthralgias and joint stiffness occurs in 25% to 50% of patients with breast cancer treated with aromatase inhibitors. Symptoms tend to occur within 1 to 3 months of starting therapy and affect hands, wrists, and knees most commonly. Magnetic resonance imaging shows intraarticular fluid and tenosynovitis in the hands. NSAIDs are of limited benefit. Changing from one aromatase inhibitor to another may lessen the symptoms. Patients with severe arthralgias may need to be switched to tamoxifen which may cause fewer musculoskeletal symptoms.
    - **Bleomycin**—may cause Raynaud's phenomenon.
    - **Taxanes**—can cause arthralgias, myalgias, and skin rash similar to subacute cutaneous lupus in breast cancer-treated patients.
    - **Interferon-α**—can cause arthralgias, positive autoantibodies, systemic lupus erythematosus-like syndrome, and autoimmune thyroid disease.

BIBLIOGRAPHY

Amoura Z, Duhaut P, Huong DL, et al: Tumor antigen markers for the detection of solid cancers in inflammatory myopathies, Cancer Epidemiol Biomarkers Prev 14:1279, 2005.

Andras C, Ponyi A, Constantin T, et al: Dermatomyositis and polymyositis associated malignancy: a 21-year retrospective study, J Rheumatol 35:438–444, 2008.

Ashouri JF, Daikh DI: Rheumatic manifestations of cancer, Rheum Dis Clin N Am 37:489–505, 2011.

Askling J, Baecklund E, Granath F, et al: Anti-tumour necrosis factor therapy in rheumatoid arthritis and risk of malignant lymphomas: relative risks and time trends in the Swedish Biologics Register, Ann Rheum Dis 68:648–653, 2009.

Baecklund E, Iliadou A, Askling J, et al: Association of chronic inflammation, not its treatment with increased lymphoma risk in rheumatoid arthritis, Arthritis Rheum 54:692–701, 2006.

Bongartz T, Sutton AJ, Sweeting MJ, et al: Anti-TNF antibody therapy in rheumatoid arthritis and the risks of serious infections and malignancies: systematic review and meta-analysis of rare harmful effects of randomized controlled trials, JAMA 295:2275–2285, 2006.

Buchbinder R, Forbes A, Hall S, et al: Incidence of malignant disease in biopsy-proven inflammatory myopathy. A population-based cohort study, Ann Intern Med 134:1087–1095, 2001.

Buggaini G, Krysenka A, Grazzini M, et al: Paraneoplastic vasculitis and paraneoplastic vascular syndromes, Dermatol Ther 23:597–605, 2010.

Cush JJ, Dao KH: Malignancy risks with biologic therapies, Rheum Dis Clin N Am 38:761–770, 2012.

Fain O, Hamidou M, Cacoub P, et al: Vasculitides associated with malignancies: analysis of sixty patients, Arthritis Rheum 57:1473, 2007.

Fudman EJ, Schnitzer TJ: Dermatomyositis without creatine kinase elevation, Am J Med 80:329–332, 1986.

Kim MJ, Ye YM, Park HS, et al: Chemotherapy-related arthropathy, J Rheumatol 33:1364, 2006.

Martinez-Lavin M, Vargas A, Rivera-Vinas M: Hypertrophic osteoarthropathy: a palindrome with a pathogenic connotation, Curr Opin Rheumatol 20:88–91, 2008.

Naschitz JE, Rosner I: Musculoskeletal syndromes associated with malignancy (excluding hypertrophic osteoarthropathy), Curr Opin Rheumatol 20:100–105, 2008.

Racanelli V, Prete M, Minoia C, et al: Rheumatic disorders as paraneoplastic syndromes, Autoimmun Rev 7:352–358, 2008.

Selva-O'Callaghan A, Grau JM, Gamez-Cenzano C, et al: Conventional cancer screening versus PET/CT in dermatomyositis/polymyositis, Am J Med 123:558, 2010.

Singer O, Ciglar T, Moore AB, et al: Defining the aromatase inhibitor musculoskeletal syndrome: a prospective study, Arthritis Care Res (Hoboken) 64:1910–1918, 2012.

Targoff IN, Mamyrova G, Trieu EP, et al: A novel autoantibody to a 155-kd protein is associated with dermatomyositis, Arthritis Rheum 54:3682, 2006.

Thomas E, Brewster DH, Black RJ, et al: Risk of malignancy among patients with rheumatic conditions, Int J Cancer 88:497–502, 2000.

FURTHER READING

www.fda.gov/Drugs/DrugSafety/PostmarketDrugSafetyInformationforPatientsandProviders/DrugSafetyInformationforHeathcare-Professionals/ucm174474.htm

VIII
Bone and Cartilage Disorders

I cannot conceive why we who are composed of over 90 percent water should suffer from rheumatism with a slight rise in the humidity of the atmosphere.

John W. Strutt (Baron Rayleigh) (1842–1919)
British physicist, discoverer of argon

OSTEOARTHRITIS

Scott Vogelgesang, MD

> **KEY POINTS**
> 1. Osteoarthritis is the most common articular disorder.
> 2. Obesity is a modifiable risk factor most closely associated with osteoarthritis.
> 3. The joints typically involved are: distal interphalangeal joints, proximal interphalangeal joints, first carpometacarpal joints, hips, knees, first metatarsophalangeal joint, cervical spine, and lumbosacral spine.
> 4. Typical radiologic findings include normal bony mineralization, nonuniform joint space narrowing, osteophytes, and sclerosis.
> 5. There are two indications for joint replacement surgery: (1) pain unresponsive to medical therapy and (2) loss of joint function.

1. What is osteoarthritis?

A slowly progressive, noninflammatory musculoskeletal disorder that typically affects the joints of the hand (especially those involved with a pinch grip), spine, and weight-bearing joints (hips, knees, first metatarsophalangeal [MTP] joint) of the lower extremity. It is the most common articular disorder and accounts for more disability among the elderly than any other disease. It is characterized by joint pain, particularly after activity, crepitus, stiffness after immobility, and limitation of motion. The clinical joint symptoms are pathologically associated with defects in the articular cartilage, osteophytes, and subchondral sclerosis. There are no systemic symptoms, and joint inflammation, when present, is mild.

2. Give other names for osteoarthritis.

- Osteoarthrosis.
- Degenerative joint disease.
- Hypertrophic arthritis.
- Degenerative disc disease (in the spine).
- Generalized osteoarthritis (Kellgren's syndrome).
- Erosive osteoarthritis (EOA) (Crain's disease).

3. Under what circumstances can osteoarthritis develop?

Osteoarthritis can develop when **excessive loads** (i.e., trauma) across the joint cause the normal articular cartilage or subchondral bone to fail. Alternatively, osteoarthritis may develop under **normal loads** if the cartilage, bone, synovium, or supporting ligaments and muscles are abnormal because of any one of a number of secondary causes. Damaged cartilage releases damage (danger)-associated molecular patterns (e.g., breakdown products of extracellular matrix) that can activate the innate immune system with subsequent release of cytokines and other mediators leading to synovitis, which can contribute to subsequent cartilage damage.

4. What are the pathologic features of osteoarthritis?

- Early:
  - Swelling of articular cartilage.
  - Loosening of collagen framework.
  - Chondrocytes increase proteoglycan synthesis but also release more degradative enzymes.
  - Increased cartilage water content.
- Later:
  - Degradative enzymes break down proteoglycan faster than it can be produced by chondrocytes, resulting in diminished proteoglycan content in cartilage.
  - Articular cartilage thins and softens (joint space narrowing on radiographs will be seen eventually).
  - Fissuring and cracking of cartilage. Repair is attempted but inadequate.
  - Underlying bone is exposed, allowing synovial fluid to be forced by the pressure of weight into the bone. This shows up as subchondral cysts or geodes on radiographs.
  - Remodeling and hypertrophy of the subchondral bone results in subchondral sclerosis and osteophyte ("spur") formation.

This pathology explains the joint space narrowing, subchondral sclerosis, cysts/geodes, and osteophytes seen on radiographs in patients with osteoarthritis.

5. List the clinical features of osteoarthritis.
1. Pain in involved joints.
2. Pain worse with activity, better with rest.
3. Morning stiffness (if present) <30 minutes.
4. Stiffness after periods of immobility (gelling).
5. Bony joint enlargement.
6. Joint instability.
7. Limitation of joint mobility.
8. Periarticular muscle atrophy.
9. Crepitus.

6. What is crepitus?
A creaking, cracking, or grinding noise made by joints having irregular cartilage that moves against a similar surface. Crepitus may be painless but most often is uncomfortable.

7. Name the joints typically involved in primary (idiopathic) osteoarthritis.
- Distal interphalangeal (DIP) joints of the hands.
- Proximal interphalangeal (PIP) joints of the hands.
- First carpometacarpal (CMC) joints of the hands.
- Acromioclavicular joint of shoulder.
- Hips.
- Knees.
- First metatarsophalangeal (MTP) joints of the feet.
- Facet (apophyseal) joints of the cervical spine and lumbosacral spine.

8. Name some joints *not* typically involved in primary (idiopathic) osteoarthritis.
- Wrists.
- Elbows.
- Shoulders (glenohumeral joint).
- Ankles.
- Metacarpophalangeal (MCP) joints of the hands.
- Second to fifth MTP joints of the feet.

PEARL: involvement of these atypical joints should prompt a search for secondary causes of osteoarthritis (see Question 23).

9. What laboratory features are seen in osteoarthritis?
Laboratory findings are nonspecific:
- Erythrocyte sedimentation rate (ESR) typically within normal limits.
- Rheumatoid factor (RF) is negative.
- Antinuclear antibodies (ANAs) are not present.
- Synovial fluid.
  - Normal viscosity with good string sign.
  - Color is clear and yellow.
  - White blood cell counts typically <1000/mm^3 to 2000/mm^3.
  - No crystals and negative cultures.

10. What are the radiographic "ABCDES" of osteoarthritis?
A—No ankylosis.
  Alignment may be abnormal.
B—Bone mineralization is normal.
  Bony subchondral sclerosis.
  Bony spurs (osteophytes).
C—No calcifications in cartilage.
  Cartilage space narrowing that is nonuniform (occurs in area of maximal stress in weight-bearing joints).
D—Deformities of Heberden's/Bouchard's nodes.
  Distribution: involvement of typical joints (see Questions 7 and 8).
E—No erosions.
  ("Gull wing" sign in "erosive" osteoarthritis—see Question 18).
S—Slow progression over years.
  No specific nail or soft tissue abnormalities.
  Vacuum sign in degenerative disc disease (a collection of nitrogen in a degenerated disc space).
Always obtain weight-bearing radiographs when evaluating for joint space narrowing of lower extremity large joints (Figure 51-1).

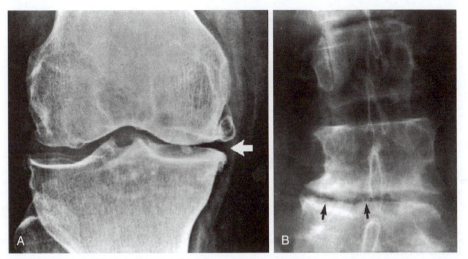

Figure 51-1. A, Radiograph of knee osteoarthritis, showing sclerosis, cysts, osteophytes, and medial joint space narrowing (*arrow*). B, Anterior radiograph of the lumbar spine with disc disease/osteoarthritis. Note disc space narrowing, osteophytes, and vacuum sign (*arrows*).

11. How is osteoarthritis classified?
- Primary, idiopathic osteoarthritis.
  - Localized.
    - Hands (DIP joints, PIP joints, and first CMC joints): nodal osteoarthritis.
    - Hands (DIP joints, PIP joints, and first CMC joints): erosive, inflammatory osteoarthritis.
    - Feet (first MTP joint).
    - Hip.
    - Knee.
    - Spine.
  - Generalized (also called Kellgren's syndrome).
- Secondary osteoarthritis.

12. Discuss the epidemiologic features of primary (idiopathic) osteoarthritis.
- More common in men than women <age 45 years; more common in women than men >age 45 years.
- Association with increased age.
- Osteoarthritis in an estimated 12% of the adult population (>age 25 years) overall.
- *Symptomatic* knee osteoarthritis in 7% to 24%: hip osteoarthritis in 8% to 11% of those >45 years of age.
- *Radiographic* knee osteoarthritis in 14% to 37%; hip osteoarthritis in 11% to 27%; first MTP osteoarthritis in 12% to 35% of U.S. adults depending on age studied. Radiographic hand osteoarthritis in 67% of women and 55% men over age 55 years.
- Between 10% and 30% of patients with osteoarthritis are significantly disabled.
- Annual cost for medical care for patients with osteoarthritis is $185.5 billion a year.

PEARL: radiographic osteoarthritis is at least twice more common than symptomatic osteoarthritis. Therefore, changes in osteoarthritis on radiographs do not prove that osteoarthritis is the cause of that patient's musculoskeletal pain.

13. Where do Heberden's nodes and Bouchard's nodes occur?
Bony articular nodules (osteophytes or "spurs") located on the DIP joints are called **Heberden's** nodes. Such nodules on the PIP joints are **Bouchard's** nodes (Figure 51-2). They can occur on the fingers and toes. Palmar and lateral deviation of the distal phalanx as a result of these nodules is not uncommon. Heberden's nodes are 10 times more frequent in women than in men. The tendency to develop Heberden's nodes may be familial, with one estimate suggesting that a woman whose mother has Heberden's nodes is twice as likely to develop similar joint changes as a woman without such a family history. The clinical importance of Heberden's and Bouchard's nodes is that they usually signify that the patient has primary nodal osteoarthritis and does not have a secondary etiology for the osteoarthritis.

14. Who was Heberden? Who was Bouchard?
William Heberden was an 18th century British physician who made substantial contributions to cardiology, preventive medicine, and rheumatology. He identified the interphalangeal nodular swellings seen in the DIP

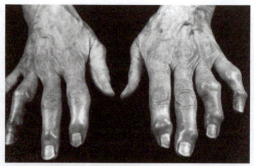

Figure 51-2. Heberden's (distal interphalangeal joints) nodes and Bouchard's (proximal interphalangeal joints) nodes in a woman with osteoarthritis. *(Copyright 2014 American College of Rheumatology. Used with permission.)*

joints in osteoarthritis. Heberden collected a set of clinical observations that became one of the first systems of differentiation of the arthritides.

Charles-Joseph Bouchard was a 19th century French pathologist who described the interphalangeal nodular swellings of the PIP joints seen in osteoarthritis.

15. List the risk factors for osteoarthritis.
- Age: strongest risk factor associated with osteoarthritis.
- Heredity: family risk studies estimate a 50% to 65% heritable component in primary osteoarthritis. There are multiple candidate genes.
- Gender: prevalence of osteoarthritis increases in women after age 50 years. Chondrocytes have functional estrogen receptors. Women on estrogen replacement therapy have less hip osteoarthritis and knee osteoarthritis.
- Obesity (see Question 16).
- Previous joint trauma: meniscal and ligament injuries, as well as fractures, can lead to altered joint biomechanics and articular incongruence leading to osteoarthritis.
- Abnormal joint mechanics (i.e., excessive knee varus or valgus; hip dysplasia).
- Smoking (may contribute to degenerative disc disease).
- Certain occupations/sports causing repetitive high impact loading: pneumatic drill operators (shoulders, elbows), ballet dancers (ankles), boxers (MCP joints), basketball players (knees), and others.

16. How does obesity predispose to osteoarthritis?
Obesity is a clear risk factor for the development of osteoarthritis, especially of the knee and, to a lesser degree, of the hand and the hip. The risk for knee osteoarthritis increases by 36% for every 5 kg (11 pounds) of weight gain, whereas the risk for osteoarthritis decreases by 50% for every 5 kg of weight loss in patients with a body mass index >25. One theory to explain this association is that obesity increases the forces across weight-bearing joints and alters joint mechanics by causing varus stress at the knee and changes in posture and gait. Another theory postulates that adipose tissue is a source of proinflammatory cytokines including leptin, adiponectin, resistin, interleukin-1 (IL-1), IL-6, and tumor necrosis factor-α (TNF-α). These cytokines can have negative effects on chondrocyte function. Because women have more adipose tissue, this helps to explain the increased prevalence of osteoarthritis in women and the involvement of nonweight-bearing joints such as the DIP joints.

17. Does running or jogging predispose to osteoarthritis?
Previous joint injury and repetitive impact loading predispose to the development of osteoarthritis, raising the question of whether runners are at increased risk for developing osteoarthritis in the knee and hip. Although there is some disagreement in the literature, most of the present data suggest that in the absence of previous joint injury, recreational runners do not develop osteoarthritis in the knee or hip at higher rates than others. However, highly competitive, elite runners may have an increased risk.

18. What is erosive (inflammatory) osteoarthritis (EOA)?
EOA, sometimes called Crain's disease, is an aggressive subset (5% to 10%) of primary osteoarthritis. EOA primarily occurs in Caucasian women 40 to 50 years of age. It is rare in men. The involved joints include the DIP joints, PIP joints, and first CMC joints, which are usually bilaterally affected. The first MTP joints are rarely involved. In EOA, there is a component of joint inflammation that is superimposed on the degenerative osteoarthritic symptoms. The clinical course of EOA usually waxes and wanes for up to 5 years with painful inflammatory "flares" leading to joint deformities. Radiographs are characteristic, showing osteophytes and central "erosions" with a hallmark "gull wing" or "inverted T" appearance (Figure 51-3). Subchondral

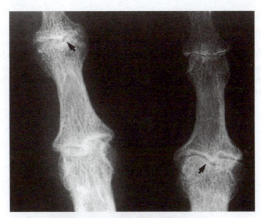

Figure 51-3. Radiograph of hands of a patient with "erosive" osteoarthritis of the distal interphalangeal joints and proximal interphalangeal joints. Note "gull wing" sign *(arrows)*, which is the hallmark of this disease.

pseudocysts can occur under the central "erosions." Joint ankylosis occurs in 15% of cases. Hand disability in patients with EOA is worse than typical nodal osteoarthritis.

Patients with EOA may be misdiagnosed as having rheumatoid arthritis (RA) or psoriatic arthritis. However, unlike RA, EOA is not accompanied by systemic symptoms; does not involve the MCP joints, wrists, or second to fifth MTP joints; and serologically has a normal ESR and C-reactive protein, and negative RF and ANA. Additionally, radiographs in RA and psoriatic arthritis show synovial-based erosions, which occur in the periarticular "bare areas" and not centrally as seen in EOA (see Chapters 8 and 15). However, patients with EOA do need to have superimposed gout and pseudogout ruled out when they have "flares."

The etiology of EOA is unknown. There is a strong family history in 66% of patients. Genetic studies have reported an association of EOA with a particular IL-1 genotype on chromosome 2. Synovial biopsies show synovial changes similar to RA with synovial hypertrophy and lymphocytic/neutrophilic infiltration. The centrally eroded cartilage is not caused by synovial pannus invasion. One theory is that cytokines such as IL-1 from the synovium may signal chondrocyte release of matrix metalloproteinases leading to cartilage destruction. This may be centrally accelerated where the cartilage is thinner. Another proposed etiology of EOA suggests a pathologic role of hydroxyapatite crystals and calcium pyrophosphate dihydrate (CPPD) crystals.

Multiple therapies have been used to control symptoms in patients with EOA. Topical and oral nonsteroidal antiinflammatory drugs (NSAIDs) are typically tried first. Intraarticular steroid injections have proven effective in some patients. Because of the synovial inflammation resembling RA, hydroxychloroquine, methotrexate, and anti-TNF agents have been tried with varying success. Recently, based on the theories that IL-1 polymorphisms and/or crystals may play a pathogenic role in EOA, anakinra has been used with a reported 70% reduction in pain.

19. **Define generalized osteoarthritis.**

A variant of osteoarthritis, sometimes called Kellgren's syndrome, in which individuals have several affected joints in the typical distribution for osteoarthritis. Although there is no universally accepted definition, most patients with generalized osteoarthritis typically have ≥4 joint sites symmetrically involved. The most commonly involved joints are the hand interphalangeal joints (DIP joints, PIP joints) and first CMC joints with the spine, knees, hips, and first MTP involved in descending frequency. The disease frequently becomes manifest before age 40 to 50 years. Radiographic findings may be more severe than symptoms. Generalized osteoarthritis may simply be a more severe form of common osteoarthritis, although some researchers have reported various associations with genetic polymorphisms or mutations that could contribute to more rapid cartilage degeneration.

20. **What is diffuse idiopathic skeletal hyperostosis?**

Diffuse idiopathic skeletal hyperostosis (DISH) has also been called Forestier's disease and ankylosing hyperostosis. DISH can be confused with ankylosing spondylitis or osteoarthritis of the spine. It is, however, not an arthropathy in that there is no abnormality of articular cartilage, adjacent bone margins, or synovium. Instead, it is a bone-forming condition in which ossification occurs at skeletal sites subjected to stress. It occurs most frequently in the thoracic spine and can be clinically associated with stiffness or decreased motion. Pain is usually not a significant symptom and if severe the patient should be evaluated for other causes of pain. Involvement of the cervical spine can cause dysphagia. DISH occurs in approximately 12% of the elderly population and may coexist with other disorders, particularly type 2 diabetes mellitus.

21. **Describe the radiographic findings in DISH.**

   Normal bone mineralization is seen in addition to "flowing" ossification of the anterior longitudinal ligament connecting at least *four* contiguous vertebral bodies. The calcification of the anterior longitudinal ligament is seen as a radiodense band separated from the anterior aspect of the vertebral bodies by a thin radiolucent line similar to flowing candle wax (Figure 51-4). Ossification of multiple tendinous or ligamentous sites in the appendicular skeleton may also be seen. Disc spaces, apophyseal joints, and sacroiliac joints are radiographically normal, helping to separate DISH from osteoarthritis and ankylosing spondylitis.

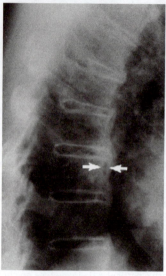

Figure 51-4. Lateral radiograph of thoracic spine showing calcification of the anterior longitudinal ligament connecting four vertebrae. Note the space between this calcified ligament and the anterior borders of vertebral bodies *(arrows)*.

22. **How does secondary osteoarthritis differ from primary osteoarthritis?**

   Secondary osteoarthritis has the same clinical features as idiopathic osteoarthritis except that it has an identifiable etiologic factor and may have a different joint distribution. **Atypical joint involvement** (MCP joints, wrists, elbows, shoulders, ankles, MTP joints) or early age onset of osteoarthritis should prompt a search for an underlying disease process. A classic example is osteoarthritis seen in the MCP joints of the hands in association with hemochromatosis (young patients) and CPPD disease (older patients).

23. **List some causes of secondary osteoarthritis.**
    - Congenital disorders
        - Hip
            - Legg–Calvé–Perthes disease
            - Congenital hip dislocation
            - Slipped capital femoral epiphysis
            - Congenital shallow acetabulum
            - Femoroacetabular impingement
        - Dysplasias
            - Epiphyseal dysplasia
            - Spondyloepiphyseal dysplasia
        - Mechanical features
            - Joint hypermobility syndromes
            - Leg length discrepancy
            - Varus/valgus deformity
            - Scoliosis
    - **Trauma**: anterior cruciate ligament tear; fracture through joint; meniscectomy
    - Metabolic diseases
        - Hemochromatosis
        - Ochronosis
        - Gaucher's disease
        - Hemoglobinopathy
        - Crystal deposition disorders

- Endocrine disorders
  - Acromegaly
    - Hypothyroidism
    - Hyperparathyroidism
- Neuropathic joints
  - Diabetes mellitus
  - Syphilis
- Other
  - End result of any infectious or inflammatory arthropathy
  - Osteonecrosis
  - Paget's disease
  - Kashin–Beck disease: osteochondropathy in China as a result of mycotoxins and selenium deficiency.

24. **Does "cracking" one's knuckles lead to osteoarthritis of the fingers?**
    The joint cavity is a potential space with a negative pressure compared with ambient atmospheric pressure. Joint synovial fluid acts as an adhesive seal that permits sliding motion between cartilage surfaces while effectively resisting distracting forces. During knuckle cracking or popping, there is a fracture of this adhesive bond. A gas bubble is created within the joint, which cavitates with a cracking sound, liberating energy in the form of heat and sound. This radiologically obvious bubble of gas can require up to 30 minutes to dissolve before the synovial fluid adhesive bond can be reestablished and the joint can be "cracked" again. Although knuckle cracking may look and sound obnoxious, there are no data to support that it leads to osteoarthritis of the finger joints. The evidence for this is a report by a physician who cracked the knuckles of his left hand twice a day for 50 years (36,500 times total) while not cracking the knuckles of his right hand. Symptom evaluation and radiographs showed that no arthritis developed in either hand. This is a classic example of a "two arm trial without randomization." (Unger DL: Does knuckle cracking lead to arthritis of the fingers? Arthritis Rheum 41:949-950, 1998.)

25. **What is the manual labor metacarpal arthropathy syndrome?**
    Primary osteoarthritis typically does not involve the MCP joints and when involved patients should be evaluated for secondary causes such as hemochromatosis and CPPD. Rarely, osteoarthritis of the MCP joints (worse in the dominant hand) has been described in male patients over the age of 50 years who have engaged in heavy manual labor (truck drivers, farmers, heavy machine operators) involving their hands for several decades. It is hypothesized that repetitive power gripping of both hands during heavy labor increases the load across the joints' articular surface leading to MCP joint degeneration.

26. **What is the relationship between femoroacetabular impingement and osteoarthritis?**
    Patients with femoroacetabular impingement (FAI) present with groin pain exacerbated by sitting or athletics. Hip flexion is limited to 90 degrees. They have limitation in internal rotation at the 90 degree flexed position with pain at the extreme (*impingement sign*). They may have a click/snap with hip rotation as a result of a labral lesion or chondral lesion. The mechanism underlying FAI is that normal motion such as flexion results in abnormal contact between the femoral head or proximal femur at the head–neck junction and anterior rim of the acetabulum. This can lead to labral tears and early osteoarthritis. Two types of FAI are recognized:
    - **Cam impingement** is caused by any deformity of the proximal femur or femoral head resulting in an aspherical femoral head with loss of the normal femoral head–neck offset (pistol grip deformity). Flexion of the hip causes the abnormal femoral head to rotate into the acetabulum causing stress on the labrum and cartilage of the anterosuperior acetabular rim. A cross-table lateral radiograph, computed tomography scan, or magnetic resonance imaging (MRI) may show a cam lesion on the femoral head–neck junction.
    - **Pincer impingement** is caused by local or global overcoverage of the femoral head by the acetabulum. Hip flexion compresses the labrum against the acetabular rim cartilage. Radiographs show a deep acetabular socket (Figure 51-5).

    The treatment is surgical removal of bony factors contributing to abutment of the femoral head and/or neck with the acetabular ring.

27. **What MRI findings in the knee are associated with pain?**
    Bone marrow edema lesions under thinned cartilage correlate with pain. Notably, meniscal degenerative lesions are common but do not correlate with symptoms. This explains why knee arthroscopy to repair meniscal abnormalities rarely improves symptoms unless there are clear mechanical symptoms such as locking.

28. **Can pes planus cause knee problems?**
    Yes. Pes planus (flat feet) morphology with pronation causes rotational stress on the medial compartment of knee leading to osteoarthritis. In addition, the patella tracks laterally causing patellofemoral osteoarthritis. Patients presenting with knee pain should have their foot morphology and gait analyzed. If ples planus is present, foot orthotics may help relieve the knee pain.

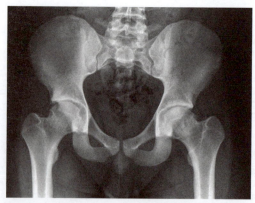

Figure 51-5. Radiograph of pelvis with bilateral cam deformities causing femoroacetabular impingement.

29. **Why is primary osteoarthritis of the ankle uncommon?**
    Primary osteoarthritis of the ankle is nine times less common than osteoarthritis of the knee or hip and usually a result of trauma (i.e., secondary osteoarthritis). Because the weighted load (five times body weight when walking) on the ankle exceeds that of the knee (four times body weight) and hip (three times body weight), it is surprising that primary osteoarthritis is so uncommon in the ankle. The reason for this is not entirely clear. However, there are clear anatomical and biomechanical differences between the ankle and the knee or the hip. For instance, the ankle is mainly a rolling joint with congruent surfaces at high load, whereas the knee joint is a mixture of sliding, rolling, and rotation with less congruent surfaces resulting in more stress on the knee cartilage. There are also differences in thickness and composition of ankle cartilage, which increases its tensile strength and gives it more resistance to catabolic cytokines such as IL-1β.

30. **A 72-year-old grandmother with generalized osteoarthritis complains that she can predict changes in the weather better than the weatherman on television. Can weather changes affect patients with arthritis?**
    Yes. It does not matter so much whether it is hot, cold, dry, or humid. Many patients with arthritis (66%) are affected by changes in barometric pressure and temperature as weather fronts are moving in or out of an area. It is hypothesized that changes in barometric pressure and temperature increase stiffness of joints, which can heighten a nociceptive response. Consequently, the myth that patients with arthritis should move to a warm climate is unlikely to be helpful because changes in weather and barometric pressure occur everywhere. (Sibley JT: Weather and arthritis symptoms, J Rheum 12:707-710, 1985.)

31. **List nonpharmacologic interventions for osteoarthritis that should be tried first and/or added to medications.**
    - Patient education and Arthritis Foundation self-help courses.
    - Weight loss: every 1 lb (0.45 kg) lost results in a fourfold reduction in load per step on the knee. Weight loss of 5% results in 18% to 24% improvement in function in patients with knee osteoarthritis.
    - Occupational therapy assistive aids/devices, joint protection, and modification of activities of daily living.
    - Exercise for muscle strengthening/flexibility and aerobic conditioning: proven for knee osteoarthritis more than hip osteoarthritis.
    - Medial taping of patella for patellofemoral disease.
    - Unloader/off-load knee brace.
    - Optimal footwear (athletic shoe) with shock-absorbing insoles: medial knee osteoarthritis may be symptomatically improved and progression potentially slowed by biomechanical interventions to unweight the knee. The use of clogs, dress shoes, and high heels increase medial compartment loading of the knee by 15% compared with flat shoes, flip flops, or bare feet.
    - Foot orthotics: orthotics for pes planus/foot pronation to help knee and patellofemoral symptoms and heel lifts to alter forces causing pain in hip osteoarthritis appear useful. Although in many clinical guidelines, lateral wedge insoles to unweight and help medial knee joint osteoarthritis have not been shown to be beneficial (controversial).
    - Ambulatory aids (canes, crutches, walkers): cane can unload hip by 25% to 40% if used in hand opposite the hip.
    - Splinting (CMC splints, knee sleeves).
    - Paraffin baths for hands (may be done at home).
    - Cervical collar.

- Cervical traction or distraction.
- Topical lidocaine.
- Topical capsaicin (works by depleting nerve terminal of substance P, thereby decreasing pain).
- Transcutaneous electrical nerve stimulator (TENS) (controversial but may help individual patients).
- Superficial heat and cold.
- Hydrotherapy.
- Unconventional: acupuncture (controversial); spa.
- Not effective: pulsed electromagnetic fields; static magnets.

32. What is the role of exercise in osteoarthritis therapy?

A specific exercise program can play a significant role in improving joint range of motion and function and reducing pain. Several studies have shown that a supervised program of fitness walking resulted in improvement of pain and joint function. Other studies have shown that participants also have improved psychological well-being. Caution is advised, however. Weight-bearing exercise may worsen the articular cartilage and subchondral bone.

The compromise should be an exercise that does not involve weight-bearing but does provide joint range of motion, muscle strengthening, and aerobic fitness. It is important that the individual selects an exercise program that is enjoyable, easily done, and possible to accomplish. An ideal exercise for some is swimming. When done in a warm pool, the individual can move affected joints, strengthen periarticular muscles, and improve cardiovascular fitness, all without bearing weight on diseased joints. Other good options include bicycling, walking, elliptical training, and cross-country skiing.

33. How would you initiate and advance medical treatment in a typical patient with osteoarthritis?

No medication or intervention has been shown to stop or reverse the disease process underlying osteoarthritis. Medications are used, therefore, to alleviate symptoms and increase function with the least toxicity. A reasonable approach to therapy is to start with **acetaminophen**, 650 mg every 6 to 8 hours as needed (maximum total dose ≤3-4 g/day), which can decrease osteoarthritis pain by approximately 30%. If this is unsuccessful, a trial of nonacetylated salicylates is warranted. **Salsalate** can be used in typical doses of 1000 mg twice or three times a day. If unsuccessful, less-expensive, short-acting **NSAIDs** may be added to the acetaminophen, such as ibuprofen or naproxen sodium. NSAIDs are more effective than acetaminophen in patients with osteoarthritis with an inflammatory component (knee effusion, EOA). In these patients, using the smallest effective dose and/or intermittent dosing is prudent if possible. Further protection against gastrointestinal ulceration and bleeding may be accomplished with proton-pump inhibitors. For those at high risk of gastrointestinal ulceration and/or for whom gastroprotective therapy is contraindicated and who also have a low risk of cardiovascular disease, NSAIDs with specificity for cyclooxygenase 2 (**celecoxib**) may be considered. In patients who are considered high risk for oral NSAID use, **topical NSAIDs, tramadol**, or **duloxetine** may be effective. Notably, there is no role for oral corticosteroids. However, in a single joint with an inflammatory component, **intraarticular corticosteroids** (see Chapter 82) can be helpful. **Narcotic analgesics** are reserved for patients who have failed or cannot tolerate standard medical therapy and who are awaiting surgery or who are not a surgical candidate.

34. Are glucosamine and chondroitin effective in treating osteoarthritis?

Glucosamine sulfate (or hydrochloride) and chondroitin sulfate (so-called nutraceuticals) are classified as dietary supplements and as such are not regulated by the federal government (i.e., the Food and Drug Administration [FDA]). Consequently, compound amount, purity, long-term safety, and product labeling are not guaranteed. Absorption of both of these molecules varies greatly between individuals. Approximately 90% of glucosamine sulfate is initially absorbed with half of that being removed by the liver leaving a bioavailable dose for distribution to joints of only 45% with only half of this (i.e., 20% to 25%) actually getting into the joint. Gastrointestinal absorption of chondroitin sulfate is worse with only 15% to 24% being bioavailable. Glucosamine is the principal component of glycosaminoglycans, which form the matrix of all connective tissue including cartilage. In vitro studies show that glucosamine is incorporated into and increases synthesis of proteoglycans by chondrocytes. Glucosamine may also have some mild antiinflammatory effects. In vitro, chondroitin sulfate has a tropism for cartilage and can stimulate proteoglycan synthesis and block certain proteases.

Published studies are conflicting on the effectiveness of glucosamine and chondroitin sulfate in reducing pain and increasing function in patients with osteoarthritis. There are some data supporting a decreased rate of joint space narrowing in patients with osteoarthritis who took either of these nutraceuticals compared with placebo. Guidelines for patients who wish to take these medications are as follows:

- Glucosamine sulfate is three times better absorbed than glucosamine hydrochloride. The DONA brand of glucosamine sulfate is the brand used in most controlled studies ($38.00/month).
- Dose of glucosamine is 1500 mg daily. It should be taken all at once and not in divided doses.
- Dose of chondroitin sulfate is 1200 mg daily.
- Symptomatic relief should be noted within 2 months if it is going to be effective.
- Side effects are minimal. Patients with shellfish allergies may have a reaction to glucosamine. May increase warfarin effect.

35. What is viscosupplementation?

Viscosupplementation is a therapy for moderate (not end stage) osteoarthritis for which standard medical management fails. The therapy consists of injecting hyaluronan into the affected joint. It is FDA-approved only for the knee but has been used successfully in the temporomandibular joint, shoulder, hip, and ankle. Hyaluronan (sodium hyaluronate) is a glycosaminoglycan found in synovial fluid that allows viscous lubrication at low loads and shock absorbency at high loads. In the synovial fluid of a normal joint, there is 4 to 8 mg of hyaluronan with a molecular weight of 5 million daltons. In the synovial fluid of an osteoarthritic joint, there is less hyaluronan with a molecular weight of 2 to 3 million daltons, making it less effective for lubrication/shock absorbency. There are several different formulations with varying molecular weights, composition, side effect profiles, and frequency of injections. None are superior to another:

- **Hyalgan** (sodium hyaluronate): made from rooster coombs. Requires 3 to 5 weekly injections. Lasts 26 weeks.
- **Synvisc** and **Synvisc-One** (Hylan G-F 20): hylan A and B polymers produced from chicken coombs and chemically cross-linked. Synvisc-One requires one injection. Regular Synvisc requires 3 weekly injections. Lasts 26 weeks. Owing to polymer composition, synvisc is more highly associated with postinjection "pseudoseptic" flares. Should not be used in patients with CPPD disease.
- **Orthovisc** (high molecular weight hyaluronan): made from rooster coombs. Requires 3 to 4 weekly injections. Lasts 26 weeks.
- **Supartz** (sodium hyaluronate): made from chicken coombs. Requires 3 to 5 weekly injections. Lasts 18 weeks.
- **Gel-One** (sodium hyaluronate): made from chicken coombs by the same company that produces Supartz. Requires one injection. Lasts 18 to 26 weeks.
- **Euflexxa** (highly purified hyaluronan): made by bacterial fermentation. Can use this in patients who have allergies to birds or eggs. Requires 3 weekly injections. Lasts 12 weeks.

PEARL: all viscosupplementation therapy is more effective if joint effusion is aspirated dry before the hyaluronan is injected.

Intraarticular hyaluronan appears to be safe and can be repeated in patients who get prolonged improvement (>18 to 26 weeks). Reported side effects include local injection reactions, systemic allergic reactions (especially in patients allergic to avian proteins, feathers, or eggs), and "pseudoseptic" reactions often times resulting from pseudogout. This injection therapy can be repeated. Hyaluronan may have some chondroprotective (stimulates proteoglycan synthesis), antiinflammatory (scavenger sink for inflammatory mediators), and antinociceptive effects, which may explain its prolonged symptomatic benefit, even though the hyaluronan can only be detected for a few days (intraarticular half-life is 17 to 36 hours) in the joint after the injection. Cost for medication and injection is approximately $1000 per knee injected.

36. How does viscosupplementation compare with NSAIDs or intraarticular corticosteroid injections?

Most clinical trials suggest that pain relief is equivalent to NSAIDs without the gastrointestinal side effects. A direct comparison to intraarticular corticosteroids shows that they are equivalent to each other for knee osteoarthritis. Because of a difference in cost, many physicians will use intraarticular corticosteroids before going to viscosupplementation. Intraarticular corticosteroids are particularly effective in patients with knee osteoarthritis causing an effusion ("wet osteoarthritis"), which suggests a mild inflammatory component. It also has a more rapid onset of response. Intraarticular corticosteroids can be repeated as frequently as once every 3 to 4 months (no more than four injections a year and never within 2 to 3 months of a previous injection). If intraarticular corticosteroids become ineffective, viscosupplementation can then be tried. Some physicians use a combination of intraarticular corticosteroids and viscosupplementation to get a more rapid response. One key to success is to only use viscosupplementation in patients with osteoarthritis pain and radiographs showing mild to moderate joint space narrowing. Patients with end stage osteoarthritis with "bone on bone" radiographs should be sent for total knee arthroplasty.

37. List the indications for total joint replacement for osteoarthritis of the hip or knee.

- Severe pain unresponsive to medical therapy. For example:
  - Consistently awakens from sleep as a result of pain.
  - Cannot stand in one place for >20 to 30 minutes as a result of pain.
- Loss of joint function. For example:
  - Cannot walk more than one block.
  - Had to move to single story house or apartment because of inability to climb stairs.

38. What other therapies are being used or developed for osteoarthritis?

- **Botulinum toxin A**: has been used in patients with severe osteoarthritis of the knee, shoulder, and ankle who are poor surgical candidates. Intraarticular botulinum toxin A (100 units) is a neurotoxin that decreases pain an average of 30%. (Boon AJ, Smith J, Dahm DL et al: Efficacy of intra-articular botulinum toxin type A in painful knee osteoarthritis: a pilot study, PMR 2:268-276, 2010. Mahowald ML, Krug HE, Singh JA et al: Intra-articular botulinum toxin type A: a new approach to treat arthritis joint pain, Toxicon 54:658-667, 2009.)

- **Strontium ranelate** (Protelos): recent clinical trial showed that 2 g/day improved pain and decreased radiographic progression of knee osteoarthritis. Mechanism of action suggested to be strengthening of subchondral bone and stimulation of cartilage matrix formation. (Reginster JY, Badurski J, Bellamy N et al: Efficacy and safety of strontium ranelate in the treatment of knee osteoarthritis: results of a double-blind, randomised placebo-controlled trial, Ann Rheum Dis 72:179-186, 2013.)
- **Antibodies to nerve growth factor** (NGF) (Tanezumab): NGF is a neurotrophin involved in the structure and function of sensory nerves and is able to sensitize nociceptors. Clinical trials using an intravenous infusion of tanezumab every 8 weeks reduced pain in patients with osteoarthritis. Paresthesias were common and some patients developed accelerated knee degeneration. (Lane NE, Schnitzer TJ, Birbara CA et al: Tanezumab for the treatment of pain from osteoarthritis of the knee, N Engl J Med 363:1521-1531, 2010.)
- **Cartilage transplant**: cartilage is taken from nonweight-bearing surface of femur and transplanted into an isolated cartilage defect. Results have varied. Cost $20,000 to $35,000.
- **Autologous chondrocyte grafts and mesenchymal stem cell transplants**: (Koga H, Engebretsen L, Brinchmann JE et al: Mesenchymal stem cell-based therapy for cartilage repair: a review, Knee Surg Sports Traumatol Arthrosc 17:1289-1297, 2009.)
- **Abrasion and microfracture surgery**: microdrilling of subchondral bone releases autologous mesenchymal stem cells from the bone marrow that attempt to repair the osteoarthritic cartilage.

Unfortunately, many compounds (tetracyclines, rumalon, diacerein, anakinra, adalimumab) have been tried and much research has been devoted to finding a disease-modifying osteoarthritis drug with little success.

39. What is the natural history of osteoarthritis?

It is likely that the cartilage changes of osteoarthritis are asymptomatic for years. Despite this, osteoarthritis progresses with time in most individuals. The rate of progression, however, can be variable and, once symptomatic, the disease may seem to progress quickly. There may be rare individuals in whom the disease may remain stable or even improve somewhat. Nevertheless, osteoarthritis can lead to severe limitations in motion and eventual disability. Limitation in usual activities was noted by 60% to 80% of patients who reported having osteoarthritis according to the National Health Interview Survey.

BIBLIOGRAPHY

Avouac J, Vicaut E, Bardin T, et al: Efficacy of joint lavage in knee osteoarthritis: meta-analysis of randomized controlled studies, Rheumatology 49:334–340, 2010.

Bacconnier L, Jorgensen C, Fabre S: Erosive osteoarthritis of the hand: clinical experience with anakinra, Ann Rheum Dis 68:1078–1079, 2009.

Banks SE: Erosive osteoarthritis: a current review of a clinical challenge, Clin Rheumatol 29:697–706, 2010.

Bellamy N, Campbell J, Robinson V, et al: Intraarticular corticosteroid for treatment of osteoarthritis of the knee, Cochrane Database Syst Rev 2:CD005328, 2006a.

Bellamy N, Campbell J, Robinson V, et al: Viscosupplementation for the treatment of osteoarthritis of the knee, Cochrane Database Syst Rev 2:CD005321, 2006b.

Boon AJ, Smith J, Dahm DL, et al: Efficacy of intra-articular botulinum toxin type A in painful knee osteoarthritis: a pilot study, PM R 2:268–276, 2010.

Bryant LR, des Rosier KF, Carpenter MT: Hydroxychloroquine in the treatment of erosive osteoarthritis, J Rheumatol 22:1527–1531, 1995.

Clegg DO, Reda DJ, Harris CL, et al: Glucosamine, chondroitin sulfate and the two in combination for painful knee osteoarthritis, N Engl J Med 354:795–808, 2006.

Collins N, Crossley K, Beller E, et al: Foot orthoses and physiotherapy in the treatment of patellofemoral pain syndrome: randomized clinical trial, Br J Sports Med 43:169–171, 2009.

Emary PC: Manual labor metacarpal arthropathy in a truck driver: a case report, J Chiropractic Med 9:193–199, 2010.

Englund M, Guermazi A, Gale D, et al: Incidental meniscal findings on knee MRI in middle-aged and elderly persons, N Engl J Med 359:1108–1115, 2008.

Felson DT, Niu J, Guermazi A, et al: Correlation of the development of knee pain with enlarging bone marrow lesions on magnetic resonance imaging, Arthritis Rheum 56:2986–2992, 2007.

Fernandes L, Hagen KB, Bijlsma JWJ, et al: EULAR recommendations for the non-pharmacological core management of hip and knee osteoarthritis, Ann Rheum Dis 72:1125–1135, 2013.

Gross KD, Felson DT, Niu J, et al: Association of flat feet with knee pain and cartilage damage in older adults, Arthritis Care Res 63:937–944, 2011.

Hochberg MC, Altman RD, April KT, et al: American College of Rheumatology 2012 recommendations for the use of nonpharmacologic and pharmacologic therapies in osteoarthritis of the hand, hip, and knee, Arthritis Care Res 64:465–474, 2012.

Katz JN, Earp BE, Gomoll AH: Surgical management of osteoarthritis, Arthritis Care Res 62:1220–1228, 2010.

Koga H, Engebretsen L, Brinchmann JE, et al: Mesenchymal stem cell-based therapy for cartilage repair: a review, Knee Surg Sports Traumatol Arthrosc 17:1289–1297, 2009.

Kraus VB, Jordan JM, Doherty M, et al: The genetics of generalized osteoarthritis (GOGO) study: study design and evaluation of osteoarthritis phenotypes, Osteoarthritis Cartil 15:120–127, 2007.

Lane NE, Schnitzer TJ, Birbara CA, et al: Tanezumab for the treatment of pain from osteoarthritis of the knee, N Engl J Med 363:1521, 2010.

Lawrence RC, Felson DT, Helmick CG, et al: Estimates of the prevalence of arthritis and other rheumatic condition in the United States. Part II, Arthritis Rheum 58:26–35, 2008.

Lementowski PW, Zelicof SB: Obesity and osteoarthritis, Am J Orthop 37:148–151, 2008.

Mahowald ML, Krug HE, Singh JA, et al: Intra-articular botulinum toxin type A: a new approach to treat arthritis joint pain, Toxicon 54:658–667, 2009.

Niethard FU, Gold MS, Solomon GS, et al: Efficacy of topical diclofenac diethylamine gel in osteoarthritis of the knee, J Rheumatol 32:2384–2392, 2005.

Reginster JY, Badurski J, Bellamy N, et al: Efficacy and safety of strontium ranelate in the treatment of knee osteoarthritis: results of a double-blind, randomised placebo-controlled trial, Ann Rheum Dis 72:179–186, 2013.

Reid GD, Reid CG, Widmer N, et al: Femoroacetabular impingement syndrome: an underrecognized cause of hip pain and premature osteoarthritis? J Rheumatol 37:1395–1404, 2010.

Roddy E, Zhang W, Doherty M: Aerobic walking and strengthening exercise for osteoarthritis of the knee? A systemic review, Ann Rheum Dis 64:544–548, 2005.

Sibley JT: Weather and arthritis symptoms, J Rheum 12:707–710, 1985.

Sokolove J, Lepus CM: Role of inflammation in the pathogenesis of osteoarthritis, Ther Adv Musculoskel Dis 5:77–94, 2013.

Towheed TE, Maxwell L, Judd MG, et al: Acetaminophen for osteoarthritis, Cochrane Database Syst Rev 1:CD004257, 2006.

Unger DL: Does knuckle cracking lead to arthritis of the fingers? Arthritis Rheum 41:949–950, 1998.

Wu D, Huang Y, Gu Y, et al: Efficacies of different preparations of glucosamine for the treatment of osteoarthritis: a meta-analysis of randomized, double-blind, placebo-controlled trials, Int J Clin Pract 67:585–594, 2013.

METABOLIC BONE DISEASE

Michael T. McDermott, MD

CHAPTER 52

KEY POINTS

1. The major risk factors for fragility fractures (fx) are low bone mass, advancing age, previous fragility fracture, corticosteroid use, and the propensity for falling.
2. Disorders causing secondary bone loss are present in approximately one third of women and two thirds of men who have osteoporosis.
3. Patients with osteoporosis should have a complete history, physical examination, and key, cost-effective laboratory tests performed to identify any underlying disorders.
4. High doses and prolonged use of glucocorticoids produce greater risk, but all doses of oral glucocorticoids and even inhaled steroids increase the risk of osteoporotic fractures.
5. Glucocorticoid-induced osteoporosis (GIOP) results from a combination of suppressed bone formation and enhanced bone resorption accounting for the rapid bone loss often seen in patients treated with glucocorticoids.

1. What is osteoporosis?
Osteoporosis is a skeletal disorder characterized by compromised bone strength, which predisposes to the development of fragility fracture. Bone strength is determined by both **bone mass** and **bone quality**. The diagnosis of osteoporosis is established by the presence of a true fragility fracture or, in patients who have never sustained an fragility fracture, by measuring bone mineral density (BMD).

2. What are fragility fractures?
Fragility fractures are those that occur spontaneously or following minimal trauma, defined as falling from a standing height or less. Fractures of the vertebrae, hips, and distal radius (Colles' fracture) are the most characteristic fragility fracture, but patients with osteoporosis are prone to all types of fractures. Up to 40% of women and 13% of men develop one or more osteoporotic fractures during their lifetime. Osteoporosis accounts for approximately 1.5 million fractures in the United States each year.

3. What are the complications of osteoporotic fractures?
Vertebral fractures cause loss of height, anterior kyphosis (dowager's hump), reduced pulmonary function (each fracture decreases FVC by 9%), and an increased mortality rate. Approximately one third of all vertebral fractures are painful but two thirds are asymptomatic. Hip fractures are associated with permanent disability in nearly 50% of patients and with a 20% excess mortality rate compared to the age-matched nonfracture population.

4. What factors contribute most to the risk of developing an osteoporotic fracture?
- Low BMD (twofold increased risk for every one standard deviation [SD; T-score] decrease of BMD)
- Age (twofold increased risk for every decade of age above 60 years)
- Previous fragility fracture (fivefold increased risk for a subsequent fracture)
- Frequent falls
- Corticosteroid use

5. What are the currently accepted indications for BMD measurement?
- Age ≥65 years (women); age ≥70 years (men).
- Estrogen deficiency plus one risk factor for osteoporosis.
- Vertebral deformity, fracture, or osteopenia by x-ray.
- Primary hyperparathyroidism.
- Glucocorticoid therapy, ≥5 mg/day of prednisone for ≥3 months.
- Monitoring the response to a Food and Drug Administration (FDA)-approved osteoporosis medication.

6. How is BMD currently measured?
Dual energy x-ray absorptiometry (DXA) is the most accurate and widely used method in current practice. The radiation exposure is minimal with only 1 to 3 microsieverts (μSv)/site compared with 50 to 100 μSv for one chest radiograph. BMD can also be measured by computed tomography (CT) (50 μSv) and ultrasound (US) (no radiation). Central densitometry (DXA) measurements (spine and hip) are

the best predictors of fracture risk and have the best precision for longitudinal monitoring. Peripheral densitometry measurements (heel, radius, hands) are more widely available and less expensive but less accurate.

7. **How do you read a bone densitometry report?**
   T-score: the number of SD the patient is below or above the mean value for young (30 year old) normal subjects (peak bone mass). The T-score is a good predictor of the fracture risk.
   Z-score: the number of SD the patient is below or above the mean value for age-matched normal subjects. The Z-score indicates whether or not the BMD is appropriate for a particular age. A low Z-score is predictive of an underlying secondary cause other than age or menopause (Figure 52-1).
   Absolute BMD: the actual BMD expressed in g/cm². This is the value that should be used to calculate changes in BMD during longitudinal follow-up.

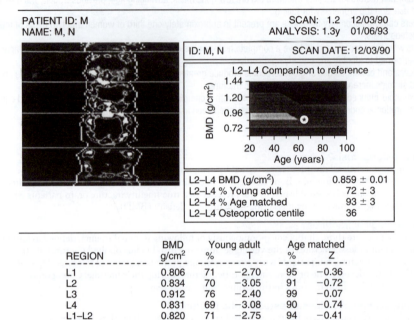

Figure 52-1. Bone density report for a dual energy x-ray absorptiometry (DXA) study of the spine. The L2–L4 region, the most frequently evaluated, shows a bone mineral density (BMD) of 0.859 g/cm², a T-score of −2.84, and a Z-score of −0.51. The very low T-score indicates osteoporosis with a significant fracture risk. The relatively normal Z-score indicates that age and menopause are likely to be the most important factors causing the low BMD.

8. **How is the diagnosis of osteoporosis made?**
   - Osteoporosis should be diagnosed in any patient who sustains a fragility fracture regardless of BMD T-score.
   - In a patient over the age of 50 years without fractures, the diagnosis can be made based on the BMD T-score at the lowest skeletal site, using the following criteria:

T-score ≥ −1	Normal
T-score between −1 and −2.5	Osteopenia
T-score ≤ −2.5	Osteoporosis

   - In a premenopausal woman or man under the age of 50 years, the diagnosis can be made based on a BMD Z-score of ≤ −2.0 at the lowest skeletal site.

9. **What estimates of bone loss and fracture risk can be made from a patient's BMD measurement by DXA?**

T-Score	Percentage Bone Loss*	Increased Fracture Risk
−1	12%	Twofold
−2	24%	Fourfold
−3	36%	Eightfold
−4	48%	Sixteenfold

*Note that one has to lose 30% BMD to see osteopenia on a routine radiograph, which suggests a T-score of −2.5.
PEARL: An older patient is more likely to suffer a fracture compared to a younger individual with the same T-score.

10. **What are the major risk factors for the development of osteoporosis?**

Nonmodifiable	Modifiable
Advanced age	Low calcium intake
Race (white, Asian)	Low vitamin D intake
Female gender	Estrogen deficiency
Early menopause	Sedentary lifestyle
Slender build (<127 lb)	Cigarette smoking
Positive family history (hip fragility fracture)	Alcohol excess (>two drinks/day)
	Caffeine excess (>two servings/day)

11. **What other conditions must be considered as causes of low BMD?**

Osteomalacia	Celiac disease
Osteogenesis imperfecta	Inflammatory bowel disease
Ehlers-Danlos syndrome	Gastrectomy/bowel bypass surgery
Hyperparathyroidism	Primary biliary cirrhosis
Hyperthyroidism	Multiple myeloma
Hyperprolactinemia	Rheumatoid arthritis/SLE
Alcoholism	Ankylosing spondylitis
Hypogonadism	Renal failure
Cushing's syndrome	Renal tubular acidosis
Eating/exercise disorders	Idiopathic hypercalciuria
High risk medications*	Systemic mastocytosis

*Glucocorticoids, excess thyroid hormone, anticonvulsants, heparin, lithium, SSRIs, aromatase inhibitors, premenopausal tamoxifen, leuprolide, cyclosporine. Probable/Possible: Thiazolidinediones, proton pump inhibitors, hypervitaminosis A.

12. **Outline a cost-effective evaluation to rule out other causes of low bone mass.**
    Calcium (albumin), phosphorous, creatinine, CO_2
    Alkaline phosphatase
    25-hydroxy (OH) vitamin D
    Testosterone (men)
    Thyroid stimulating hormone (TSH), if clinically hyperthyroid
    Celiac disease antibody testing (if white with symptoms or low 25-OH vitamin D level)
    Urine (24 hour) calcium, sodium, creatinine
    Serum protein electrophoresis (SPEP; if over the age of 50 years with abnormal complete blood count [CBC])
    PEARL: A patient needs a calcium (corrected for albumin level) × phosphorous product of 24 to properly mineralize bone.
    Approximately one third of women and two thirds of men will have an abnormality detected with this evaluation. A low Z-score suggests that an underlying secondary cause is more likely to be present.

13. **How do you determine if a patient has had a previous vertebral fracture?**
    Back pain or tenderness are helpful clues but may be absent because two thirds of vertebral fractures are asymptomatic. A height loss of ≥2 inches or dorsal kyphosis are highly suggestive clinical findings. Lateral spine films or DXA vertebral fracture assessment (VFA) are the most accurate ways to detect existing vertebral fractures.

14. What are the most significant risk factors for frequent falls?
Frailty
Use of sedatives
Visual impairment
Cognitive impairment
Lower extremity disability
Obstacles to ambulation in the home
PEARL: The most predictive factor for a future fall is a previous fall within the past 6 months. Almost all hip fractures occur as a result of falls.

15. What is the FRAX tool?
The Fracture Risk Assessment (FRAX) tool (www.shef.ac.uk/FRAX/) is a free computer-based program developed by the World Health Organization (WHO). It uses clinical risk factors with or without femoral neck BMD to provide a 10-year absolute risk estimate for developing a hip or another major osteoporotic fracture (wrist, proximal humerus, etc.). It is recommended to be used for making treatment decisions in patients who are drug-naïve and over the age of 40 years with osteopenia. Treatment is advised for those who have a 10-year risk ≥3% for hip fracture or ≥20% for other major osteoporosis fractures.

16. How does osteoporosis differ in men?
Approximately 1 to 2 million men in the United States have osteoporosis. The diagnostic criteria are the same in men as in women (fragility fracture or T-score ≤ −2.5). Nearly two thirds of osteoporotic men have an identifiable secondary cause of bone loss, most often alcohol abuse, glucocorticoid use, and hypogonadism, including gonadotropin-releasing hormone (GnRH) analog use for prostate cancer. Treatment is generally the same in men as in women although testosterone replacement in hypogonadal men is an effective adjunctive strategy.

17. When should pharmacological therapy be initiated for osteoporosis? (see Chapter 87)
Pharmacological therapy should be advised for patients who have any **one** of the following:
- a history of vertebral or hip fragility fracture,
- a T-score < −2.5,
- are drug-naïve and over the age of 40 years with osteopenia, and have a 10-year risk ≥3% for hip fracture or ≥20% for other major osteoporosis fractures according to the FRAX tool.

18. How do glucocorticoids cause osteoporosis?
Glucocorticoids adversely affect both phases of bone remodeling leading to rapid loss of bone. They impair bone formation by promoting apoptosis of existing osteoblasts and reducing the development of new osteoblasts. They increase bone resorption by decreasing the production of sex steroids and osteoprotegerin, an endogenous inhibitor of bone resorption. Osteocytes are also affected and undergo apoptosis.
PEARL: Patients on glucocorticoids fracture at higher/better BMD values (T-scores) than do patients with other types of osteoporosis.

19. How should patients on glucocorticoids be monitored?
Patients starting glucocorticoid therapy (prednisone dose ≥5 mg/day or equivalent) with a planned duration of treatment ≥3 months or on existing treatment for ≥3 months should have their BMD tested and FRAX score calculated at the start of therapy and preferably every 12 months for as long as glucocorticoid therapy is continued.

20. When should osteoporosis medications be instituted in patients over age 50 years who are taking glucocorticoid therapy? Which medications are effective?
The decision to initiate a bone-active agent is based on risk stratification using the WHO FRAX tool, the lowest T-score value, and history of fragility fracture:
- **Low risk**: FRAX 10-year risk for a major osteoporotic fracture of <10%
- **Medium risk**: FRAX 10-year risk of 10% to 20%
- **High risk**: FRAX 10-year risk >20%, **or** T-score below −2.5 at any site, **or** a history of a previous fragility fracture.

Bisphosphonates and teriparatide have been shown in randomized controlled trials to significantly improve BMD and reduce fractures in patients treated with glucocorticoids.
Pharmacologic recommendations for postmenopausal women and men over age 50 years either starting or currently on glucocorticoids with an anticipated duration of therapy of 3 or more months are as follows:
- Low-risk patients on prednisone (or equivalent) ≥7.5 mg/day should start one of the following bisphosphonates (alendronate, risedronate, or zoledronic acid).
- Medium-risk patients on any dose (including prednisone <7.5 mg/day) of glucocorticoids should start a bisphosphonate.
- High-risk patients on any dose or duration (including <3 months) of glucocorticoids should start a bisphosphonate. Teriparatide is an option for high-risk patients who have the lowest T-scores (below −2.5) and/or history of fragility fracture.
- In clinical practice, any patient not on a bone-active agent with a T-score below −1.5 and a loss of 4% or more of their BMD after 1 year on glucocorticoids should be evaluated for more aggressive therapy.

21. **How should patients under 50 years old be treated for GIOP?**
Premenopausal women and men less than age 50 years who have had a previous fragility fracture and are on prednisone ≥5 mg/day should receive a bisphosphonate regardless of their FRAX score or T-score. Zoledronic acid or teriparatide are the best options for patients who are on higher doses (≥7.5 mg/day), longer duration (≥3 months), and have the worst T-scores (below −2.5). Therapeutic guidelines for premenopausal women with childbearing potential who have had a previous fragility fracture recommend a bisphosphonate only if taking ≥7.5 mg/day. Oral risedronate theoretically may be the safest in this circumstance because of its potentially reduced fetal toxicity should the patient become pregnant. Teriparatide is an alternative option.

22. **Are there any guidelines for patients on intermittent pulses of intravenous glucocorticoids? How about inhaled steroids?**
Therapeutic guidelines for prevention and treatment of GIOP in patients receiving intermittent pulse glucocorticoids without daily therapy are lacking. Patients receiving four or more monthly intravenous pulses (1 g methylprednisolone equivalent) or high-dose oral pulses (prednisone ≥60 mg/day with tapering over 2 to 4 weeks) within a 12-month period are at risk and should be treated based on the risk stratification outlined above. Patients on daily inhaled steroids (equivalent or higher dose than Advair 200 μg/day) for a prolonged period of time (20 years) can lose bone (one T-score = 12% bone loss) and should be periodically monitored.

23. **Describe vitamin D metabolism and action.**
There are two natural forms of vitamin D: cholecalciferol (D3) and ergocalciferol (D2). Humans acquire vitamin D by two routes: endogenous synthesis in the skin during sunlight exposure (D3) and dietary intake (D2 and D3). Vitamin D from either source is converted in the liver by 25-hydroxylase to 25-OH vitamin D and fluticasone propionate - salmeterol xinafoate (Advair) then by 1-alpha-hydroxylase in the kidney to 1,25-dihydroxy $(OH)_2$ vitamin D. The latter binds to intestinal vitamin D receptors to promote calcium and phosphorous absorption. Parathyroid hormone (PTH) and hypophosphatemia are major inducers of 1-alpha-hydroxylase activity. As a patient becomes vitamin D deficient and serum calcium decreases, the PTH level increases inducing the 1-alpha-hydroxylase enzyme to convert 25-OH vitamin D into 1,25 $(OH)_2$ vitamin D. Therefore, the 25-OH vitamin D level will decrease before the 1,25 $(OH)_2$ vitamin D level. **For this reason, measuring the 25-OH vitamin D level is the best measure of vitamin D stores.**

24. **What causes osteomalacia?**
Osteomalacia, which means "soft bones," results from impaired mineralization of bone matrix as a result of inadequate concentrations of serum phosphate and/or calcium or from a circulating inhibitor of mineralization.

Box 52-1. Major Causes of Osteomalacia

Vitamin D deficiency	Hypophosphatemia
Low oral intake plus inadequate sunlight exposure	Low oral phosphate intake
Intestinal malabsorption	Phosphate-binding antacids
Abnormal vitamin D metabolism	Excess renal phosphate loss
Liver disease	Inhibitors of mineralization
Renal disease	Aluminum
Drugs (anticonvulsants, antituberculous drugs, ketoconazole)	Bisphosphonates
	Fluoride
	Hypophosphatasia

25. **Describe the clinical manifestations of osteomalacia and rickets.**
Osteomalacia/rickets causes pain and deformity in the long bones and pelvis. Laboratory features of those with osteomalacia resulting from vitamin D deficiency include low or low/normal serum calcium and phosphate levels, low 25-OH vitamin D levels, elevated serum alkaline phosphatase, elevated PTH levels, and low 24-hour urinary calcium excretion. Laboratory features of those with osteomalacia caused by renal phosphate wasting (familial hypophosphatemic rickets/adult-onset vitamin D-resistant osteomalacia and oncogenic osteomalacia) include low serum phosphate, high serum alkaline phosphatase, high urinary phosphate (low tubular reabsorption of phosphate), and inappropriately normal or low 1,25 $(OH)_2$ vitamin D for the degree of hypophosphatemia. In adults, radiographs may show characteristic pseudofractures (milkman's fractures, Looser's zones) where large arteries cross bones; in children, radiographs may show changes consistent with, rickets (see Question 27). Bone biopsies show increased osteoid seams but with reduced hydroxyapatite deposition.

26. **What causes rickets?**
Rickets results from impaired skeletal mineralization during childhood. It has the same etiologies as osteomalacia in adults in addition to three congenital disorders:
1. Hypophosphatemic rickets: deficient renal tubular phosphate reabsorption results in low serum phosphate levels that are inadequate to promote bone mineralization. This is usually X-linked and associated with the *PHEX* gene. Rarely it can be autosomal dominant and associated with the *FGF-23* gene (encoding fibroblast growth factor 23).

2. Congenital 1-alpha-hydroxylase deficiency: impaired conversion of 25-OH vitamin D into 1,25 (OH)$_2$ vitamin D causes intestinal calcium and phosphate malabsorption.
3. Congenital vitamin D resistance: defective or absent vitamin D receptors result in impaired vitamin D action causing intestinal calcium and phosphate malabsorption.

27. What are the clinical manifestations of rickets?

Clinical features include bone pain, deformities, fractures, muscle weakness, and growth retardation. Laboratory findings are similar to those in osteomalacia. x-rays may show delayed opacification of the epiphyses, widened growth plates, widened and irregular metaphyses, and thin cortices with sparse, coarse trabeculae in the diaphyses. Deformities differ depending on the time of onset (Table 52-1).

Table 52-1.

FIRST YEAR OF LIFE	AFTER FIRST YEAR OF LIFE
Widened cranial sutures	Flared ends of long bones
Frontal bossing	Bowing of long bones
Craniotabes	Sabre shins
Rachitic rosary	Coxa vara
Harrison's groove	Genu varum
Flared wrists	Genu valgum

28. What is oncogenic osteomalacia?

Oncogenic (tumor-induced) osteomalacia is a rare cause of osteomalacia in adults and rickets in children. It is most commonly caused by benign (rarely malignant) mesenchymal or endodermal tumors that secrete FGF-23 and other proteins that can cause hypophosphatemia. Serum FGF-23 can be measured and is a known inhibitor of phosphate transport in the renal tubule and the 1-alpha-hydroxylase enzyme in the kidney resulting in decreased 1,25 (OH)$_2$ vitamin D production. Patients present with myalgias and bone pain as a result of osteomalacia. Laboratory features include low serum phosphate, high serum alkaline phosphatase, high urinary phosphate, high FGF-23 level, and low 1,25 (OH)$_2$ vitamin D. The tumors tend to be small and best localized by gallium-68-1,4,7,10-tetraazacyclododecane-N,N',N'',N'''-tetraacetic acid-octreotate (gallium-68-DOTA-octreotate) positron emission tomography (PET) scanning. Surgical removal of the tumor is curative.

29. How are osteomalacia and rickets treated? (Table 52-2)

Table 52-2.

ETIOLOGY	TREATMENT
Nutritional vitamin D deficiency	Vitamin D, 5000 U/day until healing, then maintain 1000-2000 U/day
Malabsorption	Vitamin D, 50,000-100,000 U/day
Renal disease	Calcitriol, 0.25-1.0 µg/day
Hypophosphatemic rickets	Calcitriol, 0.25-1.0 µg/day, and oral phosphate
1-Alpha-hydroxylase deficiency	Calcitriol, 0.25-1.0 µg/day, and oral phosphate
Vitamin D resistance	Vitamin D, 100,000-200,000 U/day or calcitriol, 5-60 µg/day, or IV calcium infusions

30. What is hypophosphatasia?

Mutations in the gene for the bone/cartilage isoform of alkaline phosphatase result in deficient or defective enzyme activity causing inability to break down pyrophosphate, an inhibitor of mineralization. Affected patients present with rickets or osteomalacia and low serum alkaline phosphatase levels. The disorder is frequently severe and often fatal. Patients with milder forms may be relatively asymptomatic until adulthood. There is no known effective treatment.

31. **Define osteopetrosis.**
    Osteopetrosis (marble bone disease) results from defective osteoclast function. Mutations have been identified in the following genes: *TCIRG1* (proton pump), *CLCN7* (chloride channel), *CAII* (carbonic anhydrase II), and *gl/gl* (unknown function). Each of these gene abnormalities lead to the inability of osteoclasts to create an acidic environment in the resorption pit under its ruffled border, which is needed for the dissociation of calcium hydroxyapatite from bone matrix. The impaired bone resorption produces dense, chalky, fragile bones and bone marrow replacement. Skeletal x-rays show generalized osteosclerosis. The diagnosis is made by genetic testing. Bone marrow transplantation to provide normal osteoclasts may be needed in severe cases whereas high-dose calcitriol to stimulate osteoclasts can be effective in the milder forms.

BIBLIOGRAPHY

Chong WH, Molinolo AA, Chen CC, et al: Tumor-induced osteomalacia, Endocr Relat Cancer 18:R53–R77, 2011.
Damilakis J, Adams JE, Guglielmi G, et al: Radiation exposure in x-ray-based imaging techniques used in osteoporosis, Eur Radiol 20:2707–2714, 2010.
Drake MT, Murad MH, Mauck KF, et al: Clinical Review. Risk factors for low bone mass-related fractures in men: a systemic review and meta-analysis, J Clin Endo Metab 97:1861–1870, 2012.
Grossman JM, Gordon R, Ranganath VK, et al: American College of Rheumatology 2010 recommendations for the prevention and treatment of glucocorticoid-induced osteoporosis, Arthritis Care Res 62:1515–1526, 2010.
Holick MF: Vitamin D deficiency, N Engl J Med 357:266–281, 2007.
Jones G, Horst R, Carter G, et al: Contemporary diagnosis and treatment of vitamin D related disorders, J Bone Min Res 22:V11–V15, 2007.
Khosla S, Melton LJ: Osteopenia, N Engl J Med 356:2293–2300, 2007.
Liewiecki EM: In the clinic. Osteoporosis, Ann Int Med 155: ITC, 1–15, 2011.
Lindsay R, Silverman SL, Cooper C, et al: Risk of new vertebral fracture in the year following a fracture, JAMA 285:320–323, 2001.
Lips P, van Schoor NM, Bravenboer N: Vitamin D-related disorders. In Rosen CJ, editor: Primer on the metabolic bone diseases and disorders of mineral metabolism, ed 7, Washington DC, 2008, American Society for Bone and Mineral Research.
Lorente-Ramos R, Azpeitia-Armán J, Muñoz-Hernández A, et al: Dual-energy x-ray absorptiometry in the diagnosis of osteoporosis: a practical guide, AJR Am J Roentgenol 196:897–904, 2011.
Marini JC: Osteogenesis imperfecta. In Rosen CJ, editor: Primer on the metabolic bone diseases and disorders of mineral metabolism, ed 7, Washington DC, 2008, American Society for Bone and Mineral Research.
McCloskey E, Kanis JA: FRAX updates 2012, Curr Opin Rheumatol 24:554–560, 2012.
Mittan D, Lee S, Miller E, et al: Bone loss following hypogonadism in men with prostate cancer treated with GnRH analogs, J Clin Endocrinol Metab 87:3656–3661, 2002.
Painter SE, Kleerekoper M, Camacho PM: Secondary osteoporosis: a review of the recent evidence, Endocr Pract 12:436–445, 2006.
Ruppe MD, Jan de Beur SM: Disorders of phosphate homeostasis. In Rosen CJ, editor: Primer on the metabolic bone diseases and disorders of mineral metabolism, ed 7, Washington DC, 2008, American Society for Bone and Mineral Research.
Ryan CS, Pefkov VI, Adler RA: Osteoporosis in men: the value of laboratory testing, Osteoporosis Int 22:1845–1853, 2011.
Targownik LE, Lix LM, Tetge CJ, et al: Use of proton pump inhibitors and risk of osteoporosis-related fractures, CMAJ 179:319–326, 2008.
Tolar J, Teitelbaum SL, Orchard PJ: Osteopetrosis, N Engl J Med 351:2839–2848, 2004.
Weinstein RS: Clinical Practice. Glucocorticoid-induced bone disease, New Engl J Med 365:62–70, 2011.
Whyte MP: Enzyme defects and the skeleton. In Rosen CJ, editor: Primer on the metabolic bone diseases and disorders of mineral metabolism, ed 7, Washington DC, 2008, American Society for Bone and Mineral Research.
Whyte MP: Sclerosing disorders of bone. In Rosen CJ, editor: Primer on the metabolic bone diseases and disorders of mineral metabolism, ed 7, Washington DC, 2008, American Society for Bone and Mineral Research.

FURTHER READING

The National Osteoporosis Foundation: www.nof.org
NIH Osteoporosis and Related Bone Diseases – National Resource Center: www.osteo.org
American Society for Bone and Mineral Research: www.asbmr.org
The International Society for Clinical Densitometry: www.iscd.org

CHAPTER 53

PAGET'S DISEASE OF BONE
David R. Finger, MD

KEY POINTS

1. Paget's disease of bone is an osteoclastic disease of unknown etiology resulting in abnormal bone remodeling and deformity.
2. Paget's disease can be mono- or polyostotic with a predilection for pelvis, spine, femur, skull, tibia, and humerus resulting in pain, deformity, nerve compression, fracture, and rarely sarcomas.
3. Intravenous bisphosphonate therapy is the most effective therapy.

1. **What is Paget's disease?**
   Although evidence supports the existence of this disease in prehistoric times, it was not until 1877 that Sir James Paget first described chronic inflammation of bone, using the term **osteitis deformans**. Paget's disease is a disorder of bone remodeling, with increased osteoclast-mediated bone resorption followed by increased bone formation. This process leads to a disorganized, mosaic pattern of woven and lamellar bone often associated with increased vascularity, marrow fibrosis, and mechanical weakness.

2. **Who gets Paget's disease?**
   Paget's disease affects all races. This disease is rare in the Far East, India, Africa, and the Middle East and more common in whites of northern European ancestry. It appears to be more common in England, with a prevalence of 5% compared to 1% to 3% in the United States. Men have a slightly higher risk (2:1) than women.

3. **How frequently does this disease occur?**
   The incidence increases with age, occurring in 2% to 3% of patients over age 50 to 55 years and in up to 10% of persons older than 80 years. It is uncommon in people less than age 40 years. There is a juvenile form of Paget's disease, which is very different from the adult form in that it is more widespread and has different histologic and radiologic features.

4. **What is the evidence that Paget's disease is genetic?**
   Paget's disease may be a genetic disorder that is autosomal dominant with incomplete penetrance affected by aging and the environment. It occurs seven times more often in relatives of patients than in controls. This risk is further increased if the affected relative has severe disease or was diagnosed at an early age. A positive family history is reported in 10% to 40% of patients. Investigators have described a mutation in the ubiquitin binding region of the gene sequestosome I (*SQSTM1*) on chromosome 5q in up to 46% of patients with familial Paget's and 16% of patients with sporadic Paget's. This encodes a 62-kilodalton protein that is implicated in the signal pathways (nuclear factor-kappa-B [NFκB], autophagy) mediating osteoclastogenesis. Other genetic loci have been described.

5. **Do we know what triggers the onset of Paget's disease?**
   Many investigators suspect a viral infection, particularly exposure to the RNA paramyxoviruses (measles, respiratory syncytial, and canine distemper). Pagetic osteoclasts have been shown to contain intranuclear inclusions resembling nucleocapsids of the Paramyxoviridae family. Studies have linked canine distemper virus to Paget's disease, noting a threefold higher incidence of Paget's disease in owners of unvaccinated dogs compared with owners whose dogs are vaccinated.

6. **Describe the clinical features of this disease.**
   Only 10% to 30% of patients are symptomatic. **Bone pain** is the most common symptom (80%), followed by **joint pain** (50%) resulting from secondary osteoarthritis usually involving the knee, hip, or spine. Affected areas may feel **warm** to palpation as a result of increased blood flow. **Bone deformities**, such as tibial bowing and skull thickening, may occur in advanced cases. **Neurologic complications** can be caused by enlarging bone compressing neural tissue. Spontaneous **fractures**, most commonly in the femur, tibia, humerus, and forearm, may also occur.

7. **Which part of the skeleton is most likely to be involved?**
   Paget's disease can be polyostotic (80%) or monostotic (20%) and has been noted to occur in every bone in the skeleton but has a predilection for the axial skeleton. The most common locations for monostotic disease

include the tibia and iliac bones. Overall, the most common sites (in descending order) include the pelvis, lumbar spine, femur, thoracic spine, sacrum, skull, tibia, and humerus.

8. **List some potential complications of Paget's disease.**
   Skeletal
   Bone pain
   Bone and joint deformities (bowing, frontal bossing)
   Fractures (7% of patients)
   Neurologic
   Deafness (auditory nerve entrapment or involvement of bones of the inner ear) (13%)
   Nerve entrapment (cranial nerves, spinal nerve roots)
   Spinal stenosis
   Basilar invagination
   Headaches, vertigo, tinnitus
   Stroke (blood vessel compression)
   Vascular
   Hyperthermia
   Vascular steal syndrome (external carotid blood flow to the skull at the expense of the brain)
   Cardiac
   High-output congestive heart failure (as a result of increased Pagetic bone vascularity when over 40% of the skeleton is involved)
   Hypertension
   Cardiomegaly
   Angina
   Malignancy
   Osteogenic sarcomas (most commonly in the humerus) (1%)
   Fibrosarcomas, chondrosarcomas
   Benign giant cell tumors
   Metabolic
   Hypercalcemia
   Hypercalcuria
   Nephrocalcinosis

9. **How is Paget's disease usually diagnosed?**
   Asymptomatic patients are usually identified by an elevated alkaline phosphatase obtained on routine chemistry panels or by typical radiographic abnormalities noted on examination for some other complaint.

10. **Which laboratory tests are abnormal in Paget's disease?**
    Paget's is characterized by accelerated bone turnover (up to 20 times normal), with bone resorption and formation occurring simultaneously. Biochemical markers of each have been used in Paget's disease, but the most reproducible is **serum alkaline phosphatase**. These levels are more often extremely elevated in patients with skull involvement and high cardiac output, whereas other bony involvement (pelvis, sacrum, lumbar spine, femoral head) seems to be associated with lower levels. **Bone-specific alkaline phosphatase** is a marker of new **bone formation**. The level correlates with the extent and activity of the disease process and is useful in monitoring the response to bisphosphonate therapy. Markers of **bone resorption** from osteoclast activity are the urinary **N-telopeptide** of type I collagen and the serum alpha-alpha type I **C-telopeptide** fragments, which are elevated in Paget's disease and are the earliest markers to respond to therapy. Serum calcium, phosphorous, and parathyroid hormone (PTH) levels are usually normal although **hypercalcemia** can be seen in the presence of fracture or immobilization. Hyperuricemia and hypercalciuria have been reported in patients with polyostotic disease.

11. **Identify the characteristic radiographic and scintigraphic findings seen in Paget's disease.**
    Paget's can be evaluated both by plain radiography and technetium bone scanning (^{99m}Tc-bisphosphonate); however, there is some discordance. Approximately 12% of the lesions seen on a bone scan will not be seen on a radiograph, and 6% of radiographic abnormalities are absent on bone scanning.
    Plain radiographs reveal osteolytic, osteoblastic, or mixed lesions. Cortical thickening is usually present, along with adjacent trabecular thickening. The edge of lytic fronts extending from the subchondral region in long bones gives a "blade of grass" appearance. Lytic lesions can progress, but usually at a rate of less than 1 cm/year. Significant trabecular thickening of the iliopubic and ilioischial lines may be seen along the inner aspect of the pelvis in a "brim sign" or "pelvic ring" (Figure 53-1). Lytic involvement of the skull is called "osteoporosis circumscripta." This is followed by excessive new bone formation leading to cortical thickening and the "cotton wool" appearance (Figure 53-1). When atraumatic fractures of long bones occur they typically are transverse ("chalk stick") and not spiral, reflecting the weakened bony microarchitecture of Pagetic woven bone. Paget's disease classically produces regions of focal increased uptake on **bone scanning** (Figure 53-1). Scintigraphy is useful for evaluating the extent of disease, response to therapy, and for detecting relapses following treatment. Notably, Paget's disease does not spread to adjacent bones or "metastasize" to distant regions.

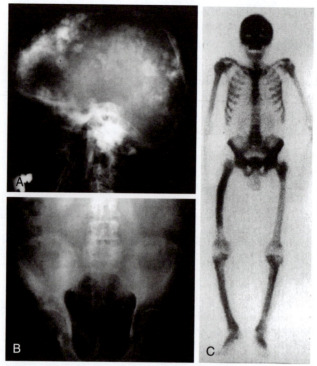

Figure 53-1. The characteristic radiographic and scintigraphic findings seen in Paget's disease. **A**, A skull radiograph showing a thickened cranium with regions of dense sclerosis and osteopenia resulting in a "cotton wool" appearance. **B**, A pelvic radiograph showing right hemipelvic loss of normal trabeculation, sclerosis, and cortical thickening, along with sclerosis of the iliopectineal line. **C**, Full-body scintigraphy showing increased uptake in the skull, pelvis, lumbar spine, bilateral femurs with bowing of the right, tibias, scapula, and bilateral proximal humerus.

12. What is the differential diagnosis of Paget's disease?

Pagetic vertebrae may resemble lymphoma and metastatic cancers, especially adenocarcinoma of the prostate, but Pagetic vertebrae are usually **enlarged**. In other affected bones, Paget's is often distinguished by the characteristic cortical thickening and adjacent thickened trabeculae. The progression of Paget's through different stages (lytic to sclerotic) also helps to differentiate it from osteoblastic metastatic lesions. Focal increased uptake on scintigraphy can be seen in many conditions besides Paget's disease, including osteomyelitis, arthritis, metastases, and fractures.

13. Describe the histopathologic findings seen in Pagetic bone.

Three phases of Paget's disease have been described. **Lytic**: initially there is increased bone resorption, mediated by giant multinucleated (up to 100 nuclei) osteoclasts. **Mixed lytic and blastic**: the osteolytic phase is followed by a compensatory increase in bone formation, associated with accelerated lamellar and woven bone deposition in a disorganized fashion, producing the characteristic mosaic pattern. **Sclerotic**: the areas of resorbed bone are replaced with fibrous tissue, and vascular hypertrophy occurs.

14. What are the indications to treat Paget's disease?

Bone or joint pain
Bone deformity
Bone, joint or neurologic complications
High-output cardiac failure
Preparation for orthopedic surgery (treat for at least 6 weeks before the procedure)
Immobilization hypercalcemia
Young patients
Active asymptomatic disease in sites at high risk for complication:
- Skull (hearing loss, other neurologic)
- Spine (neurologic)
- Lower extremity long bones or areas adjacent to major joints (fracture, osteoarthritis)

Note: because therapy is effective and safe, treatment should be withheld only in asymptomatic patients with disease located only in areas with no risk of complications.

15. What treatments are available for Paget's disease?
Nonsteroidal antiinflammatory drugs (NSAIDs), calcitonin, bisphosphonates, and surgery have all been used successfully. **NSAIDs** are used to treat pain associated with osteoarthritis when Paget's occurs near joints. **Surgery** is sometimes needed to relieve nerve compression and increase joint mobility. Specific antipagetic therapy, however, consists primarily of **calcitonin** and **bisphosphonates**. Bisphosphonates are currently the treatment of choice because they are extremely effective, relatively inexpensive, and well tolerated. **Calcitonin** (injection of 50 to 100 IU daily) is an alternative agent that is typically used when there is extensive lytic disease, severe pain, when a rapid response is desired (neurologic symptoms, high-output heart failure), or when bisphosphonates do not work, are poorly tolerated, or contraindicated (renal disease with creatinine clearance [CrCl] < 30 mL/min).

16. How are bisphosphonates used in the treatment of Paget's disease?
There are several bisphosphonates approved for treatment of Paget's disease. Zoledronate is most effective and clearly superior to intravenous pamidronate. Oral bisphosphonates including alendronate and risedronate are most commonly used. Bisphosphonates work by inhibiting osteoclastic activity, resulting in significant and prolonged inhibition of bone resorption. The vast majority of patients will experience a rapid reduction in symptoms as well as improvement in biochemical markers. Use of oral agents can cause gastric symptoms (ulcerations, esophagitis, dyspepsia) whereas intravenous agents can cause a flu-like illness for 2 to 3 days post infusion consisting of low-grade fever, transient leukopenia, and myalgias/arthralgias (pamidronate, zoledronate). Calcium (1500 mg) and vitamin D (800 IU) should be supplemented daily to prevent the development of secondary hyperparathyroidism and/or hypocalcemia.

17. List the bisphosphonates most commonly used for treating Paget's disease.
The bisphosphonates most commonly used in the treatment of Paget's disease are shown in Table 53-1.

Table 53-1. Bisphosphonates Most Commonly Used in the Treatment of Paget's Disease

DRUG	TRADE NAME	DOSE/TABLET	DOSAGE
Oral			
Alendronate	Fosamax	40 mg	40 mg/day for 6 mo
Risedronate	Actonel	30 mg	30 mg/day for 2 mo
Intravenous			
Pamidronate	Aredia	Vials of 30, 60, 90 mg	30 mg daily for 3 days; retreat if necessary
			60 mg every 2 wk for three doses
			90 mg/week for 2 wk
Zoledronic acid	Reclast	5 mg in 100 mL	5 mg infused over 15-30 min as one dose

18. How can you tell if a patient's pain is attributable to Paget's disease of bone or secondary osteoarthritis?
In patients with Paget's who have joint involvement, bone pain from Paget's usually responds to bisphosphonate therapy (especially intravenous) but secondary osteoarthritis will not respond. Alternatively, an injection of lidocaine into the affected joint (usually the hip) will transiently eliminate pain resulting from osteoarthritis but not Paget's disease.

19. How do you follow a patient who has been treated for Paget's?
Symptomatic patients should be monitored every 3 to 6 months for changes in symptoms. Disease activity can be effectively monitored by measurement of serum alkaline phosphatase and urinary N-telopeptide or serum C-telopeptide. Failure to normalize these markers results in development of new complications of Paget's in 60% to 70% of patients despite a favorable effect on pain. Therefore, therapy should be aimed at normalizing these markers, which usually occurs several months after the end of therapy. Recurrence of biochemical markers 20% to 30% above the upper limit of normal may justify retreatment although a recent trial supported retreatment only with recurrence of symptoms. Some patients may develop resistance to the bisphosphonate therapy they are on. This can be overcome by switching to another bisphosphonate. Patients with osteolytic lesions should have annual radiographs to document healing. Patients with increased localized pain should be evaluated for malignant transformation or fracture.

Bibliography

Mankin HJ, Hornicek FJ: Paget's sarcoma: a historical and outcome review, Clin Orthop Relat Res 438:97–102, 2005.

Merlotti D, et al: Comparison of different intravenous bisphosphonate regimens for Paget's disease of bone, J Bone Miner Res 22:1510–1517, 2007.

Langston AL, et al: Randomized trial of intensive bisphosphonate treatment versus symptomatic management in Paget's disease of bone, J Bone Miner Res 25:20–31, 2010.

Reid IR, et al: A single infusion of zoledronic acid produces sustained remissions in Paget disease: data to 6.5 years, J Bone Miner Res 26:2261–2270, 2011.

Rhodes EC, et al: Sequestosome 1 (SQSTM1) mutations in Paget's disease of bone from the United States, Calcif Tissue Int 82:271–277, 2008.

Seton M: Diagnosis, complications, and treatment of Paget's disease of bone, Aging Health 5:497–508, 2009.

Seton M, et al: Analysis of environmental factors in familial versus sporadic Paget's disease of bone. The New England Registry for Paget's Disease of Bone, J Bone Miner Res 18:1519–1524, 2003.

Siris ES, Roodman GD: Paget's disease of bone. In Rosen CJ, editor: Primer on the metabolic bone diseases and disorders of mineral metabolism, ed 7, Washington DC, 2008, American Society for Bone and Mineral Research.

Further Reading

www.nlm.nih.gov/medlineplus/pagetsdiseaseofbone.html

OSTEONECROSIS
Robert T. Spencer, MD

KEY POINTS
1. Osteonecrosis (ON) most commonly involves the femoral head.
2. The most common risk factors for ON are glucocorticoid (GC) use and alcohol abuse.
3. Nonoperative therapy for early disease include protected weight-bearing, bisphosphonates, statins, and anticoagulants.
4. Operative therapy includes core decompression with or without grafting and total joint replacement.

1. **List some synonyms for ON.**
   Avascular necrosis (AVN), aseptic necrosis, and ischemic necrosis.

2. **How is ON defined?**
   ON refers to death of the cellular component of bone (osteocytes) and contiguous bone marrow resulting from ischemia. Although inciting factors for such ischemia are varied, their end results are clinically indistinguishable.

3. **What skeletal regions are predisposed to developing ON?**
   Bones are most vulnerable in those areas having both limited vascular supply and restricted collateral circulation, which are areas that are also typically covered by articular cartilage. The area most frequently affected is the **femoral head**. At risk areas include: femoral head, carpal bones (scaphoid, lunate), humeral head, talus, femoral condyles, tarsal navicular, proximal tibia, and metatarsals.

4. **Name some other common spontaneous ON syndromes.**
   - Scaphoid (Preiser's disease)
   - Lunate (Kienböck's disease)
   - Basal phalanges (Thiemann's disease)
   - Capitulum of humerus (Panner's disease)
   - Vertebral body (Kummell's disease)
   - Femoral epiphysis (Legg–Calvé–Perthes)
   - Tarsal navicular (Köhler's disease)
   - Second metatarsal head (Freiberg's disease)

5. **What is the etiology of this disorder?**
   The etiology of ON is most obvious and best understood in posttraumatic disruption of the arterial blood supply. Fractures of the femoral neck have been associated with ON in 15% of nondisplaced and 25% to 50% of displaced fractures. Hip dislocation causes ON in 10% to 25% of cases.
   In ON cases that develop in the absence of trauma, various pathologic processes are capable of inducing hemostasis and, in turn, ischemia. Potential mechanisms include:
   - occlusion of blood vessels from sickled red blood cells, thrombophilia/coagulation disorders, and fat emboli (long bone fractures, fatty liver, hyperlipidemia);
   - bone marrow hypertrophy/infiltration and increased pressure in the bony compartment that compromises blood flow can occur in Gaucher's, leukemia, myeloproliferative disorders, and corticosteroids (fat hypertrophy);
   - bone marrow cellular toxicity and death as a result of external factors such as radiation, chemotherapy, and thermal injury.

6. **What clinical conditions are associated with ON?**
   The conditions associated with ON are shown in Box 54-1.

7. **Briefly describe the pathogenesis of ON and the resulting symptoms.**
   Etiologic factors initiate hemostasis directly or trigger a cascade resulting in hemostasis. Histologic findings indicate that the final common pathway for the various inciting factors involves local intravascular coagulation and resultant tissue ischemia. The end result is that of cancellous bone and bone marrow death. With subchondral cancellous bone death, collapse of the articular surface may or may not occur, depending on the extent of involvement.

> **Box 54-1.** Conditions Associated With Osteonecrosis (ON)
>
> **Nontraumatic**
> *Juvenile*
> Slipped capital femoral epiphysis
> Legg–Calvé–Perthes
>
> *Adult*
> Corticosteroid administration (Cushing's disease)
> Alcohol abuse
> Sickle cell anemia
> Hemoglobinopathies (thalassemia, hemoglobin C disease [Hgb C])
> Dysbaric ON
> Gaucher's disease/Fabry's disease
> Radiotherapy/chemotherapy
> Cushing's disease
> Diabetes mellitus
> Hyperlipidemia
> Hypercoagulable states/thrombophilia/disseminated intravascular coagulation (DIC)
> Pancreatitis
> Pregnancy
> Oral contraceptive use
> Systemic lupus erythematosus (SLE), primary antiphospholipid syndrome (PAPS), and other connective tissue disorders
> Organ transplantation
> Fat embolism
> Severe acute respiratory syndrome (SARS)
> Carbon tetrachloride/lead poisoning
> Tumor infiltration of marrow
> Arteriosclerosis/vaso-occlusive disorders
> Others: human immunodeficiency virus (HIV)/highly active antiretroviral therapy (HAART), smoking, idiopathic
>
> **Traumatic**
> Fracture of the femoral neck
> Dislocation or fracture/dislocation of the hip
> Hip trauma without fracture or dislocation
> Hip surgery

Pain, the earliest symptom of ON, may occur in the early stages of involvement, before any radiographic changes are noted. This pain is likely to be the result of elevated intraosseous pressure, because such pain can be relieved by decompression. In some individuals, no symptoms develop until the late stages of the disease process when collapse of the articular surface occurs and secondary degenerative changes develop. Others, in whom the area of infarction is small enough that collapse does not occur, may never develop symptoms. Radiographs in these patients reveal sclerotic areas often referred to as "bone islands" or "bone infarcts."

8. **What are the epidemiologic features of ON?**
   - An estimated 10,000 to 30,000 new cases develop each year in the United States. Femoral head ON accounts for 10% of all total hip arthroplasties.
   - In cases of nontraumatic ON, corticosteroid use and alcohol abuse may be responsible for 50% to 70% of cases; in up to 10% to 15% of cases, there is no identifiable risk factor (idiopathic).
   - Males are affected more frequently than females at a ratio of approximately 8:1, possibly reflecting a higher incidence of trauma in males.
   - Most cases develop in the <50-year-old age group. One exception to this observation is seen in ON of the knee (femoral condyles, proximal tibia), to which women over the age of 50 years are predisposed (female:male ratio of approximately 3:1).

9. **What clinical features would lead to suspicion of this disorder?**
   The signs and symptoms stemming from ON are nonspecific. **Pain** is what leads affected individuals to seek medical evaluation. For the hip, the joint most commonly involved, pain is unilateral at onset and localizes to the groin, buttock, medial thigh, and medial aspect of the knee. Pain occurs with weight-bearing but can be present at rest (66%) and at night (33%) as a result of elevated intraosseous pressure. Occasionally, knee pain is the major complaint in an individual with late-stage ON of the hip. Typically, morning stiffness is absent or of short duration (<1 hour), allowing differentiation from inflammatory monoarticular arthritides. Range of motion is not affected, except as limited by discomfort, until late degenerative changes develop. Although

these findings are common to other potential etiologies, their occurrence in the setting of a patient with a predisposing risk (e.g., recent trauma, high-dose steroid use) should suggest underlying ON.

10. **How much corticosteroid puts a patient at risk for ON?**
    Overall, 10% to 30% of patients on GCs develop ON. A previous review estimated a 4.6-fold increase in the rate of ON for every 10 mg/day increase in the mean daily dose of prednisone during the first 6 months of therapy. More recent reports suggest that the risk of ON is increased in patients who are on greater than 20 mg/day of prednisone for over a month or receive >2 g total over 2 to 3 months. **The risk of ON increases by 5% for every 20-mg increase in prednisone dose.** Although controversial, high-dose pulse corticosteroids alone (i.e., 1 g methylprednisolone monthly) does not increase risk unless followed by high-dose daily oral prednisone. Patients who smoke or have systemic lupus erythematosus (SLE), antiphospholipid antibodies, or rapidly develop profound Cushingoid features are particularly likely to develop ON.

11. **How do corticosteroids cause ON?**
    Glucocorticoids (GCs) cause ON by both direct and indirect effects on cells. Direct effects include increased apoptosis of osteoblasts, osteocytes, and endothelial cells. Indirect effects include increased hypercoagulability, decreased angiogenesis, and modulated local vasoactive amine production, which can contribute to the ischemia. Finally, increased intraosseous pressure as a result of adipogenesis and fat hypertrophy in the bone marrow can decrease blood flow to the area. However, because all patients who receive steroids do not get ON, genetic factors are thought to play a role. Genetic differences in the affinity of GCs to bind to their receptors as well as the speed of metabolism of GCs to their inactive forms at the local tissue level may account for why less than half of GC-treated patients get ON.

12. **How much alcohol intake does it take to be at risk for ON?**
    Overall, 2% to 5% of alcohol abusers will develop ON. It is estimated that a total of 150 L of 100% alcohol at a rate of 400 mL/week (i.e., one pint/week) increases the risk 9.8-fold for developing ON. The risk of ON increases with the amount of alcohol consumed weekly: threefold if <400 mL/week, tenfold if 400 to 1000 mL/week, and eighteenfold if >1000 mL/week. Susceptibility may be partly determined by genetics. Certain polymorphisms of alcohol-metabolizing enzymes may contribute to ON risk. Smoking also increases the risk.

13. **What is the suspected cause of idiopathic ON?**
    ON without an identifiable cause accounts for 10% to 15% of all cases. Extensive analysis supports that many of these patients may have a hypercoagulable state as evidenced by elevated lipoprotein(a), low tissue plasminogen activator activity, and/or high plasminogen activator inhibitor levels. Others have been found to have high homocysteine levels, elevated antiphospholipid antibodies, low protein C or protein S levels, or the presence of Factor V Leiden.

14. **Are there any other medications that are associated with ON?**
    Recently, **protease inhibitors**, used to treat human immunodeficiency virus (HIV) infections, have been implicated in causing ON. These medications have caused lipodystrophy, diabetes mellitus, hyperlipidemia, and hypercoagulability. Hyperlipidemia and hypercoagulable states may lead to ON. **Bisphosphonates** have been associated with ON of the jaw.

15. **What is SONK?**
    Spontaneous osteonecrosis of the knee (SONK) is an idiopathic form of ON that affects primarily women (female:male = 3:1) over the age of 50 years. Patients present with knee pain. Magnetic resonance imaging (MRI) shows lesions that tend to be small on the medial more often than the lateral femoral condyle.

16. **What is the role of plain radiographs in the diagnosis of ON?**
    Initially, plain films are normal. Later, a region of generalized osteopenia may develop (a nonspecific finding). Eventually, after bone repair mechanisms have had time to work, a mottled appearance develops in the affected area as a result of the presence of "cysts" (regions of dead bone resorption) and contiguous sclerosis (regions of bone repair).
    Early collapse of the cancellous bone beneath the subchondral plate is apparent as a pathognomonic radiolucent line frequently referred to as the **crescent sign** (Figure 54-1). Once in this stage, further collapse is almost inevitable, and it thus represents the earliest irreversible lesion of ON. Once the articular surface has collapsed and flattened, secondary degenerative changes develop, resulting in joint-space narrowing and secondary involvement of other bones within the articulation (e.g., acetabulum).

17. **How good is MRI in the diagnosis of ON? What about other imaging studies?**
    Compared with other diagnostic studies, MRI has been found to have the highest sensitivity and best diagnostic accuracy, thus obviating invasive diagnostic procedures such as biopsy and bone marrow pressure determinations. Sensitivity and diagnostic accuracy appear to be 95% to 99%. The characteristic MRI finding is an area or **line of decreased signal** on both T1 and T2 images (Figure 54-2). This area appears to correspond with the demarcation between live regenerating bone and necrotic tissue. In patients who cannot undergo an MRI, **radionuclide bone scanning** can show a subchondral "cold spot" (avascular necrosis) surrounded by a

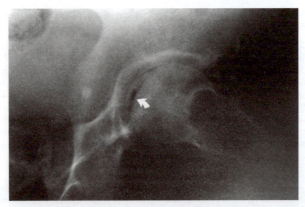

Figure 54-1. A plain radiograph of the hip showing the crescent sign (*arrow*) of osteonecrosis (ON).

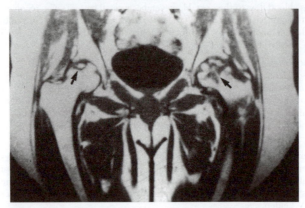

Figure 54-2. Magnetic resonance imaging (MRI) of bilateral hips showing necrotic bone (*arrows*) in both femoral heads consistent with osteonecrosis (ON).

"hot" area (donut sign) where there is increased osteoblastic activity at the interface with the necrotic bone. A **computed tomography (CT) scan** will show necrotic and reactive bone.

18. **How often does ON occur in a bilateral fashion?**
Approximately 50% of patients with symptomatic hip ON have asymptomatic disease in the contralateral hip at the time of initial presentation. Two thirds of these asymptomatic hips will eventually progress to late-stage ON. Consequently, bilateral hip MRI at time of presentation is recommended. Similar frequencies would be expected in ON of humeral head and knee. It is not uncommon to have multiple bony areas involved.

19. **Describe the staging scheme for ON of the femoral head. (Table 54-1)**

20. **Describe the medical management of ON.**
The goal in treating ON is to prevent bony collapse and subsequent deformity. Thus, effective treatment is contingent upon diagnosis while ON is still in its early stages (stage II and less). Recommended medical management is limited to having the patient **discontinue weight-bearing** on the affected side for 4 to 8 weeks and administering **analgesics** for relief of associated pain. Unfortunately, hip survival rates with nonoperative management are only in the 13% to 35% range for stage I to IV disease. Therefore, nonsurgical management does not change the natural course of the disease. Recently there have been promising reports with pharmacologic therapies including lipid-lowering drugs, bisphosphonates, and anticoagulants, which should be considered. Hyperbaric oxygen, pulsed electromagnetic field therapy, and extracorporeal shock therapy are being investigated. The best results with any of these therapies are achieved in patients where the area of involvement of the femoral head is ≤15% and not involving the weight-bearing surface.

21. **Describe the surgical management for this disorder.**
In **early, reversible stages** of ON, several surgical procedures have been developed with the aim of preventing progression. Of these, **core decompression** of the femoral head has been most commonly performed and investigated. The rationale for this operation is that if increased intraosseous pressure can be relieved, vascular

Table 54-1. University of Pennsylvania (Steinberg) System of Staging of Osteonecrosis (ON) of the Femoral Head

STAGE	PLAIN RADIOGRAPHIC FINDINGS	MRI*
0†	Normal	Normal
I	Normal	Abnormal
II	Osteopenia, bony sclerosis, cystic changes	Abnormal
III	Subchondral collapse ("crescent sign") without articular surface flattening	Abnormal
IV	Flattening of the articular surface without joint-space narrowing	Abnormal
V	Flattening of the articular surface with joint-space narrowing and/or acetabular involvement	Abnormal
VI	Advanced degenerative changes	Abnormal

*Each stage is further divided into three subclasses: A = small (<15% femoral head involvement, <2 mm depression of femoral head); B = moderate (15% to 30%, 2 to 4 mm); C = large (>30%, >4 mm) depending on the size of the lesion on magnetic resonance imaging (MRI).
†Stage 0 refers to an "at risk" asymptomatic, uninvolved hip in an individual with avascular necrosis (AVN) on the contralateral side.

perfusion can then be enhanced and help prevent progression of the lesion. Several studies comparing core decompression to nonoperative management have shown favorable results, with success rates in the range of 47% to 84% for stage I to III disease. Core decompression has also shown some benefit when used to treat knee and humerus ON. **Vascularized fibula grafting** into the femoral head has been shown in several studies to be extremely promising, with 5-year hip survival rates of 81% to 89% for stage II to IV disease. However, there is a high complication rate (19%) so this procedure is a consideration only in medical communities in which a skilled surgeon with experience in this technique is available. In general, lesions smaller than 30% of the femoral head have the best results. Initial studies using **autologous mesenchymal stem cells** inserted into the femoral head after core decompression have shown encouraging results.

In the **nonreversible stages** of ON (particularly stages V to VI), the goal of surgical intervention is to restore joint function and relieve associated pain. The effectiveness and reliability of **total hip arthroplasty** (replacement) have made earlier procedures attempting to achieve these goals obsolete.

22. **Can ON be prevented?**
Yes, to some degree. Modifiable risk factors can be manipulated—e.g., steroid dose, alcohol intake, and control of diabetes and hyperlipidemia. As an example, the vast majority of cases of corticosteroid-related ON occur in patients who have received the equivalent of ≥20 mg of prednisone/day, especially for prolonged periods. In rheumatoid arthritis (RA), where prednisone doses rarely exceed 10 mg/day, ON is uncommon. By contrast, in SLE, in which higher doses of steroids are frequently used, 30% to 50% of patients may develop some degree of ON. Early use of lipid-lowering drugs, bisphosphonates, antioxidants (vitamin E), and anticoagulants may be preventative.

23. **What is bone marrow edema syndrome (BMES)?**
BMES, also known as **transient osteoporosis of the hip**, is a self-limited transitory clinical entity characterized by hip pain, osteopenia on radiographs, and bone marrow edema of femoral head and neck on MRI. This disorder typically affects women in the third trimester of pregnancy and middle-aged men. Usually one hip is involved, but 40% to 80% can have bilateral involvement or involvement of other joints (knee, ankle, etc.). Symptoms last an average of 6 months. Up to 40% can have recurrences. Treatment is with analgesics and protective weight-bearing. Intravenous bisphosphonates have been used with success and should be considered. Core decompression is not indicated. **BMES differs from ON on MRI because it has both femoral head and neck abnormalities whereas ON only involves the femoral head.**

BIBLIOGRAPHY

Bonfonti P, Gabbut A, Carradori S, et al: Osteonecrosis in protease inhibitor-treated patients, Orthopedics 24:271–272, 2001.
Felson DT, Anderson JJ: A cross-study evaluation of association between steroid dose and bolus steroids and avascular necrosis of bone, Lancet 1:902–906, 1987.
Glueck CJ, Freiberg RA, Sieve L, et al: Enoxaparin prevents progression of stages I and II osteonecrosis of the hip, Clin Orthop Relat Res 435:164–170, 2005.
Glueck CJ, Freiberg R, Tracy T, et al: Thrombophilia and hypofibrinolysis: pathophysiologies of osteonecrosis, Clin Orthop Rel Res 334:43–56, 1997.
Hamilton TW, Goodman SM, Figgie M: SAS weekly rounds: avascular necrosis, HSS J 5:99–113, 2009.
Kerachian MA, Seguin C, Harvey EJ: Glucocorticoids in osteonecrosis of the femoral head: a new understanding of the mechanism of action, J Steroid Biochem Mol Biol 114:121–128, 2009.

Lai KA, Shen WJ, Yang CY, et al: The use of alendronate to prevent early collapse of the femoral head in patients with nontraumatic osteonecrosis. A randomized clinical study, J Bone Joint Surg Am 87:2155–2159, 2005.
Mont MA, Carbone JJ, Fairbank AC: Core decompression versus nonoperative management for osteonecrosis of the hip, Clin Orthop 324:169–178, 1996.
Mont MA, Marker DR, Zywiel MG, et al: Osteonecrosis of the knee and related conditions, J Am Acad Ortho Surg 19: 482–494, 2011.
Papadopoulos EC, Papagelopoulos PJ, Boscainos PJ, et al: Bone marrow edema syndrome, Orthopedics 24:69–73, 2001.
Pritchett JW: Statin therapy decreases risk of osteonecrosis in patients receiving steroids, Clin Orthop Relat Res 386:173–178, 2001.
Rajpura A, Wright AC, Board TN: Medical management of osteonecrosis of the hip: a review, Hip Int 21:385–392, 2011.
Shigemura T, Nakamura J, Kishida S, et al: Incidence of osteonecrosis associated with corticosteroid therapy among different underlying diseases: prospective MRI study, Rheumatology 50:2023–2028, 2011.
Urbaniak JR, Harvey EJ: Revascularization of the femoral head in osteonecrosis, J Am Acad Ortho Surg 6:44–54, 1998.
Zalavras CG, Lieberman JR: Osteonecrosis of the femoral head: Evaluation and treatment, J Am Acad Ortho Surg 22:455–464, 2014.

Further Reading

http://www.orthoinfo.aaos.org

IX
HEREDITARY, CONGENITAL, AND INBORN ERRORS OF METABOLISM ASSOCIATED WITH RHEUMATIC SYNDROMES

The law of heredity is that all undesirable traits come from the other parent.
Anonymous

HERITABLE CONNECTIVE TISSUE DISEASES

John K. Jenkins, MD

CHAPTER 55

> **KEY POINTS**
> 1. Osteogenesis imperfecta (OI) is a genetic defect of collagen type I that causes brittle bones, blue sclera, and abnormal teeth.
> 2. Ehlers–Danlos syndrome (EDS) is a genetic defect of multiple extracellular matrix (ECM) proteins causing joint hypermobility, skin hyperelasticity, and fragile blood vessel walls.
> 3. Marfan syndrome is a genetic defect of fibrillin-1 leading to marfanoid habitus, aortic root dilatation, and an ectopic lens.

1. **Discuss the characteristics of the heritable connective tissue diseases (HCTDs).**
   HCTDs are a heterogeneous group of disorders that result from genetic defects that alter the quantity or structure of ECM proteins including collagens, fibrillins, elastin, and noncollagenous matrix proteins (tenascin, fibronectin, proteoglycans in the interstitial space and integrins on cell surfaces). Depending on the ECM protein involved, the tissues most likely to be affected can be predicted, including bone, cartilage, tendon, ligament, muscle, skin, eye, heart valves, blood vessels, and lung. There are over 300 well-characterized HCTDs. Although each is relatively rare, as a group they affect 1 in 5000 individuals. This chapter discusses only the most common of these disorders.

2. **What is the classification of the HCTDs?**
   Several different classifications have been proposed. One classification is by the main collagenous structural property that is altered:
   - **Tensile HCTDs** affect primarily type I or other (III, V) collagens, ECM proteins associated with these collagens, or elastin, all of which are important for the strength of bone, ligaments, tendons, skin, heart valves, and blood vessels. The disorders include OI (collagen type I defect), EDS (collagen type I, III, or V defects; fibronectin defects, or enzyme deficiency), Marfan syndrome (fibrillin-1 defect), congenital contractural arachnodactyly (fibrillin-2 defect), pseudoxanthoma elasticum, cutis laxis, and supravalvular aortic stenosis (William syndrome caused by an elastin gene defect).
   - **Compressive HCTDs** affect multiple collagens and/or ECM proteins important for compression of cartilage and growth. Gene discovery has defined over 100 genes with various defects leading to abnormal collagens (types II, IX, X, and XI), ECM proteins, defects in metabolic pathways (enzymes), and defects in signal transduction and receptors, among others. The disorders include achondroplasias, epiphyseal chondrodysplasias (Stickler syndrome, spondyloepiphyseal dysplasia, multiple epiphyseal dysplasia), and metaphyseal chondrodysplasias, among others.
   - **Barrier HCTDs** affect type IV collagen (Alport syndrome) and type VII collagen (epidermolysis bullosa), which form barriers known as basement membranes.

TENSILE HEREDITARY CONNECTIVE TISSUE DISEASES

1. **What is osteogenesis imperfecta? What organs are involved and why?**
   OI, also known as brittle bone disease, is actually a group of diseases defined by similar clinical manifestations (brittle bones and blue sclerae) occurring to various degrees with a similar etiology. OI affects 1 in 20,000 individuals. The inheritance pattern and penetrance are variable. Most cases involve autosomal dominant (AD) inheritance, although 35% involve sporadic mutations. Most patients with OI have an AD defect in one of the genes encoding type I collagen (*COL1A1*, *COL1A2*), which is necessary for the structure and physical properties of bone. The genetic defect causes low production (50% of normal) of type I collagen, which results in osteopenia and brittleness, leading to frequent fractures. Diminished type I collagen in the sclerae leads to translucency and apparent blueness, and causes dentinogenesis imperfecta (opalescent teeth). Hearing loss can also occur.
   Clinical syndromes of brittle bone disease are variable. Affected individuals may experience in utero death from fractures, a live birth with wormian bones, short stature, and multiple fractures, or a live birth with mildly brittle bones and normal stature. The most severe forms of OI typically involve spontaneous mutations

or autosomal recessive (AR) genetic defects affecting other proteins or enzymes that regulate type I collagen folding, resulting in a more severe phenotype, whereas the milder presentations are AD defects of one of the COL1A genes described above.

2. What is the Sillence classification of OI?

The original Sillence classification grouped OI into four clinical categories of severity, which has since been expanded to seven types. Multiple different type I collagen mutations may be responsible for each Sillence type.

Type I OI (mild) (50%): bone fragility, little or no deformity, normal stature, triangular facies with frontal bossing, blue sclerae, osteopenia, and hearing loss. Affected individuals may (type IA) or may not (type IB) have dentinogenesis imperfecta, which is due to mutation of COL1A1 or COL1A2 with consequent underproduction (50%) of normal type I collagen and hypomineralization. Bone density T scores are often −2.5 to −4.0. Inheritance is AD.

Type II OI (usually lethal) (5%): multiple in utero fractures and blue or gray sclerae; in utero/neonatal death is common. Inheritance is AD or AR.

Type III OI (severe deforming) (20%): multiple fractures before age 3 years, fractures heal with major skeletal deformities, short stature, scoliosis, joint laxity, gray or blue sclerae, and hearing loss. Affected individuals are not usually ambulatory. Pulmonary insufficiency from thoracic deformity is a major cause of death before age 35 years. The condition usually results from a spontaneous mutation although AD or AR inheritance can occur.

Type IV OI (moderate severity) (25%): variable short stature, variable bone fragility with a moderate number of fractures by age 10 years, wormian bones, normal (white) or gray sclerae, dentinogenesis imperfecta, some hearing loss, ambulation. Inheritance is AD.

Types V, VI, VII OI (rare): similar to type IV but with some different manifestations. No type I collagen mutations have been identified.

Diagnosis of OI is primarily clinical. Several laboratories can perform collagen biochemical and molecular (DNA sequencing) analysis from a skin biopsy (cost $2000 to $4000). A list of laboratories can be provided by the OI foundation. Bisphosphonate therapy may be beneficial, especially intravenous pamidronate and zoledronic acid. Teriparatide and denosumab are being tested in adult patients with OI. Teriparatide is not considered safe for children because of the risk of osteosarcoma. Corrective surgery, bracing, and physical therapy are also important.

3. What is the significance of increased joint mobility? How is it diagnosed?

Hyperflexible joints are common and do not necessarily indicate that an individual has a HCTD. Joint hypermobility decreases with age. Some studies suggest that 10% to 25% of the population may have hyperflexible joints and that 5% of individuals with hypermobility have symptoms. Symptoms caused by increased joint mobility can range from arthralgias to dislocation or injury. Individuals with severe hypermobility and recurrent dislocations may have EDS.

The **Beighton score** for joint laxity and hypermobility uses a simple 9-point system. A score of 5 or more indicates hypermobility:

1. Knee extension more than 10 degrees past 180 degrees: 1 point for each knee
2. Extension of the elbow 10 degrees or more past 180 degrees: 1 point for each elbow
3. Extension of the thumb to touch the flexor aspect of the forearm: 1 point for each thumb.
4. Extension of the little (5th) fingers backward so that they are beyond parallel (over 90°) with the posterior forearm: 1 point for each little finger
5. Forward trunk flexion (knees fully extended) so that the palms of the hands can be placed flat on the ground: 1 point

4. Describe the clinical manifestations of EDS.

EDS comprises a group of uncommon disorders of connective tissue primarily involving joint and skin laxity and arterial wall abnormalities. As a group such disorders affect 1 in 20,000 individuals. **Increased joint mobility** and **increased skin fragility and hyperextensibility** occur (Figure 55-1), although there is wide variability in joint, skin, and internal organ involvement. Hyperextensibility in patients with EDS may be greater in the small than the large joints and may diminish with age. Laxity/hyperextensibility in other organs include the Gorlin sign (ability to touch the nose with the tip of the tongue). Skin laxity and fragility may be manifest as easy bruisability, inability of stretched skin to return to normal, resulting in a "cigarette paper" or papyraceous skin appearance over the knees, gaping wounds from minor trauma, or an inability of skin to retain sutures. Arteries may develop aneurysms or rupture because of elastic tissue laxity. There are several recognized clinical types of EDS. Most involve some abnormality in collagen synthesis or enzymatic modification of collagen. Direct sequencing of genomic DNA for diagnosis is available for EDS types I, II, IV, VI, and VII.

- **Classic type** (formerly EDS I and II): parrot-like facies, floppy ears, hypermobility with joint dislocations, soft skin with "fish mouth" scars, and easy bruising ranging from mild to severe. Spontaneous pneumothorax, molluscoid pseudotumors of skin, aortic root dilation, mitral valve prolapse, kyphoscoliosis, osteopenia, and varicose veins are common. Up to 30% to 50% of cases are associated with a null allele for **collagen type V** (COL5A1 or COL5A2) and have AD inheritance. Less than 10% of cases are due to tenascin X

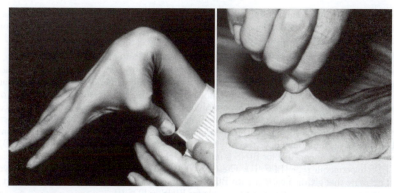

Figure 55-1. Patient with Ehlers–Danlos syndrome demonstrating hyperextensibility of joints and skin. (*Copyright 2014 American College of Rheumatology. Used with permission.*)

(ECM glycoprotein) deficiency and have AR inheritance. Both collagen type V and tenascin X associate with type I collagen and are important for its stability and deposition.
- **Hypermobile type** (formerly EDS III): **marked** hypermobility of large and small joints with soft skin but no scars. The collagen/ECM protein defect unknown. Inheritance is AD. Hypermobile joints are found in 65% of first-degree relatives.
- **Vascular type** (formerly EDS IV): normal joint mobility, translucent skin (China-doll appearance), marked bruising, aortic/arterial aneurysms, arterial rupture/dissections, and rupture of uterus/bowel (sigmoid colon). Spontaneous hemopneumothorax and mitral vave prolapse can occur. Various mutations of **type III collagen** (**COL3A1**), found in the skin, blood vessels, and the walls of hollow viscera, have been observed. Affected individuals do not have hyperelastic skin. Inheritance is AD. Pregnancy is discouraged. Surgery can be difficult because of friable arteries and organ tissue.
- **Kyphoscoliosis type** (formerly type VI): severe kyphoscoliosis noted at birth, recurrent joint dislocation, and hyperextensible fragile skin that develops gaping wounds on minor trauma that heal poorly. Unlike other EDS types, these patients have ocular fragility and rupture that can lead to blindness. Mutations of the lysyl hydroxylase gene results in deficiency. This enzyme is necessary for conversion of lysyl residues to hydroxylysine on procollagen peptides, which is important for crosslinking to stabilize the collagen. Inheritance is AR. Some clinicians advocate treatment with pharmacologic doses of vitamin C because this vitamin is a cofactor for lysl hydroxylase.
- **Arthrochalasia type** (formerly EDS VII A and VII B): significant hypermobility with dislocation of the large joints starting in the newborn period (congenital hip dislocation), moderate skin hyperlasticity and bruising, kyphoscoliosis, and short stature. The defect in type I collagen involves lack of an N-proteinase cleavage site so type I collagen retains its N-terminal peptide, resulting in abnormal collagen fibrils. Inheritance is AD.
- **Dermatosparaxis type** (formerly EDS VII C): marked joint hypermobility, micrognathia, extremely fragile skin with bruising but no scars, and blue sclerae. Large umbilical hernias are common. Deficiency of procollagen N-propeptidase enzyme results in retained N-terminal peptide and abnormal type I collagen. Inheritance is AR, unlike the arthrochalasia type.
- **Other types:** rare types include the peridontitis type (formerly EDS VIII), causing hypermobility and generalized peridontitis; the fibronectin type (formerly type X), causing easy bruising due to abnormal platelet aggregation and abnormal fibronectin; and the X-linked type (formerly EDS type V), which is similar to the mild classic type with X-linked inheritance.

5. **What are the Brighton diagnostic criteria for benign joint hypermobility syndrome (BJHS)?**
   Major criteria
   1. Beighton score of 4/9 or higher (see Question 5)
   2. Arthralgia for longer than 3 months in four or more joints

   Minor criteria
   1. Beighton score of 1, 2, or 3/9
   2. Arthralgia (≥3 months) in one to three joints or back pain (≥3 months), spondylosis, spondylolysis/spondylolisthesis
   3. Dislocation/subluxation in more than one joint, or in one joint on more than one occasion
   4. Three or more soft-tissue lesions (epicondylitis, tenosynovitis, bursitis)
   5. Marfanoid habitus
   6. Abnormal skin: striae, hyperextensibility, thin, papyraceous scarring
   7. Eye signs: drooping eyelids, myopia, or antimongoloid slant
   8. Varicose veins or hernia or uterine/rectal prolapse

BJHS is diagnosed if an individual exhibits two major criteria, or one major and two minor criteria, or four minor criteria. Note that major and minor criteria 1 are mutually exclusive, as are major and minor criteria 2 because they measure the same manifestation.

6. Are BJHS and EDS hypermobile type the same disease? (Controversial)

BJHS has a familial predisposition (70%) and occurs most commonly in young females. It is characterized by varying degrees of joint laxity without instability or disability and is an important cause of periarticular complaints. Arthralgias (hands, knees, and hips), knee effusions from patellar malalignment due to laxity, daily headaches arising from cervical spine hypermobility, and frequent ankle or wrist sprains are common. In addition to the clinical manifestations listed for the Brighton criteria, mitral valve prolapse and osteopenia (relative risk 1.8) have been associated with hypermobility. Chronic fatigue and pain amplification (fibromyalgia-like) due to dysautonomia have recently been reported more frequently in patients with BJHS. The connective tissue defect responsible for BJHS is unknown. The benign hypermobility syndrome was formerly known as EDS hypermobile type (EDS III). These two diseases likely represent a continuum. However, clinicians must be aware that giving a patient with BJHS a diagnosis of EDS is likely to affect the ability to obtain medical insurance. There is no genetic test available for BJHS or EDS III.

7. What are the revised Ghent criteria for the diagnosis of Marfan syndrome?

Marfan syndrome occurs in 1 in 10,000 to 12,000 individuals. The diagnosis can be difficult because of multiple clinical manifestations. An erroneous diagnosis can mean that an individual is uninsurable. Therefore diagnostic criteria have been established to help in making a confident diagnosis.

- In the absence of a family history, a diagnosis of Marfan syndrome can be made in a patient with any one of the following:
1. Aortic root dilatation and ectopia lentis (bilateral upward)
2. Aortic root dilatation and fibrillin-1 gene (*FBN1*) mutation
3. Ectopia lentis and *FBN1* mutation known to predispose to aortic root aneurysm/dissection
4. Aortic root dilatation and evidence of systemic features (≥7 out of 20 points)
    - The 20-point scoring system for systemic features is as follows: wrist and thumb sign, 3 points; pectus deformity, 2 points for carinatum, 1 point for excavatum; hindfoot deformirty, 2 points; pneumothorax, 2 points; dural ectasia, 2 points; protrusio acetabuli, 2 points; reduced upper segment/lower segment ratio, 1 point; scoliosis or thoracolumbar kyphoscoliosis, 1 point; reduced elbow extension <170 degrees, 1 point; facial features, 1 point; skin striae, 1 point; myopia, 1 point; mitral valve prolapse, 1 point.
- In the presence of a family history in a first-degree relative, a diagnosis of Marfan syndrome can be made in a patient with any one of the following:
1. Ectopia lentis and family history of Marfan syndrome
2. Systemic features (≥7 points) and family history of Marfan syndrome
3. Aortic root dilatation and family history of Marfan syndrome

8. What is the genetic defect in Marfan syndrome and how does it contribute to the clinical manifestations?

Classic Marfan syndrome is caused by mutations in the **fibrillin-1 gene** on chromosome 15 in all patients. Over 600 mutations of this gene have been reported. The inheritance pattern is AD, although 25% of cases are due to sporadic mutations. Fibrillin-1 is normally produced by fibroblasts and forms a scaffold for the deposition of elastin. In addition to being a connective protein important in structural support for tissues, the normal fibrillin-1 protein also binds to another protein, TGF-β. Researchers now believe that mutated fibrillin-1 cannot bind to TGF-β, resulting in excessive accumulation of free TGF-β in certain tissues. Excess TGF-β can have deleterious effects on vascular smooth muscle development and ECM integrity by binding to its receptor and upregulating TGF-β–responsive genes such as those that regulate the production of matrix metalloproteinases. Excess matrix metalloproteinases can interfere with tissue development and weaken the tissue. Therefore organs that contain a lot of fibrillin-1 and elastin are most likely to be involved in Marfan syndrome, including the elastic walls of arteries (especially aorta), heart valves, zonula fibers of the eye, ligaments, skin, and lung parenchyma. Notably, different mutations of fibrillin-1 dictate which tissues are involved and the severity of the clinical manifestations. Many laboratories can test for the most common mutations.

9. Describe the phenotype and skeletal manifestations of Marfan syndrome.

Patients with Marfan syndrome have a characteristic phenotype that is easily recognized: tall stature, long, thin extremities (arm span/height ratio >1.05), dolichostenomelia (abnormally low upper/lower body segment ratio of <0.85, compared to normal ratios of ≥0.93 for whites and ≥0.87 for blacks), and diminished subcutaneous fat. Skeletal manifestations include arachnodactyly (spider digits), pectus excavatum or carinatum, loss of thoracic kyphosis, scoliosis (>20 degrees), reduced elbow extension (<170 degrees), and pes planus. Facial manifestations include a gothic (high, arched) palate, dolichocephaly (long, narrow face), malar hypoplasia, retrognathia, enophthalmos, and downslanting palpebral fissures.

Several prominent athletes, as well as Abraham Lincoln, are said to have had Marfan syndrome. Olympic sports in which individuals with Marfan syndrome are said to excel are volleyball and basketball. In fact, a

U.S. Olympic volleyball star, Flo Hyman, is said to have died in 1986 of vascular complications of Marfan syndrome. Michael Phelps, a U.S. Olympic swimmer, does not have Marfan syndrome.

10. How is arachnodactyly (spider digits) recognized?

Arachnodactyly can be recognized from the appearance of the hands. There are three simple methods to definitively determine if arachnodactyly is present.
- The **thumb sign**, or Steinberg sign, is protrusion of the thumb past the hypothenar border when the hand is clenched in a fist (Figure 55-2).
- The **wrist sign**, or Walker–Murdoch sign, is overlap of the fifth finger and thumb when they encircle the wrist of the opposite hand.
- The **metacarpal index** is a radiographic measure of arachnodactyly. It is the average of the length divided by the midpoint width for the second through fourth metacarpals (a value of 5.4 to 7.9 is normal, whereas >8.4 occurs in Marfan syndrome).

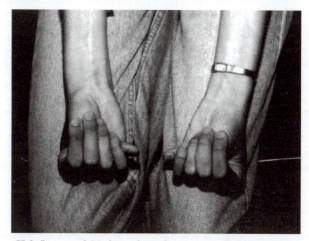

Figure 55-2. Patient with Marfan syndrome demonstrating the Steinberg thumb sign.

11. Does the presence of arachnodactyly mean a patient has Marfan syndrome? What is the differential diagnosis of arachnodactyly?

Arachnodactyly is present in approximately 90% of cases of Marfan syndrome but is not diagnostic and may be seen in other diseases. **Nonasthenic Marfan syndrome** may be a *forme fruste* of the disease; patients have a more normal-appearing phenotype with arachnodactyly but may have the same mutation as in other, more severely affected family members. The **MASS phenotype** comprises mitral valve prolapse, myopia, borderline and nonprogressive aortic root dilatation, skeletal findings, and striae. **Marfanoid hypermobility syndrome** involves skeletal features of the Marfan phenotype, such as arachnodactyly, but also comprises hyperelastic skin and hyperextensible joints as in EDS. **Congenital contractural arachnodactyly** is described in Question 17. **Homocystinuria** is an AR disease caused by cystathionine β synthase deficiency and characterized by tallness, arachnodactyly, lens dislocation (downward dislocation), and spinal abnormalities coupled with vascular thrombosis and mild mental retardation.

12. What are the nonmusculoskeletal manifestations of Marfan syndrome? Which cause significant morbidity and mortality?

Ectopia lentis (upward dislocation) occurs in over half (50% to 80%) of patients. Cardiovascular complications are multiple and common. Aneurysmal dilatation of the ascending aorta with dissection is the most common cause of death in patients. Mitral valve prolapse with regurgitation or aortic insufficiency is detectable in 60% of patients by auscultation and in >80% by echocardiography. Pulmonary manifestations include cystic disease and spontaneous pneumothorax. The primary cause of morbidity is skeletal disease of the spine. Scoliosis is a major management problem and may be rapidly progressive during adolescence, requiring surgery.

13. What other genetic diseases should be considered in a patient with aortic aneurym or dissection?

In general, the younger the age of a person in whom an aneurysm has been identified, the greater is the likelihood of a genetic cause. The following have been described and are AD, except pseudoxanthoma elasticum:
- Diseases associated with defects in extracellular matrix proteins
  - EDS vascular type: type III collagen
  - EDS kyphoscoliosis type: lysl hydroxylase deficiency
  - Menkes syndrome: copper deficiency

- Diseases caused by matrix cell signalling defects
  - Marfan syndrome: *FBN1* mutation
  - Loeys–Dietz syndrome: TGFβ receptor 1 and 2 defects
- Diseases associated with intracellular protein defects
  - Familial aortic aneurysm: smooth muscle gene mutations (*ACTA2, MYH11*, myosin light chain kinase)
  - Arterial tortuosity syndrome: glucose transporter 10 mutation (*SLC2A10*)
  - Pseudoxanthoma elasticum: mutations in the *ABCC6* gene

14. How is Marfan syndrome treated?

Genetic counseling is indicated because 50% of offspring are likely to be affected. Pregnancy is generally safe unless aortic dilatation is present. Annual ophthalmologic and orthopedic evaluations are recommended. Surgery may be needed if scoliosis exceeds 45 degrees.

Measures are taken to monitor and prevent cardiovascular problems. β-Adrenergic blockade and angiotensin-converting enzyme inhibitors have been used to prevent aortic root dilatation/dissection with unclear results. Angiotensin receptor blockers (ARBs) have recently shown promising benefits in mouse models and early human studies. Theoretically, ARBs should be effective by selectively blocking the angiotensin II type 1 receptor (AT1R). AT1R signaling can increase TGF-β production. Therefore, AT1R blockade by ARBs induces a clinically relevant (50%) decrease in TGF-β ligands and receptors. This results in reduced levels of TGF-β signaling, which should delay aortic root dilatation (see Question 10). In addition, AT1R blockade should result in overactivation of the AT2R pathway by angiotensin II. The AT2R pathway has antiproliferative and antiinflammatory effects that are beneficial in aortic-wall homeostasis. Echocardiography is needed to determine the presence of mitral and aortic valvular disease. Infective endocarditis occurs in patients with mitral or tricuspid disease, and prophylaxis is recommended for such patients. Echocardiography is performed yearly to follow aortic dilatation; when the size exceeds 50% of normal (>45 mm), echocardiography is recommended at 6-month intervals. Vigorous exercise is contraindicated. Surgery is indicated when the aortic root exceeds 50 to 55 mm.

15. What is congenital contractural arachnodactyly (CCA)?

CCA is an AD disease caused by mutations of the **fibrillin-2 gene** on chromosome 5. Patients have a marfanoid habitus but unlike Marfan syndrome have stiff joints, multiple contractures of large joints, "crumpled" ears, severe thoracic deformities, and no cardiac or eye abnormalities.

16. What are the clinical features of pseudoxanthoma elasticum?

Pseudoxanthoma elasticum is a rare (1 in 25,000 individuals) AR disease that involves degeneration and calcification of elastic fibers in the eyes, skin, and arteries. The molecular defect is mutations of the **ABCC6 gene** on chromosome 16 encoding the MRP6 protein, which is a membrane transporter protein. How this causes the disease is unknown. There is moderate heterogeneity in the clinical findings, depending on the gene mutation. **Xanthomatoid papules** occur in flexural skinfolds and are the classic finding. **Angioid streaks** occur in the fundus owing to a break in the Bruch membrane. Visual loss may occur from maculopathy and retinal lesions. **Calcific deposits** in the lungs and cardiac involvement mimicking cardiomyopathy may occur. **Arterial rupture** occurs in the gastrointestinal and genitourinary tracts. Joints can be hypermobile. Abnormal elastic fibers usually do not impair wound healing until late in life. Patients die of coronary artery fibrosis and calcification.

17. What is cutis laxa?

Cutis laxa refers to a group of inherited or acquired disorders with a common finding of lax, redundant skin. One of the inherited forms (AR) may be due to a mutation of the **fibulin-5 gene**. The skin may appear wrinkled, aged, or sagging in loose folds. A similar skin appearance may occur after penicillamine use or subsequent to inflammatory skin diseases. The skin appears to have lost elasticity and does not recoil when stretched. In EDS the skin does recoil. Cardiopulmonary manifestations may occur, including bronchiectasis and emphysema. There is no abnormality of skin fragility with bleeding, so surgery can be safely performed (again, unlike EDS).

COMPRESSIVE HEREDITARY CONNECTIVE TISSUE DISEASES

1. What is Stickler syndrome?

Stickler syndrome is a relatively common (1 in 10,000) AD disease characterized by premature and severe osteoarthritis developing in the third decade of life. The diagnosis should be suspected in any young adult with degenerative hip arthritis or any infant with congenitally swollen joints (especially wrists). Other manifestations include myopia, retinal detachment, progressive sensorineural hearing loss, cleft palate, mandibular hypoplasia, and epiphyseal dysplasia. There are two clinical subtypes, depending on the genetic mutation. The classic syndrome/subtype, called hereditary arthroophthalmopathy, is characterized by prominent skeletal and ocular abnormalities. These patients have a mutation in the **type II collagen gene** (*COL2A1*) resulting in abnormal type II collagen in cartilage and the vitreous body of the eye. The second subtype lacks eye involvement but affected individuals have severe hearing loss in addition to skeletal and joint manifestations. These patients have mutations in the **type XI collagen gene** (*COL11A2*) consistent with a lack of type XI collagen in the eye.

BARRIER HEREDITARY CONNECTIVE TISSUE DISEASES

1. **What is Alport syndrome?**
   Alport syndrome includes hereditary glomerulonephritis and deafness. Up to 85% of patients have mutations in the **COL4A5 gene on the X chromosome**, whereas 15% have AR defects in the COL4A3 or COL4A4 gene. The defect is in a nonfibrillar basement membrane collagen, type IV collagen, which is an important component of the kidney basement membrane. Patients present with hematuria, sensorineural hearing loss, and lenticonus. They eventually progress to renal failure.

2. **What is a disease caused by mutation of type VII collagen?**
   Epidermolysis bullosa is a skin disease leading to progressive blistering and bullae formation in the dermis. It is casued by one of over 100 mutations found in type **VII collagen** (*COL7A1* gene), which forms the anchoring fibrils that tether the dermis to the basement membrane. Different clinical subtypes are described, depending on the specific mutation.

BIBLIOGRAPHY

Beighton PH, Horan F: Orthopedic aspects of the Ehlers–Danlos syndrome, J Bone Joint Surg Br 51:444–453, 1969.
Brooke BS, Habashi JP, Judge DP, et al: Angiotensin II blockade and aortic-root dilation in Marfan's syndrome, N Engl J Med 358:2787–2795, 2008.
Grahame R, Hakim AJ: Hypermobility, Curr Opin Rheumatol 20:106–110, 2008.
Jondeau G, Michel JB, Boileau C: The translational science of Marfan syndrome, Heart 97:1206–1214, 2011.
Krakow D, Rimion DL: The skeletal dysplasias, Genet Med 12:327–341, 2010.
Loeys BL, Dietz HC, Braverman AC, et al: The revised Ghent nosology for the Marfan syndrome, J Med Genet 47:476–485, 2010.
Malfait F, Wenstrup RJ, DePaepe A: Clinical and genetic aspects of Ehlers–Danlos syndrome, classic type, Genet Med 12:597–605, 2010.
Pepin M, Schwarze U, Superti-Firga A, Byers PH: Clinical and genetic features of Ehlers–Danlos syndrome, type IV, the vascular type, N Engl J Med 342:673–680, 2000.
Phillipi CA, Remmington T, Steiner RD: Bisphosphonate therapy for osteogensis imperfecta, Cochrane Database Syst Rev 4:CD005088, 2008.
Shapiro JR, Sponsellor PD: Osteogenesis imperfecta: questions and answers, Curr Opin Pediatr 21:706–716, 2009.

FURTHER READING

www.oif.org
www.ednf.org
www.marfan.org

INBORN ERRORS OF METABOLISM AFFECTING CONNECTIVE TISSUE

CHAPTER 56

Sterling G. West, MD

> **KEY POINTS**
>
> 1. Consider homocystinuria in a patient with marfanoid habitus, stiff joints, and mental deficiency.
> 2. Attenuated forms of lysosomal storage diseases may present with rheumatic manifestations resembling juvenile idiopathic arthritis.
> 3. Suspect Fabry disease in a patient with fibromyalgia-like symptoms, acroparesthesias, angiokeratomas, and paternal history of early-onset renal failure.

1. What are the homocystinurias?

Homocystinuria refers to increased urinary excretion of the oxidized form of homocysteine called homocystine. The most common form of homocystinuria is due to an autosomal recessive defect in the enzyme cystathionine β-synthase. Over 90 mutations of this gene, located on chromosome 21, have been described. The enzyme is involved in the transsulfuration pathway from homocysteine to cystathione. Other less common forms are due to defective remethylation of homocysteine to methionine.

2. How common is homocystinuria and how is it diagnosed?

Cystathionine β-synthase deficiency probably occurs in approximately 1 in 200,000 (or less) live births in the United States, prompting some states to require newborn homocysteine screening. It is thought that heterozygotes for cystathionine β-synthase deficiency (1 in 70 in the general population) are unaffected but may be at risk of premature peripheral and cerebral vascular disease.

In the classic form of homocystinuria due to cystathionine β-synthase deficiency, homocysteine and methionine are increased in the blood, and homocysteine, homocystine, and methionine are increased in the urine. The urinary cyanide nitroprusside test detects sulfhydryl-containing amino acids in urine and is typically used as a screening test but is not specific for a particular enzymatic defect.

Patients with homocystinuria due a metabolic defect that affects the conversion of homocysteine to methionine (Figure 56-1) such as methylene tetrahydrofolate (MTHF) reductase deficiency and disorders of cobalamin (vitamin B_{12}) metabolism have a different metabolic pattern with low normal (not high) levels of plasma methionine. Consequently, patients with vitamin B_{12} or folate deficiency can have high levels of plasma homocysteine and urinary homocystine, but low normal levels of plasma methionine. These patients can develop premature vascular disease, but not the other manifestations of homocystinuria.

Therefore a combination of homocysteine and methionine levels in plasma and urine, in addition to homocystine in urine, must be measured to make an accurate diagnosis. Precise tissue (e.g., cultured skin fibroblasts) enzyme assays can also be performed to assess the activity of cystathionine β-synthase and its responsiveness to pyridoxal phosphate (vitamin B_6).

3. List the major clinical manifestations of homocystinuria.

- Ectopia lentis (lens dislocated downward); hallmark finding
- Thromboembolism (most common cause of death); both arterial and venous
- Mental retardation, seizures, ischemic strokes
- Marfanoid habitus but without joint laxity

Musculoskeletal findings include tallness, arachnodactyly (dolichostenomelia), pes cavus, genu valgum, and chest wall (pectus) and spinal deformity. Osteoporosis (generalized) and tight joints occur. Spinal osteoporosis occurs in up to 64% of affected individuals by the age of 15 years. Spinal disease is prominent and is usually a combination of osteoporotic fractures, degenerative disc/joint disease, and scoliosis.

Homocystinuria is a likely finding for patients with a mental deficiency and Marfan syndrome with stiff joints.

4. Why does homocystinuria affect connective tissue?

Cysteine is deficient in homocystinuria and this amino acid is necessary for proper crosslinking of structural proteins such as collagen and fibrillin in connective tissue and bone, the suspensory ligament of the eye, and the extracellular milieu of endothelial cells. On this basis, altered collagen may be responsible for the lens dislocation and osteoporosis, whereas altered proteins in the elastomeric complex or its substructure (fibrillin) may be responsible for the phenotypic similarity to Marfan syndrome. Altered endothelial function (from the cytotoxic effect of homocysteine) and increased platelet activation are responsible for the thrombosis and subsequent mental retardation.

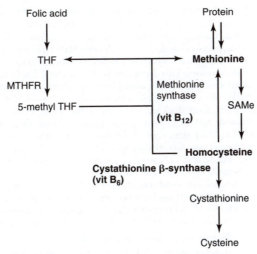

Figure 56-1. Homocysteine metabolic pathway.

5. **How is homocystinuria treated? What symptoms can be expected to respond?**
   Effective treatment requires early diagnosis to prevent mental retardation, which is the basis for newborn screening for inborn errors of metabolism. Vitamin B_6 and B_{12} and folate are cofactors for the different enzymes involved in methionine metabolism (Figure 56-1). Half of patients respond to vitamin B_6. Large doses of vitamin B_6 (300 to 600 mg of pyridoxine per day) lower blood methionine, raise blood cysteine, and improve symptoms in patients with cystathionine β-synthase deficiency, presumably by augmenting the small amount of residual enzyme activity. Development of ectopia lentis, osteoporosis, and retardation may be mitigated with therapy, but no remission of these conditions occurs if they are already present. Patients who do not respond to vitamin B_6 are treated with a low-methionine diet and betaine, which converts homocysteine back to methionine.

6. **What is Menkes disease (kinky hair syndrome) and how does it affect the musculoskeletal system?**
   Menkes disease (mild form formerly called Ehlers–Danlos IX) is a rare (1 in 300,000 individuals) X-linked recessive disorder of copper metabolism in which the clinical abnormalities are primarily neurologic and include seizures, abnormal reflexes, spasticity, and mental retardation. Patients also have occipital horns and pili torti (beaded, brittle, and sparse hair). Abnormal copper metabolism caused by a malfunction of ATPase-dependent transport of copper (*ATP7A* gene) results in poor copper distribution to cells. This lack of copper affects copper-requiring metalloenzymes (lysyl hydroxylase) involved in collagen and elastin synthesis, thereby affecting connective tissues. The rheumatic manifestations may be similar to those in either cutis laxa or Ehlers–Danlos syndrome, with highly extensible skin and joints. Death and disability occur early in life if the patient is not treated with copper supplementation.

7. **When should a rheumatologist consider a lysosomal storage disease as a cause of musculoskeletal symptoms?**
   There are over 40 lysosomal storage diseases (LSDs). Some presenting in childhood may have musculoskeletal symptoms that are initially misdiagnosed as juvenile idiopathic arthritis. However, patients with attenuated LSD forms may look "normal" and present as a teenager or adult with rheumatic symptoms. The following are a list of LSDs that can occur in a mild or attenuated form (i.e., can present with rheumatic symptoms later in life) and the unusual extraarticular manifestations that should alert a clinician that the LSD that is the cause of the symptoms:
   - **Mucopolysaccharidoses**
     - MPS I-HS (Hurler–Scheie): joint stiffness/contracture, claw-hand deformity, coarse facies, short stature, corneal clouding
     - MPS I-S (Scheie): hip dysplasia, joint stiffness/contracture, coarse facies, heart murmurs, corneal clouding
     - MPS II (Hunter): milder than Hurler–Scheie syndrome, hepatosplenomegaly, short stature, clear corneas
     - MPS VI (Maroteaux–Lamy): joint stiffness/contracture, claw-hand deformity, heart murmurs, corneal clouding
   - **Gaucher disease, type 1:** bone pain, osteonecrosis, hepatosplenomegaly, growth retardation
   - **Fabry disease:** acroparesthesia, cold/heat intolerance, angiokeratoma, cornea verticillata, paternal history of early-onset renal failure
   - **Farber disease:** periarticular subcutaneous nodules, painful swollen joints, hepatosplenomegaly, nephropathy, ceramidase deficiency.

8. What are the musculoskeletal manifestations of the mucopolysaccharidoses?

The mucopolysaccharidoses (MPS) are a group of metabolic disorders affecting 1 in 25,000 births that are caused by the absence or malfunctioning of one of the 11 lysosomal enzymes needed to break down glycosaminoglycans (formerly called mucopolysaccharides). Seven distinct MPS types have been identified. All are autosomal recessive except for MPS II (Hunter), which is X-linked recessive. Catabolites of glycosaminoglycans are progressively deposited in various tissues. This deposition leads to skeletal dysplasia, which characteristically causes short stature, joint contracture, stiff joints, carpal tunnel syndrome, and claw-hand deformity. Thick calvaria, an enlarged J-shaped sella turcica, a short and wide mandible, biconvex vertebral bodies, odontoid hypoplasia with atlantoaxial instability, short thick clavicles, coxa valga, V-shaped deformities of the distal ulna and radius, and short fingers with wide metacarpals with pointed proximal ends all occur. Many individuals affected by MPS have mental retardation, thick skin, corneal clouding, heart murmurs, and organomegaly. The Hurler, Hunter, Morquio, and Maroteaux–Lamy syndromes (types IH, II, IV, and VI) have short-trunk dwarfism, but attenuated forms (types I-HS, I-S, II, and VI) caused by varying genetic mutations can have relatively normal stature. A diagnosis of MPS is made by fractionation of urinary glycosaminoglycans, enzyme assays, and/or molecular genetics. Treatment is palliative and consists mainly of joint replacement and surgical stabilization of cervical instability. Bone marrow transplants have been successful in some forms of MPS. Enzyme replacement therapy has been beneficial for MPS I treated with α-L-iduronidase (laronidase, Aldurazyme), MPS II with iduronidase sulfatase (idursulfase, Elaprase), and MPS VI with arylsulfatase B (galsulfase, Naglazyme).

9. What are the skeletal manifestations of Gaucher disease?

Gaucher disease is caused by autosomal recessive inheritance of a deficiency of glucocerebrosidase that affects 1 in 20,000 births and is caused by one of 300 mutant alleles of the gene encoding this enzyme, located on chromosome 1. Type I (adult form) is the most common of the three forms and occurs most commonly in Ashkenazi Jews. The enzyme deficiency leads to accumulation of glucosylceramide within macrophages (Gaucher cells). Splenomegaly with hypersplenism is the most common presenting manifestation. Hepatomegaly occurs later, as does pulmonary involvement (interstitial lung disease, pulmonary hypertension). Skeletal involvement occurs in 50% to 75% of patients, including long bone or hip/shoulder pain from osteonecrosis and bony infarctions, as well as back pain from osteoporosis with fractures. Bone crisis (10%) can cause acute pain and swelling associated with elevated acute-phase reactants. Radiographic abnormalities are seen in 80% to 95% of patients and include osteopenia, osteolytic lesions, bony infarcts with serpiginous osteosclerotic areas, and osteonecrosis of the femoral and humeral heads and femoral condyles. The diagnosis is suspected by demonstrating Gaucher cells on bone marrow biopsy and confirmed by measuring enzyme activity in circulating lymphocytes. Three glucocerebrosidases, imiglucerase (Cerezyme), velaglucerase alfa (VPRIV), and taliglucerase alfa (Elelyso), are available for enzyme replacement therapy. The annual cost of therapy is $200,000. Symptomatic therapy includes bisphosphonates, analgesics, splenectomy, and joint replacement. Bone marrow transplantation has been successful.

10. How does Fabry disease mimic fibromyalgia?

Most patients with hereditary lysosomal storage diseases present and are diagnosed during childhood. However, female heterozygotes and atypical variants of Fabry disease may have a milder and later-onset phenotype. Fabry disease is an X-linked lipid storage disease cause by deficiency of lysosomal α-galactosidase A (α-Gal A), with an incidence of up to 1 in 3100 live births if mild forms are included. Males with classical Fabry disease usually develop neuromuscular symptoms in childhood including painful crises with burning paresthesias of distal extremities, often accompanied by fever. Female heterozygotes and males with low residual α-Gal A levels may develop disease manifestations for the first time as adults. Neuromuscular manifestations can range from painful acroparesthesias to fibromyalgia. Progressive or isolated cardiac, cerebrovascular, and renal disease can develop later. **Diagnosis of Fabry disease should be suspected in any patient with a paternal family history of early-onset renal failure.** Patients should be examined for characteristic ocular stigmata (**cornea verticillata**) and dermal signs (**angiokeratomas**). The diagnosis is confirmed in males by determining α-Gal A activity in plasma or peripheral leukocytes. By contrast, female carriers must be tested for one of the specific gene mutations. Early diagnosis is important because enzyme replacement therapy with agalsidase alpha (Replagal) or beta (Fabrazyme) can prevent irreversible organ damage. The annual cost of therapy is $200,000.

Acknowledgment

The author would like to thank Dr. John Jenkins for his contribution to the previous edition of this chapter.

BIBLIOGRAPHY

Aldenhoven M, Sakkers RJB, Boelens J, et al: Musculoskeletal manifestations of lysosomal storage disorders, Ann Rheumatic Dis 68:1659–1665, 2009.

Desnick R, Brady R, Barranger J, et al: Fabry disease, an under-recognized multisystem disorder: expert recommendations for diagnosis, management, and enzyme replacement therapy, Ann Intern Med 138:338–346, 2003.

Eng CM, Germain DP, Banikazemi M, et al: Fabry disease: guidelines for the evaluation and management of multi-organ system involvement, Genet Med 8:539–548, 2006.

Grabowski GA: Phenotype, diagnosis, and treatment of Gaucher's disease, Lancet 372:1263–1271, 2008.

Hughes DA, Deegan PB, Milligan A, et al: A randomised, double-blind, placebo-controlled, crossover study to assess the efficacy and safety of three dosing schedules of agalsidase alfa enzyme replacement therapy for Fabry disease, Mol Genet Metab 109:269–275, 2013.
Michels H, Mengel E: Lysosomal storage diseases as differential diagnoses to rheumatic disorders, Curr Opin Rheumatol 20:76–81, 2008.
Mudd SH, Skovby F, Levy HL, et al: The natural history of homocystinuria due to cystathionine β-synthase deficiency, Am J Hum Genet 37:1–31, 1985.
Schiff M, Blom HJ: Treatment of inherited homocystinurias, Neuropediatrics 43:295–304, 2012.
Testai FD, Gorelick PB: Inherited metabolic disorders and stroke part 2, Arch Neurol 67:148–153, 2010.
Thümler A, Miebach E, Lampe C, et al: Clinical characteristics of adults with slowly progressing mucopolysaccharidosis VI: a case series, J Inherit Metab Dis 35:1071–1079, 2012.

Further Reading

www.ncbi.nlm.nih.gov
www.rarediseases.org
www.mpssociety.org
www.fabrydisease.org

CHAPTER 57

STORAGE AND DEPOSITION DISEASES
Sterling G. West, MD

KEY POINTS

1. Musculoskeletal effects can be the presenting manifestation in up to 33% of patients with hemochromatosis.
2. Symmetric degenerative arthritis of the second and third metacarpal joints and radiocarpal joints suggests hemochromatotic arthropathy.
3. Wilson disease should be considered in patients with the triad of liver disease, neurolgic disease, and a noninflammatory arthropathy of the metacarpophalangeal joints (MCPs) and wrists.
4. Ochronotic arthropathy commonly causes severe lumbar spine osteoarthritis with disc space calcifications and vacuum discs.

1. **What is the pattern of inheritance for hereditary hemochromatosis, Wilson disease, and alkaptonuria (ochronosis)?**
   These three conditions are inherited as autosomal recessive traits and heterozygotes are asymptomatic carriers. Hereditary hemochromatosis (HHC) occurs in 1 in 500 individuals (Northern European ancestry), Wilson disease in approximately 1 in 30,000, and alkaptonuria (ochronosis) in approximately 1 in 200,000. Alkaptonuria was the first human disease for which inheritance as an autosomal recessive trait was demonstrated.

2. **Describe the normal iron homeostasis in humans and how this is altered in HHC.**
   The human body normally contain 3 to 4 g of iron, two thirds of which is contained in hemoglobin, myoglobin, and a variety of enzymes, and one third as storage iron in ferritin and hemosiderin within hepatocytes and macrophages of the liver, bone marrow, spleen, and muscle. Although the typical Western diet contains 10 to 20 mg of iron a day, only 1 to 2 mg is absorbed daily by the duodenal mucosa, which balances the iron loss from exfoliated gastrointestinal epithelial cells and desquamation of the skin. Hepcidin is normally synthesized by the liver under the control of a variety of proteins and cytokines. When plasma iron is low, hepcidin is also low, allowing efflux of iron into serum through the iron exporter ferroportin (FPN) on duodenal enterocytes and macrophages. When plasma iron is elevated, hepcidin is increased and binds to FPN, causing internalization and degradation and resulting in less iron release into serum (Figure 57-1). In HHC there is an abnormality of one of the iron regulatory proteins, which leads to excess gastrointestinal iron absorption that ranges from 3 to 4 mg per day; this results in accumulation of 15 to 35 g of iron in tissues over a 35- to 60-year period.

3. **What are the genetic subtypes of HHC?**
   HHC results from mutations in one of several genes involved in regulation of iron homeostasis:
   - **Classic/HFE-related (type I):** the *HFE* gene is located on chromosome 6 near the HLA-A locus and is responsible for most cases of HHC (approximately 80% of cases in the U.S.). HFE protein is mainly expressed in crypt enterocytes of the duodenum, where it regulates brush border iron transport from the gut lumen. HFE is also found in Kupffer cells in the liver and regulates hepcidin production via unknown mechanisms. A single G→A mutation in the *HFE* gene, resulting in cysteine→tyrosine substitution at position 282 (C282Y), is found in 90% of patients with this HHC subtype. Less common mutations are aspartate substitution for histidine at position 63 (H63D) and substitution of serine by cysteine at position 65 (S65C), each of which occurs in 1% of patients who have overall milder disease. The remaining patients with classic HHC are compound heterozygotes (one C282Y and one H63D gene mutation). There are two models of how defective HFE protein leads to HHC:
     - **Crypt cell model:** postulates that abnormal HFE protein cannot incorporate into the enterocyte membrane, which impairs its ability to associate with transferrin receptor 1. This inhibits uptake of transferrin-bound iron into crypt cells and provides a false signal that total body iron stores are low. As crypt cells migrate to the villous tip, the iron transporter protein DMT1 is upregulated and dietary iron absorption is inappropriately increased.
     - **Liver model:** postulates the abnormal HFE protein interacts with hepatocytes, limiting hepcidin production. Consequently, more iron is exported into blood from enterocytes and macrophages through FPN on their membranes. Owing to the decreased level of hepcidin, FPN is not downregulated in spite of elevated plasma iron levels.

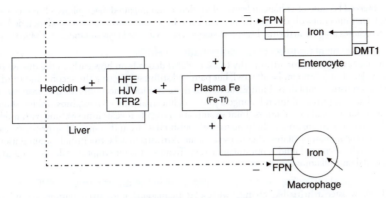

Figure 57-1. Iron homeostasis.

- **Juvenile type HHC (type II):** caused by a mutation of the hemojuvelin (*HJV*) gene on chromosome 1 (type IIA) or the hepcidin antimicrobial peptide (*HAMP*) gene on chromosome 19 (type IIB). HJV is the major modulator of hepcidin expression. A mutation in either gene means that hepcidin levels remain low, leading to excess iron export from enterocytes and macrophages via FPN into serum. Patients develop symptoms by the age of 20 years.
- **Transferrin-receptor 2–related (type III):** due to a mutation in this receptor (TFR2), the uptake of transferrin-bound iron is altered and hepcidin expression is low providing a false signal that iron stores are low.
- **Ferroportin-related HHC (type IV):** FPN mutation allows excess release of iron from enterocytes and macrophages into serum. Hepcidin is not able to cause internalization and degradation of the mutated FPN protein on cell surfaces.

4. **How common is the *HFE* gene causing classic HHC (type I)?**

Recent screening studies suggest that the *HFE* gene occurs in up to 5% of whites, giving a carrier (heterozygote) frequency of approximately 1 in 10 and a disease (homozygote) frequency of 1 in 400. There is wide variation in gene frequency. The mutation frequency is highest in individuals of northwestern European descent (1 in 200 homozygous) and less common in southern and eastern Europe populations, and is rarely found in indigenous populations of Africa, the Americas, Asia, and the Pacific Islands. The global prevalence of the gene mutation is 1.9%, making this one of the most commonly inherited metabolic diseases. Given the frequency of HHC in the general population, many physicians recommend screening iron studies in all white men by the age of 40.

The frequency of clinically significant disease (i.e., disease penetrance) in patients homozygous for the *HFE* gene is controversial. According to reports the odds ratio for developing HHC is as high as 2300 for C282Y HFE homozygotes but only 6 for H63D homozygotes. Disease penetrance is 2% to 30% in individuals homozygous for C282Y, 1.5% for compound heterozygotes, and <1% for H63D homozygotes. This low disease penetrance suggests that additional gene mutations (hepcidin gene, etc.) must be present for a homozygous patient to develop type I HHC.

5. **How does the typical patient with classic HHC (type I) present?**

Several factors, most notably physiologic blood loss in women and higher iron intake in men, modify the expression of classic HHC. Accordingly, the symptomatic stage is approximately 10 times more common in men than women, and men tend to have onset of symptoms at an earlier age. Clinical manifestations usually appear between the ages of 40 and 60 years, but the disease severity is quite variable. A few patients may develop full clinical expression as early as age 20 (rule out type II HHC), whereas 30% of *HFE* mutation homozygotes never develop clinical symptoms.

HHC typically presents with **asymptomatic abnormal liver function tests**, with 95% of patients having **hepatomegaly**. Liver disease usually progresses to hepatic cirrhosis in untreated cases. Comorbid factors that increase hepatic steatosis including obesity, diabetes, and excess alcohol consumption. Hepatocellular carcinoma risk is increased by a factor of 20 to 200. A characteristic **arthropathy** occurs in 40% to 80% of patients and may be the initial manifestation, although more often it occurs later in the disease and may even develop after treatment has been initiated. Other manifestations include slate-gray skin caused by iron in eccrine sweat glands and brown **skin pigmentation** due to melanin deposition (50%), **diabetes mellitus**, and **hypogonadism** manifest as decreased libido (20% to 40%), impotence, amenorrhea, or sparse body hair. **Constitutional symptoms** (80%) such as weakness or lethargy are also common. Cardiac involvement, manifested most commonly as **congestive heart failure**, is present in approximately 30% of patients and is a principal cause of death in untreated patients. Increased susceptibility to **infections**, particularly due to *Vibrio vulnificus* from uncooked seafood, is observed because of enhanced bacterial virulence and impaired macrophage clearance caused by high serum iron. Other infections observed at higher incidence in patients with iron overload include *Yersinia enterocolitica*, which causes a **septic arthritis**, *Listeria monocytogenes*, *Salmonella typhimurium*, and *Mucor*, among others.

6. **What are some clinical features of the arthropathy of HHC?**
   The wide frequency reported for arthropathy (40% to 80%) depends on how early in the disease the diagnosis of HHC is made. Most joints can be affected, but pain and stiffness affecting the second and third MCPs are the most characteristic complaints. Limited flexion in these two joints accounts for the "iron fist" sign. Other joints affected are the proximal interphalangeal joints, radiocarpal joints, knees, hips, ankles, shoulders, and occasionally metatarsophalangeal joints. Joint examination usually reveals firm swelling with mild tenderness, but warmth and effusions are absent, helping to distinguish HHC from rheumatoid arthritis. A few patients may suffer from inflammatory "flares" due to pseudogout. Arthritis may be the initial manifestation in 33% of patients with HHC. Synovial fluid is noninflammatory. Treatment is for symptom alleviation using analgesics and nonsteroidal antiinflammatory drugs.

7. **Describe the typical radiographic abnormalities seen in the arthropathy of HHC.**
   Radiographs show osteoarthritis-like changes with sclerotic margins, joint-space narrowing, and osteophyte formation that is characteristically hook-like when found at the MCPs (Figure 57-2). Chondrocalcinosis is present in 30% to 60% of patients and can occur without the degenerative arthropathy. The triad of subchondral lucencies (especially in the hip), chondrocalcinosis, and hook-like osteophytes of the second and third MCPs is particularly suggestive of HHC.

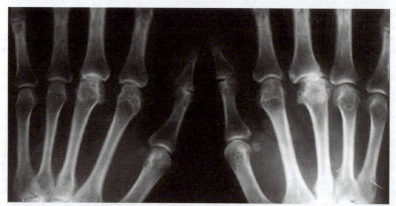

Figure 57-2. Hand radiographs for a patient with hemochromatosis. Note the degenerative arthritis of the metacarpophalangeal joints with hook-like osteophytes.

8. **Generalized osteopenia is common in HHC. What are its possible causes?**
   - Increased synovial iron (comparable to serum levels) directly inhibits bone formation.
   - Pituitary iron infiltration decreases gonadotropin levels, leading to hypogonadism (hypogonadotropic hypogonadism).
   - Hepatic cirrhosis leads to testicular atrophy and hypogonadism and poor conversion of vitamin D to 25-OH vitamin D.

9. **How is a diagnosis of hemachromatosis made?**
   In the fasting state, transferrin saturation (iron/total iron-binding capacity × 100) greater than 60% in men or 50% in women along with elevated ferritin greater than twice the normal level is 95% sensitive and 85% specific for diagnosis of hemachromatosis. Genetic screening is recommended for all patients with transferrin saturation >45% and ferritin >200 μg/L. Serum ferritin levels are an accurate measure of peripheral iron stores but may also be increased in the settings of acute liver injury, systemic inflammation, and neoplasia (i.e., lymphoma). A definitive diagnosis is made by direct measurement of iron in a liver biopsy. In addition, synovial biopsies will reveal iron deposition in type B synovial lining cells in patients with arthritis. This pattern of iron deposition is different to that seen in other diseases causing iron deposition in synovial tissue (rheumatoid arthritis, osteoarthritis, pigmented villonodular synovitis, hemophilia, and hemarthrosis). However, biopsies may not be necessary in the setting of abnormal iron studies in a patient homozygous for the C282Y HFE mutation.

10. **Once a proband case of HFE-associated HHC is identified, who should be screened and by what method?**
    All first-degree relatives of the patient should be screened for the disease using fasting transferrin saturation and testing for C282Y and H63D HFE mutations. Fasting transferrin saturation >45% and ferritin >200 μg/L

suggest HHC in an individual homozygous for the risk alleles. Liver biopsy is not necessary for diagnosis unless severe fibrosis is suspected (serum ferritin >1000 μg/L) or the diagnosis is in doubt, as in the case of individuals heterozygous for the C282Y mutation with abnormal iron indices or liver function tests. New hepatic magnetic resonance imaging techniques to quantitate hepatic iron content may replace the need for liver biopsy. Screening can be deferred until the second decade of life.

11. **Describe the treatment plan for hemochromatosis.**
Phlebotomy is performed twice weekly until transferrin saturation is <50% and ferritin is <50 μg/L (up to 2 to 3 years) and then as required (usually every 3 to 4 months) to maintain low normal serum levels (ferritin <300 μg/L in men, < 200 μg/L in women). Life expectancy of symptomatic patients is extended considerably by removal of excess iron stores (90% 5-year survival vs 33% survival without therapy). With therapy, hepatomegaly, liver function studies, and pigmentation all improve and cardiac function stabilizes or improves. Diabetes mellitus improves in approximately 50% of cases. Phlebotomy has little effect on hypogonadism or arthropathy. Hepatic fibrosis may improve, but cirrhosis is irreversible. Hepatocellular carcinoma, a late sequela in one third of those who develop hepatic cirrhosis (risk increased by a factor of 20 to 200), is not diminished by phlebotomy and is the major cause (30% to 45%) of death in treated individuals. Therefore a biannual abdominal scan (ultrasound or computed tomography) and measurement of serum α-fetoprotein levels are recommended for hepatocellular cancer screening. Because the life expectancy of homozygotes diagnosed and treated before the development of cirrhosis is the same as that of the general population, the importance of family screening and early therapy cannot be overemphasized. All patients with HHC should be advised to avoid alcohol, medicinal iron, excess vitamin C, and uncooked seafood.

12. **What are the common clinical presentations of Wilson disease (hepatolenticular degeneration)?**
Owing to multiple genetic mutations of the *ATP7B* gene, the clinical presentations can be highly variable. The hepatic form presents before age 18 years and the neuropsychiatric form in early adulthood (age 20 to 30 years); a late-onset form also exists. Manifestations include the following:
 - **Liver disease:** abnormal liver-associated enzymes are seen in over 95% of cases. Liver disease is the initial presentation in 50% of cases and can manifest as asymptomatic transient hepatitis to fulminant hepatitis, chronic active hepatitis, and cirrhosis. A clue to Wilson disease as the etiology for fulminant hepatic failure is the disproportionately low level of aminotransferases (usually <1500 μ/L) and the marked increase in bilirubin due to associated hemolytic anemia (Coombs-negative).
 - **Neuropsychiatric disease:** the most common manifestations are varying tremors, rigidity, and dystonia caused by basal ganglion degeneration. Psychiatric disorders such as mood disturbances, neurosis, hypophonia, and personality changes occur in up to 33% of cases. These manifestations tend to occur later than the hepatic presentation, but abnormal liver transaminases and Kayser–Fleischer rings are invariably seen in these patients.
 - **Eyes:** Kayser–Fleischer rings are caused by granular deposits in Descement membranes; present in 95% of patients with and 50% to 60% of patients without neurologic symptoms
 - **Hematologic:** Coombs-negative hemolytic anemia
 - **Kidneys:** tubular dysfunction, Fanconi syndrome
 - **Fertility:** amenorrhea, infertility
 - **Musculoskeletal:** osteoarthritis, osteopenia

13. **Describe the musculoskeletal manifestations of Wilson disease.**
Musculoskeletal manifestations occur in 50% of patients but are rarely the presenting symptom because all patients have other manifestations of Wilson disease. Pain and swelling of the MCPs, wrists, elbows, shoulders, knees, and hips resembling hemochromatosis may occur, although asymptomatic radiographic changes are equally as common. Radiographically, subchondral and cortical fragmentation, as well as marginal, subchondral, and central bony sclerosis of the wrist, hand, elbow, shoulder, and knee, help to distinguish this arthropathy from primary osteoarthritis. Unlike hemochromatosis, involvement of the hip and MCP joints is uncommon. Less common radiographic findings include osteochondritis dissecans, chondrocalcinosis, chondramalacia patellae, and vertebral wedging. Generalized osteoporosis or osteomalacia may be present as a result of Fanconi syndrome or renal tubular acidosis, both of which are common in Wilson disease.

14. **What is the genetic mutation leading to the biochemical defect in Wilson disease?**
The gene responsible for Wilson disease (*ATP7B*) has been localized to human chromosome 13 and encodes an abnormal P1-type ATP. This is a membrane copper transport protein localized in the trans-Golgi network in hepatocytes that normally facilitates binding of copper to ceruloplasmin and transport of hepatocellular copper into bile. The defect allows free copper to build up in hepatocytes. More than 300 mutations have been identified, although one mutation accounts for 30% to 60% of cases. Genetic testing using polymorphic DNA markers is helpful in testing presymptomatic siblings and is recommended before treatment is initiated.

15. **How is a diagnosis confirmed?**
Wilson disease results from excessive copper accumulation in association with ceruloplasmin deficiency. The capacity of hepatocytes to store copper is exceeded, and excessive free copper is deposited in the liver and at

extrahepatic sites such as the brain and kidney, where it attacks cell membranes and DNA because of its redox properties. Decreased serum ceruloplasmin (<200 mg/L) and elevated urinary copper excretion (>65 to 100 µg/day) are suggestive of Wilson disease. An elevated hepatic copper concentration (>250 µg Cu/g dry weight) is the most reliable test early in the course of the illness. Screening of first-degree relatives older than 6 years should include a physical examination, liver function tests, measurement of serum copper, ceruloplasmin, and 24-hour urine copper, and slit lamp examination. Siblings of Wilson disease patients have a 25% risk of having the disease and children of patients have a 1 in 200 risk.

16. How is Wilson disease treated?
Lifelong penicillamine chelation therapy is the preferred choice because it can prevent or improve virtually every manifestation of Wilson disease. Side effects are common (30%). Other treatment options include trientine (chelator) and zinc salts (bind copper in the gut). Foods rich in copper such as organ meats, nuts, chocolate, and mushrooms need to be avoided. With early, effective chelation, most patients can live normal, healthy lives. Patients presenting with fulminant hepatic failure do not respond well to chelation and require urgent liver transplantation.

17. What is ochronosis (alkaptonuria)?
Ochronosis (also known as alkaptonuria) is a rare autosomal recessive defect in tyrosine catabolism caused by mutations of the *HGO* gene on chromosome 3 that result in a deficiency of homogentisic acid dioxygenase (HGD). Notably, heterozygotes are unaffected even when challenged with high doses of the precursor amino acids. HGD catabolizes homogentisic acid to molecules that can be used in the tricarboxylic acid (Krebs) cycle. When HGD is absent, homogentisic acid builds up, polymerizes, and is deposited in tissue (skin, sclera, arterial walls, prostate, and ear) as a gray-brown to blue-black pigment. Microscopic visualization by Virchow demonstrated a yellowish or "ochre" tint to tissues; hence the name *ochronosis*. The urine of a patient with ochronosis darkens on addition of alkali. The original term for homogentisic acid was *alkapton*, which referred to its avidity for alkali; hence the name *alkaptonuria*.
In rare cases, exogenous ochronosis causes bluish black cartilage pigmentation in individuals exposed to phenol, benzene, hydroquinone or other noxious substances. Chronic minocycline use can also stain cartilage black.

18. How is a diagnosis of alkaptonuria made?
The clinical diagnosis is suggested by the following typical triad of findings:
- Degenerative arthritis (premature), especially in the spine with disc calcification; the earliest involvement is observed for the lumbar spine
- Abnormal pigmentation, usually occurring first in the ear cartilage and sclerae
- Urine that turns blue-black on standing (occurs in 75% of patients)

Homogentisic acid binds collagen and is therefore deposited in connective tissues throughout the body. Observation of blue-black or gray-brown pigment in tissues (skin, ears, cerumen, sclerae, cartilage) suggests ochronosis. The diagnosis can be further supported if the urine darkens on standing in air or on addition of alkali (10 drops of 10% NaOH to 20 mL of urine). However, confirmation of the diagnosis requires measurement of 24-hour urinary excretion of homogentisic acid. A specific enzyme assay for homogentisic acid dioxygenase can also be performed.

19. Describe the musculoskeletal and other manifestations of alkaptonuria.
Degenerative joint disease occurs in the third decade of life, with typical symptoms of pain, stiffness, and a limited range of motion for the large joints and spine. The most common site involved is the spine, followed by the knees, hips, and shoulders. Peripheral joint arthritis usually occurs a decade later than for the spine. Abnormal calcification and ossification occur. Tendinitis has been reported. Dense calcification of the intervertebral discs is said to be pathognomonic. The *vacuum sign* is also prominent in discs. Synovial fluid may have a characteristic **ground-pepper** appearance caused by pigmented cartilage fragments. It has been noted that calcium pyrophosphate deposition disease can coexist with ochronotic arthritis.
Patients with alkaptonuria have an increased prevalence of kidney stones (25% of patients) and also develop heart valve and coronary artery calcifications. Axillary and inguinal areas may have a brownish discoloration.

20. What are the characteristic findings for ochronosis?
Lumbosacral radiographs show premature degenerative changes, ligamentous calcifications, dense wafer-like calcifications of the intervertebral discs, vacuum discs, and narrowing of the intervertebral spaces (Figure 57-3). Sacroiliac joints are normal. Prominent intervertebral disc calcification can also be seen in hemochromatosis, hyperparathyroidism, calcium pyrophosphate deposition disease, paralytic poliomyelitis, and amyloidosis. The radiographic appearance of the large peripheral joints in ochronotic arthritis is virtually indistinguishable from that in primary osteoarthritis.

21. How is ochronotic arthritis treated?
Treatment for symptom alleviation of the arthritis as for osteoarthritis is the standard therapy and includes patient education, physical and/or local therapy, and analgesia. Dietary restriction of phenylalanine and tyrosine is indicated. Large doses of vitamin C have been used, but there are no studies of its efficacy. Total joint

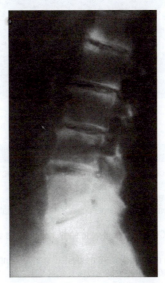

Figure 57-3. Lateral radiograph of the spine in a patient with ochronosis. Note the vertebral disc-space calcification at multiple levels.

arthroplasty is necessary in over 50% of patients by age 55. Arthroscopy has been of benefit for removal of osteochondral loose bodies in the knee. Nitisinone (Orfadin) is currently under investigation for the prevention and treatment of ochronosis. This drug inhibits the enzyme 4-hydroxyphenylpyruvic acid dioxygenase, which produces homogentisic acid. A recent trial reported that it was not effective once arthritis was established. It is unknown if earlier treatment could prevent the development of arthritis.

Acknowledgment
The author would like to thank Dr. Mark Jarek for his contribution to the previous edition of this chapter.

BIBLIOGRAPHY
Ala A, Walker AP, Ashkan K, et al: Wilson's disease, Lancet 369:397–408, 2007.
Alexander J, Kowdley KV: HFE-associated hereditary hemochromatosis, Genet Med 11:307–313, 2009.
Balaban B, Taskaynatan M, Yasar E, et al: Ochronotic spondyloarthropathy: spinal involvement resembling ankylosing spondylitis, Clin Rheumatol 25:598–601, 2006.
Carroll GJ, Breidahl WH, Olynyk JK: Characteristics of the arthropathy described in hereditary hemochromatosis, Arthritis Care Res 64:9–14, 2012.
Hunter T, Gordon D, Ogryzlo MA: The ground pepper sign of synovial fluid: a new diagnostic feature of ochronosis, J Rheumatol 1:45–53, 1974.
Huster D: Wilson disease, Best Pract Res Clin Gastroenterol 24:531–539, 2010.
Mannoni A, Selvi E, Lorenzini S, et al: Alkaptonuria, ochronosis, and ochronotic arthropathy, Semin Arthritis Rheum 33:239–248, 2004.
Perry MB, Suwannarat P, Furst GP, et al: Musculoskeletal findings and disability in alkaptonuria, J Rheumatol 33:2280–2285, 2006.
Suwannarat P, Phornphutkul C, Bernardini I, et al: Minocycline-induced hyperpigmentation masquerading as alkaptonuria in individuals with joint pain, Arthritis Rheum 50:3698–3701, 2004.

FURTHER READING
http://rarediseases.info.nih.gov/GARD

CHAPTER 58

RHEUMATOLOGIC MANIFESTATIONS OF THE PRIMARY IMMUNODEFICIENCY SYNDROMES

Sterling G. West, MD and Mark Malyak, MD

> **KEY POINTS**
>
> 1. Patients with primary immunodeficiencies (PIDs) typically present with chronic and recurring infections any time between infancy and adulthood.
> 2. Hypogammaglobulinemia occurs in over 80% of patients with a PID.
> 3. Selective IgA deficiency is the most common immunodeficiency and is associated with a variety of autoimmune manifestations.
> 4. Common variable immunodeficiency (CVID) may present in early adulthood as an aseptic polyarthritis of the large and medium joints.
> 5. Early complement protein (C1, C4, C2) deficiencies are associated with autoimmune diseases whereas late (C5 to C8) deficiencies are associated with *Neisseria* infections.

1. Why are PID syndromes of concern in rheumatology?

Although uncommon (1 in 10,000 live births), there are over 165 PID syndromes. These diseases may be associated with a variety of problems in addition to an increased risk of infection, including autoimmune and autoinflammatory manifestations, allergy, and an increased risk of lymphoid and epithelial neoplasms. Autoimmunity may manifest as a recognized autoimmune disease, such as systemic lupus erythematosus (SLE) in congenital deficiency of C4. Alternatively, various autoantibodies may be present in the absence of clinically expressed autoimmune disease, such as rheumatoid factor (RF; anti-IgG antibodies) or antinuclear antibodies (ANA) in selective IgA deficiency.

2. What components of the immune system are involved in PID syndromes?

- B cells (humoral immunodeficiency): 55% of all immunodeficiencies
- T cells and natural killer (NK) cells (cell-mediated immunodeficiency): 20%
- Phagocytes (neutrophils, macrophages, dendritic cells): 20%
- Complement proteins and mannose-binding lectin (MBL): 5%

The individual PID syndromes may be caused by dysfunction of a single component of the immune system, such as C4 deficiency, or dysfunction of multiple components, such as impairment of B-cell, T-cell, and phagocyte function in certain severe combined immunodeficiencies. Many PID syndromes are diagnosed during infancy or childhood, although the most common B-cell immunodeficiencies tend to manifest first in young adulthood. Any child with two or more sinopulmonary infections within 1 year, four or more ear infections within 1 year, or two or more deep skin or organ infections including septicemia should be evaluated for a PID disorder. The first test to order is a complete blood count with differential.

3. The types of recurrent infection in a particular patient offer a clue to the underlying PID syndrome. What microorganisms are responsible for recurrent infections in B-cell immunodeficiency syndromes?

B-cell immunodeficiency, such as X-linked (Bruton) agammaglobulinemia (XLA), results in inadequate immunoglobulin production and can lead to recurrent infection with extracellular, encapsulated, pyogenic bacteria, particularly *Streptococcus pneumoniae*, *Haemophilus influenzae*, and *Moraxella catarrhalis*. These organisms typically cause acute and chronic infections of the upper (sinusitis, otitis, bronchitis) and lower (pneumonias) respiratory tracts, meningitis, and bacteremia. Gastrointestinal (GI) infections (*Giardia*, *Cryptosporidium*) are also more prevalent.

4. What laboratory tests are performed to evaluate the integrity of the humoral immune system (B-cell function)?

A simple initial screen for hypogammaglobulinemia is to subtract the albumin from the total protein level to determine if the latter is <1.5 g/dL. A reasonable screen for evaluation of B-cell function is to determine serum IgA and perform inexpensive in vivo functional tests. If all these tests are normal, clinically significant B-cell dysfunction can be excluded. If any of these tests is abnormal, quantitation of IgG and IgM levels, IgG subclasses, and possibly in vitro testing will be necessary to determine the cause of the underlying PID syndrome (Table 58-1).

Table 58-1. Laboratory Evaluation of B-Cell Function

CATEGORY	SPECIFIC TESTS	COMMENTS
In vivo (functional tests, routine screening tests)	Isohemagglutinin titers (anti-blood group A and B)	Naturally occurring; predominantly IgM
	Diphtheria and tetanus booster immunization	Serum antibodies assayed before and 2 weeks later; assesses capacity to synthesize IgG antibodies against protein antigens
	Pneumococcal immunization	Serum antibodies assayed before and 3 weeks later; assesses capacity to synthesize antibodies against polysaccharide antigens
Immunoglobulin quantitation	IgM, IgG, IgA levels	Various immunoassays may be used; readily available
	IgG subclass, IgE levels	ELISA and RIA available (expensive)
In vitro tests (expensive)	Peripheral blood total B cells	Flow cytometry, CD19$^+$B cell numbers
	B cell subsets	Class-switched (CD27$^+$IgD$^-$) vs nonswitched (CD27$^+$IgD$^+$) memory B cells
	Genetic testing (mutation analysis)	BTK (XLA); ICOS, TACI, CD19, BAFF-R (CVID)
	In vitro immunoglobulin synthesis	Peripheral blood mononuclear cells stimulated in vitro with pokeweed mitogen

ELISA, Enzyme-linked immunosorbent assay; *RIA*, radioimmunoassay.

5. **What organisms are responsible for infections in primary T-cell immunodeficiency such as thymic hypoplasia (DiGeorge syndrome)?**
   - Viruses (e.g., herpesviruses)
   - Intracellular bacteria (e.g., mycobacteria)
   - Fungi (e.g., *Candida* species)
   - Other (*Pneumocystis jirovecii*)

   Primary T-cell immunodeficiency usually manifests during infancy and results in inadequate cell-mediated immunity, leading to infections similar to those encountered in patients with human immunodeficiency virus (HIV) infection, the prototypic acquired T-cell immunodeficiency state. CD4$^+$ helper T cells (Th2 subset) interact with B cells to facilitate immunoglobulin class switching and a productive antibody response to most protein antigens. CD4$^+$ T cells (Th1 subset) and CD8$^+$ cytotoxic T cells play a key role in detecting and eradicating intracellular organisms such as viruses, fungi, mycobacteria, and *Pneumocystis*. Regulatory T cells (CD4$^+$ CD25$^+$ FOXP3$^+$ T$_{REG}$) are important in peripheral tolerance, and absence of these cells leads to early-onset autoimmunity. It was recently shown that the Th17 subset of CD4$^+$ T helper cells are important in controlling superficial fungal infections. Patients with cellular defects (STAT1/3) or IL-17 mutations develop severe chronic mucocutaneous candidiasis.

6. **What laboratory tests can be used to evaluate the integrity of the cellular immune system (T-cell function)?**
   A reasonable screening evaluation of T-cell function is to determine the absolute lymphocyte count and perform a *Candida* skin test (Table 58-2). If these are both normal, clinically significant T-cell dysfunction can be excluded. If the *Candida* skin test is negative, negative delayed-type skin testing with at least four other antigens is necessary to demonstrate that T-cell function is inadequate. If these screening tests are abnormal, more sophisticated in vitro tests may be necessary to define the underlying PID disorder. HIV testing should be performed as part of the screening evaluation to exclude this acquired T-cell disorder.

7. **What infections are characteristic of an abnormality of phagocytic cells?**
   Phagocytic cell dysfunction can be caused by defects in neutrophil numbers (e.g., congenital or cyclic neutropenia), adherence (e.g., LAD-1 deficiency), chemotaxis, degranulation (e.g., Chédiak–Higashi syndrome), microbial

Table 58-2. Laboratory Evaluation of T-Cell Function

CATEGORY	SPECIFIC TESTS	COMMENTS
In vivo functional tests (skin testing for delayed-type hypersensitivity) (routine screening tests)	Candida skin test	Examine degree of induration 48-72 h later
	PPD, *Trichophyton*, mumps, tetanus or diphtheria toxoid, keyhole-limpet hemocyanin	If *Candida* skin test is negative, testing with at least four of these antigens must be performed to determine if cell-mediated immunity is inadequate
Absolute lymphocyte count (routine screening)	Determine from total WBC count and percentage lymphocytes	Severe cell-mediated immunity disorder unlikely in setting of normal lymphocyte count
In vitro tests (expensive)	Quantitation of total T, CD4$^+$, CD8$^+$, and NK cells	Specific monoclonal antibody may be used
	Lymphocyte blastic transformation	Assessment of radiolabeled thymidine uptake following stimulation with lectins (e.g., PHA), specific antigen (e.g., *Candida*), or one-way mixed lymphocyte reaction
	Quantitate ability of T cells to synthesize IL-2 and IL-2 receptors (CD25)	These and lymphocyte blastic transformation assays are indicators of successful T-cell activation

PHA, Phytohemagglutinin; *PPD*, purified protein derivative (for tuberculosis); *WBC*, white blood cell.

killing (e.g., chronic granulomatous disease), monocyte numbers (congenital), or macrophage dysfunction (e.g., defective IFNγ receptor or IL-12 signaling). Patients with absent pus at sites of infection and poor wound healing have defects in neutrophil numbers, adhesion, or chemotaxis. Patients with neutrophil defects of microbial killing present with lymphadenitis and visceral or perirectal abscesses with granuloma formation caused by low-virulence gram-negative organisms such as *Escherichia coli*, *Serratia*, and *Klebsiella*. Other patients will have gingivitis and skin infections or furunculosis with *Staphylococcus* or *Pseudomonas* species. Patients with macrophage defects have frequent mycobacterial infections.

8. How is neutrophil function measured?

Standard neutrophil tests include assessment of cell number, examination for giant granules on a peripheral smear (Chédiak–Higashi syndrome), and measurement of oxidative burst (chronic granulomatous disease). The flow cytometry dihydrorhodamine 123 assay is better than the nitroblue tetrazolium test for assessing neutrophil oxidative burst. If the results are normal, testing for adherence problems such as LAD-1 deficiency (measure CD11a, CD11b, and CD18), chemotaxis defects, specific granule (lactoferrin) deficiency, and phagocytosis defects can be undertaken.

9. What are the infectious manifestations of homozygous complement-deficient states?

The complement deficiencies can be divided into those of the classical pathway (C1 to C9), alternative complement pathway (factors B, D, and P), the MBL pathway and associated proteases (MASP-1 and MASP-2), and the complement regulatory proteins (C1 inhibitor, factor H, factor I, membrane cofactor protein [MCP]). Deficiency of C3 or MBL is associated with recurrent blood-borne infections with encapsulated bacteria, including *S. pneumoniae* and *H. influenza*. Deficiencies of components of the membrane attack complex (C5 to C9) or alternative complement pathway factors are associated with recurrent *Neisseria* infections (both *N. meningitidis* and *N. gonorrhoeae*). C6 deficiency is most common. **Patients with recurrent bouts of neisserial infections, particularly when systemic, should be evaluated for the presence of a complement deficiency.** All patients should be immunized with the conjugate meningococcal vaccine. Use of prophylactic antibiotics is controversial because of the risk of causing antibiotic-resistant strains of *Neisseria*.

10. What is the screening approach for homozygous complement and MBL deficiency?

In the general population, complement deficiencies are uncommon, whereas up to 3% of individuals can have MBL deficiency. The **total hemolytic complement assay (CH_{50})** assesses the integrity of the classic pathway of complement activation. Patient serum is added to a standardized suspension of sheep red blood cells (RBCs) coated with rabbit antibody. These "immune complexes" allow activation of the classic pathway, resulting in lysis of the sheep RBC. CH_{50} is the reciprocal of the serum dilution that lyses 50% of the sheep RBC. Because specific deficiencies that lead to rheumatologic manifestations are usually in the classical rather that

11. **What organisms are responsible for septic arthritis in patients with hypogammaglobulinemia due to primary B-cell immunodeficiency?**
Selective IgA deficiency, XLA, CVID, and Ig deficiency with increased IgM (hyper-IgM) account for >99% of the primary hypogammaglobulinemic states (B-cell immunodeficiency). These patients are susceptible to septic arthritis caused by the usual organisms encountered in B-cell immunodeficiency states: S. pneumoniae, H. influenzae, and Staphylococcus aureus. In addition to these typical infectious agents, patients are also susceptible to joint infections with Ureaplasma urealyticum and other Mycoplasma organisms. The incidence of septic arthritis in these B-cell disorders is unknown but is less than that for the more frequently encountered infections of the upper and lower respiratory tract and GI tract.

12. **What PID syndromes are most commonly associated with autoimmune phenomena?**
    - Selective IgA deficiency, CVID, XLA, and hyper-IgM syndrome are the B-cell immunodeficiency syndromes commonly associated with autoimmune phenomena.
    - Complete absence of certain early complement components (C1, C2, C4) is also associated with autoimmune phenomena, particularly SLE.
    - Chronic granulomatous disease, a primary disorder of neutrophils, is associated with the presence of ANA (less commonly, SLE) and inflammatory bowel disease.

    In general, patients with predominantly T-cell immunodeficiency do not exhibit autoimmune phenomena, at least in part because many such patients do not survive infancy. Severe combined immunodeficiency (SCID; 21 gene defects described), Omenn syndrome (RAG1 and RAG2 defects), *autoimmune polyendocrine syndrome* (AIRE defect), immune dysregulation, polyendocrinopathy, enteropathy X-linked (IPEX) syndrome (FOXP3 defect), autoimmune lymphoproliferative syndrome (FAS defect), and Wiskott–Aldrich syndrome (WASp defect) have T-cell and immune tolerance defects and can have autoimmune (hematologic [autoimmune hemolytic anemia, immune thrombocytopenia], enteropathic, arthritis, other organ-specific) and/or atopic (eczema) features among their manifestations. PIDs affecting CD8 and NK cell cytotoxicity such as perforin deficiency carry a risk of hemophagocytic syndrome development.

13. **What are the rheumatologic manifestations of XLA?**
XLA is a rare disorder characterized by absent or near-absent levels of serum IgG, IgM, and IgA, and abnormal in vivo B-cell functional tests. Less severe forms of this disease have been identified. Cell-mediated immunity is intact. The molecular defect is mutation within the Bruton tyrosine kinase (*BTK*) gene, resulting in abnormal function of this signal transduction protein, which is normally present within B cells at all stages of development. This results in characteristic cellular abnormalities: maturation failure for the B cell line and the absence of B cells. Arthritis occurs in approximately 20% of patients, with half of these cases caused by infection with the typical pyogenic bacteria. In addition, patients appear vulnerable to infections with enterovirus and *Mycoplasma* (Table 58-3). There are cases of arthritis in XLA in which an infectious agent cannot be detected despite rigorous evaluation. These cases may represent infection with a fastidious organism that cannot be identified or may represent a true autoimmune disorder, such as juvenile inflammatory arthritis. Overall, autoimmune phenomena occur much less frequently in XLA than in selective IgA deficiency or CVID.

Table 58-3. Rheumatologic Manifestations of X-Linked Agammaglobulinemia	
Septic arthritis	Occurs in 10% of patients
Extracellular, encapsulated bacteria (*S. pneumonia, H. influenzae, S. aureus*)	
Mycoplasma, particularly *Ureaplasma urealyticum*	
Enteroviruses, particularly echovirus and coxsackievirus	
Aseptic, possibly autoimmune, arthritis	Usually mono- or oligoarticular; involves large joints; rarely destructive; RF and ANA absent; occurs in 10% of patients
Dermatomyositis-like syndrome associated with progressive enterovirus (ECHO) central nervous system infection	Presents with rash and muscle weakness

ANA, Antinuclear antibody; *RF*, rheumatoid factor.

14. **What are the various rheumatologic manifestations of selective IgA deficiency?**
    - Autoantibodies, particularly RF and ANA, in the absence of clinically expressed autoimmune disease
    - Systemic autoimmune disorders (SLE, aseptic arthritis, etc.) occur in 7% to 36% of patients (fourfold increased risk)
    - Organ-specific autoimmune disorders (diabetes mellitus type I, myasthenia gravis, etc.)

    IgA deficiency is the most common PID syndrome, with a prevalence of 1 in 333 to 1 in 700 in whites. Some 20% of cases are familial. The deficiency is characterized by very low levels (<5 mg/dL) of serum and secretory IgA, accompanied by normal serum levels of IgG and IgM. Cell-mediated immunity is intact. Patients may be asymptomatic (most patients), have recurrent respiratory and GI tract infections (especially if associated with IgG2/IgG4 subclass deficiency), or exhibit autoimmune phenomena. In most cases, IgA deficiency is likely a genetic disorder that is present at birth and remains persistent. Various molecular defects have been proposed. Some cases may be acquired later in life, often associated with drug therapy or viral infection, and are often transient.

15. **List the autoantibodies seen in patients with selective IgA deficiency without clinically expressed autoimmune disease.**

    The presence of autoantibodies in the absence of clinically expressed autoimmune disease commonly occurs in IgA deficiency. RF and ANA are most consistently observed. Other autoantibodies that may be present include antibodies against double- and single-stranded DNA, cardiolipin, thyroglobulin, thyroid microsomes, smooth muscle, gastric parietal cells, striated muscle, acetylcholine receptor, and bile canaliculi. IgG and IgE autoantibodies against IgA occur in 40% to 60% of patients, which puts them at risk of severe reactions to blood transfusions and intravenous immunoglobulin (IVIG).

16. **What systemic and organ-specific autoimmune diseases are associated with selective IgA deficiency?**

    Table 58-4 lists the autoimmune diseases associated with selective IgA deficiency.

Table 58-4. Autoimmune Diseases Associated With Selective IgA Deficiency

SYSTEMIC	ORGAN-SPECIFIC
Systemic lupus erythematosus*	Diabetes mellitus type I*
Juvenile idiopathic arthritis*	Myasthenia gravis*
Rheumatoid arthritis*	Inflammatory bowel disease
Sjögren's syndrome	Autoimmune hepatitis
Scleroderma	Pernicious anemia
Dermatomyositis	Primary adrenal insufficiency
Vasculitic syndromes	Autoimmune thrombocytopenia

*Most likely associations. Other conditions have been noted in case reports, but their true association with IgA deficiency remains to be proved.

17. **Describe the rheumatologic manifestations of CVID.**

    CVID is a heterogeneous group of disorders involving both B-cell and T-cell dysfunction. The predominant manifestation is IgG, IgM, and IgA hypogammaglobulinemia (Box 58-1), often resulting in the very low levels seen in XLA. Features distinguishing CVID from XLA include equal sex distribution, onset of symptoms later in life, and the presence of circulating B cells. Although the underlying immunologic defect is heterogeneous (ICOS, CD19, TACI, or BAFF-R deficiency), most patients exhibit a primary B-cell defect that results in a failure to mature into Ig-secreting plasma cells. Like selective IgA deficiency, CVID is probably a genetic disorder in most cases, although some cases may be truly acquired and secondary to a viral infection or an adverse

Box 58-1. Rheumatologic Manifestations of Common Variable Immunodeficiency

Septic arthritis
    Extracellular, and encapsulated bacteria (*S. pneumoniae, H. influenzae, S. aureus*)
    Mycoplasma, particularly *Ureaplasma urealyticum*
Aseptic, possibly autoimmune, arthritis
Sarcoid-like lesions in lung, liver, lymph node, skin; occur in 5-10% of patients
Organ-specific autoimmune disorders (pernicious anemia, autoimmune hemolytic anemia, idiopathic thrombocytopenic purpura, others); occur in 20% of patients

drug effect (i.e., cytotoxic therapy). Notably, patients with selective IgA deficiency are at increased risk of CVID evolution, which suggests that a common pathogenetic defect exists.

Septic arthritis caused by S. *aureus*, the usual extracellular encapsulated bacteria, and *Mycoplasma* species occurs at higher frequency in CVID. Because cell-mediated immunodeficiency sometimes occurs in CVID, fungi and mycobacteria must also be considered as potential pathogens.

Autoantibody presence in the absence of clinically expressed autoimmune disease occurs less often than in selective IgA deficiency. Nevertheless, autoimmune disorders are not unusual (20% to 25%) in CVID. Polyarthritis in which an infectious agent cannot be detected despite rigorous evaluation has been described. Characteristics include involvement of the large and medium joints, with sparing of the small joints of the hands and feet. Rheumatoid nodules, erosions, and significant articular cartilage destruction are not features of this syndrome. This form of arthropathy often responds to treatment with intravenous gammaglobulin. CVID should be ruled out in patients with sarcoidosis-like presentations. Organ-specific autoimmunity can also occur, including hematologic (AIHA, ITP), lung (lymphocytic interstitial pneumonitis), bowel (lymphocytic colitis), liver (autoimmune hepatitis), endocrine (thyroiditis, diabetes), and skin (psoriasis, vitiligo) manifestations.

18. What is the hyper-IgM syndrome?

The hyper-IgM immunodeficiency syndrome (type 1) is characterized by extremely low levels of IgG, IgA, and IgE, and either a normal or markedly elevated concentration of polyclonal IgM. Patients develop both recurrent pyogenic infections and opportunistic infections such as *P. jirovecii* pneumonia. There is also a higher frequency of autoimmune disorders (autoimmune cytopenias, arthritis, nephritis) and malignancy (lymphoma, GI tract tumors). The defect causing this X-linked syndrome is an abnormal gene resulting in a defective CD40 ligand (CD 154) on the surface of activated $CD4^+$ T cells. This mutation results in failure of T cells to interact with CD40 on B cells. This lack of B-cell signaling by T cells results in a failure of B cells to undergo isotype switching, so they produce only IgM. Two other types of this syndrome (types 2 and 3) have different genetic defects and inheritance patterns.

19. What mechanisms may explain the presence of aseptic arthritis and other autoimmune phenomena in PID syndromes?

The mechanisms responsible for autoimmune phenomena in PID syndromes remain unknown. The following possibilities exist:

1. Aseptic arthritis in primary B-cell immunodeficiency states may be caused by infection with a fastidious organism that cannot be identified by available methods.
2. The absence of secretory IgA in primary B-cell immunodeficiency syndromes may lead to:
   - Excessive absorption of antigen from the gut, leading to the formation of immune complexes (in disorders other than XLA) and subsequent immune complex disease. In addition, immune complexes may lead to RF formation.
   - Excessive absorption of superantigen from the gut, which may lead to activation of T cells containing particular V_β families on their T-cell receptors. If one of these clones also reacts against a self-antigen, an autoimmune state may result.
   - Excessive absorption of a particular antigen from the gut, leading to autoimmunity as a result of molecular mimicry.
3. Coexistence of PID and autoimmunity may be coincidental rather than causal. Common HLA extended haplotypes often present in selective IgA deficiency and CVID are also commonly present in autoimmune disorders such as SLE, diabetes mellitus type I, and myasthenia gravis. In fact, the prevalence of IgA deficiency in patients with SLE ranges from 1% to 5%, which is 10 to 20 times higher than in the general population.
4. Homeostatic proliferation: naïve T and B cells turn over much more rapidly in the setting of severe lymphopenia because of a functional excess of IL-7. These hyperproliferating cells are more likely to react against self-antigens without appropriate regulation.

20. Discuss the therapy for XLA, CVID, and selective IgA deficiency.

XLA: IVIG and aggressive treatment of bacterial infections with appropriate antibiotics are the recommended therapy. IVIG is usually administered at a dose of 400 to 600 mg/kg every month to maintain trough IgG levels of 500 to 800 mg/dL.

CVID: IVIG is also recommended for patients with CVID who have low IgG levels and recurrent infections. Occasionally, patients with CVID have complete absence of IgA, along with anti-IgA antibodies, placing them at risk for anaphylaxis with IVIG therapy.

Selective IgA deficiency: The mainstay of therapy is rigorous treatment of active bacterial infections with antibiotics. Prophylactic antibiotic therapy is controversial. IVIG should not be administered because many patients have autoantibodies against IgA, including IgE anti-IgA, which may result in severe anaphylaxis that is occasionally fatal. Patients should ideally receive blood products obtained from other patients with IgA deficiency.

21. What are the rheumatologic manifestations of homozygous complement-deficient states?

Deficiencies of the early components of the classic pathway (C1, C4, C2) are associated with immune complex disease, particularly SLE or a lupus-like glomerulonephritis. Dermatomyositis, vasculitis, and others have also been described. This may be caused by impaired clearance of apoptotic cells, an inability to maintain circulating immune complexes in a soluble state, and/or an inability to remove circulating immune complexes. The reported prevalence of SLE is 93% with C1q, 75% with C4, and 33% with C2 deficiency. C2 deficiency is the most common complement deficiency (1 in 20,000 individuals).

Factor H deficiency and polymorphisms have recently been associated with atypical (diarrhea-negative) hemolytic–uremic syndrome and glomerulonephritis. A similar syndrome may occur with factor I and MCP defects. These patients may be helped by treatment with eculizumab (Soliris). Factor H deficiency can also lead to secondary C3 deficiency, so patients may be at increased risk of infection.

Bibliography

Chapel H, Lucas M, Lee M, et al: Common variable immunodeficiency disorders: division into distinct clinical phenotypes, Blood 112:277–286, 2008.
Cunningham-Rundles C: Autoimmune manifestations in common variable immunodeficiency, J Clin Immunol 28(Suppl 1):S42–S45, 2008.
Fried AJ, Bonilla FA: Pathogenesis, diagnosis, and treatment of primary antibody deficiencies and infections, Clin Microbiol Rev 22:396–414, 2009.
Goyal R, Bulua AC, Nikolov NP, et al: Rheumatologic and autoimmune manifestations of primary immunodeficiency disorders, Curr Opin Rheumatol 21:78–84, 2009.
Latiff AH, Kerr MA: The clinical significance of immunoglobulin A deficiency, Ann Clin Biochem 44:131–139, 2007.
Noris M, Remuzzi G: Atypical hemolytic uremic syndrome, N Engl J Med 361:1676–1687, 2009.
Notarangelo LD: Primary immunodeficiencies, J Allergy Clin Immunol 125:S182–S194, 2010.
Rose ME, Lang DM: Evaluating and managing hypogammaglobulinemia, Clev Clin J Med 73:133–144, 2006.
Schaffer AA, Salzer U, Hammarström L, Grimbacher B: Deconstructing common variable immunodeficiency by genetic analysis, Curr Opin Genet Dev 17:201–212, 2007.
Sjoholm AG, Jonsson G, Braconier JH, et al: Complement deficiency and disease: an update, Mol Immunol 43:78–85, 2006.
Subbarayan A, Colarusso G, Hughes SM, et al: Clinical features that identify children with primary immunodeficiency diseases, Pediatrics 127:810–816, 2011.
Torgerson TR: Immunodeficiency diseases with rheumatic manifestations, Pediatr Clin North Am 59:493–507, 2012.

Further Reading

www.primaryimmune.org
http://www.nichd.nih.gov/publications/pubs/Pages/primary_immuno.aspx
www.info4pi.org

BONE AND JOINT DYSPLASIAS

Edmund H. Hornstein, DO

CHAPTER 59

KEY POINTS
1. An osteochondrodysplasia should be considered in any patient with premature osteoarthritis and/or disproportionate short stature.
2. Hypophosphatasia may mimic rickets and osteomalacia.

1. What exactly is a bone or joint dysplasia?
Dysplasia is a term literally meaning abnormal growth. Applied to the skeletal system, the term encompasses a heterogenous group of more than 350 conditions in which abnormalities of growth can affect the epiphysis, metaphysis, physis, or diaphysis of developing bone and are broadly grouped under the heading of **osteochondrodysplasias**. Although each individual syndrome is rare, collectively the overall incidence is one in 5000 births. These dysplasias are heritable and can range in severity from devastatingly symptomatic or even fatal, to mere radiologic curiosities. They should be considered in any individuals with disproportionate short stature and/or early-onset osteoarthritis. Many have head and facial dysmorphisms. Early identification allows initiation of treatment and genetic counselling.

2. How are the osteochondrodysplasias classified?
By international consensus, these disorders are formally classified based on etiopathogenetic information concerning specific gene and/or protein deficits. It is useful and practical, however, to group these disorders according to where the most prominent abnormalities in growth occur. The mnemonic **EMPD** ("empty") can help to broadly group these syndromes.

E—Epiphyseal dysplasias: the epiphysis is at the end of tubular bone and is formed as a secondary site of ossification. Normal development of the epiphysis is required if the joint surface is to be normal.

M—Metaphyseal dysplasias: the metaphysis is the wider part of a tubular bone between the diaphysis and physis.

P—Physeal dysplasias: the physis, or epiphyseal cartilage plate, separates the metaphysis from the epiphysis during growth. It is the primary site responsible for elongation of tubular bones.

D—Diaphyseal dysplasia: the diaphysis is the shaft of a long or tubular bone. It is composed of the spongiosa and cortex and is covered with periosteum.

These disorders can be further differentiated depending on whether the spine is involved: spondyloepiphyseal dysplasia (SED), spondylometaphyseal dysplasia (SMD), or spondyloepimetaphyseal dysplasia (SEMD) (Figure 59-1).

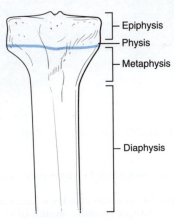

Figure 59-1. Parts of long bone.

3. What are the distinguishing features of the epiphyseal dysplasias?

Epiphyseal dysplasia is characterized by abnormal ossification of the developing epiphysis. The resulting morphologic abnormalities of the ossification centers are used to differentiate the various subtypes within this category. The most important epiphyseal dysplasias from a rheumatologic standpoint are multiple epiphyseal dysplasia (MED) and SED.

4. How does a patient with MED present clinically?

MED is primarily a group of autosomal dominant disorders. Identified gene abnormalities and associated proteins include COL9A1, COL9A2, COL9A3 (collagen 9 alpha-1, alpha-2 and alpha-3 chains), COMP (cartilage oligomeric matrix protein) and MATN3 (matrilin 3). Usually, the patient complains of symmetric joint pain in the hips, knees, wrists, and shoulders as a result of precocious osteoarthritis. Limitation in range of motion of affected joints is frequent. The spine is usually spared. Radiographs reveal irregular, flattened, small epiphyseal ossification centers during childhood and a deformed articular surface after physeal closure. The long bones of the legs and arms are most prominently affected. Adult stature is generally diminished and is proportionate to the severity of involvement. Disabling early degenerative arthritis is a common end result. Symptoms usually occur before adolescence but may not become apparent until early adulthood, depending on the severity of epiphyseal deformity.

5. What other conditions can be confused with MED?

Inflammatory arthritis: the pain and symmetry of involvement are sometimes mistaken for inflammatory arthritis. On closer evaluation, the absence of signs and symptoms of inflammation usually suffices to rule out this condition.

Hypothyroidism: occult hypothyroidism can lead to developmental skeletal abnormalities that may closely resemble some of the hereditary epiphyseal dysplasias. Thyroid function should always be checked when a diagnosis of epiphyseal dysplasia is being considered.

Juvenile osteochondrosis: these disorders, including Legg–Calvé–Perthes disease, may have a radiographic appearance similar to epiphyseal dysplasia but are usually limited to a single joint.

6. Describe the radiographic abnormalities typical for SED.

The SEDs are a diverse group of disorders linked by the radiographic findings of marked **platyspondyly** (short flat vertebrae) in association with abnormalities of **epiphyseal ossification**. Severe abnormalities in the epiphyses of long bones also occur. Spinal and long bone abnormalities often result in dwarfism with severe osteoarthritis. Genetic studies have linked this to abnormalities in the collagen type 2 gene (COL2A1) (Figure 59-2).

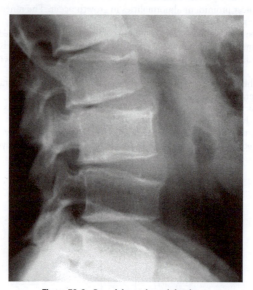

Figure 59-2. Spondyloepiphyseal dysplasia.

7. SED tarda and SED tarda with progressive arthropathy can sometimes be confused with juvenile idiopathic arthritis. Why?

Both of these X-linked recessive disorders are accompanied by enlargement of the ends of the tubular bones in the hands, which may be mistaken for juvenile idiopathic arthritis (JIA) on visual inspection. Radiographic evaluation inevitably leads to the correct diagnosis.

8. **What abnormality characterizes the metaphyseal dysplasias?**
   These dysplasias are characterized by a failure either to form or to absorb the spongiosa of developing bone. Important disorders from a rheumatologic standpoint within this category of dysplasias include the hypophosphatasias.

9. **What is the primary differential diagnosis in the hypophosphatasias?**
   The hypophosphatasias may look like **rickets** in children and **osteomalacia** in adults. Subtle radiographic findings may allow the distinction to be made, but the diagnosis of hypophosphatasia is ultimately based on the findings of an exceptionally low serum alkaline phosphatase in conjunction with high urine and serum phosphorylethanolamine levels. Mutations of *ALPL* on chromosome 1, which codes for tissue nonspecific alkaline phophatase (TNSALP), are responsible for this disease. These mutations lead to low levels of tissue alkaline phosphatase leading to less cleavage of pyrophosphate (PPi). The accumulation of PPi inhibits hydroxyapatite crystal formation. It also leads to chondrocalcinosis. Consideration of hypophosphatasia is warranted in any case of suspected rickets or osteomalacia, especially if early loss of teeth is evident.

10. **One of the most common osteochondrodysplasias is considered a physeal dysplasia and leads to dwarfism. Name this syndrome.**
    Achondroplasia is the most common skeletal dysplasia occurring in one in 20,000 live births. This physeal dysplasia is transmitted as an autosomal dominant trait, although spontaneous mutation is probably responsible for most cases. Mutations have been identified in the fibroblast growth factor (*FGFR3*) gene. It is considered a disproportionate dwarfism with rhizomelic (shorter proximal compared with distal) short limbs, macrocephaly with prominent frontal bossing, and some midface hypoplasia. An exaggerated lumbar lordosis is usually seen as well as flexion contractures at the elbows and hips. Intelligence is normal. Mean adult height is approximately 52 inches in men and 49 inches in women. Rheumatologic complaints may stem from a narrowed spinal canal and symptoms of spinal stenosis or from ligamentous laxity of the knees, leading to complaints of pain and premature degenerative disease.

11. **Where is the abnormality of bone formation found in the diaphyseal dysplasias?**
    Diaphyseal dysplasias result from abnormal formation of endosteal or periosteal bone. These dysplasias can be subclassified as hyperplasias or hypoplasias. Osteogenesis imperfecta is considered a hypoplastic diaphyseal dysplasia (see Chapter 55).

12. **A 21-year-old man complains of lower leg pain and swelling that has been gradually increasing. An x-ray is obtained (Figure 59-3). What is this disorder?**
    Melorheostosis. Melorheostosis, a nonhereditary idiopathic diaphyseal hyperplasia. Clinically, the patient complains of joint pain with onset usually in late childhood or early adulthood. Decreased range of motion, joint contracture or ankylosis, growth disturbances, foot deformities, and dystrophic skin, muscle, and soft tissue changes overlying affected bone are other features of this unusual disorder. The x-ray is characteristic and reveals dense, wavy, periosteal bony excrescences, which have been described as resembling wax flowing down the side of a candle.

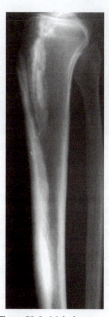

Figure 59-3. Melorheostosis.

13. **Another diaphyseal hyperplasia has radiographic and clinical features in common with hypertrophic osteoarthropathy, including clubbing of the digits, painful swollen joints, and periosteal bony apposition, but it is also associated with thickened, wrinkled elephant-like skin. Name this disorder.**
    Pachydermoperiostosis (Touraine–Solente–Gole syndrome). A literal translation of the term describes the major clinical manifestations of the disorder, which includes digital clubbing, thickening of the skin of the face and folds in the scalp, excessive sweating of hands and feet, and periostitis. It usually begins at puberty and progresses over the next 10 years. The genetic mutation responsible involves *HPGD* on chromosome 4, which encodes 15-hydroxyprostaglandin dehydrogenase and is responsible for prostaglandin degradation. The mutation leads to a lack of enzyme function resulting in persistently elevated prostaglandin E_2 (PGE2) levels.

14. **A 15-year-old boy is seen complaining of thoracic back pain with no clear history of trauma. The pain is worse with activity, improves with rest, and is not associated with significant morning stiffness. Physical exam is remarkable only for a hint of increased thoracic kyphosis with some lower thoracic tenderness to palpation in the midline and mild paravertebral muscle spasm. Workup reveals a normal erythrocyte sedimentation rate (ESR), serum chemistries, and complete blood count (CBC). An x-ray report lists that the findings are most consistent with Scheuermann's disease. What is the diagnosis?**
    Vertebral osteochondritis, or Scheuermann's disease, is a developmental abnormality of ossification of the endplates of vertebrae seen most often in the thoracic spine but also seen in the thoracolumbar and lumbar regions. It occurs during adolescence and is symptomatic in up to 60% of those affected, although it may also be found by chance on plain spine or chest x-rays requested for other reasons. The x-ray shows anterior wedging of multiple vertebrae with Schmorl's nodes and irregular vertebral endplates. Although the pathogenesis is uncertain, a hereditary weakening of the vertebral endplates present in affected patients is believed to allow disc material to encroach into the vertebral bodies. This then leads to abnormal growth and the x-ray changes described. Therapy is usually symptomatic and aimed at minimizing the tendency toward kyphosis. Occasionally, surgical intervention is required (Figure 59-4).

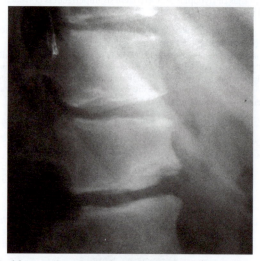

Figure 59-4. A radiograph of the spine showing irregular vertebral endplates in a patient with Scheuermann's disease.

15. **A newborn girl has a reproducible "click" as you flex and abduct her right hip (Ortolani's sign). You suspect that the child may have congenital dislocation of the hip. How can you verify this suspicion? What do you tell the parents?**
    Congenital hip dislocation or dysplasia is screened for shortly after birth using physical exam maneuvers such as Ortolani's sign and by inducing dislocation and reduction of an unstable hip (Barlow's sign). Plain films may not be easily interpretable in the first weeks of life, and modalities such as ultrasound, computed tomography (CT), or magnetic resonance imaging (MRI) generally offer better sensitivity. Congenital hip dysplasia has an excellent prognosis if recognized soon after birth. Treatment usually involves splinting the legs in abduction, thus allowing the shallow acetabulum to fully contain the femoral head. If the diagnosis is missed, however, later therapy is often much more involved and may require extensive orthopedic surgery. Untreated, this condition leads to premature osteoarthritis and may require early total hip replacement (Figure 59-5).

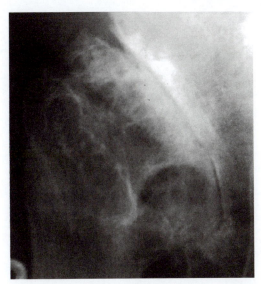

Figure 59-5. A hip radiograph from an adult with congenital hip dysplasia that was not treated during childhood. Note severe degenerative changes, shallow acetabulum, and malformed femoral head.

BIBLIOGRAPHY

Castori M, Sinibaldi L, Mingarelli R, et al: Pachydermoperiostosis: an update, Clin Genet 68:477–486, 2005.
Jain VK, Arya RF, Bharadwaj M, Kumar S: Melorheostosis: clinicopathologic features, diagnosis, and management, Orthopedics 32:512, 2009.
Krakow D, Rimoin DL: The skeletal dysplasias, Genetics in Medicine 12:327–341, 2010.
Tsirikos AI, Jain AK: Scheuermann's kyphosis: current controversies, J Bone Joint Surgery Br 93:857–864, 2011.
Warman ML, Cormier-Daire V, Hall C, et al: Nosology and classification of genetic skeletal disorders: 2010 revision, Am J Med Genet Part A 155:943–968, 2011.
Whyte MP: Enzyme defects and the skeleton. In Rosen CJ, editor: Primer on the metabolic bone diseases and disorders of mineral metabolism, ed 8, Washington DC, 2013, American Society for Bone and Mineral Research.

FURTHER READING

http://www.isds.ch
http://www.rarediseases.info.nih.gov/GARD

X
NONARTICULAR AND REGIONAL MUSCULOSKELETAL DISORDERS

The lower back is at the crossroads where the psyche meets the soma.

Voltaire (1694–1778)

APPROACH FOR THE PATIENT WITH NECK AND LOW BACK PAIN

Richard T. Meehan, MD

CHAPTER 60

KEY POINTS

1. RED FLAGS for serious pathology causing back pain: fever, bowel/bladder dysfunction, night pain unrelieved by rest, history of cancer, history of trauma in patients with osteoporosis.
2. Neurogenic claudication suggests lumbar spinal stenosis.
3. In a patient with back pain, only order magnetic resonance imaging (MRI) if the results will alter your plan of care.
4. Never advise surgery for mechanical low back pain without objective signs and symptoms of a radiculopathy unresponsive to conservative therapy.

1. **Which rheumatic disorders commonly involve the neck? (Table 60-1)**

Table 60-1. Musculoskeletal Disorders Involving the Cervical Spine

DISORDER	FEATURE
Rheumatoid arthritis	C1-C2 (atlantoaxial) subluxation, cranial settling
Juvenile idiopathic arthritis	C2-C3 fusion, C1-C2 subluxation
Ankylosing spondylitis	Ankylosis, C5-C6 fracture, C1-C2 subluxation
Diffuse idiopathic skeletal hyperostosis	Anterior longitudinal ligament ossification
Osteoarthritis	C5-C7 spondylosis
Polymyositis	Flexor muscle weakness
Polymyalgia rheumatic	Pain and stiffness
Fibromyalgia	C2, C5-C7 tender points

2. **What are the most common causes of neck pain?**
   - **Cervical strain and/or myofascial pain:** contributing causes such as sleeping difficulties, poor workplace ergonomics, and posture problems must be ruled out.
   - **Cervical spondylosis, discogenic, or facet joint pain:** there is a poor correlation between radiographic abnormalities and whether or not a patient is having neck pain. Lidocaine injection of the facet joints can determine if facet joint arthritis is the pain generator.
   - **Cervical whiplash syndrome:** caused by a traumatic event resulting in abrupt flexion/extension of the neck usually following a rear-end collision. In up to 50% of patients, pain can persist long after the acute injury in spite of no abnormality being seen on any imaging study. The exact pathology is unclear although alar ligament injury has been demonstrated in many patients. Clinical variables associated with prolonged symptoms include: female, younger age, stationary vehicle, prior history of neck pain, severity of collision, not being at fault, and bored with present job. Whether or not compensation is available also contributes to the length and severity of symptoms.

3. **When evaluating a patient with neck pain, how can you differentiate between a bony or muscular disorder?**
   Comparison of **active** and **passive** range of motion is useful for differentiating articular from soft-tissue disorders. **Passive** neck range of motion is best performed by supporting (cradling) the head while the patient is supine. The full range of the cervical spine may then be tested: flexion, extension, rotation, and lateral bending. During rotation and lateral bending, **ipsilateral** discomfort elicited in the direction of movement is suggestive of **bony** pain. Pain and/or tightness produced on the **contralateral** side usually implicates a muscular disorder. Finally, palpable tenderness of the spinous processes may indicate **bony** pathology whereas

local tenderness of paraspinous muscles usually indicates myofascial pain. **Passive range of motion (and provocative tests) should not be performed if instability or fracture of the cervical spine is suspected.**

4. **What is the value of provocative tests for diagnosing cervical radiculopathy resulting from nerve root compression within the foramina of the cervical vertebrae?**
   Provocative maneuvers vary in their sensitivity and specificity for diagnosing cervical radiculopathy. The values listed below are for **acute** cervical radiculopathy. The sensitivity for each of the tests is about 30% lower for **chronic** cervical radiculopathy.
   - **Spurling's maneuver:** with the patient seated, downward pressure is uniformly applied to the patient's cranium while the head is gently rotated or flexed toward the side of the suspected lesion. The immediate development of pain and/or paresthesias with radiation to the upper limb (see below) is indicative of cervical radiculopathy. Sensitivity 45% to 55%; specificity 85% to 93%.
   - **Shoulder abduction test:** with the patient seated, the palm of the affected extremity is actively placed on top of the head. The test is considered positive if this position **relieved** the radicular pain. Sensitivity 45% to 55%; specificity 85%.
   - **Upper limb tension test:** with the patient in supine position with affected arm placed on their body. The arm is abducted by the examiner with the forearm pronated and flexed. The forearm is then extended and supinated. Finally, the hand is extended from the wrist. The reproduction of symptoms is a positive result. Sensitivity 60% to 80%; specificity 20% to 40%.
   - **Traction/neck distraction test:** with the patient sitting, gently lift the head cephalad. The test is considered positive if radicular pain is **improved**. Sensitivity 44%; specificity 95%.
   - **Valsalva maneuver:** with the patient seated, have them take a deep breath and try to exhale it against a closed glottis for 2 to 3 seconds. The reproduction of radicular symptoms is a positive result. Sensitivity 22%; specificity 94%.

5. **What physical findings enable you to identify the approximate level of common cervical nerve root lesions?** (Table 60-2)

Table 60-2. Symptoms and Exam Findings of Cervical Nerve Root Impingement

NERVE	SENSORY LOSS	MOTOR WEAKNESS*	REFLEX
C5 (5%)	Lateral upper arm	Deltoid, biceps	Biceps
C6 (35%)	Lateral forearm, thumb, index finger	Wrist extensors, biceps	Radial[†], biceps
C7 (35%)	Middle finger	Wrist flexors, finger extensors, triceps	Triceps
C8 (25%)	Medial forearm, ring finger, little finger	Finger flexors, thumb extensor, hand intrinsics	None
T1 (rare)	Medial arm at elbow	Finger abductors	None

*Weakness of upper extremity muscles is often difficult to assess because innervations usually occur by two or more nerve roots.
[†]Radial reflex is also called the supinator jerk (tap on brachioradialis muscle near distal end of radius).

6. **What is Lhermitte's sign?**
   Lhermitte's sign is the reported sensation of an electric-like shock propagating down the spine as a result of brisk neck flexion. This maneuver may also induce limb paresthesias and weakness. Lhermitte's sign is observed is some patients with spinal cord compression but also in patients with multiple sclerosis.

7. **Compare and contrast cervical myelopathy with cervical radiculopathy.** (Table 60-3)

8. **What are the major categories of low back pain?**
   - Mechanical: degenerative disk disease, nonspecific low back pain/strain (with or without psychogenic component), pregnancy, discogenic, spondylolisthesis, facet arthritis, fractures, etc.
   - Radicular: foraminal nerve root compression, spinal stenosis
   - Inflammatory: ankylosing spondylitis
   - Infiltrative: cancer, infectious (osteomyelitis, abscess, and diskitis)
   - Referred: intra-abdominal pathology (i.e., abdominal aneurysm, nephrolithiasis)

9. **How may back pain be categorized on the basis of historical symptoms?** (Table 60-4)

10. **List the important questions that should be asked when obtaining a history from a patient with low back pain.**
    One can use the helpful mnemonic **P-Q-R-S-T** (the components of an electrocardiogram tracing) when approaching any patient with pain:

Table 60-3. Symptoms and Findings of Cervical Myelopathy vs. Radiculopathy

FEATURE	MYELOPATHY	RADICULOPATHY
Etiology	Spinal cord compression	Nerve root compression
Neck pain	Variable	Variable
Cranial nerve	Occasional	Never
Sensory loss	Stocking-glove paresthesias/numbness (all limbs)	Light touch/pinprick (upper limb dermatome)
Weakness (early)	All limbs (diffuse)	Upper limb myotome
Weakness (late)	Spastic paraparesis, quadriparesis	Upper limb myotome
Deep tendon reflexes	Upper limbs (decreased) Lower limbs (increased)	Upper limb (decreased)
Pathologic reflexes	Babinski's sign, Hoffmann's sign	None
Lhermitte's sign	Occasional	Never
Bladder disturbance	Urine retention, urine incontinence	None
Spinal automaticity	Jumping legs	None

Table 60-4. Symptoms Associated With Causes of Low Back Pain

FEATURE	MECHANICAL	INFLAMMATORY	SOFT TISSUE	INFILTRATIVE
Location	Diffuse	Diffuse	Diffuse	Focal
Symmetry	Unilateral	Bilateral	Generalized	Midline
Onset	Variable	Subacute	Acute or subacute	Insidious
Likely precipitant	Trauma Degeneration	±HLA-B27 Infection	Poor sleep Stress	Infection, cancer
Morning stiffness	30 min	>1 h	Variable	None
Activity response	↑ Symptoms	↓ Symptoms	Variable	Persistent symptoms
Rest response	↓ Symptoms	↑ Symptoms	Variable	Persistent symptoms
Nocturnal response	Mild	Moderate	Moderate	Severe
Systemic disease	No	Yes	No	Possible
Clinical conditions	Degenerative disk disease	Ankylosing spondylitis	Fibromyalgia	Cancer, infection

HLA-B27, Human leukocyte antigen B27.

P—Provocative and palliative factors: sitting (worse with diskogenic), walking (worse with spinal stenosis, relieved with forward flexion), supine (pain unrelieved if cancer or infection), Valsalva maneuver (worse with intrathecal or radicular process), lumbar extension (worse with spinal stenosis and facet arthritis) versus flexion (worse with lumbar strain or fibromyalgia). What is the position of maximal comfort, and does this reduce or eliminate pain or radicular symptoms?
Q—Quality of pain: burning/tingling, numb, sharp, or dull?
R—Radiation of pain: into leg (radicular), saddle area with bowel/bladder dysfunction (cauda equina syndrome), bilateral buttock or thigh (spinal stenosis, or referred from intra-abdominal pathology)?
S—Severity of pain or systemic symptoms: pain scale 1 to 10, fever, weight loss, change in bowel habits, etc.
T—Timing of pain: date of onset, associated trauma, and prior similar episodes?

11. **What are the potential pain generators of mechanical low back pain?**
    There are sensory nerve fibers in the disks, vertebral end plates, facet joints, ligaments, fascia, blood vessels, spinal nerve roots, and muscles surrounding the lumbar spinal column. Therefore, nonspecific mechanical low back pain could originate from any one or a combination of these sites.

12. **What are the RED FLAG signs and symptoms that indicate that a patient's low back pain may result from a serious cause?**

    Most low back pain is mechanical in nature and should slowly improve over 2 to 6 weeks. The following are symptoms or signs that suggest a more serious etiology of low back pain:
    - Unrelenting pain unaffected by change in position and not improved by supine position with hips flexed suggests infection, cancer, or infiltrative lesions.
    - Fever, chills, and weight loss suggest infection or cancer.
    - If the patient is writhing in pain on the exam table and unable to lie still as a result of pain, consider retroperitoneal pathology: aortic dissection, nephrolithiasis, pancreatitis, or a ruptured viscus unless drug-seeking behavior or psychogenic factors are present.
    - Pain and morning stiffness for >30 minutes that is improved with exercise in a patient less than 40 years of age suggest inflammatory spondyloarthropathy.
    - Bilateral radiation of pain, which is progressive, suggests cancer, central disk herniation, or spondyloarthropathy.
    - Abnormal neurological exam: sensory/motor deficit (foot drop), loss of rectal tone, urinary incontinence, saddle anesthesia, Babinski sign, or ankle clonus suggests nerve root compression, cancer, or central disk herniation.
    - Trauma or sudden onset of pain in a patient with risk factors for osteoporosis.

13. **What is sciatica?**

    The simplest definition of **sciatica** is back pain that **radiates** down one leg below the knee. The character of the pain is usually sharp or burning. Occasionally, dermatome numbness and paresthesias of the lower limb are also reported. **Valsalva** maneuvers or flexion and extension of the lumbosacral spine may exacerbate these symptoms. Sciatica pain is suggestive of nerve root irritation and usually occurs as a consequence of nerve root impingement by structures either within the central canal (disk protrusion, facet or ligament flavum hypertrophy, synovial cyst, etc.) or upon exiting the neural foramen (disk protrusion, congenital narrowing, spondylolisthesis).

14. **What physical findings enable you to identify the approximate level of common, lumbar nerve root lesions? (Table 60-5)**

Table 60-5. Physical Findings of Lower Lumbar Nerve Root Impingement

NERVE	SENSORY LOSS	MOTOR WEAKNESS	REFLEX
L4 (5%)	Anterior leg, medial foot	Tibialis anterior (ankle dorsiflexion)	Patellar
L5 (67%)	Lateral leg, web of great toe	Extensor hallucis longus (great toe extension)	None
S1 (28%)	Posterior leg, lateral foot	Peroneus muscles (foot version)	Achilles

PEARL: Note that 95% of nerve root impingement resulting from herniated disk disease occurs at the L5 or S1 level.

15. **What maneuvers on physical exam suggest lumbar spine nerve root irritation?**
    - **Femoral nerve stretch test:** performed to evaluate the upper lumbar roots (L2 to L4). With the patient prone, the examiner maximally flexes the knee (80 to 100 degrees). If there are no symptoms, then the hip is gently extended. Anterior thigh (L2, L3) or medial leg (L4) pain is suggestive of a lumbar root lesion. Pain produced in the lumbar region, posterior thigh, or between the ranges of 80 and 100 degrees of knee flexion is a positive test. Sensitivity and specificity 88%.
    - **Straight-leg raise (Lasegue's sign):** evaluates the sciatic nerve roots (L4 to S1) and is performed with the patient in a supine position. The examiner passively raises the extended leg, by the foot, to 70 degrees of elevation. Dermatome pain radiating below the knee upon raising the leg between 30 and 70 degrees of elevation is a positive test for nerve root irritation. A positive test is more convincing if passive ankle dorsiflexion reproduces the pain after the leg has been lowered to an angle that abolished the radicular pain. Sensitivity 52% to 71%; specificity 47% to 66%.
    - **Crossed-straight leg test:** this test causes contralateral radiating pain when the **unaffected** leg is elevated. It is usually is seen in patients with a herniated disk and is more specific but less sensitive than the straight-leg raise test. Sensitivity 28% to 43%; specificity 83% to 88%.
    - **Slump test:** the patient sits with the head bent forward and the leg outstretched, toes pointing upwards. The examiner gently eases the patient forward to increase stretch on the sciatic nerve. Sensitivity 44% to 87%; specificity 23% to 63%.

16. **What is Schober's test?**

    Schober's test measures mobility of the thoracolumbar spine during maximum active lumbar flexion. Two midline marks are drawn originating from dimples of Venus (which are inferior to the posterior, superior iliac spines), and 10 cm superior to that location in an upright patient. The distance between the marks is again measured with the patient's back at maximal flexion. A difference of less than 5 cm between neutral and flexion is suggestive of an inflammatory spondyloarthropathy. Limitation of lateral bending, reduced chest wall expansion during maximum inspiration, and restricted rotation of the thoracic spine with the pelvis held stable in a standing patient also support this diagnosis (see Figure 34-1).

17. **What exam suggests sacroiliitis?**
Pelvic compression, **Patrick's test**, and **Gaenslen's sign** may physically demonstrate sacroiliitis. Bilateral compression of the anterior iliac crests toward the midline, on a supine patient, may produce pathologic sacroiliac joint pain. Patrick's test (also known as the "figure of four test") is performed in a supine position by having the patient **F**lex, **AB**duct, and **E**xternally **R**otate (**FABER**) the hip such that the ipsilateral heel rests on the contralateral knee. Downward gentle pressure is then increasingly applied on the ipsilateral knee while stabilizing the contralateral anterior iliac crest. Pain arising from the contralateral pelvis is suggestive of sacroiliitis. Gaenslen's maneuver is performed with the patient supine and both hips and knees in flexion. The patient then moves one buttock off the examining table edge while extending the leg over the side. Sacroiliitis is suspected if the maneuver provokes sacroiliac discomfort on the side of the dropped leg (see figures in Chapter 34).

18. **What is lumbar spinal stenosis?**
Lumbar spinal stenosis is compression of nerve roots within the central lumbar canal that may clinically present as radiculopathy, pseudoclaudication, or cauda equina syndrome. Spinal stenosis results from narrowing of the normal oval spinal canal, which assumes a triangular appearance as a result of facet hyperostosis, ligamentum flavum hypertrophy, broad-based central disk protrusion, and spondylosis, or any combination of these. The typical patient has symptoms of lower limb claudication (neurogenic) in the absence of peripheral vascular disease. Symptoms are exacerbated by back extension and relieved with flexion, thus creating the classic simian posture. Patients will often report relief from walking-induced bilateral posterior buttock and thigh pain when they lean forward on their shopping carts. Symptoms may be produced by extending the patient's back for 30 seconds (spinal Phalen's).

19. **What is cauda equina syndrome?**
Cauda equina syndrome is a rare but serious clinical complex of low back pain, lower limb motor weakness, and saddle area anesthesia (S4) with bowel and/or bladder incontinence. The syndrome most commonly results from central intervertebral disk herniation into the sacral nerve roots. Rarely, advanced ankylosing spondylitis and malignancy may also cause cauda equina syndrome. The diagnosis of this rare syndrome requires an urgent MRI and a neurosurgical consultation.

20. **Define spondylosis, spondylitis, spondylolysis, and spondylolisthesis.**
Spondylosis refers to degenerative disease (e.g., osteoarthritis) of the intervertebral disk and/or the apophyseal (facet) joints. The natural, lordotic curves of the spinal column where maximum range of motion occurs at the C5 to C7 and L3 to L5 levels predispose these segments to accelerated degenerative changes. Spondylosis is the most common cause of neck and low back pain in patients over 40 years old.
Spondylitis literally means inflammation of the vertebral column, a classic feature of the spondyloarthropathies (e.g., ankylosing spondylitis). The inflammatory lesion of spondylitis occurs at the vertebral enthesis. It is most common in white males between 18 and 30 years old.
Spondylolysis is characterized by a defective (separated) pars interarticularis, the bony bridge joining the superior and inferior articular processes of the vertebrae. The pars defect usually results from congenital dysplasia (patients <20 years old), degenerative disease (patients >40 years old), and/or trauma.
Spondylolisthesis occurs when the pars defect (spondylolysis) allows forward displacement (subluxation) of the proximal vertebra. Clinically significant spondylolisthesis (grades 2 to 4) is best identified on lateral radiographs and instability can be documented during maximum flexion and extension. It usually occurs at the L5 to S1 level.

21. **What are the indications for obtaining a lumbosacral spine radiograph in a patient with low back pain?**
Image studies are always indicated if **RED FLAGS** (see Question 12) are present because the yield is increased if you suspect cancer, fracture, infection, or inflammatory spondyloarthropathy. Patients with back pain persisting for greater than 4 to 6 weeks despite appropriate therapy for acute lumbar strain should also have spine films.

22. **Why not obtain x-rays on all patients with low back pain?**
Always ask yourself if you would treat the patient differently based on this information. Age-related degenerative changes in the lumbar spine are often unrelated to the cause of the patient's myofascial pain. These images are often an unnecessary expense, and one lumbar series exposes the patient to the equivalent ionizing radiation dose of 40 chest x-rays.

23. **When should an MRI or computerized tomography myelogram be ordered for a patient with low back pain?**
Only if your approach will be altered. Patients with RED FLAGS for cancer or infection or patients who are surgical candidates should have an MRI. Occasionally, MRI or computerized tomography (CT) of the sacroiliac joints is needed to diagnose early ankylosing spondylitis. A CT myelogram may be necessary if the patient cannot have an MRI (pacemaker, etc.). In patients with adequate renal function, an MRI **with gadolinium** is indicated for patients who have undergone prior lumbar spine surgery to exclude infection or nerve root compression resulting from scar tissue. An MRI is not needed in a patient whose history and physical examination

are consistent with lumbar radiculopathy and is improving with conservative therapy. All imaging procedures must be interpreted in conjunction with the clinical history, physical examination, laboratory results, and electrophysiologic studies.

24. **When should an electromyogram or nerve conduction velocities be ordered for a patient with low back pain?**

    An electromyogram (EMG) is obtained in a patient with low back pain who has signs and symptoms of a radiculopathy if this information will change your approach. MRI imaging has replaced the need for an EMG or nerve conduction velocities (NCVs) in patients who have radicular symptoms/signs that correlate with the MRI findings. However, in complex cases, where the etiology of lower extremity pain or weakness is unclear despite careful neurological exam and imaging, EMG/NCV studies can be of value. The EMG is usually carried out at least 3 weeks after the onset of symptoms. The results of an EMG are helpful only when combined with the clinical presentation, physical examination, and radiographic tests (MRI). Laminectomy or microdiskectomy has the greatest likelihood of improving symptoms if the physical examination, EMG, and radiographic studies all agree on the anatomic location of the disk compressing the nerve root.

25. **When should surgery be advised for a patient with radicular symptoms resulting from a herniated disk?**

    The guidelines of the American Academy of Orthopedic Surgeons suggest that before surgical intervention patients should have failed conservative therapy for 6 weeks (physical therapy and epidural steroids), have incapacitating pain, or an increasing neurologic deficit. They should also exhibit a positive straight leg-raise and other exam findings that correlate with the same pathology identified on lumbar MRI (or CT myelogram) and EMG/NCV studies.

26. **What are the sensitivities and specificities of the various diagnostic tests used to document a herniated lumbar disk? How often are they abnormal in individuals without low back pain?**

    The diagnostic tests used to evaluate low back pain have the following sensitivity and specificity in patients with surgically documented herniated lumbar disks causing a compressive radiculopathy:

	SENSITIVITY	SPECIFICITY
EMG	92%	83%
CT scans	92%	88%
Myelography	90%	87%
MRI scans	93%	92%

    It is important to note that a significant number of asymptomatic individuals without low back pain will have an abnormal CT scan or myelogram (30% to 40%). MRI studies have shown that 25% to 50% of individuals **without** low back pain will have a disk bulge or protrusion at one or more lumbar disk levels. Consequently, disk bulges/protrusions on MRI in patients with low back pain are **usually** coincidental, whereas disk extrusion, especially with compression of the lumbar nerve, is usually a significant cause of radicular back pain.

27. **What exercises are good for patients with mechanical low back pain?**

    Exercise and weight loss are important in any rehabilitation program for mechanical low back pain. People who are more fit have fewer episodes of low back pain and recover from an episode of back pain more quickly. Exercise is important in maintaining the strength of the spinal segments.

    Flexion exercises (Williams' exercises) are prescribed to decrease the load on the posterior facet joints and to open the intervertebral foramina. Extension exercises (MacKenzie's exercises) decrease compression load on the intervertebral disk and may be useful for patients with radiculopathies resulting from a herniated or degenerative disk. Spine stabilization exercises (correct abdominal strengthening and pelvic tilt with the knees flexed) are important to decrease the load on pain-sensitive structures and may prevent recurrent episodes of mechanical low back pain/strain.

28. **What is the prognosis for patients with mechanical low back pain?**

    It is estimated that up to 80% of all individuals will develop back pain during their life. Despite the potential number of people affected, the overall prognosis is good. Within 1 week of an acute episode, 50% of patients have symptomatic improvement; 75% will improve after 1 month; and 87% improve at 3 months. By 6 months, 93% are better. However, 25% or more of patients have recurrent pain within the next year, and chronic low back pain develops in up to 7% of patients. The prognosis is less favorable among patients receiving narcotics, disability benefits, and/or workmen's compensation. Failure to return to employment within several months following an injury at work usually predicts a poor outcome.

29. **What is the best strategy to hasten recovery in a patient with mechanical low back pain?**

    It is preferable to limit bed rest to 2 days or less and refer the patient to physical therapy for instructions in the use of ice, heat, proper lifting techniques, and correct spine stabilization exercises. Limited data does not support the routine use of facet injections, acupuncture, or transcutaneous nerve stimulators. Spinal manipulation may provide some relief in the early phases of acute nonserious injuries.

30. **What are "Waddell's signs"?**

    Although most back pain is organic, some patients present with complaints of low back pain that are manifestations of a psychosomatic disorder. Other patients may be malingering for secondary gain. To distinguish behavioral (nonorganic) from organic back pain, Waddell and colleagues found eight signs that identify nonorganic back pain. Patients satisfying three or more of these signs may have a behavioral cause for their low back pain.
    - Superficial tenderness—discomfort on light touching of the skin overlying the back.
    - Nonanatomic tenderness—tenderness that crosses multiple somatic boundaries or moves to various sites during the exam.
    - Axial loading—report of low back pain when pressing down on the top of the head of a standing patient.
    - Simulated rotation—when the shoulders and pelvis are rotated in unison less than 30 degrees (i.e., acetabular rotation test) in either direction, the structures in the back are not stressed. If the patient reports pain with this maneuver, this test is considered positive.
    - Distracted straight-leg raise—report of pain in low back or posterior thigh with less than 10 degrees of elevation of leg when supine, or pain with standard straight-leg raise test when a patient is recumbent but no pain when the patient is sitting and the knee is extended so that the leg is at a 90-degree angle with the pelvis.
    - Regional sensory change—"stocking" or global distribution of numbness, not in dermatomal distribution.
    - Regional weakness—"breakaway" weakness in a patient with normal strength on muscle testing.
    - Overreaction—disproportionate grimacing, tremor, exaggerated verbalization, or collapse in a way not to hurt themselves during the exam.

31. **What other tests have been identified as suggesting a behavioral or nonorganic cause for back pain?**
    - Sit-up—a patient with significant back pain cannot do a sit-up. Patients with organic back pain will roll over to their side and push up to a sitting position. If a patient can do a sit-up, his pain is not severe.
    - Shoes and socks sign—patients with significant organic back pain should have problems putting on shoes and socks. If these actions are no problem, back pain usually is not severe.
    - Mankopf's test—pain should raise pulse rate 5% or more. Absence of this sign is a positive behavioral sign (unless on beta blockers).
    - O'Donoghue's maneuver—patients with true back pain should have greater passive range of motion than active range. If this is not the case, consider a behavioral cause of pain.

BIBLIOGRAPHY

Atlas SJ, Delitto A: Spinal stenosis: surgical versus nonsurgical treatment, Clin Orthop 443:198–207, 2006.
Awad JN, Moskovich R: Lumbar disc herniations: surgical versus nonsurgical treatment, Clin Orthop 443:183–197, 2006.
Carette S, Fehlings MG: Clinical practice. Cervical radiculopathy, N Engl J Med 353:392–399, 2005.
Carragee EJ: Clinical practice. Persistent low back pain, N Engl J Med 352:1891–1898, 2005.
Chou R, Baisden J, Carragee EJ, et al: Surgery for low back pain: a review of the evidence for an American Pain Society Clinical Practice Guideline, Spine 34:1094–1109, 2009.
Chou R, Qaseem A, Owens DK, et al: Diagnostic imaging for low back pain: advice for high-value health care from the American College of Physicians, Ann Int Med 154:181, 2011.
Chou R, Qaseem A, Snow V, et al: Diagnosis and treatment of low back pain: a joint clinical practice guideline from the American College of Physicians and the American Pain Society, Ann Int Med 147:478, 2007.
Fishbain DA, Cole B, Cutler RB, et al: A structured evidence-based review on the meaning of nonorganic physical signs: Waddell signs, Pain Med 4:141, 2003.
Guzman J, Haldeman S, Carroll LJ, et al: Clinical practice implications of the Bone and Joint Decade 2000-2010 Task Force on Neck Pain and its Associated Disorders: from concepts and findings to recommendations, Spine 33(suppl 4):S199, 2008.
Haig AJ, Tong HC, Yamakawa KSJ, et al: The sensitivity and specificity of electrodiagnostic testing for the clinical syndrome of lumbar spinal stenosis, Spine 30:2667–2676, 2005.
Hoppenfeld S, Hutton R: Physical examination of the spine and extremities, New York, 1976, Appleton-Century-Crofts.
Jensen MC, Brandt-Zawadzki MN, Obuchowski N, et al: Magnetic resonance imaging of the lumbar spine in people without back pain, N Engl J Med 331:69–73, 1994.
Katz JN, Harris MB: Clinical practice. Lumbar spinal stenosis, N Engl J Med 358:818–825, 2008.
Moffett J, McLean S: The role of physiotherapy in the management of non-specific back and neck pain, Rheumatology 45:371–378, 2006.
Rao RD, Currier BL, Albert TJ, et al: Degenerative cervical spondylosis: clinical syndromes, pathogenesis, and management, J Bone Joint Surg Am 89:1360–1378, 2007.
Roudsari B, Jarvik JG: Lumbar spine MRI for low back pain: indications and yield, Am J Roentgenol 195:550–559, 2010.
Rubenstein SM, Pool JJ, van Tulder MW, et al: A systematic review of the diagnostic accuracy of provocative tests of the neck for diagnosing cervical radiculopathy, Eur Spine J 16:307, 2007.
Staal JB, de Bie RA, de Vet HCW, et al: Injection therapy for subacute and chronic low back pain: an updated Cochrane review, Spine 34:49–59, 2009.

CHAPTER 61: FIBROMYALGIA

Mark Malyak, MD

"Take nothing on its look; take everything on evidence. There is no better rule."

Charles Dickens
Great Expectations (1861)

KEY POINTS

1. Fibromyalgia syndrome (FMS) is a chronic noninflammatory, nonautoimmune central afferent processing disorder leading to a diffuse pain syndrome as well as other symptoms.
2. Similar to patients with other chronic pain disorders, functional magnetic resonance images (MRIs) show expanded receptive fields for central pain perception and emotional modulation in patients with fibromyalgia.
3. The most effective drugs for FMS are tricyclic agents (TCAs), dual reuptake inhibitors, and anticonvulsants, which downregulate sensory processing.
4. Opioids and corticosteroids are not effective in the treatment of fibromyalgia and should be avoided.
5. Patient education, aerobic exercise, and cognitive behavioral therapy are important adjuncts to medical therapy of FMS.

1. Define soft tissue rheumatism.

Soft tissue rheumatism refers to a group of musculoskeletal pain syndromes that result from the pathology of extraarticular and extraosseous periarticular structures. These "soft tissue" structures include bursae, tendons and their synovial sheaths, entheses, muscles, and fasciae. A major point conceptually is that pain from soft tissue rheumatism is not caused by pathology of structures within the true joint (i.e., arthritis). Soft tissue rheumatism may manifest as well-defined pathology of a single periarticular site or a regional myofascial pain syndrome. Although FMS is considered a form of soft tissue rheumatism in that patients experience soft tissue pain in the absence of articular disease, the underlying pathology is probably within the central nervous system (CNS). Examples of involvement of **single periarticular sites** include bursitis, tendinitis, tenosynovitis, and enthesitis or enthesopathy (e.g., plantar fasciitis). Although diffuse connective tissue disorders, such as rheumatoid arthritis (RA) and seronegative spondyloarthropathy, may involve these soft tissue structures, involvement of a single or few periarticular sites in the absence of articular disease suggests the syndrome is attributable to chronic low-grade repetitive trauma or acute overexertion (e.g., the weekend warrior).

Regional myofascial pain syndrome is a localized soft tissue pain syndrome characterized by the presence of a **trigger** point within a muscle that upon palpation results in severe local tenderness and radiation of pain into characteristic regions. Although the discomfort of the myofascial pain syndrome remains regional, it is usually more widespread than bursitis or tendinitis. Regional myofascial pain syndrome most commonly involves the unilateral lower back, neck, shoulder, or hip region.

2. Define FMS.

FMS is a chronic (>3 months), noninflammatory, nonautoimmune central afferent processing disorder leading to a diffuse pain syndrome. The core symptoms include multifocal pain, severe fatigue, stiffness, sleep disturbance, cognitive problems (fibrofog), and oftentimes psychological distress. Physical examination and pathologic investigation reveal no evidence of articular, osseous, or soft tissue inflammation or degeneration. Patients may have tender points in characteristic areas both above and below the waist. FMS may occur alone (primary FMS) or may be associated with a number of other disorders (secondary FMS). In primary FMS, laboratory results and radiographs are normal. FMS associated with other disorders will exhibit physical exam, laboratory, and radiographic abnormalities characteristic of the associated disorder. The American College of Rheumatology (ACR) 1990 Classification Criteria for FMS used by many for diagnosis include:
- chronic widespread pain for at least 3 months **above and below the waist and on both sides of the body;**
- pain induced by palpation in at least 11 of 18 tender points;
- no other cause for symptoms based on physical examination, laboratory tests, and radiographs.

3. What are tender points and where are they located in FMS?

In normal individuals (and in patients with FMS), there exist specific regions on the surface anatomy that are more sensitive to applied pressure than other sites. These areas are primarily at musculotendinous junctions and not at tendon insertion sites into bone. FMS is a disorder of generalized pain amplification, and thus these regions are exceedingly tender, and are referred to as **tender points**. The classification criteria for FMS require chronic (>3 months) presence of at least 11 of 18 tender points existing diffusely (above and below the waist). The amount of point pressure utilized to elicit tender points is 4 kg/cm² (enough pressure to blanch your distal thumbnail) (Figure 61-1).

4. **What are control points?**
   Control points are areas that are not painful in normal individuals when point pressure (4 kg/cm²) is applied. They are located on the midforehead, thumbnail, volar surface of midforearm, and anterior midthigh. Control points are usually not as tender in patients with FMS when compared to the classic tender points. However, FMS is a generalized pain syndrome, and sites other than tender points (including control points) are more sensitive to point pressure than in normal individuals, although pressures greater than 4 kg/cm² are usually required. Many experts in FMS discount the value of testing for control points. Others feel that positive control points can identify a patient with FMS who has a worse form of the disease and a poor prognosis.

5. **List some other symptoms that commonly occur in patients with FMS.**
   - Fatigue (80%)
   - Nonrestorative sleep (80%)
   - Arthralgias/myalgias/stiffness (80%)
   - Cognitive dysfunction (20% to 30%)
   - Muscle spasms/paresthesias (20% to 30%)
   - Depression/anxiety (20% to 33%)

6. **List some other conditions that are now felt to be central pain sensitivity syndromes that are frequently seen in patients with FMS.**
   - Tension/migraine headache (50% to 60%)
   - Irritable bowel syndrome (40%)
   - Restless leg/periodic limb movement syndrome (15%)
   - Urinary frequency/urgency
   - Primary dysmenorrhea/chronic pelvic pain/urethral syndrome
   - Temporomandibular joint (TMJ) disorders
   - Hypersensitivity and multiple chemical sensitivity syndrome (odors, bright lights, loud noises, medications)
   - Many of these patients are seeing other subspecialties for their pain syndromes yet central afferent sensitization is the common pathogenesis for all these syndromes

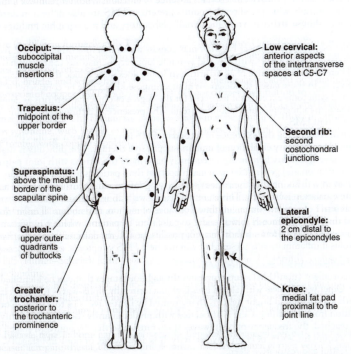

Figure 61-1. Location of the 18 (nine pairs) specific tender points in fibromyalgia patients. (From Freundlich B, Leventhal L: The fibromyalgia syndrome. In Schumacher Jr HR, Klippel JH, Koopman WJ, editors: Primer on the rheumatic diseases, ed 10, Atlanta, 1993, Arthritis Foundation, with permission.)

7. **What are the new diagnostic criteria for FMS?**
   In 2010, new diagnostic criteria were proposed for FMS. The purpose of these criteria was to recognize that fibromyalgia was a condition of widespread pain and was frequently associated with other central sensitivity syndrome symptoms. The proposed criteria are:
   - Widespread pain index (WPI) ≥ 7 and symptom severity (SS) scale score ≥ 5 **or**
   - WPI = 3 to 6 and SS scale score ≥ 9
   - Symptoms present for at least 3 months
   - No other disorder to explain symptoms

   The **WPI** is the number of areas in which the patient has had pain over the last week. There are 19 areas (bilateral TMJs [2], shoulders [2], upper arm [2], lower arm [2], hips [2], upper leg [2], lower leg [2], neck [1], chest [1], abdomen [1], upper back [1], lower back [1]), therefore 19 is the maximum score. Tender points are no longer part of the criteria because patients (especially men) can have FMS without characteristic tender points. The **SS scale score** is the sum of severity of four items over the past week. The four items are (1) fatigue, (2) waking from sleep unrefreshed, (3) cognitive disturbances, and (4) somatic symptoms. Each is subjectively scored for severity using a Likert score (0 = none, 1 = mild, 2 = moderate, 3 = severe) so that the maximum score is 12.

8. **Who generally develops FMS? At what age?**
   The prevalence of fibromyalgia in the general adult U.S. population is probably 3% to 4% (3.4% of women, 0.5% of men). **Females** account for 70% to 90% of patients. The observation that **whites** represent 90% of patients with FMS may represent selection bias. The average **age of onset** is approximately 30 to 55 years, but ranges from childhood to the elderly.
   PEARL: FMS symptoms occurring for the first time in a patient older than 55 to 60 years are usually the result of a disease other than FMS (e.g., infection, neoplasia, arthritis).

9. **How can the pain of FMS be distinguished from the pain of widespread arthritis? Why is this important?**
   Patients with FMS generally have diffuse pain that may be perceived to originate within joints, muscles, or both, and thus it may be confused with a diffuse arthritis syndrome, such as RA or ankylosing spondylitis. Pain involving the **axial skeleton** is universally present in FMS, with patients experiencing lower back, cervical spine, and/or thoracic spine pain. Patients with FMS also commonly experience **bilateral pain** in the upper and lower extremities. True arthritis may often be excluded by the physical examination, and therefore the joint exam in primary FMS reveals **absence** of effusion, synovial proliferation, deformity, and warmth. The multiple widespread **tender points** present in FMS are also helpful in distinguishing this disorder from a diffuse arthritis syndrome. Finally, laboratory and radiographic findings are normal in primary FMS.
   Fibromyalgia may occur alone (primary FMS) or may coexist with numerous other medical syndromes, including arthritis. Up to 25% of patients with RA and systemic lupus erythematosus (SLE) can have secondary fibromyalgia. Therefore, the presence of an arthritis syndrome does not exclude the presence of coexistent FMS, and vice versa. In these cases, the diagnosis of superimposed FMS may be considered if subjective pain and constitutional symptoms exceed that expected for the degree of objective arthritis as determined by physical examination, radiographs, and laboratory tests. The presence of diffuse tender points also suggests the diagnosis of coexistent FMS.
   The importance of recognizing the existence of secondary FMS in patients with an underlying inflammatory arthritis is to avoid unnecessary escalation of immunosuppressive therapy. The difficulty is that patients with RA or SLE who have secondary fibromyalgia frequently have more tenderness with joint palpation resulting from central sensitization and generalized pain magnification than patients without secondary FMS. This may fool the physician into thinking that the patient's underlying inflammatory arthritis is more active prompting an inappropriate escalation in therapy. Therefore in patients with an inflammatory arthritis who have secondary FMS, the presence of swollen joints, limitation of range of motion, and abnormal inflammatory markers is more important than the presence of joints tender to palpation. In patients where it is difficult to tell if inflammation is contributing to symptoms, a short burst of prednisone (20 mg daily, with tapering by 5 mg daily) will improve symptoms if inflammation is present but will not help FMS symptoms.

10. **Discuss the sleep disorder associated with FMS.**
    Nonrapid eye movement (nonREM) sleep progresses through four stages that can be identified by electroencephalography. Quiet wakefulness with closed eyes is characterized by alpha-waves (8 to 13 Hz), whereas alert wakefulness with eyes open and bright lights is characterized by beta-waves (14 to 25 Hz). NonREM stage I sleep is a transition from wakefulness and is associated with predominantly theta-wave activity (4 to 7 Hz). As deeper sleep is reached, the frequency of brain waves slows further, so that by nonREM stage IV sleep, delta-waves (<4 Hz) account for >50% of brain wave activity. It is delta-wave, or nonREM stage IV, sleep that is responsible for restful and restorative sleep.
    The sleep disturbance associated with FMS, termed **alpha-delta sleep**, is characterized by disruption of delta-wave sleep by frequent alpha-wave intrusion, such that nonREM stage IV sleep is significantly reduced. This

sleep pattern is not specific for FMS and may be present during periods of emotional stress, in chronic painful conditions such as RA and osteoarthritis, in sleep apnea syndrome, and in some otherwise normal individuals. Alpha-delta sleep is clinically associated with nonrestorative sleep.

PEARL: Sleep apnea needs to be considered in any patient with FMS. Patients (particularly males) may not be obese. All patients should be asked if they snore, have their neck size measured (risk increased if >17 inches in men, >16 inches women), and have an oral examination to see if the tongue obstructs the view of the posterior pharynx.

11. Outline an evaluation of a patient with suspected fibromyalgia.
- History: pain severity, fatigue severity, sleep disturbances, snoring and other symptoms of sleep apnea, mood disturbances, cognitive dysfunction, paresthesias, hypersensitivity (odors, bright lights, loud noises), other central sensitivity syndromes (see Question 6), triggers (see Question 12).
- Family history of central sensitivity syndromes: first degree relatives are eight times more likely to have FMS.
- Physical examination: general exam, joint exam including back, tender points, manual muscle strength, and neurologic exam including deep tendon reflexes (DTRs).
- Blood pressure (BP) cuff test: patients with FMS may have pain when BP is taken.
- Neck size: large necks suggest sleep apnea (>17 in males; >16 in females).
- Oral exam: receding jaw or tongue obscuring posterior pharynx increases risk of sleep apnea.
- Laboratory examination: complete blood count (CBC), erythrocyte sedimentation rate (ESR), complete metabolic panel, phosphorous, creatine phosphokinase (CPK), thyroid-stimulating hormone (TSH).
- 25-hydroxy vitamin D (25-OH vitamin D): this should be measured in patients who simultaneously have low calcium, low phosphorous, high alkaline phosphatase, which would indicate osteomalacia.
- Do **not** measure rheumatoid factor (RF) or antinuclear antibody (ANA) unless there is objective joint swelling or laboratory abnormalities suggesting inflammation.
- Radiographs: only if painful areas are out of proportion to other areas.
- Other tests: electromyography (EMG)/nerve conduction velocities (NCVs), muscle biopsy, MRI not indicated unless objective findings present suggesting a disease other than FMS.

12. What are the recognized triggers for FMS?
- Early life trauma: sexual or physical abuse
- Acute trauma especially involving the trunk (cervical whiplash)
- Infections: Epstein–Barr virus (EBV), parvovirus, Lyme, hepatitis C, West Nile virus
- Sleep apnea
- Chronic ongoing joint inflammation (secondary FMS)
- Catastrophic events: posttraumatic stress disorder following war and other major events
- Chronic psychological distress

Note: of interest is that only 5% to 10% of patients experiencing one of these triggers develop a widespread pain syndrome suggesting a biochemical predisposition.

13. What conditions other than rheumatic diseases must be considered in a patient presenting with fibromyalgia-like symptoms?
- Rheumatologic: RA, SLE, systemic sclerosis, Sjögren's, polymyositis, polymyalgia rheumatica (PMR), ankylosing spondylitis
- Endocrine: hypothyroidism, adrenal insufficiency, hyperparathyroidism, osteomalacia
- Myopathy: metabolic, statin-induced, myotonic dystrophy
- Gastrointestinal: hepatitis C, celiac, hemochromatosis, inflammatory bowel disease
- Infections: subacute bacterial endocarditis (SBE), Lyme, human immunodeficiency virus (HIV), parvovirus, brucellosis
- Neurologic: multiple sclerosis (MS), myasthenia, peripheral and small fiber neuropathy
- Malignancy: metastatic, lymphoma, others
- Sleep apnea
- Psychiatric: major depression, substance abuse, eating disorders
- Others: Chiari malformation, Fabry's disease

14. Which psychological disorders are sometimes confused with FMS? Why?
Functional psychiatric disorders, such as the somatoform disorders, often result in symptoms identical to those of FMS. The term **functional** suggests the syndrome has no organic basis and is attributable to purely psychological factors or conflicts. It is conceivable that in some patients FMS originates as a functional disorder, and subsequently the objective clinical, sleep, and neurotransmitter abnormalities become manifest as a result of neuro-psycho-immuno-endocrine interrelationships. Thus, although a "functional" psychiatric disorder may precipitate FMS, "organic" pathophysiologic mechanisms are likely to be responsible for the symptoms of FMS. The alternative possibility is that the chronic pain and fatigue of a somatoform disorder are purely functional in certain patients. It is unclear if these patients would have tender points on physical examination, alpha-delta sleep disturbance, or neurotransmitter abnormalities.

Organic psychiatric disorders, such as major depression, have also been associated with FMS, with up to 50% to 70% of patients with FMS having a history of major depression and up to 33% having major depression at the time of FMS diagnosis. Alternatively, many patients diagnosed with major depression experience sleep disturbance, fatigue, and diffuse musculoskeletal pain. Three potential explanations may account for this association. (1) Depression and FMS may both be clinical manifestations of the affective spectrum disorders, and their presence in an individual patient is coincidental rather than causal. (2) Major depression may lead to alterations of the neuro-psycho-immuno-endocrine system such that it leads to the development of FMS. In a similar fashion, FMS may lead to the development of major depression. (3) FMS and major depression may represent a single syndrome, with the diagnosis in a particular patient dependent on the major clinical manifestations present.

Finally, the **anxiety** and **mild depression** often present in FMS may be a psychological response to concerns regarding financial and personal independence in the setting of chronic pain and disability. This association may be present in any chronic pain or debilitating syndrome.

15. What variables contribute to a patient's predisposition to developing FMS?

The etiology of FMS syndrome is unknown. However, several variables probably contribute to a patient's predisposition to developing FMS as well as the severity of the symptoms:
- Biologic variables: accounts for 50% of the risk
  - Inheritance: genetic polymorphisms reported in catechol-O-methyltransferase (COMT) enzyme, serotonin transporter and receptor, and dopamine receptor genes
  - Female sex: young and middle-aged females most at risk
  - Sleep architecture abnormalities
  - Neuroendocrine response to stress: attenuated corticotropin-releasing hormone and insulin-like growth factor-1 (somatomedin-C) response
  - Autonomic dysregulation: paroxysmal orthostasis and tachycardia syndrome (POTS)
- Environmental and sociocultural variables
  - Early life developmental experiences: sexual or physical abuse in childhood
  - Family variables: spousal and family support systems
  - Work variables: job satisfaction
  - Sociocultural variables: more FMS in industrialized societies
- Psychological variables
  - Personality traits: perfectionist or self-sacrificing most common
  - Catastrophizing and negative beliefs: belief that pain cannot be controlled
  - Hypervigilance and preoccupation with pain
  - Low self-efficacy and defective coping mechanisms
  - Depression and anxiety

16. Describe the ascending pain pathways. Discuss the concept of peripheral and central sensitization in chronic pain syndromes?

Sensory fibers (nociceptor afferents) that transmit pain sensations innervate all body tissues. There are two types of sensory fibers: myelinated **A delta (δ)** and unmyelinated **C fibers**. These fibers have free nerve endings containing nociceptors that respond to noxious stimuli. There are specific nociceptors for mechanical, thermal, and chemical stimuli. Another receptor (**polymodal receptor**) responds to more than one stimuli and is only found on C fibers. Aδ fibers are rapidly conducting and respond mostly to mechanical and thermal stimuli. C fiber afferents conduct more slowly and produce perceptions of dull, aching, or burning pain. These nociceptor afferents (first order neurons) enter the spinal cord via dorsal roots and terminate in the dorsal horn of the spinal cord. These afferents release excitatory neurotransmitters that activate second order neurons. The Aδ sensory neurons mainly release glutamate that binds to the N-methyl-d-aspartate (NMDA) receptor on second order neurons that cross the cord and ascend in the neospinothalamic (lateral spinothalamic) tract and terminate in the ventroposterior basal nuclei of the thalamus. From there the neural input is relayed to the somatosensory cortex, which is important for sensory discrimination, location, and anticipation of the pain. The C fiber sensory neurons release substance P and other neurotransmitters that stimulate second order neurons in the dorsal horn of the spinal cord. Also located in this area are the **wide dynamic range (WDR) neurons** that are stimulated by both noxious and nonnoxious stimuli transmitted from the periphery by C fibers with polymodal nociceptors. The second order neurons including the WDR neurons activated by C fiber stimulation ascend in the paleospinothalamic tracts that terminate in the thalamus (anterior spinothalamic tract), periaqueductal gray (PAG) and reticular formation/nuclei (spinoreticular tract), and the medullary and tectal areas (spinotectal tract). See figure in Question 19.

From the thalamus, PAG, and other gray matter areas, third order neurons transmit to other areas of the brain and spinal cord. Spinothalamic projections facilitate nociceptive input to the insular cortex, which has interconnections with the amygdala, prefrontal cortex, and anterior cingulate cortex. These regions form a network involved in emotional, cognitive, and autonomic responses to pain. In addition, there are interconnections with the hypothalamus that is involved in stress and autonomic responses. Finally, stimulation of the PAG, hypothalamus, and other areas are important in activation of the **descending analgesia pathway**.

The concept of peripheral and central sensitization is important for an understanding of widespread chronic pain conditions such as FMS. With continuous and prolonged noxious stimulation (ex-whiplash injury), peripheral polymodal C fibers and nearby silent nociceptive neurons that were previously unresponsive to stimulation now become responsive. The nociceptors begin to initiate signals spontaneously so that nonnoxious stimuli are now perceived as noxious as a result of the lowered pain threshold (**peripheral sensitization**). The result of peripheral sensitization causes a greater and more persistent barrage of nerve impulses in the dorsal root of the spinal cord. Release of substance P by C fibers sensitizes second order neurons including wide dynamic range neurons to neurotransmitters such as glutamate. The enhanced and persistent glutamate effect on second order neurons can result in physiologic changes in the nerves so they become hyperexcitable. This is called **windup**. These hyperexcitable second order neurons transmit excessively to the brain areas described above. This results in expanded receptive fields, increased interconnectivity, and increased blood flow to the stimulated areas. The ability to expand the receptive field is called **neuroplasticity** and occurs more easily in younger brains, which may explain why painful events early in life are particularly likely to trigger FMS. Owing to these physiologic changes, **central sensitization** occurs so that the individual feels pain at a lower threshold and with increased intensity.

17. **What abnormalities in the CNS have been implicated in FMS?**
    Most investigators believe that the pathophysiology of FMS results from central sensitization within the CNS, manifesting as amplified pain perception. Thus, physical stresses to the musculoskeletal system that in the normal individual are perceived as nontender touch, position sense, and nontender temperature sensation are perceived as pain in patients with FMS. It appears that the pain threshold is lower in patients with FMS. The underlying abnormalities within the CNS leading to amplified pain perception are not completely understood, but a number of specific abnormalities have been observed in the afferent pain processing areas of the CNS in some patients with FMS:
    - Increased excitability of dorsal horn nuclei as a result of abnormal windup: increased levels of substance P, nerve growth factor, glutamate, and aspartate measured in cerebrospinal fluid (CSF) of patients with FMS.
    - Expanded receptive fields for central pain perception (central sensitization): functional MRI (fMRI) shows expanded fields in the insula, anterior cingulate cortex, and somatosensory cortex.
    - Abnormalities within the descending analgesia system: decreased levels of pain inhibitory neuro transmitters (antinociceptive) including norepinephrine, serotonin, and dopamine in the CSF of patients with FMS.
    - Suppression of normal activity of dopamine-releasing neurons in the limbic system.

    Note: the level of opioids is increased in the CSF of patients with FMS. This may explain why narcotics are not effective in controlling pain in patients with FMS.

18. **Do patients with FMS have any abnormalities on brain imaging to support a central mechanism for their amplified pain perception?**
    Brain MRIs are normal in FMS patients. However, functional imaging studies using single-photon emission computerized tomography (SPECT) scans and fMRI have shown decreased regional cerebral blood flow to the thalamus and caudate nucleus in patients with FMS compared with healthy controls. The caudate nucleus and thalamus signal noxious stimuli, and decreased blood flow to these areas has been demonstrated in other chronic pain disorders. One explanation for these findings is that the widespread pain in FMS is activating inhibitory mechanisms, which reduce the evoked activity in the thalamus in an attempt to decrease pain processing. With reduced activity the thalamus needs less blood flow. An alternative explanation is that it takes less stimulation of the thalamus in FMS to induce pain in patients with FMS or that patients with FMS have decreased gray matter density in the thalamus. The reduced blood flow to the caudate may indicate an abnormal dopaminergic system, which is important in pain modulation, pleasure perception, and motivational responses.
    More recently, fMRI has also shown increased blood flow, connectivity, and activity in the insula, anterior cingulate cortex, and primary and secondary somatosensory cortices in response to painful stimuli. These are all areas that are involved with pain perception and emotional modulation from any cause of chronic pain. These findings on fMRI support a physiologic basis causing a patient with FMS to have an increased perception of pain.

19. **Discuss the descending analgesia pathway and its potential role in the pathophysiology of FMS.**
    The descending analgesia system (also called the descending noxious inhibitory control [DNIC] pathway) is a physiologic mechanism by which the transmission of pain is inhibited at the dorsal horn and other locations within the CNS (Figure 61-2). Projections from the origin of this pathway within the hypothalamus and PAG, utilizing enkephalin as a neurotransmitter, reach the raphe magnus nucleus within the pons and medulla. The raphe nucleus sends projections into the dorsal horn, utilizing serotonin as a neurotransmitter, where they stimulate interneurons whose neurotransmitter is again enkephalin. These axons innervate the presynaptic region of incoming pain fibers, leading to the presynaptic inhibition of transmission of painful sensation to second order pain fibers, most likely through the inhibition of calcium channels.
    The implication of the descending analgesia system in the pathophysiology of FMS has been suggested by studies that have demonstrated decreased serotonin or serotonin availability within the CNS. It remains unclear if

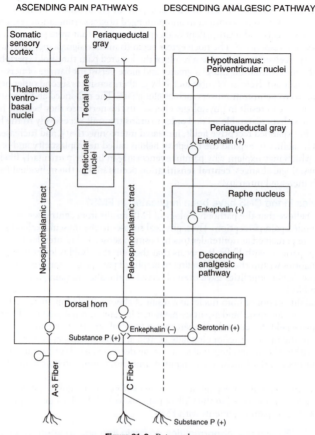

Figure 61-2. Pain pathways.

the observed serotonin abnormality is a primary dysfunction or secondary to another process within the neuro-psycho-immuno-endocrine system. It further remains unclear if the serotonin abnormality is in fact associated with dysfunction of the descending analgesia system.

Additionally, metabolites of norepinephrine and dopamine are decreased in the CSF of patients with FMS. This is important because there are norepinephrine-mediated pain-inhibitory pathways that descend to the spinal cord and dopamine-mediated pain-inhibitory pathways in the CNS that may be abnormal in patients with FMS.

20. **List the seven components of therapy for FMS.**
    - Patient education
    - Analgesia
    - Correction of sleep disturbance
    - Aerobic exercise
    - Physical therapy
    - Treatment of associated disorders
    - Cognitive behavioral therapy and/or supportive counselling for pain modification

    Although the etiology and pathophysiology of FMS remain unknown and many of the therapeutic interventions have been inadequately studied, a logical multidisciplinary approach to the treatment of this disorder is possible and necessary if meaningful results are expected.

21. **What three major points regarding the disease process should be emphasized in patient education programs?**
    1. FMS is a "real" and objective disease. This fact provides relief to the many patients whose chronic symptoms were labeled as purely psychological or imagined.
    2. A serious underlying disorder such as malignancy or destructive arthritis is not responsible for the symptoms of FMS (unless FMS is secondary to one of these disorders).

3. Although FMS is a real disease, the patient has substantial control over many components that may modulate the resultant symptoms. Discussion of an hypothesis of FMS in lay terms is appropriate, emphasizing those components that may be modified by the patient (e.g., the roles of the sleep disturbance and muscle deconditioning in the positive feedback loop resulting in amplified pain [Figure 61-2]). Provision of lay literature may also be helpful.

Two excellent education sites for patients with FMS are: www.fmaware.org and https://fibroguide.med.umich.edu/.

22. What is the goal of exercise programs in patients with FMS?

Aerobic exercise improves muscle conditioning, which may lead to less muscle microtrauma and thus may interrupt the positive feedback loop. Aerobic exercise may furthermore improve restorative sleep and increase endogenous endorphins within the CNS. Because patients with FMS often experience severe postexercise pain, the intensity of exercise must be initially low and only gradually increased as tolerated. Exercise should be aerobic and nonimpact, such as swimming, water aerobics, walking with proper footwear, or bicycling. Some patients find group exercise programs including Tai-chi and yoga to be beneficial. Physical therapy consultation may be helpful in designing the optimal exercise program for a particular patient. Isometric exercises should be avoided.

23. Which physical therapy modalities should be considered in treating a patient with FMS?

It is reasonable to try safe, relatively inexpensive interventions such as massage and the application of local heat in patients with FMS. The more expensive interventions, such as transcutaneous electrical nerve stimulation, hypnotherapy, EMG biofeedback, and acupuncture, have been inadequately tested and cannot be recommended for routine use but may be considered in patients whose symptoms are resistant to more conventional therapy. In the patient with FMS who is experiencing regional pain associated with a local very painful tender point (or trigger point) out of proportion to generalized pain, it is reasonable to treat as one would with a myofascial pain syndrome, including trigger point injection with a local anesthetic and possibly a glucocorticoid preparation followed by stretching of the muscle.

24. What medications are Food and Drug Administration-approved for therapy of fibromyalgia? How do you choose which one to use?

There are three Food and Drug Administration (FDA)-approved medications for treatment of FMS:
- Dual reuptake inhibitors (serotonin-norepinephrine reuptake inhibitors [SNRI]): increase serotonin and norepinephrine at synapses in the descending analgesia pathways.
  - **Duloxetine** (Cymbalta): start 20 to 30 mg in am with food. Titrate monthly to 60 mg daily or effect.
  - **Milnacipran** (Savella): start 12.5 mg in am with food. Increase by 12.5 mg every week to effect or maximum dose 50 mg twice daily.
- Anticonvulsant (α2–δ ligands): bind to ligand on voltage-gated calcium channels letting less calcium in which decreases release of excitatory neurotransmitters (glutamate, substance P).
  - **Pregabalin** (Lyrica): start 50 mg with food before bed and increase weekly to at least 150 mg (maximum dose 225 mg) at bedtime (qhs) before adding a morning dose. The maximum dose is 225 mg twice daily.

Experience has shown that one of these three may be more beneficial than the others depending on the associated fibromyalgia symptoms:
- **Duloxetine**: use in patients with FMS with depressed mood and fatigue or osteoarthritis of the back and knees.
- **Milnacipran**: use in patients with FMS with cognitive dysfunction (fibrofog) and fatigue.
- **Pregabalin**: use in patients with FMS with profound sleep disturbance.

Combination therapy with milnacipran and pregabalin has been shown in a small study to be more effective than either one alone without increased side effects.

25. What other medications have shown effectiveness in therapy for FMS?

Oftentimes patients cannot afford or insurance denies the use of the FDA-approved medications to treat FMS. Several other medications can be used.

1. **SNRIs**: Venlaxafine (Effexor) is an SNRI shown to be beneficial in fibromyalgia. It could be used in someone who cannot afford duloxetine or milnacipran which are also SNRIs. Venlaxafine is started at 25 mg in AM with food and increased weekly to effect or maximum dose of 175 mg twice daily. There is an extended release form that can be used once a day starting at 37.5 mg to a maximum of 225 mg in AM.
2. **TCAs**: low-dose TCAs administered before bedtime have been objectively demonstrated to improve the sleep disturbance, pain, and tender points in a proportion of patients with fibromyalgia. An example of such a regimen is the administration of **amitriptyline** at a dosage of 10 to 25 mg 1 to 3 hours before bedtime. This dose may be increased by 10 to 25 mg increments at 2-week intervals; the usual effective dose is 25 to 100 mg daily. Adverse effects are common and are attributable to the anticholinergic and antihistamine activities of the TCA. They include morning drowsiness, dry mouth, and constipation. If amitriptyline causes too many side effects, another TCA can be tried (Table 61-1).

As shown, the secondary amines (nortriptyline, desipramine) may be better tolerated but are less strong than the tertiary amines. In addition, amitriptyline and imipramine are the most likely to cause orthostatic hypotension and cardiac toxicity (arrhythmias), although the others may also cause these problems. Cyclobenza-

Table 61-1. Side effects of tricyclic antidepressants

	SEDATIVE	ANTICHOLINERGIC
Amitriptyline (Elavil, Endep)	++++	++++
Imipramine (Tofranil)	+++	+++
Doxepin (Sinequan)	+++	+++
Nortriptyline (Pamelor)	++	+
Desipramine (Norpramin)	+	+

+ to ++++, Strength of effect.

prine (Flexeril) is a weak TCA-like drug that can also be used at doses of 10 to 40 mg at night. For patients who do not tolerate TCA, trazodone (Desyrel), clonazepam, and alprazolam have been used as alternatives. Although the mechanism of action of the TCAs in the treatment of fibromyalgia remains unclear, the small dosages used and the rapid onset of action suggest it is not caused by the treatment of underlying depression. Because TCAs inhibit the reuptake of serotonin (and norepinephrine) at synaptic junctions, it is hypothesized that the greater availability of serotonin may be responsible for improved stage IV sleep in addition to providing a central analgesic effect through potentiation of the descending analgesic pathways. TCAs may also have an effect on CNS endorphins as well as on peripheral pain receptors.

3. **Anticonvulsants:** Gabapentin (Neurontin) can be used as a less expensive substitute for pregabalin. Start at 100 mg qhs and increase by 100 mg weekly to 300 mg qhs. If that is tolerated, then a morning dose can be added. The maximum dose is 800 mg three times per day. The combination of gabapentin and venlafaxine has been used with success.
4. **Analgesia:** Tramadol (Ultram) has been shown to relieve pain in patients with FMS. Start at 25 mg daily and increase by 25 mg weekly to effect or maximum dose of 100 mg on prescription. The analgesic effect of tramadol is most likely a result of its SNRI effect and not attributable to its weak binding to the mu opioid receptor. In fact opioids are not effective in FMS and should be avoided. Likewise **acetaminophen** and nonsteroidal antiinflammatory drugs (**NSAIDs**) are not effective for analgesia unless the patient also has associated pain as a result of osteoarthritis. Trigger point injections with lidocaine +/− corticosteroid should be used sparingly and only in patients with a myofascial trigger point unresponsive to physical therapy.
5. **Other "niche" therapies:** other medications have been tried depending on the associated symptoms:
- **Selective serotonin reuptake inhibitors (SSRIs).** SSRIs may be used to treat associated depression.
- **Cyclobenzaprine:** use to treat stiffness. Start 5 to 10 mg qhs and increase slowly to 30 mg qhs or effect.
- **Modafinil** (Provigil): use to treat fatigue. Dose varies between 50 and 200 mg twice daily. Armodafinil (Nuvigil) can also be used.
- **Trazodone** (Desyrel): may help sleep disturbances. Start 25 mg qhs and titrate weekly to effect. The maximum dose is 200 mg qhs.
- **Ropinirole** (Requip): this is a dopamine (D3) receptor agonist that can help restless leg syndrome. Start 0.25 mg 1 to 3 hours before bed and titrate to effect or maximum dose 4 mg qhs.

26. **What medications have not been shown to be effective in patients with FMS?**
Opioids, corticosteroids, NSAIDs, benzodiazepine and nonbenzodiazepine hypnotics, guaifenesin, S-adenosylmethionine (SAMe), melatonin, magnesium, and dehydroepiandrosterone (DHEA) are not effective and should be avoided.

27. **List some of the potential side effects from medications used to treat FMS.**
- All SNRIs may increase risk for suicidal ideation.
- Many of the drugs (SNRIs, SSRIs, tramadol, others) can increase the chance of developing **serotonin syndrome** when used together or at high doses. Pregabalin and gabapentin do not increase this risk. Potential drug interactions need to be checked and the patient monitored. Patients who develop hyperreflexia on these medications are most at risk.
- SNRIs, milnacipran: nausea, vomiting, which are lessened by administering with food. Insomnia, dizziness, high blood pressure (HBP), liver dysfunction, and renal dysfunction can occur.
- Pregabalin, gabapentin, TCAs: fatigue, somnolence, dizziness, weight gain, dry mouth, hyponatremia (TCAs).
- Tramadol: fatigue, somnolence, dizziness, nausea, headache, HBP, liver dysfunction, and renal dysfunction.

28. **Are there any other therapies that might work in patients with FMS?**
    - **Naltrexone**: recent trials have shown that low-dose naltrexone (4.5 mg daily) improves pain and mood in 30% of patients with FMS. It does not improve fatigue or sleep. The mechanism of action is unclear but is postulated to be a result of the ability of low-dose naltrexone to attenuate the production of proinflammatory cytokines and neurotoxic superoxides via suppressive effects on CNS microglia cells. Low doses do not affect the mu opioid receptors.
    - **Transcranial direct current stimulation**: electrodes are positioned to deliver direct current stimulation to the left primary motor cortex. The direct current is administered for 20 minutes and can reduce the pain by an average of 33% in patients with FMS over the 30 minutes that follow.

29. **What is the prognosis for fibromyalgia?**
    Outcome studies suggest that the majority of patients continue to experience symptoms despite specific treatment. Overall about 30% to 40% of patients will experience 40% to 50% relief of their pain. However, this is just an average and it should be realized that some patients get excellent symptom relief whereas others will get none. The number of patients needed to treat to get a 30% reduction in pain and other symptoms varies between 7 and 19 patients, which is cost-effective.
    A sympathetic patient–physician interaction and an organized approach to therapeutic intervention will lead to substantial improvement in many patients with fibromyalgia.

30. **What is the impact of FMS on the patient and society?**
    The disease impact of fibromyalgia is not trivial and comparable to RA. On average a patient with FMS sees the doctor three to four times more often than the general population (17 vs. 4 visits/year). This contributes to average direct medical costs of $10,911/year. In addition, patients with FMS miss 16.8 days/year of work. This contributes to average indirect medical costs of $10,697/year.

31. **Should FMS patients be given disability? (controversial)**
    It is estimated that as many as 25% of FMS patients in the United States receive some form of disability or injury compensation. However, disability awards do not result in clinical improvement and may actually contribute to a patient's inability to improve. Certainly, some patients need disability compensation but there should be an effort to not label patients with FMS disabled.

BIBLIOGRAPHY

Buskila D, Sarzi-Puttini P, Ablin JN: The genetics of fibromyalgia syndrome, Pharmacogenomics 8:67–74, 2007.
Carette S, Bell MJ, Reynolds WJ, et al: Comparison of amitriptyline, cyclobenzaprine, and placebo in the treatment of fibromyalgia: a randomized, double-blind clinical trial, Arthritis Rheum 37:32–40, 1994.
Carville SF, Arendt-Nielsen S, Bliddal H, et al: EULAR evidenced-based recommendations for the management of fibromyalgia syndrome, Ann Rheum Dis 67:536–541, 2008.
Goldenberg DL, Burckhardt C, Crofford L: Management of fibromyalgia syndrome, JAMA 292:2388–2395, 2004.
Hassett AL, Gevirtz RN: Nonpharmacologic treatment for fibromyalgia: patient education, cognitive-behavioral therapy, relaxation techniques, and complementary and alternative medicine, Rheum Dis Clin North Am 35:393–407, 2009.
Huser W, Bernardy K, Arnold B, et al: Efficacy of multicomponent treatment in fibromyalgia syndrome: a meta-analysis of randomized controlled clinical trials, Arthritis Rheum 61:216–224, 2009.
Moldofsky H: The significance of dysfunctions of the sleeping/waking brain to the pathogenesis and treatment of fibromyalgia syndrome, Rheum Dis Clin North Am 35:275–283, 2009.
Smith HS, Harris R, Clauw D: Fibromyalgia: an afferent processing disorder leading to a complex pain generalized syndrome, Pain Physician 14:E217–E245, 2011.
Traynor LM, Thiessen CN, Traynor AP: Pharmacotherapy of fibromyalgia, Am J Health Syst Pharm 68:1307–1319, 2011.
Vargas A, Hernandez-Paz R, Sanchez-Huerta JM, et al: Sphygmommanometry-evoked allodynia—a simple bedside test indicative of fibromyalgia: a multicenter developmental study, J Clin Rheumatol 12:272–274, 2006.
Villamar MF, Wivatvongvana P, Patumanond J, et al: Focal modulation of the primary cortex in fibromyalgia using 4x1-ring high-definition transcranial direct current stimulation: immediate and delayed analgesic effects of cathodal and anodal stimulation, J Pain 14:371–383, 2013.
Williams DA, Gracely RH: Functional magnetic resonance imaging findings in fibromyalgia, Arthritis Res Ther 8:224, 2006.
Wolfe F: The fibromyalgia syndrome: a consensus report on fibromyalgia and disability, J Rheumatol 23:534–539, 1996.
Wolfe F, Clauw DJ, Fitzcharles MA, et al: The American College of Rheumatology preliminary diagnostic criteria for fibromyalgia and measurement of symptom severity, Arthritis Care Res 62:600–610, 2010.
Younger J, Noor N, McCue R, et al: Low-dose naltrexone for the treatment of fibromyalgia: findings of a small, randomized, double-blind, placebo-controlled, counterbalanced, crossover trial assessing daily pain levels, Arthritis Rheum 65:529–538, 2013.
Yunus MB: Central sensitivity syndromes: a new paradigm and group nosology for fibromyalgia and overlapping conditions, and the related issue of disease versus illness, Semin Arthritis Rheum 37:339–352, 2008.

FURTHER READING

http://www.fmaware.org
https://fibroguide.med.umich.edu

CHAPTER 62

REGIONAL MUSCULOSKELETAL DISORDERS
Scott Vogelgesang, MD

KEY POINTS

1. Regional musculoskeletal disorders are frequently attributable to repetitive motion or "overuse."
2. Identifying and modifying the precipitating movements or activity is the **most important therapeutic maneuver**.
3. Shoulder impingement must be ruled out in a patient with recurrent rotator cuff or bicipital tendinitis.
4. Pes anserine bursitis is an important and often misdiagnosed etiology of medial knee pain.
5. Plantar fasciitis causes inferior heel pain that is worse with the first few steps upon getting out of bed.

1. **What is bursitis?**
   - Bursitis is the condition that occurs when a bursa becomes inflamed or infected.
   - A bursa is a sac with a potential space that makes it easier for one tissue to glide over another.
   - There are approximately 160 bursae in the body but only a few of them become clinically affected.
   - Most bursae differentiate during development, but new ones may form in response to stress, inflammation, or trauma.
   - Occasionally, a bursa may communicate with a nearby joint.

2. **What are the differences between tendinitis, tendinosis, and tenosynovitis?**
   - **Tendinitis** is usually caused by tendon trauma with associated vascular disruption and acute, subacute, or chronic inflammation. Crystal deposition into the tendon (especially basic calcium phosphate [apatite] crystals) can also cause inflammation (calcific tendinitis).
   - **Tendinosis (tendinopathy)** is noninflammatory, intratendinous atrophy and degeneration that is often associated with chronic tendinitis. Tendinosis can lead to partial or complete tendon rupture.
   - **Tenosynovitis** is inflammation of the paratendon, which is the outermost sheath that is lined in some tendons by a synovial membrane (e.g., extensor tendons of the thumb in De Quervain's tenosynovitis).

   Most of these conditions can be classified as "overuse" syndromes. Aging can decrease the integrity of the tendon, making it more prone to injury.

3. **Name the three most common nonarticular causes of shoulder pain.**
   - Impingement syndrome
   - Subacromial bursitis
   - Bicipital tendinitis

4. **Describe the shoulder impingement syndrome. How does it occur?**
   The shoulder impingement syndrome is a chronic, painful condition of the shoulder that results from an encroachment of the tendons of the rotator cuff (most commonly the supraspinatus) occurring most commonly with shoulder abduction. Abduction elevates the greater tuberosity of the humerus and rotator cuff tendon insertions toward the coracoacromial arch. The coracoacromial arch is made up of the acromion, the coracoid process of the scapula, and the coracoacromial ligament. Etiologies include sporting or occupational overuse (especially when the arm is used repeatedly overhead, such as tennis players or drywall workers), degenerative changes of the tendons or surrounding skeletal structures, curved or hooked acromion, and a single traumatic episode with posttraumatic tendon inflammation. It can also be idiopathic.

   In the normal functioning shoulder, the rotator cuff serves as a dynamic stabilizer of the joint. Its principal function lies in humeral head depression during shoulder abduction. The rotator cuff also assists with early abduction (0 to 30 degrees) as well as with internal and external rotation. When the rotator cuff is inflamed secondary to chronic, repetitive, microtrauma or acute posttraumatic tendon strain, it becomes relatively ineffective at shoulder depression, a characteristic called reflex inhibition. As a result, the humeral head moves closer to the coracoacromial arch (called superior translation) during contraction of the deltoid muscle (shoulder abduction). With continued motion and increased superior translation of the humeral head, there is impingement of the tendons on the coracoacromial arch, which leads to tendon inflammation and increased reflex inhibition. This is the **vicious cycle of impingement** and can lead to rotator cuff tears or voluntary decreased motion to avoid pain with resultant adhesive capsulitis (frozen shoulder) (Figure 62-1).

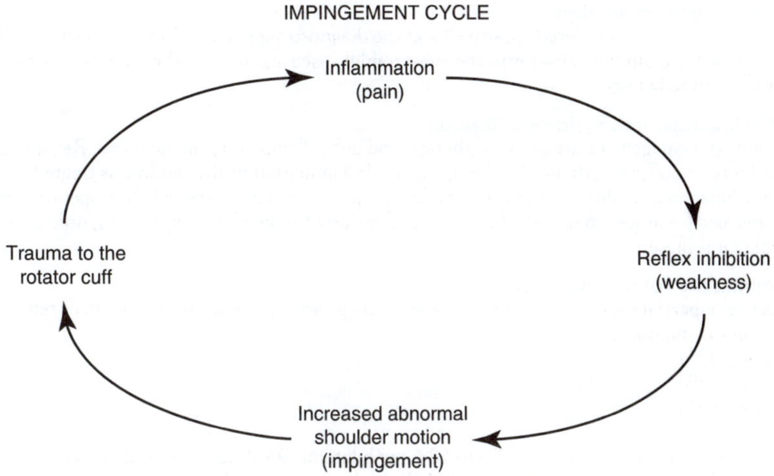

IMPINGEMENT CYCLE

```
                    Inflammation
                      (pain)

  Trauma to the                        Reflex inhibition
  rotator cuff                            (weakness)

               Increased abnormal
                 shoulder motion
                  (impingement)
```

Figure 62-1. The vicious cycle in the impingement syndrome.

5. **What are the three stages of shoulder impingement syndrome?**
   - Stage I usually occurs under 25 years of age and is characterized by tendon hemorrhage and edema.
   - Stage II usually occurs between 25 and 40 years and is characterized by tendinitis and fibrosis of the subacromial bursa.
   - Stage III usually occurs over 40 years of age and is characterized by tears of the rotator cuff and bicipital tendon.

   Stages I and II are reversible with appropriate treatment.

6. **How does the impingement syndrome present clinically?**
   - Pain with active shoulder movement (patient moves arm), especially flexion (between 60 and 120 degrees), abduction, and internal rotation
   - Much less or no pain with passive movement (examiner moves arm)
   - Absence of swelling, redness, or warmth at shoulder joint
   - Radiographically, the space between the humeral head and inferior surface of the acromion may be <8 mm

7. **What tests are done to isolate individual rotator cuff tendons that can become inflamed and cause shoulder pain?**
   - **Jobe test:** this maneuver isolates the supraspinatus, which is commonly involved in the impingement syndrome. The patient places the arm in 90 degrees of abduction, 30 degrees of forward flexion, and internal rotation with the elbow extended and arm rotated so that the thumb is pointing to the floor. The examiner pushes down on the arm as the patient resists this pressure. This will cause a worsening of the pain if the supraspinatus is inflamed or injured with a sensitivity of 86% and specificity of 50%. Further confirmation of supraspinatus pathology is obtained when the Jobe test is repeated but this time the shoulder is in external rotation (thumb pointing up), which should cause **less** pain.
   - **Infraspinatus isolation test:** this maneuver isolates the infraspinatus tendon. The arms are placed at the patient's side with elbows at the waist flexed to 90 degrees and 45 degrees of internal rotation. Shoulder external rotation is resisted and the test is positive if this results in pain. This test also tests for teres minor tendonitis because there are no tests to isolate this tendon.
   - **Gerber push with force test:** this maneuver isolates the subscapularis tendon. The patient's shoulder is placed passively in internal rotation and slight extension by placing the hand 5 to 10 cm from the lower back with the palm facing outward and the elbow flexed at 90 degrees. The examiner pushes the palms toward the patient's back while the patient resists. The test is positive if this results in pain.

8. **What are the Neer and Hawkins–Kennedy impingement tests?**
   These are provocative maneuvers that are very sensitive (80% to 90%) for impingement but not very specific (30% to 50%). The **Neer test** causes pain when the patient's shoulder is flexed forward maximally by the examiner, while the arm is internally rotated (palm down) and the shoulder is stabilized. The **Hawkins–Kennedy test** reinforces a positive Neer impingement test. The examiner puts the shoulder into 90 degrees of forward flexion and flexes the elbow to 90 degrees. The arm is internally rotated as if the patient is emptying a can of soda in front of themselves. Both these maneuvers compress the greater tuberosity of the humerus against the anterior acromion (Neer test) or coracoacromial ligament (Hawkins–Kennedy test) and elicits discomfort in patients who have a rotator cuff tear or impingement.

9. **What is the impingement sign?**
   The impingement sign is considered "positive" and the diagnosis supported when an injection of local anesthetic (10 mL of 1% plain lidocaine) into the subacromial space ameliorates the pain caused by the Jobe, Neer, and Hawkins–Kennedy tests.

10. **How is the impingement syndrome treated?**
    The mainstays of management are physical therapy and antiinflammatory medications. Regaining full shoulder motion and rotator cuff strength are the therapy goals. Inflammation in the tendons is treated with oral nonsteroidal antiinflammatory drugs (NSAIDs) or a local injection of corticosteroid. Nonoperative management should be pursued for at least 6 months before consideration of surgical decompression, unless a full-thickness rotator cuff tear is present.

11. **How common are rotator cuff tears?**
    The incidence of **partial** rotator cuff tears increases with age and can result from trauma or tendon degeneration from chronic impingement:
    - Age 40 years: 33%
    - Age 50 years: 55%
    - Age 60 years: 65%
    - Age 70 years: 80%

    Most are relatively asymptomatic and 30% to 50% are bilateral. Weakness will be demonstrated on supraspinatus testing (50% sensitivity, 60% specificity). Full thickness tears are less common (25% of individuals over age 60 years) and should be suspected in patients with shoulder muscle atrophy, those who "hike" the shoulder when asked to lift the arm, and in patients with a positive drop arm test (30% sensitivity, 90% specificity).

12. **Describe the clinical aspects of subacromial bursitis.**
    - Unusual for it to occur in the absence of the impingement syndrome
    - Primary inflammation of the bursa may occur as a result of crystal deposition or infection
    - Clinical findings similar to those of the impingement syndrome
    - Focal tenderness when the area of the bursa is palpated (Figure 62-2)

13. **Describe the clinical aspects of bicipital tendinitis.**
    - Anterior shoulder pain
    - Pain worsened with active shoulder movement
    - Positive Yergason's maneuver and/or Speed's test

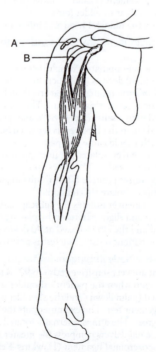

Figure 62-2. Shoulder anatomy. A, Subacromial bursa. B, Biceps tendon, long head.

- Less pain with passive movement
- Absence of swelling, redness, or warmth at shoulder joint
- Focal tenderness when area overlying long head of biceps tendon is palpated (Figure 62-2)
- Frequently accompanies the impingement syndrome

14. What are Yergason's maneuver and Speed's test?
- **Yergason's maneuver**—pain in the area of the long head of the biceps tendon is elicited by resisted supination of the forearm when the elbow is held at the side and flexed to 90 degrees. This is a difficult test to perform and interpret.
- **Speed's test**—the patient's elbow is extended, forearm supinated (palm up), and humerus flexed forward 60 to 90 degrees. Pain in the area of the biceps tendon is elicited by downward resistance applied to the forward flexed arm (63% sensitivity, 35% specificity).

15. What is a "frozen shoulder"?
Also called adhesive capsulitis or pericapsulitis, frozen shoulder can occur after **any** cause of shoulder pain that leads an affected individual to limit the motion of the shoulder because of pain. Patients with diabetes are particularly prone to develop this condition. With little movement, the shoulder joint capsule and surrounding structures contract, making the range of motion physically restricted in addition to being painful. Examination reveals at least 50% reduction in both active and passive range of motion. Arthrography shows decreased volume of the joint capsule. It is rarely seen before age 40 years. The process typically has three phases:
- Phase I: increasing pain and stiffness for 2 to 9 months
- Phase II: substantial stiffness but less pain for 4 to 12 months
- Phase III: pain resolves and function is gradually restored over 5 to 26 months

Treatment consists of NSAIDs, **supervised** physical therapy, and a single intraarticular corticosteroid injection. Physical therapy must be supervised because the patient will not be successful on his own. Viscosupplementation has been reported to be beneficial. Rarely surgical intervention is necessary.

16. List three causes of nonarticular elbow pain.
- Lateral epicondylitis (tennis elbow)
- Medial epicondylitis (golfer's/bowler's elbow)
- Olecranon bursitis

17. List the clinical features of lateral epicondylitis.
- Lateral elbow pain, especially with motions such as turning a screwdriver, shaking hands, or hitting backhand in tennis.
- Incidence is 1% to 3% of the general population. Smoking, repetitive movement for >2 hours/day, or lifting loads >20 kg are risk factors.
- Pain is worsened with extension of the wrist, especially against resistance, when the elbow is in full extension.
- Pain is elicited by palpation at the origin of the wrist extensors (Figure 62-3).
- There may be swelling and warmth at the point of maximum tenderness.
- Pain is caused by tendinitis of the wrist extensors (extensor carpi ulnaris, extensor carpi radialis longus and brevis, extensor digitorum).

18. List the clinical characteristics of medial epicondylitis.
- Medial elbow pain (much less common than in lateral epicondylitis).
- Pain is worsened with flexion of the wrist, especially against resistance, when the elbow is in full extension.
- Pain is elicited by palpation at the origin of the wrist flexors and pronator (Figure 62-3).
- There may be swelling and warmth at the point of maximum tenderness.
- Pain is caused by tendinitis of the wrist flexors and pronator (flexor carpi ulnaris, flexor carpi radialis, and pronator teres).

19. How is epicondylitis treated?
- Avoid precipitating or exacerbating actions, if possible
- Counterforce brace or strap placed 10 cm distal to the joint line
- NSAIDs
- Ice (especially when symptomatic)
- Stretching and strengthening exercises directed at affected muscle groups
- Iontophoresis with dexamethasone or NSAIDs
- Local corticosteroid injection (controversial): many experts feel that epicondylitis is a degenerative tendinopathy and not an inflammatory lesion; recent studies suggest that steroid injections help symptoms in the short term but actually make long term recovery worse
- Occasionally, splinting the wrist to prevent flexion and extension can help (**caution:** the splint should be removed two to three times a day to allow wrist movement)
- Less than 5% to 10% will need surgical debridement after 6 months of conservative therapy
- Platelet-rich plasma injections, autologous blood injections, prolotherapy, extracorporeal shock wave therapy, and percutaneous needle tenotomy

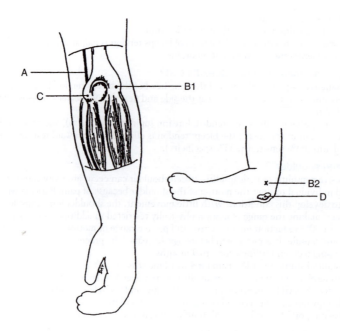

Figure 62-3. Elbow anatomy. A, Ulnar nerve. B1, B2, Lateral epicondyle. C, Medial epicondyle. D, Olecranon bursa.

20. Describe the clinical features of olecranon bursitis.
- Pain, swelling, and warmth at the location of the olecranon bursa on the extensor surface of the elbow (Figure 62-3)
- Bursa may be fluctuant and full
- Typically, elbow extension is normal but flexion may be limited
- Can be secondary to: trauma, rheumatoid arthritis (RA), crystalline arthropathies (gout, calcium pyrophosphate dihydrate deposition disease [CPPD]), dialysis, or infection (frequently caused by a break in the surrounding skin)

21. What is De Quervain's stenosing tenosynovitis?
- Tendinitis involving the abductor pollicis longus (APL) and extensor pollicis brevis (EPB) tendons
- Most frequently described as pain at the base of the thumb
- APL/EPB tendons form the palmar side of the anatomic snuffbox
- A positive Finkelstein maneuver supports the diagnosis

22. What physical examination tests are done to diagnose De Quervain's stenosing tenosynovitis?
- **Finkelstein (Eichhoff) maneuver:** the patient touches the thumb to the base of the fifth finger, then wraps the other fingers around the thumb and abducts of the wrist (the fist moves toward the ulnar side) eliciting pain (sensitivity 89%, specificity 14%).
- **Wrist hyperflexion and abduction of the thumb (WHAT) test:** the patient fully flexes his/her wrist and keeps his/her thumb fully extended and abducted while the examiner applies a gradually increasing abduction resistance to the thumb causing pain (sensitivity 99%, specificity 29%).

23. How is De Quervain's tenosynovitis treated?
- NSAIDs and ice
- Splint for the thumb and wrist called a **forearm-based thumb spica splint**
- Avoid precipitating or aggravating maneuvers
- Local corticosteroid injection
- Surgical release if conservative therapy fails

24. What is the intersection syndrome?
This is a common overuse cause of distal forearm pain that results from inflammation at the point where the APL/EPB tendons cross over the extensor carpi radialis longus and extensor carpi radialis brevis tendons in the wrist. This condition is often seen in laborers who perform repetitive dorsiflexion of the wrist or in athletes such as rowers. The area of inflammation is 6 to 8 cm proximal to the radial styloid. There may be swelling and crepitus with active wrist extension.

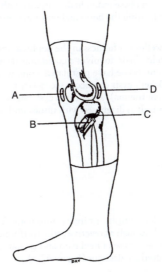

Figure 62-4. Knee anatomy. A, Prepatellar bursa. B, Conjoined tendons. C, Anserine bursa. D, Posterior fossa (where Baker's cyst will be felt).

25. **How does trochanteric bursitis present clinically?**
    Patients complain of "hip pain." When asked to localize the pain, they point to the lateral aspect of the pelvis, with the area of greatest pain typically overlying the greater trochanter on the femur. Pain is exacerbated by lying on the affected side, walking, climbing stairs, rising from a seated position, and external rotation and abduction of the hip. Iliotibial band (ITB) tightness and leg length discrepancy predisposes a person to develop trochanteric bursitis.

26. **Describe the clinical features of gluteus medius tendinopathy.**
    Gluteus medius tendinopathy can resemble trochanteric bursitis. However, tenderness on palpation is superior to the greater trochanter. With significant pathology the patient may have a positive Trendelenburg test and significant weakness or inability to complete a single repetition of the one-leg mini-squat test where the patient squats on the affected leg to 60 degrees. Failure to improve with NSAIDs, physical therapy, and corticosteroid injections should suggest a tendon tear or rupture ("rotator cuff tear of the hip").

27. **What does a "snapping hip" mean?**
    Snapping hip is characterized by a snapping sensation as hip tendons move over bony prominences. The most common site is the ITB snapping over the greater trochanter usually with walking or rotation of the hip (**iliotibial band syndrome**). Patients may subsequently develop a trochanteric bursitis. Patients usually have a positive Ober test suggesting ITB tightness or contracture. A positive "J" sign is also confirmatory. This test is performed with the patient supine and flexes the uninvolved leg to the chest. If the painful hip abducts, a restricted ITB can be diagnosed.

28. **What is "weaver's bottom"?**
    - Also called ischial bursitis
    - Bursa lies superficial to the ischial tuberosity
    - Can be caused by prolonged sitting on hard surfaces, especially in thin individuals

29. **What is prepatellar bursitis ("housemaid's knee")?**
    - Pain, swelling, and warmth in the prepatellar bursa
    - Located superficial to the patella (Figure 62-4)
    - Caused by repetitive trauma or overuse, such as kneeling
    - Can be affected in patients with gout
    - Can be infected, especially after breaks in the skin

30. **What is pes anserine bursitis?**
    Inflammation of the pes anserine ("goose's foot") bursa located at the medial aspect of the knee approximately 6 cm below the anteromedial joint line. The bursa (Figure 62-4) lies between the conjoined tendons of the sartorius/gracilis/semitendinosus muscles and the medial collateral ligament. It is frequently described as knee pain, but it is typically noticed when lying on one's side in bed when the knees are opposed. Pain is worsened

by going up stairs. It is more common in obese individuals, patients with valgus knee deformity, and patients with pes planus. Pain is elicited by palpating the bursa and may have associated warmth.

31. What is Baker's cyst?
Also called a popliteal cyst, this is swelling or fullness in the popliteal fossa with minimal tenderness (Figure 62-4). Its proposed cause, in some individuals, involves a communication between the semimembranosus/gastrocnemius bursa and the knee joint. Some have postulated a one-way valve effect in which synovial fluid moves from the knee to the bursa. Baker's cysts can occur secondary to any process that produces synovial fluid (most commonly RA, osteoarthritis, or trauma). A ruptured cyst can occasionally dissect down the calf and be confused with deep venous thrombosis. It is diagnosed with ultrasound or arthrography.

32. Name five causes of heel pain.
- Achilles enthesitis
- Achilles tendinitis
- Retrocalcaneal (Achilles) bursitis
- Plantar fasciitis
- Heel fat pad atrophy

33. What is enthesitis?
An **enthesis** is the place where a tendon or ligament inserts into bone. These areas can become inflamed (enthesitis) in the spondyloarthropathies such as reactive arthritis (formerly called Reiter's syndrome) or ankylosing spondylitis. Achilles enthesitis is a cause of heel pain and is characterized by swelling, warmth, and pain where the Achilles tendon inserts into the calcaneus (Figure 62-5).

34. Describe the clinical features of Achilles tendinitis.
- Heel pain, sometimes described as posterior leg pain
- Dorsiflexion increases the pain
- Area of most tenderness is 2 to 3 cm proximal to the insertion into the calcaneus (Figure 62-5)
- Tendon may be swollen with thickening, especially 2 to 3 cm proximal to the insertion
- May rupture spontaneously
  - Sudden onset of pain during dorsiflexion
  - Audible pop or snap
  - Positive "Thompson test"

35. How is the Thompson test performed?
The patient kneels on a chair with the feet extending back over the edge. As the examiner squeezes and pushes the calf toward the knee, normally plantarflexion of the foot should be seen; however, in rupture of the Achilles tendon, there will be no movement.

36. How does retrocalcaneal (Achilles) bursitis present clinically?
- Heel pain
- Fullness or swelling proximal and anterior to the insertion of the Achilles tendon into the calcaneus (Figure 62-5)
- Pain on palpation of the bursa

37. Describe the clinical features of plantar fasciitis.
Some may describe heel pain, but most affected individuals complain of pain along the plantar surface of the foot. The pain is worsened by pressure on the bottom of the foot (i.e., walking, running, palpation). **It is also worse with the first steps taken after getting out of bed in the morning.** There is tenderness to palpation at the attachment site of the plantar fascia to the inferior aspect of the calcaneus. Predisposing factors include obesity, pes planus, pes cavus, short Achilles tendon, and standing/running on hard surfaces.

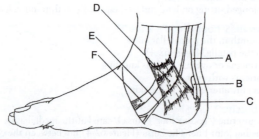

Figure 62-5. Medial ankle and foot anatomy. A, Achilles tendon. B, Achilles bursa. C, Achilles enthesitis. D, Flexor retinaculum. E, Posterior tibial nerve. F, Posterior tibial tendon.

38. **How is plantar fasciitis treated?**
    - Initial therapy:
    - Heel cup: consider custom orthotics if foot abnormalities are present
    - NSAIDs
    - Stretching exercises of the plantar fascia and Achilles tendon; soda can roll with foot
    - Avoid weight-bearing exercise
    - If no improvement after approximately 2 to 3 months, continue the plan above and add:
    - Night splint: a removable splint to hold the foot in minimal dorsiflexion while sleeping
    - Consider a local corticosteroid injection
    - Extracorporeal shock wave therapy: maximum improvement seen 3 months after treatment
    - If no improvement after approximately 6 to 12 months of conservative therapy, consider a referral for surgery (<10% of patients)

39. **What are the clinical features of heel fat pad atrophy?**
    - Pain with prolonged standing or walking
    - Pain with initial weight-bearing (i.e., in the morning)
    - Tenderness to palpation in the central, plantar region of the heel
    - Pain to palpation is improved with augmenting the fat pad (simultaneously squeezing the medial and lateral sides of the heel to force the subcutaneous tissue in a plantar direction)

40. **What is the significance of a heel spur?**
    A heel spur (osteophyte) develops at the origin of the flexor brevis muscle just superior to the plantar fascia in approximately 50% of patients with plantar fasciitis. However, the spur is not a source of pain and is present in 20% of similar-age adults who do not have plantar fasciitis.

41. **What is posterior tibial tendinitis?**
    Inflammation of the posterior tibial tendon and its synovial sheath. Pain is located more prominently on the medial side of the ankle. The pain and swelling are localized to the path of the posterior tibial tendon (Figure 62-5), with increased pain on resisted foot inversion.

42. **What are some clinical features of dysfunction or rupture of the posterior tibial tendon?**
    - **Acquired pes planus**—also called a flat foot, in which the normal contour of the longitudinal arch becomes flattened.
    - **"Too many toes" sign**—caused by hind-foot valgus and forefoot abduction. When the foot is viewed from behind the heel, you can see more toes over the lateral side of the affected foot than on the unaffected side.
    - **"Heel-rise" sign**—the inability to rise to the ball of the affected foot while lifting the unaffected foot.

43. **How can the regional musculoskeletal syndromes be treated?**
    - **Identify, modify, and avoid the precipitating movements or actions**: bursitis and tendinitis can frequently be caused by repetitive motions or movements (e.g., biceps tendinitis caused by carrying a heavy briefcase daily).
    - Rest the affected area: however, intermittent range of motion needs to be maintained, or the joint capsule may contract or "freeze."
    - Antiinflammatory or analgesic medications: NSAIDs probably have a more important role than just analgesia.
    - Splinting of the affected area (e.g., an elastic forearm band in epicondylitis).
    - Local corticosteroid injections (depending on area): never inject steroids for Achilles tendonitis/enthesitis because of the risk of rupture.
    - Superficial heat and cold.
    - Deep heat (ultrasound) and iontophoresis for superficial structures (Achilles enthesitis, lateral epicondylitis).
    - Range of motion/flexibility exercises.
    - Strengthening exercises.
    - Ambulatory aids (cane, crutches, or walker).
    - Surgery (bursectomy, tenosynovectomy, reattachment of ruptured tendons).

Acknowledgment

Illustrations by Debra Vogelgesang.

Bibliography

Bisset L, et al: A systemic review and meta-analysis of clinical trials on physical interventions for lateral epicondylalgia, Br J Sports Med 39:411, 2005.
Ciccotti MC, et al: Diagnosis and treatment of medial epicondylitis of the elbow, Clin Sports Med 23:693–705, 2004.
Cole C, et al: Plantar fasciitis: evidenced-based review of diagnosis and therapy, Am Fam Physician 72:2237, 2005.
Coombes BK, et al: Effect of corticosteroid injection, physiotherapy, or both on clinical outcomes in patients with unilateral lateral epicondylalgia: a randomized controlled trial, JAMA 309:461–469, 2013.

Gomoll AH, et al: Rotator cuff disorders: recognition and management among patients with shoulder pain, Arthritis Rheum 50:3751–3761, 2004.

Holtby R, Razmjou H: Accuracy of the Speed's and Yergason's tests in detecting biceps pathology and SLAP lesions: comparison with arthroscopic findings, Arthroscopy 20:231–236, 2004.

Koester MC, et al: Shoulder impingement syndrome, Am J Med 118:452–455, 2005.

Levine WN, et al: Nonoperative management of idiopathic adhesive capsulitis, J Shoulder Elbow Surg 16:569–573, 2007.

Murrell GA, Walton JR: Diagnosis of rotator cuff tears, Lancet 357:769–770, 2001.

Peerbooms JC, et al: Positive effect of an autologous platelet concentrate in lateral epicondylitis in a double-blind randomized controlled trial: platelet-rich plasma versus corticosteroid injections with a 1-year follow-up, Am J Sports Med 38:255, 2010.

Rennie WJ, Saifuddin A: Pes anserine bursitis: incidence in symptomatic knees and clinical presentation, Skeletal Radio 34:395, 2005.

Richie CA, Briner WW: Corticosteroid injection for treatment of de Quervain's tenosynovitis: a pooled quantitative literature evaluation, J Am Board Fam Pract 16:102, 2003.

Shiri R, et al: Prevalence and determinants of lateral and medial epicondylitis: a population study, Am J Epidemiol 164:1065, 2006.

Silva L, et al: Accuracy of physical examination in subacromial impingement syndrome, Rheumatology 47:679–683, 2008.

Smidt N, et al: Corticosteroid injections, physiotherapy, or a wait-and-see policy for lateral epicondylitis: a randomized controlled trial, Lancet 359:657, 2002.

Thompson CE, et al: The effectiveness of extracorporeal shock wave therapy for plantar heel pain: a systemic review and meta-analysis, BMC Musculoskelet Disord 6:19, 2005.

SPORTS MEDICINE AND OCCUPATIONAL INJURIES

Donald G. Eckhoff, MD, MS

CHAPTER 63

> **KEY POINTS**
> 1. The shoulder relies on tendons and ligaments for movement and stability. These are subject to tremendous stresses leading to injury particularly in overhead athletes.
> 2. Chondromalacia patella is a pathologic condition which can only be diagnosed at the time of surgery and is just one cause of anterior knee pain.
> 3. Most sports-related injuries can be managed with rest, nonsteroidal antiinflammatory drugs, and physical therapy.
> 4. Abnormal body position and mechanics contribute to the majority of recreational or occupational injuries and must be corrected as part of the treatment plan.

1. What is the difference between a sprain and a strain?

A **sprain** is an acute traumatic injury to a **ligament**. There are three grades of sprains:
- First-degree—mild pain due to tearing less than one third of ligamentous fibers, <5 mm laxity.
- Second-degree—moderate pain and swelling, one third to two third of fibers of ligament torn, 5 to 10 mm laxity.
- Third-degree—severe pain from a complete rupture of the ligament causing joint instability.

A **strain** is an acute traumatic injury to the **muscle–tendon junction**. It is commonly called a "pull." Strains are also classified according to three grades:
- First-degree—mild.
- Second-degree—moderate injury associated with a weak and painful contraction of the involved muscle.
- Third-degree—complete tear of the muscle–tendon junction resulting in severe pain and an inability to contract the involved muscle.

2. How do overuse injuries and a sprain or strain differ?

Strains and sprains are acute and traumatic in cause. Overuse injuries are nonacute injuries to the soft tissue structures resulting from chronic, repetitive microtrauma. Overuse injuries can involve the ligaments or the muscle–tendon junction. Microscopically, local tissue breakdown occurs with tissue lysis, lymphocytic infiltration, and blood extravasation.

Overuse injuries are reported to exist in 30% to 50% of the athletic population and are classified by four grades of injury:
- Grade I—pain after activity only.
- Grade II—pain during and after activity but that does not interfere with performance.
- Grade III—pain during and after activity with interference with performance.
- Grade IV—constant pain that interferes with activities of daily living.

3. List some common overuse injuries of ligaments and tendons occurring in athletes.

Ligaments	Tendons
Little leaguer's elbow	Achilles tendinitis (see Chapter 62)
Swimmer's knee	Suprapatellar tendinitis
Iliotibial band syndrome	Posterior tibialis tendinitis (see Chapter 62)
Jumper's knee	De Quervain's tenosynovitis
Plantar fasciitis (see Chapter 62)	Lateral epicondylitis (tennis elbow)
	Medial epicondylitis (golfer's/bowler's elbow)
	Supraspinatus (rotator cuff) tendinitis (see Chapter 62)
	Bicipital tendinitis (see Chapter 62)

4. How common is shoulder pain in athletes and manual laborers?

Shoulder pain affects all ages (older more than young) with a lifetime prevalence of 33%. It is the third most common musculoskeletal complaint for which a patient seeks care. Up to 15% of all athletic injuries involve the shoulder and it is one of the most common complaints among manual workers. Over half of the problems are related to the rotator cuff. It is most common in overhead athletes and workers. See Chapter 62 for a more comprehensive discussion of common shoulder problems.

5. **What is tennis elbow?**
   Tennis elbow, better termed **lateral epicondylitis**, is an overuse syndrome that presents with lateral elbow pain. Etiologically, few patients who have symptoms of this disorder have acquired it through playing tennis. The differential diagnosis of lateral elbow pain includes local conditions, elbow arthritis, loose body in the elbow, nerve compression of the radial nerve or posterior interosseous nerve, and cervical spondylosis with radiculitis.
   At present, most sports medicine physicians believe that lateral epicondylitis is primarily a degenerative process resulting from microtearing involving the origin of the extensor carpi radialis muscles and is less likely to be an inflammatory process. Provocative testing of forced middle-finger extension against resistance should reproduce pain, because the muscle in question inserts on the base of the middle-finger metacarpal. Treatment is conservative, with a tennis elbow band that anchors the muscle in the proximal forearm and unloads the true origin during activities; this is worn for 9 to 12 months. Oral nonsteroidal antiinflammatory drugs (NSAIDs) are also used, as is physical therapy. The value of a local corticosteroid injection is controversial and many believe it weakens the tendon and delays healing.

6. **Golfer's elbow and little leaguer's elbow both involve the medial elbow. What is the difference between them?**
   Golfer's elbow, better termed a **medial epicondylitis**, results from an overuse injury to the tendinous origin of the flexor pronator muscle mass. This area is placed under valgus stress at the top of a backswing in golfing and proceeds through the downswing until impact with the golf ball. Pain is elicited over the elbow's medial epicondyle and is increased with resisted wrist flexion and forearm pronation. Management includes rest, ice, NSAIDs, and splints. Steroid injections and surgery are rarely required.
   Little leaguer's elbow is a **medial apophysitis** seen mostly in young pitchers between ages 9 and 12 years. It occurs as a result of valgus stress, often from throwing curve balls. The person experiences microtearing of the flexor pronator muscle group and, in severe cases, fragmentation of the medial epicondylar apophysis. Treatment is 2 to 3 weeks of rest, no throwing for 6 to 12 weeks, and rarely surgery if the medial apophysis is displaced.

7. **How do you test for subscapularis tendonitis?**
   The subscapularis muscle is the biggest rotator cuff muscle and is the key to shoulder strength when weight lifting and internal rotation of the arm. Motions such as lifting arm over shoulder are most likely to cause pain. Weight lifters, tennis players, and swimmers are most likely to injure this muscle. Acute tears can occur with a single instance of heavy weight lifting. The **Gerber lift-off test** is performed by asking the patient to put their hand behind their back, palm facing away from the body with thumb pointing up, and then lift it away from the back against resistance. Pain and weakness suggest tendonitis and/or tendon tear.

8. **What is a superior labrum anterior-to-posterior lesion?**
   Superior labrum anterior-to-posterior (**SLAP**) lesions involve an injury to the superior glenoid labrum and the biceps anchor complex. The glenoid labrum is equivalent to the knee meniscus. It is a cartilaginous lining of the glenoid, which serves to deepen the glenoid resulting in increased stability of the shoulder. Injury to the labrum resulting in fraying or tear are mostly seen in overhead throwing athletes. Symptoms may include a deep shoulder aching and painful popping or catching in the shoulder with overhead activities. Provocative tests including the O'Brien active compression test, the crank test, and the clunk test all have poor sensitivity and specificity. They are designed to elicit pain when the lesion is compressed. Magnetic resonance (MR) arthrography is the gold standard with a sensitivity/specificity of over 90% in detecting SLAP lesions. Nonsurgical care includes NSAIDs, physical therapy, and 6 weeks of rest followed by gradual return to activity. If nonsurgical therapy fails, surgical arthroscopy for diagnosis and repair is done.

9. **What is a stinger (burner) injury?**
   The **stinger** is well known in football, resulting from forced lateral deviation of the neck and inferior force on the ipsilateral shoulder. This occurs with tackling, blocking, or ground contact. A traction injury to the brachial plexus results, predominately affecting the upper extremity. Players complain of significant shoulder and arm pain involving the lateral aspect of the entire upper extremity. Occasionally, shoulder pain is the only complaint. Motor weakness of the involved C5 and C6 root innervated muscles is commonly associated. A stinger should be managed by rest and avoidance of sports participation until normal strength has returned.

10. **What is a hip pointer?**
    A hip pointer refers to a contusion of the iliac crest that usually results from a direct blow with a hard object (e.g., football helmet) to the iliac crest during a contact sport crushing the soft tissue. The athlete experiences severe localized pain, and an audible pop or snap commonly occurs at the time of injury. Frequently, the athlete cannot walk. Physical examination reveals tenderness, swelling, and often ecchymosis that can migrate down the leg. Treatment is ice, analgesics, and a supervised stretching program.

11. **Is a snapping hip the same as iliotibial band friction syndrome?**
    A **snapping hip** occurs when the patient reports sounds or sensations of internal hip clicking with flexion and extension. This may reflect a torn acetabular labrum, or it may occur as the iliopsoas passes over the pelvic brim or as the iliotibial band moves over the greater trochanter. The patient usually does not have pain unless there is an associated bursitis. This usually occurs as a result of a tight iliotibial band (see Ober's test below) or muscle imbalance.
    The **iliotibial band (ITB) friction syndrome** causes lateral knee pain and is related to irritation and inflammation at the distal portion of the iliotibial band as it courses over the lateral femoral condyle. The **Noble test** is performed with patient supine and the knee flexed to 90 degrees. The examiner grasps behind the knee and with their thumb applies pressure to the ITB over the lateral femoral condyle. The ankle is grasped with the other hand and the knee extended. Tenderness at the lateral femoral condyle elicited between 30 degrees and 40 degrees of knee flexion is a positive sign. The **Ober test** is done by placing the patient on his or her side with the affected leg upward. The injured leg is flexed to 90 degrees at the knee and fully abducted, following which the hip is hyperextended while stabilizing the pelvis. The leg is then slowly lowered as far as possible. Inability of the extremity to drop below horizontal to the level of the table indicates a tight ITB, which is frequently seen in patients with ITB friction syndrome. The ITB syndrome is usually caused by running excessively or running uphill or on slanted surfaces. Treatment consists of stretching the ITB, ice, modalities, NSAIDs, better training techniques, and rarely corticosteroid injections.

12. **What is a sportsman's hernia?**
    A sportsman's hernia is a controversial cause of chronic groin pain in athletes, particularly soccer and hockey players. It occurs almost exclusively in males at all ages. Physical examination findings are subtle showing a dilated and tender superficial inguinal ring in the absence of a hernia and a tender pubic tubercle where the conjoined tendon inserts. Ultrasound may show posterior inguinal wall deficiency, whereas bone scan and magnetic resonance imaging (MRI) can show abnormalities at the symptomatic pubic tubercle. Conservative treatment often fails and laparoscopic surgical repair is usually required and successful (77% to 100%).

13. **How do swimmer's knee, jumper's knee, and runner's knee differ from each other?**
    Swimmer's knee (breaststroker's knee) is knee pain resulting from valgus stress placed on the knee by the whip kick used in swimming the breaststroke. This usually results in medial collateral ligament stress/strain causing pain.
    Jumper's knee is an accepted term for **patellar tendinitis**. It is common in high jumpers and volleyball or basketball players. This injury is characterized by pain at the inferior pole of the patella at its attachment to the patellar tendon. It is as a result of repetitive stress whose frequency of occurrence exceeds the body's rate of natural repair or healing.
    Runner's knee is more correctly called **patellofemoral syndrome**. This is the most common injury in runners and accounts for >30% of running injuries. Pain is caused by compression of nerve fibers in the retinaculum or in the subchondral bone of the patella or from a synovitis. It is not as a result of chondromalacia patellae (softening of the cartilage).

14. **How is a diagnosis of chondromalacia patellae made?**
    By visually inspecting the cartilage surface of the patella at the time of surgery. The term *chondromalacia patellae* refers to a degenerative condition of the articular surface of the patella that progresses from softening, through fibrillar changes and full-thickness cracks, to exposed subchondral bone. It is graded from I to IV, according to the Outerbridge classification system, using the above descriptors, as well as the size of the lesion.

15. **List the differential diagnosis for anterior knee pain.**
    For many years, chondromalacia patellae was used as a catch-all term for patients with anterior knee pain. Patellofemoral syndrome was the next generalized name that evolved for this group of patients. The current accepted diagnosis is **anterior knee pain**. The differential diagnosis is extensive:

    Chondromalacia patellae
    Patellar malalignment
    Patellar tracking abnormality
    Tendinitis quadriceps/patellae
    Tight iliotibial band
    Meniscal pathology
    Painful bipartite patella
    Blunt trauma, occult fracture
    Osteochondritis dissecans (patella)
    Sinding–Larsen–Johansson syndrome

    Symptomatic plica of the knee
    Fat pad syndrome (Hoffa's disease)
    Bursitis, infrapatellar/prepatellar
    Pes anserine bursitis
    Retinacular neuroma
    Tight lateral retinaculum
    Postsurgical neuroma
    Referred pain from hip
    Radicular pain from lumbosacral spine

16. **What is the most common condition giving rise to anterior knee pain?**
    Patellar maltracking resulting from a relative weakness of the vastus medialis portion of the quadriceps. This maltracking leads to increased pressure on the lateral facet of the patella and pain. With time, it can lead to

chondromalacia. The patellar grind and apprehension tests are often positive. It is common in young adults and responds to directed rehabilitation of the quadriceps and stretching of the hamstrings. Adjunctive modalities of oral NSAIDs and patellar centralizing bracing or taping can also be effective.

Other common conditions that affect the patella and give rise to anterior knee pain are true patellar malalignment, limb malrotation, and tendinitis. One should always evaluate the patient for pes planus with foot pronation to see if this is contributing to patellar maltracking. If present, foot orthotics can help the anterior knee pain.

17. What physical examination tests are most sensitive and specific for the diagnosis of an anterior cruciate ligament injury?

The anterior cruciate ligament (ACL) is the primary stabilizer of the knee. A tear results from twisting or hyperextension injury. Approximately half the time it is accompanied by a meniscal tear. Overall, young female athletes are four to six times more likely to sustain an ACL injury than male athletes, partly owing to females having weak hamstrings leading to neuromuscular imbalance.

The best-known test for ACL deficiency is the **anterior drawer sign**. It is performed with the patient supine and the knee flexed to 90 degrees. The leg is stabilized by the examiner sitting on the patient's foot. With the hamstrings relaxed the examiner grasps the proximal tibia with both hands and attempts to slide the tibia anteriorly. The degree of tibial translation is compared with the uninjured knee. This is a subjective test with a sensitivity of only 50%.

The most sensitive test is the **Lachman test**. With the thigh supported, muscles relaxed, and femur stabilized by one of the examiner's hands, the knee is placed in 20 degrees to 25 degrees of flexion, and the proximal tibia is then translated anteriorly by the examiner's other hand. ACL-deficient knees exhibit increased translation and a soft or mushy endpoint, as compared with the opposite, uninjured knee.

The most specific test is the **pivot shift test**. It is performed by applying a valgus and internal rotation force on the tibia with the knee in full extension and hip abducted 10 degrees to 20 degrees. The knee is then gently flexed. A clunk of tibial rotation is appreciated as the knee passes 20 degrees to 40 degrees of flexion. This must be compared with the opposite side. The appreciable clunk occurs when the tibia, which is abnormally subluxated (anterior and internally rotated secondary to ACL absence), is pulled back into its normal position by the secondary restraints. This test is highly dependent on patient relaxation and is not recommended in the acutely injured, unanesthetized knee.

18. How will a meniscal tear present, and what is the best test?

The meniscus functions as a cushion between the femur and tibia on the medial and lateral sides of the knee. It is well suited to compression but tears when subjected to shear stress with a turning or twisting motion. The nutrition of the inner two thirds of the meniscus is limited and predisposes the torn tissue to not heal once torn, a factor reflected by the typical chronic recurring history of symptoms. The torn tissue may create a mechanical block to the free motion of the knee, which will symptomatically manifest as clicking, popping, and locking, and is associated with pain and swelling at the joint line. These symptoms correlate, but often unreliably, to an audible/palpable pop with flexion/extension of the knee with the patient supine (**McMurray's test**) and prone (**Apley's test**) on physical examination. Joint line tenderness is the best clinical sign of a meniscal tear with 74% sensitivity and 50% specificity. Increased pain at the joint line with standing on one leg with knee flexed 30 degrees increases the accuracy of diagnosis in the young athlete. The history and physical findings; however, can be confused with patellofemoral pathology, particularly in the absence of a single precipitating event. Diagnosis is reliably confirmed by MRI or arthroscopy, and the problem is most efficiently remedied by arthroscopic repair or partial meniscectomy.

19. What is the "terrible triad" of knee injury?

An ACL tear, complete medial collateral ligament tear, and a tear of the medial meniscus. This combination is almost always a result of sporting activities, particularly football. The knee in these injuries exhibits a markedly positive anterior drawer test, a positive Lachman test and pivot shift test, and marked valgus angulation with applied stress in full extension. The knee will be stable to varus stress testing because the lateral collateral ligament and posterior cruciate ligament remain intact. Effusion from hemarthrosis may be mild secondary to medial capsular tearing, which allows the traumatic bleeding to exit the knee joint. Suspicion of an injury of this magnitude should lead to the prompt referral to an orthopedic surgeon. Prophylactic knee bracing may help prevent this injury in football linemen but not in players at other positions.

20. What is the difference between a low ankle sprain and high ankle sprain?

Ankle sprains are a very common injury. Residual symptoms can occur in up to 40% of patients. The most common sprain is a low ankle sprain resulting from an inversion injury. The lateral ligaments (anterior talofibular and calcaneofibular) are the most commonly involved. An injury to the anterior tibiofibular syndesmosis is referred to as a "high ankle sprain" and is more severe requiring more time for recovery. Eversion injuries are less common but involve injury to the medial deltoid ligament. The goal of treatment is to prevent chronic pain and instability. Initially patients are treated with ice, NSAIDs, and a brace. When the patient can bear weight without increased pain (2 to 4 weeks) exercises are started to increase strength.

21. **Name two lower extremity tendon injuries commonly occurring in runners.**
    - Achilles tendinitis (see Chapter 62).
    - Posterior tibialis tendinitis (see Chapter 62).

22. **What is the best treatment for acute rupture of the Achilles tendon?**
    Acute Achilles tendon rupture usually results from a forced contraction of the gastrocnemius muscle against resistance, which occurs either during sports participation or from a fall. It is not rare, and these are not subtle injuries. The patient usually has symptoms of pain, most notable in walking, and weakness in the push-off phase of gait. A positive **Thompson test** is common.
    The best treatment remains controversial. Options include closed treatment with placement in a long or short leg cast with the foot in equinus (plantar-flexed by gravity). A percutaneous suture repair has been reported with good results but may risk some injury to the sural nerve. The third option is open direct primary surgical repair.
    Many long-term studies have compared surgical versus nonsurgical treatment. The healing rate is excellent with all techniques. The closed technique requires longer cast immobilization and results in more ankle stiffness in the short-term. The biggest question revolves around the rate of rerupture. Rerupture rates are reported to be 1% to 5% with surgical treatment and 8% to 16% with closed-cast treatment. Therefore, selection of the best treatment option is individualized, with age, activity level, patient and surgeon interests, and experience as guiding parameters. The best treatment for rerupture is not controversial and universally accepted to be open surgical repair.

23. **What is a "turf toe"?**
    Turf toe is a sprain of the plantar capsule ligament complex of the metatarsophalangeal joint of the great toe. It is more common on artificial turf and results from a hyperextension injury. Hyperflexion and valgus injuries to this toe can cause similar symptoms. Treatment includes rest, taping of the toe to restrict dorsiflexion, and stiffening of the sole of the shoe to prevent motion. Without proper therapy, hallux rigidus can result.

24. **How does a "shin splint" differ from a stress fracture?**
    Shin splint is an overuse injury caused by chronic traction and inflammation of the tibial periosteum. It may involve either tibialis muscles or the soleus muscle and is characterized by anteromedial or posteromedial leg pain of gradual onset. Pain occurs at the start of running, then decreases, and returns after the athlete stops running. Tenderness is found on palpation of the posterior medial border of the tibia, usually at the junction of the middle and distal thirds. Pain is increased with resisted dorsiflexion. Radiographs are normal, but a bone scan shows fusiform uptake of tracer. Shin splint is sometimes called **medial tibial stress syndrome**.
    A **stress fracture** is an overuse injury that occurs when periosteal resorption exceeds bone formation. The tibia is the most common site for stress fractures (30%) in runners, but other areas can be affected depending on the activity or sport. A tibial stress fracture causes pain in runners the entire time they are running as well as afterward. There is often a focal area of tenderness along the anterior tibia. The pain is increased if a vibrating 128-Hz tuning fork is placed on the site (75% sensitivity). Radiographs are usually negative at onset but become abnormal after 5 or more weeks. A bone scan shows uptake, and computerized tomography scan/MRI scans are abnormal. Avoidance of activity is necessary to permit repair and to prevent progression to complete fracture.

25. **What are some hand injuries that can occur in athletes?**
    1. **Mallet finger.** Extensor tendon avulsion with or without fracture involving the distal interphalangeal (DIP) joint. The athlete cannot extend the DIP joint.
    2. **Jersey finger.** Avulsion of the flexor digitorum profundus tendon causing inability to flex the DIP joint. Usually occurs from grabbing a jersey when tackling in football.
    3. **Gamekeeper's thumb.** Rupture of the ulnar collateral ligament of the first metacarpophalangeal (MCP) joint. Frequent in skiing injuries.
    4. **Boxer's knuckle.** Longitudinal tear of the extensor digitorum communis tendon or sagittal bands overlying the metacarpal head (usually the third MCP), resulting in extensor weakness of that finger.

26. **How common are occupational overuse injuries?**
    Repetitive movements for prolonged periods can lead to overuse injuries in several professions resulting in work-related disability with costs approaching 1% of the U.S. gross national product. For example, 10% to 20% of musicians, typists, keypunch/calculator/cash register operators, and assembly-line workers will experience a repetitive strain syndrome. The most common problems are bicipital tendinitis, carpal tunnel syndrome, and De Quervain's tendinitis. Patients with tendinitis need to have a complete occupational history obtained to determine if their work is causing their problems. It should be noted that there is much controversy and debate over the scientific evidence supporting the relationship between cumulative trauma/repetitive strain disorders and many occupations.

27. **What occupations are associated with osteoarthritis?**
    Several occupations can cause stress and trauma to joints, leading to early osteoarthritis. This most likely occurs in joints that have been previously injured, have an abnormal joint alignment, or are unstable as a result of ligamentous injury. Examples include ballet dancers (ankle, feet); farmers (hips, knees); miners

(elbow/knees/spine), riveters, or metal workers (elbows); pneumatic tool operators (upper extremity joints); coal miners (knees); and cotton mill workers (hands). The relationship between osteoarthritis and sporting activities is less clear, owing to repeated joint injuries in addition to repetitive loading.

28. Discuss the principles of treatment of tendinitis and overuse injuries.
The general principles of management can be remembered with the mnemonic **PRICES**:

Primary therapies	Secondary therapies
P—Protection	Physical modalities
R—Rest	Rehabilitation
I—Ice	Injections
C—Compression	Cross-training
E—Elevation	Evaluation and reevaluation
S—Support	Salicylates and steroids

Treatment of soft tissue injuries with early control of pain and inflammation is critical. Sustained inflammation decreases soft tissue healing and leads to gradual deconditioning and functional disability. With acute problems, relative rest is important. Ice is an effective antiinflammatory in the first hours after an injury. Heat is often preferred after the acute injury. Orthotics, splinting, braces, or taping may be used to facilitate protected motion.

29. When are medications useful?
NSAIDs are often used, and all NSAIDs are equally effective. After acute injuries, there is little evidence to support using them for longer than 72 hours. More prolonged use is recommended for chronic overuse conditions.

Corticosteroid injections for chronic conditions are not definitive treatment but can be used to facilitate rehabilitation. Injections should be performed by clinicians experienced in performing these procedures and who are familiar with the side effects. Corticosteroids can increase the rate of collagen degradation, decrease new collagen formation, lower tendon tensile strength, and lead to tendon rupture if the procedure is performed incorrectly or too often. The patient should be advised to restrict activity of the affected area for 2 to 3 weeks after an injection.

30. How can injuries be prevented?
Part of the responsibility of the physician is to educate the athlete or worker on how to prevent further injury. Just treating the acute or chronic injury is not enough. Emphasizing the importance of stretching and warming up before participation should always be done. Other measures include recommendations for limiting pitches in high school pitchers (less than 80), instructing female athletes in how to pivot, jump, and land to prevent ACL injuries, or having an ergonomic evaluation of a patient's worksite. Unfortunately, many coaches and companies are resistant to this intervention.

BIBLIOGRAPHY

Burton AK, Kendall N, Pearce BG, et al: Management of work-relevant upper limb disorders: a review, Occup Med 59:44–52, 2009.
Dye SF: The pathophysiology of patellofemoral pain: a tissue homeostasis perspective, Clin Orthop Relat Res 436:100–110, 2005.
Foxman I, Burgel BJ: Musician health and safety: preventing playing-related musculoskeletal disorders, AAOHN J 54:309–316, 2006.
Moeller JL: Sportsman's hernia, Curr Sports Med Rep 6:111–114, 2007.
Sarwark JF, editor: Essentials of musculoskeletal care, ed 4, AAOS, 2010.
Spindler KP, Wright RW: Anterior cruciate ligament tear, N Engl J Med 359:2135–2142, 2008.
Weinberg J, Rokito S, Silber JS: Etiology, treatment, and prevention of athletic "stingers," Clin Sports Med 22:493–500, 2003.

FURTHER READING

www.orthoinfo.aaos.org

CHAPTER 64

ENTRAPMENT NEUROPATHIES

David R. Finger, MD

> **KEY POINTS**
>
> 1. Carpal tunnel syndrome is the most common entrapment neuropathy.
> 2. Knowledge of anatomy and predisposing factors are necessary for the accurate diagnosis of the entrapment neuropathies.
> 3. Most entrapment neuropathies of short duration can be treated conservatively.

1. **What are entrapment neuropathies and how do they occur?**
   Entrapment neuropathies occur when a peripheral nerve is compressed within an enclosed anatomic space. Entrapment can occur from increased pressure, stretch, angulation, ischemia, or friction; previously compromised nerves, such as from alcoholism or diabetes, are more vulnerable. The nerve damage is characterized by physiologic slowing, demyelination, and remyelination; intraoperative exposure of the involved nerve often reveals swelling proximal to the site of entrapment.

2. **Do entrapment neuropathies occur in rheumatoid arthritis?**
   Inflammation and swelling of synovium, bursae, ligaments, or tendon sheaths can cause pressure on adjacent nerves. Entrapment neuropathies have been reported to occur in nearly half of patients with chronic rheumatoid arthritis (RA) at some point in their lifetime. Interestingly, there does not appear to be any correlation with duration of disease, positive rheumatoid factor, level of acute phase reactants (sedimentation rate), functional class, or extraarticular disease. Carpal tunnel syndrome (CTS) occurs with a reported frequency of 23% to 69% in RA.

3. **What are some other etiologies that should be considered when evaluating entrapment neuropathies?**
   - Polyneuropathies.
   - Brachial plexopathy.
   - Radiculopathy.
   - Raynaud's phenomenon.
   - Chronic regional pain syndrome.
   - Vasculitis.
   - Tendinitis.

4. **How are entrapment neuropathies usually diagnosed?**
   The presence of characteristic symptoms along with provocative maneuvers (Tinel's sign) is usually adequate to support the diagnosis. Electrodiagnostic studies (nerve conduction velocities and electromyography) are often used to confirm and localize the site of entrapment, although this study can be normal in 10% to 25% of patients who have a definite entrapment neuropathy.

5. **When are electrodiagnostic studies indicated?**
   - When the diagnosis is uncertain.
   - To exclude radiculopathy or polyneuropathy.
   - To follow the course of patients being treated conservatively.
   - Before surgery.

6. **Describe characteristic clinical features of entrapment neuropathies.**
   - Dysesthesias, usually localized to the sensory distribution of the involved nerve.
   - Symptoms described as burning, tingling, pain, or "pins and needles."
   - Symptoms not use-related.
   - Tenderness of the involved area is usually *not* a feature.
   - Symptoms usually worse at night and while at rest.
   - Muscle weakness and atrophy are severe and late findings indicating denervation.
   - Usually unilateral, with the exception of idiopathic CTS.
   - Swelling or vasomotor abnormalities absent.

7. **What is the CTS?**
    CTS is easily the most common entrapment neuropathy, with a prevalence of 0.2% to 1%. Nine flexor tendons and the median nerve pass through the carpal tunnel, which is narrowest at its mid-portion. CTS occurs when the median nerve is compressed by the flexor retinaculum/transverse carpal ligament at the wrist, producing characteristic nocturnal dysesthesias (70%), but occasionally progressing to sensory loss and weakness of thumb abduction (Figure 64-1). Pain can radiate into the proximal arm (40%). This condition is bilateral in half of patients and occurs with increased frequency in occupations associated with high levels of repetition and force (meatpackers, shellfish packing, musicians).

8. **Describe physical examination signs indicative of CTS. How do they compare with other diagnostic testing?**
    In CTS, numbness commonly affects the index, middle, and radial side of the ring finger. The thumb is less often symptomatic. A positive Tinel's sign occurs when tapping the nerve at the site of entrapment produces pain and dysesthesias radiating into the sensory distribution of the nerve distally. In CTS, this test has a pooled sensitivity of 50% and specificity of 77%. Phalen's test is positive when passive wrist flexion to 90 degrees for 1 minute produces or worsens paresthesias in the median nerve distribution. It has a pooled sensitivity of 68% and specificity of 73% for CTS. The direct median nerve compression test is positive when pain and paresthesias occur within 30 seconds of pressure exerted over the carpal tunnel by the examiner's thumb. A recently described sign, the volar hot dog (swelling at the wrist on the ulnar side of the palmaris longus tendon), has been reported in over 90% of patients with CTS. In addition to provocative maneuvers, two-point discrimination (sensitivity 25%, specificity 90%), grip strength, and thenar muscle function and atrophy should be examined. Electrodiagnostic studies have a sensitivity of 85% and specificity of 95% for CTS. Ultrasonography and magnetic resonance imaging (MRI) can be useful in patients with equivocal electrodiagnostic studies.

9. **List some diseases associated with CTS.**
    Use the mnemonic **PRAGMATIC**.
    Pregnancy (20%).
    Rheumatoid arthritis (any inflammatory arthritis).
    Acromegaly.
    Glucose (diabetes).
    Mechanical (overuse, occupational).
    Amyloid.
    Thyroid (myxedema).
    Infection (TB, fungal).
    Crystals (gout, pseudogout).

10. **What are the treatment options for CTS?**
    Nonsurgical therapy consists of avoidance of repetitive wrist motion, cock-up wrist splints at night (and for work), along with antiinflammatory medications. Ergonomic evaluation of the patients' workplace may be beneficial. In patients with less than 6 months of symptoms, a local corticosteroid injection results in excellent short-term relief in 80% of cases. Indications for **surgical therapy** (sectioning of the transverse carpal ligament) include failure of conservative therapy, lifestyle limiting symptoms, and muscle weakness or atrophy. Long-term surgical results are favorable in over 75% of patients. Complete recovery of nerve function occurs only if surgery is performed before evidence of denervation on electromyography/*nerve conduction velocity*.

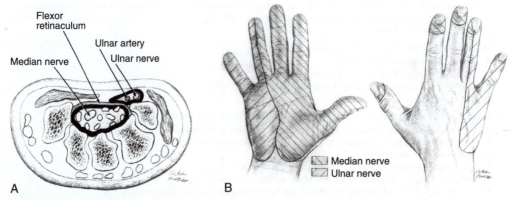

Figure 64-1. **A**, Wrist anatomy showing the median nerve through the carpal tunnel in close proximity to Guyon's canal, where the ulnar nerve passes. **B**, Median and ulnar nerve sensory distributions. (*Illustration by Victor Powell.*)

11. **Where else can median nerve entrapment occur?**
    The **anterior interosseous nerve syndrome** occurs when this nerve, a purely motor branch of the median nerve, is compressed 6 cm distal to the lateral epicondyle. The resulting loss of distal thumb and index finger flexion produces a characteristic flattened pinch sign (inability to form an "O") with normal sensation. The **pronator teres syndrome** occurs when the median nerve is compressed by the pronator teres muscle at the forearm, resulting in proximal volar forearm pain that is worsened by grasping and resistive pronation of the forearm. Patients may have numbness of the thumb and the index finger, thumb weakness, and writer's cramp.

12. **Describe the various ulnar nerve entrapment syndromes.**
    Ulnar nerve compression at (or above and below) the elbow, the second most common entrapment neuropathy of the upper extremity, can occur from external pressure at the medial epicondylar groove (synovitis, osteophytes, anesthetized patients with prolonged resting of the elbow on a flat surface), flexion dislocation, and compression at the aponeurosis of the flexor carpi ulnaris and Osborne's ligament, the so-called cubital tunnel (Figure 64-2). **Cubital tunnel syndrome** results in paresthesias in an ulnar nerve distribution (the little finger and ulnar side of the ring finger), weakness in grasping and pinching, catching the little finger on the edge of the pants' pocket when putting the hand into the pocket (weak interossei and finger adduction), and hypothenar atrophy. Ulnar nerve entrapment is often exacerbated by elbow flexion and by elevating the hand by resting the forearm on the head for 1 minute. Therapy consists of avoidance of prolonged elbow flexion, local steroid injections (in RA), and surgical release in severe cases. **Ulnar tunnel syndrome** occurs when the ulnar nerve is compressed in Guyon's canal at the wrist (Figure 64-1), resulting in symptoms similar to those seen in the cubital tunnel syndrome. Direct pressure over Guyon's canal causes paresthesias. When ulnar nerve symptoms (weakness more than sensory changes) appear late (months) after trauma to the cubital tunnel, it is referred to as **tardy ulnar nerve palsy**.

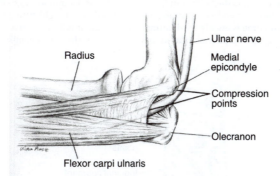

Figure 64-2. Anatomy of the ulnar nerve at the elbow, showing sites of common entrapment at the medial epicondyle and the cubital tunnel. *(Illustration by Victor Powell.)*

13. **What is thoracic outlet syndrome?**
    This syndrome, which is often difficult to diagnose, can occur from either vascular (5% of cases) or neurologic compression (95% of cases). It can be static or positional. Thoracic outlet syndrome (TOS) is most likely to occur in patients who have had trauma (clavicular fracture), repetitive strain injury (poor ergonomics at desk worksite), sports-related activities (overhead sports, baseball pitchers, swimmers, volleyball, etc.), or anatomic abnormalities (cervical rib, Pancoast tumor). Vasogenic TOS occurs when occlusion of the subclavian artery results in ischemic symptoms, or when venous occlusion results in edema, engorged superficial veins, and thrombosis (Paget–Schroetter disease). Neurogenic TOS occurs when there is brachial plexus impingement from a cervical rib (35%), fibrous tissue bands, scalene muscles, or an elongated transverse process of C7. This results in weakness of the intrinsic muscles of the hand along with sensory loss in the ulnar distribution over the hand and forearm. The **Adson maneuver** is performed with the patient in a sitting position by palpating the radial pulse while the patient inhales deeply and extends the neck, turning the head to the side being examined (cervical rib) and then turned away from the side being examined (scalenus anticus syndrome). A positive Adson maneuver occurs when there is diminution of the radial pulse **and** *reproduction of symptoms*. Another provocation test, the **hyperabduction maneuver** ("hands up test"), is performed with the shoulder placed in abduction and external rotation to 90 degrees, elbows flexed at 45 degrees, and palms facing forward for 1 minute to determine if this causes unilateral TOS symptoms, indicating pectoralis minor impingement. If this does not cause symptoms then the test is repeated with the patient's arm hyperabducted to 180 degrees and extended to see if that causes unilateral symptoms due to costoclavicular compression of the neurovascular bundle. The **costoclavicular maneuver** is performed by the patient assuming an exaggerated military posture with shoulders back and downward. This positioning causes compression between the clavicle and first rib (may be positive in

patients with a history of clavicular fracture). Note that in TOS, electrodiagnostic studies are usually normal, and many normal people have false-positive physical examination provocation tests (especially decreased pulse). Treatment consists of range of motion and strengthening exercises to improve posture, avoidance of hyperabduction, botulinum toxin injections, and surgery for those patients with severe, refractory symptoms (cervical rib or fibrous band resection).

14. How does radial nerve entrapment occur?

Improper positioning during anesthesia, sleeping (or laying) on the arm, or improperly fitting crutches can result in prolonged compression of the nerve along the radial groove on the humerus. This results in wrist-drop, referred to as **Saturday night palsy** because it often occurs while the patient is intoxicated. Decreased sensation in dorsal web space can also occur. The **posterior interosseous nerve**, a motor branch of the radial nerve, can be impinged at the elbow (RA synovitis) with resulting weakness in finger extension at the *metacarpophalangeal* joints.

15. How does a patient with suprascapular nerve entrapment present?

The suprascapular nerve innervates the supraspinatus and infraspinatus muscles. The nerve can become compressed in the suprascapular notch usually from carrying heavy loads on the shoulder. Patients have weakness on abduction and external rotation of the shoulder. Atrophy of the supraspinatus muscle can occur. Electromyography can confirm the diagnosis. Physical therapy, local corticosteroid injection, or surgical decompression can be helpful.

16. What is meralgia paresthetica?

Meralgia (Greek for "pain in the thigh") paresthetica results when the lateral cutaneous nerve of the thigh, a sensory nerve (L-2 and L-3), is compressed at the inguinal ligament just medial to the anterior superior iliac spine. This syndrome results in burning pain and dysesthesia over the anterolateral thigh (Figure 64-3). Direct pressure of the nerve where it exits the pelvis can increase symptoms. Common causes include obesity, pregnancy, trauma, surgical injury (appendectomy or inguinal herniorrhaphy), tight-fitting clothing (belts), and diabetes mellitus. This syndrome is usually self-limiting, and treatment is conservative, involving weight loss, avoidance of tight clothing, and occasional local steroid injections at the site of compression.

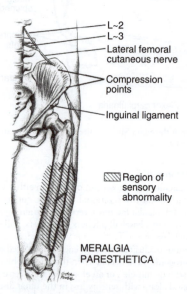

Figure 64-3. Anatomy of the lateral femoral cutaneous nerve. The inguinal ligament and the anterior superior iliac spine are the most likely points of entrapment. *(Illustration by Victor Powell.)*

17. Describe piriformis syndrome.

This controversial syndrome refers to sciatica that arises from entrapment of the sciatic nerve by the piriformis muscle. Overuse injury (running, bicycling), weak gluteals, and compression by an oversized wallet ("fat wallet syndrome") can cause this syndrome. Symptoms include pain over the buttocks (50% to 95%) radiating down the back of the leg and aggravation of pain with sitting (39% to 97%). It occurs more commonly in women and is usually precipitated by trauma. Physical examination reveals external tenderness over greater sciatic notch (59% to 92%) and buttock pain on resisted hip abduction and external rotation when the patient is seated (32% to 74%). With the patient supine, buttock pain with hip flexion, adduction, and internal rotation (FAIR) is also seen along with tenderness of the piriformis muscle on rectal or vaginal examination. Physical therapy (lateral stretching and strengthening), nonsteroidal antiinflammatory drugs, local steroid injections, and botulinum toxin injections can be beneficial. Nerve compression from herniated disc or facet arthropathy should be ruled out.

18. **Which nerve is most likely to be compressed in a patient with a painless foot-drop?**
The common peroneal nerve. **Peroneal nerve palsy** usually occurs following compression over the head of the fibula from prolonged leg crossing, squatting, leg casts and braces. The distal lateral leg often has decreased sensation, and foot eversion (superficial peroneal nerve) and dorsiflexion (deep peroneal nerve) (foot drop) are affected because the lesion occurs proximally in the common peroneal nerve.

19. **A patient with RA has symptoms of burning dysesthesias of toes and sole of foot extending proximally to the medial malleolus; it is worse at night but somewhat relieved by walking. What syndrome does this patient most likely have?**
Tarsal tunnel syndrome. This syndrome occurs when the posterior tibial nerve is compressed at the flexor retinaculum, located posterior and inferior to the medial malleolus (Figure 64-4). A positive **Tinel's sign** (obtained by percussing posterior to the medial malleolus) and a positive **tourniquet test** (applying pressure over the flexor retinaculum) will often reproduce the symptoms. Holding the ankle for 10 seconds in dorsiflexion and eversion will also exacerbate symptoms. This occurs more often in women and is associated with trauma, fracture, valgus deformity, hypermobility, inflammatory arthritis (up to 25% of patients with RA), diabetes, and occupational factors. Treatment consists of antiinflammatory medications, local steroid injection, and orthotics. Surgical release is indicated when conservative measures fail.

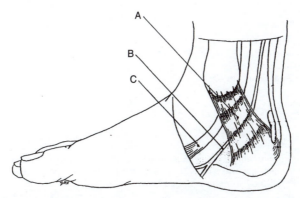

Figure 64-4. Diagram showing the posterior tibial nerve (B) and posterior tibialis tendon (C) as they descend inferior to the medial malleolus and underneath the flexor retinaculum (A). *(Illustration by Debra Vogelgesang.)*

20. **A 50-year-old woman presents with pain and burning between her third and fourth toe. Symptoms are worsened by walking on hard surfaces and wearing high heels. The region between her third and fourth metatarsal heads is tender to palpation. What is the most likely diagnosis?**
Morton's neuroma, caused by entrapment of the interdigital plantar nerve most commonly by the transverse metatarsal ligament, usually located between the third and fourth or second and third metatarsal heads. This occurs more commonly in women who wear tight-fitting shoes or high heels. Patients complain of dysesthesias between the two toes and state they feel like they are walking on a marble or wrinkled sock. Metatarsal compression may cause a palpable click (**Mulder click**) as the neuroma is forced downward, where it may be felt on the plantar surface. Ultrasound and MRI can confirm the diagnosis. Treatment consists of wearing more supportive shoes, padding the metatarsal heads, and local steroid injections. Surgical removal is done if conservative therapy fails.

BIBLIOGRAPHY

Elhassan B, Steinmann SP: Entrapment neuropathy of the ulnar nerve, J Am Acad Orthop Surg 15:672–681, 2007.
Franson J, Baravarian B: Tarsal tunnel syndrome: a compression neuropathy involving four distinct tunnels, Clin Podiatr Med-Surg 23:597–607, 2006.
Hochman MG, Zilberfarb JL: Nerves in a pinch: imaging of nerve compression syndromes, Radiol Clin North Am 42:221–245, 2004.
Hopayian K, Song F, Riera R, et al: The clinical features of the pyriformis syndrome: a systemic review, Eur Spine J 19:2095, 2010.
Huang JH, Zagler EL: Thoracic outlet syndrome, Neurosurgery 55:897–903, 2004.

Kwon BC, Jung KI, Baek GH: Comparison of sonography and electrodiagnostic testing in the diagnosis of carpal tunnel syndrome, J Hand Surg Am 33:65–71, 2008.

MacDermid JC, Wessel J: Clinical diagnosis of carpal tunnel syndrome: a systematic review, J Hand Ther 17:309–319, 2004.

Marshall S, Tardif G, Ashworth N: Local corticosteroid injection for carpal tunnel syndrome, Cochrane Database Syst Rev CD001554, 2007.

McGann SA, Flores RH, Nashel DJ: Entrapment neuropathies and compartment syndromes. In Hochberg MC, et al: editors: Rheumatology, ed 5, Philadelphia, 2011, Mosby Elsevier.

Piazzini DB, Aprile I, Ferrara PE, et al: A systematic review of conservative treatment of carpal tunnel syndrome, Clin Rehabil 21:299–314, 2007.

Shapiro B, Preston D: Entrapment and compressive neuropathies, Med Clin North Am 93:285–315, 2009.

Scholten RJ, Mink van der Molen A, Uitdehaag BM, et al: Surgical treatment options for carpal tunnel syndrome, Cochrane Database Syst Rev CD003905, 2007.

Thomas JL, Blitch 4th EL, Chaney DM, et al: Diagnosis and treatment of forefoot disorders: Morton's intermetatarsal neuroma, J Foot Ankle Surg 48:251, 2009.

Further Reading

www.orthoinfo.aaos.org

COMPLEX REGIONAL PAIN SYNDROME
Julia J. Rhiannon, MD, MSW

CHAPTER 65

TOP SECRETS
1. Complex regional pain syndrome (CRPS) is a syndrome typically occurring in a single extremity following trauma and is characterized by allodynia, hyperalgesia, and vasomotor signs.
2. A characteristic three-phase bone scan has moderate sensitivity (50% to 80%) but high specificity for the diagnosis of CRPS and predicts a better response to corticosteroid therapy.
3. A spinal cord stimulator reduces pain approximately 50% in 50% of patients with severe CRPS.

1. **How is CRPS (formerly *reflex sympathetic dystrophy*) defined?**
   In the early 1990s, a consensus statement was developed by the International Association for the Study of Pain (IASP) establishing that what had been referred to as reflex sympathetic dystrophy (RSD) may not necessarily involve abnormal sympathetic behavior. The name was therefore changed to CRPS and the syndrome was divided into two types: CRPS type I and CRPS type II. These were defined as:
   CRPS type I (RSD)
   - A syndrome that develops after an initiating noxious event (injury, surgery, or infarction) or a cause of immobilization.
   - Spontaneous and continuing pain, allodynia, or hyperalgesia occurs, is not limited to the territory of a single peripheral nerve, and is disproportionate to the inciting event.
   - There is or has been evidence of edema, skin blood flow abnormality, or abnormal sudomotor activity (i.e., sweating) in the region of the pain since the inciting event.
   - This diagnosis is excluded by the existence of conditions that would otherwise account for the degree of pain and dysfunction.
   CRPS type II (causalgia)
   - Type II is a syndrome that develops after a nerve injury.
   - All of the above findings for CRPS type I.

2. **What are the new IASP-revised CRPS clinical diagnostic criteria (Budapest criteria)?**
   To better discriminate CRPS and non-CRPS neuropathic pain, the diagnosis of CRPS is made when the following criteria are met:
   - Continuing pain that is disproportionate to any inciting event.
   - At least one symptom reported in at least three of the following categories:
     - Sensory: hyperesthesia or allodynia.
     - Vasomotor: asymmetry of temperature and/or skin color changes.
     - Sudomotor/edema: edema, sweating changes, or sweating asymmetry.
     - Motor/trophic: decreased range of motion, motor dysfunction (tremor, weakness, dystonia), or trophic changes (hair, nail, skin).
   - At least one sign at the time of evaluation in at least two of the following categories:
     - Sensory: evidence of hyperalgesia (to pinprick) and allodynia (to light touch, temperature sensation, deep somatic pressure, or joint movement).
     - Vasomotor: asymmetry of temperature (>1°C) and/or skin color changes.
     - Sudomotor/edema: evidence of edema, sweating changes, or sweating asymmetry.
     - Motor/trophic: evidence of decreased range of motion, motor dysfunction (tremor, weakness, dystonia), or trophic changes (hair, nail, skin).
   - No other diagnosis better explaining the signs and symptoms.
   NOTE: The above criteria give a sensitivity of 85% and specificity of 69%. If a patient meets one symptom from all four symptom categories and one sign from two of the four sign categories the sensitivity is 70% and specificity is 94%.

3. **What are the classic signs and symptoms of CRPS?**
   - Pain and swelling in an extremity.
   - Trophic skin changes in the same extremity.
     - Skin atrophy or pigmentary changes.
     - Hypertrichosis.

- Hyperhidrosis.
- Nail changes.
- Signs and symptoms of vasomotor instability.
- Pain and/or limited motion of the ipsilateral limb including proximal joints (e.g., shoulder–hand syndrome).
- Neglect-like symptoms concerning the extremity.

The pain is often described as burning and severe. It generally involves an entire area such as a hand or foot, although any site on the body can be involved. **Allodynia**, pain from a usually nonnoxious stimulation such as light touch or even a breeze, is commonly present. **Hyperpathia**, prolonged pain on stimulation, is also usually present. The **vasomotor instability** is manifested by a blue and cool area (but occasionally can be warm and erythematous) along with unusual sweating in the area (but occasionally can be dry and scaly). Dystrophic skin changes, such as atrophy of subcutaneous tissue with overlying tight, shiny, hairless skin, may develop later during the evolution of CRPS. Contractures of the flexor surface of the hand may occur in the late stage of this disease, leaving a claw-like, nonfunctional hand.

4. What are some synonyms for CRPS?

Causalgia (now CRPS II)	Shoulder–hand syndrome	Acute atrophy of bone
Reflex dystrophy	Sudeck's atrophy	Reflex sympathetic dystrophy
Transient osteoporosis	Algodystrophy	Algoneurodystrophy
Posttraumatic osteoporosis		

5. Who was Silas Mitchell?

Silas Mitchell was a neurologist and an assistant surgeon in the U.S. Army during the Civil War. He was in charge of Turner's Lane Hospital, in Philadelphia, to which war-wounded with neurologic injuries were brought. In October 1864, Dr. Mitchell and two colleagues published one of the classics in medical literature, *Gunshot Wounds and Other Injuries of Nerves*, with clear detailed descriptions of CRPS. He emphasized the association with trauma, the lack of direct injury to the nerve, and the articular nature of this syndrome. In 1867, Dr. Mitchell coined the word *causalgia* (from the Greek words for heat and pain) for this illness in an article in the *United States Sanitary Commission Memoirs*.

6. Who gets CRPS?

CRPS occurs in women more than men (2 to 4:1). It affects all races. Adults get CRPS much more often than children. The highest incidence is in the 40- to 60-year age group with a mean age of 50 years. In children it is more common in adolescence (mean age 12 to 13 years). The incidence in children is thought to be underreported because it often goes unrecognized, usually affects the lower extremity, and oftentimes is diagnosed as a psychiatric condition. It is, in general, a more benign disease in children.

7. What are some precipitating factors for the development of CRPS?

Approximately 65% to 75% of the time, there is a clear precipitating factor that causes the development of CRPS. It occurs most commonly after fractures (1% to 2%), peripheral nerve injury (1% to 5%), and strokes/myocardial infarctions (5%).

Inciting factors	
Trauma (common cause)	Chemical burns
Fractures	Electrical burns
Lacerations	Postherpetic neuralgia
Crush injuries	Cervical spine pathology
Contusions	Subcutaneous injections
Sprains	Drugs (barbiturates)
Immobilization in a cast	Malignancies (ovarian)
Myocardial infarctions	Pregnancy
Strokes and other central nervous system (CNS) injury (common cause)	Peripheral nerve diseases
Pleuropulmonary diseases	Emotional stress
Surgery, especially *carpal tunnel syndrome* and foot surgery (common cause)	

Predisposing factors	
Diabetes mellitus	Neurovegetative dystonia
Hyperparathyroidism	Hypertriglyceridemia
Hyperthyroidism	Alcohol abuse
Multiple sclerosis	Tobacco use
Use of angiotensin converting enzyme (ACE) inhibitors	

8. **How soon after a precipitating event, such as trauma, will a patient develop CRPS?**
   CRPS usually begins days to weeks after the inciting event. In approximately 80% of cases, it occurs within 3 months of a traumatic episode. Note that 5% to 7% of patients will develop CRPS in the contralateral (nontraumatized) limb during the course of their disease.

9. **What is shoulder–hand syndrome?**
   This term was coined by Dr. Otto Steinbrocker in 1947 to describe the concomitant shoulder involvement seen with hand CRPS. The ipsilateral shoulder may become diffusely painful, develop limited range of motion in all directions, and may progress to adhesive capsulitis.

10. **What are the stages of CRPS?**
    Stage 1 (acute stage): typically lasts 6–12 months, characterized by:
      Pain in the extremity or shoulder.
      Swelling in the extremity.
      Color change of the extremity (red or blue).
      Movement painful and tendency for immobilization.
      Early osteoporosis on X-rays.
    Stage 2 (dystrophic phase): persists an additional 1–2 years, characterized by:
      Pain usually continues.
      Swelling changes to brawny hard edema.
      Beginning of atrophy of subcutaneous tissue and intrinsic muscles.
      Cooler extremity, can be mottled or cyanotic.
      Progression of osteoporosis.
    Stage 3 (atrophic stage): persists up to several years, characterized by:
      Pain remains constant or diminishes.
      Extremity becomes stiff.
      Swelling changes to periarticular thickening.
      Skin becomes smooth, glossy, and drawn.
      Brittle nails.
      May see muscle spasm, dystonia, tremor.
      Progression of osteoporosis with pathologic fractures.
      Ankylosis in some patients.
    Some have additionally postulated a *fourth stage* (psychological stage), characterized by loss of job, unnecessary surgery, orthostatic hypotension or hypertension, neurodermatitis, depression. Although these stages can be useful, it is often difficult to place an individual patient into one of them. Most often, stages 1 and 2 are merged or fluctuate back and forth. A patient may stay in one stage for months or years, and another patient may progress rapidly through the stages. The earlier stages are much easier to treat than the later stages.

11. **What other motor and movement disorders have been reported in recent series looking at CRPS?**
    Incoordination, tremor (25% to 60%), involuntary movement (myoclonus), dystonia, muscle spasms, paresis, pseudoparalysis.

12. **Present a differential diagnosis for the patient with a tender and swollen limb.**

Inflammatory arthritis	Malignancy	Angioedema
Cellulitis	Fracture	Peripheral neuropathy
Deep venous thrombosis	Systemic sclerosis	CRPS
Osteomyelitis	Osteonecrosis	Pancoast's tumor

13. **Are there notable plain radiographic findings in CRPS?**
    The characteristic radiologic appearance is soft tissue swelling and regional patchy or mottled osteopenia (Figure 65-1). This appearance is especially evident when comparing the involved side with the contralateral side. This X-ray pattern was first described by Sudeck in 1900 and is often referred to as **Sudeck's atrophy**. This patchy osteopenia is helpful in making the diagnosis but is actually seen in less than half the patients in most series.

14. **What are the scintigraphic findings in CRPS? What other radiographic tests are used?**
    The *three-phase bone scan* (TPBS) has emerged as an objective diagnostic test, with poor sensitivity but good specificity. The results of a TPBS can vary greatly depending on how early in the course of the disease the study is performed. In **stage 1**, there is an increase in blood velocity and blood pooling with early and delayed hyperfixation. The bone scan is abnormal approximately 80% of the time in this stage. In **stage 2**, there is normalization of blood velocity and blood pooling but a persistence of early and delayed hyperfixation. The bone scan is abnormal approximately half the time in this stage. In **stage 3**, there is reduced blood velocity and blood pooling, and a minority of patients have early and delayed hyperfixation. Thus, a bone scan performed early in the disease is usually abnormal, but as the disease progresses, scans can be normal. A normal bone scan

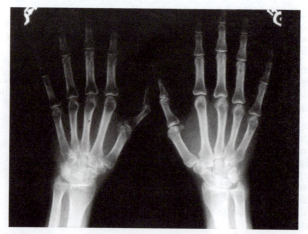

Figure 65-1. Radiograph of the hands showing reflex sympathetic dystrophy of left hand. Note marked periarticular osteoporosis compared with right hand.

does not exclude the diagnosis of CRPS. An abnormal (i.e., hot) bone scan may predict response to corticosteroids. Note that bone scans can show bilateral involvement in 22% of cases of CRPS.

Thermography and contrast-enhanced magnetic resonance imaging are similar to TPBS with poor sensitivity (<50%) but good specificity making them poor screening tests.

15. Does synovial biopsy yield any typical findings in CRPS?
CRPS is an arthritic problem. The involved joints tend to be more tender than the periarticular areas. The synovium has been shown to be clearly abnormal. Findings include synovial edema, proliferation and disarray of synovial lining cells, proliferation of capillaries, fibrosis in the deep synovial layers, and occasional infiltration with chronic inflammatory cells (primarily lymphocytes).

16. What is the current consensus on the pathophysiology of CRPS?
CRPS is hypothesized to develop when persistent noxious stimuli lead to peripheral and central nervous system sensitization. This leads to an abnormally heightened sensation of pain. The initial changes are mediated by nociceptive (Aδ and polymodal C) fibers which transmit to the spinal cord causing a release of excitatory amino acids (glutamate, asparagine), which act on the NMDA receptors causing a release of inflammatory neuropeptides, substance P, and calcitonin gene-related peptide (CGRP). These neuropeptides lower the synaptic excitability of the normally silent second-order interspinal synapses making them hyperexcitable (i.e., *wind-up*). The persistently noxious stimuli leads to peripheral sensitization and further release of inflammatory neuropeptides at the dorsal root ganglion, causing abnormal connections with the sympathetic nervous system, which may potentiate sympathetic mediation of pain. These early changes also cause abnormalities of blood flow which are responsible for some of the signs/symptoms (vasomotor instability) of CRPS. Notably, patients treated with ACE inhibitors have an increased risk of developing CRPS possibly resulting from ACE inhibitors blocking the normal metabolism of neuropeptides such as substance P and CGRP.

Chronic CNS sensitization occurs through afferent processing of the persistent peripheral noxious stimuli by the second-order neurons including wide dynamic range (WDR) neurons in the spinal cord. The WDR neurons transmit signals centrally leading to an enlarged perceptive field for pain corresponding with central sensitization. Later changes in CRPS include long-term modifications in the production of neuropeptides and derangements in both excitatory and inhibitory supraspinal and spinal pathways, which also potentiate further blood flow abnormalities. Finally, autoantibodies against neuronal antigens have recently been demonstrated in patients with late CRPS and are thought to result from neuronal damage. These autoantibodies and the inflammatory neuropeptides may contribute to neurogenically induced inflammation.

17. Describe a rational approach to the treatment of CRPS (* denotes stronger recent evidence)
- Stimulation of inhibitory neurons
  - Spinal cord stimulation*
- Physical therapy*
  - Massage, counterirritants
  - Ultrasound
  - Electroacupuncture
  - Transcutaneous nerve stimulators

- Antiinflammatory agents
  - Nonsteroidal antiinflammatory drugs (NSAIDs)
  - Ketorolac in an intravenous (IV) regional block
  - Corticosteroids*
- Sympathetic blocks
  - Lidocaine, mepivacaine, bupivacaine, etc., into sympathetic ganglion
  - Bier block with IV guanethidine, bretylium, reserpine (depletes norepinephrine) (not very effective)
  - Oral β-blockers (not very effective)
  - Prazosin, phenoxybenzamine, terazosin (α-1 adrenergic blockers)
  - IV phentolamine (α-1 adrenergic blocker)
  - Oral, patch, or epidural clonidine
  - Sympathectomy (surgical)
  - Injection of opioid into sympathetic ganglion
  - Depletion of substance P in peripheral nerves
  - Topical capsaicin
- Anticonvulsants
  - Phenytoin
  - Carbamazepine
  - Gabapentin and pregabalin
  - Valproic acid
- Antiosteoporotic therapy
  - Calcitonin*
  - IV bisphosphonates*
  - High dose oral alendronate (40 mg/day)
- Treatment of dystonia
  - Intrathecal baclofen (GABA agonist)
- Immune modulation (new)
  - IV immunoglobulin (IVIG)*
- Other treatments
  - IV lidocaine and 5% lidoderm patches (sodium channel blocking agents)
  - IV ketamine (block NMDA receptor)*
  - Stop ACE inhibitors
  - Tricyclic antidepressants and serotonin and norepinephrine reuptake *inhibitors*
  - Calcium channel blockers
  - Dimethyl sulfoxide (DMSO) topically
- Psychological therapy
  - Establish rapport with the patient, provide emotional support, assess for depression, and treat with psychotherapy and medications if a problem
  - Thermal biofeedback, relaxation training, alcohol and tobacco cessation
  - Cognitive behavioral therapy*

18. Outline an approach to therapy for CRPS?
    - All patients should be treated with a multidisciplinary approach.
    - All patients should receive information explaining their disease.
    - All patients should receive physical therapy (PT), occupational therapy, and psychological support throughout their disease course. PT should be instituted slowly and under the supervision of a therapist because a patient is unlikely to do it on his/her own. PT needs to be tailored to the severity of symptoms. During the acute stage when the patient has pain at rest, the PT program should be less aggressive (skin desensitization, gentle passive mobilization). As the pain subsides PT can be progressed to active isometric strengthening and finally isotonic training.
    - Patients with early CRPS (<3 to 6 months of symptoms), pain and swelling, and a positive TPBS should be treated with prednisone (60 to 80 mg/day for 2 weeks with taper over next 4 weeks). Corticosteroids can modulate the effect of the inflammatory neuropeptides.
    - Analgesics: opioids, NSAIDs, tricyclic antidepressants, gabapentin (or pregabalin), and/or carbamazepine. Choice depends on severity (opioids versus NSAIDs) and quality (somatic, neuropathic) of pain. Many patients develop a small fiber neuropathy with a decrease in epidermal nerve fiber density in the affected limb. These patients can benefit from neuroleptics.
    - If pain is severe (i.e., pain at rest and with movement) then more aggressive therapy should be instituted early. It is clinically impossible to know if the patient's pain is or is not sympathetically mediated but CRPS is more likely to be as a result of abnormal sympathetic nerve activity early in the disease course. In these patients, sympathetic blocks can be effective. Up to 50% of patients with symptoms less than 1 year can improve with these blocks. However, recurrent sympathetic blocks do not prolong the analgesic effect. Patients who fail to respond to sympathetic blocks are more likely to have their pain mediated by CNS sensitization.

- The following therapies have been most effective for treatment-resistant and/or cases with prolonged symptoms:
  - An epidural spinal cord stimulator can be used and will reduce pain approximately 50% in 50% of patients.
  - IV ketamine: because of the importance of the NMDA receptor some patients with CRPS type I benefit from these infusions (5-day inpatient versus 10-day outpatient infusion with slow tapering to maintenance therapy; one infusion every 3 months).
  - Patients who fail to respond to one of the above therapies may benefit from IVIG which reportedly can improve pain 50% in at least 25% of patients with chronic CRPS possibly by modulating autoantibody effects.

19. **What is the prognosis for CRPS?**
    All therapies work best when instituted early (<2 to 3 months) in the course of CRPS. In adults, up to 85% improve during the first year. Only 30% are cured by 5 years, whereas 2% to 3% have a relapsing course. In children, up to 95% resolve their symptoms within the first year.

20. **How might you prevent CRPS from occurring postsurgically?**
    Vitamin C, 500 mg daily for 50 days has been clearly demonstrated in a randomized, controlled, multicenter dose–response study to reduce the prevalence of CRPS in patients who had wrist fractures. In patients with a previous history of CRPS, perioperative stellate ganglion block has been shown to significantly reduce the recurrence rate of CRPS.

Acknowledgment

The editor and author wish to thank Dr. David Collier for his contributions to this chapter in the previous edition.

BIBLIOGRAPHY

Alexander GM, van Rijn MA, van Hilten JJ, et al: Changes in cerebrospinal fluid levels of pro-inflammatory cytokines in CRPS, Pain 116:213, 2005.
Baron R, Schattschneider J, Binder A, et al: Relation between sympathetic vasoconstrictor activity and pain and hyperalgesia in complex regional pain syndromes: a case-control study, Lancet 359:1655, 2002.
Blaes F, Schmitz K, Tschernatsch M, et al: Autoimmune etiology of complex regional pain syndrome (M. Sudeck), Neurology 63:1734–1736, 2004.
Bruehl S: An update on the pathophysiology of complex regional pain syndrome, Anesthesiology 113:713–725, 2010.
Bruehl S, Chung OY: Psychological and behavioral aspects of complex regional pain syndrome management, Clin J Pain 22:430, 2006.
Brunner F, Schmid A, Kissling R, et al: Bisphosphonates for the therapy of complex regional pain syndrome I – systemic review, Eur J Pain 13:17–21, 2009.
Cepeda MS, Carr DB, Lau J: Local anesthetic sympathetic blockade for complex regional pain syndrome, Cochrane Database Syst Rev 2005:CD004598, 2005.
Goebel A, Baranowski A, Maurer K, et al: Intravenous immunoglobulin treatment of the complex regional pain syndrome: a randomized trial, Ann Intern Med 152:152–158, 2010.
Gorodkin R, Herrick A: Complex regional pain syndrome (reflex sympathetic dystrophy). In Hochberg M, Silman AJ, Smolen JS, et al: editors: Rheumatology, ed 5, Philadelphia, 2011, Mosby Elsevier.
Harden RN: Complex regional pain syndrome, Br J Anaesth 87:99–106, 2001.
Harden RN, Bruehl S, Stanton-Hicks M, et al: Proposed new diagnostic criteria for complex regional pain syndrome, Pain Med 6:326–331, 2007.
Hsu ES: Practical management of complex regional pain syndrome, Am J Ther 16:147–154, 2009.
Kachko L, Efrat R, Ben Ami S, et al: Complex regional pain syndromes in children and adolescents, Pediatr Int 50:523–527, 2008.
Kalita J, Vajpayee A, Misra UK: Comparison of prednisolone with piroxicam in complex regional pain syndrome following stroke: a randomized controlled trial, QJM 99:89, 2006.
Kemler MA, de Vet HC, Barendse GA, et al: Spinal cord stimulation for chronic reflex sympathetic dystrophy – five-year follow-up, N Engl J Med 354:2394, 2006.
Kozin F, McCarty DJ, Sims J, et al: The reflex sympathetic dystrophy syndrome: I. Clinical and histologic studies: evidence for bilaterality, response to corticosteroids and articular involvement, Am J Med 60:321–331, 1976a.
Kozin F, Genant HK, Bekerman C, et al: The reflex sympathetic dystrophy syndrome: II. Roentgenographic and scintigraphic evidence of bilaterality and of periarticular accentuation, Am J Med 60:332–338, 1976b.
Kozin F, Ryan LM, Carerra GF, et al: The reflex sympathetic dystrophy syndrome (RSDS): III. Scintigraphic studies, further evidence for the therapeutic efficacy of systemic corticosteroids, and proposed diagnostic criteria, Am J Med 70:23–30, 1981.
Maihöfner C, Handwerker HO, Neundörfer B, et al: Cortical reorganization during recovery from complex regional pain syndrome, Neurology 63:693, 2004.
Munnikes RJ, Muis C, Boersma M, et al: Intermediate stage complex regional pain syndrome type 1 is unrelated to proinflammatory cytokines, Mediators Inflamm 366:2005, 2005.
Schürmann M, Zaspel J, Löhr P, et al: Imaging in early posttraumatic complex regional pain syndrome: a comparison of diagnostic methods, Clin J Pain 23:449, 2007.
Schwartzman RJ, Alexander GM, Grothusen JR: The use of ketamine in complex regional pain syndrome: possible mechanisms, Expert Rev Neurother 11:719–734, 2011.
Schwartzman RJ, Erwin KL, Alexander GM: The natural history of complex regional pain syndrome, Clin J Pain 25:273–280, 2009.

Stanton-Hicks M: Complex regional pain syndrome: manifestations and the role of neurostimulation in its management, J Pain Symptom Manage 31:S20–S24, 2006.
Steinbrocker O: The shoulder-hand syndrome, Am J Med 3:402–407, 1947.
Zollinger PE, Tuinebreijer WE, Breederveld RS, et al: Can vitamin C prevent complex regional pain syndrome in patients with wrist fractures? A randomized, controlled, multicenter dose-response study, J Bone Joint Surg Am 89:1424, 2007.

FURTHER READING

www.rsds.org

XI
NEOPLASMS AND TUMORLIKE LESIONS

While there are several chronic diseases more destructive to life than cancer, none is more feared.

Charles H. Mayo (1865–1939), 1926

BENIGN AND MALIGNANT TUMORS OF JOINTS AND SYNOVIUM

Edmund H. Hornstein, DO

CHAPTER 66

> **TOP SECRETS**
> 1. The most common benign joint neoplasms are tenosynovial giant cell tumors and synovial chondromatosis. Both are best diagnosed by magnetic resonance imaging followed by biopsy.
> 2. The most common malignant tumor of the joint is synovial sarcoma.
> 3. A benign or malignant neoplasm of the joint should be considered in any patient with a nontraumatic hemarthrosis.

1. **Why should practicing physicians be concerned with tumors that affect the joints and synovium?**
   Benign and malignant neoplasms affecting articular and periarticular structures may mimic inflammatory arthritis. Awareness of these conditions is crucial to prevent diagnostic delay and to avoid the initiation of ineffective and/or inappropriate therapy. Fortunately, primary neoplasms of the joint are rare.

2. **A young adult presents with a solitary, painless mass adjacent to a finger joint that has been slowly enlarging. What tumor is suggested by this scenario?**
   This presentation would be typical for a **localized tenosynovial giant cell tumor (TGCT) of the tendon sheath**. This benign condition, which occurs with a slightly increased predilection for females, is second only to the ganglion as a source of localized swelling in the hand and wrist. It occurs less frequently (3% to 10%) in the ankle and foot. These nodular lesions usually occur in association with a tendon sheath (formerly called giant cell tumor of tendon sheath). Excision is curative and recurrences are rare.

3. **TGCT exists in three forms: diffuse, localized, and localized TGCT of tendon sheath. How do these forms differ?**
   - **TGCT of joints and tendon sheaths: diffuse type** (also called pigmented villonodular synovitis [PVNS])—the entire synovium of an affected joint or tendon sheath is involved. It affects individuals in their 30s and 40s with equal sex distribution. Grossly, the synovium is red-brown to mottled orange-yellow and prolific with coarse villi, finer fronds, and diffuse nodularity resembling an Angora rug. It is almost always monoarticular. The most common locations include the knee (80%), hip (15%), and ankle. Swelling and effusion accompanied by moderate discomfort, decreased range of motion, and increased warmth to palpation are typical. Pain is frequently less than anticipated from the degree of swelling.
   - **Localized TGCT of the joint** (also called benign giant cell synovioma or localized nodular synovitis)—involves only a portion of a synovial surface in a joint, and the lesion is often pedunculated. It presents with symptoms similar to a loose body. It tends not to be as darkly pigmented and has less villous proliferation than is seen in the diffuse form.
   - **Localized TGCT of the tendon sheath** (also called giant cell tumor of tendon sheath or fibroxanthoma of tendon sheath) has been discussed in Question 2 above. Histologically, all three forms of villonodular synovitis are remarkably similar.

   The etiology of TGCT is a result of a translocation between chromosomes 1p13 and 2q35 in which the gene coding for colony-stimulating factor-1 (CSF-1) is fused to the collagen VI alpha-3 gene. Up to 15% of cells in the TGCT over-express CSF-1. The remaining cells in the tumor are inflammatory cells recruited into the tumor because they contain the receptor for CSF-1.

4. **What does the synovial fluid analysis reveal in the diffuse type of TGCT (PVNS)?**
   Typically, the fluid is brown or grossly **hemorrhagic**. This finding on joint aspiration should raise diffuse TGCT (PVNS) as a diagnostic consideration. However, up to 50% of cases will not have a hemorrhagic synovial fluid. Additionally, similar hemorrhagic fluid can be seen in trauma, Charcot's joint, bleeding disorders, sickle cell disease, and Ehlers–Danlos syndrome.

5. **What are the characteristic radiographic findings in a patient with the diffuse type of TGCT (PVNS)?**
   Plain radiographs are usually nonspecific except for mild increased density of the soft tissue of the joint resulting from blood and hemosiderin deposits. The tumor may invade into bone causing cysts or scalloped erosive changes with sclerotic borders mimicking gout or tuberculosis. The magnetic resonance imaging (MRI)

appearance of PVNS is diagnostic in most cases. Nodules with sufficient hemosiderin appear dark on both T1-weighted and T2-weighted images.

6. **Describe the histologic characteristics of TGCT.**
Grossly, the synovium looks like a tan to red-brown "shaggy carpet." Microscopically, TGCT is distinctive. It is characterized by a dense cellular infiltrate composed of synovial cell hyperplasia with surface and subsynovial invasion of mitotically active cells with eosinophilic cytoplasm. Other invading cells are fibroblasts, lipid-laden macrophages (xanthoma cells), hemosiderin-containing macrophages, and scattered, frequent, multinucleated giant cells. Although TGCT is locally aggressive, it rarely metastasizes.

7. **How is TGCT treated?**
Surgical treatment with complete synovectomy is standard, either via open or arthroscopic approaches. Recurrences, particularly in diffuse type TGCT (PVNS), are not uncommon, occurring in 20% to 40% of cases. Intraarticular installation of radioisotopes or low-dose external beam radiation are used in refractory cases. Total joint arthroplasty may be necessary for cure.

8. **What is synovial chondromatosis and how does it present?**
Synovial chondromatosis is characterized by the development of multiple foci of cartilaginous metaplasia (? neoplasia) in the subsynovial compartment. These foci form nodules that may be invaded by blood vessels leading to endochondral ossification (termed osteochondromatosis). The chondral nodules are frequently released as free bodies (**joint mice**) into the joint space. It most commonly affects men in their 40s. It is almost always monoarticular affecting the knee (50%) more than hip, shoulder, ankle, elbow, or other joints. Clinically, there is an increasingly compromised range of motion with crepitus and often with unexpected locking. Effusion may occur.

9. **How is synovial chondromatosis diagnosed?**
The X-ray examination may be diagnostic if the chondroid bodies are calcified (33% of cases), resembling a calcified mulberry or popcorn (Figure 66-1). If plain X-ray is nondiagnostic, an MRI will show nodules of cartilage in the synovium, which are dark on T1-weighted images and bright (white) on T2-weighted images owing to water content in hyaline cartilage. Loose bodies can be seen. Arthroscopic biopsy is diagnostic if performed.

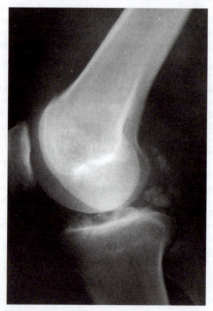

Figure 66-1. Synovial chondromatosis of the knee demonstrating multiple, calcified chondroid bodies.

10. **How is synovial chondromatosis managed?**
Treatment is via synovectomy. Recurrences occur in up to 11% of cases. Although considered benign, this condition can result in extensive local joint destruction if left untreated. Synovial chondromatosis never metastasizes but may undergo malignant transformation into a chondrosarcoma (5% of cases).

11. **What other benign tumor-like lesions can involve the joints?**
    - **Lipomas** may occur within the joint capsule or synovium, but true intraarticular lesions are rare.
    - **Lipoma arborescens** is a diffuse increase in subsynovial fat causing chronic effusions usually in the suprapatellar portion of the knee.

- **Chondroma** is an isolated mass of benign cartilage, usually in the knee.
- **Hemangiomas** are unusual intraarticular lesions that occur most frequently in the joints of children and young adults. The knee is the most common site. Recurrent hemarthrosis may occur. Diagnosis can be made by computed tomography, MRI, or angiography.
- **Osteoid osteomas**, when occurring within the joint, have less of the "classic" pattern of nocturnal pain relieved by nonsteroidal antiinflammatory drugs, and tend to involute spontaneously after 5 to 10 years.

12. **What is the most common primary malignant neoplasm involving the joints?**
    Synovial sarcoma. This tumor constitutes up to 10% of all soft tissue sarcomas. It is a highly malignant neoplasm and generally occurs in the lower extremities (70%) of young people. The tumor usually arises in the periarticular tissues of the knee or ankle. Only 10% of these malignancies arise directly within the joint itself.

13. **How does this tumor present clinically?**
    A slowly growing, often minimally symptomatic mass adjacent to the joint is the typical presentation. Pain is reported by approximately 50% of patients with this tumor. Soft tissue calcification on plain X-ray occurs in 30% to 50% of cases, and this finding serves to provide a clue as to the underlying diagnosis (Figure 66-2). MRI is the imaging procedure of choice because it defines the extent of the lesion.

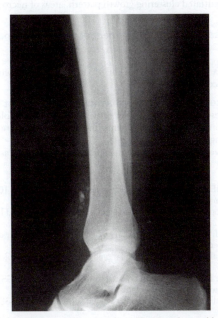

Figure 66-2. Synovial sarcoma adjacent to the ankle. Note the speckled calcifications.

14. **What is the cell of origin for synovial sarcoma?**
    The histology of this tumor may be **biphasic**, in which epithelial cells arranged in clusters, tubules, and acini are interspersed in a spindle cell stroma; or **monophasic**, in which either the epithelial or spindle cells predominate. Other morphologic types are recognized, however, including mixed and hemangiopericytic. Behavioral features include calcifying, ossifying, and poorly differentiated types. Although this tumor is called synovial sarcoma, ultrastructural and immunohistochemical studies have implicated an epithelial origin. SYT-SSX2 is the fusion product of translocation, which is found in the majority of these tumors and regulates cell adhesion. This fusion protein is identified for diagnosis of this sarcoma.

15. **How is synovial sarcoma treated? What is the prognosis?**
    Treatment is an aggressive combination of radical surgery, radiation therapy, and chemotherapy. Prognosis depends, in large part, on tumor size at the time of discovery, age of patient (<age 25 years do better), and whether or not the tumor is poorly differentiated. The cause of death in progressive disease is usually as a result of extensive pulmonary metastasis. Other common sites of metastasis include regional lymph nodes, bones, skin, and brain. A 5-year survival in synovial sarcoma is presented in Box 66-1.

Box 66-1. Five-Year Survival in Synovial Sarcoma

All tumors	50%
Tumor < 5 cm	86%
Tumor > 10 cm	22%

16. **Clear cell sarcoma is a rare highly malignant tumor of tendons, ligaments, and fascial aponeuroses. It usually presents as a slowly growing mass about the foot. What is its association with a malignancy more commonly thought of as a skin cancer?**
There are multiple lines of evidence suggesting, rather convincingly, that clear cell sarcoma is a representation of **malignant melanoma**. This evidence includes an immunohistochemical staining pattern with S-100 and HMB-45, which are considered specific for melanoma, evidence of melanin by special staining, and the presence of characteristic premelanosomes by electron microscopy. Prognosis is generally poor.

17. **Which primary malignant tumor of joints may be difficult to differentiate from the benign cartilaginous metaplasia of synovial chondromatosis?**
Occasionally arising from synovial chondromatosis, **synovial chondrosarcoma** is an exceedingly rare malignancy that may be histologically difficult to differentiate from its benign cousin. Favoring a diagnosis of sarcoma is the loss of a differentiated clustering growth pattern, areas of necrosis, and spindling of cells in the periphery.

18. **In which malignant diseases can joint involvement occur as a secondary feature?**
    - Metastatic carcinoma.
    - Lymphoma/myeloma.
    - Leukemic infiltration (12% to 65% of children and 4% to 13% of adults with leukemia).
    - Contiguous spread of adjacent bone sarcomas.

19. **What is the "classic" presentation of carcinoma metastatic to a joint?**
    - Advanced lung, gastrointestinal, or breast cancer is the most common etiology.
    - Involvement is usually monoarticular, with the knee the most common site.
    - Effusion is often hemorrhagic.
    - Synovial fluid cytology reveals the malignancy in approximately 50% of cases.

BIBLIOGRAPHY

Al-Hussaini H, Hogg D, Blackstein ME, et al: Clinical features, treatment, and outcome in 102 adult and pediatric patients with localized high-grade synovial sarcoma, Sarcoma 231789, 2011.

Cooper AJ, Reeves JD, Scully SP: Neoplasms of the joint. In Klippel JH, Stone JH, Crofford LeJ, et al (editors): Primer on the rheumatic diseases, ed 13, Atlanta, 2007, Springer.

Moller E, Mandahl N, Mertens F, et al: Molecular identification of COL6A3-CSF1 fusion transcripts in tenosynovial giant cell tumors, Genes Chromosomes Cancer 47:21, 2008.

Murphey MD, Rhee JH, Lewis RB, et al: Pigmented villonodular synovitis: radiologic-pathologic correlation, Radiographics 28:1493, 2008.

Rosenberg AE: Tumors and tumor-like lesions of joints and related structures. In Firestein GS, Budd RC, Gabriel SE, et al: editors Kelley's textbook of rheumatology, ed 9, Philadelphia, 2013, Elsevier Saunders.

Tyler WK, Vidal AF, Williams RJ, et al: Pigmented villonodular synovitis, JAAOS 14:376–385, 2006.

FURTHER READING

www.cancer.gov

CHAPTER 67

COMMON BONY LESIONS: RADIOGRAPHIC FEATURES

Brian D. Petersen, MD

1. **How should a bone lesion be characterized radiographically?**
   Bone lesions should not be defined radiographically as malignant or benign, but rather aggressive or nonaggressive. Some malignant lesions can have a nonaggressive appearance (myeloma typically has a well-circumscribed nonaggressive appearance) and many benign lesions (osteomyelitis, Langerhans cell histiocytosis of bone) can have a very aggressive appearance. There are a number of criteria that should be assessed when evaluating a bony lesion.
   - **Demographics:** lesions of bone have a specific propensity based on age and occasionally gender. It is imperative to know the age of the patient before giving a differential diagnosis.
   - **Location:** the location of the lesion within the skeleton is critical because specific lesions have a propensity to affect certain locations in the skeleton.
     - *Longitudinal location:* the location of the lesion as it relates to the diaphysis, metaphysis, or epiphysis of long bones should be defined. Special consideration should be given to flat bones (pelvis, ribs) and epiphyseal or metaphyseal equivalents (around apophyses or in flat bones that form by membranous ossification). Most common tumor sites:
       - *Epiphysis:* chondroblastoma, giant cell tumor (GCT), aneurysmal bone cyst (ABC). GCT and ABC usually arise from the metaphysis and extend into the epiphysis.
       - *Metaphysis:* osteochondroma, chondrosarcoma, nonossifying fibroma, enchondroma (long bones), osteosarcoma, chondromyxoid fibroma, ABC, GCT.
       - *Diaphysis:* enchondroma (phalanges), osteoid osteoma, osteoblastoma, Ewing's sarcoma, fibrous dysplasia.
     - *Axial location:* The location of the lesion should be defined as central intramedullary, eccentric intramedullary, cortically based, or surface (periosteal) centered.
   - **Zone of transition:** the transition zone between the lesion and the adjacent uninvolved bone should be classified as:
     - *Narrow:* well-defined margins that can be traced out with a pencil. This is a nonaggressive feature.
     - *Wide or ill-defined:* poorly defined margins, not easily traceable with a pencil. This is an aggressive feature.
   - **Pattern of bone destruction:** the pattern of bone replacement should be assessed and characterized as:
     - *Geographic:* well-defined lesion of bone. Geographic lesions have a narrow zone of transition by definition. This is a nonaggressive feature.
     - *Blastic or sclerotic:* densely sclerotic lesion of bone. Can be aggressive or nonaggressive.
     - *Permeative:* ill-defined bony destruction. This is an aggressive feature.
     - *Bubbly:* multilocular lucencies, with or without expansile appearance. This is usually a nonaggressive feature.
   - **Presence of matrix:** this is one of the most critical and difficult decisions in the radiographic assessment of a bone lesion. The confident presence of matrix can narrow the differential markedly. If present, matrix falls into one of following categories (Table 67-1):
     - *Clear or cystic* (Figure 67-1).
     - *Fibrous:* uniform intermediate density described as "ground glass" in appearance. Lesions producing fibrous matrix are usually (but not always) nonaggressive (Figure 67-2).
     - *Chondroid:* punctate matrix described as "rings and arcs" or "Cs and Js." Usually equal or greater density to cortical bone. Can be associated with either aggressive or nonaggressive lesions (Figure 67-3).
     - *Osteoid:* amorphous, fluffy, cloudy appearing matrix, usually less dense than cortical bone. Osteoid matrix can be immature and fluffy favoring an aggressive lesion or more mature, resembling bone, and favor a nonaggressive lesion (Figure 67-4).
   - **Periosteal reaction:** the response of the body to osseous insult is to produce callous and lay down new bone. The periosteum is a remarkable combination of tissues that has progenitor cells ready to differentiate into osteoblasts and chondroblasts. This allows the rapid formation of new bone producing the radiographically visible periosteal reaction. Pathologic processes that are aggressive and rapidly growing produce periosteal reaction indicative of ongoing attempts to wall off the expanding lesion. Periosteal reaction can be described in one of four typical patterns:
     - *Smooth:* favors a nonaggressive, slow growing, or reactive process allowing the formation of solid periosteal new bone (Figure 67-5).

498 XI NEOPLASMS AND TUMORLIKE LESIONS

Table 67-1. Types of Nonaggressive Primary Bone Tumors by Matrix Appearance

CLEAR	FIBROUS	CHONDROID	OSTEOID
Unicameral bone cyst	Fibroxanthoma	Enchondroma	Osteoma
Aneurysmal bone cyst	Fibrous dysplasia	Osteochondroma	Osteoid osteoma
Giant cell tumor		Chondroblastoma	Osteoblastoma
Eosinophilic granuloma		Chondromyxoid fibroma	

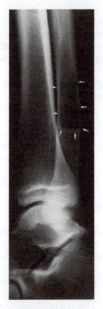

Figure 67-1.

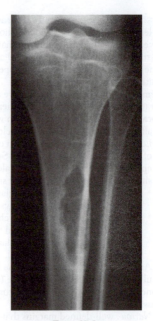

Figure 67-2.

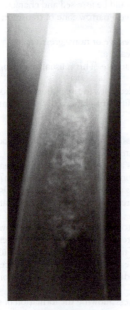

Figure 67-3.

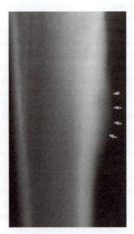

Figure 67-4.

- Lamellated (onion skin): layers of periosteal new bone laid down on one another. Indicative of an aggressive or fast growing lesion as the new periosteal layers are not allowed sufficient time to mature before another is laid down on top (Figure 67-6).
- Codman's triangle: a very aggressive appearance, indicative of osseous soft tissue mass expanding at such a rate that the adjacent margin of periosteal new bone is lifted up, forming a triangle with the underlying cortex (Figure 67-7).
- Sun burst: the most aggressive form of periosteal reaction is seen exclusively in very aggressive lesions. Has classically been described in osteosarcoma (Figure 67-8).

- **Presence or absence of a soft tissue mass/cortical breakthrough:** visible cortical breakthrough and/or soft tissue mass are hallmarks of an aggressive lesion of bone. One might logically think that a soft tissue mass is not possible without cortical breakthrough; however, there are several entities (lymphoma and Ewing's

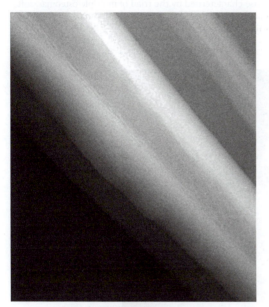

Figure 67-5.

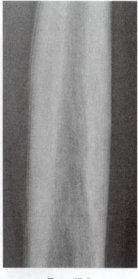

Figure 67-6.

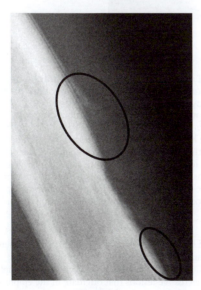

Figure 67-7.

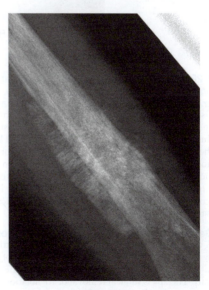

Figure 67-8.

sarcoma) that characteristically spread through cortical tunnels, resulting in an appearance of intact cortex with large surrounding soft tissue mass.
- **Polyostotic versus monostotic:** this alters the differential significantly. Although metastases are the most common malignant lesion of bone, they are uncommonly monostotic. Whole body bone scan, positron emission tomography-computed tomography (PET-CT) scan, or whole body magnetic resonance imaging (MRI) may help clarify this issue.

2. **A 30-year-old man presents with rectal bleeding and a well-circumscribed, geographic area of increased bone density seen on skull films in the left frontal sinus. What bone lesion is this?**
   Osteoma (Figure 67-9). These tumors usually arise from areas of membranous bone formation such as the paranasal sinuses, skull, and mandible. The lesions are smooth, rounded, and often <1 cm in size. Although they have no malignant potential, the tumors may become symptomatic according to their site of origin. *Gardner's syndrome* is an autosomal dominant disease characterized by the triad of multiple osteomas, soft tissue tumors, and colonic polyps. It is linked to mutations of the APC gene on chromosome 5, which is responsible for familial adenomatous polyposis which predisposes to colon cancer.

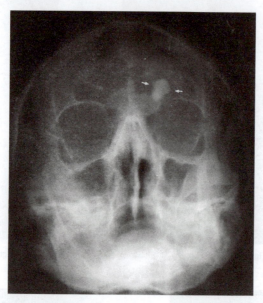

Figure 67-9.

3. **A 20-year-old man with leg pain, greater at night, and relieved with aspirin. Radiographs demonstrate a subtle cortically based lucency, with surrounding smooth periosteal reaction, on his anterior tibia. CT confirms the cortically based lucency. What might this lesion be?**
   Osteoid osteoma (Figure 67-10). The round, sharply delineated radiolucent center or nidus measuring <1.5 cm with a wide zone of uniform reactive sclerosis is characteristic of this lesion. Over 90% of patients with this lesion complain of nighttime pain relieved by aspirin. The area overlying the lesion is often tender to the touch. CT scan is the modality of choice for demonstrating the nidus when it is obscured by the perilesional reactive zone. Although surgical excision is curative, less invasive and equally successful, is CT-guided radiofrequency (RF) ablation of the lesion. Osteoid osteomas are classically cortically based and are commonly seen in the lower extremity (around the knee) and posterior elements of the spine. New onset, painful scoliosis in an age-appropriate patient is a clinical scenario occasionally encountered with spinal osteoid osteomas.

4. **Describe the characteristics of a chondroblastoma.**
   A **chondroblastoma** (Figure 67-11) is an eccentric, lobulated lesion with a smooth geographic contour defined by a thin, discrete, marginal sclerosis. It is one of the few primary bone lesions that arise in the epiphysis. Internal chondroid matrix can help to make the diagnosis, but matrix is occasionally not visible radiographically. Therapy is surgical removal or RF ablation. Other nonaggressive lesions that originate in the epiphysis or that cross the physis to involve the epiphysis include aneurysmal bone cysts and giant cell tumors.

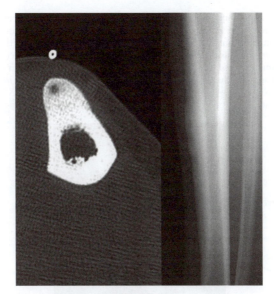

Figure 67-10.

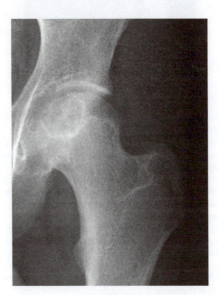

Figure 67-11.

5. A 31-year-old man with leg pain presented with an osseous tumor on the tibia, as seen in the radiograph (Figure 67-12). What bone lesion does this represent?

Osteochondroma (also known as *exostosis*) is the most common bone tumor and is more accurately described as a developmental lesion rather than a tumor. This osseous excrescence often arises from the metaphyseal region of a long tubular bone, such as the femur (70%) and tibia. This lesion can be pedunculated or sessile in morphology. Pedunculated osteochondromas typically grow to point away from the adjacent joint. An osteochondroma characteristically demonstrates marrow continuity with the underlying bone. Exostoses are rarely symptomatic in an adult and are usually an incidental finding radiographically.

All osteochondromas have a cartilage cap, although this is typically thin. This cartilage cap provides the source of malignant degeneration and can be accurately assessed by MRI. A cartilage cap of >2 cm is indicative of malignant transformation and should be surgically resected. Radiographically, an interval increase in chondroid matrix, or the dissipation of previously seen chondroid matrix can indicate malignant transformation.

Growth of a known osteochondroma after skeletal maturity is reached, pain or a palpable new soft tissue mass overlying an osteochondroma can indicate malignant transformation and should be investigated with MRI. Although pain may be an indication of malignant transformation, pain associated with overlying soft tissue irritation, development of overlying bursitis, fracture of the osteochondroma, or adjacent compression of neurovascular structures are more commonly the source. The incidence of malignant transformation to chondrosarcoma is rare ranging from 1% in solitary osteochondromas to 5% in cases of autosomal dominant *multiple hereditary exostoses*, which has been linked to mutations in three genes, *EXT1*, *EXT2*, and *EXT3*. The EXT protein is important in the synthesis of heparan sulfate. Axial or central lesions degenerate at a greater frequency than appendicular lesions.

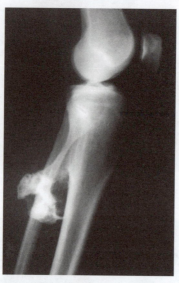

Figure 67-12.

6. **A 30-year-old woman has a painless soft tissue swelling of the finger as seen on the radiograph (Figure 67-13). What bone lesion is this?**
   Enchondroma. This well-circumscribed, geographic lucency arises eccentrically within the diaphysis of the proximal phalanx. The lobulated contour is characteristic of cartilaginous lesions, as are the punctate, sharply defined calcifications. Endosteal erosion and bulging of the cortex are common.
   Enchondromas are the most common, nonaggressive lesions of the hands. More than 50% of enchondromas occur in the diaphyses of the short, tubular bones of the hands and feet. The metaphysis is the site of origin when the long tubular bones are affected. Malignant transformation occurs in 1% of solitary enchondromas, usually arising in lesions of the long, tubular or flat bones and is not a valid concern in phalangeal enchondromas. *Enchondromatosis (Ollier's disease)* is a rare, nonhereditary disorder consisting of widespread involvement of predominantly one side of the body with multiple, asymmetrically distributed enchondromas. Often there is associated shortening and deformity of the long bones affected. Malignant transformation of an individual lesion in Ollier's disease is common, occurring in one third to one half of patients. *Maffucci's syndrome* is a rare, congenital disorder of mesodermal dysplasia characterized by enchondromatosis and soft tissue hemangiomas. Malignant transformation is common.

7. **A 16-year-old male with fall on outstretched hand. Incidental osseous finding in the distal radius demonstrates a cortically based bubbly, mildly expansile lesion of bone with narrow zone of transition and sclerotic margins located in the metaphysis of the radius (Figure 67-14). What bone lesion is this?**
   Nonossifying fibroma (NOF). NOF is commonly used interchangeably with *fibrous cortical defect* or *fibroxanthoma*. NOF is a common (30% to 40%) finding in children and adolescents. As the skeleton matures, these typically in-fill with bone and can occasionally remain radiographically visible. The characteristic nonaggressive appearance, cortical, and metaphyseal based location can all suggest the appropriate and reassuring diagnosis. Progressive in-filling of bone is the typical fate of NOF and this may produce radiographically confusing areas of focal metaphyseal sclerosis with the unfortunate descriptive name of an ossifying nonossifying fibroma.

8. **A 27-year-old woman with a previous history of precocious puberty presents with femur radiographs (Figure 67-15). What does this bone lesion represent?**
   Fibrous dysplasia (FD). These nonaggressive, ground glass density, long lesions of bone are classic for FD. As in this case, medullary expansion and deformities of bone, such as bowing or varus angulation at the

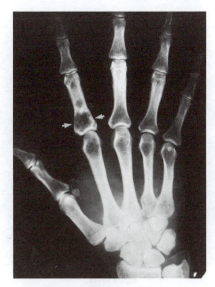

Figure 67-13.

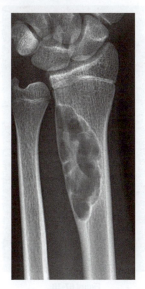

Figure 67-14.

hip (shepherd's crook deformity), are common. Histologically, FD represents a fibroosseous lesion. Normal bone is replaced by abnormal fibrous tissue within an abnormally arranged trabecular pattern. This has led to speculation that FD may be a growth or developmental aberration rather than a true neoplasm. Approximately 20% to 25% of patients with FD have multiple sites of involvement. The femur and tibia, skull and mandible, and ribs are commonly affected. *McCune–Albright syndrome* is identified by the triad of polyostotic, predominantly unilateral FD, café-au-lait macular lesions with irregular "coast of Maine" margins, and endocrine dysfunction, particularly precocious puberty, which is a result of a mutation of the gene, *GNAS1*, on chromosome 20, which is involved in G-protein signaling and prevents downregulation of cAMP signaling.

9. **A 12-year-old boy was injured during soccer practice and presented with arm pain. Radiographs demonstrate an expansile, radiolucent lesion of the mid-humeral diaphysis, with a narrow zone of transition, pathologic fracture, and linear density in the dependent portion (Figure 67-16, *arrow*). What bone lesion is this?**
Unicameral (simple) bone cyst (UBC). On the radiograph, there is a narrow zone of transition. A thin bony density in the dependent portion of the lesion represents a "fallen fragment" (Figure 67-16, *arrow*) secondary

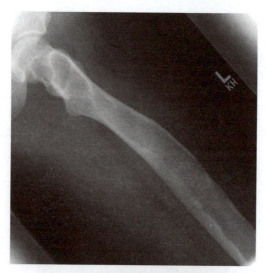

Figure 67-15.

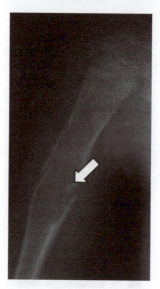

Figure 67-16.

to a pathologic fracture. Unicameral bone cysts generally occur in the long tubular bones, especially the proximal ends of the humerus and femur (up to 90%), and may represent a disturbance of growth at the physeal plate rather than a true neoplasm. These are asymptomatic lesions unless traumatized. Pathologic fracture of a UBC can lead to in-filling of the lesion with healing bone. Surgical intervention, either with surgical curettage and bone packing, steroid injection, or injection of cement or ablative material may be pursued to prevent a multiplicity of pathologic fractures and subsequent bone deformity and shortening. On radiographs, a favorable response is noted by a decrease in lesion size and an increase in radiodensity with adjacent cortical thickening.

10. **A 32-year-old man presents with a tender wrist. Radiographs show an expansile, lytic lesion that extends to the articular surface, involving both the epiphysis and metaphysis of the distal radius (Figure 67-17). The cortex is thinned. There is no visible calcified matrix. Any ideas?**
    GCT. GCTs may be differentiated from aneurysmal bone cysts because they tend to occur in the skeletally mature individual, after physeal closure, and, although they originate in the metaphysis of the bone, commonly extend to a subarticular location within the epiphysis. Soft tissue extension can be suggested on plain films, but CT or MRI is most helpful to map the extent of bone and soft tissue involvement before resection.

The vast majority of GCTs are histologically benign, with approximately 5% deemed malignant. Despite their benign histologic pattern, GCTs can be locally very aggressive and destructive. Wide resection is typically curative, but given the subarticular location of the GCT, joint sparing surgery is typically performed with local resection and curettage with bone graft or cementation. The recurrence rate after local excision is rather variable, ranging from 25% to 60%. GCT is one of the few tumors that can produce benign metastases.

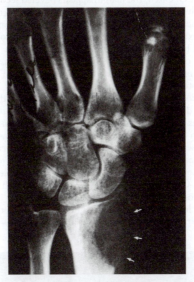

Figure 67-17.

11. **A 6-year-old boy presents with wrist pain. A radiograph shows ballooning of the cortical surface of the ulnar metaphysis (Figure 67-18). MRI shows fluid–fluid levels. What bone lesion does this represent?**
    Aneurysmal bone cyst (ABC). This osteolytic lesion with occasional trabeculation arises from the fibular metaphysis. The cortical surface is markedly expanded or ballooned. The loss of cortical definition and suggestion of extension into the soft tissues are alarming features of a rapidly expansile lesion. Although histologically benign, ABCs often simulate malignant tumors. They may be posttraumatic or reactive responses to preexisting bony lesions, possibly related to local alterations in hemodynamics (i.e., venous obstruction and arteriovenous fistulas). The blood-filled cavities of an ABC are exquisitely demonstrated by MRI, which delineates the fluid–fluid levels caused by the settling of red blood cells from the fluid blood. Approximately 60% to 70% of ABCs occur within the long tubular bones, usually originating from the metaphysis. These cysts also

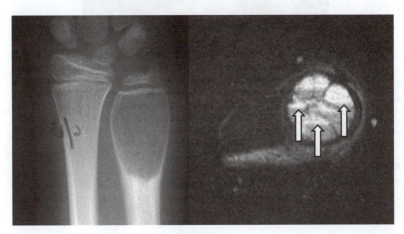

Figure 67-18.

have a predilection for the posterior elements of the vertebral bodies, where they can be difficult to distinguish from other nonaggressive lesions that occur in this location (e.g., osteoblastomas and GCTs).

12. **A 20-year-old man with head pain shows a single, lytic, "punched out" lesion on a skull film (Figure 67-19). What lesion is this?**

    Eosinophilic granuloma (EG). The exquisitely well-circumscribed, "punched out" lesion in the skull with a clear matrix is characteristic of EG. Often, the margin appears beveled secondary to involvement of both the inner and outer tables of the calvarium. In the mandible, the loss of supporting bone results in the appearance of "floating teeth." When the metaphysis or diaphysis of the long bones is affected, the lesion is associated with both endosteal scalloping and extensive, thick, laminated periosteal reaction. EG is also one of the causes of complete collapse of a vertebral body, a condition known as *vertebra plana*.

    Plain film remains the modality of choice for documentation of EG lesions, because 30% to 35% of lesions have no uptake of radionuclide on bone scan and up to 10% result in "cold" areas of abnormally decreased uptake. Lesions can be monostotic or polyostotic.

    Langerhans cell histiocytosis (Histiocytosis X) is a group of diseases caused by the clonal proliferation of Langerhans cells, which are epidermal dendritic cells. An activating mutation of the *BRAF* gene is commonly found. When it is unifocal and involves only bone without extraskeletal involvement it is called *eosinophilic granuloma*. When it is multifocal with both bone and visceral involvement, it has been called Letterer–Siwe disease or Hand–Christian–Schüller disease depending on the presentation. *Letterer–Siwe* disease is marked by rapid dissemination and a poor prognosis. It tends to appear in children under 2 to 3 years old, causing bone lesions, hepatosplenomegaly, and occasionally "honeycomb" interstitial lung disease. With chemotherapy the 5-year survival rate is only 50%. *Hand–Christian–Schüller* disease is associated with the chronic dissemination of osseous lesions, fever, and skin lesions usually in the scalp and ears. Peak onset is 3 to 10 years old. Up to 50% of cases involve the pituitary stalk leading to diabetes insipidus. The characteristic triad is bone lesions, diabetes insipidus, and exophthalmos. Ten percent to 30% of cases are fatal.

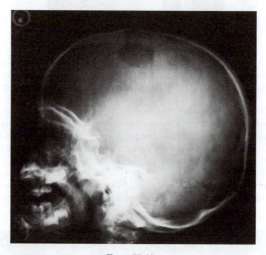

Figure 67-19.

Bibliography

Hudson TM: Radiologic-pathologic correlation of musculoskeletal lesions, Baltimore, 1987, Williams & Wilkins.
Miller T: Bone tumor and tumor-like conditions: analysis with conventional radiography, Radiology 246:662–674, 2008.
Resnick D: Diagnosis of bone and joint disorders, ed 4, Philadelphia, 2002, WB Saunders.
Resnick D, Kransdorf MJ: Bone and joint imaging, ed 3, Philadelphia, 2005, Elsevier Saunders.
Wilner D: Radiology of bone tumors and allied disorders, Philadelphia, 1981, WB Saunders.

Further Reading

www.bonetumor.org

XII
PEDIATRIC RHEUMATIC DISEASES

Parents learn a lot from their children about coping with life.

Muriel Spark
(1918–2006)
The Comforter

APPROACH TO THE CHILD WITH JOINT PAIN

CHAPTER 68

Esi Morgan DeWitt, MD, MSCE and Randy Q. Cron, MD, PhD

KEY POINTS

1. Growing pains do not occur during the daytime.
2. A limp in a child is pathologic until proven otherwise.
3. Malignancy is more likely than systemic juvenile idiopathic arthritis (JIA) in any child who has fever, a painful arthritis, an elevated lactate dehydrogenase (LDH), and/or a low platelet count.
4. Neck or back pain in a young child is never normal and demands an extensive workup.

1. **What is the differential diagnosis of joint pain in childhood?**
   There are at least 110 illnesses associated with arthritis or related musculoskeletal syndromes in childhood. The broad differential diagnosis can be remembered with the mnemonic **PRIME BONE PAIN**:
   P—Pharmacologic: serum sickness; drug-induced lupus
   R—Rheumatologic: juvenile idiopathic arthritis; systemic lupus erythematosus (SLE); Sjögren's syndrome; systemic sclerosis/mixed connective tissue disease (MCTD); vasculitis; dermatomyositis; sarcoidosis
   I—Infectious/postinfectious: bacterial (osteomyelitis, discitis, septic arthritis, rheumatic fever, reactive arthritis, Lyme disease); viral ("toxic/transient" synovitis, human immunodeficiency virus [HIV], hepatitis B [Hep B] or hepatitis C [Hep C], parvo, Epstein–Barr virus [EBV], Herpes, rubella vaccination)
   M—Metabolic/genetic: mucopolysaccharidoses; mucolipidoses; heritable collagen disorders (Marfan, etc.); pseudorheumatoid chondrodysplasia
   E—Episodic: autoinflammatory syndromes (FMF, HIDS, TRAPS, CAPS, BLAU, PAPA, DIRA). See Chapter 79.
   B—Blood/hematologic: sickle cell anemia; hemophilia
   O—Orthopedic: chondromalacia patellae; Osgood–Schlatter disease; osteochondritis dissecans; Legg–Calve–Perthes disease; slipped capital femoral epiphysis
   N—Neoplastic: neuroblastoma; leukemia/lymphoma; bone tumors (osteoid osteoma, osteochondroma, osteosarcoma, Ewing's sarcoma); pigmented villonodular synovitis; metastases
   E—Endocrine: hypercortisolism; hypothyroidism; rickets; diabetes mellitus
   P—Pain amplification syndromes/psychosomatic: complex regional pain syndrome (CRPS); fibromyalgia; conversion reactions
   A—Accidental/trauma
   I—Inflammatory: inflammatory bowel disease
   N—"Normal variants": "growing pains"; benign hypermobility

2. **What are the characteristics of an organic versus a nonorganic cause for joint pain?**

Organic	*Nonorganic*
Occurs day and night	Occurs only at night
Occurs during weekends and on vacation	Occurs primarily on school days
Severe enough to interrupt play and other pleasant activities	Child is able to carry out normal daily activities
Located in joint	Located between joints
Unilateral	Bilateral
Child limps or refuses to walk	Child has unusual/bizarre gait
Description fits with logical anatomic explanation	Description is illogical, often dramatically stated, and not consistent with known anatomic or physical process

3. **What are the historical clues of an organic versus a nonorganic cause for joint pain?**
   Organic: signs of systemic illness, including weight loss, fever, night sweats, rash, and diarrhea.
   Nonorganic: isolated pain in an otherwise healthy child; may have history of depression or anxiety; can occur in the setting of chronic disease, but with pain amplified above the usual disease process.

4. **List the physical signs that suggest an inflammatory cause for joint pain.**
   Point tenderness; redness; swelling; limitation of movement of affected extremity, secondary to pain or anatomic restriction; objective muscle weakness or atrophy; signs of systemic illness: fever, rash, lymphadenopathy, and organomegaly.

5. **Which laboratory tests are helpful in differentiating causes of joint pain?**

Test	Conditions in which test may be helpful
Complete blood count (CBC), differential, platelets	Leukemia (if blasts on smear)
Sedimentation rate	Infections in bones, joints, muscles Systemic connective tissue diseases Infections Systemic connective tissue diseases Inflammatory bowel disease Tumors
Radiographs	All bone tumors, malignant and benign Osteomyelitis (chronic) Discitis (late) Fractures Scoliosis Rickets Slipped capital femoral epiphysis Legg–Calvé–Perthes disease Leukemia
Bone scan	Osteomyelitis (acute and chronic) Discitis Osteoid osteoma Malignancies (leukemia, bone tumors, and metastases) Infarction of bone Complex regional pain syndrome
Muscle enzymes	Inflammatory muscle disease Muscular dystrophy Rhabdomyolysis

6. **How does the number of affected joints help in sorting through the differential diagnosis of arthritis?**
   Factors helpful in assessing the cause of arthritis are the duration of disease at the time the child is evaluated, the sex and age of the child, and the onset type and pattern of joint involvement. The differential diagnosis of polyarthritis is considerably different from that of monoarthritis or oligoarthritis. Juvenile idiopathic arthritis (JIA) is the most common cause of chronic monoarthritis, especially in girls younger than 5 years of age (Box 68-1).

7. **How does the diurnal variation in joint pain aid in diagnosis?**
   Stiffness and pain on range of motion (ROM) immediately upon rising in the morning (morning stiffness) and after periods of inactivity ("gelling") are classic findings for the inflammatory arthritides. Morning stiffness is relieved by heat and ROM exercises. The duration of morning stiffness is an excellent gauge of the severity of the arthritis and the efficacy of therapy. By contrast, mechanical joint pain worsens over the course of the day and with activity. Finally, night time pain and/or awakening with pain are red flags for neoplasia or, on a less serious level, for "growing pains."

8. **In which rheumatic conditions are the affected joints erythematous?**
   Septic arthritis, rheumatic fever, and neoplasia.
   Red joints are very rare in JIA and in most other rheumatic conditions, and they should be a "red flag" for the above diagnoses. The arthritis of rheumatic fever is also characterized by its migratory nature and by pain often out of proportion to the apparent severity of findings on joint examination (e.g., degree of swelling).

9. **In a child with a swollen joint, how is joint fluid helpful in determining the cause of joint pain? (Table 68-1)**

10. **How is leg length assessed in a child? Why is the affected leg often longer in a child with oligoarticular JIA?**
    Leg length is measured from the anterior superior iliac spine to the medial malleolus. In a child with a joint contracture, the functional leg length may be shorter than the actual leg length, and therefore both must be measured.

Box 68-1. Differential Diagnosis of Childhood Mono- and Polyarthritis

MONOARTHRITIS		POLYARTHRITIS
Acute monoarthritis Early rheumatic disease - Oligoarticular JIA - ERA Arthritis related to infection - Septic arthritis - Reactive arthritis - Lyme disease Malignancy - Leukemia - Neuroblastoma Hemophilia Traumatic Gout	**Chronic monoarthritis** JIA - ERA - Juvenile psoriatic arthritis - Oligoarticular Sarcoidosis Infection - Tuberculosis - Lyme disease Hemarthrosis - PVNS - Hemophilia - Hemangioma Noninflammatory - Synovial chondromatosis - Internal derangement - Lipomatosis arborescens - Lymphangioma	Polyarticular JIA (RF+, RF−) ERA Juvenile psoriatic arthritis SLE MCTD Sjögren's syndrome Polyarthritis related to infection - Rheumatic fever - Reactive arthritis - Lyme disease (rarely) Mucopolysaccharidoses Pseudorheumatoid chondrodysplasia Sarcoidosis

Adapted from Cassidy JT et al: Textbook of pediatric rheumatology, ed 6, Philadelphia, 2011, WB Saunders.
ERA, Enthesitis-related arthritis; JIA, juvenile idiopathic arthritis; MCTD, mixed connective tissue disease; PVNS, pigmented villonodular synovitis; RF, rheumatoid factor; SLE, systemic lupus erythematosus.

Table 68-1. Utility of synovial fluid count in the differential diagnosis of childhood arthritis

GROUP/CONDITION*	WBC COUNT (/ML)	PMN (%)	MISCELLANEOUS FINDINGS
Noninflammatory			
Normal	<200	<25	—
Traumatic arthritis	<2000	<25	Debris
Osteoarthritis	1000	<25	—
Inflammatory			
SLE	5000	10	LE cells
Rheumatic fever	5000	10-50	—
JIA	15,000-20,000	75	—
Reactive arthritis	20,000	80	Reiter cells
Pyogenic			
Tuberculous arthritis	25,000	50-60	Acid-fast bacteria
Septic arthritis	50,000-300,000	>75	Low glucose, bacteria

Adapted from Cassidy JT et al: Textbook of pediatric rheumatology, ed 6, Philadelphia, 2011, WB Saunders.
JIA, Juvenile idiopathic arthritis; PMN, polymorphonuclear leukocyte; SLE, systemic lupus erythematosus; WBC, white blood cell.
*Note that crystal-induced synovitis is rare in childhood apart from genetic (familial hyperuricemia, FMF), neoplastic (leukemia), enzymatic (Lesch–Nyan), and nephropathy. Note that these are guidelines and some inflammatory arthritides like JIA can have a synovial fluid WBC count >100,000/mL (pseudoseptic).

Leg-length discrepancy reflects a chronic disease process. The affected leg is often longer in a child with chronic arthritis (in particular, that affecting the knee) as a result of increased blood flow to the joint in response to localized inflammation and cytokine release. This increased blood flow may also lead to development of "macroepiphysis." A leg-length discrepancy may result in an abnormal gait, and correction with a lift on the bottom of the shoe of the shorter leg is recommended. The shorter, unaffected leg will usually "catch up" to the affected leg and may overgrow the affected leg because the epiphysis of the inflamed joint will undergo accelerated fusion. In addition, muscle bulk of the thigh or the calf may be reduced in the affected leg, and will rarely "catch up" to that of the unaffected leg, particularly if the arthritis has an onset at <6 years of age.

11. **What are "red flags" for neoplasia as the cause of joint pain?**
    - Joint redness
    - Fever, weight loss, night sweats

- Night time pain
- Adenopathy
- Associated bone pain (i.e., pain between joints and on direct palpation) out of proportion to physical findings

Malignancy must be considered in any child in whom a diagnosis of systemic JIA is entertained because the classic features of systemic JIA (i.e., fever, rash, and arthritis) are also seen in malignancy. Malignant infiltration of bone or synovium may mimic polyarthritis. In addition, joint effusions occur in children with malignancy, possibly owing to antigen–antibody complex deposition producing a serum sickness-like picture. This may also be responsible for the tremendous inflammatory response (high erythrocyte sedimentation rate [ESR] and anemia) seen in some children with malignancy, again mimicking systemic JIA.

Acute leukemia causing polyarthritis should be suspected in children with an elevated ESR but low platelet counts. Other frequent laboratory abnormalities are an elevated LDH (more than two times the upper limit of normal), elevated uric acid, and abnormal peripheral blood smear. Notably, the white blood cell (WBC) count and differential may initially be normal. Blasts on blood smear may be a later finding.

Radiographs of affected joints and/or whole body bone scans may be helpful in diagnosis. Bone marrow examination is recommended before initiation of high-dose corticosteroid therapy for systemic JIA in which the diagnosis is not clear, because inappropriate use of corticosteroids in malignancy can worsen the prognosis.

12. **What neoplasms are most likely to result in musculoskeletal complaints upon presentation in childhood?**
    - Acute leukemia (especially acute lymphoblastic leukemia [ALL])—consider in any child with "painful" JIA.
    - Neuroblastoma—70% of cases occur in children, with 85% of patients less than 5 years old. Many have systemic symptoms.
    - Ewing's sarcoma—monoarticular pain.
    - Lymphoma.

13. **Describe the characteristics of the childhood "pain amplification" syndromes: growing pains, primary fibromyalgia, and CRPS. (Table 68-2)**

Table 68-2. Characteristics of childhood musculoskeletal amplification syndromes

	GROWING PAINS	FIBROMYALGIA	CRPS
Age at onset	4-12 yr	Adolescence	Late childhood and adolescence
Sex ratio	Equal	Female >> male	Female >> male
Symptoms	Deep aching, cramping pain in thigh or calf Usually in evening or during the night; never present in morning Bilateral Responds to massage and analgesia	Fatigue Anxiety, depression Disturbed, sleep patterns Headaches Abdominal pain Dizziness, paresthesias Widespread MSK pain (>3 mo)	Exquisite superficial and deep pain in the distal part of an extremity Exacerbated by passive or active movement
Signs	Physical exam normal	Tender points at characteristic sites	Diffuse swelling, tenderness, coolness and mottling Bizarre posturing of affected part
Investigations	Laboratory exam normal	Laboratory exam normal	Osteoporosis, bone scan abnormalities Laboratory exam normal

Adapted from Cassidy JT et al: Textbook of pediatric rheumatology, ed 6, Philadelphia, 2011, WB Saunders.
CRPS, Complex regional pain syndrome; MSK, musculoskeletal.

14. **How does CRPS in childhood differ from adult CRPS?**
    - Less likely to have trauma as a precipitating cause compared to adults
    - Leg is most often involved, skin temperature is cooler, and fewer neurologic symptoms
    - Psychologic issues more common
    - Frequently does not progress through three stages (see Chapter 69)
    - Children have better outcomes and response to physical/occupational therapy

15. **Describe the characteristics of the common nonrheumatic pain syndromes in childhood: patellofemoral pain syndrome (chondromalacia) and Osgood–Schlatter disease. (Table 68-3)**

Table 68-3.

	CHONDROMALACIA	OSGOOD–SCHLATTER
Age at onset	Adolescence to young adulthood	Athletic adolescents
Sex ratio	Female > male	Male > female
Symptoms	Insidious onset of exertional knee pain, pain with knee flexion Difficulty going up and down stairs; need to sit with legs straight	Pain over tibial tubercle exacerbated by exercise
Signs	Patellar tenderness on compression Quadriceps weakness Inhibition sign Joint effusion	Tenderness and swelling over attachment of patellar tendon
Investigations	—	Radiograph shows soft tissue swelling, enlarged and sometimes fragmented tubercle

Adapted from Cassidy JT et al: Textbook of pediatric rheumatology, ed 6, Philadelphia, 2011, WB Saunders.

16. **What are the causes of hip pain in childhood?**
    - Transient synovitis, malignancy—local, benign (e.g., osteoid osteoma), malignant (e.g., Ewing's sarcoma), generalized, leukemia, neuroblastoma
    - Septic arthritis
    - Avascular necrosis (Legg–Calvé–Perthes disease)
    - Slipped capital femoral epiphysis (SCFE)
    - Protrusio acetabuli
    - Osteomyelitis (femur, pelvis)
    - JIA (including enthesitis-related arthritis [ERA]/spondyloarthropathy)
    - Rheumatic fever

    PEARL: Arthritis of the hip joint is **rare** at the onset of oligoarticular JIA. The onset of apparent arthritis in the hip in a young child should be considered first to be a septic process. The presence of (1) fever (≥38.5° C); (2) WBC count > 12,000/μL; (3) ESR ≥ 40 mm/h; (4) CRP ≥ 20 mg/L; (5) inability to bear weight predicts septic arthritis is more likely than transient synovitis of the hip. Without these systemic symptoms, congenital dislocation should be considered. Transient synovitis of the hip may cause very severe pain, but the process is self-limiting, lasting one to a few weeks, and all laboratory and radiologic studies are normal. In the older child and adolescent, avascular necrosis (Legg–Calvé–Perthes disease) and SCFE should be considered. In older boys, ERA/juvenile spondyloarthropathy (JAS) may present with unilateral or bilateral hip involvement, although distal joints are affected more commonly than proximal joints. Be aware that hip pain may be referred to the knee.

17. **What causes back pain in childhood?**
    Back and neck pain are relatively rare complaints in young children (unlike the situation in adolescents and adults) and should be taken very seriously. Although infection of an intervertebral disc space is rare secondary to osteomyelitis of an adjoining vertebral body, acute discitis should be considered. Discitis is an inflammatory process that occurs throughout childhood, with a peak at age 1 to 3 years and most cases occur before the age of 8 years. It may be caused by pathogens of low virulence (e.g., viruses, *Staphylococcus aureus*, Enterobacteriaceae, or *Moraxella*), although bacteria or viruses are seldom recovered by aspiration. Fever, refusal to walk, unusual posturing, stiffness, and point tenderness over the lumbar region are characteristic. The ESR is usually moderately elevated. Plain radiographs may show disc-space narrowing, although often not until late in the disease. Earlier in the course, magnetic resonance imaging (MRI) or technetium-99m (Tc-99m) bone scan are abnormal and valuable diagnostically at the time of presentation.
    In addition, malignancy (e.g., metastases, primary bone tumors, or leukemia) should be considered, as well as ERA/JAS. However, JAS generally presents as peripheral arthritis (75% of children at presentation), with back complaints (pain, stiffness, or limitation of motion of the lumbosacral spine or sacroiliac joints) only reported by 25% of affected children before the third decade. Back pain is uncommon in JIA before adolescence. Spondylolysis, with or without spondylolisthesis, may cause chronic back pain. Scheuermann's disease or, rarely, herniation of an intervertebral disc results in pain in the lower thoracic or lumbar region.

18. **List the nonsteroidal antiinflammatory drugs (NSAIDs) that are used to treat arthritis in childhood. (Table 68-4)**

Table 68-4.

MEDICATION*	DAILY DOSE (MG/KG/DAY)
Salicylate	<25 kg: 80-100 divided three times a day >25 kg: 2.5 gm/m²/day divided three times a day (max 4000 mg/day)
Choline magnesium trisalicylate	50-65 divided twice a day (max 4500 mg/day)
Ibuprofen	30-50 divided twice a day (max 3200 mg/day)
Naproxen (>2 yrs old)	10-20 divided twice a day (max 1 g/day)
Indomethacin	0.5-3 divided three times a day (max 150 mg/day); SR divided twice a day
Tolmetin (>2 yrs old)	15-30 divided three times a day (max 1800 mg/day)
Meloxicam (>2 yrs old)	0.125-0.25 daily (max 15 mg/day)
Etodolac SR (>6 yrs old)	20-30 daily (max 1200 mg/day); 400 mg daily (wt 20-30 kg); 600 mg daily (31-45 kg); 800 mg daily (46-60 kg)
Oxaprozin (>6 yrs old)	10-20 daily (max 1200 mg/day); 600 mg daily (wt 22-31 kg); 900 mg daily (wt 32-54 kg); 1200 mg daily (wt ≥ 55 kg)
Celecoxib (>2 yrs old)	6-7 divided twice a day (max 400 mg/day); 50 mg twice a day (wt 10-25 kg); 100 mg twice a day (wt > 25 kg)
Piroxicam	0.25-0.45 daily (max 20 mg/day); 5-10 mg daily (wt < 25 kg); 5-20 mg daily (wt ≥ 25 kg)
Sulindac	4-6 divided twice a day (max 400 mg/day)
Nabumetone	20-30 divided twice a day (max 2000 mg/day)
Diclofenac	1-3 divided twice a day (max 150 mg/day)

FDA, Food and Drug Administration; JIA, juvenile idiopathic arthritis; NSAID, nonsteroidal antiinflammatory drug; SR, sustained release.

*The last four on the list (piroxicam, sulindac, nabumetone, and diclofenac) are not FDA-approved and have little safety data for use in children. Owing to the concern of possible Reye syndrome, salicylate is less often used, especially during the influenza season and varicella outbreaks. NSAIDs are also available in liquid form (naproxen, ibuprofen, meloxicam, and indomethacin), which are easier to administer to children < age 5 years old. Naproxen, tolmetin meloxicam, and celecoxib are FDA-approved for JIA patients over the age of 2 years; ibuprofen is FDA-approved for JIA patients over 12 years old; indomethacin is FDA-approved for JIA patients over 14 years old.

19. **A child presents with a 1-week history of a single, hot, red, swollen, painful joint. The child is febrile and refuses to bear weight on the affected leg. Describe the work-up.**

    Immediate joint aspiration is always indicated in such a patient to exclude septic arthritis or osteomyelitis. Gram stain should be performed; WBC and differential counts, glucose, and protein levels should be determined; and the synovial fluid should be cultured for *Haemophilus influenzae*, *Neisseria gonorrhoeae*, and other aerobic organisms. Special media and conditions are required if anaerobic organisms or mycobacteria are suspected. Cultures of blood and suspected sources of infection (e.g., cellulitis, otitis) are required in a child with suspected septic arthritis. Although an organism can be identified in approximately two thirds of children, no causative organism is identified in approximately one third, with the diagnosis being made on the basis of a consistent history and the presence of pus on arthrocentesis. However, synovial fluid WBC counts may be low (<25,000/mm³) in up to one third of patients with septic arthritis. Conversely, WBC counts in noninfectious chronic inflammatory arthritis can exceed 50,000/mm³. Identification of an organism is particularly difficult in those patients who have received antibiotics. Supportive laboratory studies are an elevated WBC count with a predominance of polymorphonuclear leukocytes (PMNs) and bands, and a markedly elevated ESR or C-reactive protein.

20. **A child has an 8-week history of a single warm, swollen joint that is not very painful, tender, or red. The child has been afebrile and, with the exception of a mild upper respiratory infection, has been otherwise well. Describe the work-up.**

    Whereas any history of antecedent trauma should be elicited, trauma is very unlikely to cause a swollen joint persisting 8 weeks in the absence of significant pain. Interestingly, parents often link joint swelling to an acute event (such as a fall), although the event may serve only to bring their attention to an already swollen joint. The 8-week history of swelling meets the criteria of >6 weeks required for a diagnosis of JIA (see Chapter 73).

The first episode of JIA, and subsequent flares of arthritis, are often precipitated by intercurrent illness such as an upper respiratory infection.

The most useful finding on physical exam in this case would be the presence of a second (or more) affected joint(s), because this would argue strongly for a diagnosis of a chronic (JIA) and noninfectious arthritis. In particular, the small joints of the hands and feet should be examined carefully. If the knee is involved, a Baker's cyst would strongly indicate a diagnosis of JIA. Involvement of the wrists by JIA would be suggested if the child holds the hands still in the lap, supinated, with the wrists slightly flexed. Lack of neck movement, using only the eyes to follow the examiner, is a clue for neck involvement. Circumduction of the affected leg on gait examination may suggest a leg-length discrepancy, indicating a longer duration of arthritis than 8 weeks. Similarly, the presence of joint contractures would suggest a longer duration of arthritis.

In oligoarticular JIA, the CBC and ESR are often entirely normal. Tests for Lyme disease in endemic areas should be negative. Radiographs, other than confirming the presence of effusion, also are normal, without evidence of loss of joint space or bony erosion. This form of JIA does not generally lead to joint destruction, and even in the more destructive forms (e.g., a subgroup of polyarticular JIA), bony erosion is rarely seen until after 2 years of disease. The antinuclear antibody (ANA) test is the most helpful laboratory test in suspected oligoarticular JIA. One half of children with this diagnosis have a positive ANA, and one half of children with a positive ANA have chronic anterior uveitis, a potentially blinding (yet almost invariably asymptomatic) inflammation of the eyes. Children with JIA only rarely have a positive rheumatoid factor.

Acknowledgement

The authors and editor thank Terri H. Finkel, MD, PhD, for her contribution to this chapter in previous editions.

BIBLIOGRAPHY

Berent P, Salvatore A, Alberto M: Juvenile idiopathic arthritis, Lancet 377:2138–2149, 2011.
Beukelman T, Patkar NM, Saag KG, et al: 2011 American College of Rheumatology recommendations for the treatment of juvenile idiopathic arthritis: initiation and safety monitoring of therapeutic agents for the treatment of arthritis and systemic features, Arthritis Care Res 63:465–482, 2011.
Cabral DA, Tucker LB: Malignancies in children who initially present with rheumatic complaints, J Pediatr 134:53–57, 1999.
Cassidy JT, Laxer RM, Petty RE, Lindsley CB: Textbook of pediatric rheumatology, ed 6, Philadelphia, 2011, WB Saunders.
Clinch J, Eccleston C: Chronic musculoskeletal pain in children: assessment and management, Rheumatology 48:466–474, 2009.
Evans AM: Growing pains: contemporary knowledge and recommended practice, J Foot Ankle Res, 2008. http://dx.doi.org/10.1186/1757-1146-1-4.
Fernandez M, Carrol CL, Baker CJ: Discitis and vertebral osteomyelitis in children: an 18-year review, Pediatrics 105:1299, 2000.
Houghton KM: Review for the generalist: evaluation of anterior knee pain, Pediatr Rheumatol Online J, 2007. http://dx.doi.org/10.1186/1546-0096-5-8.
Junnila JL, Cartwright VW: Chronic musculoskeletal pain in children. Part I. Initial evaluation, AFP 74:115–122, 2006.
Junnila JL, Cartwright VW: Chronic musculoskeletal pain in children. Part II. Rheumatic causes, AFP 74:293–300, 2006.
King S, Chambers CT, Huguet A, et al: The epidemiology of chronic pain in children and adolescents revisited: a systematic review, Pain 152:2729–2738, 2011.
Sherry DD, Malleson PN: The idiopathic musculoskeletal syndromes in childhood, Rheum Dis Clin North Am 28:669–685, 2002.
Sultan J, Hughes PJ: Septic arthritis or transient synovitis of the hip in children: the value of clinical prediction algorithms, J Bone Joint Surg Br 92:1289–1293, 2010.
Trapani S, Grisolia F, Simonini G, et al: Incidence of occult cancer in children presenting with musculoskeletal symptoms: a 10-year survey in a pediatric rheumatology unit, Semin Arthritis Rheum 29:348, 2000.

FURTHER READING

http://www.arthritis.org/conditions-treatments/disease-center/juvenile-arthritis/
https://www.carragroup.org
http://www.printo.it/pediatric-rheumatology/
http://www.ped-rheum.com
http://www.childhoodrnd.org/

CHAPTER 69

JUVENILE IDIOPATHIC ARTHRITIS

J. Roger Hollister, MD

KEY POINTS

1. Juvenile idiopathic arthritis (JIA) consists of several subgroups with different clinical characteristics, pathogenesis, and responses to therapy.
2. Systemic JIA symptoms include quotidian fever, rash, and arthritis, which responds best to interleukin (IL)-1 and IL-6 inhibition.
3. Oligoarticular JIA is characterized by young age of onset, female predominance, positive antinuclear antibody (ANA), and chronic anterior uveitis.
4. Polyarticular JIA with a positive rheumatoid factor (RF) resembles adult seropositive rheumatoid arthritis (RA).
5. ANA positivity, female sex, and age less than 6 years old increase the risk of chronic uveitis regardless of the JIA subgroup.
6. Enthesitis-related arthritis (ERA) is characterized by lower extremity enthesitis, male sex, human leukocyte antigen-B27 (HLA-B27), acute anterior uveitis, and sometimes the later development of sacroiliitis.

---

1. **Based on the International League of Associations for Rheumatology (ILAR) classification, what are the main types of JIA? What percentage of JIA does each comprise?**
   JIA is an arthritis of unknown cause, beginning before age 16 years, and lasting for at least 6 weeks. It affects 1 in 1000 children. The subgroups are:
   - Systemic JIA (10% to 15% of all JIA)
   - Oligoarthritis (30% to 60%)
   - Polyarthritis, RF positive (5% to 10%)
   - Polyarthritis, RF negative (10% to 30%)
   - Psoriatic arthritis (2% to 15%)
   - Enthesitis-related arthritis (ERA)/juvenile spondyloarthropathy (JAS) (20%)
   - Undifferentiated arthritis

2. **In the differential diagnosis of arthritis in childhood, what is the significance of a migratory versus summating pattern of onset?**
   A **migratory pattern**—i.e., one joint is subsiding as another becomes inflamed—is seen in rheumatic fever, poststreptococcal arthritis, and gonococcal arthritis. A **summating (additive) pattern**—i.e., adding one inflamed joint to another—is characteristic of JIA.

3. **Which rashes are specific to causes of juvenile arthritis?**
   The rash of **erythema marginatum** is pathognomonic of acute rheumatic fever, a condition that has diminished in frequency over the past several decades for unknown reasons. This circinate rash with central clearing appears at the time of the migratory arthritis, heart murmur, and subcutaneous nodules. It is one of the five major criteria for diagnosis of rheumatic fever.
   The **ecchymotic, lower-extremity rash** characteristic of Henoch–Schönlein purpura may start as a maculopapular or even urticarial lesion. The rash usually precedes joint swelling but may follow it by a few days. It leaves no residue and rarely needs treatment.
   The **"Still's" rash** of systemic JIA is present in 90% of cases. The pink macules are evanescent, migratory, salmon pink, and sometimes urticarial. The face is spared and rash is most common on the trunk and proximal extremities. It is rarely pruritic. The rash may be elicited by the Koebner phenomenon (scratching the skin) or by warming the skin (hot shower, heating blanket). The rash is frequently present during fever spikes (80%). If the lesions are present for 24 hours at a single location, they are not the lesions of Still's rash (Figure 69-1).

4. **What are the demographic and clinical characteristics of systemic JIA (sJIA)?**
   Systemic JIA is also called Still's disease, named after the English pediatrician, Sir George Frederic Still (1861–1941), who first described the disease.
   - Peak age of onset: 2 to 5 years
   - Sex ratio: equal

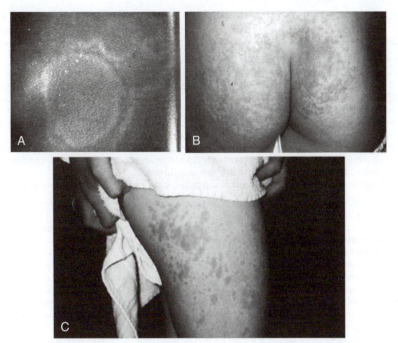

Figure 69-1. A, Erythema marginatum. B, Henoch–Schönlein purpura. C, Systemic juvenile idiopathic arthritis (JIA).

- More frequent in Asian countries (India)
- Arthritis of one or more joints: can be minimal synovitis to severe polyarticular disease
- Fever for at least 2 weeks that is documented to occur daily for at least 3 days (see Question 5)
- One or more of the following:
  - Evanescent rash (see Question 3)
  - Generalized lymph node enlargement
  - Hepatomegaly and/or splenomegaly
  - Serositis (pleural/pericardial 10%)
  - Sore throat is common

5. **Two fever patterns are represented below that may aid in the diagnosis of a fever of unknown origin (FUO). Which is characteristic of systemic JIA?**
The fever pattern of systemic JIA is characterized by fever spikes (frequently to 39° C) occurring once (quotidian) or twice (double quotidian) a day. The fever usually occurs at the same time each day, with spontaneous defervescence to normal or **subnormal** levels. During the fever, the child is irritable but often feels normal between fevers. By contrast, the fever spikes of bacterial sepsis are hectic and occur on an elevated temperature base. Normal temperatures and the child feeling better do not occur until adequate antibacterial treatment is initiated (Figure 69-2).

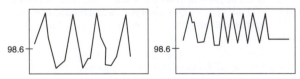

Figure 69-2. The fever pattern of systemic juvenile idiopathic arthritis (JIA) (left) compared to bacterial sepsis (right).

6. **In the diagnosis of FUO, what laboratory tests are specific for systemic JIA (Still's disease)?**
None. The laboratory tests demonstrate a chronic inflammatory process, and a normal erythrocyte sedimentation rate (ESR) excludes the diagnosis of systemic JIA. The leukocyte count is often elevated to extraordinary, even leukemoid levels, with a significant left shift (bandemia). Platelet counts are often equally elevated, and thrombocytopenia is inconsistent with the diagnosis. A mild/moderate anemia of chronic disease is often present. Other acute-phase reactants, such as ferritin (>1000 μg/L) and C-reactive protein (CRP) are frequently

increased. Liver enzymes and aldolase can be elevated. Notably the aldolase is coming from the liver and not muscle. Creatine phosphokinase (CPK) is normal. ANA and RF are negative. In perplexing cases, a normal lactate dehydrogenase (LDH) level can add reassurance that a malignancy is not the cause of the FUO.

7. **What is the differential diagnosis for systemic JIA?**
   - Infection: any infection.
     - Infections causing double quotidian fevers: kala-azar, right-sided gonococcal/meningococcal endocarditis, miliary tuberculosis (TB), mixed malaria.
   - Kawasaki's syndrome.
   - Malignancy: leukemia and neuroblastoma.
     - LDH is elevated usually to high levels (more than twice the upper limit of normal).
     - White blood cell (WBC) count and differential is usually abnormal in leukemia but not always.
     - Urinary catecholamines [vanillylmandelic acid (VMA), homovanillic acid {HVA}] are elevated in neuroblastoma.
   - Other childhood rheumatic diseases: systemic lupus erythematosus (SLE).
   - Autoinflammatory diseases: the fever pattern and rashes are persistent and differ from sJIA.

8. **What is the most feared life-threatening complication seen in systemic JIA?**
   Macrophage activation syndrome (MAS). MAS occurs in up to 10% of sJIA patients. The most common manifestations are persistently high fevers, hepatosplenomegaly, lymphadenopathy, severe cytopenias, liver dysfunction, hypertriglyceridemia, central nervous system (CNS) symptoms including seizures and coma, coagulopathy (elevated prothrombin time [PT] and partial thromboplastin time [PTT] as a result of low fibrinogen), and purpura. MAS should be considered in any sJIA patient who develops a precipitous decrease in ESR (resulting from low fibrinogen), decrease in leukocyte and platelet counts, liver dysfunction, and hypertriglyceridemia. Ferritin level is usually greater than 3000-10,000 ng/mL and fibrin degradation products are increased. Soluble IL-2 receptor alpha (sCD25) is elevated and correlates closely with disease activity. Biopsies show macrophages (CD163+) exhibiting hemophagocytosis in the bone marrow, lymph node, or liver. The cause or trigger of MAS is unknown. Sometimes an infection, particularly Epstein–Barr virus (EBV) or cytomegalovirus (CMV) virus, can be a trigger for MAS. Treatment of patients with impending MAS includes pulse methylprednisolone coupled with IL-1ra (anakinra) or IL-6R inhibition (tocilizumab) therapy. If MAS continues, treatment with cyclosporine (especially if triggered by a virus), etoposide (VP-16), or another immunosuppressive agent is tried. Recent studies show that MAS is associated with diminished natural killer (NK) (CD56+) cell function and low perforin expression caused by mutations in the perforin gene.

9. **What is the current therapy for systemic JIA? What is the prognosis?**
   IL-1, IL-6, and IL-18 appear to have a key role in the pathogenesis of sJIA. Therefore, inhibitors of these cytokines are highly effective therapies. Antitumor necrosis factor (TNF) agents appear to be less effective. Therapy of systemic JIA should be tailored to severity of presentation:
   - Severe systemic symptoms, impending MAS, or pleuropericardial effusions: pulse intravenous (IV) methylprednisolone followed by prednisone 2 mg/kg/day split dose plus anakinra (2 mg/kg [max 100 mg] subcutaneous [SQ] daily), canakinumab (4 mg/kg every 4 weeks), or tocilizumab (12 mg/kg IV every 2 weeks if <30 kg; 8 mg/kg IV every 2 weeks if >30 kg). A clinical trial of rilonacept is in progress.
   - Moderate systemic symptoms with/without synovitis: nonsteroidal antiinflammatory drugs (NSAIDs) and prednisone, 1 mg/kg/day split dose, plus anakinra or tocilizumab. If synovitis predominates, add methotrexate and intraarticular steroids.
   - Synovitis with mild systemic symptoms: NSAIDs and methotrexate. Failure to respond in 2 months, add anakinra, tocilizumab, or anti-TNF agent.
   - Resistant systemic disease: intravenous immunoglobulin (IVIG), cyclosporine, abatacept, and stem cell transplant have been used with success.

   Systemic JIA patients can have a monocyclic (lasts 2 to 4 years), relapsing, or chronic progressive course. Growth retardation and steroid side effects such as osteoporosis and cataracts are frequent (less likely to occur if prednisone doses can be tapered to ≤5 mg/day). Chronic uveitis is rare. Amyloidosis and rarely pulmonary hypertension can occur.

10. **What are the demographics and clinical characteristics of oligoarticular JIA?**
    Oligoarticular JIA is defined as the involvement of one to four joints during the first 6 months of disease. It usually presents as an asymmetric large joint arthritis with the knee most commonly involved. It is the most common subcategory of JIA in North America/Europe. Notably, this disease is unique to pediatric patients because there is no adult equivalent.
    - Peak age of onset in whites: 2 to 4 years
    - Sex ratio: female > male 3:1
    - Genetic associations: HLA-DRB1*0801, DRB1*1103/04, and DRB1*1301 (ANA positive)
    - Two subgroups of arthritis defined after 6 months:
      - Persistent: never more than one to four joints involved. Knee > ankle, wrist. Joint may be swollen but does not have much inflammation. Child may not complain of pain and only present with a limp (25%). If the hand is involved, the patient is more likely to develop psoriatic arthritis. The hip and back are not involved; any child complaining of pain in these areas needs an extensive workup to rule out other causes.

- Extended: more than four joints involved after the first 6 months of disease. This develops in 30% to 50% of patients especially in those with symmetric joint involvement and an elevated ESR at onset.
- Laboratory abnormalities: ANA is positive in 75% to 85% of cases. It is low titer, ≤1:320. More commonly positive in young girls. RF is negative, WBC count is normal, and acute phase reactants are only mildly elevated. Any fever, iron deficiency anemia, or significantly elevated ESR/CRP should suggest septic arthritis, inflammatory bowel disease arthritis, or malignancy.
- **Chronic nongranulomatous anterior uveitis**: occurs in 17% to 26% of patients overall. Most common in ANA-positive girls (30%) less than age 6 years. Most likely to occur in the first 4 years of disease. Uveitis usually starts in one eye, and then goes to the other. Uveitis can precede arthritis in 5% of cases. Because uveitis is **asymptomatic** and can lead to blindness, patients need a baseline eye exam and frequent follow-up screens based on ANA status, age of onset, and disease duration.

11. **What types of anterior uveitis are associated with JIA? (Table 69-1)**

Table 69-1. Anterior Uveitis in Juvenile Idiopathic Arthritis

	ACUTE UVEITIS	CHRONIC UVEITIS
Disease association	Spondyloarthropathy	Oligoarticular JIA
Lab markers	HLA-B27 antigen	Positive ANA
Symptoms	Hot, red, photophobic eye	None
Complications (if untreated)	Few	Synechiae, cataract, glaucoma, band keratopathy
Necessity of slit-lamp screening	No	Yes

ANA, Antinuclear antibody; HLA-B27, human leukocyte antigen-B27; JIA, juvenile idiopathic arthritis.

12. **How frequent and how long should slit-lamp screening be continued in patients with JIA?**
Half of the children who will develop chronic uveitis will have it present at the first eye appointment. Uveitis incidence diminishes with each subsequent year after joint swelling develops. By 5 to 7 years after joint swelling develops, the risk of new-onset uveitis is quite low. However, slit-lamp screening is necessary within the first 5 to 7 years, even when the joint disease is in remission. The following are guidelines:
- **High risk group:** ANA-positive children (especially girls) with oligoarticular or polyarticular disease with age at disease onset <7 years old should have a baseline eye exam and then a repeat eye exam every 3 months until they have had their disease for 4 (some say 7) years total. They should then have an eye exam every 6 months for an additional 3 years. After that, they should have annual exams.
- **Moderate risk group:** ANA-positive children with oligoarticular or polyarticular disease with age at disease onset ≥7 years old and ANA-negative children with age at disease onset <7 years old should have a baseline eye exam and then a repeat eye exam every 6 months for 4 years. After that, they should have annual exams.
- **Low risk group:** ANA-negative children with oligoarticular or polyarticular disease with age at disease onset ≥7 years old **or** who have had their disease over 7 years should get annual eye exams. Systemic onset JIA should get annual eye exams regardless of age at disease onset or duration (Table 69-2).

Table 69-2. The Frequency and Recommended Length of Time for Slit-Lamp Screening in Patients With JIA

JIA CATEGORY	<7 YR AT DISEASE ONSET	≥7 YR AT DISEASE ONSET
ANA+ poly or oligo	Every 3 mo for 4-7 yr, then every 6 mo for 3 yr, then yearly	Every 6 mo for 4 yr, then yearly
ANA– poly or oligo	Every 6 mo for 4 yr, then yearly	Yearly
Systemic JIA	Yearly	Yearly

ANA, Antinuclear antibody; JIA, juvenile idiopathic arthritis; oligo, oligoarticular; poly, polyarticular.

13. **A patient presents with poorly localized leg pain sufficient to interrupt sleep and cause a limp. Which malignancies must be considered in the differential diagnosis?**
Leukemia and stage IV **neuroblastoma** are the two neoplasms that can involve bone and simulate arthritis, even to the point of producing joint swelling, elevated sedimentation rate, and increased platelet counts. If an isolated LDH level is elevated while other liver functions tests are normal, additional tests such as bone scans, ultrasound, or bone marrow biopsy may be warranted to rule out malignancy.

14. **What is the treatment and prognosis for oligoarticular JIA?**
Patients with persistent oligoarticular JIA are treated with NSAIDs and intraarticular steroids. **Triamcinolone hexacetonide (Aristospan)** is most efficacious at a dose of 1 mg/kg up to 40 mg. EMLA cream can be used as a topical anesthetic. Methotrexate is added for patients who continue with arthritis. A TNF inhibitor or abatacept is added in the case of methotrexate failure.

Remission off medication occurs in 68% of patients in the persistent oligoarticular subgroup and only 31% of children in the extended oligoarticular subgroup. However, up to 50% to 67% of patients will have a relapse within 2 years of stopping therapy. Chronic sequellae include leg length discrepancy, joint contractures, and blindness.

15. Compare RF-negative to RF-positive polyarthritis. (Table 69-3)

Table 69-3. Comparison Between RF-Negative and RF-Positive Polyarticular JIA

	RF NEGATIVE	RF POSITIVE
Peak age of onset (yr)	1-4; 10-12	>12
Sex ratio, female:male	3:1	6:1 to 12:1
HLA associations	DRB*0801, *1401	DRB*0401
Serologies	ANA (40%), ACPA (50% to 80%)	ANA (55%), ACPA (57% to 73%)
EAMs	Chronic anterior uveitis (4% to 25%)	RA nodules (10%), uveitis (0% to 2%)

ACPA, Anticitrullinated protein antibodies; ANA, antinuclear antibody; EAMs, extraarticular manifestations; HLA, human leukocyte antigen; RA, rheumatoid arthritis; RF, rheumatoid factor.

16. What are the differences in arthritic manifestations between RF-negative polyarthritis compared to extended oligoarthritis or RF-positive polyarthritis? How does it compare to adult RA?
RF-negative polyarthritis can be subdivided into:
- ANA-positive subgroup in girls <age 6 years that resembles oligoarthritis except for the fact that the number of joints involved in the first 6 months is more than four. These patients have an asymmetric onset of arthritis and a higher risk of developing chronic uveitis, similar to that seen in extended oligoarthritis patients.
- ANA-negative subgroup in children older than 7 to 9 years that has a symmetric polyarthritis similar but not as severe as RF-positive polyarthritis JIA. Children in this subgroup of RF-negative polyarthritis as well as children with RF-positive polyarthritis have an arthritis that is similar to adult RA with both large and small joint involvement. However, they tend to have more hip, shoulder, C-spine, and distal interphalangeal (DIP) joint involvement. The classic radiographic changes are fusion of the carpal bones, micrognathia, and fusion of the C-spine apophyseal joints.

17. List the treatments used in the polyarticular subgroup of JIA.
Patients are initially treated with NSAIDs and intraarticular steroids. Methotrexate or another synthetic disease-modifying antirheumatic drug (DMARD) and later biologics are added as necessary to control the arthritis. The following are typical doses for patients over 2 years of age:
- Methotrexate: start at 5 to 7.5 mg/week. Increase to maximum oral or SQ dose of 0.6 mg/kg/week (equivalent to 15 mg/m²/week), not to exceed 25 mg/week. Children require and tolerate higher doses than adults owing to differences in metabolism.
- Sulfasalazine: 50 mg/kg/day (max 2 g) orally. Divide dose to twice a day.
- Hydroxychloroquine: 6 mg/kg/day. Based on ideal body weight.
- Leflunomide: <40 kg (10 mg daily, orally); >40 kg (20 mg daily, orally).
- Etanercept: 0.8 mg/kg/week SQ weekly (max 50 mg).
- Adalimumab: <30 kg (20 mg SQ every 2 weeks); >30 kg (40 mg SQ every 2 weeks).
- Abatacept: (≥6 years): 10 mg/kg (max 1000 mg) IV at 0, 2, 4 weeks, then every 4 weeks.
- Tocilizumab: <30 kg (10 mg/kg IV every 4 weeks); >30 kg (8 mg/kg IV every 4 weeks).
- Rituximab: 750 mg/m² (max 1000 mg) IV at 0 and 2 weeks.

18. What are the demographic and clinical characteristics of juvenile psoriatic arthritis?
- Peak age of onset: bimodal 2 to 4 years and 7 to 10 years.
- Sex ratio: equal.
- Psoriatic skin lesions are frequently **not** present at arthritis onset but usually occur within 2 years.
- Arthritis can be oligoarticular (60% to 70%) or polyarticular. May be difficult to separate from other subgroups of JIA if psoriatic skin lesions are not present. The presence of dactylitis (15% to 37%) and a family history of psoriasis are important clues that the child has psoriatic arthritis.
- Children (especially girls) <4 to 6 years of age with juvenile psoriatic arthritis are more likely to be ANA positive (15% to 20%) and are at risk for developing subacute anterior uveitis that can cause blindness similar to the oligoarticular JIA subgroup.
- Juvenile psoriatic arthritis is more likely to progress than the oligoarticular JIA subgroup.
- Treatment similar to oligoarticular and polyarticular JIA subgroups depending on presentation and severity.

19. What are the demographic and clinical manifestations of the ERA subgroup of JIA?
The ERA subgroup includes: juvenile ankylosing spondylitis (JAS); spondylitis, enthesitis, arthritis (SEA) syndrome; reactive arthritis; and arthritis associated with inflammatory bowel disease.

- Peak age of onset: >6 years.
- Sex ratio: male > female 7:1.
- Genetics: HLA-B27 positive in 80% to 90% depending on ethnicity.
- The hallmark of the ERA subgroup is the presence of **enthesitis** (inflammation of tendon/ligament insertion sites into bone). The most common sites are patella tendon, Achilles' tendon, plantar fascia insertions into calcaneous and metatarsal heads, greater trochanter, and tibial tuberosity (may mimic Osgood-Schlatter disease).
- Classic arthritis is subtalar synovitis with inflammation of surrounding tendon sheaths.
- Spinal symptoms are rare at onset but a subset (about 30%) will develop sacroiliitis and spondylitis during adolescence. Modified Schober's test is abnormal if the change is <6 cm and thoracic excursion <5 cm in adolescents. Risk factors for progression to the adult form of AS are age of onset >8 years old, HLA-B27 positive, and early-onset hip disease.
- Extraarticular manifestations:
  - Uveitis: **acute** anterior uveitis in 6% to 27% of patients (see Question 11).
  - Aortitis: rare but aortic insufficiency can occur.
- Laboratory: ESR elevated; ANA and RF negative.
- Treatment: NSAIDs and intraarticular steroids. Severe disease treated with methotrexate, sulfasalazine, and anti-TNF agents. Most patients require therapy because spontaneous remission rates are less than 50%.
- Reactive arthritis and inflammatory bowel disease-associated arthritis can occur and resembles their adult counterparts. Because children may have few abdominal symptoms, any child with iron-deficiency anemia and arthritis should have inflammatory bowel disease ruled out.

20. **In a child with JIA, what is the risk that a sibling will develop the same illness?**

    In several published series, there is a remarkable agreement that the risk is 1 in 100. The prevalence of the disease in the normal population is 1 in 1000. Therefore, there may be a genetic predisposition, although it clearly is not as strong as that for diseases such as hemophilia, cystic fibrosis, or diabetes. These facts suggest that an unidentified environmental agent may also be necessary for disease expression.

21. **School-aged children with JIA have legal rights to therapeutic resources in school. What are they?**

    Under P.L. 94-142 (the Education for All Handicapped Act), children with arthritis are entitled to a free, public education that may require "special related services." These services may include physical and occupational therapy through the school system. This requirement depends on the financial status of the individual school district. However, if the school system provides such services for developmentally disabled children or those with cerebral palsy, they must provide them to children with arthritis.

BIBLIOGRAPHY

Albers HM, Brinkman DMC, Kamphuis SSM, et al: Clinical course and prognostic value of disease activity in the first two years in different subtypes of juvenile idiopathic arthritis, Arthritis Care Res 62:204-212, 2010.

Beukelman T, Patkar N, Saag K, et al: 2010 American College of Rheumatology recommendations for the treatment of juvenile idiopathic arthritis: initiation and safety monitoring of therapeutic agents for the treatment of arthritis and systemic features, Arthritis Care Res 62:1515-1526, 2010.

Flato B, Lien G, Smerdel-Ramoya A, et al: Juvenile psoriatic arthritis longterm outcome and differentiation from other subtypes of juvenile idiopathic arthritis, J Rheumatol 36:642-650, 2009.

Grom AA, Mellins ED: Macrophage activation syndrome: advances towards understanding pathogenesis, Curr Opin Rheumatol 22:561-566, 2010.

Jones OY, Spencer CH, Bowyer SL, et al: A multicenter case-control study on predictive factors distinguishing childhood leukemia from juvenile rheumatoid arthritis, Pediatrics 117:840-844, 2006.

Kelly A, Ramanan AV: Recognition and management of macrophage activation syndrome in juvenile arthritis, Curr Opin Rheumatol 19:477-481, 2007.

Kemper AR, Van Mater HA, Coeytaux RR, et al: Systemic review of disease-modifying antirheumatic drugs for juvenile idiopathic arthritis, BMC Pediatrics 12:29, 2012.

Macaubas C, Nguyen K, Milojevic D, et al: Oligoarticular and polyarticular JIA: epidemiology and pathogenesis, Nat Rev Rheumatol 5:616-626, 2009.

Nigrovic PA, Mannion M, Prince FHM, et al: Anakinra as first-line disease modifying therapy in systemic juvenile idiopathic arthritis, Arthritis Rheum 63:545-555, 2011.

Oen K, Duffy CM, Tse SML, et al: Early outcomes and improvement of patients with juvenile idiopathic arthritis enrolled in a Canadian multicenter inception cohort, Arthritis Care Res 62:527-536, 2010.

Petty RE, Southwood TR, Manners P, et al: International League of Associations for Rheumatology classification of juvenile idiopathic arthritis: second revision, Edmonton, 2001, J Rheumatol 31:390-392, 2004.

Ravelli A, Martini A: Juvenile idiopathic arthritis, Lancet 369:767-778, 2007.

Saurenmann RK, Levin AV, Feldman BM, et al: Risk factors for development of uveitis differ between girls and boys with juvenile idiopathic arthritis, Arthritis Rheum 62:1824-1828, 2010.

Tse SML, Burgos-Vargas R, Laxer RM: Anti-tumor necrosis factor alpha blockade in the treatment of juvenile spondylarthropathy, Arthritis Rheum 52:2103-2108, 2005.

Woo P, Colbert RA: An overview of genetics of paediatric rheumatic diseases, Best Pract Res Clin Rheumatol 23:589-597, 2009.

Yokota S, Imagawa T, Mori M, et al: Efficacy and safety of tocilizumab in patients with systemic-onset juvenile idiopathic arthritis: a randomized, double-blind, placebo-controlled, withdrawal phase III trial, Lancet 371:998-1006, 2008.

CHAPTER 70: JUVENILE SYSTEMIC CONNECTIVE TISSUE DISEASES

Esi Morgan DeWitt, MD, MSCE and Randy Q. Cron, MD, PhD

KEY POINTS

1. Childhood-onset systemic lupus erythematosus (SLE) is more severe, has more nephritis, and has a worse prognosis compared to adult-onset SLE.
2. Inflammatory myositis in childhood is almost always dermatomyositis and not polymyositis.
3. Henoch–Schönlein purpura is an immunoglobulin A (IgA)-mediated process and the most common small-vessel vasculitis in childhood.
4. Localized scleroderma is the predominant childhood form of scleroderma and may respond to early aggressive immunosuppressive therapy.

1. **What are the juvenile systemic connective tissue diseases?**
   SLE; juvenile dermatomyositis (JDM); overlap syndromes, including mixed connective tissue disease (MCTD); systemic sclerosis (SSc, scleroderma); vasculitis; juvenile Sjögren's syndrome.

2. **Discuss the epidemiology of pediatric SLE.**
   SLE is the most common CTD of childhood. The proportion of all patients with SLE showing symptoms of SLE before the age of 18 years is 20%. In childhood, the disease generally occurs after age 10 years (60%) and rarely before the age of 5 years (5%). The ratio of girls to boys is about 2:1 before age 10 years and then, in adolescents, is similar to the ratio of adult women to men (5:1 to 10:1). SLE appears to be more common in nonwhite children. About 10% have one or more affected relatives, including siblings and twins.

3. **What are the criteria for the diagnosis of SLE in children?**
   The same as in adults (Chapter 16). A child is considered to have SLE if any four or more of the 11 criteria are present (96% sensitivity, 96% specificity). Childhood-onset SLE is generally more severe than in adults, with a higher incidence of nephritis, fever, hepatosplenomegaly, and lymphadenopathy at presentation, and a higher prevalence of malar rash and chorea (associated with antiphospholipid antibodies) over time. Childhood-onset SLE has an increased mortality risk (hazard ratio [HR 3.1]) compared with adult SLE.

4. **What are the clinical manifestations of SLE? How commonly do they occur?**
   SLE is characterized by multiple autoantibodies and multisystem involvement. An easy way to remember the complex array of systemic manifestations of SLE is to think from head to toe (Table 70-1).
   PEARL: A child with SLE who develops psychosis while on prednisone is much more likely to have neuropsychiatric lupus than steroid psychosis, which is very rare in childhood. Avascular necrosis as a result of steroid usage rarely occurs in children less than age 14 years.

5. **How does the antinuclear antibody pattern and titer aid in the diagnosis and management of SLE?**
   Antinuclear antibodies (ANAs) are present in the sera of almost all children with active SLE. In fact, the absence of ANAs, particularly at the time of symptomatic disease, essentially eliminates SLE as a diagnostic consideration. The average ANA titer in individuals with SLE is 1:320, although in active disease it may be considerably higher. Changes in the ANA titer are not a useful indicator of disease activity and are not followed subsequent to diagnosis. By contrast, the anti-double-stranded DNA (anti-dsDNA) antibody titer, which is found in >80% of patients, often correlates with disease activity.
   The "rim" pattern on the ANA, in which fluorescence is seen rimming the nuclear membrane, is pathognomonic of SLE, although rarely seen. The "homogeneous" pattern, in which fluorescence is seen uniformly over the nucleus, is the pattern most commonly seen in SLE, while the "speckled" pattern is the least specific. The ANA is a highly subjective test, and the pattern and titer vary greatly among laboratories. Low titer false-positives are not uncommon (5% to 30% of the healthy population). False negatives are rare, but if you are convinced of the diagnosis of SLE in a patient, the ANA should be repeated in a different laboratory and/or at a future date.

Table 70-1. Systemic Manifestations of Systemic Lupus Erythematosus

General (90%)	Malaise, weight loss, fever
Skin (55-70%)	Butterfly rash, discoid lupus, vasculitic skin lesions, alopecia, photosensitivity
Brain (25%)	Headache, blurred vision, psychosis, chorea, seizures, neuropathies, cerebrovascular accident, transverse myelitis
Eye	Cotton-wool spots, retinitis, episcleritis, iritis (rarely)
Mouth (20-50%)	Oral ulcers
Chest (15-20%)	Pleuritis, basilar pneumonitis, pulmonary hemorrhage, shrinking lung syndrome
Heart (15-20%)	Pericarditis, myocarditis, Libman–Sacks endocarditis
Digestive system	Hepatosplenomegaly, mesenteric arteritis, colitis, hepatitis
Kidneys (>50%)	Glomerulonephritis, nephrotic syndrome, hypertension
Extremities (60-80%)	Arthralgia or arthritis, myalgia or myositis, Raynaud phenomenon, thrombophlebitis, aseptic necrosis (6-10% of patients, often associated with corticosteroids)

Table 70-2. ANA Subtypes in Juvenile Systemic Connective Tissue Disease

	ACTIVE SLE	MCTD	SSc	CREST	PRIMARY SJÖGREN'S	JIA (POLY)
ANA	99%	100%	70-90%	60-90%	>70%	40-50%
Anti-native DNA	80%	Neg	Neg	Neg	Neg	Neg
Anti-Sm	30%	Neg	Neg	Neg	Neg	Neg
Anti-RNP	30%	>95% titer >1:10,000	Common (low titer)	Neg (low titer)	Rare	Rare
Anti-centromere	Rare	Rare	10-15%	60-90%	Neg	Neg
Anti-Ro (SS-A)	30%	Rare	Rare	Neg	70%	Rare
Anti-La (SS-B)	15%	Rare	Rare	Neg	60%	Rare

ANA, Antinuclear antibody; Anti-RNP, anti-ribonucleoprotein; Anti-Sm, anti-Smith antibody; CREST, calcinosis, Raynaud phenomenon, esophageal dysmotility, sclerodactyly, telangiectasias; JIA, juvenile idiopathic arthritis; MCTD, mixed connective tissue disease; SLE, systemic lupus erythematosus; SSc, systemic sclerosis (scleroderma).

6. **How does the ANA profile aid in the diagnosis and management of SLE and related juvenile systemic CTDs?**
   As detailed in Table 70-2, although a negative ANA profile does not rule out any of the juvenile systemic CTDs, a positive ANA profile can be extremely useful in making a specific diagnosis. In particular, anti-dsDNA and anti-Smith (anti-Sm) antibodies are specific for SLE; high titers of anti-ribonucleoprotein (anti-RNP) antibody are suggestive of MCTD; and anti-Ro (SS-A) and/or anti-La (SS-B) antibodies are found in Sjögren's syndrome, although this syndrome and antibodies against Ro (SS-A) are most commonly seen as a part of SLE. In addition, antihistone antibodies may be seen in SLE and in drug-induced lupus. These two diagnoses may be distinguished by the presence of antibodies to specific histones. Finally, a positive ANA is essentially never found in systemic juvenile idiopathic arthritis (JIA, Still disease).

7. **Which other autoantibodies (other than ANA and ANA profile) can be helpful in the diagnosis of systemic juvenile CTD?**
   Antibodies reactive with Scl-70 are not typically measured in the standard ANA profile but are found in 15% to 20% of individuals with SSc. Myositis-associated and myositis-specific antibodies are found in only a small minority of children with JDM. If present, their clinical associations are the same as adults, such as anti-Jo-1 identifying those children at increased risk for developing interstitial lung disease. Vasculitic syndromes associated with the presence of antineutrophil cytoplasmic antibodies (C-ANCA or P-ANCA) are granulomatosis polyangiitis (GPA, Wegener), microscopic polyangiitis (MPA), Churg–Strauss syndrome, and crescentic glomerulonephritis. Rheumatoid factor (RF) is frequently positive in Sjögren's syndrome as well as MCTD.

8. **Describe the management of children with SLE.**
    - General
        - Counseling, education
        - Adequate rest
        - Use of sunscreens
        - Immunizations, especially pneumococcal
        - Management of infection
    - Nonsteroidal antiinflammatory drugs (NSAIDs) for musculoskeletal signs and symptoms (caution if renal disease is present)
    - Hydroxychloroquine (5 to 6 mg/kg/day) for cutaneous disease and as adjunct to glucocorticoids for systemic disease
    - Glucocorticoids
        - Oral prednisone, 1 to 2 mg/kg/day divided twice daily
        - Intravenous (IV) methylprednisolone initially for severe disease
    - Immunosuppressives
        - Azathioprine, 1 to 2 mg/kg/day divided twice daily
        - Cyclophosphamide: oral 1 to 2 mg/kg/day; IV 500 to 1000 mg/m^2/month or Euro-Lupus protocol (500 mg/m^2 every 2 weeks × six doses)
        - Mycophenolate mofetil, 1200 mg/m^2/day divided twice daily (max 1000 mg twice a day)
        - Cyclosporine, 6 mg/kg/day divided twice daily
    - Anti-B cell therapy: off label use of rituximab, belimumab
    - Plasmapharesis: indicated for thrombotic thrombocytopenic purpura (TTP), catastrophic antiphospholipid syndrome (CAPS), transverse myelitis (antineuromyelitis optica, anti-NMO)
    - Intravenous immunoglobulin (IVIG): used for CAPS, macrophage activation syndrome (MAS), immune hemolytic anemia/thrombocytopenia

9. **Discuss the pathophysiology of neonatal lupus.**
    Neonatal lupus is associated with the transplacental passage of maternal anti-Ro/SS-A and anti-La/SS-B IgG antibodies. It occurs in 25% to 30% of infants whose mothers have one or both of these antibodies regardless of their underlying disease. The most frequent abnormalities are rash (lesions of discoid lupus or subacute cutaneous lupus), hepatic dysfunction, and thrombocytopenia, which are more often associated with anti-La/SS-B antibodies. Congenital heart block (CHB) is of most concern and is associated with anti-Ro/SS-A antibodies. The cutaneous and hematologic manifestations are transient, generally resolving within 2 to 6 months after delivery, whereas heart block is frequently permanent and may require a pacemaker. The overall risk of CHB is 2% to 5% but is increased to 20% in an anti-Ro/SS-A positive mother who had a previous child with CHB. Mothers with these antibodies are screened with serial biweekly echocardiograms/obstetric ultrasounds starting at 16 weeks' gestation. Development of first-degree heart block or a pericardial effusion in the fetus is treated with fluorinated steroids that cross the placenta (dexamethasone, betamethasone). Once third-degree heart block has developed, it cannot be reversed with medications and the infant will require a pacemaker. Fetal mortality is 20% in those that develop CHB and a cardiomyopathy (fetal hydrops) in utero.

10. **What is the differential diagnosis of Sjögren syndrome in childhood?**
    Sjögren's syndrome is characterized by dry eyes (keratoconjunctivitis sicca), dry mouth and carious teeth, and parotitis. Differentiating children with **benign recurrent parotid swelling, mumps, lymphoma, sarcoidosis, tuberculosis**, or **acquired immunodeficiency syndrome (AIDS)** from children with Sjögren's syndrome is important. As in adults, salivary gland biopsy of the lip is often helpful to confirm a suspected diagnosis of Sjögren's syndrome. Sjögren's syndrome is uncommon in childhood and is usually found in association with other CTDs.

11. **What forms of systemic vasculitis occur in childhood?**
    The most common small-vessel vasculitis in childhood is **Henoch–Schönlein purpura (HSP)**. Small-vessel vasculitis can also be a component of many of the juvenile systemic CTDs including systemic JIA, JDM, and SLE. ANCA-associated small-vessel vasculitis (GPA, MPA, Churg–Strauss) may present initially mimicking HSP. **Primary central nervous system (CNS) vasculitis** may involve small- or medium-sized vessels of the brain and spinal cord. Five percent of cases of **polyarteritis nodosa (PAN)**, which is a medium-vessel vasculitis, occurs in childhood and, as in adults, is characterized by rash, fever, weight loss, myositis, and cutaneous nodules. Life-threatening renal, gastrointestinal (GI), cardiac, and CNS involvement is often seen. **Cutaneous PAN** has also been reported. **Kawasaki disease** is a uniquely pediatric vasculitis and is discussed in Chapter 71. Large-vessel vasculitis is unusual in childhood, however, up to 30% of all **Takayasu's arteritis** cases occur in childhood, typically developing in adolescent females.

12. **What triad of signs and symptoms is associated with HSP in children?**
    - Purpura
    - Colicky abdominal pain
    - Arthritis

HSP (anaphylactoid purpura) is an IgA-mediated small-vessel leukocytoclastic vasculitis. It is the most common vasculitis of childhood and rare in adults. The median age at presentation is 4 to 6 years, and the male to female ratio is about 1.8:1. Approximately 50% of children have a history of preceding upper respiratory tract infection with a variety of organisms. Purpura is usually the initial manifestation but can be preceded by arthritis, edema, testicular swelling, and abdominal pain. Renal disease occurs in 40% to 50% usually within the first 2 months of vasculitis onset. Laboratory abnormalities include an elevated erythrocyte sedimentation rate (ESR; >50%) and elevated serum IgA (37%), and occasionally a positive IgA ANCA. Complement levels are normal but there is evidence of alternate complement pathway activation. Over 95% of children with HSP have a self-limiting course, lasting 2 to 6 weeks. Recurrence is seen overall in 33% with 20% recurring during the first year. Children with renal disease and those >8 years of age are more likely to have recurrences. Up to 5% of children will suffer persistent purpura with or without persistent renal disease. In patients who have renal involvement, 30% develop renal insufficiency and 5% progress to renal failure, especially those who are nephrotic.

13. **List the clinical manifestations of HSP. (Table 70-3)**

Table 70-3. Clinical Manifestations of HSP

	% AT ONSET	% POST ONSET	NOTES
Purpura	50-100	100	Normal platelet count
Edema	10-20	20-50	Painful, scrotal edema (13%)
Arthritis	25-70	60-85	Large joints
GI	30	85	Volvulus (<1%), ileal infarcation
Renal	15	40-50	Renal failure (2%)
GU	2	2-35	Differential is testicular torsion
Pulmonary	?	95 (by DL_{CO})	Abnormal CO diffusion
Hemorrhage	?	Rare	Fatal
CNS	?	Very rare	Headache, encephalitis, seizures

CNS, Central nervous system; DL_{CO}, carbon monoxide diffusing capacity; GI, gastrointestinal; GU, genitourinary.

14. **How is the diagnosis confirmed? What role does IgA play in the pathogenesis?**
A skin biopsy with immunofluorescence showing a leukocytoclastic vasculitis with predominantly IgA vessel wall deposition in the appropriate clinical setting is diagnostic of HSP. Notably HSP has been reported most often to occur following an upper respiratory infection. It also can occur before or during the course of ANCA-associated vasculitis or Crohn disease. Each of these triggers involve inflammation at mucosal surfaces where IgA plays a role in mucosal immunity. In patients with HSP, serum IgA1 has been shown to be galactose-deficient at the hinge region O-linked glycan causing it to form aggregates that interact with IgG forming IgA–IgG immune complexes that deposit in tissues.

15. **What are poor prognostic factors in HSP at onset? (Table 70-4)**

Table 70-4. Poor Prognostic Factors at Onset of HSP

MANIFESTATION	COMMENT
Melena	7.5-fold increase in renal disease
Persistent rash for 2-3 months	Associated with glomerulonephritis
Hematuria with proteinuria >1 g/day	15% progress to renal insufficiency
Nephrosis with renal insufficiency	50% renal insufficiency in 10 years

16. **How should HSP be treated?**
- Arthritis responds to NSAIDs
- Edema responds to steroids
- Abdominal pain with positive test for blood in stool should be treated with steroids
- Evaluate for and treat infection (e.g., group A β-hemolytic streptococci, *Helicobacter pylori*)
- Recurrent skin purpura may respond to dapsone

- Aggressive treatment (high-dose or IV pulse corticosteroids) for children with poor prognostic signs
- Severe nephritis: high-dose IV pulse methylprednisolone plus azathioprine or cyclophosphamide; angiotensin-converting enzyme (ACE) inhibitors for proteinuria

PEARL: Corticosteroid therapy helps arthritic and abdominal symptoms but may not prevent nephritis or subsequent recurrences.

17. Describe the physical examination of a child presenting with JDM.

JDM is a an immune-mediated vasculitis that presents with an inflammatory myositis and a characteristic skin rash. The mean age of onset is 6 to 9 years old with 25% occurring in children less than the age of 4 years. In whites it is associated with human leukocyte antigen (HLA)-DRB1*0301. Muscle weakness, in particular of the proximal musculature (limbs, girdle, neck), is prominent (80% to 100% of patients). The Gower maneuver is abnormal, and the child will be unable to do a sit-up as a result of weakness. The head may hang back as the child is lifted from a lying position, owing to weakness of the neck muscles. Skin manifestations are characteristic. The eyelids and face are edematous, and a heliotrope or mauvish rash is noted around the eyes (75%). Deep red patches (66% to 95%), known as Gottron papules, will be found over the extensor surfaces of the finger joints, as well as over the elbows, knees, and ankle joints. These patches may ulcerate as a result of vasculitis. Telangiectasias may be found around the eyelids and capillary dilatation and dropout can be found around nailfolds (see Chapter 74). GI manifestations include dysphagia (18% to 44%) and intestinal vasculitis causing abdominal pain, lower GI bleeding, and bowel perforation. Arthralgia or arthritis may occur (20% to 60%), sometimes with swelling and contractures of the fingers resulting from tenosynovitis. The most common lung finding is a decreased carbon monoxide diffusing capacity (DL_{CO}) in 50% of patients. Cardiac involvement is uncommon.

18. How can the muscle weakness of JDM be differentiated from that of other causes of weakness?

The muscle weakness of JDM predominantly involves the proximal musculature, and in general, the involvement is symmetric. The child gives a history of difficulty in climbing stairs or riding a bicycle. Some of the maneuvers detailed in the previous question (e.g., Gower maneuver) can discriminate true muscle weakness from, for example, inanition. The palate and swallowing musculature may be weak in JDM and may lead to choking, cough, or aspiration pneumonia. Serum muscle enzymes are elevated, but not to the degree seen in the muscular dystrophies. Assays for all muscle-derived enzymes are required (aldolase, creatine kinase, aspartate aminotransferase [AST], lactate dehydrogenase [LDH]) because only one may be elevated. ANA is positive in 10% to 85% of patients. Myositis-associated and myositis-specific antibodies are rare although anti-p155/140 has been identified in 29% of patients. In patients who have symptoms such as "classic" skin rash, muscle weakness, and elevated muscle enzymes, the diagnosis can be made clinically. A magnetic resonance imaging (MRI) scan of shoulder or thigh muscles can preclude the need for electromyography (EMG) and/or muscle biopsy if short tau inversion recovery (STIR) or T2-weighted images of the muscle shows increased signal, indicative of muscle edema and active inflammation. In atypical cases, an EMG and muscle biopsy may be necessary and the MRI can determine the best site for biopsy. In JDM, the EMG will show spontaneous fibrillations, increased insertional activity, and small muscle unit action potentials whereas the muscle biopsy will show inflammation and/or fiber necrosis, perifascicular atrophy, and small-vessel vasculitis.

19. How is JDM different from adult dermatomyositis or polymyositis?

In children:
- Dermatomyositis is distinguished by being a generalized vasculitis.
- Polymyositis is **exceedingly rare** in childhood. In a child with progressive weakness, other muscle diseases are more likely than polymyositis.
- Unlike adults, malignancy is rarely associated with childhood dermatomyositis.

20. Can a patient have just skin involvement and no muscle disease in JDM?

Yes. Patients with clinically amyotrophic JDM (**CAJDM**) can have skin without muscle involvement. Over time (2 years), 25% to 30% will develop muscle involvement.

21. What chronic sequellae can be seen in patients with JDM?

- In severe chronic JDM, nodules resulting from subcutaneous calcinosis may be found (up to 40%). Mobility may be impaired because of calcinotic lesions at the joints or as a result of involvement of musculature.
- Partial or generalized lipodystrophy can develop in 30% to 40% of patients with JDM. The face is frequently involved. It is frequently associated with the metabolic syndrome, insulin resistance, hirsuitism, cliteromegaly, and acanthosis nigricans.

22. Compare the occurrence and frequency of Raynaud phenomenon and Raynaud disease in children and adults.

Raynaud phenomenon should be distinguished from normal vasomotor instability, particularly in young girls. It should also be distinguished from acrocyanosis, a rare vasospastic disorder of persistent coldness and bluish discoloration of the hands and feet, which may follow a viral infection. Patients with Raynaud phenomenon associated with digital ulcers, nailfold capillary abnormalities, and/or an ANA with a nucleolar or centromere pattern are more likely to have or to develop a systemic CTD (Table 70-5).

Table 70-5. Raynaud's in Children and Adults

CATEGORY	CHILDREN	ADULTS
Raynaud disease	5%	70%
Raynaud phenomenon with		
Nonconnective tissue disease	1	15
JIA	1	7
SLE	60	4
SSc	30	3
Dermatomyositis	3	1

Adapted from Cassidy JT et al: Textbook of pediatric rheumatology, ed 6, Philadelphia, 2011, WB Saunders.
JIA, Juvenile idiopathic arthritis; SLE, systemic lupus erythematosus; SSc, systemic sclerosis (scleroderma).

23. Describe the types of scleroderma that occur in childhood.
- Scleroderma is characterized by abnormally increased collagen deposition in the skin and occasionally in the internal organs.
- **Localized scleroderma** is three times more common than diffuse scleroderma in childhood. It occurs more commonly in children than adults. Localized scleroderma may take the form of morphea, with a single patch or multiple patches. Linear scleroderma may occur on the face, forehead, and scalp (en coup de sabre), or in the form of progressive hemifacial atrophy (Parry–Romberg syndrome). It can also occur on the limb (en bande). ANA (50%), RF (10% to 25%), and hypergammaglobulinemia can be seen. Treatment includes high-dose IV methylprednisolone initially followed by prednisone with tapering over 3 to 6 months. Methotrexate is coadministered with the steroids and continued for at least 2 years. There is a 30% recurrence rate after methotrexate is stopped.
- **Diffuse scleroderma** (SSc) may be limited in its involvement, with a prolonged interval before the appearance of visceral stigmata, or as part of the CREST syndrome (calcinosis, Raynaud phenomenon, esophageal dysmotility, sclerodactyly, and telangiectasias). Myositis occurs in 25% of patients and may be the presenting manifestation.

24. What laboratory abnormalities are seen in the juvenile systemic CTDs? (Table 70-6)

Table 70-6. Laboratory Abnormalities in Childhood Systemic Connective Tissue Diseases

	SYSTEMIC JIA	SLE	JDM	SSc	VASCULITIS	ARF
Anemia	++	+++	+	+	++	+
Leukopenia	—	+++	—	—	—	—
Thrombocytopenia	—	++	—	—	—	—
Leukocytosis	+++	—	+	—	+++	+
Thrombocytosis	++	—	+	—	+	+
ANAs	—	+++	+	++	—	—
Anti-DNA antibodies	—	+++	—	—	—	—
RFs	—	++	—	+	+	—
Antistreptococcal antibodies	+	—	—	—	—	+++
Hypocomplementemia	—	+++	—	—	++	—
Elevated hepatic enzymes	++	+	+	+	+	—
Elevated muscle enzymes	—	+	+++	++	+	—
Abnormal urinalysis	+	+++	+	+	++	—

Adapted from Cassidy JT et al: Textbook of pediatric rheumatology, ed 6, Philadelphia, 2011, WB Saunders.
ANA, Antinuclear antibodies; ARF, acute rheumatic fever; JDM, juvenile dermatomyositis; JIA, juvenile idiopathic arthritis; RF, rheumatoid factor; SLE, systemic lupus erythematosus; SSc, systemic sclerosis (scleroderma).

25. **List some infections that can mimic childhood CTD.**
    - Acute rheumatic fever—rare before age 4 years. Severely painful, migratory polyarthritis with fever (Chapter 44).
    - Parvovirus infection—young children get erythema infectiosum ("slapped cheeks"). Older children and adults can get fever (50%), polyarthritis, and rash. Can mimic systemic or polyarticular JIA. IgM antiparvovirus antibodies can be negative for the first 2 to 3 weeks, but polymerase chain reaction for parvovirus B19 DNA will be positive. Arthritis can last over 4 months (50%) (Chapter 41).
    - Epstein–Barr virus (EBV) infection—can mimic SLE. Monospot negative in children under 4 years old. Diagnose with IgM antibodies to viral capsid antigen (VCA) and negative antibodies to EBV nuclear antigen (EBNA) during initial acute infection.
    - Immunodeficiency—humoral and combined immunodeficiency can present as infections including septic joints. Echovirus can cause a myositis and mycoplasma a chronic monoarticular arthritis. Consider immunodeficiency in any child with history of two previous bacterial pneumonias (Chapter 58).
    - Lyme disease—can mimic oligoarticular JIA (Chapter 39). May start out as migratory arthritis.
    - HIV infection—can present as muscle, skin, or joint problems in children. Generalized adenopathy, fever of unknown origin (FUO) with organomegaly, and thrombocytopenia are other presentations (Chapter 42).

26. **What bowel disease is most likely to occur with arthritis and systemic symptoms?**
    Up to 20% of children with Crohn disease have arthritis, which is usually monoarticular or oligoarticular. Children will not volunteer information about their bowel habits, so they must be asked. Furthermore, some children with arthritis attributable to Crohn disease will not have bowel symptoms or a positive stool guaiac. Consequently, inflammatory bowel disease needs to be considered in any child with arthritis, weight loss, halt in linear growth, iron-deficiency anemia, and elevated sedimentation rate.

27. **What are the general principles of therapy for the juvenile CTDs?**
    Although therapy for the juvenile CTDs must clearly be tailored to the specific diagnosis, certain therapeutic principles can be stressed. The principal drugs used are those that suppress the inflammatory and immune responses. The arachidonic acid metabolic pathways and the cells of the immune system are the primary targets of their therapeutic effects. Childhood and adult CTD are treated similarly. An obvious difference in the use of these drugs in children, as compared with adults, is dosing on the basis of the weight of the child. Additionally the effects of therapy, particularly corticosteroids, on growth, osteoporosis, dyslipidemia, and infection must be considered.

Acknowledgement

The authors and editor thank Terri H. Finkel, MD, PhD, for her contributions to this chapter in previous editions.

Bibliography

Brunner J, Feldman BM, Tyrell PN, et al: Takayasu's arteritis in children and adolescents, Rheumatology 49:1806–1814, 2010.
Cabral DA, Uribe AG, Benseler S, et al: Classification, presentation, and initial treatment of Wegener's granulomatosis in childhood, Arthritis Rheum 60:3413–3424, 2009.
Cassidy JT, Petty RE, Laxer R, Lindsley C, et al: Textbook of pediatric rheumatology, ed 6, Philadelphia, 2011, WB Saunders.
Jauhola O, Ronkainen J, Koskimies O, et al: Renal manifestations of Henoch–Schönlein purpura in a 6 month prospective study of 223 children, Arch Dis Child 95:877–882, 2010.
Khanna S, Reed AM: Immunopathogenesis of juvenile dermatomyositis, Muscle Nerve 41:581–592, 2010.
Kim S, El-Hallack M, Dedeoglu F, et al: Complete and sustained remission of juvenile dermatomyositis resulting from aggressive treatment, Arthritis Rheum 60:1825–1830, 2009.
Lehman TJ: SLE in childhood and adolescence. In Wallace DJ, Hahn BH, editors: Dubois' lupus erythematosus and related syndromes, ed 8, Philadelphia, 2013, Elsevier Saunders.
Livingston B, Bonner A, Pope J: Differences in clinical manifestations between childhood-onset lupus and adult-onset lupus: a meta-analysis, Lupus 20:1345, 2011.
Marks SD, Tullus K: Modern therapeutic strategies for pediatric systemic lupus erythematosus and lupus nephritis, Acta Paediatr 99:967, 2010.
Martini G, Foeldvari I, Russo R, et al: Systemic sclerosis in childhood: clinical and immunologic features of 153 patients in an international database, Arthritis Rheum 54:3971–3978, 2006.
Singer NG, Tomanova-Soltys I, Lowe R: Sjögren's syndrome in childhood, Curr Rheumatol Rep 10:147–155, 2008.
Stringer E, Singh-Grewal D, Feldman BM: Predicting the course of juvenile dermatomyositis: significance of early clinical and laboratory features, Arthritis Rheum 58:3585–3592, 2008.
Takehara K, Sato S: Localized scleroderma is an autoimmune disorder, Rheumatology 44:274–279, 2005.
Trapani S, Micheli A, Grisolia F, et al: Henoch Schönlein purpura in childhood: epidemiological and clinical analysis of 150 cases over a 5-year period and review of literature, Semin Arthritis Rheum 35:143–153, 2005.
Wahren-Herelenius M, Sonesson SE, Clowse ME: Neonatal lupus erythematosus. In Wallace DJ, Hahn BH, editors: Dubois' lupus erythematosus and related syndromes, ed 8, Philadelphia, 2013, Elsevier Saunders.
Watson L, leone V, Pilkington C, et al: Disease activity, severity, and damage in UK juvenile-onset systemic lupus erythematosus cohort, Arthritis Rheum 64:2356, 2012.
Weibel L, Sampaio MC, Vinsentin MT, et al: Evaluation of methotrexate and corticosteroids for the treatment of localized scleroderma in children, Br J Dermatol 155:1013–1020, 2006.
Weiss PF, Klink AJ, Localio R, et al: Corticosteroids may improve outcomes during hospitalization for Henoch–Schönlein purpura, Pediatrics 126:674–681, 2010.

Further Reading

http://www.lupus.org/
https://www.carragroup.org
http://www.printo.it/pediatric-rheumatology/
http://www.curejm.com/
http://www.myositis.org
http://www.scleroderma.org/medical/juvenile.shtm

CHAPTER 71

KAWASAKI DISEASE
J. Roger Hollister, MD

KEY POINTS
1. Kawasaki disease (KD) is the most common vasculitis and cause of acquired heart disease in children.
2. Consider KD in any child under the age of 5 years presenting with prolonged high fevers and conjunctivitis.
3. Intravenous immunoglobulin (IVIG) within 10 days of disease onset is the treatment of choice for KD.

1. **What are the diagnostic criteria for KD?**
   Fever is present in 100% of patients. It is usually high grade (frequently >40° C), unresponsive to antibiotics, and lasts an average of 10 days (range 5 to 25 days). The diagnostic criteria for KD are one of the following:
   - Fever for >5 consecutive days, with four of the following five criteria:
     1. Bilateral conjunctivitis, nonexudative, often dramatic (85% to 92%).
     2. Oropharyngeal manifestations: vertical cracking and fissuring of lips, red pharynx without exudate; "strawberry" tongue (90%).
     3. Cervical lymphadenopathy (33% to 66%)—one or more enlarged (>1.5 cm) nodes, usually unilateral and painful.
     4. Polymorphic rash involving trunk and extremities (80% to 90%) accentuated in groin (50%)—may be pruritic, never vesicular or bullous.
     5. Erythema (painful) of palms and soles, progressing to edema dorsum of hands and feet, and finally periungual desquamation usually 2 to 3 weeks after fever onset (65% to 80%).
   - Fever plus echocardiographic/angiographic demonstration of coronary artery aneurysms or stenoses.

2. **Does incomplete KD exist?**
   Yes. Up to 10% of patients with KD have prolonged fever (>5 days) but do not meet four or more of the mucocutaneous criteria. This is particularly common in infants less than 6 to 12 months old. Most of these (90%) patients will have oropharyngeal manifestations and conjunctivitis. However, cervical adenopathy (10%), extremity swelling and erythema (40%), and rash (50%) are less likely to occur in patients with incomplete KD. Therefore, infants/young children with prolonged fever, one or more mucocutaneous manifestations, and three or more supplemental laboratory abnormalities (erythrocyte sedimentation rate [ESR] > 40 mm/h or C-reactive protein [CRP] > 3 mg/dL, anemia of chronic disease, white blood cell [WBC] count > 15,000/mm^3, platelets > 450,000/mm^3, albumin < 3 g/dL, alanine aminotransferase [ALT] > 50 U/L, or urine WBC > 10/high power field [HPF]) should have an echocardiogram and be considered for IVIG therapy to prevent coronary aneurysms.

3. **What epidemiologic facts are known about KD?**
   - It is a disease of young children:
     - Peak incidence at 9 to 12 months of age.
     - 50% cases in children < 2 years old.
     - 80% in children < 5 years old; disease is rare after age 11 years.
     - Males > females up to 1.9:1.
   - There is a 1% to 2% incidence in siblings.
   - There is a 3% to 4% recurrence rate.
   - Epidemics appear to be cyclic, occurring at approximately 2 to 3 year intervals, particularly in late winter/early spring and mid summer.
   - More common among Japanese people and those of Japanese ancestry (17×).
   - Most common vasculitis of childhood (previously called infantile polyarteritis nodosa).
   - Rarely has been reported in adults (Gomard-Mennesson et al, 2010).

4. **What other complications may occur in the acute phase of the illness?**
   Cardiac—myocarditis, pericarditis, and arteritis predispose to aneurysms in approximately 20% of patients.
   Arthritis—short-lived, may involve small joints of hands and feet (7% to 20%); can have very high synovial fluid WBCs.
   Uveitis—acute, anterior (80%).
   Respiratory—cough (35%).

Hydrops of gallbladder—produces abdominal pain and jaundice.
Gastrointestinal—vomiting and diarrhea with abdominal pain (60%).
Skin—previous Bacillus Calmette–Guérin (BCG) immunization site becomes inflamed.
Others—meningitis, pneumonitis, sterile pyuria, transaminitis (40%), facial nerve palsy, sensorineural hearing loss (<1%), macrophage activation syndrome.

5. **Is there a diagnostic test for KD?**
   No. Laboratory tests show the findings of acute inflammation (80% have CRP > 3.5 mg/dL). However, a progressive increase in the platelet count, often to thrombocytotic levels (>10^6/mm^3), is characteristic and is not seen in many other causes of fever of unknown origin (FUO).

6. **Name a streptococcal illness in the differential diagnosis of KD. What other diseases need to be considered?**
   Scarlet fever shares many of the features, including fever, conjunctivitis, mucous membrane involvement, and desquamating skin rash. Some authorities suggest that scarlet fever must be ruled out by appropriate cultures of streptococci before concluding that the diagnosis is KD. Other infections (Epstein–Barr virus [EBV], adenovirus, echovirus, measles, Rocky Mountain spotted fever [RMSF], leptospirosis), Steven's Johnson syndrome, and Still's disease can mimic KD.

7. **Name the epidemiologic and clinical factors associated with a poor prognosis in KD.**
   Age < 1 year or > 9 years; male sex; Asian ancestry; fever > 14 days; WBC count > 12,000/mm^3. Patients with these characteristics are more likely to develop coronary aneurysms (50%).

8. **What symptoms and findings present in the acute phase of KD suggest cardiac involvement?**
   Obviously, in preverbal children, it may be difficult to communicate ischemic myocardial pain. Symptoms that may be helpful include restlessness, pallor, weak pulse, abdominal pain, and vomiting. A gallop rhythm with a third heart sound may be heard in 70% of cases. Friction rubs indicative of pericarditis are much less common. Coronary artery aneurysms are more common in patients with pericarditis. In one series, palpable axillary artery aneurysms were highly predictive of coronary artery aneurysms.

9. **What tests are helpful in assessing cardiac involvement?**
   Electrocardiograms may show ST–T wave changes indicative of pericarditis or myocarditis. Chest x-rays may show cardiomegaly. However, an echocardiogram is most useful to assess myocardial function, rarely valvular regurgitation, and most commonly coronary arterial dilatation and aneurysm formation (20% of all patients). Echocardiography should be done immediately on all children suspected of having KD and should be repeated at 1 to 2, 6, and 12 weeks. Patients should have echocardiograms every 5 years thereafter due to recognition of cardiac complications manifesting during adulthood.

10. **Besides the fact that "giant" coronary aneurysms sound bad, what is the significance of finding coronary artery dilatations ≥ 8 mm on echocardiography?**
    "Giant" coronary artery aneurysms are the most prone to thrombosis and the least likely to regress with time. Their presence requires anticoagulation with warfarin (international normalized ratio [INR] 2.0 to 2.5) and very close follow-up by a pediatric cardiologist. A recent study found that abciximab, a monoclonal antibody against glycoprotein GPIIb/IIIa on platelets improved vascular remodeling in these patients.

11. **What is the natural history of these coronary aneurysms?**
    From a peak incidence of 20% in the first 1 to 2 weeks of illness, most of the vascular dilatations will regress, so that only 2% to 5% can be found on echocardiography 1 year later. Antiplatelet therapy should begin with high-dose aspirin (80 to 100 mg/kg/day) split into three doses in the acute phase of the illness. This is followed by low-dose aspirin (3 to 5 mg/kg/day) once a day in the convalescent phase for an additional 2 months. In patients with aneurysms, low-dose aspirin or clopidogrel should be continued indefinitely.

12. **What causes KD?**
    Unknown. It is believed that it is caused by an infectious agent in a genetically predisposed host. Many infections (bacterial, viral) and toxins (staphylococcal enterotoxins, toxic shock syndrome toxin 1, or streptococcal pyrogenic exotoxins) have been proposed but none proven. Recently a functional polymorphism in the inositol-triphosphate 3-kinase C (*ITPKC*) gene that is a negative regulator of T cell activation and a polymorphism of the proinflammatory caspase 3 (*CASP3*) gene have been found to confer increased susceptibility to developing KD.

13. **Is there an effective treatment for KD?**
    Conclusive evidence from numerous multicenter, double-blind, placebo-controlled series shows that IVIG at a dose of 2 g/kg given over 12 hours within the first 10 days of illness is the treatment of choice in KD. This is given in conjunction with high-dose aspirin (30 to 50 or 80 to 100 mg/kg/day) (Table 71-1). Two parameters have repeatedly been shown to be responsive to IVIG: resolution of the acute symptoms and prevention of coronary aneurysm formation. It is commonly observed that the fever lyses, the rash regresses, and the toxicity of the illness improves within 12 hours of IVIG administration. Once the fever has resolved, the dose of aspirin is decreased to 3 to 5 mg/kg/day for its antiplatelet effect. In those who do not develop aneurysms, the aspirin

Table 71-1.

	ANEURYSM AT 14 DAYS	ANEURYSM AT 30 MONTHS
Aspirin alone	23%	11%
Aspirin and IVIG	5%	2%

IVIG, Intravenous immunoglobulin.

can be discontinued after the ESR/CRP and platelet counts return to normal. The implementation of this approach within 10 days of disease onset reduces the incidence of coronary aneurysms from 20% to 25% to 3% to 5%. Notably, one recent study (Kobayashi et al, 2012) suggested that earlier use of prednisolone (2 mg/kg/day for 2 to 3 weeks) in conjunction with the initial IVIG dose may prevent coronary aneurysms better than the standard regimen of IVIG plus aspirin. Patients with persistent aneurysms are at risk for accelerated atherosclerosis and/or stenoses requiring stents or bypass surgery.

14. **What is unique about IVIG that might explain its usefulness in KD?**
    IVIG is pooled immunoglobulin from 10,000 donors. When the antibody profile of IVIG was examined, it was found to have extraordinarily high titers of antistaphylococcal, antistreptococcal, and antitoxic shock toxin antibodies. Many of the features of KD (fever, rash, etc.) are reminiscent of toxin-mediated diseases.

15. **Are any patients with KD resistant to IVIG therapy? Can steroids be used to treat acute, refractory KD?**
    Between 15% and 30% of KD patients are resistant to one course of IVIG. It is recommended to give these patients a second course of IVIG from a different manufacturer. Patients who fail a second IVIG course should be treated with IV solumedrol followed by oral prednisone. Patients who fail to respond to steroids have been empirically treated successfully with infliximab.

BIBLIOGRAPHY

Burns JC, Kushner HI, Bastian JF, et al: Kawasaki disease: a brief history, Pediatrics 106:E27, 2000.
Burns JC, Cayan DR, Tong G, et al: Seasonality and temporal clustering of Kawasaki syndrome, Epidemiology 16:220–225, 2005.
Gomard-Mennesson E, Landron C, Dauphin C, et al: Kawasaki disease in adults: report of 10 cases, Medicine 89:149–158, 2010.
Ha KS, Jang G, Lee J, et al: Incomplete clinical manifestation as a risk factor for coronary artery abnormalities in Kawasaki's disease: a metaanalysis, Eur J Pediatr 172:343–349, 2013.
Kawasaki T, Kosaki F, Okawa S, et al: A new infantile acute febrile mucocutaneous lymph node syndrome (MLNS) prevailing in Japan, Pediatrics 54:271–276, 1974.
Kobayashi T, Saji T, Otani T, et al: Efficacy of immunoglobulin plus prednisone for prevention of coronary artery abnormalities in severe Kawasaki disease (RAISE study): a randomised, open-label, blinded-endpoints trial, Lancet 379:1613, 2012.
Newburger JW, Takahashi M, Burns JC, et al: The treatment of Kawasaki syndrome with intravenous gammaglobulin, N Engl J Med 315:341–347, 1986.
Newburger JW, Takahashi M, Gerber MA, et al: Diagnosis, treatment, and long term management of Kawasaki disease, Circulation 110:2747–2771, 2004.
Rowley AH: Kawasaki disease: novel insights into etiology and genetic susceptibility, Ann Rev Med 62:69–77, 2011.
Sugahara Y, Ishii M, Muta H, et al: Warfarin therapy for giant aneurysm prevents myocardial infarction in Kawasaki disease, Pediatr Cardiol 29:398–401, 2008.
Tremoulet AH, Best BM, Song S, et al: Resistance to intravenous immunoglobulin in children with Kawasaki disease, J Pediatr 153:117–121, 2008.
Yellen ES, Gauvreau K, Takahashi M, et al: Performance of 2004 American Heart Association recommendations for treatment of Kawasaki Disease, Pediatrics 125:e234–241, 2010.

FURTHER READING

http://www.kdfoundation.org

XIII
Miscellaneous Rheumatic Disorders

Sickness is a place, more instructive than a long trip to Europe, and it is a place where there's no company, where nobody can follow.

Flannery O'Connor
(1925–1963)

METABOLIC AND OTHER GENETIC MYOPATHIES

CHAPTER 72

Ramon A. Arroyo, MD

KEY POINTS

1. Muscle cramps, pain, or myoglobinuria brought on by exercise suggests a metabolic myopathy.
2. Muscle symptoms with short bursts of high-intensity exercise and the second wind phenomenon are characteristic of a glycogen storage disease (GSD). McArdle's disease and acid maltase deficiency are most common.
3. Muscle symptoms with prolonged low-intensity exercise and/or prolonged fasting suggests a defect in fatty acid oxidation. Carnitine palmitoyltransferase (CPT) II deficiency is most common.
4. Elevated resting lactate level and/or ragged red fibers on muscle biopsy are characteristic of a mitochondrial myopathy.
5. The most common metabolic myopathies associated with myoglobinuria are CPT II deficiency and McArdle's disease.
6. The most common myopathies that are confused with polymyositis are acid maltase deficiency and limb-girdle muscular dystrophy.
7. Children with symptoms of a muscle disease without rash almost always have a metabolic or genetic myopathy and not primary polymyositis.

1. What are metabolic myopathies?

Metabolic myopathies are conditions that have in common abnormalities in muscle energy metabolism that result in skeletal muscle dysfunction. **Primary metabolic myopathies** are associated with biochemical defects that affect the ability of the muscle fibers to maintain adequate levels of adenosine triphosphate (ATP). The three main categories of primary metabolic myopathies are *glycogen storage diseases, fatty acid oxidation defects*, and *mitochondrial disorders* as a result of respiratory chain impairment. Because many of the enzyme defects are partial, these diseases can manifest at various ages from infancy to adulthood. **Secondary metabolic myopathies** are attributed to various endocrine and electrolyte abnormalities.

Metabolic myopathies can be categorized into two groups based on clinical presentation: (1) patients with dynamic symptoms such as muscle pain, cramps, or myoglobinuria caused by exercise but have a normal examination between episodes; and (2) patients with static symptoms such as fixed or progressive weakness often associated with systemic symptoms such as an endocrinopathy or encephalopathy.

2. Which conditions are considered primary metabolic myopathies?

A. Defects of glycogen metabolism (GSD type)	B. Defects in lipid metabolism that affect muscle
Acid maltase deficiency (Pompe disease, II)	Carnitine deficiency (CD) syndromes
Debrancher enzyme deficiency (Cori–Forbes disease, III)	—Primary muscle carnitine deficiency
Brancher enzyme deficiency (Andersen disease, IV)	—Systemic CD with hepatic encephalopathy
Myophosphorylase deficiency (McArdle's disease, V)	—Systemic CD associated with cardiomyopathy
Phosphofructokinase deficiency (Tarui's disease, VII)	Fatty acid transport defects
Phosphorylase b kinase deficiency (VIII)	—CPT defects I and II
Phosphoglycerate kinase deficiency (IX)	—Carnitine-acylcarnitine translocase deficiency
Phosphoglycerate mutase deficiency (X)	β-oxidation mutations
Lactate dehydrogenase deficiency (XI)	

C. Mitochondrial myopathies	D. Disorders of purine metabolism
Electron transport chain protein deficiency (Complex I to IV mutations)	Myoadenylate deaminase deficiency
Mitochondrial ATP synthase deficiency (Complex V mutations)	
Coenzyme Q10 gene mutation	

535

3. What are secondary causes of metabolic myopathies?

A. Endocrine myopathies

Acromegaly	Cushing's disease and Addison's disease
Hyperthyroidism and hypothyroidism	Hyperaldosteronism
Hyperparathyroidism	Carcinoid syndrome

B. Metabolic nutritional myopathies

Uremia	Vitamin D and vitamin E deficiencies
Hepatic failure	Malabsorption and periodic paralysis

C. Electrolyte disorders

Elevated or decreased levels of sodium, potassium, or calcium	Hypophosphatemia
	Hypomagnesemia

4. What is the source of energy for muscle contraction?

Hydrolysis of ATP. Intracellular concentrations of ATP are maintained by the action of enzymes such as creatine kinase, adenylate cyclase, and myoadenylate deaminase. The energy to replenish ATP after it is consumed during muscle contraction is provided by intermediary metabolism of carbohydrates and lipids by pathways of glycolysis, the Krebs cycle, β-oxidation, and oxidative phosphorylation (see Chapter 3).

5. How does ATP provide the energy for muscle contraction?

The immediate source of energy for skeletal muscle during work is found in preformed organic compounds containing high-energy phosphates, such as ATP and creatine phosphate. Creatine kinase (CK or CPK) helps maintain intracellular ATP concentrations by catalyzing the reversible transphosphorylation of creatine and adenine nucleotides and by modulating changes in cytosolic ATP concentrations.

At rest, when there is excess ATP, the terminal phosphate of ATP is transferred to creatine, forming creatine phosphate (CrP) and adenosine diphosphate (ADP) in a reaction catalyzed by CK. The CrP serves as a reservoir of high-energy phosphate. With muscle activity and ATP utilization, CK catalyzes the transfer of those phosphates from CrP to rapidly restore ATP levels to normal. The stores of CrP are sufficient to allow the rephosphorylation of ADP to ATP for only a few minutes of exercise.

Thus, CK along with its products, creatine and creatine phosphate, serve as a shuttle mechanism for energy transport between mitochondria, where ATP is generated by oxidative metabolism (Krebs cycle and respiratory/cytochrome chain), and the myofibrils, where ATP is consumed during muscle contraction and relaxation (Figure 72-1).

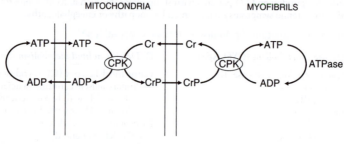

Figure 72-1.

6. What is the purine nucleotide cycle?

When approximately 50% of creatine phosphate has been used during exercise, ATP levels in muscle begin to fall. When this occurs, the purine nucleotide cycle is activated.

During exercise, as ATP is hydrolyzed to ADP by ATPase and then to adenosine monophosphate (AMP) by adenylate kinase, AMP accumulates. The first step of the purine nucleotide cycle is catalyzed by *myoadenylate deaminase*, which converts AMP to inosine monophosphate (IMP) with release of ammonia (NH_3) (Figure 72-2). Both IMP and ammonia stimulate glycolytic activity in an attempt to generate more energy. As ATP levels fall, IMP levels rise until muscle activity decreases and recovery can occur. During recovery, oxidative pathways function and AMP is regenerated from IMP with the liberation of fumarate. Fumarate is converted to malate, which enters the mitochondria and participates in the tricarboxylic acid (TCA) (Krebs) cycle. This helps to regenerate ATP by oxidative phosphorylation within the mitochondria.

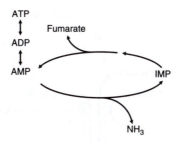

Figure 72-2.

7. What is the role of carbohydrate metabolism during muscle work?

Glycogen, the major storage form of carbohydrate, is the major source of ATP generation when physical activity is of short duration and high intensity (lifting heavy weight) or when anaerobic conditions exist (sustained running). Glycogen is mobilized to form glucose-6-phosphate (G-6-P) by glycogenolysis in a process started by the enzyme *myophosphorylase*. Glucose and glucose-6-phosphate are metabolized through a series of reactions in the glycolytic pathway to pyruvate. Under aerobic conditions, pyruvate enters the Krebs (TCA) cycle and is metabolized to carbon dioxide and water (Figure 72-3). Under aerobic conditions a net of 36 molecules of ATP are generated for each molecule of glucose. However, under anaerobic conditions, pyruvate is converted to lactate and does not enter the Krebs cycle. Under these conditions, only two molecules of ATP are generated for each glucose molecule. Anaerobic glycogenolysis can supply energy to muscle for only several minutes until the muscle fatigues, whereas there are sufficient muscle glycogen stores to supply energy for up to 90 minutes under aerobic conditions.

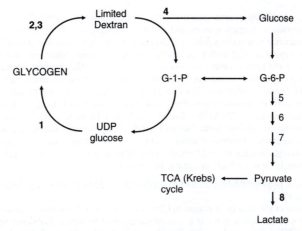

Figure 72-3. Catalyst enzymes: *1*, Brancher enzyme; *2*, phosphorylase b kinase; *3*, myophosphorylase; *4*, debrancher enzyme; *5*, phosphofructokinase; *6*, phosphoglycerate kinase; *7*, phosphoglycerate mutase; *8*, lactate dehydrogenase; *9* (not shown), acid maltase, which catalyzes release of glucose from glycogen and maltase in lysosomes.

8. What is the role of lipid metabolism during muscle work?

Lipids, especially long-chain fatty acids (L-cFAs), constitute the major substrate for energy production (ATP) during fasting intervals, at rest, and with muscular activities of low intensity and long duration (more than 40 to 50 minutes).

L-cFAs from adipose tissues move through the bloodstream bound to albumin. These, plus medium-chain and short-chain fatty acids, move across endothelial cells and into the muscle cells (called fibers), where they are available for energy production, storage, or synthesis into membrane components. To be processed for energy, the free fatty acid must enter the mitochondria. Short-chain and medium-chain fatty acids cross freely into the mitochondria. L-cFAs must combine with carnitine to enter the mitochondrial matrix. The combination of L-cFAs with carnitine and their release into the mitochondrial matrix are catalyzed by CPT I and CPT II, respectively (circled 1 and 2 in Figure 72-4), which are located on the outer (OM) and inner mitochondrial membrane (IM) respectively. Once in the mitochondria, the fatty acids are converted to their respective coenzyme A (CoA) esters and sequentially shortened by the process of β-oxidation, which releases acetyl CoA that then enters the TCA (Krebs) cycle. At present, carnitine deficiency, CPT deficiency, and mutations in enzymes involved in β-oxidation (acylCoA synthetase deficiency) have been described in patients with abnormal muscle function.

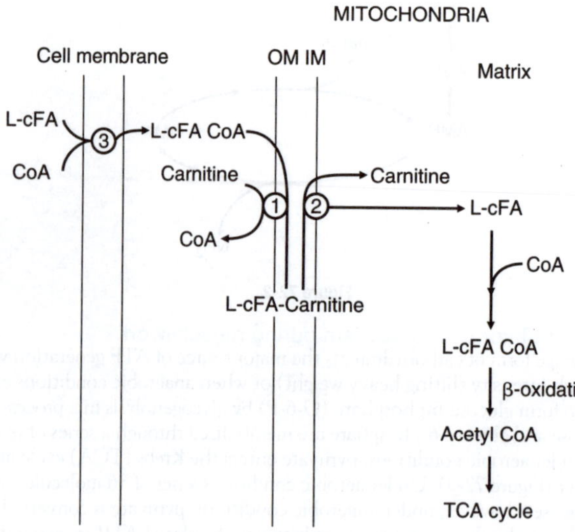

```
                           MITOCHONDRIA
    Cell membrane      OM IM
                                          Matrix

    L-cFA      ③   → L-cFA CoA ─┐
     ↓                           │
    CoA            Carnitine    │    → Carnitine
                         ① ②─────────────→ L-cFA
                    CoA ←                      ↑
                                              CoA
                    L-cFA-Carnitine
                                          L-cFA CoA
                                              │
                                              ↓ β-oxidation
                                          Acetyl CoA
                                              │
                                              ↓
                                          TCA cycle
```

Figure 72-4.

9. How do disorders of glycogen and glucose metabolism present clinically?

Patients who develop muscle cramps, spasms, and/or myoglobinuria with short bursts of high-intensity exercise (weight lifting or sprinting) may have a defect of glycogen metabolism known as a GSD. There are 12 types of GSDs (glycogenoses, types I to XII) with nine having muscle symptoms. Most are autosomal recessive. These patients are well at rest and perform low-intensity exercise without difficulty, because free fatty acids are the major source of energy under these conditions. The enzymatic block that interferes with the use of carbohydrates to generate ATP causes problems only when exercise reaches a level that produces anaerobic conditions. Typically, the patient starts exercising and within a few minutes the muscle fatigues (patients describe this as "hitting the wall"). In some cases (McArdle's disease and Tarui's disease), continued exertion can result in improved exercise tolerance, referred as the **"second wind"** phenomenon. However, in many patients if they continue exercising, the muscle becomes painful and may develop a firm cramp. This could result in severe muscle damage and myoglobinuria. In children, defects in glycogenolysis may also occur with liver dysfunction, hepatosplenomegaly, or neurologic or cardiac involvement.

10. Describe the clinical presentation seen in myophosphorylase deficiency (McArdle's disease; glycogenosis type V).

McArdle's disease is one of the two most common GSDs. It is autosomal recessive and attributable to one of 30 mutations of the myophosphorylase gene. It is a common cause of recurrent rhabdomyolysis and myoglobinuria, second only to CPT deficiency. Myophosphorylase degrades glycogen to glucose-1-phosphate and hence is important in calling up stored energy for muscle use. The cardinal manifestation of this deficiency is exercise intolerance associated with pain, fatigue, or weakness. The degree of intolerance varies among affected individuals. Symptoms can follow activities of high intensity and short duration or those that requires less intense effort for longer intervals. Symptoms should resolve with rest. In fact, at rest, affected individuals function well and adjust their activities to a level below their threshold for symptoms. Some individuals experience the "second wind" phenomenon, which is a marked improvement in exercise tolerance approximately 10 minutes into aerobic exercise involving large muscle masses (jogging or cycling). For unknown reasons, severe cramps and myoglobinuria are rare before adolescence. Elevated CK at rest is a common finding. The forearm ischemic test is usually diagnostic, showing a flat venous lactate curve. Definitive diagnosis requires histochemical and biochemical testing showing the enzyme deficiency in muscle. Low-dose creatine monohydrate and a diet high in complex carbohydrates may improve exercise performance and tolerance in patients with this condition.

11. How does phosphofructokinase deficiency (Tarui's disease; glycogenosis type VII) present?

The clinical manifestations of phosphofructokinase (fructose-6-phosphate to fructose-1,6-phosphate) deficiency can be identical to those of McArdle's disease. Glucose or sucrose intake before exercise may exacerbate the muscle symptoms. The second wind phenomenon is less common, and the exercise intolerance is likely to be associated with nausea and vomiting. Approximately one third of affected individuals develop myoglobinuria, and most have elevated CK at rest. The disease can also cause hemolytic anemia.
PEARL: consider this diagnosis in any patient with exercised-induced muscle symptoms, elevated CK, and a hemolytic anemia.

12. **How does acid maltase deficiency (Pompe disease; glycogenosis type II) present?**
    Acid maltase deficiency is one of the two most common GSDs. It is caused by one of 200 mutations of the gene that codes for the intralysosomal enzyme acid alpha-glucosidase (GAA) that catalyzes the release of glucose from maltose, oligosaccharide, and glycogen in lysosomes. Its deficiency is transmitted by autosomal recessive inheritance and produces three different clinical syndromes depending on the severity of the enzyme deficiency.
    1. The infantile form causes symptoms of muscle weakness, hypotonia, and congestive heart failure that begins shortly after birth and progresses to death within the first 2 years of life.
    2. The juvenile form presents in early childhood with progressive proximal muscle weakness. Death is usually from respiratory failure and occurs before age 30 years.
    3. The adult form presents in the third to fifth decades of life with insidious, painless limb-girdle weakness, and an elevated CK. The respiratory muscles are usually affected and 30% have respiratory failure. This form is frequently misdiagnosed as polymyositis or limb-girdle muscular dystrophy, and a muscle biopsy is most helpful in differentiating them. Characteristically, there are muscle fibers with vacuoles filled with periodic acid Schiff-positive material and stain intensely for acid phosphatase, another lysosomal enzyme. The electromyogram (EMG) shows myopathic changes, electrical irritability, and pseudomyotonic discharges without clinical evidence of myotonia. The diagnosis is confirmed by biochemical analysis of GAA enzyme activity in skin fibroblasts or muscle tissue. Therapy consists of a high protein diet, physical training, and in selective cases enzyme replacement therapy with recombinant human GAA (Myozyme, Lumizyme).

    PEARL: consider this diagnosis in any patient that appears to have polymyositis with *significant respiratory insufficiency*.

13. **How do disorders of lipid metabolism present clinically?**
    In patients with disorders of lipid metabolism, symptoms such as muscle pain, stiffness/tightness, or myoglobinuria are usually induced by events such as prolonged low-intensity exercise (hiking, soccer), prolonged fasting, infection, general anesthesia, exposure to cold, and low carbohydrate high-fat diets. The heart, skeletal muscle, and liver depend on fatty acid oxidation for energy. Metabolic blocks in fatty acid oxidation result in accumulation of abnormal amounts of fatty acid in those tissues, leading to cardiomyopathy, weakness, and fatty liver. An increasing number of neurologic diseases have been associated with defects in fatty acid metabolism. Many of them cause abnormalities in the central nervous system (CNS).
    Few disorders of lipid metabolism present as isolated exercise intolerance without other organ involvement. Primary muscle *carnitine deficiency* and *CPT II deficiency* are the two that can occur with predominantly muscle disease. In contrast to patients with glycogen metabolic defects, patients with these lipid metabolism defects do not experience muscle cramps or the second wind phenomenon. CK levels at rest and EMG are usually normal or only show mild abnormalities.

14. **What is the syndrome of CPT deficiency?**
    CPT II deficiency is an autosomal recessive disorder characterized by attacks of exertional myalgias and myoglobinuria (80%). Patients, most of whom are male, experience no difficulty with short bursts of strenuous activity. Indeed, the favorite recreational sport of the patient is often weight lifting. When prolonged exercise is demanded, particularly in the fasting state (when the body is dependent on fatty acid metabolism as a source of energy), muscle pain, fatigue, and myoglobinuria may occur. Patients do not experience the "second wind phenomenon." CPT II deficiency is the most common genetic metabolic myopathy causing recurrent rhabdomyolysis. The resultant myoglobinuria can cause renal failure. The diagnosis is made by measuring CPT activity in biopsied muscle or by identification of the genetic defect on chromosome 1. Treatment consists of education about avoidance of prolonged strenuous exercise and fasting. Frequent small meals and a low-fat, high-carbohydrate diet may improve exercise tolerance.

15. **What are mitochondrial myopathies?**
    These are a clinically and biochemically heterogeneous group of disorders that have morphologic abnormalities in the number, size, and structure of the mitochondria. As a group they are the most common cause of a genetic metabolic myopathy. However, most have symptoms other than a myopathy (stroke, encephalopathy). The most typical morphologic change on muscle biopsy is the **ragged red fiber**, a distorted-appearing muscle fiber that contains large peripheral and intermyofibrillar aggregates of abnormal mitochondria. These appear as red deposits on modified Gomori staining. Most mitochondrial myopathies are attributed to defects in maternally transmitted mitochondrial DNA that codes for proteins important for mitochondrial function. More than 25 enzyme defects have been described.
    The syndromes associated with abnormalities of mitochondria have a variety of clinical manifestations. Many have multisystem problems with involvement of the CNS, heart, and skeletal muscle. The skeletal muscle involvement is manifested by progressive proximal muscle weakness, external ophthalmoplegia, and exercise intolerance attributable to premature fatigue out of proportion to weakness. Mild activity such as walking up one flight of stairs can cause symptoms that resolve with a short rest but recur with activity. Patients complain of heaviness or burning in muscles but do not have cramps. Serum CK levels are usually normal. Lactate levels

are elevated at rest (70% of cases) or with trivial exercise. Dietary supplement with creatine monohydrate, high-dose coenzyme Q10, and L-carnitine may be of benefit for some patients with mitochondrial myopathies.

16. Are disorders in purine metabolism associated with any problems besides gout?

Yes, myoadenylate deaminase is an isoenzyme that catalyzes the irreversible deamination of AMP to IMP favoring the formation of ATP and plays an important role in the purine nucleotide cycle. Individuals with myoadenylate deaminase deficiency may complain of exercise intolerance, postexertional cramps, and myalgias. Myoadenylate deaminase deficiency caused by a gene mutation (*AMPD1* mutation) occurs in up to 2% of the population and is therefore the most common metabolic abnormality of muscle. However, the precise relationship between myoadenylate deaminase deficiency and muscular symptoms is controversial. ATP is rapidly consumed during exercise in these patients, and the time to replenish ATP to normal concentration is prolonged. The expected rise in lactate during exercise occurs, but the corresponding increase in ammonia concentration does not. CK and aldolase are usually normal in myoadenylate deaminase deficiency, as are EMG and muscle biopsy findings. Histochemical techniques are useful in establishing this deficiency. Creatine monohydrate supplementation has been used to improve symptoms.

17. How do you clinically evaluate patients with suspected metabolic muscle disease?

The evaluation begins with a careful history and thorough physical examination. The problem of diagnosing metabolic myopathies is confounded because at rest patients are usually asymptomatic and have normal physical findings. The importance of the physical examination is to pick up any additional abnormalities, such as neurologic defects, which might indicate a mitochondrial myopathy. Patients with metabolic myopathies typically have one of the following symptoms:

- Metabolic myopathies presenting with exercise intolerance, severe prolonged cramps, and **red wine-colored or cola-colored urine** (indicating myoglobinuria). If symptoms occur during strenuous *brief* exercise then a GSD is most likely (e.g., McArdle's disease) because glycogen is the main source of energy during brief exercise. If symptoms (usually myalgias and myoglobinuria without cramps) occur only after *prolonged* exercise and are worse during *fasting*, then lipid storage disease (e.g., CPT II deficiency) is more likely because free fatty acids are the most important source of fuel during prolonged exercise.
- Metabolic myopathies presenting with progressive muscle weakness that may mimic limb-girdle dystrophy or polymyositis include acid maltase, debrancher enzyme, or carnitine deficiency.

18. How are the metabolic myopathies diagnosed?

Once a detailed history and physical examination are done, measurement of muscle enzymes and electrodiagnostic studies follow if complaints are suspicious for myopathy. Increased levels of CK, aldolase, liver transaminases, lactate dehydrogenase, carnitine, potassium, phosphorous, creatinine, lactate, ammonia, and myoglobin may be observed in the blood of patients depending on the metabolic myopathy. Of these, CK is the most sensitive. Levels are usually increased in patients with glycogen storage disease but are usually normal in CPT or myoadenylate deaminase deficiency.

The EMG is useful in excluding a neuropathic process, demonstrating myopathic changes and indicating a preferential site for muscle biopsy. Elevated muscle enzymes and myopathic changes on EMG are variable and nondiagnostic. A normal EMG does **not** exclude a metabolic myopathy. Measurement of venous lactate and ammonia before and after forearm ischemic exercise provides a useful tool for ruling out myoadenylate deaminase deficiency and all myopathic forms of GSD except acid maltase deficiency, phosphorylase kinase b deficiency, and brancher disease. A positive result should be confirmed by tissue analysis. Enzyme analysis in muscle tissue or skin fibroblast and/or genetic testing provide the most important diagnostic information in the evaluation of a patient with suspected metabolic myopathy.

19. What is the forearm ischemic test? How it is performed?

The forearm ischemic test is a nonspecific tool used in individuals suspected of having myophosphorylase deficiency or a block anywhere along the glycogenolytic or glycolytic pathway. This test exploits the abnormal biochemistry that results in the absence of those enzymes. Normal muscle generates lactate from the degradation of glycogen when it exercises under ischemic or anaerobic conditions. When these pathways are blocked, no lactate is released into the circulation. In addition, ammonia, inosine, and hypoxanthine concentrations increase significantly. A protocol for forearm ischemic testing follows:

1. A blood sample for analysis of baseline lactate and ammonia concentrations is drawn through an indwelling catheter in an antecubital vein, preferably without use of a tourniquet. Pyruvate can also be measured.
2. A sphygmomanometer cuff is placed on the upper arm of the side with the indwelling catheter and inflated. It is maintained at least 20 mm Hg above systolic pressure while the subject squeezes a tennis ball, or similar object, at a rate of one squeeze every 2 seconds for 60 to 90 seconds.
3. After 60 to 90 seconds, the cuff is deflated and additional venous samples are obtained at 1, 3, 6, and 10 minutes thereafter.

In normal individuals, lactate and ammonia increase at least threefold from baseline values in the first two samples after exercise and then gradually decrease to baseline. The major reason for a false-positive result is insufficient work by the individual while exercising. This should be suspected if both lactate and ammonia fail to rise. If lactate (and pyruvate) does not rise but ammonia does, the patient may have a defect in glycolysis, such as McArdle's disease. If lactate rises but ammonia does not, the patient has myoadenylate deaminase deficiency. If pyruvate rises but lactate does not, the patient has lactate dehydrogenase-M subunit deficiency. In CPT II deficiency both lactate and ammonium rise appropriately. This test has been superseded by muscle enzyme analysis and genetic testing.

20. **Why is muscle biopsy the most important diagnostic tool in the evaluation of metabolic myopathies?**

    Muscle biopsy for routine histologic, histochemical, and ultrastructural analysis (electron microscopy) is the most helpful tool in evaluating a suspected metabolic myopathy, primarily because it helps rule out other conditions that can cause muscle dysfunction and allows the specific enzyme defect to be determined. However, biopsy should be the final step in the clinical evaluation, done only after a preliminary diagnosis has been made. Specific enzymes can be tested for in muscle tissue by immunohistochemistry. The most important studies are listed in Table 72-1.

Table 72-1. Enzyme Analysis of Muscle Tissue

STAIN	CONDITION
Periodic acid Schiff	Glycogen storage diseases
Sudan black or Oil red O	Lipid storage diseases
Gomori	Mitochondrial myopathy
Acid phosphatase	Acid maltase deficiency
Histochemical for specific enzymes	Myophosphorylase, phosphofructokinase, lactate dehydrogenase, cytochromes, myoadenylate deaminase

21. **Describe the common muscular dystrophies that may be confused with childhood or adult polymyositis.**
    - **Dystrophinopathies:**
    —**Duchenne dystrophy**: X-linked disease caused by a mutation of the *dystrophin* gene. **Dystrophin** is part of a protein complex that connects the cytoskeleton of a muscle fiber with the extracellular matrix through the cell membrane. Onset of shoulder and pelvic girdle muscle weakness occurs by age 5 years. Elevated CK can be 50 to 100 times the upper limit of normal at rest. Myopathic EMG and abnormal muscle biopsy show fat and occasionally inflammation. Pseudohypertrophy of calf muscles, scoliosis, inability to walk by age 13 years, and death from respiratory failure or cardiomyopathy by age 20 years. Corticosteroids can delay progression of muscle and cardiac disease.
    —**Becker dystrophy**: X-linked disease attributable to a less severe mutation of the *dystrophin* gene resulting in a partially functional protein complex. Similar to Duchenne dystrophy but milder, with patients able to walk beyond age 16 years.
    - **Facioscapulohumeral dystrophy.** Autosomal dominant disease attributable to a partial deletion located on chromosome 4. Variable disease expression with disease onset between adolescence and middle-adult years. Facial muscle weakness (cannot whistle) occurs first. Scapulohumeral weakness leading to winged scapulae is a prominent feature. Lower extremities are less involved. CK is elevated up to five times normal, and inflammation can be seen on muscle biopsy.
    - **Dysferlinopathies**: there are 19 dysferlinopathies. The most common type that can be confused with polymyositis is:
    —**Limb-girdle muscular dystrophy (type 2B).** Autosomal recessive disease. This type is caused by a mutation of the *dysferlin* gene on chromosome 2 that codes for a protein important in muscle repair. Patients have progressive lower extremity followed by upper extremity proximal muscle weakness beginning in second to fourth decades. Facial muscles and heart are spared and winged scapulae are not seen. The disease slowly progresses leading to being wheelchair-bound in 10 to 30 years. This dystrophy is the one most readily confused with adult polymyositis because CK is elevated and inflammatory infiltrates may be seen on muscle biopsy. Does not respond to corticosteroids.
    - **Sarcoglycanopathy.** Autosomal recessive disease caused by mutations of sarcoglycans in the sarcolemma. The sarcoglycans are a family of transmembrane proteins ($\alpha, \beta, \gamma, \delta$, or ε) involved in the protein complex responsible for connecting the muscle fiber cytoskeleton to the extracellular matrix, preventing damage to the muscle fiber sarcolemma through shearing forces. Patients have a limb-girdle and Duchenne-like dystrophy by age 6 to 8 years old. Progression of weakness can be rapid. Cardiomyopathy occurs in 30%. Serum CK levels are high. Does not respond to corticosteroids.
    - **Myotonic dystrophies.** Autosomal dominant diseases. **Type 1** has temporal atrophy, sternocleidomastoid muscle wasting, ptosis, distal limb weakness, and systemic features (balding, cataracts,

cardiorespiratory, and gastrointestinal involvement). Characteristic physical finding is delayed relaxation and muscle stiffness (myotonia). Inability to relax handgrip when shaking hands and myotonic contraction of thumb when thenar eminence musculature is hit with a reflex hammer are commonly observed. EMG shows excessive insertional activity and a "dive bomber" sound with contraction of muscle. Ringed myofibers seen in 70% on muscle biopsy and atrophy of type 1 fibers is prominent.
Type 2 has proximal muscle weakness, muscle pain, cataracts, intermittent and asymmetric myotonia, tremors, cardiac disturbances (heart block), and hypogonadism. Neck flexors, hip flexors, and triceps are affected most commonly. CK is elevated up to four times normal.
- **Congenital myopathies** (e.g., central core, nemaline rod, etc.): attributable to multiple different protein polymorphisms.

BIBLIOGRAPHY

Albert DA, Cohen JA, Burns CM, et al: When should a rheumatologist suspect a mitochondrial myopathy? Arth Care Res 63:1497–1502, 2011.
Berardo A, DiMauro S, Hirano M: A diagnostic algorithm for metabolic myopathies, Curr Neurol Neurosci Rep 10:118–126, 2010.
Cardamone M, Darras B, Monique M: Inherited myopathies and muscular dystrophies, Semin Neurol 28:250–259, 2008.
DiMauro S, Garone C, Naini A: Metabolic myopathies, Curr Rheumatol Rep 12:386, 2010.
Devries M, Tarnopolsky M: Muscle physiology in healthy men and women and those with metabolic myopathies, Phys Med Rehabil Clin N Amer 20:101–131, 2009.
Manzur AY, Muntoni F: Diagnosis and new treatments in muscular dystrophies, J Neurol Neurosurg Psychiatry 80:706–714, 2009.
van Adel B, Tarnopolsky M: Metabolic myopathies: update 2009, J Clin Neuromusc Dis 10:97–121, 2009..

FURTHER READING

www.mda.org
www.neuro.wustl.edu/neuromuscular/index.htlm

CHAPTER 73

AMYLOIDOSIS

James D. Singleton, MD

KEY POINTS

1. Systemic amyloidosis is protean in its manifestations and frequently mimics more common rheumatic conditions.
2. Abdominal fat pad aspiration is the easiest and most sensitive method of obtaining tissue to examine for amyloid deposition.
3. Diagnosis is established by tissue biopsy and polarized microscopy of Congo red-stained tissue.
4. Treatment varies depending on type of amyloidosis: AL by eliminating clonal B cells; AA by controlling chronic inflammation; ATTR by liver transplantation.

1. What is amyloidosis?

Amyloidosis is a disorder of protein folding in which normally soluble proteins are deposited as an insoluble proteinaceous material in the extracellular matrix of tissue. At least 27 precursor proteins can form amyloid. The deposits may be localized to one organ or may be systemic. Amyloid deposition may be subclinical or may produce a diverse array of clinical manifestations.

2. Why is it called amyloid? How does its deposition result in clinical disease?

In 1854, Rudolph Virchow coined the term *amyloid* (starchlike) owing to the reaction of the material with iodine and sulfuric acid. This designation has been retained despite the recognition of the proteinaceous nature of amyloid. Amyloid deposits encroach on parenchymal tissues, compromising their function. Organ compromise is related to the location, quantity, and rate of deposition which varies within and between types of amyloid.

3. Describe the structure of amyloid.

All amyloid shares a unique ultrastructure as seen by electron microscopy. Thin, nonbranching protein fibrils constitute approximately 90% of amyloid deposits. Fibrils tend to aggregate laterally to form fibers. X-Ray diffraction studies show that the polypeptide chains are oriented perpendicularly to the long axis of the fibril, forming a cross β-pleated sheet conformation. Serum amyloid P-component (SAP), a protein composed of two pentagonal subunits forming a doughnutlike structure, makes up 5%. SAP is 50% homologous to C-reactive protein but not an acute phase reactant. The remainder of amyloid is composed of small amounts of certain glycosaminoglycans (GAGs) including heparan sulfate and dermatan sulfate.

4. Describe the light microscopic appearance of amyloid.

Without staining, amyloid appears as a homogeneous, amorphous, hyaline extracellular material. It is eosinophilic when stained with hematoxylin–eosin and metachromatic with crystal violet. Amyloid stains homogeneously with *Congo red* (congophilic) as a result of its β-pleated sheet configuration. Viewing of Congo red-stained tissue under polarized microscopy yields the pathognomonic *apple green birefringence*.

5. Where do the amyloid proteins come from and why does amyloid deposition occur?

Fibrillar amyloid proteins are derived from either an intact protein or a fragment of a larger precursor molecule. There are four circumstances that predispose to amyloid deposition:
- Sustained high concentrations of normal proteins (i.e., serum amyloid A in chronic inflammation and β2-microglobulin in renal failure).
- Exposure to normal concentrations of a weakly amyloidogenic protein over a prolonged period (i.e., β-protein in Alzheimer's disease).
- Acquired protein with an amyloidogenic structure (i.e., monoclonal immunoglobulin light chains in AL amyloid).
- Inherited variant protein with an amyloidogenic structure (i.e., transthyretin, others).

The pathogenesis of why certain proteins are capable of depositing as amyloid fibrils is unclear. Notably, little tissue reaction occurs around amyloid and, once deposited, amyloid resists proteolysis and phagocytosis. Features of the precursor proteins and/or host factors could result in abnormal processing by mononuclear phagocytic cells or ineffective degradation. Certain protein variants are "amyloidogenic," and may be more susceptible to the processing that leads to amyloidosis. For example, in systemic AL amyloidosis, the immunoglobulin light chain λ VI is highly associated with amyloidosis, whereas the more common κ light chains are not. In systemic AA amyloid, certain phenotypes of SAA are more likely to form amyloid, whereas in hereditary systemic amyloidosis single amino acid variants of transthyretin (TTR) are most commonly found. Finally, in addition to these amyloidogenic precursor proteins undergoing misfolding, SAP and certain GAGs may contribute to the seeding, aggregation, and deposition of amyloid in tissues.

6. How are the amyloidoses classified?
By the major protein component of the fibril. This has also become the basis for defining the clinical syndromes with certainty. However, routine stains do not identify the major fibril protein, and specific immunohistochemical stains are needed for identification (Table 73-1).

Table 73-1. Classification of Amyloidoses

CLINICAL CATEGORIES	MAJOR PROTEIN TYPES	RELATIVE FREQUENCIES
Systemic AL amyloidosis	AL	50% to 70%
Systemic AA amyloidosis	AA	3% to 18%
Senile transthyretin amyloidosis	AATR	8% to 32%
Localized amyloidosis	AL and others*	–
Dialysis-related amyloidosis	Aβ$_2$M	–
Hereditary systemic amyloidosis	ATTR and others†	1%

*Other localized: Aβ, amyloid β protein – Alzheimer's disease, Down syndrome; AIAPP, islet amyloid polypeptide – type 2 diabetes, insulinoma; ACal, calcitonin – medullary thyroid cancer; AANF, atrial natriuretic factor – atrial amyloid; AMed, lactadherin – aortic media; ALac, lactoferrin – cornea; others.
†Other hereditary (familial): AApoA, apolipoprotein A; AGel, gelsolin; AFib, fibrinogen A alpha; ALys, lysozyme; ACys, cystatin C.

7. What is systemic AL amyloidosis?
Systemic AL amyloidosis in the absence of multiple myeloma was formerly called idiopathic or primary amyloidosis. It is now recognized that this amyloid, similar to that associated with myeloma, is composed of whole or fragments of immunoglobulin light chains. The designation AL was given to reflect the light chain source of this amyloid. AL amyloid appears to represent a spectrum of disease. At one end, the source of light chains is a malignant clone of plasma cells (myeloma-associated). At the other extreme, light chains are derived from a small, nonproliferative plasma cell population (immunocyte dyscrasia).

8. Describe the epidemiology of systemic AL amyloidosis.
Systemic AL amyloidosis occurs in 2% of individuals with monoclonal B cell dyscrasias. Over 80% of cases are associated with "benign" monoclonal gammopathies with the remainder having myeloma or Waldenstrom's disease. Men and women are equally affected. The median age at diagnosis is 65 years, and 99% of patients are >40 years of age. Whites are more frequently affected than other races.

9. What are the most common initial symptoms in patients with systemic AL amyloidosis?
- Fatigue (54%).
- Weight loss (42%).
- Pain (15%).
- Purpura (16%).
- Gross bleeding (8%).

Diagnosis is often delayed as a result of the nonspecific nature of the symptoms. Weight loss can be striking, exceeding 40 lbs (18.1 kg) in some patients and prompting a search for occult malignancy. Pain is more common in those with myeloma (40%) than those without (8%). In those without myeloma, pain is frequently attributable to peripheral neuropathy (10%) and/or carpal tunnel syndrome (20%). Other symptoms are often present in patients with specific organ involvement (dyspnea on exertion and pedal edema with congestive heart failure; paresthesias with peripheral neuropathy; orthostasis, syncope, impotence, and gut dysmotility resulting from autonomic neuropathy).

10. What physical findings are common in patients with systemic AL amyloidosis?
- Edema (most common).
- Palpable liver (34%).
- Macroglossia (10% to 20%) (pathognomonic when present).
- Purpura (16%).
- Carpal tunnel syndrome (10% to 20%): can cause claw hand due to clumping of tendons together.

Edema may occur as a result of nephrotic syndrome, congestive heart failure, and rarely, protein-losing enteropathy. Hepatomegaly is usually of only modest degree. Macroglossia and purpura should particularly raise suspicion of systemic AL amyloidosis; both may be a source of patient complaints and are easily overlooked. Increased firmness of the tongue and dental indentations are helpful in determining the presence of macroglossia. Cutaneous purpura is generally localized to the upper chest, neck, and face. Purpura of the eyelids is a clue that is seen only when the patient's eyes are closed. Gentle pinching of the eyelids may cause bruising (pinch purpura) due to vascular fragility caused by amyloid deposition in blood vessels. Purpura around the eyes is called the "raccoon eyes" sign. Other findings include arthropathy ("shoulder pad" sign), nail dystrophy, adenopathy, and submandibular enlargement.

11. Because symptoms are nonspecific and physical findings insensitive, what clinical syndromes should suggest the presence of systemic AL amyloidosis?

Nephrotic syndrome	Autonomic neuropathy (orthostatic hypotension, gastric atony)
Congestive heart failure	Carpal tunnel syndrome (especially if claw hand)
Peripheral neuropathy	Hepatic disease

The most common initial clinical manifestation is nephrotic syndrome. The major sign distinguishing it from other causes of nephrosis is the finding of a monoclonal protein in the serum or urine (electrophoresis *and* immunofixation should be done). Although overt congestive heart failure can occur in up to one third of patients, amyloid deposits in the heart are eventually seen on imaging in 90%. Peripheral neuropathy clinically resembles the neuropathy seen in diabetes, including the chronic course. Autonomic neuropathy may be superimposed on peripheral neuropathy or occur alone. A history of carpal tunnel syndrome is a very important clue to the presence of amyloidosis. It is typically bilateral, and surgical release may not provide complete relief.

12. What clues should alert you to the presence of hepatic amyloidosis?
- Proteinuria—high association with nephrotic syndrome.
- Monoclonal protein in serum and/or urine.
- Howell–Jolly bodies in the peripheral blood smear resulting from splenic infiltration causing hyposplenism.
- Hepatomegaly (>15 cm) out of proportion to liver function tests (one third with hepatomegaly will have normal test results).
- Elevated alkaline phosphatase >1.5 times greater than upper limit of normal.

13. Describe some of the characteristic findings in amyloid cardiomyopathy?
- N-terminal pro brain natriuretic peptide (NT-proBNP): normal levels exclude cardiac amyloid. Elevated levels of NT-proBNP and cardiac troponin are predictors of poor survival, especially if they do not decrease with therapy.
- Electrocardiogram: reduced voltage as a result of replacement of myocardium by amyloid.
- Two-dimensional echocardiography has a high sensitivity for detecting amyloid deposits, which can cause a restrictive cardiomyopathy. Symmetric thickening of the left ventricular wall (>12 mm) or thickening of the interventricular septum may lead to an erroneous diagnosis of concentric left ventricular hypertrophy or asymmetric septal hypertrophy. Hypokinesis may suggest prior "silent" infarction. The combination of increased myocardial "sparkling" echogenicity and increased septal thickness (>6 mm) is 60% sensitive and 100% specific for the diagnosis of amyloidosis.
- Cardiac magnetic resonance imaging (MRI) shows diffuse subendocardial late gadolinium enhancement.

14. Name three presentations of amyloidosis that mimic other rheumatic diseases.
Vascular involvement by amyloid can lead to claudication of the extremities and jaw as seen in temporal arteritis. Amyloid arthropathy can mimic rheumatoid arthritis. Clues are the lack of inflammation and frequent hip and shoulder involvement with periarticular amyloid infiltration, which leads to enlargement of the pelvic or shoulder girdle (shoulder pad sign). Synovial fluid analysis can be helpful in detecting amyloid deposits. Infiltration of amyloid into muscle may lead to weakness or pain, simulating polymyositis. Enlargement of involved muscles (pseudohypertrophy) can be striking and may not be associated with other symptoms.

15. Why does amyloid cause bruising and bleeding?
Amyloid deposition in blood vessels can lead to weakening of the vessel wall and easy bruising. A rare manifestation (8%) of AL amyloid is a bleeding diathesis as a result of an acquired factor X deficiency caused by factor X binding to widely deposited amyloid fibrils.

16. Do most patients with systemic AL amyloidosis display only one syndrome?
No. Most patients have widespread disease and more than one syndrome. Carpal tunnel syndrome is seen more often in those with peripheral neuropathy and cardiomyopathy than in other syndromes.

17. What is systemic AA amyloidosis?
Systemic AA amyloidosis was formerly called secondary or reactive amyloidosis. It is attributable to deposition of amyloid A (AA) and can complicate any chronic inflammatory disorder, whether infectious, neoplastic, rheumatic, or familial Mediterranean fever. Notably, up to 7% of patients with AA amyloidosis have no clinically

obvious chronic inflammatory disease. Some of these may have an undiagnosed autoinflammatory syndrome (see Chapter 79) or Castleman's disease. The clinical feature most common in AA amyloidosis is renal involvement (70% to 90%) followed by hepatosplenomegaly. Clinical cardiac disease and autonomic nerve involvement are less common than in AL amyloidosis. Patients with AA amyloidosis attributable to a chronic inflammatory (rheumatic, Crohn's) disease have a slow progression, whereas AA amyloid attributable to an untreated chronic infection can be rapidly progressive.

18. **Name the infectious and neoplastic disorders most commonly associated with systemic AA amyloidosis.**

Infections	Neoplasms
Tuberculosis	Hodgkin's disease
Leprosy	Non-Hodgkin's lymphoma
Chronic pyelonephritis	Renal cell carcinoma
Bronchiectasis	Melanoma
Osteomyelitis	Cancers of gastrointestinal tract, genitourinary tract, lung
Paraplegia complications	
Parenteral drug abuse	

19. **What three rheumatic diseases are most commonly complicated by systemic AA amyloidosis?**
Older studies reported a 5% to 15% overall incidence of amyloidosis in rheumatoid arthritis, juvenile idiopathic arthritis, and ankylosing spondylitis. With the new therapies available for rheumatoid arthritis, juvenile idiopathic arthritis, and ankylosing spondylitis, the frequency of systemic AA amyloidosis is much less today (<1%).

20. **Other than systemic AL amyloidosis, name two amyloidoses that occur more commonly in the elderly.**
    - **Senile transthyretin (ATTR) amyloidosis**: deposits of normal transthyretin amyloid are common in patients over age 70 years. Males are more commonly affected. The most commonly involved organ is the heart and patients have a restrictive cardiomyopathy.
    - **Aβ protein amyloidosis**: deposits of β-protein in Alzheimer's plaques. It can also be deposited in cerebral blood vessels (cerebral amyloid angiopathy) leading to strokes and hemorrhage which can mimic central nervous system vasculitis.

21. **What is localized AL amyloidosis and how does it present?**
Amyloid may occur in localized deposits, resembling tumors. The lung, skin, larynx, eye, and bladder are common sites. The deposits are attributable to a focal infiltrate of monoclonal B cells that produce amyloidogenic light chains. Progression of this form of localized amyloid to systemic disease or to myeloma is exceedingly rare.

22. **Name three forms of amyloid localized to endocrine tissue.**
ACal (calcitonin)—medullary carcinoma of the thyroid.
AANP (atrial natriuretic factor)—isolated atrial amyloid.
AIAPP (islet amyloid polypeptide)—type 2 diabetes mellitus, insulinoma.

23. **Describe the features of dialysis-related amyloidosis.**
Dialysis-associated amyloidosis is caused by $β_2$-microglobulin amyloid deposits. Serum $β_2$-microglobulin levels are elevated 50 to 100 times normal in patients on long-term dialysis. However, high levels alone do not predict the development of amyloid. Generally, patients with amyloidosis will have been on hemodialysis for at least 5 years. Up to 80% of patients who undergo dialysis for more than 15 years will have evidence of amyloidosis. Carpal tunnel syndrome is the first and most common clinical presentation. Chronic arthralgias, especially of the shoulders, may also occur. Patients can have the shoulder pad sign with inability to raise arms over their head. Persistent noninflammatory joint effusions in large joints can occur in up to 50% of patients. $β_2$-Microglobulin amyloid deposits can be found in the synovial fluid sediment with Congo red staining. A spondyloarthropathy with intervertebral disc destruction (mimics infection) and paravertebral erosions from amyloid deposits has been described. Cystic bone changes (carpals and other bones) can occur due to advanced glycation end products stimulating osteoclasts resulting in cyst formation. Rarely, other areas (skin, gastrointestinal tract, heart) are involved. The treatment is renal transplantation.

24. **Study of many types of hereditary amyloidosis has shown them to be attributable to single amino acid variants of transthyretin (ATTR). What is their pattern of inheritance? How is it treated?**
Familial amyloid polyneuropathy is an autosomal dominant disease with peak onset between 20 and 60 years old. The clinical features are similar to AL amyloidosis. A family history of amyloidosis should be sought and may or may not be present because spontaneous ATTR mutations can occur sporadically. Patients typically have a progressive peripheral and autonomic neuropathy. The heart and conduction system can also be involved. Treatment is liver transplantation, which removes the source of the variant TTR production and replaces it with normal TTR. Death occurs within 5 to 15 years without liver transplantation. A medical

treatment, tafamidis meglumine, is presently in clinical trials. It binds to and stabilizes TTR preventing fibril formation and amyloid deposition.

25. What other forms of hereditary systemic amyloidosis have been reported?
In addition to the 100 variant forms of TTR that have been reported to cause amyloidosis, other variant proteins that can cause amyloid deposits include mutations in genes for cystatin C, gelsolin, lysozyme, fibrinogen A α-chain, and apolipoprotein AI and AII. Due to causing a nephropathy, these autosomal dominant forms of amyloidosis have a worse prognosis than familial amyloidotic polyneuropathy (TTR mutations).

26. How is the diagnosis of amyloidosis established?
Polarized light microscopy showing the characteristic apple green birefringence of Congo red-stained tissue. Immunohistochemical staining of tissue can be done to characterize the amyloid fibril protein type.

27. Which tissue should be biopsied?
A screening biopsy should be performed first, because the sensitivity is good and complications are few. Screening sites and their yields are:

Abdominal fat pad	75% to 90%
Bone marrow	30% to 50%
Rectal mucosa	50% to 84%
Gingiva/labial salivary gland	60%
Skin	50%

Abdominal fat pad aspirate is done by injecting saline into the abdominal wall fat through a 16-gauge needle attached to a 20-mL syringe and sucking back. Fat obtained is processed for Congo red staining. It is positive in 80% to 90% of patients with AL or ATTR amyloidosis and 60% to 70% with AA amyloidosis. Note that 15% of patients with systemic AL amyloidosis will have both a negative abdominal fat pad and bone marrow biopsy.

28. What if the screening biopsies are negative?
If screens are negative, biopsy of a clinically involved site may be undertaken, realizing that the risk of bleeding may be substantial. For this reason, do not biopsy a liver that is grossly enlarged. Yields for clinically involved sites are:

Kidney	90% to 98%
Carpal ligament	90% to 95%
Liver	92% to 96%
Sural nerve	100%
Skin	45% to 83%

29. What additional laboratory and imaging studies should be performed?
- All patients with systemic amyloidosis should be evaluated for evidence of an associated plasma cell dyscrasia by ordering serum and urine protein electrophoresis *and* immunoelectrophoresis *and* free light chains. If all of these tests are negative then it is unlikely that the amyloidosis is attributable to a plasma cell dyscrasia.
- In patients with symptoms consistent with a hereditary systemic amyloidosis, DNA analysis to identify the amyloidogenic variant protein should be performed.
- MRI or ultrasound of involved joints (especially shoulders): ultrasound showing rotator cuff >8 mm thick with echogenic deposits (sensitivity 72%, specificity 97%).
- Radiolabeled (I^{123}) SAP scintigraphy: if available, radioiodine-labeled SAP can be used for establishing extent of disease and monitoring response to therapy.

30. How is systemic AL amyloidosis treated?
The control of light chain production by proliferating plasma cells has been the rationale for the use of cytotoxic agents. Melphalan-containing regimens have been shown to be effective. Dexamethasone is more effective than prednisone in these regimens. Bortezomib and lenalidomide-containing regimens are being investigated and show great promise. High-dose chemotherapy with autologous peripheral blood stem cell transplantation can result in improvement of the patient's clinical condition, but treatment-related toxicity can be high, particularly in patients with cardiac involvement. Any of these therapies need to decrease the serum/urine levels of free light chains by over 50% to increase survival. Digitalis, calcium channel blocker, and β blockers should be avoided in patients with cardiac involvement due to causing adverse cardiac events.

31. What factors are prognostic in systemic AL amyloidosis?
The overall median survival for systemic AL amyloidosis is 12 to 15 months. The most common cause of death is attributable to cardiac involvement. The presence of multiple myeloma reduces the median survival significantly. Grouping of patients by clinical symptoms (heart failure, nephrotic syndrome, peripheral neuropathy, and others) is a useful guide to long-term prognosis. The presence of heart failure is associated with the worst prognosis (median survival, 6 months). The best prognosis is in patients with peripheral neuropathy when it

occurs as the sole manifestation (median survival, 56 months). Although the 24-hour urinary total protein excretion does not affect survival, the presence of an increased serum creatinine and failure of serum/urine free light chains to decrease with therapy are poor prognostic signs.

32. **Describe the treatment and prognosis of systemic AA amyloidosis.**
   Mobilization and clearance of amyloid deposits are possible and are best recognized for patients with AA. A basic tenet is to control the underlying inflammatory disease. Potent biologic agents are available to control the inflammatory arthritides (rheumatoid arthritis, juvenile idiopathic arthritis, and ankylosing spondylitis) and the autoinflammatory syndromes. Prophylactic colchicine (1.2 to 1.8 mg/day) is effective in suppressing the inflammatory episodes and subsequent amyloidosis seen in familial Mediterranean fever. Surgical treatment of osteomyelitis with amputation and aggressive surgical therapy for Crohn's disease has been reported to reverse or resolve nephrotic syndrome. Measurement of SAA levels can monitor success of therapy. Median survival in patients with AA amyloidosis whose underlying inflammatory disease is not suppressed is 5 to 10 years with 40% to 60% dying of renal failure. Eprodisate (Kiacta) is a new antiamyloid drug currently in clinical trials. It is a sulfonated molecule which competitively binds to the GAG-binding sites on SAA and inhibits fibril polymerization and amyloid deposition in tissues such as the kidneys.

BIBLIOGRAPHY

Blancas-Mejia LM, Ramirez-Alvarado M: Systemic amyloidoses, Annu Rev Biochem 82:745–774, 2013.
Dubrey SW, Hawkins PN, Falk RH: Amyloid diseases of the heart: assessment, diagnosis, and referral, Heart 97:75–84, 2011.
Lachmann HJ, Goodman HJB, Gilbertson JA, et al: Natural history and outcome in systemic AA amyloidosis, N Engl J Med 356:2361–2371, 2007.
Merlini G, Seldin DC, Gertz MA: Amyloidosis: pathogenesis and new therapeutic options, J Clin Oncol 29:1924–1933, 2011.
Pepys MB: Amyloidosis, Annu Rev Med 57:223–241, 2006.
Simmons Z, Specht CS: The neuromuscular manifestations of amyloidosis, J Clin Neuromusc Dis 11:145–157, 2010.
Straub JE, Thirumalai D: Toward a molecular theory of early and late events in monomer to amyloid fibril formation, Annu Rev Phys Chem 62:437–463, 2011.

FURTHER READING

www.amyloidosis.org

CHAPTER 74

RAYNAUD'S PHENOMENON
Marc D. Cohen, MD

KEY POINTS

1. Vasospasm of the digital arteries and cutaneous arterioles causes Raynaud's phenomenon (RP).
2. The sequential color changes of RP are white to blue to red.
3. Nailfold capillary microscopy and specific autoantibodies predict which patients with RP are likely to develop a rheumatic disorder.
4. Calcium channel blockers are most efficacious and best tolerated in patients who require therapy.

1. What is RP?
Maurice Raynaud in 1862 described RP, which is a vasospastic disorder characterized by episodic attacks of well-demarcated color changes with numbness and pain of the digits on exposure to cold. It may be primary (idiopathic) or secondary to an underlying condition. Primary RP is also called Raynaud's disease (RD).

2. How common is primary RP? Who gets it?
The prevalence of primary RP (i.e., RD) is estimated to be 3% to 4% in most studies, although it may be higher (up to 30%) in colder climates and more common in women, younger age groups, and in patients with a family history of the phenomenon. The female/male ratio ranges from 4:1 to 9:1. RP appears to be equally distributed among ethnic groups.

3. Which conditions are associated with secondary RP?
Conditions associated with secondary RP may be grouped into seven broad categories: (1) systemic, (2) traumatic (vibration) injury, (3) drugs or chemicals, (4) occlusive arterial disease, (5) hyperviscosity syndromes, (6) endocrine disorders, and (7) miscellaneous causes (Table 74-1).

Table 74-1. Causes of Secondary Raynaud's Phenomenon

CATEGORY	CONDITION
Systemic rheumatic disorder	Systemic sclerosis, limited scleroderma (CREST), mixed connective tissue disease, systemic lupus erythematosus, polymyositis/dermatomyositis, Sjögren's syndrome, rheumatoid arthritis, Buerger's disease, vasculitis, chronic active hepatitis, primary pulmonary hypertension
Traumatic	Rock drillers, lumberjacks, grinders, riveters, pneumatic hammer operators, frostbite
Drugs or chemicals	β Blockers, ergots, methysergide, vinblastine, bleomycin, bromocriptine, cisplatin, tegafur, cocaine, interferon-α, vinyl chloride
Occlusive arterial disease	Postembolic/thrombotic arterial occlusion, carpal tunnel syndrome, thoracic outlet syndromes, crutch pressure
Hyperviscosity diseases	Polycythemia, cryoglobulinemia, paraproteinemia, thrombocytosis, leukemia, cold agglutinins, cryofibrinogen
Endocrine disorders	Carcinoid, pheochromocytoma, hypothyroidism
Miscellaneous	Infections (bacterial endocarditis, Lyme borreliosis, infectious mononucleosis, viral hepatitis), complex regional pain syndrome, peripheral arteriovenous fistula, carcinoma (ovarian, angiocentric lymphoma)

4. **Discuss the relevant pathophysiology of RP.**
   Digital artery blood flow is dependent on a pressure gradient that, in turn, is dependent on vessel length, blood viscosity, and vessel radius. The radius of a vessel is most subject to change and may be altered by variations in wall thickness, intrinsic smooth muscle tone, and sympathetic nervous system activity. A given reduction in radius results in a *fourfold* decrease in blood flow (law of Poiseuille).
   Vasospasm of the digital arteries and cutaneous arterioles causes RP. Neural signals, circulating hormones, and mediators from immunomodulatory cells and endothelial cells all interact to control blood vessel reactivity. Neural signals from sympathetic, parasympathetic, and sensory motor fibers include epinephrine, vasopressin, bradykinin, histamine, leukotrienes, norepinephrine, acetylcholine, substance P, and calcitonin gene-related peptide. Mediators from circulating cells include serotonin and adenosine triphosphate/adenosine diphosphate (ATP/ADP). Mediators from endothelial cells include prostacyclin, endothelin, and other contractile factors.
   Epinephrine directly acts on α-2 adrenoreceptors on the smooth muscle cells of small arteries causing vasoconstriction. A defect allowing activation of cold sensitive α-2 receptors on vascular smooth muscle may be present. Other substances may indirectly act by activating endothelial cells to produce vasodilators (e.g., nitric oxide) or vasoconstrictors (e.g., endothelin-1). Vascular smooth muscle may also directly react to circulating hormonal or environmental stimuli.

5. **Compare the pathophysiology of primary RP to secondary RP.**
   - **Primary RP**: increased sensitivity to cold temperatures is attributable to a defect causing an increase in α-2 adrenergic responses in the digital and cutaneous vessels. It has not been determined if this is due to an increase in expression or sensitivity of the α-2 adrenergic receptors. Notably the blood vessel is structurally normal.
   - **Secondary RP**: the underlying vascular disease disrupts the normal mechanisms responsible for control of vessel reactivity. For example, in scleroderma significant endothelial cell dysfunction and apoptosis associated with increased platelet adhesion results in intimal proliferation causing reduced vessel lumen size. Increased activity of reactive oxygen species that follows ischemic reperfusion injury may then alter smooth muscle α-2 adrenergic receptor expression increasing vessel reactivity to cold, emotion, and pain.

6. **Describe the triphasic color response of RP and briefly explain the pathophysiology of each phase.**
   The sequential color changes of RP are *white to blue to red*. Initial digital artery vasospasm causes a **pallor** (blanching) of the digit (Figure 74-1), which gives way to **cyanosis** as static venous blood deoxygenates. With rewarming, the ischemic phase lasts 15 to 20 minutes followed by reactive hyperemia which causes the final stage, **rubor**. The classic triad in the classic order may not be seen in all patients. *Pallor is the most definitive phase.*

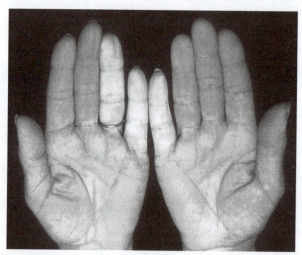

Figure 74-1. The pallor (blanching) stage of Raynaud's phenomenon. (*Copyright 2014 American College of Rheumatology. Used with permission.*)

7. **Contrast the clinical presentations of primary RP and secondary. RP.**
   The onset of primary RP usually occurs in women between the ages of 15 and 30 years. The fingers are most commonly affected, but 40% of patients also have attacks in the toes. Ears, nose, tongue, lips, and nipples may also be involved. For reasons unexplained, the thumbs are frequently spared. The well-demarcated color changes

involve part or all of one or more digits (never the "whole hand") on exposure to cold. The color changes may be accompanied by numbness during the ischemic phase and by a throbbing pain during the reactive hyperemic phase. The frequency, duration, and severity of attacks vary widely, with some patients having several attacks per day and other having two or three per winter. Primary RP patients should not develop trophic complications such as digital ulceration, pitting, fissuring, and gangrene. Nailfold capillary examination and serologies are normal/negative.

The onset of secondary RP is usually in the third and fourth decades and may be seen in either men or women depending on the underlying condition. The symptoms of digital vasospasm are the same as those of primary RP; however, secondary RP patients are more prone to trophic complications. Signs and symptoms related to an underlying condition may be seen on careful history and physical examination. Nailfold capillary examination and serologies can be abnormal depending on the underlying disease.

8. **Is cold the only precipitant of RP?**

    Cold exposure is by far the most common precipitating cause of RP, especially when accompanied by pressure. Typical examples would be the gripping of a cold steering wheel, holding a cold soft drink can, or grasping items in the frozen food section of a grocery store. An attack of RP can also occur after stimulation of the sympathetic nervous system such as with pain and emotional distress. Other potential stimuli include trauma, hormones, and certain chemicals such as those found in cigarette smoke. Additional "causes" such as vibration injury are more correctly attributed to the associated conditions of secondary RP.

9. **Is the vasospasm of RP restricted to digital vessels?**

    A large case-control study has demonstrated an increased frequency of migraine headaches and chest pain in patients with primary RP. Reversible livedo reticularis (cutis marmorata), which is a violaceous mottling of the skin of the arms and legs, sometimes with regular unbroken circles, can be seen. Other studies have implicated vasospasm of the myocardium, lungs, kidneys, esophagus, and placenta. Although definitive proof is lacking, RP is probably a systemic vasospastic disorder.

10. **In the evaluation of a patient with RP, what abnormalities may be noted on physical examination?**

    Patients may occasionally come to the clinic with an ongoing attack of RP, thereby allowing a definitive diagnosis. Induction of an attack in the physician's office by submergence of hands in an ice water bath is frequently unsuccessful, seldom necessary, and sometimes dangerous.

    The physical examination in primary RP is normal. The real goal in patients with RP is to discern the presence or absence of findings attributable to an underlying condition of secondary RP. A careful search for evidence of an underlying rheumatologic disease is required. Abnormal peripheral pulses or asymmetric involvement suggests peripheral vascular disease or perhaps thromboembolic disease. Puffy hands, tendon friction rubs, sclerodactyly, or telangiectasia suggest scleroderma or its variants. Examination for thoracic outlet syndrome (Adson's test) should be performed. Nailfold capillary microscopy may be useful.

11. **Describe the technique, clinical findings, and prognostic value of nailfold capillary microscopy.**

    Along with the retina, the nailfold represents one of the only sites in the body where direct visualization of the vasculature is possible. Nailfold capillary microscopy (NCM) involves the placement of a drop of immersion oil or surgical lubricant on the cuticle of one or more digits (usually the ring or middle fingers), and visualization of the capillaries through an ophthalmoscope set at 40 diopters.

    The normal nailbed demonstrates a confluent distribution of fine capillary loops (Figure 74-2). Dilated tortuous capillary loops and areas of avascularity ("dropout") are often demonstrated in patients with underlying rheumatologic diseases such as systemic sclerosis, dermatomyositis, and mixed connective tissue disease. Up to 1% of patients initially diagnosed with primary RP will transition to a connective tissue disease (usually CREST) each year. NCM is the best test to predict which patients with primary RP are at risk. A normal NCM connotes an excellent prognosis and rheumatologic disease rarely develops in these patients.

12. **Which laboratory studies are worthwhile in the evaluation of a patient with RP?**

    To date, no laboratory test is pathognomonic of RP. In primary RP, laboratory tests should be normal or negative, although up to one third of patients will exhibit low titer antinuclear antibodies in their serum. Less than 25% of these patients develop an autoimmune disorder unless they have a nucleolar pattern. In patients with clinical evidence suggestive of an underlying collagen vascular disease, appropriate studies for the presence of a hypercoagulable state, cryoglobulins, hypothyroidism, and anticentromere, anti Th/To, and antitopoisomerase antibodies should be considered. The presence of an abnormal NCM and abnormal serology (anticentromere, etc.) is more predictive of developing a rheumatic disease than either one alone.

13. **Describe the usefulness of vascular or other studies in the diagnosis of RP.**

    Doppler studies of vessels in the palmar arch may be helpful. Finger photoplethysmography and blood pressure studies at ambient temperature may also be useful, with abnormal waveforms or brachial-finger pressure gradients over 20 mm Hg suggesting a proximal fixed obstruction.

    Arteriography or magnetic resonance arteriography may reveal an embolic source but is usually not necessary. Similarly, nerve conduction studies may suggest a nerve compression syndrome and a chest radiography may demonstrate a cervical rib.

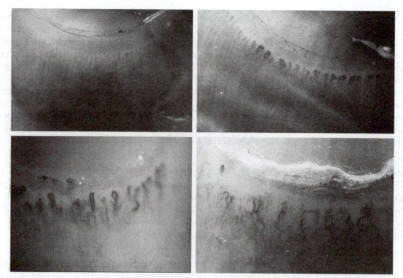

Figure 74-2. Nailfold capillary microscopy. Normal pattern (*upper left*). Dilated capillary loops in systemic sclerosis (*upper right*). Dilated loops and avascularity in adult dermatomyositis (*lower left*). Childhood dermatomyositis (*lower right*). (*Copyright 2014 American College of Rheumatology. Used with permission.*)

14. **List the "red flags" that would be worrisome for the potential presence or later development of a disease associated with secondary RP.**
    - Onset of digital vasospasm after age 40 years.
    - Male gender.
    - Asymmetric attacks.
    - Trophic changes in the digits (ulcers, pits, gangrene).
    - Ischemic signs/symptoms proximal to fingers or toes.
    - Abnormal NCM.
    - Sclerodactyly, rashes, or other obvious evidence of an underlying condition.
    - Serologic presence of autoantibodies, especially anticentromere antibodies or antibodies against a specific nuclear antigen (SCL-70, Th/To, RNP, Sm, SS-A, SS-B).

15. **Which general measures are important in the treatment of patients with RP?**
    The majority of RP patients respond best to simple prevention measures. Careful planning of one's activities of daily living minimizes unnecessary exposure to cold. Because reductions in core temperature as well as peripheral temperature may induce digital vasospasm, it is important to promote "total body" heat conservation. Loose-fitting, layered clothing, warm socks, hats, and scarves should be worn in addition to gloves or mittens. Tobacco, sympathomimetic drugs (decongestants, amphetamines, diet pills), and β blockers must be avoided. Temperature biofeedback training is also effective in some patients with primary RP.

16. **When is pharmacologic intervention indicated in the management of RP?**
    Most patients with primary RP will not require pharmacologic therapy. Those with secondary RP more often require (but less often respond to) medication. Therapy of secondary RP should address the underlying disorder and the vasospasm. Pharmacologic intervention is indicated in patients who suffer frequent, prolonged, and/or severe episodes of RP in the setting of adequate preventative measure or with minimal provocation. Patients who manifest evidence of ischemic injury (digital pitting, etc.) should definitely be considered for medical management. Many patients who do require medication may only need it during the colder months of the year. β Blockers and smoking should be discontinued. Any evidence of digital infection should be treated with antibiotics. Analgesics may be necessary to reduce pain, which can contribute to vasospasm.

17. **Which medications have been useful in the management of the vasospastic component of RP?**
    All available therapies work better in primary RP than secondary RP.
    Calcium channel blockers: nifedipine, amlodipine, diltiazem, felodipine, nisoldipine, and isradipine are best tolerated and most efficacious as vasodilators. As a group they improve symptoms in 35% of patients with primary RP. Verapamil and nicardipine are not effective. Nifedipine also inhibits platelet activation, which may increase its effectiveness. Slow-release preparations are most commonly used. Potential side effects include edema, constipation, lightheadedness, and worsening gastroesophageal reflux. These drugs should not be used

in pregnancy. Patients with compromised left ventricular function should use a calcium channel blocker of the dihydropyridine class (i.e., nifedipine, amlodipine).
Sympatholytic agents: prazosin or phenoxybenzamine have been beneficial particularly with short-term use. They lose their effectiveness with long-term use. Postural hypotension may limit their usefulness. Presynaptic sympathetic inhibitors such as reserpine and guanethidine are rarely used because the other drugs are more effective and better tolerated.
Direct vasodilators: these are used if patients fail to respond to or tolerate calcium channel blockers. Topical nitrates may be helpful. Patients use a quarter to a half an inch of topical 2% nitroglycerin ointment applied two times daily: once in the morning on arising and repeated 6 hours later. A rest from nitrates for 12 hours is necessary to prevent development of a refractory state. The dose can be increased. It is best to use topical therapy on only a few digits that are most severely involved. It is important to warn patients not to touch their eyes while it is on. Alternatively, a nitrate patch can be used. Headache is a common limiting side effect. Nitrates can be used in combination with calcium channel blockers. Other direct vasodilators include hydralazine, minoxidil, and niacin.
Indirect vasodilators: fluoxetine (20 mg/day), losartan, sildenafil (50 mg two times daily), and bosentan have all been reported in some trials to be effective.
Prostaglandins: PGI_2 (epoprostenol), PGI_2 analog (iloprost), and PGE_1 (alprostadil) are vasodilators and platelet aggregation inhibitors. They are only available intravenously and, overall, their availability is limited, expensive, and not widely studied in RP. Iloprost (an analog of prostacyclin) is beneficial in patients with severe RP and may be tried to prevent severe vasospastic digital damage. Toxicity is common and includes chest pain, headache, and nausea. Oral iloprost and misoprostol (oral PGE_1) are no better than placebo.
Others: antiplatelet drugs (aspirin, dipyridamole) and pentoxifylline (Trental) have demonstrated minimal benefit, particularly in severe RP. Full anticoagulation is not recommended unless there is embolization or new thrombosis, although low-dose anticoagulation may be helpful in patients with systemic sclerosis. Thrombolytic therapy needs to be further studied.
Note that all vasodilators are nonselective and may vasodilate healthy vessels, stealing blood flow from diseased vessels and making RP worse in some digits. This must be monitored, especially in patients with secondary RP.

18. **Describe an approach to treatment of patients with RP.**
    - Step 1—make sure to institute general measures. Heat conservation and cold protection.
    - If general measures are not significantly effective, use medications. Try to use only during cold months.
    - Step 2—start nifedipine XL 30 mg/day, amlodipine 5 mg/day, or diltiazem (Cardiazem CD, Dilacor XR) 120 mg/day. If no response in 2 weeks, increase dose every 2 to 4 weeks until the maximum is reached (nifedipine XL 180 mg/day, amlodipine 20 mg/day, Cardiazem CD 360 mg/day, or Dilacor XR 480 mg/day) or side effects develop.
    - Step 3—add topical nitrates, sildenafil, or prazosin. If prazosin is used start with 1 mg test dose while lying down and increase it slowly to as high as 5 mg three times daily or side effects develop.

19. **What can be done medically in patients with acute ischemic crisis that is digit threatening?**
    - Step 1—put to rest in a warm and quiet environment in the hospital.
    - Step 2—control pain. Chemical digital or limb sympathectomy preferable over narcotics, which can cause vasospasm. Chemical sympathectomy helps open blood vessels so medication can get to the digits. Narcotics can be used if needed.
    - Step 3—start one of following vasodilator therapies:
        - Calcium channel blocker—start amlodipine (5 mg to 10 mg) or nifedipine XL (30 mg to 60 mg) and titrate.
        - Intravenous prostaglandins—epoprostenol (PGI_2), alprostadil (PGE_1), or iloprost (PGI_2) if available.
    - Step 4—antiplatelet therapy with aspirin 81 mg/day.
    - Step 5—anticoagulation with heparin during acute crisis can be considered especially if antiphospholipid antibodies are present.

20. **What surgical options can be done for patients who are refractory to standard therapy?**
    Surgical sympathectomy may be considered in patients in whom more conservative measures have failed and who present with impending digital necrosis or evidence of recurrent ischemic complications. It can be performed at the cervical, lumbar, or digital levels. Permanent surgical ablation may be preceded by demonstrating efficacy using a bupivacaine stellate ganglion block or epidural infusion. Sympathectomies may not provide long-term benefits, although digital sympathectomy may restore blood flow to fingers immediately. In patients with infarcted digits unresponsive to treatment, amputation for pain control is the best option.

21. **What is the prognosis for patients with RP?**
    The prognosis for patients with primary RP is excellent. In 10% of patients, attacks disappear completely. Digital vascular complications rarely occur. The vast majority of patients with primary RP never develop an

underlying condition such as those associated with secondary RP. This is especially true if NCM and autoantibody testing are negative.

The prognosis for patients with secondary RP is generally dependent on the underlying condition. Intrinsic vascular disease is often present. Complications arising from vasospasm such as digital ulcerations are common.

BIBLIOGRAPHY

Chikura B, Moore TL, Manning JB, et al: Sparing of the thumb in Raynaud's phenomenon, Rheumatology (Oxford) 47:219, 2008.
De LaVega AJ, Derk CT: Phosphodiesterase-5 inhibitors for treatment of Raynaud's: a novel indication, Expert Opin Investig Drugs 18:23, 2009.
Henness S, Wigley FM: Current drug therapy for scleroderma and secondary Raynaud's phenomenon: evidence-based review, Curr Opin Rheumatol 19:611, 2007.
Herrick AL: Pathogenesis of Raynaud's phenomenon, Rheumatology (Oxford) 44:587, 2005.
Hirschl M, Hirschl K, Lenz M, et al: Transition from primary Raynaud's phenomenon to secondary Raynaud's phenomenon identified by diagnosis of an associated disease: results of ten years of prospective surveillance, Arthritis Rheum 54:1974, 2006.
Ingegnoli F, Boracchi P, Gualtierotti R, et al: Prognostic model based on nailfold capillaroscopy for identifying Raynaud's phenomenon patients at high risk for development of a scleroderma spectrum disorder: PRINCE, Arthritis Rheum 58:2174, 2008.
Koenig M, Joyal F, Fritzler MJ, et al: Autoantibodies and microvascular damage are independent predictive factors for progression of Raynaud's phenomenon to systemic sclerosis: a twenty-year prospective study of 586 patients, with validation of proposed criteria for early systemic sclerosis, Arthritis Rheum 58:3902, 2008.
Korn JH, Mayes M, Matucci Cerinic M, et al: Digital ulcers in systemic sclerosis: prevention by treatment with bosentan, an oral endothelin receptor antagonist, Arthritis Rheum 50:3985, 2004.
Lambova SN, Muller-Ladner U: The role of capillaroscopy in differentiation of primary and secondary Raynaud's phenomenon in rheumatic diseases: a review of the literature and two case reports, Rheumatol Int 29:1263, 2009.
Scorza R, Caronni M, Mascagni B, et al: Effects of long term cyclic iloprost therapy in systemic sclerosis with Raynaud's phenomenon. A randomized, controlled study, Clin Exp Rheumatol 19:503, 2001.
Thompson AE, Pope JE: Calcium channel blockers for primary Raynaud's phenomenon: a meta-analysis, Rheumatology (Oxford) 44:145, 2005.
Vinjar B, Stewart M: Oral vasodilators for primary Raynaud's phenomenon, Cochrane Database Syst Rev 2:CD006687, 2008.
Wigley FM: Clinical practice. Raynaud's phenomenon, N Engl J Med 347:1001, 2002.
Yee AM, Hotchkiss RN, Paget SA: Adventitial stripping: a digit saving procedure in refractory Raynaud's phenomenon, J Rheumatol 25:269, 1998.

CHAPTER 75

AUTOIMMUNE EYE AND EAR DISORDERS

Korey R. Ullrich, MD

KEY POINTS

1. Ophthalmologic manifestations are common in patients with rheumatologic disease, and causes including uveitis, episcleritis, scleritis, and retinal vasculitis should be considered in any patient with a red eye or ocular symptoms.
2. Infectious causes are in the differential diagnosis of all the common ophthalmologic diseases listed above, and they are particularly important to keep in mind given the immune dysregulation and immunosuppression that is characteristic of this patient population.
3. The various causes of eye disease in the patient with rheumatologic disease can be difficult to distinguish, and urgent referral to an ophthalmologist is necessary for appropriate evaluation and assistance with management.

UVEITIS

1. **What is uveitis and how is it anatomically classified?**
   Inflammation of the middle portion of the eye, which includes the iris, ciliary body, choroid, and vitreous humor (Figure 75-1). Uveitis and iritis are used interchangeably.
   - Anterior uveitis: iris and ciliary body.
   - Posterior uveitis: choroid, with possible extension into the retina (retinochoroiditis).
   - Intermediate uveitis: anterior vitreous, peripheral retina, and pars plana.
   - Panuveitis: when there is no predominant site and all segments are affected.

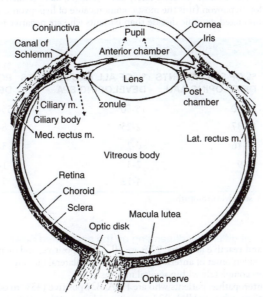

Figure 75-1. Diagram of a human eyeball. (*From Stedman, T: Stedman's medical dictionary, ed 23, Baltimore, 1976, Williams & Wilkins. With permission.*)

2. **List the primary parameters used to characterize subsets of uveitis.**
   1. Anatomic location of inflammation: anterior, intermediate, posterior, or panuveitis.
   2. Laterality: unilateral (can be asynchronous) or bilateral (occurring in both eyes simultaneously).

3. Onset: sudden or insidious.
   4. Duration: limited (≤3 months) or persistent (>3 months).
   5. Course: acute (sudden onset and limited duration), recurrent (repeat episodes separated by ≥3 months), chronic (persistent disease with relapse within 3 months of discontinuation of therapy).

3. **How do the typical presenting symptoms differ among anterior, intermediate, and posterior uveitis?**
   - **Anterior uveitis:** patients usually have complaints of **pain, redness,** and **photophobia.** There may be a variable degree of visual disturbance. Perilimbal injection (ciliary flush) may be present when onset is acute.
   - **Intermediate uveitis:** patients usually complain of **blurry vision, floaters,** and **distortion of central vision.** Typically, the anterior chamber is quiet (i.e., no inflammation), and there is **no pain or photophobia.** Although initial complaints may be unilateral, evidence of mild inflammation in the contralateral eye is common (bilateral disease occurs in 80% of cases).
   - **Posterior uveitis:** patients usually complain of the insidious onset of **blurred vision, floaters,** and **scotomata.** As in intermediate uveitis, the external eye is quiet, and there is **no pain or photophobia.**

4. **List the differential diagnosis of anterior uveitis.**
   Anterior uveitis accounts for 50% to 92% of all cases of uveitis. The most common associations are idiopathic and **HLA-B27-associated** with or without an associated spondyloarthropathy (accounts for 18% to 32% of cases). Other causes include sarcoidosis, Behçet's disease, infectious (bacterial or fungal endophthalmitis, herpes simplex virus [HSV], varicella zoster virus [VZV], cytomegalovirus [CMV], Epstein–Barr virus [EBV], tuberculosis, syphilis, Lyme disease), multiple sclerosis, Posner–Schlossman syndrome, sympathetic ophthalmia, drugs (e.g., intravenous bisphosphonates, rifabutin, cidofovir, sulfonamides), and trauma.
   Juvenile idiopathic arthritis (JIA), tubulointerstitial nephritis and uveitis (TINU), and **Kawasaki disease** are the most common associations in the pediatric population.
   Fuchs' heterochromic iridiocyclitis is a common cause of chronic, unilateral anterior uveitis characterized by iris heterochromia.

5. **How is HLA-B27 associated with uveitis?**
   In Western populations, acute anterior uveitis (AAU) is associated with HLA-B27 in 50% of cases. Over half of the patients with uveitis who are HLA-B27-positive will have or develop a spondyloarthropathy (SpA). Patients with HLA-B27-positive AAU are more likely to be younger, male gender, have an acute course, experience recurrences, develop hypopyon (it is the most common cause of hypopyon-complicated uveitis in North America), and have an associated systemic disease than patients who are negative for HLA-B27 (Table 75-1).

Table 75-1. Association Between HLA-B27 and Uveitis

HLA-B27-ASSOCIATED DISEASE	% OF SPA PATIENTS DEVELOPING AAU	% OF ALL AAU PATIENTS DEVELOPING SPA	% OF HLA-B27-POSITIVE AAU PATIENTS DEVELOPING SPA
Ankylosing spondylitis	20-30	15-50	55-90
Reactive arthritis	12-37	2-25	8-21
Psoriatic arthritis	7-16	0-2	3-4
Enteropathic arthropathy	2-9	2-3	1-7
Undifferentiated SpA	–	4-12	5-21

AAU, Acute anterior uveitis; SpA, spondyloarthropathy.

6. **How does uveitis present differently depending on the associated SpA?**
   Ankylosing spondylitis and reactive arthritis: 90% are HLA-B27 positive, and men are affected more often than women. Typically, sudden onset of **anterior uveitis** that is unilateral but alternating has a recurrent course and usually resolves completely within several months.
   Psoriatic arthritis and enteropathic: patients who are HLA-B27 positive (45% to 60%) can have acute anterior uveitis. However, patients who are HLA-B27 negative with one of these diseases can have the insidious onset of bilateral **posterior uveitis** with a chronic course.

7. **How is the uveitis of JIA unique?**
   Unlike patients with almost all other causes of anterior uveitis, JIA patients with anterior uveitis (15% of all patients with JIA) are usually **asymptomatic** and can have a **normal appearing eye.** As a result, complications of uveitis may develop before the inflammation is detected, so close monitoring is required. Risk factors include young age, female gender, antinuclear antibody (ANA) positivity, and pauciarticular disease.

8. **Define intermediate uveitis and pars planitis.**
   Intermediate uveitis refers to ocular inflammation primarily affecting the anterior vitreous, pars plana, and peripheral retina. It typically affects children and young adults, is bilateral in 80% of cases, and tends to be chronic with periods of exacerbations and remissions. The hallmark finding is **vitritis** that can be associated with aggregates of exudates referred to as "snowballs" or "snowbanks." When anterior segment inflammation is present, it is typically only mild to moderate. Peripheral retinal vasculitis and cystoid macular edema resulting in visual loss may occur. When the condition is idiopathic and pars plana exudation ("snowball" or "snowbank") occurs, it is referred to as **pars planitis**, which accounts for >50% of intermediate uveitis cases.

9. **What systemic diseases have been associated with intermediate uveitis?**
   Sarcoidosis, multiple sclerosis, infection (Lyme disease, syphilis, herpes family viruses, tuberculosis [TB], Whipple's disease, rickettsiosis, human T cell lymphotropic virus [HTLV1], HIV, toxocara), Behçet's disease, and thyroid disease.

10. **Define posterior uveitis and list the differential diagnosis.**
    Posterior uveitis describes inflammation of the choroid, with possible extension into the retina and posterior vitreous. **Toxoplasmosis** is the most common identifiable cause. Other causes include Behçet's disease, sarcoidosis, Vogt–Koyanagi–Harada (VKH) disease, birdshot retinochoroidopathy, serpiginous choroiditis, sympathetic ophthalmia, presumed ocular histoplasmosis syndrome, herpes family viruses, TB, and syphilis. TORCH organisms and toxocariasis may be causes in the pediatric population.
    Birdshot retinochoroidopathy is an idiopathic cause of posterior uveitis that is characterized by multiple, discrete cream-colored spots throughout the retina and choroid (primarily distributed around the optic nerve). It is highly associated with **HLA-A29**.

11. **List the common causes of panuveitis.**
    Behçet's disease, sarcoidosis, toxoplasmosis, VKH disease, herpes family viruses, and TB.

12. **Describe the typical features of VKH disease.**
    It is an idiopathic, bilateral, chronic panuveitis more commonly occurring in **pigmented** races that progresses over phases (prodromal, uveitic, convalescent, and chronic/recurrent). Other features include an aseptic meningitis-like prodrome (lymphocytic pleocytosis of lumbar puncture) and other **neurologic deficits**, **auditory symptoms**, and **cutaneous findings** (vitiligo, poliosis, alopecia). During the convalescent phase, the fundus demonstrates the characteristic **"sunset glow"** appearance resulting from choroid depigmentation. Skin changes do not appear until the convalescent phase and thus cannot be relied on to make an early diagnosis. **Exudative retinal detachments** are a characteristic complication. It must be distinguished from sympathetic ophthalmia, which is a bilateral, autoimmune uveitis resulting from trauma to one eye.

13. **Describe some features that may be useful for distinguishing HSV and VZV from other causes of uveitis.**
    Uveitis caused by HSV and VZV may not be associated with other characteristic ocular, cutaneous, or systemic manifestations, making the diagnosis difficult to establish. An accurate and timely diagnosis is critical so appropriate treatment can be instituted. Suggestive findings include unilateral involvement, marked anterior chamber inflammation, elevated intraocular pressure, iris atrophy or nodules, iris transillumination, and corneal hypoesthesia. Polymerase chain reaction of the aqueous humor may be required for definitive diagnosis.

14. **What masquerade syndromes mimic uveitis? How can they be clinically distinguished?**
    The most common is ocular or central nervous system (CNS) **lymphoma**, but other causes include leukemia, retinitis pigmentosa, melanoma, and retinoblastoma. The diagnosis of a masquerade syndrome may be suggested by the appearance of the eye, age of the patient (e.g., malignancy in a patient >45 years of age with unilateral disease, retinoblastoma in children), presence of neurologic signs or symptoms, or a lack of response to standard uveitis therapy.

15. **List the rheumatic diseases most likely to be associated with uveitis. Compare their typical onset, laterality, and location.**
    A list of the rheumatic diseases most likely to be associated with uveitis is presented in Table 75-2.

Table 75-2. Rheumatic Diseases Most Likely to Be Associated With Uveitis

RHEUMATOLOGIC DISEASE	ONSET	LATERALITY	LOCATION
HLA-B27-positive spondyloarthropathy	Sudden	Unilateral	Anterior
Psoriatic arthritis, enteropathic (non-B27 positive)	Insidious	Bilateral	Posterior
Juvenile idiopathic arthritis	Insidious	Bilateral	Anterior
Sarcoidosis	Sudden	Bilateral	Anterior
Behçet's disease	Sudden	Bilateral	Panuveitis

16. **List some common causes of uveitis based on the pattern of disease.**
    A list of some common causes of uveitis based on the pattern of disease is given in Table 75-3.

Table 75-3. Common Causes of Uveitis Based on the Pattern of Disease*

Anterior	
—Acute recurrent unilateral	SpA (B27 positive), idiopathic (HLA-B27 and non-HLA-B27-associated), herpes viruses (HSV, VZV)
—Acute nonrecurrent unilateral	Idiopathic (HLA-B27 and non-HLA-B27 associated), SpA, herpes viruses
—Acute bilateral	Idiopathic non-HLA-B27-associated, **TINU**, Behçet's disease, Sjögren's syndrome
—Chronic	Idiopathic non-HLA-B27-associated, JIA, Sjögren's syndrome, sarcoidosis, SpA, Lyme disease, syphilis, TB
Intermediate	**Pars planitis**, sarcoidosis, multiple sclerosis, Behçet's disease, Lyme disease
Posterior	**Toxoplasmosis, VKH disease, Behçet's disease, sarcoidosis**, herpes viruses, TB, Lyme disease, SpA (PsA, IBD)
Panuveitis	**Toxoplasmosis, VKH disease, Behçet's disease, sarcoidosis**, IBD, herpes viruses, TB, bacterial, fungal

HSV, Herpes simplex virus; IBD, inflammatory bowel disease; JIA, juvenile idiopathic arthritis; PsA, psoriatic arthritis; SpA, spondyloarthropathy; TB, tuberculosis; TINU, tubulointerstitial nephritis and uveitis; VKH, Vogt–Koyanagi–Harada; VZV, varicella zoster virus.
* Behçet's disease, sarcoidosis, Lyme disease, syphilis, and **herpes viruses** can present with any form of uveitis. Various ophthalmologic syndromes (e.g., Fuchs' heterochromic cyclitis, birdshot retinochoroidopathy) are also common causes. No etiology is identified in ~30% of cases.

17. **Which causes of uveitis have been associated with specific HLA types?**

Seronegative SpA	HLA-B27
Behçet's disease	HLA-B51
Birdshot retinochoroidopathy	HLA-A29
Pars planitis	HLA-DR2, HLA-DR15
VKH disease	HLA-DRB1, HLA-DR4, HLA-DQA1
TINU	HLA-DRB1, HLA-DQB1, HLA-DQA1

18. **Which diagnostic workup is of value for a patient with unclassified uveitis?**
    History and physical examination should be used to guide further workup in all cases of uveitis. Routine laboratory tests including complete blood count (CBC), comprehensive metabolic panel, urinalysis, erythrocyte sedimentation rate (ESR), and C-reactive protein (CRP) should also be performed. The need for further workup (e.g., infectious disease studies, imaging, autoantibodies) will depend on the results.
    Chest X-ray: sarcoidosis is part of the differential diagnosis of all patterns of uveitis, and a chest X-ray should be performed in all patients with unexplained disease. It is also a useful screen for TB.
    Syphilis testing: similar to sarcoidosis, syphilis can cause any type of uveitis in the absence of characteristic systemic manifestations. Therefore, serologic testing should be performed on all patients with uveitis of unknown etiology.
    PPD test: positive results do not indicate active disease and can be misleading, so PPD testing should be reserved for cases where there is suspicion for infection (exposure history, chest X-ray findings).
    ANA: indicated only in the evaluation of pediatric patients with pauciarticular onset JIA and uveitis, as it has prognostic implications in these patients. It is not indicated for routine screening of adult patients with unclassified uveitis because it has an extremely low diagnostic and prognostic value unless other features of systemic lupus erythematosus (SLE), Sjögren's syndrome, anti-C1q disease, or another ANA-associated disease are present.
    HLA-B27: only appropriate for patients with acute anterior uveitis, even in the absence of a demonstrable SpA given its prognostic implications.
    Medication history: certain medications such as bisphosphonates, moxifloxacin, and sulfonamides can cause uveitis.
    The following are *not* recommended as part of the initial evaluation:
    ACE level: elevations are a nonspecific finding, and may be seen in sarcoidosis, liver disease, granulomatous infections (TB, leprosy), Gaucher's disease, hyperthyroidism, Hodgkin's disease, and various causes of lung disease.
    Antineutrophil cytoplasmic antibody (ANCA): ANCA-associated vasculitis is an extremely rare cause of uveitis and thus routine testing is not recommended.

19. **Describe general treatment principles of uveitis.**
    Infectious causes should be treated accordingly. Mydriatic and cycloplegic agents are used to alleviate pain and prevent synechiae. Oral nonsteroidal antiinflammatory drugs (NSAIDs) have a limited role in HLA-B27-associated and idiopathic disease. Topical corticosteroids are the hallmark of therapy, but have limited efficacy in posterior disease. Periocular or intravitreal corticosteroids may be useful for more severe cases, or when posterior disease is prominent.
    When the above measures fail, or when disease onset is severe, systemic corticosteroids are indicated (usually started at a dose of 1 mg/kg/day). When systemic steroids are inadequate, not tolerated, or cannot be tapered, steroid-sparing immunosuppressive agents are required. Methotrexate, leflunomide, azathioprine, mycophenolate mofetil, calcineurin inhibitors, cyclophosphamide, chlorambucil, antitumor necrosis factor (anti-TNF) therapy (monoclonals > etanercept), rituximab, and daclizumab have all demonstrated efficacy in the treatment of uveitis.
    In most cases, management strategies for uveitis parallel those of the systemic disease. Cyclosporine, chlorambucil, azathioprine, and infliximab are particularly beneficial in Behçet's disease; rituximab may be a useful alternative to cyclophosphamide in ANCA-associated vasculitis; and infliximab may be efficacious in refractory cases of sarcoidosis and HLA-B27-positive uveitis. Gevokizumab, an antiinterleukin-1 monoclonal antibody, is in clinical trials for treatment of resistant uveitis attributable to Behçet's disease and for treatment of acute, nonanterior, noninfectious uveitis.

EPISCLERITIS/SCLERITIS

20. **What is the clinical classification of episcleritis and scleritis?**
    - Episcleritis (30% to 40% of cases)
      - Simple (78%)
      - Nodular (22%)
    - Scleritis (60% to 70% of cases)
      - Anterior (98%)
        - Diffuse (40%)
        - Nodular (44%)
        - Necrotizing (14%)
          - With inflammation (10%)
          - Without inflammation (4%) (scleromalacia perforans)
      - Posterior (2%)

21. **What are the typical features of episcleritis?**
    Typically acute onset of erythema and discomfort **without pain**. Affects women in two thirds of cases, is bilateral at some point over the course of disease in 50% of cases, and is associated with a systemic autoimmune disorder in 30% of cases. Tends to have a good prognosis, typically resolving in 2 to 3 weeks without complications, but may recur at 1-month to 3-month intervals for several years in up to 60% of cases. Rarely progresses to scleritis (~5%).

22. **What are the typical features of scleritis?**
    Patients typically have **severe, boring**, and **persistent pain** (except with scleromalacia perforans), with associated erythema, photophobia, and tearing. Less commonly, there can be a reduction in visual acuity. Affects women in two thirds of cases. Bilateral disease develops in 30% to 70% of cases, with recurrence rates of up to 70%. Most patients (~95%) maintain the same clinical subtype. Associated with a systemic disease in ~50% of cases, with frequency depending on the subtype (see below). Complications include keratitis, uveitis, glaucoma, cystoid macular edema, and exudative retinal detachment.
    Diffuse scleritis is the most benign form, with ocular complications occurring in 50% of cases, but only 18% experiencing a decrease in visual acuity. Approximately 60% of patients have an associated systemic disease, with rheumatoid arthritis being the most common.
    Nodular scleritis is characterized by local inflammation with a tender immobile nodule. Nodules may have a dark red or violaceous hue. Ocular complications occur in 50% of cases, with <10% experiencing decreased visual acuity. Approximately 45% of patients have an associated systemic disorder such as rheumatoid arthritis.
    Necrotizing scleritis is the most destructive form and can progress rapidly to scleral necrosis. Up to 95% of patients have an associated systemic disorder and ocular complications are common. Its presence may indicate increased activity of systemic vasculitis, and 45% of untreated patients will die from vasculitis complications within 5 years. Can be insidious when not associated with visible inflammation (scleromalacia perforans), and pain and globe perforation are rare in this setting.
    Posterior scleritis may be difficult to diagnose because redness may be absent (unless anterior involvement is also present), and pain and visual disturbance may be minimal. A clue on history and examination may be pain with eye accommodation. Orbital ultrasonography may demonstrate scleral thickening, and magnetic resonance imaging (MRI) and computed tomography scans can also be helpful. Ocular complications occur in

85% of cases, with retinal pathology (cystoid macular edema, exudative retinal detachment) being the most common. Associated with systemic disease in less than one third of patients when posterior involvement is isolated.

23. **How are episcleritis and scleritis differentiated?**
    The superficial inflammation of the loose vascular connective tissue overlying the sclera that characterizes episcleritis explains the historical and examination features that may distinguish it from scleritis. The significant pain associated with scleritis is the primary distinguishing feature. A blue/purple hue, rather than bright red discoloration, may be seen with scleritis; and the presence of avascular areas within the regions of vascular engorgement is highly suggestive of scleromalacia perforans. In episcleritis, application of **phenylephrine** results in rapid resolution of erythema. Episcleritis and scleritis can coexist, which must be remembered when interpreting these results. Urgent evaluation by an ophthalmologist is necessary for an accurate diagnosis.

24. **What systemic autoimmune/autoinflammatory diseases are associated with episcleritis?**
    Association in ~30% of cases: rheumatoid arthritis (11%), inflammatory bowel disease (8%), vasculitis (5%), SLE (3%), other rheumatologic diseases (3%).

25. **What systemic autoimmune/autoinflammatory diseases are associated with scleritis?**
    Association in up to 50% of patients (Table 75-4). **RA is the most common**, usually occurring in the setting of severely disabling and well-established disease. Joint inflammation may be "burnt out," and patients often have other extraarticular manifestations (e.g., systemic vasculitis) seen in this population. When associated with peripheral ulcerative keratitis, RA, granulomatosis with polyangiitis (formally known as Wegener's granulomatosis), relapsing polychondritis, and SLE are most common. Necrotizing scleritis without inflammation (scleromalacia perforans) is seen almost exclusively in RA.

Table 75-4. Systemic Autoimmune/Autoinflammatory Diseases That Are Associated With Scleritis

ASSOCIATED CONDITION	% OF ALL CASES
Rheumatoid arthritis	10.3% to 18.6%
Granulomatosis with polyangiitis	3.8% to 8.1%
Relapsing polychondritis	1.6% to 6.4%
Systemic lupus erythematosus	1.0% to 4.1%
Inflammatory bowel disease	2.1% to 4.1%
Seronegative spondyloarthropathies	0.3% to 3.5%
Other*	≤1%

*Other: Behçet's disease, Takayasu's disease, giant cell arteritis, hypersensitivity urticarial vasculitis, cutaneous vasculitis, hepatitis C virus-associated vasculitis, undifferentiated connective tissue disease, polymyalgia rheumatica, pyoderma gangrenosum, sarcoidosis, and Cogan's syndrome.

26. **What nonrheumatologic diseases should be considered in a patient with episcleritis or scleritis?**
    Infections such as herpes zoster, herpes simplex, aspergillus, TB, syphilis, Lyme disease, pseudomonas, and other bacterial infections account for ~5% of episcleritis and 5% to 10% of scleritis cases. A high index of suspicion must be maintained for infectious causes in the setting of the chronic immunosuppression typical of rheumatology patients.
    Oral and intravenous bisphosphonates, trauma, and malignancies (penetration by ocular adnexal lymphoproliferative lesions and intraocular tumors) are rare causes.

27. **What workup is indicated for a patient with episcleritis or scleritis?**
    A history, medication history, physical examination, chest X-ray, and routine laboratory tests (CBC, comprehensive metabolic panel, urinalysis, ESR, and CRP) evaluating for associated diseases are necessary, with further workup (e.g., ANA, rheumatoid factor [RF], anticyclic citrullinated peptides, imaging, and microbiology studies) depending on clinical suspicion. Routine testing for ANCA should be performed in all patients with scleritis, as positivity may be seen when other manifestations of ANCA-associated vasculitis are absent, and positive results tend to indicate more aggressive disease.

28. **How is episcleritis treated?**
    Initial symptomatic treatment includes cold compresses and topical lubricants. If frequent or prolonged use of topical lubricants is required, preservative-free formulations should be used to prevent irritation. If these measures fail, topical NSAIDs may be tried, but data suggest that they are no more effective than lubricants alone. **Topical corticosteroids** are extremely effective and should be considered the next line of therapy. Oral NSAIDs may be used if there is no response to local therapies, but systemic corticosteroids are rarely required.

29. **How is scleritis treated?**
    Systemic therapy is required for scleritis whether it is isolated or in the setting of systemic disease, and pain is often the best indicator of inflammation control. The selection of therapy is based on the subtype of the disease and any associated systemic features. Oral NSAIDs are generally used as first-line therapy for nonnecrotizing anterior scleritis and may occasionally be effective for idiopathic posterior scleritis.
    If inflammation is not controlled, or in necrotizing and most cases of posterior scleritis, systemic corticosteroids should be used. Subconjunctival corticosteroid injections are a good option for nonnecrotizing scleritis, but should be considered with caution in necrotizing disease because of the risk of scleral melting and globe perforation.
    In cases unresponsive to oral corticosteroids, or when the dose cannot be tapered to an acceptable level, the use of steroid-sparing immunosuppressive agents such as methotrexate, mycophenolate mofetil, azathioprine, cyclosporine, or cyclophosphamide may be required. In one study, additional immunosuppression was required in 23% of diffuse anterior cases, 7% of nodular anterior cases, 70% of necrotizing cases, and 17% of posterior scleritis cases. There are reports of the successful use of anti-TNF therapies and rituximab. Ultimately, the immunosuppressive regimen should be based on the requirements of any associated systemic illness.

RETINAL VASCULITIS

30. **Define retinal vasculitis.**
    Inflammation of retinal vessel walls or perivascular spaces affecting veins more commonly than arterioles (except in polyarteritis nodosa and SLE), and occurring bilaterally in almost all cases. Can be complicated by occlusive disease secondary to obliterative or thrombotic processes. Can be primary or secondary to other ocular inflammatory processes (e.g., posterior uveitis).

31. **What are the symptoms of retinal vasculitis?**
    Painless blurred vision, scotomata, and floaters are most common. Less frequently, dyschromatopsia (difficulty perceiving colors) and metamorphopsia (distorted vision where straight lines appear wavy) may be present. **Pain and redness are uncommon** if vasculitis is not associated with other ocular inflammatory conditions. Can be asymptomatic if only the peripheral vasculature is affected.

32. **What ocular findings are seen in patients with retinal vasculitis?**
    Ophthalmoscopic examination and **fluorescein angiography** are required for the diagnosis. **Vascular sheathing** is the most characteristic feature and correlates with a perivascular infiltrate of inflammatory cells seen on pathologic specimens. Other findings may include cotton wool spots, retinal hemorrhages, retinal or optic disc edema, vitritis, vascular leakage, capillary dropout, and neovascularization.

33. **What is the differential diagnosis of retinal vasculitis?**
    May be inflammatory (vasculitis) or noninflammatory (vasculopathy), with atherosclerosis being the most common cause of abnormal retinal vessels. Otherwise, causes are generally grouped into three categories:
    1. Systemic diseases: **Behçet's disease**, **SLE**, **sarcoidosis**, and **multiple sclerosis** are the most common. It is less frequently associated with nearly every rheumatic disease, including ANCA-associated vasculitides, large and medium vessel vasculitides (e.g., giant cell arteritis), and antiphospholipid syndrome. Primary CNS lymphoma, acute leukemia, paraproteinemias, and cancer-associated retinopathy are other rare causes.
    2. Infectious diseases: toxoplasmosis, TB, Lyme disease, syphilis, cat scratch disease, herpes simplex, and varicella zoster are the most common. Less frequent associations include CMV, HIV, Whipple's disease, HTLV1, brucellosis, and leptospirosis.
    3. Ocular syndromes: idiopathic retinopathy, birdshot retinochoroidopathy, frosted branch angiitis, Susac's syndrome, VKH disease, Eales' disease, frosted branch angiitis, sympathetic ophthalmia, and IRVAN syndrome.

34. **Briefly describe the defining features of Susac's syndrome, frosted branch angiitis, and Eales' disease.**
    Susac's syndrome: a microangiopathy of unclear etiology causing encephalopathy (corpus callosum involvement is prominent), branch retinal artery occlusions, and hearing loss. Headache can be a prominent feature. Diagnosis is based on characteristic clinical features and MRI findings.
    Frosted branch angiitis: an idiopathic cause of diffuse retinal vasculitis with characteristic perivascular translucent sheathing giving a "frosted branch" appearance.
    Eales' disease: peripheral retinal vasculitis affecting young adults, with a higher prevalence in India. A role of TB in the pathogenesis is suspected but not proven.

35. **What laboratory evaluation is indicated in the evaluation of retinal vasculitis?**
    Initial evaluation should include a CBC, comprehensive metabolic panel, urinalysis, ESR, CRP, HIV screening, syphilis serology, chest radiograph, and TB screening (PPD test or interferon-γ release assay). Further evaluation is determined by the results of the history, physical examination, and initial screening studies and is guided by the diagnosis suspected.

36. **Describe the treatment of retinal vasculitis.**
   The treatment of retinal vasculitis depends on the underlying diagnosis, the severity of the disease, and whether the process is unilateral or bilateral. If its cause is infectious, appropriate antibiotic therapy should be initiated. Corticosteroids are needed in almost all cases, including those secondary to infection. Periocular steroids may be used in patients with moderate to severe disease, or in those with unilateral involvement. Systemic steroids are needed when bilateral involvement is present, or in cases of moderate to severe inflammation with a marked decrease in visual acuity.
   Steroid-sparing agents may be needed if there is an inadequate response to steroids or they cannot be tapered, and selection should be based on the underlying disease. Cyclosporine and azathioprine have been used with success, but mycophenolate mofetil, anti-TNF drugs, rituximab, and interferon α-2a may also be effective. Laser photocoagulation and vitreoretinal procedures may also play a role.

IMMUNE-MEDIATED INNER EAR DISEASE

37. **Define immune-mediated inner ear disease (also known as autoimmune inner ear disease).**
   Immune-mediated inner ear disease (IMIED) is a syndrome characterized by *rapidly progressive, bilateral* sensorineural hearing loss (SNHL) that can be responsive to immunosuppressive therapy. It is often accompanied by vertigo (50%), tinnitus, and a sense of aural fullness. It may exist as a primary illness or be associated with a systemic autoimmune disease (30% of cases). Although believed to be autoimmune, definitive evidence of an autoimmune etiology is lacking.
   Caution should be taken to distinguish IMIED from **idiopathic sudden SNHL**, a much more common (85%) cause of SNHL that is *unilateral*, rapidly progresses over 72 hours, usually not associated with vestibular symptoms, and commonly improves within 2 weeks (65% of cases) irrespective of treatment, although corticosteroids are frequently used. Approximately 5% develop Ménière's disease years later. All patients with sudden SNHL should be evaluated for secondary causes including infection (HSV, VZV), vascular (vasculitis, antiphospholipid syndrome, hypercoagulable diseases), medications, neoplasm, and other immune-mediated diseases. Patients with unilateral SNHL cannot hear a tuning fork and localizes the Weber test (tuning fork on forehead) sound to good ear. When they hum the sound localizes to the good ear.

38. **What is the differential diagnosis of IMIED?**
   Ménière's disease, infection (syphilis, Lyme disease, viral, TB, fungal, or bacterial labrynthitis), acoustic or barotrauma, perilymph fistula, hereditary hearing loss, drugs (e.g., aminoglycosides, hydroxychloroquine, NSAIDs, loop diuretics), mass effect from a tumor (acoustic neuroma, metastatic disease, lymphoma) or an abscess, presbycusis, ischemia, multiple sclerosis, basilar migraine, endocrine disease (diabetes mellitus, hypothyroid), and sarcoidosis.

39. **What characteristics help distinguish IMIED from other causes of inner ear dysfunction?**
   - *Relatively rapid time course*, with progression to severe irreversible damage within weeks to months of onset.
   - *Bilateral disease* that may be asymmetric and asynchronous.
   - *Fluctuating course*.
   - *Vestibular symptoms* may be prominent (50%).

40. **How is Ménière's disease distinguished from IMIED?**
   Time course. Hearing loss typically occurs over several years in Ménière's disease rather than the weeks or months in IMIED. These two disease entities may be impossible to differentiate early in the disease course. Some data suggest that a subset of Ménière's disease may be autoimmune in nature, and possibly part of a spectrum of disease including IMIED.

41. **What systemic autoimmune diseases are associated with SNHL?**
   Cogan's syndrome, ANCA-associated vasculitides, relapsing polychondritis, polyarteritis nodosa and other vasculitides, SLE, Sjögren's syndrome, rheumatoid arthritis, Susac's syndrome, antiphospholipid antibody syndrome, Behçet's disease, and sarcoidosis.

42. **What diagnostic workup is indicated in a patient suspected of having IMIED?**
   Immediate referral to an otolaryngologist is necessary. Routine history, physical examination, and diagnostic tests including a CBC, comprehensive metabolic panel, ESR, CRP, testing for syphilis, and an MRI to exclude a retrocochlear lesion should be performed to evaluate for other causes of SNHL or an associated systemic process. Disease severity should be measured at baseline and followed serially with audiograms.
   The role of testing for ANCA, ANA, RF, complement levels, and antiphospholipid studies in patients with no other evidence of a systemic autoimmune illness is unclear. ANA, RF, low to moderate titer antiphospholipid antibodies, and antithyroid antibodies are frequently detected in patients with IMIED and no other features of systemic disease, and they do not seem to have prognostic relevance in this setting.

43. **Are there any specific diagnostic tests for IMIED?**
    Antibodies to a **68-kDa inner ear antigen**, which is a heat shock protein (HSP-70), are seen in up to 70% of patients with IMIED. Owing to low sensitivity, this test is unreliable to establish or exclude a diagnosis of IMIED. However, studies suggest that their presence may have a prognostic role, predicting both a more aggressive course and a more favorable response to steroids. Patients with Cogan's syndrome and other autoimmune diseases associated with SNHL can also have these antibodies (less than 50%). The value of testing for antibodies to **myelin P0 protein** (30 kDa) is controversial but has been detected in 30% of patients with bilateral SNHL.

44. **What is the treatment for IMIED?**
    Corticosteroids should be started at a dose of 1 mg/kg and continued for 2 to 4 weeks. If there is no response they should be tapered off quickly, with tapering at a slower rate (over 1 to 2 months) if a response is noted. Otherwise, there is no consensus regarding treatment because data from clinical trials are limited. In the only randomized, placebo-controlled trial of treatment of IMIED, methotrexate was shown to be ineffective. Cyclophosphamide has been employed for resistant cases, and azathioprine, mycophenolate mofetil, anti-TNF drugs (systemic and intratympanic), rituximab, and intratympanic steroids have also been used with some success (interpretation of these results is limited given the lack of systematic studies). Given the toxicities of these therapies, cochlear implants should be considered as an alternative in severe cases.

COGAN'S SYNDROME

45. **What are the ocular and auricular manifestations of Cogan's syndrome?**
    Nonsyphilitic interstitial keratitis (IK) is the classic ocular manifestation and typically presents as the acute onset of unilateral or bilateral redness, pain, photophobia, and increased lacrimation. Other forms of ocular inflammation, including uveitis, scleritis, choroiditis, and retinal artery occlusion, can occur with or without concomitant keratitis. **Vestibuloauditory dysfunction** is usually acute in onset and presents in a **Ménière-like** manner, with episodes of tinnitus, vertigo, and sensorineural hearing loss. Hearing loss is fluctuating, but progressive, leading to deafness in >50% of cases. Unilateral involvement is typical, but bilateral disease can occur. Vestibular dysfunction may be prominent, manifesting as vertigo, ataxia, and nausea.
    Eye and ear involvement usually occur within 1 to 6 months of each other, but can be separated by years.
    Atypical Cogan's syndrome is defined as non-IK inflammatory ocular manifestations, typical or atypical ocular manifestations with audiovestibular symptoms different from Ménière-like episodes, or >2 years between the onset of eye and ear manifestations.

46. **What is the epidemiology of Cogan's syndrome?**
    Only approximately 250 cases have been reported. The mean age of onset is 30 years, although cases in children and the elderly have been reported. Distribution is equal between males and females, and there are no racial differences. An upper respiratory syndrome precedes the onset in many cases, but no definite infectious etiology has been identified.

47. **What are other common manifestations of Cogan's syndrome?**
    Systemic vasculitis occurs in 15% to 20% of cases, usually affecting the **large-sized and medium-sized vessels**. Involvement of the aorta and its major branches is well described and manifests in a **Takayasu-like** manner. Musculoskeletal complaints are seen in up to one third of patients and include arthralgias, myalgias, and inflammatory arthritis. Constitutional symptoms occur in 50% of cases, mostly when systemic disease is present. Other organ involvement includes gastrointestinal (pain, bleeding, hepatomegaly), cardiac (pericarditis, aortic insufficiency), pulmonary (pleuritis), neurologic (headache, peripheral neuropathy, mononeuritis multiplex, meningitis), dermatologic (nodules, rash), and lymphatic (lymphadenopathy, splenomegaly). Laboratory findings suggestive of inflammation, including elevated CRP and ESR, leukocytosis, thrombocytosis, and anemia, may be present. ANCA, ANA, RF, antiphospholipid antibody tests, and complement levels are usually absent/normal.

48. **What is the differential diagnosis of Cogan's syndrome?**
    Infection (syphilis, chlamydia, TB, viral infection, Whipple's disease), rheumatologic diseases (rheumatoid arthritis, SLE, Sjögren's syndrome, ankylosing spondylitis, systemic vasculitides, relapsing polychondritis, Behçet's disease), sarcoidosis, toxins, Ménière's disease, and VKH disease.

49. **How is the diagnosis of Cogan's syndrome established?**
    It is a **clinical diagnosis** and should be suspected when IK or other ocular manifestations are accompanied by audiovestibular disease in the absence of another underlying disorder (see differential diagnosis above). The presence of either ocular or ear manifestations in isolation can make the diagnosis extremely challenging. Slit lamp examination and audiovestibular testing are necessary. Laboratory evidence of systemic inflammation may be present. There is no role for checking autoantibodies unless clinical suspicion exists for a particular associated disorder. Microbiologic testing and MRI of the brain to evaluate for a tumor causing inner ear disease can be considered.

50. How is Cogan's syndrome treated?

Keratitis almost always responds to **topical corticosteroid therapy**. Topical cyclosporine is sometimes required, but the need for systemic steroids is rare (unless other ocular manifestations are present and dictate therapy). Note that keratitis resolves quickly on systemic corticosteroids. Therefore, immediate eye examination is needed to document keratitis if the patient has other manifestations requiring high dose corticosteroids. Otherwise, keratitis will be missed.

Vestibuloauditory dysfunction is less responsive to therapy in general. Oral **prednisone** is required and should be started at a dose of 1 mg/kg/day immediately. The usual tapering schedule is by 5 to 10 mg every 2 to 4 weeks, with a total duration of 4 to 6 months. Audiovestibular testing should be repeated 2 to 4 weeks after the initiation of treatment, and prednisone should be tapered quickly if no response is noted. A response to additional immunosuppression is unlikely if prednisone has failed. If an initial response is noted, but flares occur as prednisone is tapered, a steroid-sparing agent should be initiated. Cochlear implantation can be considered for end-stage hearing loss.

Systemic manifestations such as vasculitis should be treated by standard immunosuppressants (e.g., cytotoxic agents, mycophenolate mofetil, azathioprine, methotrexate, and cyclosporine).

Bibliography

Albini TA, Rao NA, Smith RA: The diagnosis and management of anterior scleritis, Int Ophthalmol Clin 45:191–204, 2005.
Andreoli CM, Foster CS: Vogt–Koyanagi–Harada disease, Int Ophthalmol Clin 46:111–122, 2006.
Bañares A, Jover J, Fernández-Gutiérrez B, et al: Patterns of uveitis as a guide in making rheumatologic and immunologic diagnoses, Arthritis Rheum 40:358–370, 1997.
Bodaghi B, Cassoux N, Wechsler B, et al: Chronic severe uveitis: etiology and visual outcome in 927 patients from a single center, Medicine 80:263–270, 2001.
Bonfioli AA, Damico FM, Curi AL, et al: Intermediate uveitis, Semin Ophthalmol 20:147–154, 2005.
Chang JH, McCluskey PJ, Franzco F, et al: Acute anterior uveitis and HLA-B27, Surv Ophthalmol 50:364–388, 2005.
Hooper C, McCluskey P, Franzco F: Intraocular inflammation: its causes and investigations, Curr Allergy Asthma Rep 8:331–338, 2008.
Jabs DA, Mudun A, Dunn JP, et al: Episcleritis and scleritis: clinical features and treatment results, Am J Ophthalmol 130:469–476, 2000.
Jabs DA, Nussenblatt RB, Rosenbaum JT: Standardization of Uveitis Nomenclature Working Group: Standardization of uveitis nomenclature for reporting clinical data. Results of the first international workshop, Am J Ophthalmol 140:509–516, 2005.
Jabs DA, Rosenbaum JT, Foster CS, et al: Guidelines for the use of immunosuppressive drugs in patients with ocular inflammatory disorders: recommendations of an expert panel, Am J Ophthalmol 130:492–513, 2000.
Jakob E, Reuland MS, Mackensen F, et al: Uveitis subtypes in a German interdisciplinary uveitis center – analysis of 1916 patients, J Rheumatol 36:127–136, 2009.
Mazlumzadeh M, Matteson EL: Cogan's syndrome: an audiovestibular, ocular, and systemic autoimmune disease, Rheum Dis Clin N Am 33:855–874, 2007.
Miserocchi E, Waheed NK, Dios E, et al: Visual outcome in herpes simplex virus and varicella zoster virus uveitis: a clinical evaluation and comparison, Ophthalmology 109:1532–1537, 2002.
Okada A: Immunomodulatory therapy for ocular inflammatory disease: a basic manual and review of the literature, Ocul Immunol Inflamm 13:335–351, 2005.
Pavesio CE, Meier FM: Systemic disorders associated with episcleritis and scleritis, Curr Opin Ophthalmol 12:471–478, 2001.
Rachitskaya A, Mandelcorn ED, Albini TA: An update on the cause and treatment of scleritis, Curr Opin Ophthalmol 21:463–467, 2010.
Rauch SD: Idiopathic sudden sensorineural hearing loss, N Engl J Med 359:833–840, 2008.
Schreiber BE, Agrup C, Haskard DO, et al: Sudden sensorineural hearing loss, Lancet 375:1203–1211, 2010.
Smith JR, Mackensen F, Rosenbaum JT: Therapy insight: scleritis and its relationship to systemic autoimmune disease, Nat Clin Pract Rheumatol 3:219–226, 2007.
Stacher RJ, Chandrasekhar SS, Archer SM, et al: Clinical practice guideline: sudden hearing loss, Otolaryngol Head Neck Surg 146(Suppl):S1–S35, 2012.
Stone JH, Francis HW: Immune-mediated inner ear disease, Curr Opin Rheumatol 12:32–40, 2000.
Suhler EB, Martin TM, Rosenbaum JT: HLA-B27-associated uveitis: overview and current perspectives, Curr Opin Ophthalmol 14:378–383, 2003.
Walton RC, Ashmore ED: Retinal vasculitis, Curr Opin Ophthalmol 14:413–419, 2003.
Watson PG, Hayreh SS: Scleritis and episcleritis, Br J Ophthalmol 60:163–191, 1976.
Zamecki KJ, Jabs DA: HLA typing in uveitis: use and misuse, Am J Ophthalmol 149:189–193, 2010.

Further Reading

www.uveitissociety.org/pages/index.html
www.uveitis.org/default.html

RHEUMATIC SYNDROMES ASSOCIATED WITH SARCOIDOSIS

CHAPTER 76

Daniel F. Battafarano, DO, MACP

KEY POINTS

1. Sarcoidosis can have a variety of rheumatic manifestations and should be included in the differential diagnosis for inflammatory arthritis, myopathic syndromes, vasculitis, neurologic disease, and uveitis.
2. A patient with acute, inflammatory arthritis involving bilateral ankles should always be evaluated for sarcoidosis.
3. Antitumor necrosis factor (TNF)-α therapy is effective for treatment-resistant cases of sarcoidosis.

1. What is sarcoidosis?
Sarcoidosis derives from Greek "*sarco*," meaning flesh, "*eidos*" meaning like, and "*osis*," meaning condition. The first case was described in 1877 by Dr. Jonathan Hutchinson at King's College Hospital in London. It is a systemic inflammatory disorder characterized by **noncaseating granulomas** that classically involve the lungs but can affect any organ. Because there is no specific test for sarcoidosis, the diagnosis is established when the following criteria are met:
- a consistent clinical and radiographic presentation;
- histologic evidence of widespread noncaseating epithelioid granulomata in more than one organ system;
- exclusion of other granulomatous diseases caused by mycobacterial infection, fungal infection, berylliosis, drugs, and local reactions to tumors or lymphoma.

2. Who is affected by sarcoidosis?
Sarcoidosis occurs worldwide but most frequently among African-Americans and northern Europeans. It typically appears in the third or fourth decade of life, and sex varies among ethnic groups. There is a higher prevalence of disease in first-generation relatives of those with sarcoidosis. The disease is less likely to occur in people who smoke cigarettes.

3. What are the immunopathologic features of sarcoidosis?
Although the antigen(s) responsible for sarcoidosis is unknown, it is generally accepted that this disease occurs in response to an antigen-driven cell-mediated immune response. Genetic factors also play a role in the racial and ethnic variations in prevalence, clinical presentations, and severity of sarcoidosis. Classically, a lymphocytic alveolitis is the first step in pathogenesis. Antigen(s) are processed and presented by antigen presenting cells (type II alveolar epithelial cells, alveolar macrophages, and dendritic cells) bearing human leucocyte antigen (HLA) Class II molecules that are then recognized by CD4+ T cells (Th1). This results in an augmented immune response, increased tissue permeability and cell migration, and production of proinflammatory cytokines. Ultimately, there is clonal expansion of T cells in response to the antigen(s) resulting in persistent inflammation, noncaseating granuloma formation, and potential fibrosis of involved organs. In early and active disease there is an elevated lymphocyte count and increase in macrophage number with a marked increase in CD4/CD8 T lymphocyte ratio in the bronchoalveolar lavage (BAL) fluid. Additionally, there is depression of delayed-type hypersensitivity, imbalance of CD4/CD8 T cell subsets, an influx of T helper cells to sites of activity, hyperactivity of B cells, and circulation of immune complexes. Typical clinical observations related to these immunologic events include peripheral lymphopenia and a low CD4/CD8 T cell ratio (0.8/1.0), cutaneous anergy (70%), polyclonal gammopathy (30% to 80%), and autoantibody production (low titer rheumatoid factor [RF] and/or antinuclear antibody [ANA] in up to 35%).

4. What is the typical clinical presentation of sarcoidosis?
The clinical spectrum is protean, ranging from an abnormal chest radiograph in an asymptomatic individual (up to 50% of patients) to severe multiorgan involvement. A recent large trial (ACCESS trial) confirmed that 95% of patients will have thoracic involvement (an abnormal chest roentgenogram revealing hilar adenopathy, pulmonary infiltrates, or both), 50% have extrathoracic involvement, and only 2% have isolated extrathoracic sarcoidosis. Notably there are significant differences in clinical findings between groups on the basis of race, sex, and age.

5. Describe the respiratory tract manifestations of sarcoidosis.
The entire respiratory tract from sinuses (2% to 18%) to lungs can be involved. Pulmonary involvement is the most common visceral manifestation occurring in 95% of patients. The clinical spectrum ranges from

asymptomatic hilar adenopathy (50%) to interstitial lung disease with alveolitis. Pleural effusions are rare (<5%). Symptoms include dry cough (30%), dyspnea (28%), and chest pain (15%). Lung crackles (20%) and pulmonary hypertension (5% to 15%) are uncommon. Wheezing can occur when there is endobronchial involvement. Hemoptysis and clubbing are rare.

6. **Describe the chest radiographic stages of sarcoidosis and their prognoses.**
   For chest radiographs the **Scadding staging system** is used (Table 76-1). Some investigators add a stage IV for end-stage pulmonary fibrosis. Notably, the stages are not chronologic, do not indicate disease chronicity, and do not correlate with pulmonary function testing. High-resolution computed tomography of the chest can show abnormalities when chest radiographs are normal. The chest radiographic stage at presentation can be used to predict the probability of future spontaneous remission, which can help guide therapy.

Table 76-1. Scadding Chest X-ray Staging System

STAGE	CHEST RADIOGRAPHIC FINDINGS	SPONTANEOUS REMISSION RATE (%)
0	Normal	–
1	Bilateral hilar adenopathy	60-80
2	Bilateral hilar adenopathy with pulmonary infiltrates	30-50
3	Pulmonary infiltrates with lung insufficiency	<20

7. **What are the extrathoracic clinical manifestations of sarcoidosis?**
   The most common extrathoracic manifestations are **cutaneous** and **ocular involvement**. Cutaneous involvement occurs in 30% of patients and they may have the following symptoms: erythema nodosum in early sarcoidosis or subcutaneous nodules, papules, plaques, and lupus pernio in chronic disease. Eye involvement (25%) is typically bilateral and can be the initial manifestation (5%) or occur anytime during the disease. Any area of the eye may be involved but acute anterior uveitis is the most common manifestation. Because eye involvement may be asymptomatic, all patients with sarcoidosis should have a baseline slit lamp examination. **Arthritis** (4% to 38%) and arthralgias are present in up to 50%. Involvement of **skeletal muscle** occurs in 50% to 80%, although most patients are asymptomatic. **Hepatomegaly** (20%) and **splenomegaly** (10%) are common findings but rarely cause significant complications. Bilateral parotid enlargement is seen in 10% and is associated with xerostomia. **Neurologic** findings are observed in 5%, with unilateral facial nerve palsy being most common. Encephalopathy, mass lesions, basilar meningitis, and peripheral neuropathy can also occur. Up to 33% of patients who develop neurosarcoidosis have neurologic manifestations as their initial manifestation of sarcoidosis. **Heart** involvement (5%) presents with arrhythmias, left ventricular dysfunction, and pericarditis. The hypothalamic–pituitary axis may be involved and classically presents as diabetes insipidus. Kidney and gastrointestinal organs are rarely affected. Vasculitis of any size vessel has been described.

8. **Where are granulomas most commonly found on biopsy in sarcoidosis?**
   Tissue biopsy is the gold standard for confirming a clinicoradiographic diagnosis of sarcoidosis. Well-circumscribed, noncaseating granulomas of the epithelioid type are widely distributed and have been reported in many organs. They are most commonly found in the lung (90% if abnormal chest x-ray, 40% if normal chest x-ray, 83% using endobronchial ultrasound-guided transbronchial fine needle aspiration of intrathoracic lymph nodes), liver (50% to 80%), muscle (50% to 80%), minor salivary gland (36%), and bone marrow (17%). When the following organs are clinically abnormal, granulomas can be demonstrated in skin (90%), parotid (90%), lymph node (90%), synovium (80%), and heart (20%). Granulomas may produce elevated serum angiotensin-converting enzyme (ACE) levels and may significantly enhance production of 1,25-dihydrocholecalciferol, which is responsible for clinical hypercalcemia and hypercalciuria.

9. **List the initial evaluation of a patient with sarcoidosis.**
   - Environmental/occupational/medication exposure
   - Physical examination
   - Chest radiography
   - Pulmonary function testing
   - Complete blood count (CBC), complete metabolic profile, creatine phosphokinase (CPK), urinalysis
   - 24-Hour urine for calcium and creatinine
   - Electrocardiogram

- Ophthalmological evaluation including slit-lamp examination
- Tuberculin skin testing
- Biopsies of affected organs with special stains and cultures

10. Is the serum ACE level useful for the diagnosis of sarcoidosis?

The ACE level is elevated in 40% to 90% of all patients with sarcoidosis. Elevations correlate with active pulmonary disease and can normalize with therapy. This enzyme is produced by epithelioid cells and alveolar macrophages at the periphery of granuloma in response to an ACE-inducing factor released by T cells. Elevated ACE levels are not specific for sarcoidosis. Other diseases in which ACE levels can also be elevated include miliary tuberculosis, histoplasmosis, Gaucher's disease, α1 antitrypsin deficiency, hypersensitivity pneumonitis, silicosis, asbestosis, leprosy, Kaposi's sarcoma with human immunodeficiency virus (HIV) infection, cirrhosis, hyperthyroidism, and diabetes mellitus. Additionally, ACE levels are influenced by ACE gene polymorphisms (DD allele). Therefore, an elevated ACE level may be supportive (especially if more than twice the upper limit of normal), but not diagnostic, of sarcoidosis.

11. What are the rheumatic manifestations of sarcoidosis? (Table 76-2)

Table 76-2. Rheumatic Manifestations of Sarcoidosis

MANIFESTATION	FREQUENCY IN SARCOIDOSIS (% OF PATIENTS)	DIFFERENTIAL DIAGNOSIS
Arthritis	4-38	RA, gonococcal arthritis, rheumatic fever, SLE, gout, spondyloarthropathies
Parotid gland enlargement	5	Sjögren's syndrome
Upper airway disease (sinusitis, laryngeal inflammation, saddle nose deformity)	3	Granulomatosis polyangiitis (Wegener's)
Uveitis	19	
Anterior	18	Spondyloarthropathies
Posterior	7	Behçet's
Keratoconjunctivitis	5	Sjögren's syndrome
Proptosis	1	Granulomatosis polyangiitis (Wegener's)
Myositis	3	Polymyositis
Mononeuritis multiplex	1	Systemic vasculitis
Facial nerve palsy	2	Lyme disease

Modified from Hellman DB: Sarcoidosis. In Schumacher HR et al, editors: Primer on the rheumatic diseases, ed 10, Atlanta, 1993, Arthritis Foundation.
RA, Rheumatoid arthritis; SLE, systemic lupus erythematosus.

12. What is Lofgren's syndrome? What is Heerfordt's syndrome?

Lofgren's syndrome is a triad of acute arthritis, erythema nodosum, and bilateral hilar adenopathy in a patient with sarcoidosis. This can be associated with fever and uveitis. The arthritis typically involves the ankles and knees. The acute arthritis usually resolves within weeks but may persist for months (average 3 months). The ACE level is normal in most patients (70% to 85%). Those patients with elevated ACE level are more likely to have recurrence or persistence of the arthritis. Overall, these patients have an excellent response to corticosteroid therapy and have a greater than 90% remission rate. Acute histoplasmosis may simulate Lofgren's syndrome and must be excluded by serologies and cultures.

Heerfordt's syndrome (uveoparotid fever) is a combination of fever, parotid enlargement, uveitis, arthritis, and facial nerve palsy. It occurs most commonly in males and usually has a poor prognosis.

13. How do acute and chronic sarcoid arthritis differ clinically? (Table 76-3)

14. How does sarcoid myopathy present clinically?

Sarcoid myopathy most commonly occurs in patients with multiorgan involvement. Although muscle involvement in sarcoidosis is usually asymptomatic, there are three clinical presentations: nodular, acute myositic,

Table 76-3. Comparison of Acute and Chronic Sarcoid Arthritis

FEATURES	ACUTE	CHRONIC
Initial clinical manifestation	Common	Not seen
Joint involvement	Symmetrical; ankles, knees, wrists, PIP joints	Same as acute, dactylitis
Hilar adenopathy	Common, no pulmonary infiltrates	May be seen with pulmonary disease
HLA association	DR3, DQ2 in whites of northern European ancestry	Not known
Synovial fluid	Usually not obtainable	Inflammatory; <5000 cells/mm^3 (lymphocyte predominance)
Synovial biopsy	Synovial hyperplasia, no inflammatory infiltrate	Sarcoid granuloma
Destructive bony lesions	Absent	Present
Clinical course	Benign, self-limited	Chronic

Modified from Mathur A, Kremer JM: Immunology, rheumatic features, and therapy of sarcoidosis, Curr Opin Rheumatol 4:76–80, 1992.
HLA, Human leucocyte antigen; PIP, Proximal interphalangeal.

and chronic myopathic. The nodular presentation is the least common type, involving the musculotendinous junctions. Acute granulomatous inflammatory myositis is rare, occurs mainly in African-American females, and is indistinguishable clinically from polymyositis. Chronic myopathy is the most common form and is manifested by an insidious onset of proximal symmetrical muscle weakness and wasting. Neurogenic atrophy as a result of granulomatous infiltration of nerves can occur. Muscle enzyme levels, electromyography, and muscle biopsies are necessary to differentiate the different types of muscle involvement. The acute myositis will respond to corticosteroids whereas the nodular and chronic myopathic forms are less likely to respond.

15. **What osseous changes occur in patients with sarcoidosis?**
    The overall incidence of osseous sarcoid is reported in 3% to 13%. Bony lesions are associated with chronic skin and multiorgan involvement. The phalanges of the hands and feet are most commonly involved. The metacarpophalangeal joints, metacarpals, and wrists are usually spared. Radiographic findings include soft tissue swelling, periarticular osteopenia, joint-space narrowing, cyst formation, eccentric/punched-out erosions, sclerosis and periosteal reactions, pathologic fractures, and phalangeal fragmentation (Fig 76-1). Bone scans, magnetic resonance imaging (MRI), and 18-fluoro-deoxyglucose positron emission tomography (FDG-PET) scans may detect unsuspected osseous involvement given that 50% of bony lesions are asymptomatic.

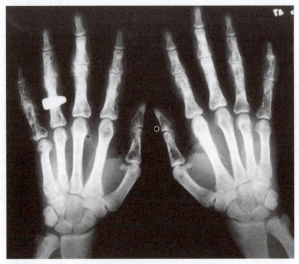

Figure 76-1. Osseous sarcoid involving the hands. The phalanges demonstrate a coarsened, reticulated, or lacelike trabecular pattern seen in chronic sarcoid bone involvement.

16. **Can sarcoidosis and other connective tissue diseases coexist? What other diseases can it associate with?**
    Yes. Several reports have described sarcoidosis in patients with other rheumatic diseases, including systemic lupus erythematosus (SLE), rheumatoid arthritis (RA), systemic sclerosis, Sjögren's syndrome, polymyositis, and spondyloarthropathies. This is most often discovered on biopsy to exclude a lymphoproliferative malignancy in a patient with a primary rheumatic disease. The occurrence is believed to be a coincidence because a common etiopathogenesis is not known. In addition to rheumatic diseases, sarcoidosis has been reported in patients with inflammatory bowel disease, primary biliary cirrhosis, autoimmune endocrine disorders, various malignancies, and common variable immunodeficiency. Medication-induced sarcoidosis has been described following therapy with interferon (IFN)-α, IFN-γ, interleukin-2 (IL-2), and anti-TNF-α.

17. **How is sarcoidosis usually treated?**
    Because the cause of sarcoidosis is unknown, therapy is empirical. Whenever possible, patients with good prognostic signs should be observed for the first 3 to 6 months without immunosuppressive therapy because of the potential for spontaneous resolution. In patients with progressive disease, the recommended doses of corticosteroids and adjunctive therapies vary, depending on the organ system involved. There have been few controlled, randomized trials to establish the appropriate dose and duration of any therapy for sarcoidosis. Despite a lack of well-controlled clinical trials proving that corticosteroids improve long-term outcome, oral corticosteroids (up to 1 mg/kg/day) are used as first-line treatment for symptomatic and progressive stage II and III lung disease, malignant hypercalcemia, and severe ocular, neurologic, and cardiac involvement. Nonsteroidal antiinflammatory drugs (NSAIDs) and/or lower corticosteroids dosages (less than 0.5 mg/kg/day) are used for joint and muscle involvement. Chloroquine/hydroxychloroquine and low-dose methotrexate have been effective for long-term management of musculoskeletal involvement in selected patients. Cutaneous disease is typically treated with corticosteroids (topical or oral), but antimalarials, low-dose methotrexate, and azathioprine have been useful for chronic lesions. Cyclophosphamide (oral and intravenous) has been beneficial in treating cardiac sarcoidosis or neurosarcoidosis that have failed combination corticosteroid and methotrexate treatment. Recently, the monoclonal anti-TNF-α agents, particularly infliximab, have been effective for various disease manifestations refractory to standard immunosuppressive therapy. In case reports, rituximab has been used successfully for refractory disease particularly when granulomatous mass lesions are present. Implantable pacemakers are inserted in patients with cardiac involvement and arrhythmias. Solid organ transplantation can be life-saving in patients who have failed all medical therapies.
    Patients must be monitored for side effects and prophylactic measures used to prevent toxicities. Patients on high-dose corticosteroids should receive prophylaxis against *Pneumocystis jirovecii*. Osteopenia and osteoporosis resulting from dysregulated calcium metabolism and medications used in therapy can occur in up to two thirds of patients. All sarcoidosis patients on corticosteroids or who are postmenopausal should have bone density measurements and bisphosphonate therapy started in those at risk for fractures. Although calcium is given to patients on corticosteroids to prevent osteoporosis, vitamin D therapy is usually avoided because of the tendency to cause hypercalcemia. Vaccinations should be kept up to date. Depression is common (46% to 66%) and should be screened for and treated. Fatigue is common (50% to 70%), can be disabling, and may respond to armodafinil or dexmethylphenidate. Hypothyroidism, hypoxemia, depression, and sleep apnea are potential and correctable causes of fatigue.

18. **Discuss the prognostic factors in sarcoidosis?**
    The extent of organ involvement in most cases is defined at presentation with less than 25% of patients developing new organ involvement during follow-up. Most patients (60%) undergo spontaneous remission with an additional 10% to 20% resolving with corticosteroid therapy. However, in 10% to 30% the course is chronic. Of those having a chronic course, half will have progressive pulmonary disease and half will display involvement of critical extrapulmonary organs, such as the eye, brain, and heart. In general, the more severe the involvement and the more organ systems (more than three) involved at the time of diagnosis, the worse the prognosis. Cutaneous sarcoidosis, pulmonary hypertension, African-American race, disease onset after age 40 years, and symptoms lasting over 6 months are poor prognostic signs.

BIBLIOGRAPHY

Fayad F, et al: Muscle involvement in sarcoidosis: a retrospective and followup studies, J Rheumatol 33:98–103, 2006.
Fernandes SRM, Singsen BH, Hoffman GS: Sarcoidosis and systemic vasculitis, Semin Arthritis Rheum 30:33–46, 2000.
Grunewald J, Ecklund A: Sex-specific manifestations of Lofgren's syndrome, Am J Respir Crit Care Med 175:40–44, 2007.
Hamzeh N: Sarcoidosis, Med Clin N Am 95:1223–1234, 2011.
Iannuzzi MC, Rybicki BA, Teirstein AS: Medical progress: sarcoidosis, N Engl J Med 357:2153–2165, 2007.
Judson MA: Extrapulmonary sarcoidosis, Semin Resp Crit Care Med 28:83–101, 2007.
Judson MA, et al: Efficacy of infliximab in extrapulmonary sarcoidosis: results from a randomized trial, Eur Respir J 31:1189–1196, 2008.
Lazar CA, Culver DA: Treatment of sarcoidosis, Semin Respir Crit Care Med 31:501–518, 2010.
Noor A, Knox KS: Immunopathogenesis of sarcoidosis, Clin Dermatol 25:250–258, 2007.
O'Regan A, Berman JS: Sarcoidosis, Ann Int Med 156, 2012. ITC5-1-ITC5-16.
Paramothayan S, Jones PW: Corticosteroid therapy in pulmonary sarcoidosis: a systemic review, JAMA 287:1301–1307, 2002.

Paramothayan S, et al: Immunosuppressive and cytotoxic therapy for pulmonary sarcoidosis, Cochrane Database Syst Rev(issue 3) CD003536, 2003.
Rosen Y: Pathology of sarcoidosis, Semin Respir Crit Care Med 28:36–52, 2007.
Rossman MA, et al: A double-blinded, randomized placebo-controlled trial of infliximab in subjects with active pulmonary sarcoidosis, Sarcoidosis Vasc Diffuse Lung Dis 23:201–208, 2006.
Sweiss NJ, et al: Rheumatologic manifestations of sarcoidosis, Semin Respir Crit Care Med 31:463–473, 2010.
Theiler N, et al: Osteoarticular involvement in a series of 100 patients with sarcoidosis referred to rheumatology departments, J Rheumatol 35:1622–1628, 2008.
West SG: Sarcoidosis. In Hochberg MC, et al: Rheumatology, ed 5, Philadelphia, 2011, Mosby (Elsevier).

Further Reading

http://www.stopsarcoidosis.org
http://www.LungUSA.org

RHEUMATIC DISORDERS IN PATIENTS ON DIALYSIS

Mark Jarek, MD

> **KEY POINTS**
> 1. Renal osteodystrophy includes osteitis fibrosa, osteomalacia, and adynamic bone disease.
> 2. Osteitis fibrosa is a manifestation of secondary hyperparathyroidism caused by chronic renal failure.
> 3. Osteomalacia in chronic renal failure is most often attributed to aluminum toxicity.
> 4. Adynamic bone disease is the most common form of renal osteodystrophy and results from oversuppression of parathyroid hormone (PTH).
> 5. Dialysis-associated amyloidosis is caused by nondialyzable β2-microglobulin accumulation in tissues.

1. **What are the rheumatologic complications that can occur in patients with end-stage renal disease?**
   Rheumatologic complications occur in up to 70% of patients with end-stage renal disease (ESRD). There is a temporal relationship between the frequency of these disorders and the length of kidney disease. Some of the musculoskeletal disorders that develop in chronic renal failure and dialysis can be recalled with the mnemonic **VITAMINS ABCDE**:
   V—Vascular calcification
   I—Infections (osteomyelitis, septic arthritis)
   T—Tumoral calcifications and tendon ruptures
   A—Amyloid arthropathy (β2-microglobulin)
   M—Metabolic bone disease (osteomalacia, osteoporosis)
   I—Infarction (osteonecrosis)
   N—Nodules (tophi)
   S—Secondary hyperparathyroidism
   A—Aluminum toxicity
   B—Bursitis (olecranon)
   C—Crystal arthropathy (gout, calcium pyrophosphate deposition disease [CPDD], hydroxyapatite)
   D—Digital clubbing
   E—Erosive spondyloarthropathy

2. **What is renal osteodystrophy?**
   The term **renal osteodystrophy**, which was introduced by Liu and Chu in 1943, refers to the full spectrum of musculoskeletal disorders associated with renal failure. Because the kidney plays a critical role in the overall regulation of mineral homeostasis, the development of renal failure has widespread consequences for the skeleton. The four principal types of renal osteodystrophy are:
   - **Osteitis fibrosa:** bony lesions caused by accelerated bone turnover as a result of secondary hyperparathyroidism.
   - **Osteomalacia:** reduced rate of bone turnover with increased osteoid volume and defective mineralization often associated with aluminum toxicity.
   - **Adynamic bone disease:** bone turnover is markedly decreased as a result of excessive suppression of PTH. Unlike osteomalacia, there is no increase in osteoid volume.
   - **Mixed disease:** combined osteitis fibrosa and osteomalacia with marrow fibrosis.

   The only way to separate these and definitively establish a diagnosis is by a dual-labeled bone biopsy.

3. **Why does secondary hyperparathyroidism develop in chronic renal failure? How does this lead to bone disease?**
   Secondary hyperparathyroidism starts relatively early, when the glomerular filtration rate (GFR) drops below 60 mL/min, as evidenced by increased levels of PTH and histological changes in bone. As renal function deteriorates, these changes become more dramatic. Several factors in patients with chronic renal failure contribute to the sustained increases in PTH secretion and, ultimately, to parathyroid gland hyperplasia.
   - Relative hyperphosphatemia resulting from impaired renal excretion occurs early and becomes overt as GFR drops to below 20 mL/min.

- Impaired renal hydroxylation of 25-hydroxyvitamin D to 1,25-dihydroxyvitamin D (calcitriol) attributable to reduced 1-α hydroxylase activity occurs early even before hyperphosphatemia develops as a result of the diseased kidney parenchyma. This enzyme is further inhibited by hyperphosphatemia and by increased fibroblast growth factor-23 (FGF-23) levels caused by reduced GFR. Notably, 1,25-dihydroxyvitamin D normally inhibits both parathyroid gland growth and PTH secretion, therefore low levels cause secondary hyperparathyroidism.
- Decreased free calcium owing to poor gastrointestinal (GI) absorption resulting from reduced 1,25-dihydroxyvitamin D levels, skeletal resistance to PTH, and calcium deposition into vasculature, soft tissues, and viscera as a result of high calcium–phosphate product caused by hyperphosphatemia.
- Insensitivity of the parathyroid gland to the suppressive effects of calcium on PTH secretion.

The end result of each of these defects (high phosphate, reduced calcitriol, and decreased free calcium) is stimulation of the parathyroid chief cell causing a sustained increase in PTH release. This increase in PTH (and FGF-23) is attempting to decrease phosphorous levels by reducing the renal reabsorption of phosphate as well as trying to stimulate 1-α hydroxylase activity. However, as kidney disease worsens and GFR decreases, this becomes ineffective and the resulting high PTH levels stimulate osteoclast activation and rapid bone resorption leading to osteitis fibrosa. This is usually asymptomatic but can be associated with bone pain/tenderness and proximal muscle weakness.

4. **List the characteristic radiographic features of osteitis fibrosa attributable to secondary hyperparathyroidism.**

   Early: subperiosteal resorption in the hands, wrists, feet, and medial tibia, particularly on the radial side of the middle phalanx of the index and middle fingers (see Chapter 48); osteoporosis.

   Intermediate: subchondral resorption of sternoclavicular, acromioclavicular, discovertebral, and sacroiliac joints and symphysis pubis; loss of the lamina dura around teeth; acro-osteolysis of the phalangeal tufts; chondrocalcinosis of knees, wrists, and symphysis pubis (see Chapter 46); periarticular and soft tissue calcification; osteosclerosis.

   Late: bone cysts (single or multiple) (Figure 77-1).

   Brown tumor: osteoclastomas with dried blood (brown); typically occur at the medial end of clavicles or skull, long bones, sternum, and spine.

   Subligamentous bone resorption: of trochanters, ischial tuberosities, humeral tuberosities, and calcanei.

5. **What is a "salt and pepper" skull? What is "rugger-jersey spine"?**

   Trabecular bone resorption in hyperparathyroidism creates a characteristic mottling of the cranial vault with alternating areas of lucency and sclerosis, producing the **salt and pepper** radiographic appearance (Figure 77-1). **Rugger-jersey spine** refers to the bandlike osteosclerosis of the superior and inferior margins of the vertebral bodies that is only seen in patients with secondary (not primary) hyperparathyroidism (Figure 77-2).

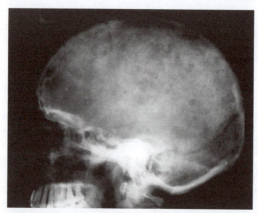

Figure 77-1. Skull radiograph of a patient with renal failure and secondary hyperparathyroidism. Note the bone cysts ("brown tumors") superimposed on a "salt and pepper" skull.

6. **Outline the prevention and treatment of secondary hyperparathyroidism.**
   - Dietary phosphate restriction (800 to 1000 mg/day). Avoid colas.
   - Calcium-based phosphate binders (calcium carbonate or calcium acetate limited to <1.5 g/day) or a noncalcium-based phosphate-binding resin (sevelamer, lanthanum) before meals if dietary restriction alone is unable to maintain serum phosphorous between 3.5 and 5.5 mg/dL (if on dialysis). If corrected total calcium is greater than 9.5 mg/dL or vascular calcifications are present, a noncalcium-based phosphate-binding resin is preferred.

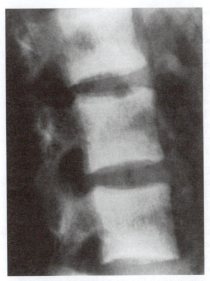

Figure 77-2. Rugger-jersey spine.

- Vitamin D derivatives (paricalcitol, doxercalciferol, calcitriol, others): if corrected total calcium is less than 9.5 mg/dL and PTH level are still greater than 300 pg/mL. There is a need to monitor for hypercalcemia causing a high calcium–phosphate product, which ideally should be <55 to prevent vascular calcifications.
- Calcimimetics (cinacalcet): if vitamin D derivatives are ineffective, corrected total calcium >8.4 mg/dL, and PTH > 300 pg/mL. Use before vitamin D derivatives if calcium–phosphate product above 55.
- Once hyperparathyroidism has advanced, it may be refractory to these interventions, at which time subtotal parathyroidectomy is indicated to correct symptomatic hyperparathyroidism. Subtotal parathyroidectomy is also indicated in patients who develop **tertiary hyperparathyroidism**, which have symptoms such as high PTH levels (>800 pg/mL) and hypercalcemia in spite of being off all calcium and vitamin D therapies.

7. **How does osteomalacia present? What role does aluminum play in this type of renal osteodystrophy?**

In renal failure or hemodialysis, dietary aluminum is not adequately cleared and deposits in the osteoid lamellae of newly formed bone, inhibiting mineralization, which leads to osteomalacia. Therefore in patients with ESRD, osteomalacia may be related to aluminum toxicity although it can occur without aluminum toxicity. Therefore, other common causes of osteomalacia, such as vitamin D deficiency, need to be considered, although this is now uncommon with the routine supplementation of vitamin D in patients on dialysis. Chronic hypophosphatemia and metabolic acidosis can also cause osteomalacia in some patients. Clinically, aluminum-induced osteomalacia presents as diffuse bone pain and predisposes to insufficiency fractures. Aluminum levels, PTH, and bone-specific alkaline phosphatase levels are increased. Radiographic findings are osteopenia and Looser's zones. Bone biopsy with aluminum staining is diagnostic and should be done for confirmation. Other manifestations of aluminum toxicity include an acute or chronic encephalopathy. Deferoxamine chelation therapy may be beneficial. This type of renal bone disease is becoming less common because aluminum-containing phosphate binders and antacids (including sucralfate) are now avoided and aluminum levels are monitored in patients on dialysis.

8. **What is adynamic bone disease?**

Adynamic bone disease is the most common type of renal osteodystrophy and can lead to fragility fractures. Patients with ESRD who are older and diabetic are most at risk. The pathogenesis is unclear, but excessive suppression of PTH (<100 to 150 pg/mL) plays a major role. There is no diagnostic biochemical profile that can establish the diagnosis of adynamic bone disease. Recently, a ratio of 1-84/7-84 PTH of less than one correlated with a bone biopsy showing adynamic bone disease. However, in most cases a bone biopsy is necessary to establish a definitive diagnosis and will show a markedly reduced bone turnover resulting from lack of osteoblast and osteoclast activity. The suppressed PTH is often a result of excessive use of calcium-based phosphate binders, vitamin D analogues, or cinacalcet. Patients can be asymptomatic or have symptoms such as hypercalcemia and fractures. Treatment is aimed at eliminating PTH suppression to allow the PTH to rise to the recommended level of 150 to 300 pg/mL for patients on dialysis. Bisphosphonates should never be used to treat osteoporosis or fragility fractures in a patient with ESRD without first having a bone biopsy to rule out adynamic bone disease.

9. **What is amyloid arthropathy of renal failure?**

   β2-Microglobulin is an endogenous structural protein (molecular weight = 11.8 kDa) that is poorly cleared by standard dialysis membranes and accumulates to extremely high levels in patients on long-term hemodialysis. Owing to its high affinity for collagen, β2-microglobulin deposits in bones, joints, and synovium. These deposits can lead to chronic arthralgias and carpal tunnel syndrome. This chronic arthropathy most commonly involves the shoulder, hip, wrist and finger tendon sheaths, and rarely the spine (especially cervical). Rotator cuff and subacromial bursae deposition leads to impingement syndrome.

   Synovial fluid is noninflammatory but may be hemorrhagic as a result of anticoagulation use during dialysis. Synovial fluid or biopsy will identify amyloid fibrils when stained with Congo red. Radiographs are notable for erosions and large subchondral bony cysts that tend to occur at the ends of long bones (humerus, femur, tibia, and carpals). The use of more permeable, high-flux membranes may delay the onset of disease but does not prevent disease development (see Chapter 73).

10. **Which spondyloarthropathy is unique to dialysis patients?**

    A **destructive spondyloarthropathy** (DSA) is found only in long-term patients on dialysis and is defined by its radiologic picture. It can mimick an infectious discitis. There is multilevel disk-space narrowing with erosions and cysts of adjacent vertebral endplates without significant osteophytosis or sclerosis. Calcification of surrounding vertebral discs is common. The cervical and lumbar spine are most frequently involved. The erosions progress radiographically over a few weeks or more, followed by reactive endplate sclerosis. Diffuse spinal involvement is unusual, although multisegment involvement has been described.

    This entity has been reported occasionally in patients who are uremic before dialysis but has not been reported following renal transplantation. Most patients are asymptomatic, which accounts for the rarity of its description. Neck pain or cervical radiculopathy is the most common complaint in symptomatic patients. Despite the severe radiologic picture, medullary compression is rare. Biopsies reveal calcium crystals (CPDD or hydroxyapatite) and/or β2-microglobulin. Hyperparathyroidism is usually also present and appears to play a role in the pathogenesis of DSA. Control of hyperparathyroidism, including subtotal parathyroidectomy, helps to slow progression of DSA.

11. **What types of crystal deposition diseases occur in patients with renal disease?**
    - **Monosodium urate arthritis (gouty arthritis)** occurs occasionally, although less frequently than one would expect considering how common hyperuricemia is in patients with chronic renal failure. There is increased GI excretion of uric acid when patients are in renal failure. Uric acid is extensively removed during hemodialysis.
    - **CPDD** is seen occasionally in secondary hyperparathyroidism (although less common than in primary hyperparathyroidism). CPDD is manifested by chondrocalcinosis (knee, wrist, symphysis pubis), acute pseudogout, and/or a degenerative arthritis.
    - **Hydroxyapatite arthropathy** can present as acute episodes of joint pain or as a chronic periarthropathy resulting from calcium hydroxyapatite deposits. This arthropathy is strongly correlated with a high calcium–phosphate product. Periarticular and subcutaneous deposits may become quite large (tumoral calcinosis), particularly around the hips, knees, shoulders, and wrists, where they may cause pain, reduce range of motion, and predispose to infection.
    - **Secondary oxalosis** rarely develops in long-standing renal failure. It is marked by oxalate deposition in visceral organs, blood vessels, bones, and articular cartilage, where it may contribute to chronic polyarthralgias. Oxalate is produced from ascorbic acid and is cleared very poorly in chronic renal failure and dialysis. Most cases of oxalosis can be prevented by limiting ascorbic acid (vitamin C) and oxalate intake (tea, spinach, okra, sweet potatoes, nuts, and soy products). Treatment of established calcium oxalate arthropathy with nonsteroidal antiinflammatory drugs (NSAIDs), colchicine, intraarticular corticosteroids, or increased dialysis has produced only slight improvement.

12. **Where do soft tissue calcifications occur in renal osteodystrophy?**

    Soft tissue calcification is common in renal osteodystrophy. Sites of soft tissue deposition are multiple, including the cornea and conjunctiva, viscera, vasculature, and subcutaneous and periarticular tissues. Calcification consistently occurs in chronic renal failure when the concentration (mg/dL) product of plasma calcium and phosphorus exceeds 70. It can also occur at lesser levels. Of particular concern is the high incidence of coronary artery calcification in patients on hemodialysis, which can predispose them to coronary events. Additionally, vascular calcification may compromise blood flow leading to ischemic necrosis of skin and muscle, which is called **calciphylaxis**. The chemical composition of the calcium depends on the site of deposition. In subcutaneous, vascular, and periarticular sites, hydroxyapatite is observed, whereas in viscera, a magnesium whitlockite-like material is found.

13. **A patient who is 3 months' postrenal transplant develops an acute knee arthritis. Current medications include cyclosporine, mycophenylate mofetil, and prednisone. What is the most likely etiology for the knee pain?**

    This is a common presentation of **acute gouty arthritis** associated with **cyclosporine** use. Cyclosporine blocks renal uric acid clearance, leading to marked hyperuricemia and gout. Polarized microscopy of the synovial fluid may identify numerous intracellular, negatively birefrigent, needle-shaped crystals, confirming the diagnosis of gout (see Chapter 45). Positively birefrigent rhomboid crystals of pseudogout also may be seen because of the association of secondary hyperparathyroidism and CPDD disease. Septic arthritis needs to be considered in the differential diagnosis because of the potent immunosuppressive therapy used in this posttransplant patient. Therefore, joint fluid should be sent for Gram stain and cultures to include bacteria, fungi, and mycobacteria. Note, when determining acute and long-term therapy, colchicine should not be used in patients taking cyclosporine owing to the risk of myotoxicity.

14. **What other musculoskeletal problems are increased in patients on dialysis?**
    - Erosive osteoarthritis
    - Tendinitis and tendon ruptures (quadriceps, patellar, Achilles, triceps, finger extensors): attributable to secondary hyperparathyroidism
    - Osteonecrosis (avascular necrosis): does not improve with core decompression (see Chapter 54)
    - Osteopenia: especially after renal transplantation (see Chapter 52)
    - Nephrogenic systemic fibrosis (see Chapter 19)

15. **What dose adjustments are needed for antirheumatic drugs in patients with renal insufficiency?**
    Serum creatinine may be an inaccurate measurement of renal function because as renal function declines, less creatinine is excreted by glomerular filtration and more is excreted by tubular secretion. The use of cimetidine (400 mg four times a day for 2 days) blocks tubular secretion of creatinine and may improve accuracy of creatinine clearance measurements. After determining the correct creatinine clearance, the following guidelines can be used:
    - Anakinra—GFR <30 mL/min, decrease frequency from daily to 100 mg subcutaneously (SC) every other day.
    - Antimalarials—40% to 50% excreted by kidneys. Reduce dose 50% or do not use at all in severe renal insufficiency GFR <30 mL/min. Neuromyopathy, cardiomyopathy, and retinal toxicity increases with renal insufficiency. Cannot be hemodialyzed.
    - Allopurinol—GFR 30 mL/min, use 100 mg; GFR 60 mL/min, use 200 mg; GFR 90 mL/min, use 300 mg daily. In patients on hemodialysis, give 100 mg daily after dialysis. Dialysis usually lowers uric acid without the need for allopurinol.
    - Azathioprine—GFR 10–50 mL/min, reduce dose by 25%; GFR <10 mL/min, cut dose 50%. Give after hemodialysis.
    - Biologics (monoclonal antibodies, decoy receptors, receptor antagonists)—most not tested but probably do not need dose adjustment. Chronic kidney disease is a risk factor for increased infections on biologic therapy.
    - Bisphosphonates—avoid in ESRD. Use half oral dose or not at all in severe renal insufficiency (<30 mL/min). Risedronate may be safer than alendronate. Intravenous (IV) bisphosphonates need to be administered more slowly with IV ibandronate safer than IV zoledronic acid in patients with moderate renal insufficiency (<50 mL/min). Denosumab may be a better alternative.
    - Colchicine—avoid prolonged use in patients with GFR less than 50 mL/min if possible. Use 0.6 mg daily for GFR <50 mL/min and 0.3 mg daily for GFR <30 mL/min. Do not use if GFR <10 mL/min or on hemodialysis unless no other alternative. Watch for cytopenias and neuromyopathy. Cannot be hemodialyzed.
    - Corticosteroids—no change in dose.
    - Cyclophosphamide—GFR <25 mL/min, reduce dose to 25% usual dose; GFR 25–50 mL/min, reduce dose to 50%. If patient has ESRD, give the dose after hemodialysis.
    - Cyclosporine—no dose adjustment for renal insufficiency. However, use of cyclosporine can worsen renal insufficiency. If creatinine rises, the cyclosporine dose needs to be lowered. Cannot be hemodialyzed.
    - Dapsone—GFR <50 mL/min, give every other day.
    - Leflunomide—insufficient data. The drug (40% to 50%) is eliminated by the kidneys although the active metabolite is not increased in renal insufficiency that occurs as a result of increased enterohepatic excretion. Cannot be hemodialyzed.
    - Methotrexate—reduce dose 50% with renal insufficiency. Should not be used or used with extreme caution owing to hematologic toxicity when GFR <50 mL/min (max dose 5 mg weekly). Cannot be hemodialyzed.
    - Mycophenolate mofetil—hepatic metabolism with 90% renally excreted. Enterohepatic circulation can be safety valve with renal insufficiency. Do not exceed 1 g twice daily for GFR <25 mL/min or on peritoneal dialysis. Do not exceed 500 mg twice daily if on hemodialysis.
    - Narcotics—GFR 10 to 50 mL/min, use 75% usual dose; GFR <10 mL/min, cut dose 50%. Avoid meperidine. Fentanyl is safest.
    - NSAIDs—most are metabolized by liver except for diflunisal. All NSAIDs except salsalate can make renal insufficiency worse. No need for dose adjustment for NSAIDs in ESRD except for diflunisal (decrease dose 50%). Avoid sulindac, owing to renal stone formation in patients with low urine output. Also avoid ketoprofen, because it will be metabolized back to active drug if it cannot be renally excreted.
    - Probenecid—does not work if GFR <50 to 60 mL/min. No dosage change for mild renal insufficiency.
    - Sulfasalazine—no change in dose.

- Tacrolimus—same as cyclosporine.
- Teriparatide—no change in dose. Teriparatide effective for osteoporosis in patients with GFR as low as 30 mL/min even if PTH mildly elevated (100 pg/mL) as long as vitamin D is abundant.
- Tramadol—give dose (50 to 100 mg) every 12 hours instead of every 6 hours if GFR <30 mL/min or on hemodialysis. Give after dialysis.

16. **Which antirheumatic drugs are removed by hemodialysis?**
    - Allopurinol—removes 50%
    - Azathioprine
    - Prednisolone
    - Cyclophosphamide—removes 50%
    - Tramadol—removes 70%

    These drugs should be given after hemodialysis. Other antirheumatic drugs are either not removed by hemodialysis (NSAIDs, narcotics, cyclosporine, methotrexate, leflunomide, colchicine, antimalarials, tacrolimus) or it is unknown if they are.

BIBLIOGRAPHY

Alteri P, Sau G, Cao R, et al: Immunosuppressive treatment in dialysis patients, Nephrol Dial Transplant 17(suppl 8):2–9, 2002.
Andress DL: Adynamic bone in patients with chronic kidney disease, Kidney Int 73:1345–1354, 2008.
Bardin T, Richette P: Rheumatic manifestations of renal disease, Curr Opin Rheumatol 21:55–61, 2009.
Cho SK, Sung YK, Park S, et al: Etanercept treatment in rheumatoid arthritis patients with chronic kidney failure on predialysis, Rheumatol Int 30:1519–1522, 2010.
Cunningham J, Locatelli F, Rodriguez M: Secondary hyperparathyroidism: pathogenesis, disease progression, and therapeutic options, Clin J Am Soc Nephrol 6:913, 2011.
Dember LM, Jaber BL: Dialysis-related amyloidosis: late finding or hidden epidemic? Semin Dial 19:105, 2006.
Hruska KA, Mathew S: Chronic kidney disease mineral bone disorder. In Rosen CJ, editor: Primer on the Metabolic Bone Diseases and Disorders of Mineral Metabolism, ed 7, Washington DC, 2008, American Society for Bone and Mineral Research (ASBMR).
Kidney Disease: Improving Global Outcomes (KDIGO) CKD-MBD Work Group: KDIGO clinical practice guidelines for the diagnosis, evaluation, prevention, and treatment of chronic kidney disease-mineral and bone disorder (CKD-MBD), Kidney Int 76(suppl 113):S1–S130, 2009.
Mehdi S, Prete P, Hashimzadeh M, et al: A study of musculoskeletal disease in two chronic hemodialysis populations and its impact on quality of life, J Clin Rheumatol 15:405–407, 2009.
Miller PD: Diagnosis and treatment of osteoporosis in chronic renal disease, Semin Nephrol 29:144–155, 2009.
Moe S, Drueke T, Cunningham J, et al: Definition, evaluation, and classification of renal osteodystrophy: a position statement from Kidney Disease: Improving Global Outcomes (KDIGO), Kidney Int 69:1945–1953, 2006.
Rafto SE, Dalinka MK, Schieber ML, et al: Spondyloarthropathy of the cervical spine in long-term hemodialysis, Radiology 166:201–204, 1988.
Swarup A, Sachdeva N, Schumacher Jr HR: Dosing of antirheumatic drugs in renal disease and dialysis, J Clin Rheumatol 10:190–204, 2004.

FURTHER READING

http://www.kidney.org
http://www.kdigo.org

CHAPTER 78

RHEUMATIC DISEASE AND THE PREGNANT PATIENT

Sterling G. West, MD and Mark Jarek, MD

> **KEY POINTS**
>
> 1. Up to 50% to 75% of patients with rheumatoid arthritis (RA) improve during pregnancy.
> 2. Patients with systemic lupus erythematosus (SLE) who have anti-Ro (SS-A) and anti-La (SS-B) antibodies are at increased risk for having infants who develop neonatal lupus syndrome.
> 3. Patients with SLE should attempt to become pregnant only when their disease is controlled for over 6 months.
> 4. Hydroxychloroquine offers more benefit than risk when used in a pregnant patient with SLE.
> 5. Azathioprine is the safest nonbiologic disease-modifying agent to use in a patient who requires additional immunosuppressive therapy.

1. **List some of the physiologic changes that occur during pregnancy and their possible effects on patients with rheumatic diseases?**
    - The T helper 2 (TH2) cytokine profile is dominant during pregnancy. TH2-dominant diseases such as SLE have a propensity to flare whereas T helper 1 (TH1)-dominant diseases such as RA tend to improve.
    - Patients with rheumatic diseases should have the disease well controlled for at least 6 months before becoming pregnant.
    - Transplacental passage of immunoglobulin G (IgG) starts from 16 weeks' gestation. Potentially pathogenic antibodies (e.g., anti-SS-A) and biologics (e.g., rituximab) do not cross until then. IgG does not get into breast milk.
    - There is a significant increase in intravascular volume with pregnancy, which can affect patients with cardiac, pulmonary, and renal diseases.
    - Hypertension may get worse. Anemia may get worse as a result of hemodilution.
    - Patients with significant cardiac disease (cardiomyopathy, valve disease), renal failure, pulmonary hypertension, and interstitial lung disease should be counseled on the risk of pregnancy to them and their fetus. Avoiding pregnancy may be the best option. Adoption and in vitro fertilization with surrogate pregnancy may be better options.
    - The glomerular filtration rate (GFR) increases 50% during pregnancy.
    - Patients with proteinuria will have an increase in proteinuria.
    - The erythrocyte sedimentation rate (ESR) will increase during pregnancy as a result of the increase in fibrinogen.
    - You cannot follow disease activity with ESR. C-reactive protein (CRP) may be reliable depending on rheumatic disease.
    - Pregnancy increases the risk of thrombosis.
    - Patients with antiphospholipid antibodies (aPLAs) and/or history of a previous clot are at increased risk for thrombosis.
    - Pregnancy and lactation increase the risk of reversible bone loss.
    - Patients with severe osteoporosis may be at increased risk for fragility fractures.
    - Pregnancy-related conditions may mimic a rheumatic disease exacerbation: facial flushing (mimics SLE malar rash), preeclampsia and eclampsia (mimics lupus nephritis, scleroderma renal crisis), HELLP syndrome (mimics SLE flare), low back pain (mimics ankylosing spondylitis [AS] exacerbation), gastroesophageal reflux (mimics worsening scleroderma), arthralgia and carpal tunnel syndrome (mimics arthritis exacerbation).

2. **A young patient with recently diagnosed SLE is currently being treated with low-dose prednisone, hydroxychloroquine, and occasional nonsteroidal antiinflammatory drugs with good disease control. She is considering pregnancy and asks about the optimal timing of a pregnancy and the potential maternal and fetal complications. What advice do you give her?**
Patients with SLE should be advised to conceive while SLE is quiescent or at least under good control for 6 to 12 months. There is no increased rate of infertility for patients with SLE as long as the disease is under control. The PROMISSE (Predictors of pRegnancy Outcome: bioMarkers In antiphospholipid antibody Syndrome and Systemic lupus Erythematosus) trial recently reported that 80% of patients with SLE who conceive with low disease activity (average SLE Disease Activity Index [SLEDAI] ≤3) have a good

pregnancy outcome. However, adverse pregnancy outcomes (20%) were still twice the general population and four times a healthy population who were pregnant. There was an increased risk for intrauterine growth retardation (IUGR) (9%), prematurity (9%), fetal death (6%), and toxemia of pregnancy (10%). There was a 20% to 25% likelihood of stable SLE relapsing (18% moderate flare, 4% severe flare) during pregnancy. Patients with SLEDAI >4, lupus anticoagulant, and/or high titer IgG anticardiolipin antibodies (aCLs) were most likely to flare and have adverse fetal outcomes. Most children born to women with SLE will have normal development and intelligence. Less than 10% will develop an autoimmune disease at some time during their life.

Patients who decide to become pregnant should continue hydroxychloroquine throughout pregnancy. Low-dose aspirin should be started to decrease thrombotic and toxemia risks regardless of aPLA status. Notably, several medications are contraindicated during pregnancy including cyclophosphamide, mycophenylate mofetil (MMF), angiotensin-converting enzyme (ACE) inhibitors/angiotensin receptor blockers (ARBs), and warfarin. Calcium channel blockers and labetalol can be used to treat hypertension. All patients should be managed in collaboration with an obstetrician who specializes in cases of high risk.

3. A patient with SLE and active lupus nephritis wants to become pregnant. Current medications include prednisone, 20 mg/day. What do you recommend?

The PROMISSE trial specifically excluded patients with an elevated creatinine or who were on greater than 20 mg of prednisone daily. Therefore, the pregnancy outcomes cited in the above question do not apply to this patient. In contrast to a patient with SLE with quiescent disease, this patient should be counseled against becoming pregnant at this time. There is an increased chance of worsening disease activity that could result in renal function deterioration, IUGR, hypertension, and preeclampsia. Patients with creatinine greater than 1.6 mg/dL, hypertension, and nephrosis are at particular risk for renal function deterioration during pregnancy. It has been estimated that patients with active lupus nephritis have a 50% to 60% chance of nephritis exacerbation during pregnancy or immediately postpartum. By contrast, for patients with quiescent disease, the risk of nephritis exacerbation is <10%.

Flares of lupus nephritis during pregnancy can be very severe. In patients with active lupus, there is also a high chance for problems in the fetus. For example, the risk of prematurity may be as high as 60%. Furthermore, if the renal disease should worsen, certain therapies such as cyclophosphamide and MMF are contraindicated. This would limit therapeutic options, although azathioprine (up to 2 mg/kg/day) has been used successfully because it is metabolized by the placenta and little gets into the fetal circulation. In patients with a lupus flare in the late third trimester, intravenous cyclophosphamide can be used, if necessary.

4. How can you distinguish lupus nephritis from toxemia of pregnancy?

The **toxemia syndrome** (preeclampsia–eclampsia) usually occurs in the third trimester of primigravidas. **Preeclampsia** occurs after the twentieth week of gestation and is manifested by hypertension (>140/90), proteinuria (>300 mg/24 hours), and edema. The **HELLP syndrome** is a severe form of preeclampsia and includes microangiopathic **h**emolytic anemia, **e**levated **l**iver tests, and a consumptive coagulopathy with **l**ow **p**latelets. **Eclampsia** is the addition of grand mal seizures. The distinction between severe toxemia of pregnancy and active lupus nephritis can be difficult because both diseases can cause thrombocytopenia, hemolytic anemia, hypertension, seizures, and renal insufficiency with proteinuria. The absence of other clinical manifestations of SLE, such as arthritis, rash, and leukopenia, as well as the lack of red cell casts, stable anti-DNA antibodies, and decreased urine calcium, make the diagnosis of eclampsia more likely. (Table 78-1)

Complement values usually rise during a normal pregnancy. Complement levels frequently decrease during a lupus flare and may decrease during toxemia. Therefore, complement values may not be helpful in distinguishing the two diseases. The ESR is usually elevated in both conditions and therefore is of no value. Proteinuria can occur during a normal pregnancy as a result of the physiologic increased renal blood flow but should be accompanied by a normal, pregnancy-associated rise in creatinine clearance and a corresponding fall in serum creatinine. Toxemia of pregnancy remits immediately following delivery and therefore usually requires no further therapy, whereas lupus nephritis requires high-dose corticosteroids frequently in combination with azathioprine during pregnancy or cyclophosphamide or MMF after completion of pregnancy.

5. What is the significance of SLE developing during pregnancy?

Fetal outcome is very poor when SLE develops during pregnancy, with a fetal death rate as high as 45%. In addition, the maternal course is frequently severe if lupus nephritis occurs for the first time during pregnancy. Patients with severe SLE, particularly active lupus nephritis, are at particularly high risk for maternal and fetal complications and should be cautioned strongly against conception. Fetal mortality in this group is increased at least threefold, and prematurity occurs in most of the successful pregnancies. In some studies, the fetal mortality rate did not improve even when the SLE nephritis was inactive.

6. In an SLE patient who is pregnant, which lupus-related autoantibodies can cause problems for the fetus?

- **Antibodies to Ro/SS-A**, especially when directed against the 52-kDa component and in conjunction with antibodies to **La/SS-B**, have been associated with neonatal lupus syndrome. This can also occur in pregnant patients with primary Sjögren's syndrome who have these antibodies. See Question 7.

Table 78-1. Clinical Findings Distinguishing Toxemia of Pregnancy from a Lupus Flare

ABNORMALITY	TOXEMIA	SLE
Blood pressure	High	Normal or high
Platelets	Low or normal	Low or normal
Complement	Variable*	Normal or low
Uric acid	High	High or normal
Proteinuria	Present	Present
Hematuria	Macroscopic, no casts	Microscopic, with casts
24-Hour urine calcium	Low	Normal
Anti-DNA antibody	Normal or stable	Rising or high
Other SLE symptoms	Absent	Present

SLE, Systemic lupus erythematosus.
*Patients with preeclampsia and eclampsia can develop low complement levels.

- **aPLAs** have been associated with recurrent first trimester spontaneous abortion, stillbirths (fetal wastage), pre-eclampsia, IUGR, and preterm birth. One hypothesis for this complication is complement activation leading to influx of inflammatory cells resulting in thrombosis and placental insufficiency. Anticoagulation can dramatically improve obstetric outcomes (70% live birth rates). See Chapter 23 for management. Rarely, neonatal antiphospholipid antibody syndrome (APS) attributed to transplacental passage of aPLAs may occur. Evaluation of long-term complications supports an increased risk of learning disabilities in infants born to mothers with aPLAs.
- **Antiplatelet antibodies** can occasionally cause autoimmune thrombocytopenia in the fetus with associated hemorrhage, especially at the time of delivery. The management of this complication can be difficult.

7. **Describe the typical clinical presentation of infants with neonatal lupus erythematosus and speculate on pathogenesis. What treatment options exist?**
The major clinical manifestations of neonatal lupus erythematosus (NLE) are dermatologic (35%), cardiac (60%), and hepatic. Hemolytic anemia, thrombocytopenia, and neurologic symptoms occur less commonly. The skin rash is photosensitive and similar to that of subacute cutaneous lupus erythematosus. Most noncardiac manifestations are self-limited because the maternal autoantibodies clear the neonatal circulation in 6 months.
Congenital heart block (CHB) is the most common cardiac manifestation and the accompanying myocarditis accounts for the major morbidity and mortality. CHB is usually irreversible and permanent pacemaker therapy is required in 50% of cases. Despite pacemaker placement, 10% of these children develop a subsequent cardiomyopathy with 20% to 30% mortality before the age of 10 years. The conduction defect is attributed to maternal IgG anti-Ro (SS-A) and anti-La (SS-B) antibodies that cross the placenta and bind to fetal cardiocytes and heart conducting cells, eliciting an inflammatory injury during the second trimester of pregnancy. Clinical manifestations of NLE occur in 5% to 20% of offspring of mothers with high circulating levels of these antibodies. The risk of CHB is 2% overall but may be as high as 5% in patients with high titer anti-Ro/SS-A antibodies.
Mothers with antibodies to Ro/SS-A or La/SS-B should have serial fetal echocardiography weekly from 16 to 26 weeks and every 2 weeks thereafter until 34 weeks of gestation to measure the mechanical PR interval. If complications such as recent onset complete heart block, incomplete heart block, or if signs of myocarditis, congestive heart failure, or hydrops are present, treatment should be considered. High-dose prednisone and immunosuppressive medications do not lower maternal autoantibody titers, are ineffective, and should be avoided. Removal of maternal autoantibodies with plasmapheresis has been reported to successfully prevent CHB in small series and anecdotal case reports. Treatment with fluorinated steroids may offer benefit. Dexamethasone (4 mg/day) or betamethasone (4 mg/day) are not metabolized substantially by the placenta and therefore cross into the fetal circulation. Studies have shown that neonates with first and second degree heart block can respond to this therapy and not progress to CHB. Fluorinated steroids are also helpful to treat myocarditis. Postnatal treatment with high-dose corticosteroids may prevent progression to complete heart block. No therapy has been proven effective in reversing complete heart block once it is established. The risk of another fetus developing CHB in a mother with anti-SS-A antibodies if a previous baby had CHB is 15% to 20%. Intravenous immunoglobulin (IVIG) has not been shown to treat or prevent autoimmune heart block. A prospective trial (PATCH), is in progress evaluating the effectiveness of hydroxychloroquine therapy during pregnancy to prevent fetal heart block in high-risk patients.

8. **Are combined oral contraceptives safe in patients with SLE? Are intrauterine contraceptive devices safe?**
With 50% of pregnancies unplanned in the general population, effective contraception is important in all female patients with rheumatic diseases, especially SLE. Recent trials including the SELENA trial have shown

that combined oral contraceptives (COCs; estrogen-containing) are not associated with an increased flare rate in patients who have inactive lupus and no or low titer aPLAs. The safety of COCs has not been tested in patients with SLE with active disease. Therefore, most authorities recommend that COCs be avoided in patients with active SLE and/or moderate/high titer aPLAs to lessen the chance for disease flare and thromboembolic complications. In these high-risk patients, **progestin-only** contraceptive therapy (progestin-only pills, Depo-Provera injectable, progestin-releasing intrauterine device [IUD]) and barrier methods (IUD, diaphragm) lack the risks associated with estrogen and therefore are considered safer. Drawbacks unique to the progestin-only agents include reduction in high-density lipoprotein (HDL) and lack of osteoporosis prevention. Both of these are frequently already present in women with long-standing SLE. The lower doses of estrogens used as **hormone replacement therapy (HRT)** in postmenopausal women have not been proven to exacerbate SLE and therefore are recommended as long as there are no contraindication to their use (blood clots, etc.).

There has been a concern that IUDs (Copper 7, levonorgestrel-releasing) are less effective and predispose to intrauterine infections and pelvic inflammatory disease in immunocompromised patients. Experience in patients with human immunodeficiency virus (HIV) infection and renal transplants shows that IUDs do not increase the risk of pelvic infections. Immunosuppressive medications may blunt the inflammatory response caused by a Copper 7 IUD making it less effective. Therefore, using a progestin-secreting IUD is felt to be safe and effective in patients who are immunocompromised. These IUDs also reduce menstrual blood flow helping to lessen the chance of anemia in these patients.

9. **What is the value of the anti-Mullerian hormone test in an patient with SLE who has previously received cyclophosphamide for lupus nephritis and wants to become pregnant?**
The anti-Mullerian hormone (AMH) is secreted by the granulosa cells of ovarian follicles during the reproductive years and controls the formation of primary follicles by inhibiting excessive follicular recruitment by follicle-stimulating hormone (FSH). The AMH level is a measure of ovarian reserve, which peaks at age 25 years and decreases with age. Notably, many patients with SLE appear to have a lower level than normal even when they have not previously received cyclophosphamide. In patients less than the age of 30 years who have received 6 g of cyclophosphamide, there is a 75% chance for them to have an undetectable AMH level indicating no ovarian reserve. Notably, AMH levels are not affected by azathioprine, MMF, or cyclosporine.

10. **Should patients without a history of clot or pregnancy loss be screened for aPLAs when they become pregnant?**
Studies have found that at least one aPLA can be present in 8% to 24% of low-risk patients at the first prenatal visit. It is impossible to tell which patients will have thrombotic or pregnancy problems in the absence of a prior history of a clinical event. There is no increase in maternal complications, low birth weight, or low Apgar scores in mothers who just had aCLs without a lupus anticoagulant. Therefore, routine screening in asymptomatic healthy patients is currently not recommended. Patients without a history of clot or previous pregnancy loss but who have an autoimmune disease like SLE, in which aPLAs are increased, should be screened at the time of their first pregnancy because of the prognostic significance of these antibodies. Patients with lupus anticoagulant (LA), triple positive (LA, aCL, and anti-β2 glycoprotein-I [anti-β2GPI]), and/or SLE are at increased risk for poor pregnancy outcomes. Many clinicians treat pregnant primigravidas with one of these risk factors with low-dose aspirin.

Primiparas and women who have had previous live births who are found to have aPLAs need not be treated prophylactically with heparin, especially if they do not have one of the above risk factors for adverse pregnancy outcome. Although there are no data, many patients are put on low-dose aspirin and, if they have SLE, they are put on acetylsalicylic acid (ASA) and hydroxychloroquine. In all patients, the progress of their pregnancies (fetal growth and activity) should be monitored closely including using serial human chorionic gonadotropin levels and nonstress tests from week 30 onward. Slowing of fetal growth or reduction in amniotic fluid volume may be warning signs. Although its prognostic value is less certain, a falling platelet count is taken by some authorities to indicate fetal involvement. In the presence of slow fetal growth or thrombocytopenia not explained by toxemia or SLE, prophylaxis treatment with aspirin (81 mg/day) and subcutaneous heparin or low molecular weight heparin (LMWH) is recommended. Patients with positive aPLA but no history of thrombosis should receive up to 6 weeks of prophylactic heparin postpartum to prevent clots (see Chapter 23).

11. **How does APS affect pregnancy outcome? How is it best treated?**
Patients with APS with or without SLE are at risk for poor pregnancy outcomes. Up to 40% will have premature babies and/or IUGR. Patients with the LA, triple positive aPLA, SLE, and/or history of prior thrombosis are most at risk (odds ratio [OR] > 12). Patients who are pregnant and have APS and a history of arterial or venous clot are at risk for maternal thrombosis and fetal demise. These patients should be treated with low-dose aspirin and full anticoagulant doses of LMWH (e.g., enoxaparin 1 mg/kg subcutaneously [sc] every 12 hours) throughout pregnancy. Because most are on coumadin before getting pregnant, they should be switched to LMWH before conception and aspirin added once pregnancy is confirmed.

Patients who are pregnant and have APS and a prior history of pregnancy loss without a personal history of thrombosis (i.e., obstetrical APS criteria) should be treated with low-dose aspirin plus prophylactic doses of unfractionated heparin (5000 to 10,000 units sc twice daily) or LMWH (e.g., enoxaparin 40 mg sc daily). Typically, aspirin is started before conception and heparin added once pregnancy is confirmed. High-dose (≥40 mg/day) prednisone is not beneficial for APS uncomplicated by active SLE, is associated with numerous potential side effects, and should be avoided. Overall, live-birth rates are 70% to 75% with this approach. See Chapter 23.

Whereas, warfarin crosses the placenta and cannot be used during pregnancy, it can be used postpartum and does not get into breast milk, therefore it is allowed in patients who are breast feeding. Heparin and LMWH do not cross the placenta or get into breast milk, so they are safe during pregnancy and breast feeding.

12. **How does pregnancy affect the course of RA? How does RA affect the course of pregnancy?**
RA and polyarticular juvenile inflammatory arthritis (JIA) improves during pregnancy, possibly owing to immunomodulating effects of the gravid state. Between 50% and 75% of women with RA experience improvement in disease activity during pregnancy, and thus treatment should be minimized to avoid unnecessary fetal exposure to medications. This improvement is unfortunately short-lived because 40% to 90% develop a relapse by 6 months postpartum. This remission recurs with subsequent pregnancies especially in those who have seronegative RA. Rarely, RA presents during pregnancy, although up to 10% of patients with RA have initial onset within 6 months postpartum. The relationship between RA and pregnancy, along with the female predominance of the disease during reproductive years (4:1), suggests a hormonal influence. Recent data suggest that COCs may protect against developing RA and decrease symptoms in women who have established RA.

Infertility is not increased in patients with well-controlled RA, and there is no significant increase in fetal or maternal complications except for risks associated with its therapy. Patients with active disease during the third trimester are more likely to have preterm births and/or small for gestational age babies. In patients with long-standing RA, joint involvement should be assessed before delivery. If the cervical spine is involved, care should be taken to not hyperextend the neck, and vaginal delivery may be precluded by significant hip involvement.

13. **What effect does pregnancy have on the spondyloarthropathies and vice versa?**
Fertility is not affected by the spondyloarthropathies. Fetal outcomes are similar to the general population. The course of ankylosing spondylitis varies during pregnancy (33% improve, 33% worsen) and up to 60% worsen postpartum (mostly low back pain). Notably, up to 50% of patients with psoriatic arthritis improve. Patients with severe back and/or hip disease should be assessed for their capability to deliver vaginally.

14. **How does systemic sclerosis affect fertility and pregnancy complications? What about inflammatory myositis?**
Systemic sclerosis was once considered to be associated with reduced fertility, but more recent data contradict this. Some (7% to 20%) women experience a worsening of their disease during pregnancy. The most feared complication, scleroderma renal crisis, does not appear to be increased (2% to 3%) during pregnancy. During pregnancy, Raynaud's symptoms often improve and gastrointestinal reflux and arthralgias often worsen. Fetal complications, such as miscarriage (15%), prematurity (25% to 40%), and IUGR can occur. Patients with pulmonary hypertension have a high rate of adverse maternal and fetal outcomes and should not get pregnant.

Patients with new onset of poly/dermatomyositis during pregnancy have a high risk of fetal loss. In patients with controlled disease, maternal and fetal outcomes are good with 80% fetal survival.

15. **Should patients with a history of vasculitis get pregnant?**
    - **Takayasu's arteritis:** based on a case series, 80% of pregnancies do well if the disease is controlled. Most adverse effects are not attributed to disease flares but to vascular sequelae from previously active disease. Fetal demise (8%), IUGR (20% to 85%), and premature delivery (40%) are increased as is preeclampsia (20%) and hypertension (30%). Hypertension must be controlled.
    - **Antineutrophil cytoplasmic antibodies (ANCA)-associated vasculitis:** preterm delivery and miscarriage are common especially during active disease. Up to 25% of patients may have a relapse of their vasculitis during pregnancy.
    - **Behçet's disease:** miscarriages and thromboses are increased. Up to 30% have disease relapse during pregnancy.

16. **What are the Food and Drug Administration categories for drug risks during pregnancy?**
Major congenital malformations occur in 2% to 3% of pregnancies of healthy women with less than 10% resulting from exposure to a drug. To lessen that risk further, the Food and Drug Administration (FDA) has assigned drug risk categories to medications.
    - **Category A**: controlled studies in women failed to demonstrate risk to the fetus in the first trimester and the possibility of fetal harm is remote.
    - **Category B**: either animal reproduction studies have not demonstrated a fetal risk but there are no controlled studies in pregnant women, or animal reproduction studies have shown an adverse effect that was not confirmed in controlled studies in pregnant women during any time in pregnancy.
    - **Category C**: either studies in animals have revealed adverse effects on the fetus and there are no controlled studies in women, or studies in women and animals are not available. Drugs in this class should be given only if potential benefit justifies the potential risk to the fetus.
    - **Category D**: there is positive evidence of human fetal risk, but the benefits from use in pregnant women may be acceptable despite the risk if needed in a life-threatening or serious disease without a safer alternative available.

- **Category X:** studies in animals or humans have demonstrated fetal abnormalities, or there is evidence of fetal risk based on human experience, and the use of the drug in pregnant women clearly outweighs any possible benefit. The drug is contraindicated in women who are or may become pregnant.

17. **A patient whose SLE is well controlled on prednisone (5 mg/day), a nonsteroidal antiinflammatory drug, and hydroxychloroquine (400 mg/day) informs you that she is pregnant. What should you recommend regarding the current medications?**

    Corticosteroids, such as prednisone and methylprednisone, are classified as FDA category B (low-dose) and C (high-dose) drugs. Placental enzymes (11-beta hydroxylase) metabolize 90% of these corticosteroids, and therefore low doses of prednisone (5 to 10 mg/day) are generally well tolerated during pregnancy and probably are protective against a flare of SLE during pregnancy or postpartum. Doses greater than 20 mg of prednisone daily increase risk of preeclampsia, gestational diabetes, and premature rupture of membranes. Cleft lip and palate (<1% to 4%), congenital cataracts, and premature birth are fetal effects that can occur with high-dose corticosteroids.

    Nonsteroidal antiinflammatory drugs (NSAIDs; FDA category C during the first two trimesters; category D during the third trimester). NSAIDs may have an effect on fertility as a result of the importance of cyclooxygenase (COX)-1 and COX-2 in ovulation and implantation. Similarly, miscarriage may be increased (twofold to eightfold) in chronic NSAID users. Therefore, it is recommended that NSAIDs be discontinued or used sparingly during conception. Although congenital malformations, particularly cleft lip and palate, have been seen in animal studies, there is no evidence to suggest that aspirin, indomethacin, diclofenac, ibuprofen, or sulindac causes human fetal abnormalities. There are insufficient data on the newer NSAIDs to include COX-2-specific NSAIDs. There are a few reports of premature ductus arteriosus closure, oligohydramnios, respiratory distress syndrome, pulmonary hypertension, and fetal death associated with indomethacin, therefore this should be avoided. Premature ductus arteriosus closure is a concern with all the NSAIDs after the twenty-seventh week. Therefore, NSAIDs should be used sparingly during the first and second trimesters and stopped completely during the third trimester. One exception would be short-term (<48 hours) use as a tocolytic agent.

    Low-dose **aspirin** (81 mg/day) appears safe and may lessen the risk for preeclampsia in those at high risk (SLE, antiphospholipid antibody syndrome [APAb], systemic sclerosis, vasculitis). Full-dose aspirin (>1 g/day) use at the time of delivery is associated with prolonged labor, anemia, and increased maternal blood loss, along with a possible increased risk of neonatal hemorrhage in premature infants (FDA category D).

    Hydroxychloroquine and **chloroquine** (FDA category C). The blood level in the fetus is similar to the maternal level. There are numerous reports of increased risk of miscarriages, retinal damage, and ototoxicity with high doses of chloroquine. However, recent studies with hydroxychloroquine (400 mg/day) have suggested the risk is relatively low (4.5%) for these complications and therefore the risk may be outweighed by potential benefits. It is generally accepted that patients with SLE who are controlled on hydroxychloroquine should **not** be taken off it during pregnancy.

18. **Can aspirin, NSAIDs, corticosteroids, and antimalarial medications be used during breast feeding?**
    - **Aspirin** in doses greater than one 325-mg tablet results in high infant plasma salicylate levels and should be used cautiously during breast feeding.
    - **NSAIDs** are weak acids and only a small amount gets into breast milk. The American Academy of Pediatrics (AAP) considers ibuprofen, naproxen, diclofenac, tolmetin, piroxicam, and ketorolac compatible with breast feeding. Of these, ibuprofen is the safest option.
    - **Corticosteroids** are excreted in the breast milk at a rate of 0.1% of the total maternal dose, which is less than 10% of the infant's daily endogenous cortisol production and therefore unlikely to be toxic. Peak steroid levels in breast milk occur 2 hours after a dose is taken and have been eliminated by 3 to 4 hours. Therefore, some clinicians recommend that mothers wait 3 to 4 hours before nursing if the dose is greater than 20 to 30 mg.
    - **Antimalarials** (chloroquine/hydroxychloroquine) are compatible with breast feeding according to the AAP. Only 0.2 mg/kg/day gets into breast milk. This is thought to be very low and unlikely to cause retinal toxicity in the infant.

19. **Which nonbiologic disease-modifying antirheumatic drugs can be considered relatively safe for use during pregnancy and lactation?**

    Data on the use of nonbiologic disease-modifying antirheumatic drugs (DMARDs) are limited. Much of the information that is available is derived from anecdotal reports, not prospective studies.

    Sulfasalazine (FDA category B) has been used safely throughout pregnancy and lactation in the treatment of inflammatory bowel disease. Therefore, although its safety in pregnant patients with rheumatic diseases has not been extensively studied, it is probably safe and can be used with caution during pregnancy and lactation. Folate supplementation (800 μg/day) is recommended to prevent neural tube defects because sulfasalazine can cause folate deficiency. Premature infants at risk for hyperbilirubinemia should not be exposed to sulfasalazine, which can potentially displace bilirubin from albumin. Sulfasalazine can cause reversible oligospermia, making conception difficult for up to 2 months after discontinuation. Sulfasalazine is considered safe during lactation in a healthy full term infant. Prematurity and jaundice are contraindications.

Cyclosporine (FDA category C) crosses the placenta and has been associated with IUGR and prematurity (40% rate). More serious effects such as teratogenesis have not been seen despite frequent use in pregnant transplant patients. Cyclosporine is secreted into breast milk. Owing to theoretical risks for immune suppression and growth retardation, use during lactation is not recommended.

Azathioprine (FDA category D) has been used in patients with renal transplants, hematologic malignancies, inflammatory bowel disease, and lupus nephritis during pregnancy. Although placental metabolism may offer some protection to the fetus, various adverse effects to include fetal growth retardation, cytopenias, and opportunistic infections have been identified. Therefore, azathioprine should be reserved for patients whose rheumatic disease is severe and life threatening (such as lupus nephritis). Close prenatal monitoring and long-term evaluation of the offspring are essential. Less than 10% of an azathioprine dose is detected in breast milk and considered safe during lactation although many recommend not breast feeding within 4 hours of a dose in order to lessen exposure. Azathioprine seems to be safe for men who are attempting to father children.

20. **Which nonbiologic DMARDs must be avoided during pregnancy and lactation?**
    - **Methotrexate (MTX)** (FDA category X) is associated with increased spontaneous abortions and birth anomalies. Men and women on MTX should discontinue the drug at least 3 months before conception, owing to prolonged retention of MTX in tissues after discontinuation. Even after discontinuation, female patients should stay on folic acid supplementation (800 µg/day) to lessen the risk of a neural tube defect. Patients who become pregnant while on MTX should discontinue the drug, have the folic acid dose doubled, and have ultrasound screening for fetal anomalies. Breast milk appears to be a minor route of excretion of MTX, but most physicians would recommend against breast feeding if a patient is on MTX.
    - **Leflunomide** (FDA category X) is associated with increased fetal death and teratogenesis. Men and women on leflunomide desiring pregnancy should receive the standard protocol with cholestyramine (8 g three times a day for 11 days) for drug elimination followed by two separate tests to verify negligible (<0.03 mg/L) plasma levels. Without this elimination method, leflunomide remains at unsafe levels for up to 2 years. Consequently, any patient who has taken leflunomide within the previous 2 years should have a blood level check before conception. Patients who become pregnant while taking leflunomide and are treated early with cholestyramine have a 5% to 6% rate of having an infant with a major birth defect, which is only slightly greater than the general population (3% to 4%). Consequently, pregnancy termination is not mandatory and ultrasound screening for fetal anomalies can be done. Little data is available concerning breast feeding so this should be avoided in patients on leflunomide.
    - Mycophenolate mofetil (MMF) (FDA category D) has been shown to be teratogenic in animals and humans with a 22% to 26% rate of congenital malformations. An MMF embryopathy has been identified as the EMFO (Ears, Mouth, Fingers, Organs) tetrad. Women taking MMF who want to get pregnant should be taken off the drug for at least 6 weeks before conception. Many are switched to azathioprine, which is considered safer. Breast feeding is contraindicated in a patient on MMF.
    - **Cyclophosphamide** and **chlorambucil** (both FDA category D) are contraindicated during pregnancy because of the high risks of congenital malformation (22% and 33%, respectively) if used during the first trimester. In extreme situations, cyclophosphamide can be used in the second half of pregnancy. Neonatal bone marrow suppression, infection, and hemorrhage are concerns if used later in pregnancy. Cyclophosphamide is secreted into breast milk and has been associated with leukopenia in the offspring and therefore is not recommended for use during lactation. Chlorambucil has not been shown to pass into breast milk, but data are insufficient to recommend its use during lactation.

21. **Is biologic therapy safe to use during pregnancy and breast feeding?**
    Most biologics are IgG antibodies or receptors attached to the Fc portion of IgG. As such, they will not cross the placenta until after the sixteenth week of gestation. Also, because IgG does not get into breast milk, these biologics are unlikely to get into breast milk. Even if they did, the infant's gastrointestinal (GI) tract should digest them. However, because the safety of these biologics during pregnancy and lactation is not proven, their routine use cannot be recommended.
    Tumor necrosis factor (TNF) inhibitors (FDA category B): animal and small series of human subjects suggest that conception and early pregnancy are not adversely affected by use of TNF inhibitors. One report suggested that VACTERL embryopathy may be increased but this awaits confirmation. All TNF inhibitors cross the placenta but not until after 16 weeks' gestation. Certolizumab lacks an Fc fragment and is the least likely to cross the placenta. Any infant born to a mother who has received TNF inhibitors (especially infliximab) during the third trimester should not be given live vaccines for the first 6 months postpartum until the anti-TNF-α antibodies have been cleared from the neonate's circulation. Breast feeding is permissible.
    Anakinra (FDA category B): animal and small series of human subjects suggest that conception and early pregnancy are not adversely affected. It should only be used in pregnancy when benefits outweigh the risks. Safety in breast feeding is unknown.
    Rituximab (FDA category C) has been shown to cause transient cytopenias and B cell depletion in fetus and infants. Owing to its long half-life, it is recommended to stop 6 months before conception. It is unknown if it is transmitted in breast milk.

Abatacept (FDA category C): animal studies have not shown teratogenicity. Abatacept does cross the placenta. There is no human data, therefore it is recommended that abatacept be discontinued 10 weeks before conception. It is unknown if it gets into breast milk.

Tocilizumab (FDA category C): animal studies have not shown adverse effects during pregnancy. Tocilizumab does cross the placenta after 16 weeks of gestation. There is no human data, therefore it is recommended that tocilizumab be stopped 10 weeks before conception. It is unknown if it gets into breast milk. Notably, tocilizumab may decrease the effectiveness of birth control pills.

Belimumab (FDA category C): animal studies have not shown teratogenicity. Belimumab does cross the placenta in the latter half of pregnancy. There is no human data, therefore it is recommended that belimumab be discontinued 10 weeks before conception. It is unknown if it gets into breast milk.

Tofacitinib (FDA category C): animal studies have shown adverse effects. Therefore, tofacitinib should be stopped before pregnancy. In spite of its short half-life, it should be stopped 1 month before conception. It gets into breast milk so breast feeding is contraindicated.

22. **Who is collecting data on the outcome of patients who are pregnant and fetuses exposed to these antirheumatic medications?**
   Organization of Teratology Information Specialists (OTIS). This organization is collecting data on autoimmune diseases and pregnancy as well as autoimmune disease treatments and pregnancy. They can be reached at http://www.otispregnancy.org and by calling 1-877-311-8972.

BIBLIOGRAPHY

Ali YM, Kuriya B, Orozco C: Can tumor necrosis factor inhibitors be safely used in pregnancy? J Rheumatol 37:9–17, 2010.
American Academy of Pediatrics Committee on Drugs: Transfer of drugs and other chemicals into human milk, Pediatrics 108:776–789, 2001.
Anderka MT, Lin AE, Abuelo DN, et al: Reviewing the evidence for mycophenylate mofetil as a new teratogen: a case report and review of the literature, Am J Med Genet A 149A:1241–1248, 2009.
Branch DW, Khamashata MA: Antiphospholipid syndrome. In Queenan JT, editor: High-risk pregnancy, Washington DC, 2007, American College of Obstetricians and Gynecologists.
Browne H, Manipalviratn S, Armstrong A: Using an intrauterine device in immunocompromised women, Obstet Gynecol 112:667–669, 2008.
Cassina M, Johnson DL, Robinson LK, et al: Pregnancy outcome in women exposed to leflunomide before or during pregnancy, Arthritis Rheum 64:2085–2094, 2012.
Cleary BJ, Kallen B: Early pregnancy azathioprine use and pregnancy outcomes, Birth Defects Res A Clin Mol Teratol 85:647–654, 2009.
Clowse ME, Magder LS, Witter F, Petri M: The impact of increased lupus activity on obstetric outcomes, Arthritis Rheum 52:514–521, 2005.
Clowse MEB, Magder L, Petri M: Cyclophosphamide for lupus during pregnancy, Lupus 14:593–597, 2006.
Clowse MEB, Magder L, Witter F, Petri M: Hydroxychloroquine in lupus pregnancy, Arthritis Rheum 54:3640–3647, 2006.
Costedoat-Chalumeau N, Amoura Z, Huong DLT, et al: Safety of hydroxychloroquine in pregnant patients with connective tissue diseases. Review of the literature, Autoimmunity Rev 4:111–115, 2005.
Friedman DM, Kim MY, Copel JA, et al: Prospective evaluation of fetuses with autoimmune-associated congenital heart block: the PR Interval and Dexamethasone Evaluation (PRIDE) study, Am J Cardiol 103:1102–1106, 2009.
Friedman DM, Rupel A, Buyon JP: Epidemiology, etiology, detection, and treatment of autoantibody-associated congenital heart block in neonatal lupus, Curr Rheumatol Rep 9:101–108, 2007.
Golding A, Haque UJ, Giles JT: Rheumatoid arthritis and reproduction, Rheum Dis Clin North Am 33:319–343, 2007.
Hazes JMW, Coulie PG, Geenen V, et al: Rheumatoid arthritis and pregnancy: evolution of disease activity and pathophysiological considerations for drug use, Rheumatology 50:1955–1968, 2011.
Ingec M, Nazik H, Kadanali S: Urinary calcium excretion in severe preeclampsia and eclampsia, Clin Chem Lab Med 44:51–53, 2006.
Lockshin MD, Kim M, Laskin CA, et al: Prediction of adverse pregnancy outcome by the presence of lupus anticoagulant, but not anticardiolipin antibody, in patients with antiphospholipid antibody, Arthritis Rheum 64:2311–2318, 2012.
Mok CC, Chan PT, To CH: Anti-mullerian hormone and ovarian reserve in systemic lupus erythematosus, Arthritis Rheum 65:206–210, 2013.
Park-Wyllie L, Mazzotta P, Pastuszak A, et al: Birth defects after maternal exposure to corticosteroids, Teratology 62:385–392, 2000.
Petri M, Kim MY, Kalunian KC, et al: Combined oral contraceptives in women with systemic lupus erythematosus, N Engl J Med 353:2550–2558, 2005.
Pisoni CN, Brucato A, Ruffatti A, et al: Failure of intravenous immunoglobulin to prevent congenital heart block: findings of a multicenter, prospective, observational study, Arthritis Rheum 62:1147–1152, 2010.
Saha SP, Bhattacharjee N, Ganguli RP, et al: Prevalence and significance of antiphospholipid antibodies in selected at-risk obstetric cases: a comparative prospective study, J Obstet Gynecol 29:614–618, 2009.
Sammaritano LR: Pregnancy in rheumatic disease patients, J Clin Rheumatol 19:259–266, 2013.
Sammaritano LR, Bermas BL: Rheumatoid arthritis medications and lactation, Curr Opin Rheumatol 26:354–360, 2014.
Sánchez-Guerrero J, Uribe AG, Jiménez-Santana L, et al: A trial of contraceptive methods in women with systemic lupus erythematosus, N Engl J Med 353:2539–2549, 2005.
Shim L, Eslick GD, Simring AA, et al: The effects of azathioprine on birth outcomes in women with inflammatory bowel disease, J Crohns Colitis 5:234–238, 2011.
Smyth A, Oliveira GH, Lahr BD, et al: A systemic review and meta-analysis of pregnancy outcomes in patients with systemic lupus erythematosus and lupus nephritis, Clin J Am Soc Nephrol 5:2060–2068, 2010.

Steen VD: Fertility and pregnancy outcome in women with systemic sclerosis, Arthritis Rheum 42:763–768, 1999.
Temprano KK, Brandlamudi R, Moore TL: Antirheumatic drugs in pregnancy and lactation, Semin Arthritis Rheum 35:112–121, 2005.

Further Reading

http://www.otispregnancy.org
http://toxnet.nlm.nih.gov/

CHAPTER 79: FAMILIAL AUTOINFLAMMATORY SYNDROMES

M. Kristen Demoruelle, MD and Christina M. Bright, MD

KEY POINTS

1. Autoinflammatory syndromes present as recurrent episodes of inflammation without evidence of infection or autoantibodies.
2. Autoinflammatory syndromes are characterized by episodes of fever, rash, arthritis, peritonitis, eye inflammation, and elevated acute phase reactants in various combinations that normalize between flares.
3. Familial Mediterranean fever (FMF) is the only autoinflammatory syndrome responsive to colchicine.
4. In the cryopyrin-associated periodic syndromes (CAPS), nucleotide-binding oligomerization domain, leucine-rich repeat, and pyrin domain containing 3 (NLRP3) mutations cause dysfunction of the inflammasome leading to abnormal interleukin-1β (IL-1β) production.
5. Amyloidosis (AA) can lead to renal failure in untreated patients.
6. IL-1β inhibitors are the most effective therapy for many of these diseases.

1. What characterizes the familial autoinflammatory syndromes?
The familial autoinflammatory syndromes (FAS) are characterized as follows:
- Recurrent (not necessarily periodic) episodes of antigen-independent inflammation
- Involvement of the innate immune system mediated primarily by IL-1β
- Absence of infection or autoimmunity (no autoantibodies)

2. What are the characteristic clinical features of FAS?
Typically, acute unprovoked attacks are characterized by fever and elevated inflammatory markers (e.g., erythrocyte sedimentation rate [ESR], C-reactive protein [CRP], white blood cell [WBC], and serum amyloid A) associated with additional symptoms involving joints, abdomen, skin, and eyes. Acute attacks resolve spontaneously, and between acute attacks patients are usually asymptomatic with normal laboratory values.

3. What are the FAS?
The FAS are listed in Table 79-1.

4. What nonhereditary diseases need to be ruled out in patients with prolonged (>2 years), recurrent fever syndromes?
- Infectious
  - Hidden infectious focus (aortoenteric fistula, Caroli's disease)
  - Recurrent reinfection (chronic meningococcemia, host defense defect)
  - Specific infection (Whipple's disease, malaria)
- Noninfectious inflammatory disorders
  - Adult-onset Still's disease
  - Juvenile idiopathic arthritis (JIA)
  - Schnitzler syndrome
  - Behçet's syndrome
  - Inflammatory bowel disease (usually Crohn's disease)
  - Sarcoidosis
  - Extrinsic alveoliits
  - Humidifier lung, polymer fume fever
- Neoplastic
  - Lymphoma (Hodgkin's disease, angioimmunoblastic lymphoma)
  - Solid tumor (pheochromocytoma, myxoma, colon carcinoma, renal cell carcinoma)
- Vascular (recurrent pulmonary embolism)
- Hypothalamic
- Psychogenic periodic fever
- Factitious
- Cyclic neutropenia

Table 79-1. Familial Autoinflammatory Syndromes (FAS)

CLASSIFICATION	SYNDROME	AGE AT ONSET (YEARS)	DURATION OF ATTACK (DAYS)	CLINICAL FEATURES	AMYLOID RISK	GENE	PROTEIN
Periodic fever syndromes	FMF	<20	1-3	Erysipelas-like rash, sterile peritonitis, monoarthritis, pleuritis	+++	MEFV	Pyrin
	TRAPS	<20	>14	Myalgias with overlying rash, conjunctivitis or periorbital edema, abdominal pain, monoarthritis	++	TNFRSF1A	TNF receptor type 1
	HIDS	<1	3-7	Maculopapular rash, abdominal pain, splenomegaly, cervical lymphadenopathy, aphthous ulcers	−	MVK	Mevalonate kinase
Cryopyrin-associated periodic syndromes (CAPS)	FCAS	<1	<2	Cold-induced urticaria, arthralgia, conjunctivitis	−	CIAS1 (NLRP3)	Cryopyrin
	MWS	<20	1-2	Urticarial rash, arthralgia/arthritis, conjunctivitis, sensorineural hearing loss	++	CIAS1 (NLRP3)	Cryopyrin
	CINCA or NOMID	<1	Continuous	Epiphyseal bone formation, chronic aseptic meningitis, arthopathy, hepatosplenomegaly	+	CIAS1 (NLRP3)	Cryopyrin
Other	PAPA	<10	Variable	Pyogenic sterile arthritis, pyoderma gangrenosum, acne	Unknown	CD2BP1/PSTPIP1	CD2-binding protein
	Blau	<3-5	Variable	Polyarthritis, tenosynovitis, anterior or panuveitis	Unknown	NOD2/CARD15	NOD2
	DIRA	<4 weeks	Variable	Skin rash (pustulosis), sterile osteomyelitis	Unknown	IL-1RN	IL-1 RA

CINCA, Chronic infantile neurologic, cutaneous, and articular syndrome; DIRA, deficiency of the IL-1 receptor antagonist; FCAS, familial cold autoinflammatory syndrome; FMF, familial Mediterranean fever; HIDS, hyperimmunoglobulin D syndrome; MWS, Muckle–Wells syndrome; NOMID, neonatal-onset multisystem inflammatory disease; PAPA, pyogenic sterile arthritis, pyoderma gangrenosum, and acne syndrome; TRAPS, tumor necrosis factor-α receptor autoinflammatory periodic syndrome.

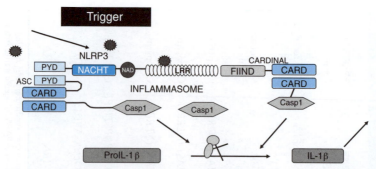

Figure 79-1. The importance of the inflammasome and IL-1β in the pathogenesis of FAS. *CARD*, Caspase activation and recruitment domain; *Casp1*, caspase 1; *FAS*, familial autoinflammatory syndromes; *FIIND*, function to find domain; *IL-1β*, interleukin-1β; *LRR*, leucine-rich repeat; *NACHT*, also called NOD (nucleotide-binding oligomerization) domain; *NLRP3*, nucleotide-binding oligomerization domain, leucine-rich repeat, and pyrin domain containing 3; *PYD*, pyrin domain.

5. Discuss the importance of the inflammasome and IL-1β in the pathogenesis of FAS.

The gene *CIAS1* on chromosome 1 encodes for the protein previously called **cryopyrin** but is now known as NLRP3 (or NALP3). NLRP3 is a member of the nucleotide-binding oligomerization domain-leucine-rich repeat (NOD-LRR) protein family. It consists of a pyrin domain (PYD), a NOD (also called NACHT), and an LRR domain. NLRP3 is primarily found in neutrophils and monocytes and is an intracellular sensor of pathogens and danger signals. Upon stimulation, NLRP3 interacts with adaptor proteins ASC and Cardinal forming a multiprotein complex called the **NLRP3 inflammasome**. ASC contains a PYD and a caspase activation and recruitment domain (CARD) whereas Cardinal contains a function to find (FIIND) domain and a CARD domain. The PYD of NLRP3 interacts with PYD of ASC whereas the LRR domain of NLRP3 interacts with FIIND of Cardinal. This activates both CARDs, which then interact with CARD on procaspase 1, therein activating it to caspase 1 (also called the IL-1β converting enzyme [ICE]). Caspase 1 can activate pro-IL-1β to be released as the proinflammatory cytokine IL-1β. Genetic mutations of any of these proteins can contribute to development of the FAS (Figure 79-1).

PERIODIC FEVER SYNDROMES

6. What is the most common FAS?

Familial Mediterranean fever (FMF). Note there are two presentations of FMF. Type 1 is characterized by recurrent episodes of inflammation and serositis. Patients can develop AA and renal failure. Type 2, where there is no previous history of inflammatory episodes, is characterized by AA (especially renal) as the first manifestation of FMF. Both types of FMF respond to colchicine therapy.

7. What clinical features are characteristic of an acute episode of FMF?

- Children <20 years of age (90% of cases) of Eastern Mediterranean ancestry (Armenian, Jewish, Arabian, and Turkish origin)
- **Fever lasting 12 to 72 hours** (100%)
- Serositis: **generalized peritonitis** (85% to 95%), unilateral pleuritis (33% to 66%)
- Typically nondestructive **large joint monoarticular arthritis** (hip, knee, ankle, wrist) (50% to 77%): severe pain out of proportion to swelling; absence of erythema and warmth; **poorly responsive to prednisone**
- **Erysipelas-like rash** (30%)
- **Attacks responsive to colchicine**
- Recurrence of attacks: average every 2 to 4 weeks
- Uncommon manifestations: polyarthritis, prolonged arthritis, severe lower extremity myalgias, aseptic meningitis, pericarditis, scrotal swelling, lymphadenopathy, Henoch–Schönlein purpura, infertility as a result of peritoneal adhesions

8. What is the genetic mutation associated with FMF?

A mutation of the Mediterranean fever (*MEFV*) gene on the short arm of chromosome 16 that encodes the **pyrin** protein. The pattern of inheritance in FMF is primarily autosomal recessive. There are over 80 mutations with six being most common. Notably, in 30% of patients only one or no mutations are found.

9. What is the role of IL-1 in FMF?

FMF is an IL-1-dependent inflammatory process. Pyrin is one protein component of the NLRP3 inflammasome (see Question 5). Mutations of pyrin lead to increased IL-1 β production.

10. **What is the treatment and prognosis for FMF?**
    Renal AA leading to renal failure occurs commonly in untreated patients. The prevalence of renal AA is more common in certain ethnic populations, increases with age, and is not associated with the severity or frequency of acute attacks. Daily colchicine prevents both acute attacks of FMF and subsequent development of renal AA. IL-1 inhibitors including anakinra can be used if intolerant or unresponsive to colchicine (5% to 10% of patients with FMF are unresponsive to colchicine). Thalidomide and tumor necrosis factor-α (TNFα) antagonists have also shown some benefit. End-stage renal disease as a result of AA is treated with renal transplantation with continuing colchicine therapy.

11. **What clinical features are characteristic of an acute episode of TNFα receptor autoinflammatory periodic syndrome?**
    The features of TNFα receptor autoinflammatory periodic syndrome (TRAPS) are as follows:
    - Formerly called **familial Hibernian fever**; most common in Northwestern Europeans.
    - Primarily children, but age of onset can vary up to middle-aged adults.
    - High, spiking **fever varies in duration but always >5 days**, averages 3 to 4 weeks.
    - **Centrifugal, migratory, erythematous patch** or urticarial plaque overlying area of myalgia.
    - **Arthralgias** (hip, knee, ankle, wrist); synovitis rare and monoarticular if it occurs.
    - Myalgias of thighs that migrate to other areas.
    - **Ocular inflammation common**: conjunctivitis, perorbital pain/edema.
    - **Peritonitis** (92%), pleuritis.
    - Responsive to glucocorticoids. **No response to colchicine.**
    - Recurrence of attacks: average two to six attacks per year.
    - Uncommon manifestations (<5%): pericarditis, scrotal swelling, uveitis.

12. **What is the genetic mutation in TRAPS?**
    Mutations are in the gene for type I (55 kDa) TNFα receptor (*TNFRSF1A*) on the short arm of chromosome 12. Most mutations are single-nucleotide missense mutations and affect the extracellular domain of the TNF receptor. The pattern of inheritance is autosomal dominant.

13. **What are the theories behind the pathogenesis of TRAPS?**
    There are two main theories to explain how the mutation in TRAPS causes increased inflammation. One theory is that mutated TNF receptor molecules interact with each other in the absence of TNF binding. This interaction allows for ligand-independent signaling, which increases cytokine release and leads to fever and cachexia. A second theory is that the mutation in the extracellular domain of the TNF receptor prevents it from shedding into the extracellular space and therefore there is less receptor to bind excess TNF.

14. **What is the prognosis and treatment for TRAPS?**
    AA occurs in 15% to 25% of patients with TRAPS and its primary complication is renal dysfunction with proteinuria. Therefore, patients should be periodically screened with a urinalysis. Treatment lessens the chance of developing AA. First-line therapy consists of nonsteroidal antiinflammatory drugs (NSAIDs) and glucocorticoids. Prednisone is typically started at doses >20 mg/day and then tapered over several weeks. Etanercept is more effective than monoclonal antibodies because it is a fusion protein of the receptor. The overall response rate is 66%. There is evidence that anti-IL-1 therapy (anakinra) is also effective and should be used in patients who are not responsive to etanercept.

15. **What clinical features are characteristic of an acute episode of hyper hyperimmunoglobulin D syndrome?**
    The features of hyperimmunoglobulin D syndrome (HIDS) are as follows:
    - Also known as **mevalonate kinase deficiency.**
    - Onset in infants <1 year old (90% of cases); median 4 months; episodes become more frequent in childhood; mostly whites.
    - Rare onset in adolescence or young adults.
    - Fever lasting 1 to 10 days (100%); median **3 to 5 days**; acute onset with chills.
    - Fever associated with **cervical adenopathy, abdominal pain** with nausea and vomiting, and splenomegaly.
    - **Skin rash with erythematous macules,** papules, petechiae that can affect anywhere including face, palms, and soles.
    - Other frequent manifestations: headache, myalgias, arthralgias, painful **orogenital ulcers** (40%), large joint arthritis.
    - Recurrence of attacks: average every 4 to 6 weeks; can vary in severity and frequency.

16. **Are there any triggers for acute attacks in a patient with HIDS?**
    HIDS can be induced by immunizations, surgery, minor trauma, and physical or emotional stress.

17. **What laboratory abnormalities are constantly present in HIDS, even between acute episodes? How about during episodes of flare?**
    Elevated immunoglobulin D (IgD) levels (>100 U/mL) are constantly present. IgD levels can rarely be normal (<2 U/mL) in some patients with HIDS (usually <3 years of age). Note that IgD levels can be elevated in other

inflammatory diseases but never greater than 100 U/mL. Patients with HIDS can also have elevated IgA levels (>2.6 g/L) in 80% of cases. ESR, CRP, WBC, and **urinary mevalonic acid** are increased only during flares.

18. **What is the genetic mutation associated with HIDS? How does it lead to recurrent febrile episodes?**

    An autosomal recessive mutation of the mevalonate kinase (MVK) gene on chromosome 12 that encodes the MVK enzyme. MVK is involved in the cholesterol synthesis pathway. Through this pathway, MVK mutations lead to decreased production of geranylgeranyl pyrophosphate (GGPP), and decreased geranylgeranylation of GTPase Rac1 can result in increased IL-1β production by peripheral blood mononuclear cells.

19. **Is there any treatment for HIDS? What is the prognosis?**

    NSAIDs for fever or arthralgias. There is no universally accepted therapy to prevent acute attacks, but anakinra, etanercept, and simvastatin have shown some benefit. These patients rarely have a good response to oral corticosteroids or colchicine. There are good long-term outcomes in most patients with HIDS. Half of patients experience complete or partial remission. AA is rare.

CAPS

20. **What are the CAPS?**
    - **Familial cold autoinflammatory syndrome (FCAS):** this is the mildest form of CAPS. Patients typically develop fever, chills, rash (100%), arthralgia (93%), and conjunctivitis (84%) within 1 to 3 hours after **cold exposure**. Typical attacks start with a rash on the extremities, then extend to other parts of the body. The rashes can be urticarial patches, erythematous macules, or petichiae. The subsequent fever lasts from hours to 3 days. Most patients (95%) develop symptoms within the first year of life. Symptoms become less severe as the patient gets older. AA is rare.
    - **Muckle–Wells syndrome (MWS):** this form of CAPS is of intermediate severity. Generally **starts in adolescence** and episodes can be triggered by hunger, fatigue, or cold exposure. Attacks last for 24 to 48 hours and are characterized by fever, chills, abdominal pain, myalgia, urticarial rash, macules (1 to 7 cm in diameter) and conjunctivitis. Patients can have either arthralgias or uncommonly large joint arthritis. Late-onset **development of deafness** is a common complication of MWS. Renal AA can occur.
    - **Chronic infantile neurologic, cutaneous, and articular syndrome (CINCA)/neonatal-onset multisystem inflammatory disease (NOMID):** the most severe form of CAPS. Characterized by **triad of chronic aseptic meningitis, neonatal-onset skin lesions, and arthropathy**. This triad is accompanied by recurrent fever. Onset is within the first few months of life and patients develop a generalized urticarial skin rash, fever, and often lymphadenopathy and hepatosplenomegaly. Typically, central nervous system (CNS) manifestations occur later with evidence of chronic aseptic meningitis. Late complications include headache from chronic meningitis, visual impairment, sensorineural hearing loss, hoarseness, and arthropathy with enlarged epiphysis and patellar overgrowth. Prognosis is poor with 20% mortality in childhood. AA can occur.

21. **What is the inheritance pattern and genetic mutation in CAPS?**

    CAPS has an autosomal dominant inheritance pattern, however there are also cases from sporadic mutations. The mutation in CAPS is found in the *CIAS1* gene, found on the long arm of chromosome 1. This gene codes for the protein previously called **cryopyrin** but is now known as NLRP3 (or NALP3). Most mutations occur in the NOD domain (NACHT). The severity of the mutation correlates with the progressive severity of the CAPS (also known as cryopyrinopathies). One hypothesis is that the defect prevents an intrinsic autoinhibitory mechanism in NLRP3 leading to increased inflammasome activity and ultimately increased IL-1β. See Question 5.

22. **How are the cryopyrinopathies (CAPS) diagnosed?**

    Owing to autosomal dominant transmission, family history can be elicited that is suggestive of a cryopyrinopathy. Laboratory results generally show a nonspecific elevation in inflammatory markers such as ESR and CRP and leukocytosis during attacks. Genetic testing of the *CIAS1* (NLRP3) gene can be performed; however, not all patients (only 60% of CINCA/NOMID patients) can be identified using known mutations.

23. **What is the treatment of choice for CAPS?**

    IL-1 inhibitors have become the treatment of choice for CAPS. Daily subcutaneous anakinra (1 to 2 mg/kg) has shown improvement in patients with CINCA/NOMID syndrome. Other studies have recorded benefit with **canakinumab** (anti-1L-β) every 2 months and **rilonocept** (IL-1 trap) weekly in patients with CAPS.

OTHER AUTOINFLAMMATORY SYNDROMES

24. **What are the differences between PAPA and PFAPA?**
    - **Pyogenic sterile arthritis, pyoderma gangrenosum, and acne syndrome (PAPA):** a rare autosomal dominant episodic disorder resulting from mutation of CD2-binding protein 1 (*CD2BP1*), also known as proline-serine-threonine phosphatase interacting protein 1 (PSTPIP1). This mutation results in hyperphosphorylation of PSTPIP1 resulting in a stronger interaction between PSTPIP1 and pyrin that leads to increased IL-1B production. The first episode of arthritis typically occurs between 1 and 10 years of age

and affects one joint at a time. Fever is not prominent. The skin manifestations typically occur later (at puberty). Treatment includes glucocorticoids and biologics (infliximab or anakinra).
- **Periodic fever with aphthous stomatitis, pharyngitis, and adenitis syndrome (PFAPA):** is characterized by recurrent febrile episodes beginning in early childhood. Acute episodes last 3 to 6 days and involve fever, elevated inflammatory markers, aphthous ulcers, pharyngitis, lymphadenopathy, and mild abdominal pain. Many patients outgrow the febrile episodes. The genetic mutation is currently unknown.

25. What are the differences between Blau syndrome and early-onset sarcoidosis?

Nothing. They are the same disease and are also known as **familial granulomatous arthritis**. Clinically, patients have recurrent granulomatous inflammation of the **joints** (polyarthritis or tenosynovitis), **eyes** (anterior uveitis or panuveitis), and **skin** (dermal granulomas) with onset before the age of 5 years. Other manifestations include multiple interphalangeal contractures, cranial neuropathies, fever, and large-vessel vasculitis. The disease is associated with mutations in the nucleotide-binding oligomerization domain 2/caspase recruitment domain 15 gene (*NOD2/CARD15*) on chromosome 16. Interestingly, different polymorphisms in *NOD2/CARD15* are associated with susceptibility to Crohn's disease, however, there is no bowel inflammation in Blau syndrome. Infliximab, corticosteroids, and anakinra have proven beneficial. Joint deformity and visual impairment can occur in nonresponders.

26. What are the differences between DIRA and DITRA?

- **Deficiency of the IL-1 receptor antagonist (DIRA):** patients with this autosomal recessive syndrome are homozygotes for mutations of the gene (*IL1RN*) encoding the IL-1 receptor antagonist (IL-1ra) resulting in absence of endogenous IL-1ra secretion. Onset is typically in the first month of life and patients have symptoms of cutaneous pustulosis and sterile osteomyelitis. They do not have fever. Anakinra has been used to treat this disease.
- **Deficiency of IL-36 receptor antagonist (DITRA):** patients with this syndrome have missense mutations in IL-36 receptor antagonist leading to uninhibited IL-36 signaling. Onset can be from neonate to adult. Patients have generalized pustulosis including the palms and soles. Glossitis, nail dystrophy, and oligoarthritis can occur.

27. What is the CANDLE syndrome? What is CRMO?

- **Chronic atypical neutrophilic dermatosis with lipodystrophy and elevated temperature (CANDLE):** patients have recurrent fever in infancy, almost daily, in addition to skin rash (erythematous annular plaques) and unique facial features including lipodystrophy (loss of fat on their face). It is associated with a genetic mutation in the *PSMB8* gene that encodes components of cellular proteasomes resulting in an abnormal interferon-γ (IFNγ) response.
- **Chronic recurrent multifocal osteomyelitis (CRMO):** also known as Majeed's syndrome. CRMO is an autoinflammatory osteopathy caused by mutations in the *LPIN2* gene encoding for the protein, lipin-2. Beginning in early childhood, patients have fever, bone lesions (osteolysis with surrounding sclerosis on radiograph), anemia, and rash (psoriasis, palmoplantar pustulosis, acne).

BIBLIOGRAPHY

Agostini L, Martinon F, Burns K, et al: NALP3 forms an IL-1beta-processing inflammasome with increased activity in Muckle-Wells autoinflammatory disorder, Immunity 20:319–325, 2004.
Aksentijevich I, Masters SL, Ferguson PJ, et al: An autoinflammatory disease with deficiency of the interleukin-1-receptor antagonist, N Engl J Med 360:2426–2437, 2009.
Drenth JP, van der Meer JW: The inflammasome – linebacker of innate defense, N Engl J Med 355:730–732, 2006.
Goldbach-Mansky R: Immunology in clinic review series; focus on autoinflammatory diseases: update on monogenic autoinflammatory diseases: the role of interleukin (IL)-1 and an emerging role of cytokines beyond IL-1, Clin Exp Immunol 167:391–404, 2012.
Goldbach-Mansky R, Dailey NJ, Canna SW, et al: Neonatal-onset multisystem inflammatory disease responsive to interleuking-1beta inhibition, N Engl J Med 355:581–592, 2006.
Hoffman HM: Therapy of autoinflammatory syndromes, J Allergy Clin Immunol 124:1129–1138, 2009.
Hoffman HM, Throne ML, Amar NJ, et al: Efficacy and safety of rilonacept (interleukin-1 Trap) in patients with cryopyrin-associated periodic syndromes: results from two sequential placebo-controlled studies, Arthritis Rheum 58:2443–2452, 2008.
Lachmann HJ, Kone-Paut I, Kuemmerle-Deschner JB, et al: Use of canakinumab in the cryopyrin-associated periodic syndrome, N Engl J Med 360:2416–2425, 2006.
Mankan AK, Kubarenko A, Hornung V: Immunology in clinic review series; focus on autoinflammatory diseases: update on monogenic autoinflammatory diseases: inflammasomes: mechanisms of activation, Clin Exp Immunol 167:369–381, 2012.
Masters SL, Simon A, Aksentijevich I, Kastner DL: Horror autoinflammaticus: the molecular pathophysiology of autoinflammatory disease, Annu Rev Immunol 27:621–668, 2009.
Ozen S, Bilginer Y, Ayaz NA, Calguneri M: Anti-interleukin 1 treatment for patients with familial Mediterranean fever resistant to colchicine, J Rheumatol 38:516–518, 2011.
Ozkurede VU, Franchi L: Immunology in clinic review series; focus on autoinflammatory diseases: update on monogenic autoinflammatory diseases: role of inflammasomes in autoinflammatory syndromes, Clin Exp Immunol 167:382–390, 2012.
Shohat M, Halpern GJ: Familial Mediterranean fever—a review, Genet Med 13:487–498, 2011.
van der Hilst JC, Bodar EJ, Barron KS, et al: Long-term follow-up, clinical features, and quality of life in a series of 103 patients with hyperimmunoglobulinemia D syndrome, Medicine (Baltimore) 87:301–310, 2008.

FURTHER READING

http://www.rarediseases.org

CHAPTER 80

ODDS AND ENDS

Sterling G. West, MD

> **KEY POINTS**
>
> 1. Patients with palindromic rheumatism involving small joints of hands associated with rheumatoid factor are most likely to develop rheumatoid arthritis.
> 2. Multicentric reticulohistiocytosis frequently involves the distal interphalangeal joints.
> 3. Patients with erythromelalgia who respond to aspirin therapy have an underlying myeloproliferative disorder.
> 4. Always rule out a medication as the cause of musculoskeletal symptoms.

1. **Name the nonhereditary periodic arthritis syndromes. Why are they grouped together?**
   - Intermittent hydrarthrosis.
   - Palindromic rheumatism.
   - Eosinophilic synovitis.
   - RS3PE syndrome (see Chapter 15).

   These syndromes are grouped together because they share four features: (1) intermittent arthritis followed by periods of remission; (2) complete resolution between attacks; (3) rare development of joint damage; and (4) unknown cause.

2. **Are all disorders with intermittent arthritis encompassed by the periodic syndromes?**
   No. Many other disorders may include intermittent joint swelling and other characteristics of the periodic syndromes. Among these are mechanical and inflammatory disorders. Thus, a broad differential should be kept in mind in patients with intermittent arthritis.

   Periodic syndromes
     Intermittent hydrarthrosis
     Palindromic rheumatism
     Eosinophilic synovitis
     Familial autoinflammatory syndromes
   Crystalline arthropathies
     Gout
     Calcium pyrophosphate dihydrate/pseudogout
     Hydroxyapatite
   RS3PE

   Spondyloarthropathies
     Reactive arthritis
     Enteropathic arthritis
   Sarcoidosis
   Infections
     Lyme disease
     Whipple's disease
   Mechanical
     Loose bodies
     Meniscal tears

3. **Describe the typical clinical features of intermittent hydrarthrosis.**
   Recurrent joint effusions occur at regular intervals. Males and females are equally affected. May parallel menses in females and resolve after menopause. The knee or another large joint develops an effusion over 12 to 24 hours with no or minimal discomfort or signs of inflammation. Attacks last 3 to 5 days. There are no systemic symptoms, no treatment is proven to prevent or abort attacks, and episodes may occur lifelong.

4. **What do laboratory studies and joint radiographs show in intermittent hydrarthrosis?**
   Laboratory tests, including the erythrocyte sedimentation rate (ESR), are normal, even during an attack. Synovial fluid is normal or mildly inflammatory (5000 white blood cells/mm^3) with a slight increase in polymorphonuclear leukocytes. An effusion may be seen on radiographs, but no other abnormalities are seen even after years of attacks.

5. **What is palindromic rheumatism? What does it mean?**
   Palindromic rheumatism is a recurrent syndrome of acute arthritis and periarthritis. *Palindromic* means "recurring" and is derived from a Greek word which literally means "to run back." The term *palindromic* was introduced by Hench and Rosenberg in 1944 as descriptive of the syndrome. They preferred *rheumatism* to *arthritis* because of the frequent involvement of periarticular structures and occasional presence of subcutaneous nodules.

6. **How do the clinical features of palindromic rheumatism differ from those of intermittent hydrarthrosis?**
   Palindromic rheumatism, similar to intermittent hydrarthrosis, affects both men and women, often begins in the third to fifth decade, frequently affects the knees, and is rarely associated with constitutional symptoms.

However, unlike intermittent hydrarthrosis, palindromic rheumatism attacks occur irregularly and may involve more than one joint (usually 2 to 5 joints). The pattern of joint attacks tends to be characteristic in an individual patient. Symptoms may begin in one joint while waning in another. Attacks are sudden and pain may be intense, often reaching a peak within a few hours. Signs of joint inflammation (swelling, warmth, redness) can be noted soon after pain begins. Small joints of the hands, wrist, and feet may be affected, and occasionally the temporomandibular joints. Also, unlike intermittent hydrarthrosis, periarticular attacks (occurring in one third of cases) and transient subcutaneous nodules may be seen.

7. **What do laboratory studies and joint radiographs show in palindromic rheumatism?**
The ESR and other acute phase reactants may be elevated during attacks but are normal between them. Rheumatoid factor (RF) and anticyclic citrullinated peptide (anti-CCP) are positive in 30% to 50% of cases and identify patients who will develop rheumatoid arthritis. Antinuclear antibodies (ANAs) are typically negative and serum complement levels are normal. There have been few studies of synovial fluid in palindromic rheumatism. Leukocytes may vary from a few hundred to several thousand, with the magnitude poorly correlated with symptom severity. Radiographs show only soft tissue swelling.

8. **How is palindromic rheumatism treated?**
Nonsteroidal antiinflammatory drugs (NSAIDs) may provide some relief from joint symptoms but do not reliably prevent attacks. A variety of other agents have been used including antimalarial agents, sulfasalazine, and methotrexate.

9. **Describe the course of palindromic rheumatism.**
Although the course is variable, fewer than 10% of patients experience a spontaneous remission. Some patients continue to have the disease for many years. However, 30% to 50% of cases evolve into a chronic inflammatory arthritis, usually rheumatoid arthritis. Less commonly, a diagnosis of systemic lupus erythematosus (SLE) or other connective tissue disease is eventually made. Antimalarials and methotrexate have been reported to reduce the risk of subsequent development of rheumatoid arthritis or other connective tissue disease.

10. **What features are predictive of a patient with palindromic rheumatism later developing rheumatoid arthritis?**
Female gender, proximal interphalangeal and wrist involvement, positive RF and/or anti-CCP, and HLA-DR4 positivity increase the likelihood of evolution to rheumatoid arthritis.

11. **What are the clinical characteristics of eosinophilic synovitis?**
    - History of atopy, may have dermatographism.
    - Both genders, age of onset 20 to 50 years old.
    - Minor trauma causes acute onset (within 12 to 24 hours) of painless monoarthritis (usually knee) without warmth or erythema. Trauma may activate mast cells which attract eosinophils.
    - Synovial fluid shows mildly inflammatory fluid with up to 50% eosinophils. Charcot–Leyden crystals (bipyramidal, hexagonal-shaped crystal made of products of intracellular lipases in eosinophils) may be seen.
    - Peripheral blood white blood cell normal with no eosinophilia. ESR normal.
    - Attacks last 1 to 2 weeks. Therapy is NSAIDs.

12. **How does Tietze's syndrome differ from costochondritis?**
Tietze's syndrome is a syndrome of pain, tenderness, and *swelling* of joints of the chest wall, usually the costochondral joints. Costochondritis is a much more common syndrome characterized by costochondral joint pain and tenderness without objective signs of inflammation. Tietze's syndrome is more common in women, usually (80%) involves a single joint, and is rarely bilateral. Polyarticular disease affects neighboring articulations on the same side of the sternum. It may be seen more frequently in patients with costal cartilage calcification, suggesting that hydroxylapatite may play an etiologic role.

13. **Define foreign body synovitis.**
Inflammatory reaction of synovium (from joint, bursa, or tendon sheath) attributable to the introduction of a foreign material. Most commonly, it results from a traumatic event, but it may also follow surgical introduction of foreign material.

14. **Name the foreign bodies most commonly associated with foreign body synovitis.**
Plant thorns, wood splinters, and sea urchin spines are the most common. Other recognized materials include fish bones, chitin fragments, stones, gravel, brick fragments, lead, glass, fiberglass, plastic, and rubber. Surgically implanted materials include metallic fragments, cement (methylmethacrylate), and silicone.

15. **Name five activities that are risk factors for foreign body synovitis.**
Professional fishing, professional diving, marine recreational activities, farming, and gardening.

16. **Describe the clinical, laboratory, and radiographic features of foreign body synovitis.**
The joints of the hands and knees are most commonly affected. There is sudden onset of pain at the site of injury, which may be forgotten by the patient or overlooked by the physician. The patient may be seen with

acute synovitis several days after the injury, ranging from months to years later, with chronic synovitis (particularly of the knee). The ESR is usually normal, and synovial fluid is inflammatory with a predominance of neutrophils. Radiographs may show soft tissue swelling only and can be useful to detect radiodense particles (metal, fish bones, sea urchin spines) but not wood, plastic, or plant thorns. Chronic changes of periarticular osteoporosis, osteolysis, osteosclerosis, and periosteal new bone formation can mimic osteomyelitis or bone tumors.

17. **How is foreign body synovitis diagnosed and treated?**

    In the approximately two thirds of patients with foreign body synovitis attributable to exogenous particles who develop a chronic or relapsing course, diagnosis and treatment usually necessitates excisional biopsy with synovectomy. Because of its resolution, ultrasound is better than computerized tomography scanning and magnetic resonance imaging in detecting particles that are too small or radiolucent to be seen with conventional radiography. Bacteriologic studies (including mycobacterial studies) and histopathologic examination of tissue are essential. Polarized microscopy is useful in detecting birefringent fragments of plant origin, sea urchin spines, and polymethylmethacrylate.

18. **What is multicentric reticulohistiocytosis?**

    Multicentric reticulohistiocytosis (MRH) is a rare disease with prominent skin and joint manifestations that is classified among the non-Langerhans cell histiocytoses. It affects females more than males (3:1), most commonly in the fourth decade. Most patients have symmetric polyarthritis. The cutaneous manifestations occur a mean of 3 years later (66%), although in one third of patients the skin lesions will occur before or simultaneously with the arthritis. Systemic manifestations including fever, weight loss, and fatigue commonly occur. Pulmonary, cardiac, and myopathy symptoms can occur.

19. **How does the arthritis of MRH resemble that of rheumatoid arthritis? How does it differ?**

    Similar to rheumatoid arthritis, the arthritis of MRH is inflammatory, usually chronic, symmetric, and polyarticular; it characteristically affects the interphalangeal joints of the hands and is destructive. Large joints, the feet, and occasionally C1 to C2 can also be involved. However, unlike rheumatoid arthritis, *distal interphalangeal joint* synovitis and destruction may be prominent (75%), and severely deforming arthritis mutilans occurs in 50% of patients. Fever and weight loss can occur. Glucocorticoid therapy has little, if any, effect on the arthritis. Also in contrast to rheumatoid arthritis, radiographs in MRH feature well-circumscribed erosions, widened joint spaces, and absent or disproportionately mild periarticular osteopenia for the degree of erosive change. Serologies are negative and 50% have a moderately elevated sedimentation rate. Synovial fluid can range from mildly to significantly inflammatory.

20. **Describe the cutaneous manifestations of MRH.**

    Firm papulonodules, reddish-brown or yellow, occur most commonly on the face, hands, ears, arms, scalp, neck, and chest. A classic finding is "coral beads" around the nailbeds These nodules may wax and wane and even disappear completely. They can be induced by sun exposure. The nodules may coalesce on the face leading to a "leonine facies." Lesions are less common on the legs.

21. **Several disorders have been associated with MRH. Name them.**

    - Tuberculin skin test positivity is seen in 12% to 50% of cases, but only two patients have been reported to have active tuberculosis.
    - Xanthelasma occurs in one third of patients. Up to 60% have hyperlipidemia.
    - Malignant disease of various types has been reported in approximately 15% to 30% of cases. Breast, heme, and gastric malignancies are most common. The cancer may precede, be concurrent with, or follow the development of MRH. Treatment of the malignancy can lead to improvement of the MRH.
    - Autoimmune diseases occur in 5% to 20% of cases. Multiple different autoimmune diseases have been reported.

22. **What are the typical histologic findings of MRH on biopsy of skin or synovium?**

    The characteristic finding is aggregates of multinucleated giant cells and histiocytes (i.e., tissue macrophages) having a granular, ground-glass appearance. This ground-glass cytoplasm contains a periodic acid–Schiff-reactive material thought to be attributable to a mucoprotein or glycoprotein. This cellular tissue reaction has prompted the idea that MRH represents a histiocytic granulomatous reaction to an as yet unidentified stimulus. Fat stains, such as Sudan black, are also positive. Cell markers indicate a monocyte/macrophage of the histiocytes and multinucleated giant cells. Some have osteoclast markers.

23. **How is MRH treated?**

    No treatment has consistently shown benefit. In patients with mild disease, symptomatic therapy with NSAIDs or nonnarcotic analgesics should be tried. Unfortunately, the arthritis in 40% to 50% of patients progresses to an arthritis mutilans. Methotrexate and antitumor necrosis factor (anti-TNF) agents have been effective for severe cases. Cyclophosphamide has also been reported to achieve partial and complete remissions. As a result of some of the cells exhibiting osteoclastic markers, intravenous bisphosphonates have shown efficacy in some patients. Most cases of MRH will resolve within 10 years leaving behind joint deformities.

24. **What is fibroblastic rheumatism?**

    Fibroblastic rheumatism can resemble MRH. It is a rare fibroblastic (not histiocytic) disease with at least 33% of cases occurring in children. Patients develop the rapid onset of symmetric polyarthritis mainly of the upper extremities. Palmar thickening and inability to extend fingers is seen in 80% of cases, leading to functional disability. Sclerodactyly and skin thickening of arms and trunk can be seen. Raynaud's phenomenon occurs in 50% of cases. Cutaneous manifestations start as maculopapular lesions that develop into nodules over the extensor surfaces of the metacarpophalangeal joints and fingers. They usually develop after the arthritis. There is no association with malignancy or autoimmune disease. Serologies are unremarkable. Radiographs can show joint destruction resembling MRH. Nodule and synovial biopsies show "spindle-shaped" fibroblastic cells that are myofibroblasts. Treatment with prednisone and methotrexate have had variable results.

25. **What is Erdheim–Chester disease (polyostotic sclerosing histiocytosis)?**
Similar to MRH, *Erdheim–Chester disease* is classified among the non-Langerhans cell histiocytoses. Patients usually have symptoms of bilateral, symmetric long bone pain which occurs in middle age. More than 50% of cases can have extraskeletal involvement including painless exophthalmos, brain (pituitary and cerebellum), kidney, heart, or skin involvement (xanthomas). Radiographs of involved areas show *osteosclerosis*. Bone biopsy shows xanthogranulomatous infiltration with foamy histiocytes surrounded by fibrosis. Approximately 50% of patients have a point mutation of the *BRAF* gene. These patients respond to vemurafenib therapy. Corticosteroids, interferon-α, cladribine, tyrosine kinase inhibitors, and anakinra are used for therapy of patients without the gene mutation with 50% 3-year survival.

26. **What is Kikuchi's disease?**
Kikuchi–Fujimoto disease is a histiocytic, necrotizing lymphadenitis. Most patients are less than age 40 years and previously well. The most common presentation is fever (30% to 50%) and cervical lymphadenopathy (100%). Fever is low grade and lasts 1 to 4 weeks. Cervical adenopathy is usually unilateral and affects the posterior more than the anterior lymph nodes. Up to 20% can have other nodal involvement. Nodes are usually less than 2 cm, firm, discrete, and mobile. Some patients have extranodal involvement with night sweats, joint pain (7%), rash (10%), weight loss (10%), gastrointestinal symptoms, hepatosplenomegaly (3%), as well as others. Laboratory evaluation can show an elevated ESR (40% to 70%), leukopenia (25%), and elevated liver function tests. ANA and RF are negative and if positive suggest an associated rheumatic disease. Lymph node biopsy will establish the diagnosis and exclude lymphoma, infections (tuberculosis, others), and unicentric Castleman's disease that can present with cervical adenopathy. The biopsy classically shows necrosis *without* a neutrophilic infiltrate. Histiocytes and CD8+ T cells predominate. The etiology is unknown but suspected to be an immune response to an infectious agent such as Epstein–Barr virus (EBV). Most patients (90%) improve in 1 to 4 months without treatment. Others will have relapses or persistent symptoms which can be treated with hydroxychloroquine, corticosteroids, or intravenous immunoglobulin.

27. **What is erythromelalgia?**
Erythromelalgia is a neurovascular peripheral pain disorder in which blood vessels are episodically blocked and then become hyperemic and inflamed. The attacks are episodic and characterized by red, warm, swollen, and painful (burning) extremities. Feet are affected more than hands. Attacks are triggered by exertion, heat, pressure, caffeine, and alcohol. Symptoms are bilateral but not necessarily symmetric. Rarely symptoms may progress to gangrene. Erythromelalgia is categorized as primary or secondary.
  - **Primary erythromelalgia** is autosomal dominant. It is associated with a gain-of-function mutation of the *voltage-gated sodium channel α subunit* gene (*SCN9A*) located on chromosome 2. This mutation causes hyperexcitability of dorsal root ganglion leading to symptoms similar to chronic regional pain syndrome. The severity of the mutation determines if the clinical symptoms start at puberty or later in adulthood. Elevation and cold exposure including emersion of feet in ice water give relief. There is no consistently effective therapy. It does not respond to aspirin therapy. Mexiletine may be helpful.
  - **Secondary erythromelalgia** is similar to primary erythromelalgia clinically, has its onset during adulthood, and is associated with various diseases or medications. Treatment of the underlying disease or withdrawal of the offending medication is helpful. There are two types of secondary erythromelalgia: aspirin sensitive and aspirin insensitive.
     - Erythromelalgia that is aspirin sensitive is associated with polycythemia vera, essential thrombocytosis, and other chronic myeloproliferative disorders. In 85% of patients, the cutaneous symptoms precede the myelodysplastic syndrome by months to years (median 2.5 years). Erythromelalgia is diagnosed on the basis of platelet counts exceeding 400,000, relief of symptoms lasting for days with low-dose aspirin, and histopathologic evidence of arterioles with fibromuscular proliferation. The response to aspirin suggests that platelet-derived prostaglandins cause the symptoms.
     - Erythromelalgia that is *not* aspirin sensitive is typically attributable to a medication (calcium channel blockers, bromocriptine) or another disease (small fiber neuropathy, autoimmune disease, poisoning).

28. **Discuss the differences between the various types of soft tissue calcifications?**
  - **Calcinosis cutis**: calcium deposits form in the skin. (See Question 29.)
  - **Calciphylaxis**: calcification occurs in the intima of blood vessels and subcutaneous tissue. This is primarily seen in patients with chronic renal failure, uremia, and a high calcium/phosphorous product. This frequently presents with ischemia and skin ulceration. Treatment is to control the hyperphosphatemia and uremia. In severe cases, intravenous sodium thiosulfate has been used.

- **Tumoral calcinosis**: large calcific nodules in juxtaarticular locations causing pain and limited range of motion. There are three types: primary normophosphatemic, primary hyperphosphatemic, and secondary tumoral calcinosis. The primary hyperphosphatemic subtype is autosomal recessive and tends to affect adolescents and young adults. The basic defect is thought to be in the proximal renal tubular cell with an elevated renal phosphate reabsorption threshold and increased production of 1,25-dihydroxyvitamin D. Mutations of the GALNT3 and FGF23 genes have been described. Treatment is inadequate and includes low phosphate diet, phosphate-binding antacids, and surgical excision. These tend to recur after surgical removal.
- **Heterotopic ossification**: abnormal formation of lamellar bone within soft tissues such as tendons, ligaments, or muscles. It commonly occurs in patients with traumatic brain injuries or spinal cord injuries. Patients with these neurologic problems as well as patients with diffuse idiopathic skeletal hyperostosis or ankylosing spondylitis are at risk for developing this following total joint arthroplasty. Patients have pain and a limited range of motion. Patients at high risk should receive indomethacin, intravenous bisphosphonates, or local radiation therapy before arthroplasty to prevent this complication. Recurrence is common after surgical removal.

29. What is dystrophic calcification? What connective tissue diseases are associated with it?

When calcification occurs in cutaneous tissues, it is called **calcinosis cutis** and can be divided into four categories: dystrophic, metastatic (high calcium × phosphorous product >70), idiopathic (e.g., tumoral calcinosis), and iatrogenic. *Dystrophic calcification* is the most common type and is secondary to nonmetabolic diseases such as connective tissue diseases or to deposition of calcium salts in damaged tissue. The calcium is deposited either as numerous large masses (calcinosis universalis) or a few small, localized masses (calcinosis circumscripta). Dystrophic calcifications are most commonly associated with systemic sclerosis, dermatomyositis, SLE, pseudoxanthoma elasticum, panniculitis, and trauma. Tests for serum calcium and phosphorous should be normal. Medical therapy is poor. Small lesions may be improved with intralesional corticosteroids, low dose (1 mg/day) warfarin, minocycline (50 to 100 mg/day), ceftriaxone (2 g/day intravenous for 20 days binds calcium salts), carbon dioxide laser, or surgical excision. Larger lesions may be improved by high-dose diltiazem (3 mg/kg/day), probenecid (1.5 g/day), intravenous bisphosphonates (zoledronic acid 4 mg intravenous every 3 to 4 months for a year inhibits calcium apposition onto hydroxyapatite), topical sodium thiosulfate (1.5 g/day × 6 months), or surgical excision.

30. Describe the histologic classification of the panniculitides and the most common connective tissue diseases associated with each.
- **Septal panniculitis**: erythema nodosum (R/O sarcoidosis).
- **Lobular panniculitis**: *Weber–Christian syndrome* (relapsing febrile nodular nonsuppurative panniculitis), enzymatic panniculitis attributable to pancreatic enzymes or α_1-antitrypsin deficiency, and connective tissue panniculitis.
- **Mixed panniculitis**: *lupus profundus*.

31. Describe the histologic classification and clinical associations with pyoderma gangrenosum.
- *Ulcerative pyoderma gangrenosum*: ulceration, purulent. Associated with poorly controlled rheumatoid arthritis and inflammatory bowel disease.
- *Pustular pyoderma gangrenosum*: discrete pustules. Associated with inflammatory bowel disease.
- *Bullous pyoderma gangrenosum*: superficial bullae that develop ulcerations. Associated with myeloproliferative diseases.
- *Vegetative pyoderma gangrenosum*: erosions, superficial ulcers.

32. Discuss the musculoskeletal complications of cystic fibrosis.

Cystic fibrosis is an autosomal recessive disease characterized by decreased mucous production leading to obstructive lung disease and malabsorption. Other organs, including sinuses, pancreas, liver, sweat glands, and reproductive tract, can be affected. It is attributable to a defect in the CF gene on chromosome 7, which encodes for a membrane glycoprotein (CFTR) that is a chloride ion channel. In cystic fibrosis, one of the chloride ion channels present on the apical membrane of the epithelial cell is either absent or defective. This leads to increased sodium absorption and decreased chloride secretion resulting in decreased extracellular water content. Patients have obstruction with infections in the lung and malabsorption from the gut. As a result of this, patients are susceptible to osteoporosis (up to 75% of cases) attributable to poor calcium and vitamin D absorption. Additionally, 2% to 9% of patients have an episodic nondestructive oligoarthritis most commonly involving the fingers and lower extremity large joints. The arthritis is felt to be as a result of immune complexes attributable to chronic lung infection. Attacks last for a few days (median 7 days) and may be associated with fever and painful nodular skin lesions and purpura. Rarely, hypertrophic osteoarthropathy (5%) and small vessel vasculitis can occur. Musculoskeletal symptoms are more common the longer the disease duration (adults > adolescence > children), the more severe the disease, and in patients infected with *Pseudomonas aeruginosa*.

33. What rheumatic and autoimmune syndromes have been associated with the following medications?
- Fluoroquinolones: Achilles tendinitis and rupture.
- Minocycline: drug-induced lupus, autoimmune hepatitis, perinuclear antineutrophil cytoplasmic antibody (pANCA) positivity.
- Statins: myopathy, myositis (anti-HMG-CoA reductase antibodies).
- Rifabutin: drug-induced lupus.

- Hydralazine: ANCA vasculitis, drug-induced lupus.
- Zafirlukast: Churg–Strauss syndrome.
- Antithyroid medications (propylthiouracil): ANCA vasculitis.
- Anti-TNF agents: drug-induced lupus, vasculitis.
- Interferon-α: thyroiditis, drug-induced lupus.
- Protease inhibitors (HIV): osteonecrosis, adhesive capsulitis.
- Cancer chemotherapy: isolated case reports of several rheumatic diseases caused by various chemotherapies.
- Myopathies: corticosteroids, antimalarials, colchicine, zidovudine, antifungals (triazoles, imidazoles), oncologic drugs, succinylcholine, others.
- Drug-induced antiphospholipid antibodies: procainamide, quinidine, antipsychotics, phenytoin, interferon-α, hydralazine, TNF-α antagonists.
- Bisphosphonates: uveitis, atypical femoral fractures.
- Voriconazole: nodular hypertrophic osteoarthropathy.

34. What is the ASIA syndrome?
ASIA stands for **A**utoimmune/inflammatory **S**yndrome **I**nduced by **A**djuvants. This is a controversial concept that suggests that certain environmental exposures (infections, vaccines, adjuvants, silicone, drugs) can act as an adjuvant stimulating the innate immune system resulting in symptoms and/or subsequent stimulation of the adaptive immune system resulting in autoantibodies and/or autoimmune disease. In patients who already have a defined autoimmune disease, these adjuvants may exacerbate their disease. Because this only occurs in a small fraction of patients exposed to these adjuvants, causality is difficult to prove.
The proposed diagnostic criteria are: (1) development of symptoms (muscle, joint, fatigue, demyelination, cognitive impairment, pyrexia) or (2) development of an undifferentiated connective tissue disease and/or autoantibodies within proximity to exposure to an adjuvant. Some examples are:
- Immunizations: associated with causing demyelinating syndromes, reactive arthritis, and small vessel vasculitis. Recombinant hepatitis B vaccination has been associated with a higher than expected number of rheumatic disorders including vasculitis (especially central retinal vein occlusion), rheumatoid arthritis, SLE, reactive arthritis, as well as various demyelination syndromes. These rheumatic disorders occur within 1 to 2 months of the first, second, or third vaccination. Unlike other typical side effects of an immunization, these rheumatic disorders may not resolve.
- Silicone: breast implants (especially those that ruptured) and oil injections for cosmetic purposes have been reported to cause scleroderma-like diseases. Very controversial.
- Alum adjuvant: alum in vaccines has been associated with causing the macrophage myofasciitis syndrome.
- Gulf War syndrome: soldiers exposed to multiple vaccinations in a short period of time developed fibromyalgia-like symptoms and cognitive dysfunction. All patients had antisqualene antibodies.
- Case reports of parvovirus infection with arthritis evolving into rheumatoid arthritis, EBV infection evolving into SLE, and pronestyl exposure triggering SLE that does not resolve with drug withdrawal.

35. What is the differential diagnosis of a patient with fever and generalized lymphadenopathy?
- *Infections*: toxoplasmosis, EBV, cytomegalovirus, HIV.
- *Malignancies*: lymphoma.
- **Multicentric Castleman's disease** (giant or angiofollicular lymph node hyperplasia): a lymphoproliferative disorder presenting with fever, generalized adenopathy, hepatosplenomegaly, weight loss, neutropenia, and polyclonal hypergammaglobulinemia. It is associated with a hyperproliferation of certain B cells that produce cytokines, especially interleukin-6 (IL-6). Approximately 50% are caused by the herpes virus, HHV-8. Lymph node biopsies show hyalinization of germinal centers and plasma cell infiltration of interfollicular areas. Treatment involves use of antivirals, corticosteroids, rituximab, and IL-6 inhibitors.
- *Systemic inflammatory disease*: SLE, adult-onset Still's disease, sarcoidosis.
- *Medications*: allopurinol, phenytoin.
- *Autoimmune lymphoproliferative syndrome*: see Question 36.

36. What are the genetic or immune defects in Canale–Smith syndrome and Stiff-person syndrome?
Canale–Smith syndrome (*autoimmune lymphoproliferative syndrome*): a rare autosomal dominant disorder typically presenting in childhood and characterized by generalized lymphadenopathy, hepatosplenomegaly, and autoimmune hemolytic anemia and thrombocytopenia. Rarely patients with mutations causing a milder phenotype may not have symptoms until adulthood. Patients are diagnosed by increased numbers (≥5% of all T cells) of circulating double-negative T cells (CD3$^+$, CD4$^-$, CD8$^-$) which comprise >1.5% of all circulating lymphocytes. Most (70%) patients have germline mutations in the *Fas* gene (*TNFRSF6*), leading to abnormalities in the intracellular "death domain" of the receptor Fas (APO-1, CD95). This leads to the inability of the T cell to be signaled to undergo programmed cell death (apoptosis). Consequently, autoreactive T cells will downregulate CD4 and CD8 molecules but cannot be disposed of by Fas-mediated apoptosis (similar to *lpr* mice), leading to autoimmune disease. Patients without *Fas* gene mutations have been found to have mutations in the *Fas ligand* gene (similar to *gld* mice) or enzymes involved in apoptosis (caspase 10). Corticosteroid therapy has variable effects. Mycophenolate mofetil and sirolimus have been effective steroid-sparing medications. Notably, up to 10% of patients can develop neoplasms (lymphoma).

Stiff-person syndrome: a disorder characterized by muscle rigidity and episodic muscle spasms, primarily involving the trunk. Episodes can be prolonged, painful, and precipitated by loud noises. There are three types:
- The most common (60%) type is associated with *antibodies against glutamic acid decarboxylase* (GAD65) and frequently with autoimmune diseases (e.g., type I diabetes mellitus, Graves' disease, hypothyroidism, pernicious anemia) because of its high association with HLA DQ-0201. It is postulated that the anti-GAD antibodies inhibit the enzymes in the central nervous system responsible for production of GABA, which is an inhibitory neurotransmitter. Consequently, neural transmission is unopposed and can lead to muscle rigidity. This type of Stiff-person syndrome is treated with diazepam, plasmapheresis, immunosuppressives including rituximab, and/or intravenous gammaglobulin.
- The other two types of Stiff-person syndrome are not associated with anti-GAD antibodies or a certain HLA phenotype. One type (5% of cases) is a *paraneoplastic* manifestation of cancers (lymphoma, breast, lung, colon), whereas the other type (35% of cases) is *idiopathic*. Patients with Stiff-person syndrome associated with breast cancer have recently been found to have *antiamphiphysin* (128 kd protein on surface of synaptic vesicles) antibodies. These two types do not respond to immune modulating therapies and are treated with high doses of muscle relaxants such as diazepam or baclofen.

37. Differentiate the following skin manifestations that can mimic vasculitis: livedo reticularis, livedo racemosa, livedoid vasculopathy, and malignant atrophic papulosis.
    - *Livedo reticularis*: macular, violaceous, netlike, patterned erythema of the skin. The livid rings are due to reduce blood flow and low oxygen tension at the periphery. Skin biopsy is unrevealing. There are four types:
        - Physiologic (also called cutis mamorata): mainly occurs on legs of young women. Typically worse in cold and resolves with warming.
        - Primary: has fluctuant course but does not resolve with warming.
        - Idiopathic: persistent and unresolving livedo. May be early form of livedo racemosa.
        - Amantadine-induced: occurs in 2% to 28% of patients on amantadine. Vascular reaction due to catecholamine depletion.
    - *Livedo racemosa*: resembles livedo reticularis but is persistent and more widespread. Pattern is irregular, broken circles. Associated with a secondary cause including Sneddon's syndrome, antiphospholipid antibody syndrome (APS), SLE, essential thrombocythemia, thromboangiitis obliterans, polycythemia vera, and polyarteritis nodosa. Skin biopsy shows thrombi and/or vessel inflammation. Strong association with cerebral and ocular ischemic arterial events, valve disease, and seizures in patients with APS.
    - *Livedoid vasculopathy* (atrophie blanche): is included as a cause of livedo racemosa. It is a vascular disease characterized by thrombosis and skin ulcerations on bilateral lower extremities. It occurs predominantly in middle-aged women and is not associated with another disease. Some patients are hypercoagulable (Factor V Leiden, APS, etc). Skin biopsy shows segmental hyalinization of dermal vessels and thrombi but no vasculitis. There is no internal organ manifestations unless associated with another disease. Skin lesions respond poorly to therapy and heal with characteristic stellate ivory scars.
    - *Malignant atrophic papulosis* (Kohlmeier-Degos disease): a rare thrombo-occlusive vasculopathy that presents with erythematous papular skin lesions with a porcelain depressed center. There is an average of 30 lesions scattered on trunk and extremities. Up to 33% develop systemic manifestations due to involvement of small and medium-sized arteries of the GI tract, CNS, pericardium, and bladder. Laboratory tests are nonspecific. Diagnosis is made by skin biopsy showing endothelial proliferation, thrombosis, and infarction. Vasculitis is not present. Treatment is poor and many patients die of sepsis from GI perforation. Immunosuppressives are ineffective although eculizumab has been reported to be beneficial.

Acknowledgment
The author wishes to thank Dr. James Singleton for his contributions to this chapter in the previous edition.

BIBLIOGRAPHY

Gonzales-Lopez L, Gamez-Nava JI, Jhangri GS, et al: Prognostic factors for the development of rheumatoid arthritis and other connective tissue diseases in patients with palindromic rheumatism, J Rheumatol 26:540–545, 1999.
Hench PS, Rosenberg EF: Palindromic rheumatism, Arch Intern Med 73:293–321, 1944.
Koch A-K, Bromme S, Wollschlager B, et al: Musculoskeletal manifestations and rheumatic symptoms in patients with cystic fibrosis, J Rheumatol 35:1882–1891, 2008.
Powell A, Davis P, Jones N, et al: Palindromic rheumatism is a common disease: comparison of new-onset palindromic rheumatism compared to new onset rheumatoid arthritis in a 2 year cohort of patients, J Rheumatol 35:992–994, 2008.
Schoenfeld Y, Agmon-Levin N: "ASIA"– autoimmune/inflammatory syndrome induced by adjuvants, J Autoimmun 36:4–8, 2011.
Teachey DT, Seif AE, Grupp SA: Advances in the management and understanding of autoimmune lymphoproliferative syndrome (ALPS), Br J Haematol 148:205–216, 2010.
Trotta F, Colina M: Multicentric reticulohistiocytosis and fibroblastic rheumatism, Best Pract Res Clin Rheumatol 26:543–557, 2012.
Van der Linden PD, van Puijenbroek EP, Feenstra J, et al: Tendon disorders attributed to fluoroquinolones: a study on 42 spontaneous reports in the period 1988-1998, Arthritis Care Res 45:235–239, 2001.
Young FB: When adaptive processes go awry: gain of function in SCN9A, Clin Genet 73:34–36, 2008.
Zafrir Y, Agmon-Levin N, Paz Z, et al: Autoimmunity following hepatitis B vaccine as part of the spectrum of ASIA – analysis of 93 cases, Lupus 21:146–152, 2012.

XIV
MANAGEMENT OF THE RHEUMATIC DISEASES

As to diseases, make a habit of two things—to help, or at least to do no harm.

Hippocrates
(c. 460–377 bc)

NONSTEROIDAL ANTIINFLAMMATORY DRUGS

Jason R. Kolfenbach, MD

No drug is as good as the day it is first thought of.

—Sir William Osler

KEY POINTS

1. Although nonsteroidal antiinflammatory drugs (NSAIDs) are equally effective, individual patients have varying responses and side effects depending on the NSAID structural class.
2. The cyclooxygenase (COX)-2 specific inhibitors are associated with fewer gastrointestinal adverse events.
3. All NSAIDs should be used with caution (if at all) in patients with underlying renal or cardiovascular disease.

1. Describe the general properties of NSAIDs.

NSAIDs are weak organic acids that avidly bind to serum proteins (mainly albumin). The vast majority have low ionization constants (pK_a) ranging from 3 to 5, which accounts for their accumulation at sites of inflammation such as arthritic joints (inflamed joints often have a lower pH than clinically uninvolved joints). NSAIDs have antiinflammatory properties by virtue of their inhibition of prostaglandin synthesis and a number of other mechanisms.

2. When were NSAIDs first used?

Salicylates have probably been used for centuries. In the 4th century BC, Hippocrates, Celsus, Galen, and others recorded the use of willow bark and other plants known to contain salicylates to treat fever and pain. Today, one can find numerous health food stores and herbal websites selling willow bark for use in pill form, tinctures, and a dried-form to be used in tea. Purification of the active ingredient and development of modern NSAIDs is outlined as follows:

1760s—Dr. Edward Stone publishes his experience with willow bark as an antipyretic when dried.
1829—Salicylic acid isolated from willow bark.
1853—Gerhardt buffers salicylic acid with sodium and acetyl chloride, creating acetylsalicylic acid (ASA; aspirin).
1860—ASA chemically synthesized (Kolbe and Hoffman).
1899—Aspirin introduced in the United States as a powder (Bayer Company).
1949—Phenylbutazone, the first alternative to salicylates, introduced.
1960s—Indomethacin introduced.
1970s—J.R. Vane (1971) demonstrates that ASA, indomethacin and salicylate all exert their effect by COX inhibition (Nobel Prize in Medicine, 1982).
—Ibuprofen, fenoprofen calcium, naproxen, and tolmentin introduced.
1990s—Introduction of the specific COX-2 inhibitors.

It has been reported that Felix Hoffman of Bayer Company chemically synthesized aspirin in response to complaints from his arthritic father about the bitter taste of salicylates. He gave this new medicine to his father and it helped his arthritis. This constituted the first Phase I, II, and III testing of a drug, which for new drugs today takes many millions of dollars and an average of 10 years!

3. How often are NSAIDs used?

It is estimated that >70 million prescriptions for nonsalicylate NSAIDs are given annually in the United States, with over 30 billion doses used annually (over-the-counter and prescription NSAIDs). Individuals over age 60 years, a rapidly growing segment of the population, comprise over half of regular users.

4. What are the beneficial effects of NSAIDs?

Analgesia—some studies have shown equivalent reductions in acute pain compared with narcotics.
Antipyresis—NSAIDs inhibit prostaglandins in the central nervous system (CNS), which reduces fever.
Antiinflammatory—probably achieved by a number of mechanisms (prostaglandin inhibition is the most understood and thought to represent the main mechanism of action).
Antiplatelet—most NSAIDs decrease platelet aggregation by inhibiting COX-1, thus preventing thromboxane A_2 (TXA_2) production, which is important in platelet activation and clotting.

5. **What is the structural classification of NSAIDs?**
   - *Carboxylic acids*
     - Salicylates
       - Acetylated—aspirin*
       - Nonacetylated—sodium salicylate*, choline magnesium trisalicylate*, salicylamide*, salsalate, diflunisal
     - Acetic acids
       - Indole derivatives—indomethacin, tolmentin, sulindac
       - Phenylacetic acid—diclofenac
       - Pyranocarboxylic acid—etodolac
     - Propionic acids—ibuprofen*, naproxen*, fenoprofen, ketoprofen, flurbiprofen, oxaprozin
     - Fenamic acids—mefenamic acid, meclofenamate sodium
     - Pyrrolizine carboxylic acid derivative—ketorolac
   - *Enolic acids*
     - Oxicams—piroxicam, meloxicam
     - Pyrazolones—phenylbutazone (no longer available for human use)
   - *Nonacidic compounds*—nabumetone
   - *Diaryl substituted pyrazoles* (COX-2 inhibitors)
     - Celecoxib
     - Rofecoxib and valdecoxib: withdrawn from market
     - Etoricoxib, lumiracoxib, and parecoxib (injectable prodrug of valdecoxib): not available in the United States/not FDA-approved

6. **Why should you know the structural classification of NSAIDs?**
   The drugs in each structural class tend to have similar efficacy and side effects. Therefore, if a patient fails to respond or has a side effect to a particular NSAID it may be prudent to select an NSAID from a different structural class.

7. **What is thought to be the major mechanism of action of NSAIDs?**
   The major mechanism of action is thought to be the inhibition of cyclooxygenase, causing a decrease in prostaglandin production. There are two main isoforms of cyclooxygenase: cyclooxygenase-1 (COX-1) and cyclooxygenase-2 (COX-2). They are similar in size, have 60% C-DNA homology, and have similar but slightly different active sites. **COX-1** is on chromosome 9 and lacks a TATA box and upstream transcriptional start sites. The transcriptional product (mRNA) of COX-1 enzyme activity is long-lived. These aspects suggest that the COX-1 gene is a "housekeeping gene" with constitutive expression in the stomach, intestine, kidney, platelet, and other sites. **COX-2** is on chromosome 1 and contains a TATA box as well as upstream regions that serve as binding sites for multiple transcription factors. These transcription factors include: nuclear factor κB (NF-κB), interleukin-6 (IL-6)/CCAAT-enhancer-binding protein (C-EBP), cAMP regulatory binding protein, activator protein 1 (AP-1), nuclear factor of activated T cells (NFAT), and glucocorticoid receptors. The mRNA produced by transcription is short-lived; hence, ongoing expression is dependent on continual stimulation. As such, the COX-2 gene is thought to be an inducible gene with increased expression in response to inflammatory states resulting from binding of upregulated transcription factors.
   It is this understanding of the different roles of COX-1 and COX-2 that led to the development of specific COX-2 inhibitors. The hope was that analgesic and antiinflammatory NSAIDs could be made with little or no side effects. However, COX-2 is now known to be constitutively produced in sites such as the kidney, brain, bone, and endothelium, and plays an important role in vascular and thrombotic regulation. Therefore, selective blockade in certain populations may result in deleterious side effects (discussed later).

8. **What are other mechanisms of action of NSAIDs?**
   Nonprostaglandin mediated effects of NSAIDs have been postulated, but the relative importance of each of these pathways in the clinical effectiveness of NSAIDs is uncertain. These effects include:
   - Inhibitory effects on lipoxygenase products.
   - Inhibition of superoxide formation.
   - Inhibition of neutrophil aggregation, adhesion, and enzyme release.
   - Inhibition of degradative enzymes.
   - Inhibition of cytokine production by inhibiting NF-κB.
   - Suppression of proteoglycan degradation in cartilage.

9. **Do some NSAIDs inhibit COX-1 or COX-2 preferentially?**
   Yes. A common classification system was developed by separate groups in the United States and Europe, according to the ability of NSAIDs to inhibit COX-1 and/or COX-2 in therapeutic doses. This classification is presented in Table 81-1.

---

*Available over-the-counter (nonacetylated salicylates often come in combination with other ingredients, often in tablet or powder form).

Table 81-1. The Common Classification System According to the Ability of an NSAID to Inhibit COX-1 and/or COX-2 in Therapeutic Doses

AMERICAN NOMENCLATURE	EUROPEAN NOMENCLATURE	NSAIDS IN THIS CLASSIFICATION
COX-1 specific	COX-1 selective	Low-dose aspirin (irreversibly binds to serine 530 on COX-1)
COX nonspecific	COX nonselective	Ibuprofen, naproxen, meclomen, indomethacin
COX-2 preferential	COX-2 selective	Etodolac, diclofenac, nabumetone, meloxicam
COX-2 specific	COX-2 highly selective	Celecoxib

COX, Cyclooxygenase; NSAIDs, nonsteroidal antiinflammatory drugs.

10. What is the COX-3 enzyme?

COX-3 is a unique enzyme found in several species and is derived from a splice variant of COX-1 (identical to COX-1 mRNA but with a retained intron 1). In dogs, COX-3 expression is predominantly found in the brain and it is inhibited by acetaminophen and some NSAIDs. Initially this was thought to perhaps explain the mechanism of action of acetaminophen in humans, given the analgesic and antipyretic effects of this medication (CNS action) but relatively weak antiinflammatory effects (proposed lack of peripheral action). This has been questioned more recently, however, as several researchers have demonstrated very low levels of COX-3 expression in humans. Furthermore, the COX-3 protein that is produced seems to lack cyclooxygenase activity. The current relevance of COX-3 in human biology is uncertain, but it is unlikely to explain the effects of acetaminophen or NSAIDs.

11. What factors affect the choice of NSAIDs?

Factors that affect the choice of NSAIDs are outlined in Box 81-1.

Box 81-1. Factors That Affect the Choice of Nonsteroidal Antiinflammatory Drugs

PROPERTIES OF THE DRUG	PATIENT CHARACTERISTICS
Efficacy	Individual variation
Tolerance	Disease being treated
Safety	Age
Convenience of dosage	Other diseases
Formulation	Other drugs
Cost	

12. What have efficacy studies of NSAIDs found?

In general, there are no important differences among the various NSAIDs in terms of "comparative effectiveness," although there are clear individual variations in response. In some arthritic diseases, specific NSAIDs have been traditionally used as first-line agents over others. This is typically based on evidence of clinical effectiveness of a drug for a particular condition, rather than evidence of superiority over other NSAIDs. For example, in gout and the seronegative spondyloarthropathies, indomethacin is often the initial drug of choice. There is no clear relationship between the amount of cyclooxygenase inhibition and effectiveness of a particular agent for treatment of arthritis. Although the pharmacodynamics of the drug are important in a given individual, there is no good correlation between the plasma level of the drug and efficacy except for salicylates.

13. Who is at risk for a hypersensitivity reaction to NSAIDs?

The patient most at risk is a severe asthmatic with nasal polyps: up to 78% may react to aspirin (Samter's triad = asthma, nasal polyps, aspirin sensitivity). Patients with isolated asthma (10% to 20% aspirin sensitivity overall), nasal polyps, or chronic urticaria are also mildly at risk to react to NSAIDs, usually with acute bronchospasm and shortness of breath. It is important to note that this is a sensitivity and not an allergy, because it is not immunoglobulin E-mediated.

Two theories have been proposed to explain aspirin/NSAID-sensitive asthma. One suggests that asthma is caused by cyclooxygenase inhibition resulting in decreased production of prostaglandin E_2, an important bronchodilator. A second theory proposes that this type of asthma is a consequence of the 5-fold increased bronchial expression of leukotriene C4 synthetase. When aspirin or NSAIDs block cyclooxygenase, the arachidonic acid precursors are diverted down the leukotriene pathway resulting in excessive production of leukotrienes C, D, and E (slow reacting substance of anaphylaxis). These theories are supported by: (1) salsalate does not inhibit cyclooxygenase to a large degree and has not been found to cause asthma attacks (it is the NSAID of choice for patients with asthma who are aspirin-sensitive); (2) leukotriene inhibitors block bronchospasm provoked by NSAIDs in patients who are aspirin-sensitive; and (3) NSAID-induced asthma attacks are acute in onset, severe and prolonged, and can be resistant to glucocorticoids. Small studies of patients with aspirin-sensitive asthma given celecoxib did not demonstrate an increased risk of hypersensitivity reaction, but there are no long-term studies documenting its safety in this population. As such, the selective COX-2 inhibitors have the same warning as nonselective NSAIDs in their package inserts.

14. Discuss the hepatotoxicity of NSAIDs.
The clearance of NSAIDs is predominantly by hepatic metabolism, with the production of inactive metabolites that are excreted in urine. An elevation of liver enzymes, especially the aminotransferases (aspartate aminotransferase and alanine aminotransferase), can occur with all NSAIDs (up to 15% of patients can have significant, reversible elevations). Diclofenac may cause transaminitis more commonly than other NSAIDs. The NSAID-induced hepatotoxicity is usually evident during the first 6 months of use. **Severe hepatitis** has been reported with indomethacin, diclofenac, and sulindac. **Fatal hepatotoxicity** in children using indomethacin has been noted, prompting the recommendation that children under age 11 years should not be given indomethacin for arthritis. **Cholestasis** has also been described. Liver function studies should be obtained during the first month of use and every 3 to 6 months thereafter.

15. What are the gastrointestinal side effects of NSAIDs?
- Dyspepsia, indigestion, and vomiting.
- Gastroesophageal reflux/esophagitis.
- Gastroduodenal ulcers.
- Gastrointestinal (GI) hemorrhage and perforation.
- Small and large bowel ulceration.
- Small bowel webs (especially with piroxicam).
- Colonic diverticular perforation.
- Diarrhea (especially with meclofenamate).

16. How do prostaglandins protect the gastric mucosa?
Prostaglandin E1 and E2 effects on gastric mucosa
- Induce protective superficial mucous barrier.
- Induce bicarbonate output.
- Increase mucosal blood flow in the superficial gastric cell layer.
- Inhibit gastric acid synthesis.

17. How common are NSAID-induced gastritis and peptic ulcers?
Gastritis and peptic ulcers are among the most common side effects of these drugs. NSAID injury to the GI tract is responsible for an estimated 100,000 hospitalizations and approximately 10,000 deaths annually in the United States. Approximately 1% to 2% of patients treated with NSAIDs develop serious GI complications annually (bleeding, perforation, or obstruction) with a hospitalization mortality rate of 5% to 6%. The absolute risk increases approximately 4% per year for patients over the age of 65 years. In patients using chronic aspirin and another NSAID, the annual risk increases to 6% to 8% per year.
Asymptomatic (endoscopically diagnosed) ulcers occur in 30% of chronic NSAID users. Routine stool guaiac testing for blood is insensitive in detecting these ulcers. **Unfortunately, over one half of all patients who develop significant ulcer complications do not have preceding symptoms.**

18. Who is at risk for NSAID-induced gastroduodenal ulcer disease?
- Older age (>65 to 70 years old) (relative risk [RR] 5 to 6× increased).
- Multiple NSAIDs (including ASA) (RR 9×).
- History of peptic ulcer disease, with or without NSAIDs (RR 6×).
- Higher dose, prolonged use of NSAIDs (RR 7×).
- Chronic disease status such as rheumatoid arthritis, chronic obstructive pulmonary disease, coronary artery disease, diabetes.
- Concomitant corticosteroid (prednisone ≥10 mg/day) (RR 2×), warfarin (RR 6×), clopidogrel, or low-dose aspirin.
- Suspected risk factors: tobacco, alcohol, existing infection with *Helicobacter pylori* (RR 3 to 4×).

19. How can you decrease the incidence of NSAID-induced gastric and duodenal ulcers in high-risk individuals?
1. When appropriate, use alternative analgesics or topical NSAID formulations.
2. Use the lowest dose and frequency of NSAID possible.
- Nonselective COX inhibitors, COX-2 selective inhibitors, and ASA have all demonstrated a linear dose–response relationship with GI side effects.

3. If NSAIDs are required, consider COX-2 selective inhibitors or use of a nonselective NSAID and gastric protective agent.
- Randomized controlled trials and metaanalyses have demonstrated reduced rates by 50% to 66% of ulcer bleeding and complications with COX-2 selective inhibitors compared with nonselective inhibitors.
- Proton pump inhibitors (PPIs) and misoprostol (prostaglandin E_1 analog) have each demonstrated reduced rates of bleeding and complications secondary to gastric ulcers among users of nonselective NSAIDs.
- Agents such as H2 blockers, sucralfate, and antacids may reduce dyspepsia, but have not demonstrated a protective effect against ulcer complications.
- Studies suggest that use of a PPI and a nonselective NSAID may afford similar GI protection to that of COX-2 selective inhibitors.
- Taking a COX-2 selective inhibitor and low-dose aspirin has the same GI toxicity as a nonselective NSAID without aspirin. Therefore, in high-risk patients on a COX-2 selective NSAID and low-dose aspirin, a PPI is needed for GI protection.

4. Treatment of an existing *H. pylori* infection should be done before initiation of a NSAID.
- Testing is recommended in all high-risk groups; there is no current data to support routine testing in lower risk groups

20. How nephrotoxic are NSAIDs?

Prostaglandins can vasodilate renal arteries, increase sodium loss, and increase renin release. They have relatively little impact on the renal system in euvolemic patients with normal renal function. However, in renal insufficiency or hypovolemic states, prostaglandins are important in maintaining adequate glomerular flow and pressure. Nephrotoxic effects of NSAIDs include:
- Vasoconstriction, leading to decreasing glomerular filtration rate and increasing creatinine.
- Increased sodium retention and blood volume (can be important in patients with congestive heart failure, liver disease, or other conditions leading to renal insufficiency).
- Papillary necrosis.
- Hyperkalemia.
- Hyponatremia.
- Interstitial nephritis (more common with fenoprofen).

21. What NSAIDs would you use in a patient with mild renal compromise?

The **nonacetylated salicylates** are poor prostaglandin inhibitors and may have less effect on glomerular filtration rate. The hope was that the selective COX-2 inhibitors would have less renal effects than the traditional NSAIDs. However, COX-2 is found in the glomeruli and renal vasculature in humans. COX-2 appears to be the dominant contributor to salt and water homeostasis, and COX-1 has a more dominant role in the maintenance of glomerular filtration rate. Thus, in practice, the selective COX-2 inhibitors have similar effects on blood pressure and induction of edema as traditional NSAIDs.

22. Describe the cardiovascular effects of aspirin.

Aspirin (ASA) is a well-established therapy for secondary prevention of myocardial infarction (MI) in patients with known coronary artery disease. This is accomplished through inhibition of COX-1 and subsequent decline in thromboxane A_2, a potent platelet activator. It is an ideal agent for several reasons: (1) COX-1, but not COX-2, is expressed in mature platelets; (2) ASA is a COX-1 specific inhibitor; (3) ASA works through irreversible binding to the COX-1 enzyme, providing stable suppression of enzyme activity; and (4) recent evidence demonstrates "ASA-triggered" production of antiinflammatory mediators such as lipoxins and resolvins. Other traditional NSAIDs that inhibit COX-1 can reversibly inhibit platelets, but there is no definitive evidence of cardioprotection with these agents.

23. What are the cardiovascular effects of NSAIDs?

Nonselective NSAIDs inhibit the COX-1 and COX-2 enzymes to varying degrees. However, even among those offering significant levels of COX-1 inhibition, none have consistently shown the same level of cardioprotection afforded by ASA. This may stem from concurrent inhibition of the COX-2 enzyme, unsustained COX-1 inhibition attributable to the reversible nature of NSAID binding, or inability of NSAIDs to form protective mediators (lipoxins, resolvins) as occurs with ASA. NSAIDs have been associated with sodium and fluid retention in susceptible patients (see Question 20), loss of hypotensive effects of several blood pressure medications (see Question 32), and blockage of physiologic levels of COX-2 (see Question 24), all of which could serve to increase the risk of MI, stroke, and thromboembolism.

Evidence of potential cardiovascular risk was first identified shortly after the development of COX-2 specific inhibitors. Secondary analysis of a large multicenter trial (VIGOR trial) identified a significant increase in nonfatal MI in patients on rofecoxib compared with naproxen. A second trial examining the role of rofecoxib in the prevention of adenomatous polyps in the colon (APPROVe) demonstrated an increased risk of cardiovascular events in patients taking rofecoxib compared with placebo. These studies eventually lead to the withdrawal of the drug from the market. Valdecoxib and parecoxib have also been studied in high-risk populations (patients undergoing coronary artery bypass grafting); the combined incidence of MI and stroke in patients taking these medications was significantly increased, despite small study size and short trial duration, leading to drug withdrawal from the market.

Cardiovascular risk with other COX-2 inhibitors and nonselective NSAIDs has been evaluated through secondary analysis of randomized, controlled trials and through observational studies. The data in celecoxib suggest a slight increase in cardiovascular events over time in low to moderate risk patients, although conflicting data exist. Data from large randomized trials do not exist for the older nonselective NSAIDs, but recent observational studies have demonstrated an increased cardiovascular risk among several nonselective NSAIDs, suggesting that this risk is not specific to COX-2 selective inhibitors.

24. Is the cardiovascular risk associated with NSAIDs specific to certain drugs (controversial)?

Epidemiologic data suggest that all NSAIDs may pose some level of cardiovascular risk, especially in high-risk populations. However, some studies have shown that naproxen has a neutral or even mildly protective effect on cardiovascular outcomes. This has been theorized to occur because of the strong inhibition of platelet COX-1 by naproxen (>95% reduction of COX-1 dependent TXA_2, resulting in functional platelet suppression) as well as its long half-life (>12 hours). The data on naproxen are inconsistent, however, and ASA should be considered the only *proven* cardioprotective agent.

Cardiovascular risk was first identified in studies of COX-2 selective inhibitors, and several aspects of COX-2 biology may explain some of the risk associated with its inhibition by both selective and nonselective NSAIDs. COX-2 activity in the endothelium serves as the main source of **prostacyclin (PGI_2)** production. In vitro studies have shown that COX-2 expression is turned on in response to shear stress, suggesting that expression occurs constitutively in response to laminar blood flow in the physiologic state. In the pathologic state (e.g., severe atherosclerosis, unstable MI), prostacyclin levels are further increased in an effort to inhibit vessel constriction and platelet aggregation. Inhibition of this enzyme by selective or nonselective NSAIDs, especially in high-risk patients, could lead to subsequent cardiovascular events. In addition, COX-2 specific inhibitors such as celecoxib have been shown to have no effect on in vitro platelet function nor bleeding time, perhaps serving as a "second hit" for the development of CV disease. Given these findings, one may expect the RRs for particular NSAIDs to separate according to their inhibition of the COX-2 enzyme. Currently, however, there are not enough data to support such a rigid rank-ordering of NSAIDs in terms of cardiovascular risk.

25. List some strategies to reduce cardiovascular risk from NSAIDs in high-risk patients.
- Take low-dose ASA more than 2 hours before an NSAID.
- Do not use NSAIDs for 3 to 6 months after a cardiovascular event or procedure.
- Do not use extended-release NSAID preparations.
- Control blood pressure.

26. What are some important considerations for the concurrent use of ASA and NSAIDs?
1. Increased risk of GI toxicity; risk is increased 5-fold over that with either agent alone.
2. With COX-2 selective inhibitors, concurrent use of ASA appears to abrogate the gastroprotective effects of selective COX-2 blockade.
3. Pharmacodynamic studies of ASA coadministration with ibuprofen and naproxen have demonstrated evidence of *interference* with the sustained reduction of TXA_2 of aspirin and subsequent platelet inhibition. Studies of ASA plus ibuprofen suggest that administration of ASA 2 hours before ibuprofen (rather than concurrently or following the use of ibuprofen) resulted in adequate (and sustained) suppression of TXA_2 and platelet function. Hence, the results from this study suggest that staggering the use of these medications, with use of ASA first, may be beneficial in terms of platelet suppression. Studies of ASA plus naproxen demonstrate interference with the maximal inhibition of platelet function of ASA when the two medications are given concurrently as a one-time dose. In contrast, when naproxen was given in a scheduled manner with ASA, TXA_2 and subsequent platelet inhibition remained at similar levels to ASA use alone. This is probably because when naproxen is given in a chronic manner, it results in significant (>95% reduction of TXA_2) and *sustained* platelet inhibition, thus "masking" interference with the effects of aspirin.

Other NSAID medications are not likely to result in similar reductions in TXA_2 as seen with naproxen. In addition, given the reversible nature of NSAID binding to the COX site, intermittent use may also interfere with ASA effects. As such, in patients using short half-life NSAIDs in an intermittent (PRN) manner, it may be advisable to take ASA before NSAID (controversial).

27. List some rare adverse reactions to NSAIDs.
1. Febrile reactions—ibuprofen.
2. Mediastinal lymphadenopathy—sulindac.
3. Hematologic effects: aplastic anemia, pure red cell aplasia, thrombocytopenia, neutropenia—rare; reported with most NSAIDs (phenylbutazone removed from the market as a result of its association with hematologic effects).
4. Stomatitis—most NSAIDs.
5. Cutaneous effects: photosensitivity, urticaria/angioedema, erythema multiform, toxic epidermal necrolysis—most NSAIDs, especially piroxicam.
6. Aseptic meningitis (especially patients with systemic lupus erythematosus)—ibuprofen, other NSAIDs less commonly.

Other NSAIDs have been associated with CNS effects without aseptic meningitis: headaches, dizziness, loss of concentration, depersonalization, tremor, and psychosis have been described in patients taking indomethacin and, to a lesser extent, tolmetin.
7. Small bowel webs—most NSAIDs but particularly piroxicam.
8. Sulfa allergy—celecoxib.
9. Kidney stones—sulindac.
10. Reversible infertility attributable to interference with ovulation and implantation.
11. Nonunion of fractures and bone grafts (controversial).

28. **Which of the NSAIDs have short plasma elimination half-lives and which have long half-lives?**
Classification according to plasma half-life can be problematic given that NSAIDs tend to accumulate at sites of inflammation such as arthritic joints (Table 81-2). As such, NSAIDs with a short half-life may not need to be redosed as frequently as the plasma half-life suggests. In NSAIDs with a longer half-life (>12 hours), it can take several days to a week to reach plasma steady state, but chronic use then leads to stable plasma levels between doses and eventual equilibration with synovial fluid concentration. Monthly costs range from generic naproxen (500 mg twice daily) at $4 to brand name Celebrex (400 mg daily) at $199. On average, when an NSAID has both a generic and a brand name available, the brand name will be 1.5 to 2× the cost of the generic name (e.g., generic meloxicam 15 mg daily [$148/month] versus brand name Mobic 15 mg daily [$216/month]).

29. **What are some different formulations of NSAIDs?**
    1. **Enteric-coated tablets.** Enteric-coated aspirin are supposed to have less GI symptoms than regular aspirin, but there is no evidence that the enteric coating decreases gastritis or peptic ulcers.
    2. **Liquid formulations.** Ibuprofen, naproxen, choline magnesium trisalicylate, and indomethacin are available in liquid formulations that are designed for patients who have difficulty swallowing pills and for children.
    3. **Slow release.** This formulation is designed to give a short-acting drug a longer half-life so that it can be taken only once or twice a day.
    - Diclofenac (Voltaren XR): 100 mg daily. Cost: generic $79/month, brand $235/month.
    - Etodolac (Lodine XL): 400 mg, 500 mg, 600 mg tablets. Dose: 400 to 600 mg daily. Cost: generic $42 to $81/month.
    - Indomethacin (Indocin SR): 75 mg daily to twice daily. Cost: generic $88 to $176/month.
    - Ketoprofen (Oruvail): 200 mg daily. Cost: generic $83/month.
    - Naprosyn (Naprelan): 375 mg, 500 mg, or 750 mg tablets. Dose: 750 to 1000 mg daily. Cost: generic $72/month, brand $271/month.
    4. **Topical formulations.** Salicylate containing creams (Bengay, Aspercreme) and diclofenac formulations (liquid drops, gel, and patch) are available in the United States. Topical diclofenac offers the potential for pain relief with decreased incidence of serious side effects in comparison to oral preparations. Studies involving the topical liquid diclofenac (Pennsaid) have shown low systemic absorption of the drug (6.6%; mean peak plasma concentrations nearly 100-fold less than oral formulation). Recent data have demonstrated clinical benefit in hand, hip, and knee osteoarthritis for some of these formulations.
    - Diclofenac 1% topical gel (Voltaren gel): 2 g twice daily to four times daily for small joints and 4 g twice daily to four times daily for large joints. Maximum dose 32 g/day. Cost $300/month.
    - Diclofenac 1.3% topical patch (Flector patch): two patches/day. Cost $370/month each area treated.
    - Diclofenac 1.5% topical solution (Pennsaid solution): 40 drops/knee twice daily to four times daily. Cost: $168/month per knee.
    5. **Combination medications.** NSAID combined with a gastroprotective agent.
    - Diclofenac sodium with misoprostol (Arthrotec): 50 to 75 mg/200 μg twice daily to 50 mg/200 μg four times daily. Cost: 50 mg/200 μg twice daily is $200/month.
    - Naproxen plus esomeprazole (Vimovo): 375/20 mg or 500 mg/20 mg twice daily. Cost: $112/month.
    - Ibuprofen plus famotidine (Duexis): 800 mg/26.6 mg three times daily. Cost: $167/month.

30. **One of your patients who is on chronic NSAIDs suffers a recent humeral fracture and is told by her orthopedist to stop her NSAID. Why was this suggested?**
Prostaglandins and the COX enzymes (specifically COX-2) probably play a role in fracture healing. Animal models have demonstrated impaired fracture healing in response to selective and nonselective NSAIDs. Human studies have shown conflicting results, but at least one metaanalysis has identified an increased risk for nonunion in users of NSAIDs following fracture of long bones. Studies thus far have been retrospective and therefore no causal relationship has been established, but a conservative approach would include stoppage of NSAIDs during periods of bone healing.

31. **One of your patients would like to become pregnant in the near future and wonders about the potential use of some of her medications both during pregnancy and after. She is on chronic NSAIDs for joint pain. Describe your advice to her.**
The COX-2 enzyme probably plays several roles in the female reproductive cycle leading to a successful pregnancy and birth of a child. For example: (1) COX-2 mediated prostaglandins are involved in follicle rupture

Table 81-2. Nonsteroidal Antiinflammatory Drugs That Have Short Plasma Elimination Half-Lives and Long Half-Lives

DRUG	HALF-LIFE (hours)	DOSAGE
Short half-life (<6 hours)		
Aspirin	0.25	3000 mg (maximum daily dose)
Diclofenac sodium (Voltaren)	1.1	25 to 50 mg twice daily to three times daily
Diclofenac potassium (Cataflam)		75 mg twice daily
Etodolac (Lodine)	3.0/6.5*	200 mg three times daily to four times daily
		400 mg three times daily
Fenoprofen (Nalfon)	2.5	200 to 600 mg three times daily to four times daily
Flurbiprofen (Ansaid)	3.8	50 to 100 mg twice daily to three times daily
Ibuprofen (Motrin)	2.1	400 to 800 mg three times daily to four times daily
Indomethacin (Indocin)	4.7	25 mg three times daily to four times daily
		50 mg three times daily
		75 mg SR twice daily
Ketoprofen (Orudis)	1.8	50 mg four times daily
		75 mg three times daily
		200 mg ER four times daily
Tolmetin (Tolectin)	1.0/6.8*	400 to 600 mg three times daily
Long half-life (>10 hours)		
Diflunisal (Dolobid)	13	250 to 500 mg twice daily
Nabumetone (Relafen)	26	500 to 1000 mg twice daily
		1000 to 2000 mg daily
Naproxen (Naprosyn)	14	250 to 500 mg twice daily
Naproxen sodium (Anaprox)	14	275 to 550 mg twice daily
Oxaprozin (Daypro)	58	600 to 1200 mg daily
Meloxicam (Mobic)	17	7.5 to 15 mg daily
Piroxicam (Feldene)	57	10 to 20 mg daily
Salicylate (Salsalate)	2 to 15†	750 to 1500 mg twice daily
Sulindac (Clinoril)	14	150 to 200 mg twice daily
Celecoxib (Celebrex)	11	200 mg daily to 100 to 200 mg twice daily

*Elimination of this drug occurs in two phases, of which the first is generally more important
†Elimination of this drug is dose-dependent.

and release; (2) COX-2 is important in implantation of the embryo in the uterus; and (3) prostaglandins have a well-established role in uterine contractions during labor. Overall, this enzyme is probably important for several processes in the very early and late stages of pregnancy.

There are case reports of infertility while on NSAIDs which reversed upon stoppage of the medication, but there are no strong data demonstrating this risk. It is not necessary to routinely stop NSAIDs, but if problems with fertility occur then it is recommended to hold their use. After a woman becomes pregnant, use of NSAIDs in the first and second trimester is relatively safe (category B). Use of NSAIDs after 32 weeks of gestation should be avoided, however, as prostaglandins are necessary late in pregnancy to maintain a patent ductus arteriosus, for fetal kidney development, and for progression of labor. NSAID use is compatible with breastfeeding.

Table 81-3. Drug–Drug Interactions Involving Nonsteroidal Antiinflammatory Drugs

DRUG AFFECTED	NSAID IMPLICATED	EFFECT
Warfarin	NSAIDs that inhibit COX-1	Inhibits metabolism of warfarin; increases risk of bleeding owing to inhibition of platelet function and gastric mucosal damage
Sulfonylurea	High-dose salicylate	Potentiates hypoglycemia
Beta-blocker	All PG-inhibiting NSAIDs	Blunts hypotensive but not negative chronotropic or inotropic effect
Hydralazine Prazosin ACE inhibitor	All PG-inhibiting NSAIDs	Loss of hypotensive effects
Diuretics	All PG-inhibiting NSAIDs	Loss of natriuretic, diuretic, hypotensive effects of furosemide Loss of natriuretic effect of spironolactone Loss of hypotensive but not natriuretic or diuretic effects of thiazide
Phenytoin	Other NSAIDs	Displaces phenytoin from plasma protein, reducing total concentration for the same active concentration
Lithium	Most NSAIDs	Increases plasma lithium level
Digoxin	Most NSAIDs	May increase digoxin levels
Aminoglycosides	Most NSAIDs	May increase aminoglycoside level
Methotrexate	Most NSAIDs	May increase methotrexate plasma concentration
Sodium valproate	Aspirin	Inhibits valproate metabolism, increasing plasma valproate concentration

ACE, Angiotensin-converting enzyme; COX, cyclooxygenase; NSAIDs, nonsteroidal antiinflammatory drugs; PG, prostaglandin.

32. **Why do the elderly tend to have more complications with NSAIDs?**
    The elderly have more complications from these drugs than any other group of patients, because of:
    - Altered drug absorption. The gastric pH rises with age. Active absorption and transport of drugs may be altered.
    - Reduced drug distribution.
    - Decreased protein binding. Plasma albumin decreases with aging, decreasing protein-binding sites.
    - Hepatic metabolism and renal excretion may be altered.
    - Polypharmacy. Some patients' medications may have drug interactions with NSAIDs.

33. **List some drug–drug interactions involving NSAIDs.**
    Some drug–drug interactions involving NSAIDs are outlined in Tables 81-3 and 81-4.

34. **What is flavocoxid (Limbrel)?**
    Flavocoxid (Limbrel) is classified as a "medical food" that is approved for treatment of osteoarthritis. The compound is a proprietary mixture of a flavonoid and flavan (baicalcin and catechin) and zinc. It is marketed as a dual inhibitor of cyclooxygenase (COX-1, COX-2) and 5-lipoxygenase (5-LOX) and comes in 250-mg and 500-mg capsules. Studies have shown that flavocoxid inhibits prostaglandin production through inhibition of phospholipase A2 and inhibition of the peroxidase activity of the COX enzymes. This differs from NSAIDs which inhibits the cyclooxygenase activity of the COX enzymes. In vitro studies also suggest that flavocoxid inhibits 5-LOX, resulting in less leukotriene production and reduces NF-κB stimulation through inhibition of reactive oxygen species. The sum result is an antiinflammatory compound with less toxicity and few drug interactions including warfarin. The dose is 250 to 500 mg twice daily. Cost: $130/month for 250 mg twice daily.

Table 81-4. Other Drugs Affecting NSAIDs

DRUG-IMPLICATED	NSAID AFFECTED	EFFECT
Antacids	Indomethacin Salicylates Other NSAIDs?	Aluminum-containing antacids reduce rate and extent of absorption Sodium bicarbonate increases rate and extent of absorption
Cimetidine	Piroxicam	Increases plasma concentrations and half-life of piroxicam
Probenecid	Most NSAIDs	Reduces metabolism and renal clearance of NSAIDs
Cholestyramine	Naproxen Probably others	Anion exchange resin binds NSAIDs in gut, reducing rate (and extent?) of absorption
Caffeine	Aspirin	Increases rate of absorption of aspirin
Metoclopramide	Aspirin and probably others	Increases rate and extent of absorption in patients with migraines

NSAIDs, Nonsteroidal antiinflammatory drugs.

Acknowledgment

The author would like to thank David Collier, MD, for his contributions to this chapter in previous editions, as well as Luke Gansen, PharmD, for his work in this edition.

BIBLIOGRAPHY

Abraham NS, Hartman C, Castillo D, et al: Effectiveness of national provider prescription of PPI gastroprotection among elderly NSAID users, Am J Gastroenterol 103:323–332, 2008.
Bresalier R, Sandler R, Quan H, et al: Adenomatous polyp prevention on Vioxx. Cardiovascular events associated with rofecoxib in a colorectal adenoma chemoprevention trial. APPROVe Trial Investigators, N Engl J Med 352:1092–1102, 2005.
Capone ML, Sciulli MG, Tacconelli S, et al: Pharmacodynamic interaction of naproxen with low-dose aspirin in healthy subjects, J Am Coll Cardiol 45:1295–1301, 2005.
Catella-Lawson F, Reilly MP, Kapoor SC, et al: Cyclooxygenase inhibitors and the antiplatelet effects of aspirin, N Engl J Med 345:1809–1817, 2001.
Chan FK, Chung SC, Suen BY, et al: Preventing recurrent upper gastrointestinal bleeding in patients with *Helicobacter pylori* infection who are taking low-dose aspirin or naproxen, N Engl J Med 344:967–973, 2001.
Chan FK, Hung LC, Suen BY, et al: Celecoxib versus diclofenac plus omeprazole in high risk patients: results of a randomized double-blind trial, Gastroenterology 127:1038–1043, 2004.
Chan FK, Wong VW, Suen BY, et al: Combination of a COX-2 inhibitor and a proton pump inhibitor for the prevention of recurrent ulcer bleeding in patients at very high risk: a double blind, randomized trial, Lancet 369:1621–1626, 2007.
Desai SP, Solomon DH, Abraham SB, et al: Recommendations for use of selective and nonselective nonsteroidal antiinflammatory drugs: an American College of Rheumatology white paper, Arthritis Rheum 59:1058–1073, 2009.
Friedewald VE, Bennett JS, Christo JP, et al: AJC Editor's Consensus: selective and nonselective nonsteroidal anti-inflammatory drugs and cardiovascular risk, Am J Cardiol 106:873–884, 2010.
Garcia Rodriquez LA, Tacconelli S: Patrignani P: Role of dose potency in the prediction of risk of myocardial infarction associated with nonsteroidal anti-inflammatory drugs in the general population, J Am Coll Cardiol 52:1628–1636, 2008.
Graham DY, Opekun AR, Willingham FF, et al: Visible small intestinal mucosal injury in chronic NSAID users, Clin Gastroenterol Hepatol 3:55–59, 2005.
Hippisley-Cox J, Coupland C: Risk of myocardial infarction in patients taking cyclo-oxygenase-2 inhibitors or conventional nonsteroidal anti-inflammatory drugs: population based nested case-control analysis, BMJ 330:1366, 2005.
Kis B, Snipes JA, Busija DW: Acetaminophen and the cyclooxygenase-3 puzzle: sorting out facts, fictions, and uncertainties, J Pharmacol Exp Ther 315:1–7, 2005.
Lanas A: Gastrointestinal injury from NSAID therapy: how to reduce the risk of complications, Postgrad Med 117:23–28, 2005.
Lanza FL, Chan FK, Quigley EM: Guidelines for prevention of NSAID-related ulcer complications, Am J Gastroenterol 104:728–738, 2009.
Levy RM, Khokhlov A, Kopenkin S, et al: Efficacy and safety of flavocoxid, a novel therapeutic, compared with naproxen: a randomized multicenter controlled trial in subjects with osteoarthritis of the knee, Adv Ther 27:731–742, 2010.
McAdam BF, Catella-Lawson F, Mardini IA, et al: Systemic biosynthesis of prostacyclin by COX-2: the human pharmacology of a selective inhibitor of COX-2, Proc Natl Acad Sci USA 96:272–277, 1999.
Moen MD: Topical diclofenac, Drugs 69:2621–2632, 2009.
Rahme E, Barkun AN, Toubouti Y, et al: Do proton-pump inhibitors confer additional gastrointestinal protection in patients given celecoxib? Arthritis Rheum 57:748–755, 2007.

Schjerning OAM, Fosbel EL, Lindhardsen J, et al: Duration of treatment with NSAIDs and impact on risk of death and recurrent myocardial infarction in patients with prior myocardial infarction: a nationwide cohort study, Circulation 123:2226–2235, 2011.

Silverstein FE, Faich G, Goldstein JL, et al: Gastrointestinal toxicity with celecoxib vs nonsteroidal anti-inflammatory drugs for osteoarthritis and rheumatoid arthritis. The CLASS study: a randomized controlled trial, JAMA 284:1247–1255, 2000.

Solomon S, McMurray J, Pfeffer M, et al: Adenoma Prevention with Celecoxib APC Study Investigators: cardiovascular risk associated with celecoxib in a clinical trial for colorectal adenoma prevention, N Engl J Med 352:1071–1080, 2005.

Steinbach G, Lynch PM, Phillips RKS, et al: The effect of celecoxib, a cyclooxygenase-2 inhibitor, in familial polyposis, N Engl J Med 342:1946–1952, 2000.

Veld BA, Ruitenberg A, Hofman A, et al: Nonsteroidal antiinflammatory drugs and the risk of Alzheimer's disease, N Engl J Med 345:1515–1521, 2001.

Woessner K, Simon R, Stevenson D: The safety of celecoxib in patients with aspirin-sensitive asthma, Arthritis Rheum 46:2201, 2002.

Wolfe MM, Lichtenstein DR, Singh G: Gastrointestinal toxicity of nonsteroidal antiinflammatory drugs, N Engl J Med 340:1888–1899, 1999.

CHAPTER 82: GLUCOCORTICOIDS—SYSTEMIC AND INJECTABLE

Puja Chitkara, MD and Gregory J. Dennis, MD

> **KEY POINTS**
> 1. Every effort should be made to taper glucocorticoids and institute measures to limit side effects.
> 2. Cortisol (Solu-Cortef) 20 mg = prednisone 5 mg = prednisolone 5 mg = Medrol 4 mg (Solu-Medrol) = Decadron 0.75 mg.
> 3. Do not inject the same joint or tendon sheath more than three times yearly.

1. **List some general indications for implementation of glucocorticoid therapy in rheumatology.**
   Glucocorticoids (GCs) are potent medications discovered in 1949 (Drs. Hench and Kendall won Nobel Prize in 1950) and since used for a variety of medical indications. In the management of rheumatic disorders, there are two primary indications for their use:
   - Suppression of the inflammatory cascade.
   - Modification of the immune response.

2. **How are the antiinflammatory effects of GCs mediated?**
   GCs have beneficial antiinflammatory effects through numerous mechanisms. Some of the most important are:
   - Genomic
     - GCs diffuse passively across cell membranes, bind to intracellular GC receptors (cGCRs), and this complex is chaperoned to the nucleus where it binds to GC response elements on DNA.
       - GCs bind and block promoter sites of proinflammatory cytokine genes: interleukin-1 (IL-1).
       - GCs recruit transcription factors to promoter sites encoding regulatory proteins and antiinflammatory molecules (IκB, lipocortin-1, IL-10, IL-1R, others).
       - GCs inhibit production of proinflammatory transcription factors (NF-κB, AP-1, others) resulting in inhibition of production of proinflammatory cytokines, adhesion molecules, and COX-2.
   - Nongenomic
     - GCs bind to cGCRs causing release of inhibitory proteins such as Src.
     - GCs bind to membrane GCRs on lymphocytes and monocytes leading to antiinflammatory effects.
     - GCs at very high doses (>100 mg/day prednisone) intercalate into cell membranes reducing calcium and sodium cycling across the membrane, which has antiinflammatory effects. This may explain differential effects of high-dose "pulse" steroids.

3. **What are the effects of GCs on the innate and adaptive immune systems?**
   - Innate immune system
     - GCs upregulate enzymes that degrade bradykinin resulting in vasoconstriction. This causes less swelling and pain.
     - GCs suppress production of prostaglandins by inducing synthesis of lipocortin-1 which inhibits phospholipase A-2 mediated liberation of arachidonic acid from cell membranes.
     - GCs inhibit NF-κB which suppresses COX-2 synthesis. Does not affect COX-1 so platelet function is preserved.
     - GCs interfere with phagocytosis and cytokine production by macrophages and neutrophils.
     - Neutrophilia occurs as a result of increased release from bone marrow and decreased migration out of vasculature resulting from inhibition of adhesion molecule production and decreased cellular adherence to vessel walls.
     - GCs decrease release of eosinophils from bone marrow and increase apoptosis (eosinopenia).
   - Adaptive (acquired) immune response
     - Dendritic cells undergo increased apoptosis.
     - T cells are redistributed to tissues (lymphopenia).
       - Inhibits T helper, type 1 (Th1) > Th2 and Th17 cytokine production. Leads to anergy.
     - B cells less affected by GCs than T cells.
       - Immunoglobulin production preserved unless prolonged high-dose GCs.
     - Monocytes redistributed to tissues (monocytopenia).

4. **Which method(s) of GC administration are effective in the treatment of rheumatic disease?**
   - Intrasynovial therapy (needle injection into joint, bursa, or tendon sheath) is generally used to control inflammatory reactions involving the synovial lining of articular surfaces.
   - Oral or alimentary therapy.
   - Parenteral: intramuscular (IM) and intravenous (IV).

5. **How may a general clinical baseline be established for potential complications before instituting GC therapy?**
   - Some **chronic infections**, that is, opportunistic, may not be immediately apparent on the initial physical examination and may progress rapidly when corticosteroid therapy is implemented. For a baseline, obtain a **chest X-ray, tuberculin skin test (or interferon release assay), and screen for hepatitis B and hepatitis C.**
   - For **glucose intolerance**, a baseline **fasting glucose** is sufficient before the implementation of therapy, with periodic monitoring, especially with longer courses of therapy.
   - To assess one's risk for **osteoporosis**-related problems, a **bone mineral densitometry** should be performed within the first few months if GC therapy will be prolonged.
   - The activity of **gastrointestinal erosive disease** may be further aggravated by corticosteroid medications. A **complete blood count** with mean cell volume should be performed before beginning therapy. In selected patients a stool guaiac should be done.
   - **Cardiovascular disease** and **hypertension** may be aggravated by corticosteroid medications. Attention should be given toward **blood pressure determination** as well as the presence of peripheral edema on physical examination, with periodic reevaluation.
   - Performing a **Mini-Mental status examination**, especially in those with a history of mental disturbance, to provide an objective baseline for future comparison may be useful.

6. **To minimize the risk of hypothalamic–pituitary–adrenal axis suppression, when should patients take their daily dose of GC medication?**
   The body makes 10 to 12 mg/day of cortisol (equivalent to 2.5 to 3 mg/day prednisone). Because natural cortisol secretion in humans has a circadian rhythm with the peak level in the morning, taking the corticosteroid at that time will have less of a suppressive effect on the release of cortisol-releasing factor. Taking the corticosteroid before approximately 10:00 AM will result in less suppression of the hypothalamic–pituitary–adrenal (HPA) axis. When taking corticosteroids long term this probably is less important.

7. **Is GC therapy the cornerstone of therapy for rheumatic disease?**
   GCs remain the cornerstone of therapy for rheumatic disease. Clinicians use them to rapidly gain control of inflammatory conditions listed in Table 82-1 and subsequently attempt to taper the medication more rapidly after the implementation of an additional agent as a steroid sparing drug. This approach is thought to minimize the potential consequences of more prolonged corticosteroid therapy.

Table 82-1. Examples of Steroid Responsive Rheumatic Diseases
A. Selective complications of connective tissue diseases: 　Rheumatoid arthritis 　Systemic lupus erythematosus 　Polymyositis/dermatomyositis 　Sjögren's extra-salivary gland manifestations
B. Vasculitis disorders (initial treatment)
C. Crystalline disease flares
D. Polymyalgia rheumatica

8. **In the treatment of rheumatic disease, what is considered to be low-dose, medium-dose, and high-dose daily prednisone therapy?**

Low dose	≤7.5 mg/day.
Medium dose	7.5 mg/day to <40 mg/day.
High dose	≥40 mg/day to 100 mg/day (2 mg/kg/day in children).
Very high dose	>100 mg/day.

9. **Does dosage scheduling influence the potency of GC therapy?**
   Yes. The potency of GC therapy roughly correlates with the duration of hypothalamic–pituitary axis suppression. Table 82-2 lists the dosage schedules from the least to the most suppressive.

Table 82-2. Relative Potency of Glucocorticoid Administration Schedules

Intermittent oral dosing	+
Alternate day	++
Single daily morning dose	+++
Intermittent intravenous pulse therapy	++++
Multiple daily dosing	+++++

10. **How might GCs be grouped in terms of biologic activity?**
    GCs may be divided into three main groups according to their duration of biologic activity. The categories are presented in Table 82-3.

Table 82-3. Glucocorticoids Grouped in Terms of Biologic Activity

SHORT-ACTING	INTERMEDIATE-ACTING	LONG-ACTING
(Half-Life 12 hours)	(Half-Life 12 to 36 hours)	(Half-Life 48 hours)
Hydrocortisone	Prednisone	Paramethasone
Cortisone	Prednisolone	Betamethasone
	Methylprednisolone	Dexamethasone
	Triamcinolone	

11. **How do the GC properties of the corticosteroids compare with cortisol?**
    The GC potency of medications correlates in part with the duration of biologic activity (Table 82-4).
    PEARL: cortisol (Solu-Cortef) 20 mg = prednisone 5 mg = prednisolone 5 mg = Medrol 4 mg (Solu-Medrol) = Decadron 0.75 mg.

Table 82-4. Glucocorticoid Properties of Corticosteroid Preparations

GLUCOCORTICOID	GLUCOCORTICOID POTENCY*
Short-acting	
Hydrocortisone (cortisol)	1
Cortisone	0.8
Intermediate-acting	
Prednisone	4
Prednisolone	4
Methylprednisolone	5
Triamcinolone	5
Long-acting	
Paramethasone	10
Betamethasone	25
Dexamethasone	30 to 40

*Potency is determined with cortisol as a reference value of 1.

12. **What factors may affect GC dose efficacy?**
    - Age
      - Children <12 years old clear GCs 33% faster.
    - Diseases
      - Severe liver disease: may not convert prednisone to prednisolone (active form).
      - Hyperthyroidism, nephrotic syndrome, and hemodialysis increases GC clearance.

- Medications
  - Aluminum/magnesium antacids reduce absorption by 40%.
  - Most anticonvulsants and rifampin enhance GC metabolism by upregulating the CYP3A4 hepatic enzyme.
  - Erythromycin and ketoconazole decrease GC metabolism.

13. **What are some of the adverse consequences of GC therapy? At what dose (prednisone) does risk increase the most?**
    - Glucose intolerance and increased triglycerides attributable to insulin resistance (doses >10 mg/day).
    - Growth suppression (less if dose ≤0.5 mg/kg).
    - Osteonecrosis (risk at dose >20 mg/day for a month).
    - Posterior subcapsular cataract formation (risk even at 5 mg/day) and glaucoma (>10 mg/day).
    - Skin disorders (bruising, striae, delayed wound repair, hirsutism).
    - Peptic ulcer disease (doses >10 mg/day with nonsteroidal antiinflammatory drugs [NSAIDs] increases risk 3×).
    - Weight gain (>5 mg/day).
    - Infection (doses >20 to 25 mg/day [≥0.3 mg/kg] cause unacceptable risk).
      - Dose-dependent increased risk starts at >10 mg/day. *Staphylococcus aureus* most common.
      - *Pneumocystis jirovecii* infection increased risk >15 mg/day.
      - Mycobacterial (especially *Mycobacterium tuberculosis*) risk increases at >10 to 15 mg/day for a month.
      - **Anergy** can occur within 2 to 4 weeks on prednisone 30 mg/day.
      - Fungal: especially *Candida*.
      - Viral infections, especially herpes (cytomegalovirus, herpes zoster).
    - Hypertension (doses >10 mg/day).
    - Abnormal menstruation (decreased follicle-stimulating hormone and luteinizing hormone) and depressed hormone levels (thyroid-stimulating hormone, testosterone).
    - Mental disturbance (doses ≥20 to 30 mg/day) – rare to occur in children.
    - Muscle weakness (doses >10 to 20 mg/day) – worse with fluorinated GCs.
    - Osteoporosis (doses ≥5 to 7.5 mg/day for 3 months).
    - Vaccinations – live vaccines safe if on <20 mg/day.
    - Response to vaccines – less response if on >40 mg/day.
    - Allergy skin test results – can be affected by 15 to 20 mg/day for 2 to 4 weeks.

14. **Which group of corticosteroid medications results in the least amount of sodium retention?**
    Sodium retention is dependent upon the mineralocorticoid effect of the preparation. It is insignificant in the usual doses of methylprednisolone, triamcinolone, paramethasone, betamethasone, and dexamethasone (Table 82-5).

Table 82-5. Mineralocorticoid Properties of Glucocorticoid Preparations

GLUCOCORTICOID	MINERALOCORTICOID POTENCY*
Short-acting	
Hydrocortisone (cortisol)	1
Cortisone	0.8
Intermediate-acting	
Prednisone	0.25
Prednisolone	0.25
Methylprednisolone	±
Triamcinolone	±
Long-acting	
Paramethasone	±
Betamethasone	±
Dexamethasone	±

*Potency is expressed in milligram comparisons to cortisol reference value of 1.

15. **How common is adrenal atrophy in patients taking GCs?**
    Exogenous administration of GCs is the most common cause of adrenal insufficiency, resulting from suppression of adrenocorticotropic hormone (ACTH). Any patient who is Cushingoid in appearance, has received more than

20 mg of daily prednisone for more than a month in the preceding year, or has been on greater than 3 to 5 mg for more than a year should be considered to have a potentially suppressed HPA axis. When patients with adrenocortical functional impairment are stressed by infection, trauma, or surgery they may not be able to respond optimally (the body's normal cortisol output when under stress is up to 200 to 300 mg/day). Proper management during periods of physiologic stress aims to mimic the normal cortisol response. Full recovery of the HPA axis may take 6 to 9 months after stopping GC therapy. The responsiveness of the adrenal gland to stress can be tested with a short ACTH (Cortrosyn) stimulation test (250 μg [40 international units] IM, measure baseline and 60 minute plasma cortisol levels). A normal response is doubling of baseline cortisol and a 60-minute level >16 μg/dL. In patients at risk for adrenal insufficiency who are undergoing surgery or experiencing a severe infection, "stress dose steroids" may be needed to prevent hemodynamic instability. (Refer to Chapter 18 and Question 15 for a recommended regimen.)

16. List seven basic measures that should be done routinely for patients receiving GCs to lessen the chance of an adverse reaction.
1. Prescribe corticosteroids at the lowest possible dose and discontinue as soon as the disease activity permits.
2. Encourage physical activities and avoid immobilization (helps prevent myopathy).
3. Implement fall prevention program.
4. Prescribe dietary and supplemental calcium to achieve intake of 1000-1500 mg/day.
5. Supply vitamin D at a minimum of 1000 international units per day.
6. Consider bisphosphonate therapy implementation (if >7.5 mg/day for >3 months) particularly if postmenopausal. (See Chapter 52).
7. Document patient education concerning the adverse effects of therapy particularly risk of osteonecrosis.

17. Outline a tapering schedule for GCs.
There are many methods to taper GCs after the disease manifestations are brought under control. In some diseases GCs can be tapered rapidly. In other chronic inflammatory diseases such as systemic lupus erythematosus (SLE) and systemic vasculitis the taper must be slower. The following is one possible taper schedule:
- Prednisone 30 mg twice daily until disease is controlled.
- 25 mg twice daily × 1 to 2 weeks, then taper to 40 mg daily (single daily dose).
- Under 40 mg daily taper by 5 mg every week.
- Under 30 mg daily taper by 5 mg every 1 to 2 weeks.
- Under 20 mg daily taper by 2.5 mg every 1 to 2 weeks.
- Under 10 mg daily taper by 1 mg every 2 to 4 weeks.
- Under 5 mg daily taper by 1 mg daily every month (if at all).

Some patients may develop a steroid withdrawal syndrome with rapid tapering including arthralgias and myalgias. These symptoms should be controllable with acetaminophen and resolve within 3 to 4 days after the dose has been lowered. If symptoms do not resolve, consider a disease flare may be causing the symptoms.

18. What is Acthar Gel? What is it used for?
Acthar Gel (Repository Corticotropin) is a purified preparation of ACTH extracted from slaughtered pigs' pituitary glands. It is in a gel form designed to provide extended release of ACTH following injection. ACTH stimulates the adrenal cortex gland to secrete cortisol, corticosterone, and aldosterone. In addition, it is postulated to have other substances (e.g,. melanocortins) from the pig's pituitary that have additional immunomodulatory effects above that of just ACTH alone. However, the substances responsible for these additional effects are unclear. Acthar Gel is FDA-approved for the treatment of a variety of autoimmune diseases (dermatomyositis/polymyositis, SLE, nephrotic syndrome, acute exacerbation of multiple sclerosis, sarcoidosis, inflammatory eye disease, Stevens–Johnson syndrome, others) as well as for infantile spasms. The dose varies depending on the disease being treated (80 units IM daily to 80 units IM twice a week). Acthar Gel is supplied in 5 mL multidose vials (80 USP units/mL). It is extremely expensive (each vial costs $28,400) because of its orphan drug status for treating infantile spasms, which is a rare disease.

19. What is Rayos?
Rayos is the brand name of delayed-release prednisone tablets (1, 2, and 5 mg). Compared with immediate-released prednisone it has a formulation that results in a 4-hour lag time for its release. Otherwise its mode of action and pharmokinetics are identical to immediate-release prednisone. Rayos is administered at 10:00 PM and the prednisone is released during the night when cytokine release is increased. This allows for improved symptoms in the morning. It is primarily for use in patients with rheumatoid arthritis, polymyalgia rheumatica, asthma, and chronic obstructive pulmonary disease. The cost is $1000/month (30, 5-mg tablets) compared with $10 for 3 months of immediate-release prednisone (90, 5-mg tablets).

20. List some of the general indications for GC injection therapy in rheumatic conditions.
- Monoarthritis or disproportionate joint inflammation (after joint infection is ruled out).
- Recurrent joint effusion.
- Tendon sheath inflammation.
- Bursitis or tendinitis refractory to NSAIDs.

Note that the effectiveness of a single GC injection ranges from 50% to 100% and lasts for days to months.

21. **Construct a summary table of GC preparations available for injection into a joint, bursa, or tendon sheath.**
    Glucocorticoid preparations suitable for joint or other injection are presented in Table 82-6.

Table 82-6. Glucocorticoid Preparations Suitable for Joint or Other Injection

PREPARATION	STRENGTHS (MG/ML)	PREDNISONE EQUIVALENT (MG)*
Short-acting, soluble		
Dexamethasone sodium phosphate (Decadron, Hexadrol)	4	40
Hydrocortisone acetate (Hydrocortone)	25, 50	5, 10
Long-acting, less soluble		
Prednisolone tebutate (Hydeltra-TBA)	20	20
Methylprednisolone acetate (Depo-Medrol)	20, 40, 80	25, 50, 100
Dexamethasone acetate (Decadron-LA)	8	80
Longest-acting, least soluble		
Triamcinolone acetonide (Kenalog, Aristocort)	10, 40	12.5, 50
Triamcinolone hexacetonide (Aristospan)	20	25
Combination		
Betamethasone sodium phosphate/acetate† (Celestone Soluspan)	6	50

*Of 1 mL of injected steroid preparation
†Has longest-acting and short-acting steroid combined.

22. **Is there any characteristic(s) of GC preparations that are important to consider when determining which to use for injection therapy?**
    Solubility of the GC preparation is an important factor when considering injection therapy. Reducing the solubility of a compound increases the duration of the local effect, because slower diffusion of the medication will occur. Thus, less soluble (i.e., fluorinated) preparations have greater potency but are also more likely to result in adverse consequences.

23. **What volume of GCs can be safely injected into a joint?**
    The volume of GCs that can be safely injected depends on the size of the joint. The provider must be aware of the volume to be injected and attempts should be made to avoid overdistention of the surrounding joint capsule (Table 82-7).

Table 82-7. Volume of Glucocorticoids Can Be Safely Injected into a Joint

SIZE OF JOINT	VOLUME (ML)
Large (knees, ankles, shoulders)	1 to 2
Medium (elbows, wrists)	0.5 to 1
Small (interphalangeal, metaphalangeal)	0.1 to 0.5

24. **How often can a joint or tendon sheath be injected with glucocorticoid medications?**
    The main concern with frequent injections is accelerated deterioration of the joint attributable to cartilage breakdown or weakening of the tendon. A single GC injection into a tendon sheath can weaken the tendon up to 40% for 3 to 12 weeks. Thus, the longer the interval between injections the better. A minimum of 4 to 6 weeks between injections is recommended. Weight-bearing joints should not be injected more frequently than every 6 to 12 weeks. A good rule of thumb is not to inject the same joint or tendon sheath more than three times yearly.

25. **Can GC preparations for injection be combined with an anesthetic to minimize the number of needle sticks to the patient?**
    Yes, anesthetic preparations can be safely mixed with GC preparations. If the GC preparation contains a paraben compound as a preservative, flocculation of the suspension is likely to occur. Immediately before injecting, shake the syringe vigorously to minimize joint precipitation.

Table 82-8. Guidelines for the Appropriate Dose of Glucocorticoid to Be Injected

SITE	PREDNISONE EQUIVALENT DOSE (MG)
Bursa	10 to 20
Tendon sheath	10 to 20
Small joints of hands and feet	5 to 15
Medium-sized joints (wrist, elbow)	15 to 25
Large joints (knee, shoulder, ankle)	20 to 50

The dose for injection into a child's knee is 1 mg/kg.

26. **Is there an optimal amount of GC that should be injected into a joint, bursa, or tendon sheath?**

    It is generally recommended that short-acting or long-acting GCs be injected into tendon sheaths, because they are more soluble and cause less soft tissue atrophy or chance of tendon rupture (Table 82-8). The longest-acting, least-soluble GC preparations are typically injected into inflamed joints because they tend to be more effective.

27. **List some concerning problems and sequelae that may occur from GC injections.**
    - Infection (1 in 50,000 injections).
    - Skin hypopigmentation.
    - Steroid crystal-induced synovitis (postinjection flare) (2%).
    - Subcutaneous tissue atrophy.
    - Tendon rupture (never inject Achilles tendon).
    - Osteonecrosis (rare).
    - Erythroderma.

28. **How might a postinjection flare be distinguished from infection after a GC injection?**

    Postinjection flares occur in 1% to 2% of patients receiving GC injections and are most likely to occur with use of least soluble (i.e., long-acting) GC preparations. Injections of the lateral epicondyle of the elbow are particularly prone to this complication. The flare occurs within 6 to 18 hours after an injection. An infection usually becomes apparent 2 to 4 days after an injection. If need be, the joint can be aspirated and will show intracellular steroid crystals in a postinjection flare (look like calcium pyrophosphate dihydrate crystals but polarize with first order red compensation like gout crystals). Treat with ice, NSAIDs, and pain medications. A postinjection flare should resolve within 24 hours, whereas an infection will not.

BIBLIOGRAPHY

Bijlsma JW, Saag KG, Buttgereit F, et al: Developments in glucocorticoid therapy, Rheum Dis Clin North Am 31:1–17, 2005.

Buttgereit F, Mehta D, Kirwan J, et al: Low-dose prednisone chronotherapy for rheumatoid arthritis: a randomized clinical trial (CAPRA-2), Ann Rheum Dis 72:204–210, 2013.

Curtis JR, Westfall AO, Allison J, et al: Population-based assessment of adverse events associated with long-term glucocorticoid use, Arthritis Rheum 55:420–426, 2006.

Hench PS, Kendall EC, Slocumb CH, et al: The effect of a hormone of the adrenal cortex (17 hydroxy-11-dehydrocorticosterone: compound E) and of pituitary adrenocorticotropic hormone on rheumatoid arthritis: preliminary report, Proc Staff Meet Mayo Clin 24:181–197, 1949.

Richter B, Neises G, Clar C: Glucocorticoid withdrawal schemes in chronic medical disorders. A systemic review, Endocrinol Metab Clin North Am 31:751–778, 2002.

Saag K, et al: Systemic glucocorticoid therapy in rheumatology. In Hochberg MC, et al, editor: Rheumatology, ed 5, Philadelphia, 2011, Mosby Elsevier.

Sabir S, Werth V: Pulse glucocorticoids, Dermatol Clin 18:437–446, 2000.

Stahn C, Buttgereit F: Genomic and nongenomic effects of glucocorticoids, Nat Clin Pract Rheumatol 4:525–533, 2008.

SYSTEMIC ANTIRHEUMATIC DRUGS

Marcus H. Snow, MD and James R. O'Dell, MD

If many drugs are used for disease, all are insufficient.

—Sir William Osler

KEY POINTS

1. Choice of disease-modifying antirheumatic drug (DMARD) therapy is based on disease severity, comorbidities, and fertility plans.
2. Hydroxychloroquine or sulfasalazine monotherapy is best used for mild rheumatoid arthritis (RA).
3. Methotrexate (MTX) is the most effective anchor drug for all combination therapies.
4. Combination DMARD therapy is more effective than monotherapy in severe RA.
5. Patients need to be screened for G6PD deficiency before dapsone use.

1. What is meant by a DMARD?
Because there is no cure for most rheumatic diseases such as RA or systemic lupus erythematosus (SLE), the goal of treatment is to put the disease into remission. A category of drugs with some ability to do this is the disease-modifying antirheumatic drugs. To be designated a DMARD, a drug must change the course of the disease for at least 1 year as evidenced by one of the following: sustained improvement in physical function, decreased inflammatory synovitis, slowing or prevention of structural joint damage.

2. When should a patient with RA be started on a DMARD?
Once the diagnosis of RA is established, all patients (with rare exception) should begin DMARD therapy. Bone erosions and joint space narrowing develop within the first 2 years of disease in most patients and are progressive from that point onward. Therefore, early, aggressive treatment with DMARDs is warranted. Additionally, patients with RA who have evidence of active disease (synovitis, morning stiffness, etc.), bony erosions or deformities, or extraarticular disease manifestations and are not already on DMARDs should begin treatment immediately.

3. How quickly can traditional nonbiologic DMARDs be expected to work?
Most nonbiologic DMARDs take several months (3 to 6) to achieve a significant response. It is important to educate patients about this time frame of response so they are not discouraged when results are not seen immediately.

4. How are antimalarials used in the treatment of rheumatic diseases such as RA or SLE?
The antimalarials are the **least toxic** of all DMARDs and can be safely combined with other DMARDs. They are particularly effective in early treatment or add-on therapy of RA patients with mild to moderate disease manifestations. Hydroxychloroquine (HCQ) is the main antimalarial used.
Dosage: Hydroxychloroquine (Plaquenil), 200 to 400 mg/day (≤6.5 mg/kg ideal body weight of HCQ base). Note that 200mg tablet contains 155mg of HCQ base.
Chloroquine (Aralen), 250 mg/day (≤3.0 mg/kg ideal body weight of chloroquine base).
- Note that 500 mg tablets have 300 mg of chloroquine base and 250 mg tablets have 150 mg of base.
Quinacrine (Atabrine), 100 to 200 mg/day. Made by compound pharmacy.
Side effects: Nausea and vomiting (less likely to occur if start at half dose and titrate up over 2 to 4 weeks). Central nervous system (CNS) effects—headache, dizziness.
Muscle—myopathy (in high doses or renal insufficiency). Creatine phosphokinase can be normal.
Cardiomyopathy and peripheral neuropathy—increased risk in patients who develop a myopathy.
Aplastic anemia (quinacrine)—especially if *lichen planus rash* develops.
Hemolysis (rare)—in patients with G6PD deficiency.
Rash, hyperpigmentation of skin (gray-black with chloroquine, yellow with quinacrine), bleaching of hair.
Retinal toxicity (rare at currently recommended doses).
Monitoring: ophthalmologic examination every 12 months depending on risk factors.

5. What is the mechanism of action of the antimalarials?
Unknown. Antimalarials are weak bases and accumulate in acidic vesicles such as lysosomes. By increasing lysosomal pH, there is a disruption in the normal assimilation of peptides with class II major histocompatibility

complex (MHC) molecules or binding of RNA/DNA to Toll-like receptors (especially TLR7, TLR9). Antimalarials have also been shown to decrease production of interleukin-1 (IL-1), IL-6, interferons (IFNs), and prostaglandins by cells.

Other cellular effects of antimalarials are beneficial. For instance, they can increase lipoprotein (low-density lipoprotein) receptors, thus helping to lower lipid levels. They also decrease degradation of insulin, helping to prevent diabetes mellitus. Finally, they can inhibit platelet aggregation and adhesion, helping to prevent thrombosis.

6. **In which rheumatic conditions has treatment with antimalarials been effective?**
   - Rheumatoid arthritis.
   - Juvenile idiopathic arthritis.
   - SLE.
   - Discoid lupus, skin rash of dermatomyositis.
   - Antiphospholipid antibody syndrome.
   - Palindromic rheumatism.
   - Psoriatic arthritis (controversial)—use with caution, because antimalarials may exacerbate psoriatic skin lesions.
   - Sjögren's syndrome—recent controlled trials question its effectiveness.
   - Sarcoidosis.
   - Erosive osteoarthritis (controversial).

7. **Discuss the use of antimalarial therapy in SLE.**
   Antimalarial therapy is very useful in treating patients with SLE. Skin manifestations, serositis, fatigue, and joint disease are especially responsive to treatment. Additionally, antimalarials are useful in **maintaining remissions** and **preventing flares** of disease. Pregnant lupus patients (anti-SS-A$^+$) on antimalarial therapy may be less likely to have a child with neonatal lupus. Antimalarials also have a mild antithrombotic effect and may decrease risk of thrombosis, especially in patients with antiphospholipid antibodies. Therefore, almost all patients with SLE should be on an antimalarial.

8. **How common is antimalarial retinopathy and what steps can be used to decrease this toxicity?**
   Chloroquine binds more avidly to corneal and retinal pigmented epithelium than hydroxychloroquine and thus causes more corneal deposits and retinopathy. Corneal deposits are not an indication to stop antimalarials, but retinopathy is an absolute indication to stop therapy. Retinopathy is very uncommon and occurs in less than 1% to 2% of individuals who have been on antimalarials for more than 5 years (or total dose >1000 mg). It is extremely rare if dosed according to ideal (lean) body weight. Consequently, patients less than 1.52 m (60 inches) should get 200-300 mg of hydroxychloroquine and not the usual 400 mg. Likewise, patients less than 1.57 m (62 inches) in height should receive less than 250 mg of chloroquine a day. These doses must be decreased further if there is renal or liver dysfunction. Notably, owing to a different chemical composition, quinacrine does not cause retinopathy. Consequently, quinacrine can be combined with chloroquine or hydroxychloroquine without added retinal toxicity.
   A baseline ophthalmologic examination should be done on all patients at 6 months after starting an antimalarial. Revised recommendations state that annual screening using Humphrey automated visual fields 10-2 perimetry as well as newer objective tests (spectral domain optical coherence tomography, electroretinography, fluorescein angiography) should begin at 5 years of usage. Patients who are at higher risk for toxicity should be examined more frequently (i.e., every year after baseline examination). These high-risk patients include those on higher than recommended doses, have coexistent eye disease, are over age 60 years, or have renal or liver dysfunction. The first evidence of toxicity is loss of red light perception. If this is detected, the antimalarial can be stopped and there will be no loss of vision. However, if toxicity is allowed to progress to decrease in visual acuity and/or macular pigmentary changes, the patient may lose further vision even if the antimalarial is discontinued. Although no longer recommended, an added inexpensive safety measure is to give a patient an Amsler grid and instruct them on how to use it monthly at home. If the lines become blurry, the patient should be examined immediately.

9. **What can interfere with antimalarial effectiveness? What drug interactions can occur?**
   Smoking can induce hepatic cytochrome P450 enzymes resulting in accelerated metabolism of antimalarials, causing them to be less effective. Cimetidine can decrease the clearance of antimalarials. Antimalarials can increase digoxin levels and add to the effectiveness of hypoglycemic agents. They can antagonize the effects of anticonvulsants and amiodarone.

10. **Discuss the use of sulfasalazine in RA.**
    Sulfasalazine (Azulfidine) is often used in early, mild disease because it acts quickly with measurable results in 4 weeks. For many years, this was the first and most commonly used DMARD in Europe. Its potential for toxicity is low and it is often combined with other DMARDs. Sulfasalazine is a two-component drug, made up of sulfapyridine and 5-aminosalicylic acid (5-ASA).
    Dosage: 1 to 3 g/day in divided doses. Start at 500 mg and increase by 500 mg each week.
    Side effects: Nausea and vomiting (less if dose is titrated up slowly, if taken with meals, and if enteric-coated tablets are used).

Rash (1% to 5%): usually within first 3 months.
Headache and dizziness.
Azoospermia (reversible on discontinuation of drug).
Neutropenia (1% to 5%): usually within first 3 months.
Hemolysis if G6PD deficient (rare).
Pulmonary infiltrates with eosinophilia.
Hepatic enzyme elevation ± fever, adenopathy, rash.
Monitoring: complete blood count (CBC) with platelets and liver enzymes at baseline and monthly for the first 3 months of therapy and then every 3 months, creatinine at 1 month and then every third month.

11. What is the metabolism and mechanism of action (MOA) of sulfasalazine?
Only 10% to 30% of sulfasalazine is ultimately absorbed in the small intestine. Most sulfasalazine is broken down by colonic bacteria to sulfapyridine, which is then 90% absorbed, and into 5-ASA, which mostly (90%) stays in the bowel. The sulfapyridine component is felt to be most effective and thus patients without a colon may not respond to sulfasalazine. Sulfasalazine has multiple antiinflammatory and immunomodulatory effects but the exact mechanism of action is unknown.

12. In what rheumatic diseases is sulfasalazine used?
- RA.
- Juvenile idiopathic arthritis.
- Reactive arthritis (Reiter's syndrome).
- Psoriatic arthritis.
- Ankylosing spondylitis (peripheral arthritis).
- Enteropathic arthritis.

13. Discuss the role of MTX in RA.
MTX (Rheumatrex, Trexall) is considered the most effective DMARD for RA. Approximately 30% of patients will achieve low disease activity on MTX monotherapy. MTX acts relatively quickly after being started, often within several weeks. In addition to providing efficacy clinically, MTX appears to retard appearance of new erosions in involved joints. Using other drugs (hydroxychloroquine, sulfasalazine) in combination with MTX has resulted in improved efficacy over MTX alone without an additive increase in side effects.

14. What dose of MTX is used to treat RA and what toxicities are associated with its use?
Dosage: 7.5 to 25 mg per os, subcutaneous, or intramuscular weekly. The absorption of oral and parenteral MTX is equivalent at doses less than 15 mg/week. At higher doses parenteral MTX gives serum levels 30% higher than oral MTX. At oral doses above 15 mg/week, better absorption is obtained if the oral dose is split or the parenteral form is used.
Parenteral forms for subcutaneous injection are supplied as:
- Generic MTX: a solution of 25 mg/mL (supplied in 2-mL and 10-mL vials). The patient must draw up the correct dose (2.5 mg per 0.1 mL). Cost of two 2 mL vials is $30 to $40.
- Fixed-dose individual syringes (Otrexup): supplied as single-dose, autoinjector (0.4 mL) with prefilled doses of 10, 15, 20, or 25 mg. Cost of four 25 mg syringes is $548.

Folic acid 1 mg/day should always be given with MTX, and the dose can be increased to 2 to 5 mg/day if symptoms of toxicity (mouth sores) develop. *Folinic acid* (leukovorin) 5 mg given as one dose 24 hours after weekly dose of MTX can sometimes help mouth sores even if folic acid fails.
Side effects: Oral ulcers (folic acid helps prevent and/or decrease symptoms); photosensitivity.
Nausea, vomiting, anorexia. Can worsen migraine headaches.
Hepatic toxicity (concern has lessened with further experience—see below).
Hematologic toxicity (leukopenia, thrombocytopenia, pancytopenia, megaloblastic anemia)—folic acid helps prevent this. Less likely to occur if renal function is normal.
Pneumonitis—occurs early (stop MTX and do not rechallenge, also need to rule out opportunistic infections such as *Pneumocystis jiroveci* pneumonia).
Flu-like symptoms of nausea, fever, chills, myalgias (MTX flu).
Worsening nodulosis (5%) and leukocytoclastic vasculitis in seropositive patients with RA.
Lymphomas— some related to Epstein–Barr virus infection. May resolve if MTX is stopped.

15. Discuss the precautions and monitoring required for patients taking MTX.
Monitoring: before starting MTX, CBC with platelets, hepatitis B and C serology, as well as aspartate aminotransferase (AST), alanine aminotransferase (ALT), alkaline phosphatase, albumin, and creatinine (creatinine clearance, CrCl) should be obtained. A chest X-ray should be done if the patient has not had one in the past year. CBC with platelets, AST, ALT, albumin, and creatinine should then be followed every 4 to 12 weeks. Monitoring can be less frequent (every 12 weeks) when on stable dose for longer than 3 to 6 months.
Precautions: MTX should be avoided (CrCl <30 mL/min) or used in reduced dose (by 25% for CrCl <80 mL/min; by 50% for CrCl <50 mL/min) in patients with renal insufficiency. Patients should also avoid alcohol and trimethoprim–sulfamethoxazole (decreases excretion). MTX is also contraindicated in pregnancy, and female

patients of child-bearing age should use a reliable form of contraception. MTX should be stopped for 3 months in both males and females before attempting to get pregnant since the normal life cycle from oocyte to mature egg is 90 days. MTX can accumulate in pleural effusions and be reabsorbed causing neutropenia. MTX should be used with caution (if at all) in patients with hepatitis B or C infections.

16. Describe the rationale and value of testing for MTX polyglutamate levels.

    MTX enters the cell via the reduced folate carrier (RFC). It is pumped out of the cell by members of the ATP-binding cassette (ABC) protein family. Intracellular MTX undergoes polyglutamation by the enzyme folylpolyglutamyl synthetase (FPGS). Polyglutamation of MTX (MTX-PG) is essential to its immune modulation effects and to prevent intracellular MTX from being transported out of the cell. Polymorphisms of RFC, ABC proteins, and FPGS account for variations in efficacy and toxicity of MTX among patients. Measurement of MTX-PG can determine if a patient is likely to respond clinically. Patients with a low MTX-PG level are either not taking the medication, not absorbing it, or has one or more polymorphisms that inhibits their ability to form MTX-PG. Patients with active disease who are unable to achieve a therapeutic MTX-PG level should be switched to another DMARD. Note that a stable MTX-PG level is not achieved for 6 to 7 months after a dosage change.

    PEARL: patients who have an increase of their red blood cell mean cell volume (MCV) value by 5 fL over baseline after starting MTX are most likely to have a clinical response to MTX and a therapeutic MTX-PG level.

17. When should a liver biopsy be done on patients receiving MTX?

    Routine baseline or periodic liver biopsies in patients receiving MTX are not recommended. However, baseline liver biopsy is recommended in patients with risk factors for cirrhosis such as significant alcohol use, positive hepatitis serology, or elevated liver transaminase levels. Liver biopsy is also recommended if AST or ALT levels are persistently elevated (>3 months) or if albumin levels decrease (not attributable to inflammation) while on MTX.

18. What is the mechanism of action for the immunologic effects of MTX at the doses currently used?

    MTX has multiple effects on the immune system. At the low doses used to treat rheumatic diseases, it is unlikely that it significantly inhibits purine synthesis through inhibition of dihydrofolate reductase (resulting in a decrease in metabolically active reduced folates). However, MTX can inhibit AICAR *transformylase*. This leads to increases in the intracellular concentration of its substrate AICAR, which stimulates the release of adenosine. Adenosine is a potent inhibitor of neutrophil function and has potent antiinflammatory properties.

19. In what rheumatologic conditions is MTX used?
    - RA.
    - Juvenile idiopathic arthritis.
    - Psoriatic arthritis.
    - Reactive arthritis (Reiter's syndrome).
    - Ankylosing spondylitis (peripheral arthritis).
    - Polymyositis/dermatomyositis.
    - Antineutrophil cytoplasmic antibody-associated vasculitides.
    - Adult-onset Still's disease.
    - SLE.
    - Polymyalgia rheumatica/giant cell arteritis.
    - Sarcoidosis.
    - Uveitis.

20. Discuss the role of leflunomide in RA.

    Leflunomide (Arava) is a novel DMARD that inhibits pyrimidine synthesis and is approved for treatment of active RA. Studies support that the efficacy of leflunomide is comparable to low-dose MTX and to sulfasalazine. Additionally, leflunomide has been shown to slow radiographic progression in RA. Leflunomide may be used when MTX is contraindicated or not tolerated. It can also be added at a reduced dose (10 mg/day) to MTX in patients who have received benefit from MTX but still have active disease, although the potential of liver toxicity is increased.

21. Discuss the dosing and side effects of leflunomide.

    Dosage: 10 to 20 mg daily. To save money, leflunomide 20 mg every other day works as well as 10 mg daily. Patients are rarely given a loading dose (100 mg daily × 3) because of gastrointestinal toxicity of the drug.
    Side effects: Nausea, vomiting, and diarrhea (17%)—can lead to significant weight loss.
    Skin rash (8%).
    Allergic reaction (usually occurs at higher doses).
    Neutropenia > thrombocytopenia.
    Alopecia (reversible) (8%).
    Hepatic enzyme elevation.

Hypertension.
Teratogenicity (Category X).
Pneumonitis less common than with MTX.

22. What is the mechanism of action of leflunomide?
The active metabolite of leflunomide, A77 1726, inhibits dihydroorotate dehydrogenase leading to a decrease in de novo synthesis of uridine resulting in a decrease in the synthesis of pyrimidines. Activated but not resting lymphocytes (B cells > T cells) have low pools of pyrimidine nucleotides, making them sensitive to this drug. When uridine is lowered below a critical level, the tumor suppressor p53 is activated, arresting lymphocyte cell division in the G1 stage of the cell cycle.

23. Is leflunomide used in diseases other than RA?
Yes. Although not FDA-approved, leflunomide has been used in most diseases where MTX is used with similar results.

24. What precautions and monitoring are required in patients taking leflunomide?
Monitoring: Hepatitis B and C serology, AST, ALT, and creatinine should be obtained at baseline and monthly thereafter. If laboratory results are stable, monitoring can be done less frequently (8 to 12 weeks) at the discretion of the clinician.

Precautions: Leflunomide should not be used in patients with hepatic impairment or positive hepatitis serology and is also contraindicated in pregnancy. Caution should be used in patients with renal impairment, because there are currently no clinical data available in this group of patients. Leflunomide has an extremely *long halflife*; in some cases, it may take up to 2 years to reach undetectable plasma concentrations. Because of this, an enhanced drug elimination procedure has been developed in cases of overdose, toxicity, or desire for pregnancy (both males and females). Cholestyramine 8 g three times daily for 11 days (does not have to be consecutive days) will rapidly reduce plasma concentrations in these situations. In patients desiring to become pregnant, the active metabolite plasma level must be documented to be less than 0.02 µg/mL on two occasions 14 days apart. This is done through the company by calling 1-800-221-4023 to get the kit and instructions for blood draw.

Drug interactions: Rifampin increases serum level of active metabolite of leflunomide, which can increase toxicity. Warfarin therapy may be potentiated by leflunomide.

25. Discuss the management of hepatotoxicity attributable to leflunomide.
There have been several reports of severe hepatotoxicity attributable to leflunomide. Some of these cases have resulted in liver failure and death. Most occurred within the first several months of initiation of therapy. Most patients were taking additional medications (such as MTX) that are known to be hepatotoxic to the liver or had coexistent hepatitis B that was reactivated. Appropriate precautions can decrease the chance of this toxicity:
- Limit use of other drugs with potential for additive liver toxicity.
- Do not use leflunomide in patients with hepatitis B or hepatitis C.
- Monitor ALT and AST monthly for first 6 months. If also on MTX or have minor elevations of liver associated enzymes (LAEs), continue monthly monitoring. Otherwise, monitor every 2 months.

The following are recommendations should LAEs become elevated:
- Minor sporadic elevations (>1× and <2× upper limit of normal [ULN])—follow with repeat testing.
- LAEs >2× ULN or persistent minor elevations—dose reduction.
- LAEs >3× ULN—stop leflunomide and consider drug elimination protocol that can be abbreviated (cholestyramine 4 g three times daily for 5 days).

26. Can combinations of two or more DMARDs be used in the treatment of RA?
The role of combination DMARD therapy in the treatment of RA continues to evolve. With the addition of new medications, more therapeutic combinations are possible than ever before. Most clinical trials of combination therapy with DMARDs have included MTX. Several studies have shown that combination therapy with MTX, whether step-up or as initial therapy, is more beneficial than MTX alone. The following are combinations that have been studied:
- MTX and hydroxychloroquine.
- MTX, hydroxychloroquine, and sulfasalazine (**triple therapy**).
- MTX and leflunomide (typically MTX plus 10 mg of leflunomide).
- MTX and azathioprine.
- MTX and cyclosporine.
- MTX and biologic agents.

27. Should patients on immunosuppressive medications be vaccinated?
- Patients on prednisone or on immunosuppressive medications listed above and in Chapter 84 and 85 can receive any of the *inactivated* vaccines. They can receive these vaccinations without an increased chance of flaring their underlying disease. However, their protective antibody titers following vaccination may be blunted as a result of being on immunosuppressive medications (especially prednisone). Patients should receive the following:

- Influenza A/B/H1N1 vaccine yearly.
- Pneumococcal vaccine (PPSV23) to all immunosuppressed patients over age 19 years at the start of therapy and 5 years later. They should receive an additional dose at age 65 years if it has been greater than 5 years since the previous two doses of PPSV23.
  - Pneumococcal conjugate 13-valent vaccine (PCV13) has recently been advised to be given to immunosuppressed patients over age 19 years. If the patient has not previously received PPSV23 they should get one dose of PCV13 followed 8 weeks later with a dose of PPSV23. If the high-risk patient has received PPSV23 previously they should get one dose of PCV13 given at least 1 year after the PPSV23 vaccination.
- Hepatitis B vaccine: at-risk patients on MTX or leflunomide.
- Age appropriate vaccinations: tetanus diphtheria/acellular pertussis (Td/Tdap), meningococcal, *Haemophilus influenzae* B (Hib).
- Other inactivated vaccines as appropriate: inactivated polio, rabies, hepatitis A, hepatitis B, human papilloma virus, typhoid polysaccharide.
- Patients on MTX (>0.4 mg/kg/wk), leflunomide, prednisone ≥20 mg/day, and/or medications listed in Chapter 84 and 85 should **not** receive *live* attenuated virus vaccines. Furthermore, they should avoid contact with children recently vaccinated with oral polio vaccine, small pox, or rotavirus, because the virus is shed in their stool. They should avoid contact with patients who received the live influenza virus intranasally and those who develop a rash following the herpes zoster vaccine. Additional guidelines for live vaccine administration:
  - Live vaccines currently available: mumps/measles/rubella (MMR), herpes zoster, live attenuated influenza (nasal), varicella zoster, yellow fever, oral typhoid, Bacillus Calmette–Guérin (BCG), rotavirus, oral adenovirus, smallpox.
  - Patients on prednisone (<20 mg/day), MTX (<0.4 mg/kg/week), azathioprine (<3 mg/kg/day), 6-mercaptopurine (<1.5 mg/kg/day) can receive live vaccines, most notably the herpes zoster vaccine. If initially on higher doses, patient must be on the lower dose (e.g., prednisone <20 mg/day) for at least 1 month before receiving the live vaccine.
  - Patients on biologics (antitumor necrosis factor [anti-TNF], tocilizumab, abatacept, tofacitinib, anakinra, belimumab, rituximab) should be off the biologic for at least three half-lives before receiving a live vaccine and not restart the biologic until 1 month after administration of the live vaccine.

28. How is dapsone used in the treatment of rheumatic diseases?

Dapsone is a sulfone. It is poorly water-soluble, poorly absorbed through the gastrointestinal tract, and metabolized by the liver. It is used as an antimicrobial for treatment of leprosy. However, it also has antiinflammatory effects and is particularly useful in dermatoses involving polymorphonuclear leukocytes. It is a free oxygen radical scavenger and impairs the myeloperoxidase system. In rheumatic diseases, it is particularly useful for skin vasculitis (leukocytoclastic, urticarial, or erythema elevatum diutinum, cutaneous polyarteritis nodosa), skin lesions of Behçet's disease, SLE rashes (particularly bullous disease and panniculitis), relapsing polychondritis, and pyoderma gangrenosum. Doses range from 50 to 200 mg with an average of 100 mg a day. The major drug interaction is probenecid, which slows its renal excretion. Dapsone is also used as *Pneumocystis jiroveci* prophylaxis in patients allergic to sulfa antibiotics.

29. What are the major toxicities of dapsone?

All patients treated with dapsone will have some degree of hemolysis and methemoglobinemia and thus should be supplemented with 1 mg of folate daily. Patients with G6PD deficiency will have severe hemolysis, so all patients should be screened, particularly those of Mediterranean or African descent. The hemolysis is attributable to a metabolite of dapsone causing oxidation of glutathione, which is essential for erythrocyte membrane integrity. G6PD is necessary to produce NADPH, which is a cofactor for glutathione reductase, which reduces the oxidized glutathione back to an active form.
Other side effects can include leukopenia, hypersensitivity syndrome, liver toxicity, nausea, and peripheral neuropathy (on high doses). Monitoring should include CBC and reticulocyte count every month for 3 months, then every 3 months with renal and liver tests.

30. How is thalidomide used in the treatment of rheumatic diseases?

Thalidomide (Thalomid) has antiinflammatory, immunomodulatory, and antiangiogenic properties. A major effect may be its ability to reduce TNF-α production by 40%. It is not immunosuppressive and has not been associated with opportunistic infections. At doses of 50 mg to 300 mg a day, it has been useful to treat inflammatory skin diseases associated with Behçet's disease and SLE that are resistant to standard therapy. It is particularly useful for severe oral and/or genital ulcerations. Major toxicities include sedation, constipation, rash, sensory polyneuropathy, blood clots, and teratogenicity (phocomelia). Owing to these toxicities, the FDA requires registration for its use and following stringent regulations and guidelines for use (call 1-888-423-5436 to get application for use). Owing to the frequency of polyneuropathy (up to 50%), which is more common in women and not related to daily or cumulative dose, it is recommended that a baseline electromyography/nerve conduction velocity be performed and repeated every 6 months. A decline in the sensory nerve action potential by 50% or development of subjective complaints at monthly follow-ups requires discontinuation of the drug, because the neuropathy is often progressive and nonreversible. Lenalidomide (Revlimid) is similar to thalidomide but potentially less toxic. Its major toxicity is thrombocytopenia more than neutropenia. It is less likely than thalidomide to cause blood clots and sensory polyneuropathy.

31. Are there any new medications recently approved for the treatment of rheumatic diseases?

Apremilast (Otezla) is a novel systemic drug with FDA approval in 2014. It is an immune modulator rather than an immunosuppressant. Apremilast is an inhibitor of phosphodiesterase 4 (PDE4) which results in an elevation of cAMP intracellularly in multiple cell types (T cells, mononuclear cells, others). The increase in intracellular cAMP decreases the production of several proinflammatory mediators (TNF-α, IL-12, IL-23, IFNγ, and inducible nitric oxide synthase) and increases the production of antiinflammatory cytokines (IL-10). Patients are started on low dose with titration to 30 mg twice daily. Modest efficacy has been shown in psoriasis, psoriatic arthritis, and Behçet's disease (oral and genital ulcers). Trials are ongoing in ankylosing spondylitis. The drug is well tolerated with diarrhea, nausea, and headache being the most common side effects. No specific lab monitoring is required. The cost of apremilast is $22,000 a year.

32. What is the American College of Rheumatology definition for improvement in RA treatment trials? What radiographic scoring system is most often used to measure radiographic progression in RA trials?

An American College of Rheumatology (ACR) study group determined that improvement for clinical trial patients with RA be defined as:

Required: ≥20% improvement in tender joint count
and
≥20% improvement in swollen joint count

Plus: ≥20% improvement in three of the following five:
- Patient pain assessment
- Patient global assessment
- Physician global assessment
- Patient self-assessed disability (Health Assessment Questionnaire, HAQ)
- Acute-phase reactant (erythrocyte sedimentation rate or C-reactive protein)

Patients who improve as defined above are said to have met criteria for ACR 20. If improved 50% or 70%, they have met criteria for ACR 50 or ACR 70. Achieving an ACR 20/50/70 is more difficult than just improving the patient's joint count by 20%, 50%, or 70%.

The most commonly used radiographic scoring system used in RA trials is the **van der Heijde modification of the Sharp scoring system**. In brief, this method scores the presence of erosions in 16 joints of hands and wrists (graded from 0 to 5), and in 6 joints of the feet (graded from 0 to 5), and the presence of joint space narrowing in 15 joints of the hands and wrists (graded from 0 to 4), and in 6 joints of the feet (graded from 0 to 4). The maximal range is 280 units for erosion and 168 units for joint space narrowing, summing up to a maximum of 448 units for the total Sharp score. Studies have shown that an increase of 5 to 6 units in total Sharp score was equivalent to destroying one small joint and correlated with a physician's desire to change therapy. An increase of 25 units of total Sharp score correlates with a 0.22 to 0.25 increase in the HAQ-DI score, which is the minimally important difference that can be detected clinically. A total Sharp score of over 50 to 100 units correlates with a HAQ-DI of 1.0 (0.0 to 3.0 total scale), which correlates with moderate functional impairment.

33. Discuss the time, cost, and success rate of developing a new drug for treating a rheumatic disease.

- It takes 10 years and 1 billion dollars from the time a new drug is tested in mice until it makes it to market.
- Preclinical phase (efficacy, toxicity, and pharmacokinetics in animals): only 2% of new drugs tested make it out of this phase.
- Phase 0 and I trials (drug metabolism [Phase 0] tested in 10 normal volunteers and dose ranging and safety [Phase I] tested in 20 to 100 normal humans): 70% of drugs make it out of this phase.
- Phase II trials (dose [Phase IIA] and efficacy/safety [Phase IIB] tested in 100 to 300 patients with disease): 33% of drugs make it out of this phase.
- Phase III trials (efficacy and safety tested in 1000 to 2000 patients with disease): 80% of drugs make it out of this phase to market.
- Overall, 1 out of 5 (20%) drugs entering Phase I make it to market.

34. What are the monthly costs for these medications when used to treat RA?

The monthly costs for these medications when used to treat RA are outlined in Table 83-1.

PEARL: Leflunomide 10 mg and 20 mg tablets cost the same. Owing to long half-life, a patient on 10 mg a day can be switched to 20 mg every other day, which is much less expensive.

Table 83-1. Monthly Cost (Dollars) of Medications to Treat Rheumatoid Arthritis

MEDICATION	GENERIC	BRAND
Hydroxychloroquine (200 mg twice daily)	25	200
Sulfasalazine (1000 mg twice daily)	20	90
Methotrexate (15 mg/week)	40	250
Leflunomide (10 or 20 mg/day)	25	820

BIBLIOGRAPHY

Bird P, Griffiths H, Tymms K, et al: The SMILE Study – safety of methotrexate in combination with leflunomide in rheumatoid arthritis, J Rheumatol 40:228–235, 2013.

Braun J, Kastner P, Flaxenberg P: Comparison of the clinical efficacy and safety of subcutaneous versus oral administration of methotrexate in patients with active rheumatoid arthritis, Arthritis Rheum 58:73–81, 2008.

Felson DT, Anderson JJ, Boers M, et al: American College of Rheumatology preliminary definition for improvement in rheumatoid arthritis, Arthritis Rheum 38:727–735, 1995.

Hoekstra M, Haagsma C, Neef C, et al: Splitting high-dose oral methotrexate improves the bioavailability: a pharmacokinetic study in patients with rheumatoid arthritis, J Rheumatol 33:481–485, 2006.

Katz SJ, Russell AS: Re-evaluation of antimalarials in treating rheumatic diseases: re-appreciation and insights into new mechanisms of action, Curr Opin Rheumatol 23:278–281, 2011.

Kremer J: Toward a better understanding of methotrexate, Arthritis Rheum 50:1370–1382, 2004.

Landewe RBM, Boers M, Verhoeven AC, et al: COBRA combination therapy in patients with early rheumatoid arthritis: long-term structural benefits of a brief intervention, Arthritis Rheum 46:347–356, 2002.

Marmor MF, Kellner U, Lai TY, et al: Revised recommendations on screening for chloroquine and hydroxychloroquine retinopathy, Ophthalmology 118:415–422, 2011.

Moreland LW, O'Dell JR, Paulus HE, et al: A randomized comparative effectiveness study of oral triple therapy versus etanercept plus methotrexate in early aggressive rheumatoid arthritis: the Treatment of Early Aggressive Rheumatoid Arthritis Trial, Arthritis Rheum 64:2824–2835, 2012.

O'Dell JR, Haire C, Erikson N, et al: Treatment of rheumatoid arthritis with methotrexate, sulfasalazine, and hydroxychloroquine, or a combination of these medications, N Engl J Med 334:1287–1291, 1996.

Plosker G, Croom K: Sulfasalazine: a review of its use in the management of rheumatoid arthritis, Drugs 65:1825–1849, 2005.

Schafer P: Apremilast mechanism of action and application to psoriasis and psoriatic arthritis, Biochem Pharmacol 83:1583–1590, 2012.

Singh JA, Furst DE, Bharat A, et al: 2012 update of the 2008 American College of Rheumatology recommendations for the use of disease-modifying antirheumatic drugs and biologic agents in the treatment of rheumatoid arthritis, Arthritis Care Res 64:625–639, 2012.

Smolen J, Kalden JR, Scott DL, et al: Efficacy and safety of leflunomide compared with placebo and sulphasalazine in active rheumatoid arthritis: a double-blind, randomized, multicentre trial, Lancet 353:259–266, 1999.

Smolen JS, Landewe R, Breedveld FC, et al: EULAR recommendations for the management of rheumatoid arthritis with synthetic and biological disease-modifying antirheumatic drugs, Ann Rheum Dis 69:964–975, 2010.

IMMUNOSUPPRESSIVE AND IMMUNOREGULATORY AGENTS

Amy C. Cannella, MD and James R. O'Dell, MD

CHAPTER 84

The physician without physiology and chemistry practices a sort of popgun pharmacy, hitting now the malady and again the patient, he himself not knowing which.

—Sir William Osler

> **KEY POINTS**
> 1. Cyclophosphamide is best used for remission induction in severe rheumatic diseases.
> 2. Azathioprine is best used for remission maintenance of rheumatic diseases.
> 3. Azathioprine-induced myelosuppression is increased in patients with low thiopurine methyltransferase enzyme activity.
> 4. Mycophenolate mofetil can be used for remission induction and maintenance for lupus nephritis.
> 5. Multiple drug and food interactions need to be screened for in patients treated with cyclosporine.

1. **How is azathioprine (Imuran, Azasan) supplied and used?**
   - Available formulations: 50 mg tablets (Imuran), 75 mg tablets (Azasan), 100 mg powder vial.
   - Side effects: bone marrow depression, nausea, vomiting, skin rash, malignancy (some studies show lymphoma is increased two times), hepatotoxicity (liver enzymes mildly increased in 33% of cases, isolated hyperbilirubinemia, severe toxicity is rare), infections (herpes zoster, cytomegalovirus), pancreatitis, hypersensitivity syndrome (rash, fever, hepatitis, renal failure within first 2 weeks of use).
   - Dosage: 50 to 200 mg/day (1 to 2.5 mg/kg/day). Start 50 mg/day and increase by 25 to 50 mg every 1 to 2 weeks to desired dose.
   - Cost (150 mg/day): generic ($50/month); Azasan ($260/month); Imuran ($500/month).
   - Follow-up: in absence of thiopurine methyltransferase (TPMT) testing, complete blood count (CBC) weekly first 3 to 4 months as dose is escalated. Liver enzymes within 2 weeks of a dosage change. CBC every 1 to 3 months with liver enzymes every 3 months once on stable dose.
   - Precautions: avoid in pregnancy unless warranted by disease severity; avoid live vaccines if dose >2.5 mg/kg/day; drastically reduce dose with allopurinol or febuxostat (reduce azathioprine dose by 75% or *do not use at all*). Sulfasalazine and bactrim/septra increase risk of leukopenia. Azathioprine may cause *warfarin resistance*. Increases risk of rash on ampicillin.

   PEARL: patients who cannot tolerate azathioprine as a result of nausea, vomiting, or rash may be able to tolerate 6-mercaptopurine (6-MP; Purinethol), which is the active product of azathioprine. However, 6-MP cannot be used in patients who develop pancreatitis or liver toxicity on azathioprine. The effective dose of 6-MP is half the dose of azathioprine (i.e., 50 mg 6-MP = 100 mg azathioprine).

2. **Describe the mechanism of action and metabolism of azathioprine.**
   Azathioprine is a prodrug converted to 6-MP. 6-MP is then converted to thiopurine nucleotides (6-TGN), which decrease de novo synthesis of purine nucleotides and are incorporated into nucleic acids of cells. This results in both cytotoxicity and decreased cellular proliferation. The patient is getting a maximum effect from azathioprine if the erythrocyte mean corpuscular volume (MCV) increases by 5 fL. Alternatively, 6-TGN metabolite levels can be measured within 4 hours of taking azathioprine with 230 to 400 pmol/8×10^8 red blood cells being therapeutic (cost: $270).

   The metabolism of 6-MP by two enzymes, xanthine oxidase and TPMT, results in formation of inactive metabolites. Inhibition of xanthine oxidase (by allopurinol, febuxostat) or of TPMT (by sulfasalazine) causes an accumulation of 6-MP resulting in toxicity. In addition, TPMT enzyme activity is affected by genetic polymorphisms with 90% having high activity, 10% intermediate activity, and 0.3% low activity. Blacks have 17% less TPMT activity than whites. Patients with low TPMT activity are at risk for the sudden onset of severe myelosuppression occurring between 4 and 10 weeks after starting azathioprine. Patients with intermediate activity have more frequent adverse side effects, particularly gastrointestinal. TPMT genotype and phenotype can be measured. Notably, the TPMT enzyme activity (i.e., phenotype) cannot always be predicted by the genotype. Therefore, the most cost-effective approach is to measure TPMT phenotype activity (cost $220 compared with $395 for gene testing). Whether or not this is necessary before starting azathioprine is controversial because over half of all cases of leukopenia are seen in patients with normal TPMT activity (Figure 84-1).

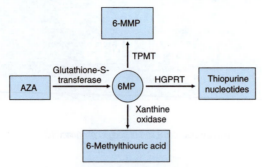

Figure 84-1. Azathioprine metabolism. *AZA,* Azathioprine; *HGPRT,* hypoxanthine-guanine-phosphoribosyl-transferase; *6-MP,* 6-mercaptopurine; *6-MMP,* 6-methylmercaptopurine; *TPMT,* thiopurine methyltransferase. *From Van Laar, JM: Immunosuppressive drugs in Kelley's textbook of rheumatology, ed 9, Philadelphia, 2013, Elsevier.*

3. What rheumatic diseases are commonly treated with azathioprine?
- Rheumatoid arthritis (less effective than methotrexate and slower onset).
- Systemic lupus erythematosus.
- Polymyositis/dermatomyositis.
- Behçet's disease.
- Antineutrophil cytoplasmic antibody (ANCA)-associated vasculitis (remission maintenance).
- Many other rheumatic diseases (in an attempt to decrease corticosteroid dosage).

PEARL: azathioprine is more effective as a maintenance therapy than for induction of remission.

4. How is mycophenolate mofetil (Cellcept) supplied and used?
- Available formulations: 250 mg, 500 mg capsules; oral suspension (200 mg/mL) and intravenous (IV) form (500 mg powder vial) available.
- Side effects: gastrointestinal (especially diarrhea, 25%), leukopenia, anemia, hepatotoxicity, infections; lymphoproliferative malignancies (Epstein–Barr virus [EBV]-associated).
- Dosage: 500 to 1500 mg twice a day on an empty stomach (1 hour before food). Decrease maximum dose to 1000 mg twice a day if severe renal insufficiency (creatinine clearance <30 mL/min).
- Cost (1000 mg twice a day): generic ($120/month); brand Cellcept ($1600/month).
- Follow-up: CBC and liver enzymes weekly with dose change and then CBC every 1 to 3 months.
- Precautions: *avoid in pregnancy and lactation*; avoid live vaccines. Cholestyramine and administration with food or antacids decrease bioavailability. Tacrolimus may potentiate effects of mycophenolate mofetil.

PEARL: good alternative to azathioprine in patients with gout who need allopurinol or febuxostat and in patients who need warfarin.

5. What is Myfortic?
Myfortic (mycophenolic acid, MPA) is enteric-coated, delayed-release mycophenolate sodium. It comes in 180-mg and 360-mg delayed-release tablets. Dose conversion is 360 mg of Myfortic is equivalent to 500 mg of mycophenolate mofetil. Some patients will tolerate Myfortic when they have experienced severe gastrointestinal side effects with mycophenolate mofetil. Cost of 720 mg twice a day is $1050/month.

6. What is the mechanism of action of mycophenolate mofetil?
Mycophenolate mofetil is an inactive prodrug that is hydrolyzed to the active MPA. MPA is a reversible inhibitor of inosine-5′-monophosphate dehydrogenase (IMPDH), which is an enzyme necessary for the de novo synthesis of the purine, guanosine. Lymphocytes (T and B cells) depend on IMPDH to generate sufficient guanosine levels to initiate a proliferative response to antigen. Cytokine production is not affected. MPA also inhibits carbohydrate (fucose, mannose) transfer to glycoproteins, resulting in less production of adhesion molecules (VLA-4, ICAM-1). In summary, MPA inhibits lymphocyte proliferation and lymphocyte migration. It also has antifibrotic activity. The enterohepatic recycling of glucuronide-conjugated MPA contributes to gastrointestinal toxicity because gastrointestinal mucosal cells are 50% dependent upon the de novo synthesis pathway of purines, which is inhibited by MPA.

7. What rheumatic diseases have been successfully treated with mycophenolate mofetil?
Use is similar to azathioprine. Good success has been seen in *lupus nephritis* (diffuse proliferative glomerulonephritis [DPGN], membranous) especially in African American and Hispanic patients. It has been successfully used for treating cutaneous lupus (discoid and subacute cutaneous lupus), systemic sclerosis, myositis, uveitis, and vasculitis (granulomatosis with polyangiitis [GPA] maintenance therapy). Because of its lymphocyte and antifibrotic effects, it has been effective in treating *interstitial lung disease associated with many rheumatic diseases*. Patients with rheumatoid arthritis and psoriatic arthritis usually do not respond.

8. **Discuss the use of cyclophosphamide (Cytoxan) in rheumatic diseases.**
   - Available formulations: 25 mg and 50 mg tablets; 500 mg, 1000 mg and 2000 mg vials.
   - Dosage: daily oral, 50 to 200 mg (0.7 to 2 mg/kg/day); monthly IV, 0.5 to 1 g/m² body surface area or 15 mg/kg; 500 mg IV every 2 weeks for 6 doses (Euro-Lupus).

   PEARL: dose of cyclophosphamide is based on actual body weight even if the patient is obese.
   - Cost (150 mg/day): oral generic tablets $270/month.
   - Follow-up: daily dosing, CBC every week until stable dose, then monthly; urinalysis monthly; urinalysis with cytology every 6 to 12 months after cessation of therapy. For monthly dosing, CBC with urinalysis before each dose, CBC 10 to 14 days after each dose to see nadir.
   - Precautions: avoid in pregnancy, avoid live vaccines, use lower doses in elderly as a result of less bone marrow reserve (cellularity = 100% − age). Cimetidine and allopurinol increase frequency of leukopenia. IV cyclophosphamide interferes with stable coumadin dosing.

9. **Describe the mechanism of action and metabolism of cyclophosphamide.**
   Cyclophosphamide is an inactive prodrug that is activated by hepatic cytochrome P450 enzymes. Genetic polymorphisms of cytochrome P450 enzymes can affect response to cyclophosphamide. The major active metabolite is phosphoramide mustard, which alkylates DNA and results in cross-linking of DNA, breaks in DNA, decreased DNA synthesis, and apoptosis. Cyclophosphamide synthesis has a marked effect on rapidly dividing cells and throughout the cell cycle, resulting in alterations in humoral and cellular immunity (B > T cells). Liver disease does not increase the toxicity of cyclophosphamide. Initial dose is decreased by 30% if creatinine clearance is less than 30 mL/min. Cyclophosphamide is dialyzable and should be administered more than 12 hours before a dialysis or administered any time after dialysis.
   Acrolein is a major metabolic product of cyclophosphamide metabolism. It is responsible for causing hemorrhagic cystitis and bladder cancer.

10. **In which rheumatic diseases is cyclophosphamide therapy indicated? How effective is it?**
    - GPA (also known as Wegener's granulomatosis).
    - Systemic lupus erythematosus (particularly lupus nephritis, severe manifestations).
    - Interstitial lung disease in patients with systemic sclerosis.
    - Other systemic vasculitis syndromes.
    - Other rheumatic diseases refractory to conventional therapy.

    Cyclophosphamide is considered to be one of the most potent immunosuppressive drugs available. Its use has succeeded in almost all rheumatic diseases, particularly when other less potent and usually less toxic forms of therapy have failed. When preservation of renal function in patients with lupus nephritis is the desired result, cyclophosphamide has superior efficacy. However, because of its potentially severe toxicity, overall improvements in mortality have been more difficult to demonstrate in some diseases (systemic sclerosis) in which it is used.

11. **What are the major toxicities of cyclophosphamide? What can be done to prevent them?**
    - *Bone marrow suppression*. The white blood cell (WBC) nadir after a dose is 8 to 14 days later. Start at 50 mg/day and increase weekly while following CBC 1 to 2 times a week initially.
    - *Infection* (all types, especially herpes viruses). Screen for hepatitis B and hepatitis C, HIV, and tuberculosis before therapy. Keep WBC nadir above 3000/mm³ and preferably above 4000/mm³. Decrease prednisone dose to less than 20 to 25 mg/day as soon as possible. Prophylaxis for *Pneumocystis jiroveci* pneumonia with bactrim/septra, dapsone, or inhaled pentamidine. Pneumococcal and flu vaccines should be administered.
    - *Hemorrhagic cystitis and bladder cancer*. Hemorrhagic cystitis is more common in patients with BK virus. Nonglomerular hematuria occurs in up to 50% of patients with 5% developing bladder cancer (31-fold increased risk). Decrease risk by using monthly IV pulse therapy instead of daily oral therapy. Also can use mesna, a sulfhydryl compound that binds and inactivates acrolein in the urine. Stop smoking, which increases risk of bladder toxicity. With daily oral therapy, give cyclophosphamide in the morning, force fluids (>2 L/day), and empty bladder frequently.
    - *Malignancy*. Risk increased 2-fold to 4-fold. Increased risk if given daily oral versus monthly IV; the higher the cumulative dose, the greater the risk (50% in patients receiving ≥80 g total dose develop a malignancy).
    - *Infertility*. The risk for ovarian failure ranges from 30% to 70% and varies depending on the age of the patient and the cumulative dose. The risk may be two times less with monthly IV than daily oral dosing. Women less than 20 years old have a 13% risk, ages 20 to 30 years a 50% risk, and over age 30 years a 100% risk of premature ovarian failure. Ovarian failure is unlikely if women receive less than 6 monthly doses and common if they receive over 15 monthly pulses (50% with 8 g/m² and 90% with 12 g/m² total dose). It is rare in patients who received the Euro-Lupus protocol (500 mg IV every 2 weeks × 6 doses). Azoospermia is found in 50% to 90% of men. Various strategies have been tried to limit this toxicity. Banking ova and sperm can be done but is expensive. In women, using gonadotropin-releasing hormone analog (Lupron depot, 3.75 mg intramuscular [IM] monthly) plus estradiol 0.05 to 0.1 mg/day In men, testosterone, 100 mg IM every 15 days, may be protective. Antimüllerian hormone levels are a good marker of ovarian reserve and can be measured at any time during the cycle.

- *Pulmonary*. Less than 1% get pneumonitis or pulmonary fibrosis.
- *Others*. Reversible alopecia, syndrome of inappropriate antidiuretic hormone secretion, nausea (use antiemetics), teratogenicity, reversible posterior leukoencephalopathy syndrome after IV administration.

12. **What other alkylating agent has been used to treat rheumatic diseases?**

    Chlorambucil has been used to treat several rheumatic diseases. The usual dose is 0.1 mg/kg/day (2 to 8 mg/day). It has primarily been used to treat the eye and neuropsychiatric complications of Behçet's disease. It has also been used in cryoglobulinemia, refractory dermatomyositis, lupus nephritis, and amyloidosis secondary to chronic inflammatory arthritis (rheumatoid arthritis, juvenile idiopathic arthritis, ankylosing spondylitis). Major toxicities are myelosuppression, infection (herpes zoster), and induction of myeloid leukemia and other malignancies.

13. **How is cyclosporine microemulsion (Gengraf, Neoral) used in the treatment of rheumatic diseases?**
    - Available formulations: 25 mg and 100 mg capsule; oral solution 100 mg/mL; IV solution 50 mg/mL.
    - Dosage: 2.5 to 4 mg/kg *ideal body weight* for most rheumatic diseases. Start low in divided doses and increase 0.5 mg/kg/day every 4 to 8 weeks.
    - Cost (200 mg/day): $350 to $400/month.
    - Follow up: monitor creatinine and blood pressure every 2 weeks for 3 months and then monthly; periodic CBC, liver function tests, magnesium, potassium, uric acid, and lipid levels.
    - Precautions. Concurrent use of nonsteroidal antiinflammatory drugs, aminoglycosides, and angiotensin-converting enzyme (ACE) inhibitors may contribute to renal insufficiency. Erythromycin/clarithromycin, azole antifungals, diltiazem/verapamil, and other CYP3A4 inhibitors increase cyclosporine levels causing toxicity. Cyclosporine is stopped if creatinine increases 30% over baseline *even if still in the normal range*. Cyclosporine can increase toxicity of statins (myopathy), colchicine (neuromyopathy), digoxin, and potassium-sparing diuretics (hyperkalemia). Do not use colchicine in patients on cyclosporine.

    Cyclosporine is a potent immunomodulating agent that works by inhibition of T cell activation. It does so by binding to a cytoplasmic protein (immunophilin) called cyclophilin, which is turn binds to calcineurin. This blocks the interaction of calcineurin with calmodulin, which is necessary to dephosphorylate nuclear factor of activated T cells (NF-AT), which is a transcription factor needed to activate interleukin-2 (IL-2) and other T cell activation genes.

14. **What affects cyclosporine absorption?**

    Cyclosporine is poorly and variably absorbed from the gut with a bioavailability of 30% but with substantial variability among individuals. A high-fat meal can increase absorption. *Grapefruit juice* and marmalade from Seville oranges contain dihydroxybergamottin, which inhibits the cytochrome P450 enzyme in the small intestine, resulting in increased absorption and decreased metabolism of cyclosporine, as well as statins and ACE inhibitors. St. John's wort decreases cyclosporine levels by inducing cytochrome P450 3A4, duodenal P-glycoprotein, and MDR-1 gene.

15. **What are tacrolimus (Prograf) and sirolimus (Rapamune)?**

    Tacrolimus is a macrolide produced by a fungus (actinomycete). It has immunosuppressive effects similar to cyclosporine but at a dose 10 to 100 times lower (0.1 to 0.25 mg/kg/day; usual dose 2 to 5 mg twice a day). Tacrolimus, similar to cyclosporine, is a potent inhibitor of T cell activation and inhibits transcription of early T cell activation genes, such as IL-2. It does so by interfering with the binding of nuclear regulatory factor, NF-AT, to its target region in the enhancer region of these inducible genes (see Question 13). Notably, tacrolimus causes less increase in uric acid than cyclosporine and it may be useful to switch from cyclosporine to tacrolimus in patients who have undergone a transplant who also have tophaceous gout. Tacrolimus has shown efficacy, particularly in treatment of refractory myositis with or without lung involvement.

    Sirolimus (rapamycin) and its derivative, everolimus (Afinitor), inhibit T cell proliferation by binding to its cytoplasmic immunophilin (FK binding protein, TOR, or FRAP) which inhibits IL-2 receptor transduction events after the receptor has bound IL-2. This blocks progression of the T cell cycle from G1 phase to S phase. Sirolimus has not been used much in the treatment of rheumatic diseases.

16. **What rheumatic syndromes have been treated with cyclosporine?**
    - Rheumatoid arthritis (especially when combined with methotrexate).
    - Polymyositis/dermatomyositis (especially with interstitial lung disease): tacrolimus may be a better drug.
    - Psoriatic arthritis and psoriasis.
    - Systemic lupus erythematosus (especially membranous glomerulonephritis as a result of its effect on podocytes).
    - Uveitis.
    - Others: Behçet's disease, macrophage-activation syndrome (Still's disease), pyoderma gangrenosum.

17. **What are the major toxicities of cyclosporine?**
    - Decreased renal function (usually reversible with discontinuation of drug).
    - Hypertension (treat with nifedipine or labetalol).
    - Anemia (note that it does not decrease WBC count).
    - Malignancies (lymphomas and skin cancers): lymphoma (EBV-related) may regress with stopping drug.
    - Hyperuricemia and gout (switch to tacrolimus which causes less hyperuricemia).

- Bone pain (treat with calcium channel blockers and lower cyclosporine dose).
- Others: infections, headaches, tremors, hyperpigmentation, hirsuitism, anorexia, hepatotoxicity (rare).

18. **Why do physicians use "pulse" corticosteroids?**
Many clinicians use IV pulse corticosteroids as the initial treatment of severe life-threatening or organ-threatening presentations of rheumatic diseases. This is typically methylprednisolone given in doses of 1 g/day for 3 to 5 consecutive days. Many physicians split the dose (500 mg IV every 12 hours or 250 mg IV every 6 hours) for inpatients to lessen potential side effects. This regimen of corticosteroid administration is felt to have more immunomodulating effects than high-dose daily oral corticosteroids through rapid (within minutes) nongenomic mechanisms including cell membrane physiochemical effects (controversial). As the sole therapeutic intervention, pulse steroids probably have no role in long-term therapy. However, in combination therapy with a cytotoxic agent, pulse steroids may provide time for a second agent to achieve its therapeutic effect. The effect of pulse steroids usually lasts 4 to 6 weeks with wide variation between patients. It has been used most often in the treatment of severe vasculitis, lupus nephritis, and neuropsychiatric lupus. Side effects include psychosis, arrhythmias (some from hypokalemia), glucose intolerance, hypertension, glaucoma, and, rarely, sudden death. The risk of these adverse effects may be lessened by using a slow rate of infusion and ensuring that the serum potassium level is normal.

19. **How is IV gammaglobulin used as an immunomodulator in rheumatic diseases?**
    - Available formulations: multiple suppliers; solution concentrations vary from 3% to 12% immunoglobulin (Ig); cost is $75/g.
    - Dosage: 1 to 2 g/kg administered over 1 to 5 days.
    - Side effects: headache (2% to 20%), flushing, chest tightness, back pain/myalgias, fever, chills, nausea, diaphoresis, hypotension, aseptic meningitis, clot, leukopenia, serum sickness.
    - Follow-up: creatinine 24 hours after infusion if baseline renal insufficiency.
    - Precautions: anaphylactic reaction in patients with hereditary IgA deficiency (1/700 patients); transmission of infectious agents (rare).

    Some side effects of gammaglobulin (IG) are avoided by premedicating patients with acetaminophen and diphenhydramine hydrochloride (Benadryl) or hydrocortisone sodium succinate (Solu-Cortef) and by slowing the rate of infusion. Infusion is started at 30 mL/h and increased to a maximum of 250 mL/h (sometimes higher). Patients who get migraine headaches may benefit from premed with sumatriptan. Avoid sucrose containing IVIG (Carimune) which can cause acute renal failure. Avoid sugar containing IVIG in diabetics. Use isoosmolar IVIG (240 to 300 mOsm/kg) to lessen chance of clot. Use IVIG preparations (Privigen, Gammagard S/D) containing low IgA levels in patients who are IgA-deficient. In a patient who is not IgA-deficient, Gamunex-C (10%) may be best tolerated.

20. **In which rheumatic diseases is IVIG indicated? How might it work in these diseases?**
    - Autoimmune thrombocytopenia: Fc portion of IVIG binds the Fc receptor on reticuloendothelial cells blocking the removal of antibody-coated cells.
    - Kawasaki's disease: IVIG reduces expression of adhesion molecules on endothelial cells, binds cytokines that cause inflammation, reduces number of activated T cells, and binds staphylococcal toxin superantigens.
    - Dermatomyositis and polymyositis: the Fc portion of IVIG can bind to C3b and C4b, decreasing complement activation.
    - Chronic inflammatory demyelinating polyneuropathy .
    - Antiphospholipid antibody syndrome (off-label).
    - Autoimmune hemolytic anemia and neutropenia (off-label).

    Other proposed mechanisms that may explain IVIG effectiveness in autoimmune diseases include:
    - Antiidiotypic antibodies bind surface Ig on B cells preventing binding to target autoantigen.
    - Saturation of neonatal Fc receptor resulting in accelerated degradation of pathogenic IgG.
    - Sialylated fraction of IVIG (5% of total IVIG) binds to the protein, DC-SIGN, on dendritic cells resulting in enhanced expression of inhibitory FcγRs (FcγRIIb) on effector macrophages which can attenuate inflammation.
    - Others: enhancement of Treg function, inhibition of dendritic cells.

21. **Why is plasma exchange used in the treatment of rheumatic diseases?**
Theoretically, plasma exchange should remove immune complexes and autoantibodies that contribute to the pathogenesis of some rheumatic diseases. It is most effective when used acutely to gain a rapid response in life-threatening situations. Plasma exchange is usually used in combination with corticosteroids and/or cytotoxic therapy to decrease the risk of a rebound flare of the underlying immunologic disease once the pheresis is stopped. Most plasma exchange protocols remove 2 to 4 L (40 mL/kg = 1 plasma volume) of plasma over a 2-hour period daily. Each exchange of 1 to 1.5 plasma volumes removes 60% to 70% of plasma constituents. Replacement fluid is generally albumin–saline or another protein-containing solution. To decrease the risk of infection and bleeding, 1 to 2 units of fresh frozen plasma (FFP) are included as part of the replacement solution. If not, monitoring of coagulation studies and Ig levels are important. If the patient develops elevated international normalized ratio/partial thromboplastin time then FFP is given. If the patient develops hypogammaglobulinemia, IVIG (0.4 g/kg × 1 dose) is given. Cost of plasma exchange: >$5000 per session.

22. In which rheumatic diseases has plasma exchange been beneficial?
- Thrombotic thrombocytopenic purpura (TTP) associated with rheumatic diseases.
- Catastrophic antiphospholipid syndrome.
- Systemic lupus erythematosus: diffuse alveolar hemorrhage; neuropsychiatric lupus with coma; TTP.
- Neuromyelitis optica spectrum disorder.
- ANCA-associated vasculitis with diffuse alveolar hemorrhage and/or rapidly progressive crescentic glomerulonephritis (creatinine >3.5).
- Hepatitis B-associated polyarteritis nodosa (combined with antiviral agent).
- Hepatitis C-associated cryoglobulinemia (combined with antiviral agent).
- Goodpasture syndrome with progressive renal failure and/or diffuse alveolar hemorrhage.
- PANDAS (pediatric autoimmune neuropsychiatric disorders associated with streptococcal infections).

23. Discuss the use of high-dose immunoablative therapy with autologous hematopoietic stem cell transplantation for the treatment of severe autoimmune disease.

Autologous (using a patient's own stem cells) hematopoietic stem cell transplantation is a method of increasing the intensity of chemotherapy that can be given to a patient with a severe autoimmune disease who is failing standard therapy. By collecting stem cells ($CD34^+$) before chemotherapy, higher doses of cyclophosphamide (200 mg/kg) can be given to ablate the immune system because the patient can be rescued from bone marrow failure by reinfusion of the patient's own stem cells. Some patients may also receive lymphoablative antibodies or total body irradiation to eradicate residual autoreactive cells. This stem cell transplantation strategy allows the patient to reconstitute their immune system without redeveloping their autoimmune disease or developing graft versus host disease. This procedure is most often used for treatment-resistant systemic lupus erythematosus, systemic sclerosis, and multiple sclerosis with varying success rates and a mortality rate as high as 8% at a cost of up to $100,000. Other immunoablative and/or transplantation strategies are also being investigated.

Bibliography

Ballow M: The IgG molecule as a biological immune response modifier: mechanisms of action of intravenous immune serum globulin in autoimmune and inflammatory disorders, J Allergy Clin Immunol 127:315–323, 2011.

Bejarano V, Conaghan PG, Proudman SM, et al: Long-term efficacy and toxicity of cyclosporine A in combination with methotrexate in poor prognosis rheumatoid arthritis, Ann Rheum Dis 68:761–763, 2009.

Blumenfeld Z, Shapiro D, Shteinberg M, et al: Preservation of fertility and ovarian function and minimizing gonadotoxicity in young women with systemic lupus erythematosus treated by chemotherapy, Lupus 9:401–405, 2000.

de Jonge ME, Huitema AD, Rodenhuis S, et al: Clinical pharmacokinetics of cyclophosphamide, Clin Pharmacokinet 44:1135–1164, 2005.

Farge D, Labopin M, Tyndall A, et al: Autologous hematopoietic stem cell transplantation for autoimmune diseases: an observational study on 12 years' experience from the European Group for Blood and Marrow Transplantation Working Party on Autoimmune Diseases, Haematologica 95:284–292, 2010.

Fields CL, Robinson JW, Roy TM, et al: Hypersensitivity reaction to azathioprine, South Med J 91:471–474, 1998.

Gaujoux-Viala C, Smolen JS, Landewe R, et al: Current evidence for the management of rheumatoid arthritis with synthetic disease-modifying antirheumatic drugs: a systemic literature review informing the EULAR recommendations for the management of rheumatoid arthritis, Ann Rheum Dis 69:1004–1009, 2010.

Gerbino AJ, Goss CH, Molitor JA: Effect of mycophenolate mofetil on pulmonary function in scleroderma-associated interstitial lung disease, Chest 133:455–460, 2008.

Haubitz M, Bohnenstengel F, Brunkhorst R, et al: Cyclophosphamide pharmakokinetics and dose adjustments in patients with renal insufficiency, Kidney Int 61:1495–1501, 2002.

Monach PA, Arnold LM, Merkel PA: Incidence and prevention of bladder toxicity from cyclophosphamide in the treatment of rheumatic diseases. A data driven review, Arthritis Rheum 62:9–21, 2010.

Pilmore HL, Faire B, Dittmer I: Tacrolimus for treatment of gout in renal transplantation, Transplantation 72:1703–1705, 2001.

Schedel J, Godde A, Schutz E, et al: Impact of thiopurine methyltransferase activity and 6-thioguanine nucleotide concentrations in patients with chronic inflammatory diseases, Ann NY Acad Sci 1069:477–491, 2006.

Sievers TM, Rossi SJ, Ghobrial RM, et al: Mycophenolate mofetil, Pharmacotherapy 17:1178–1197, 1997.

Somers EC, Marder W, Christman GM, et al: Use of a gonadotropin-releasing hormone analog for protection against premature ovarian failure during cyclophosphamide therapy in women with severe lupus, Arthritis Rheum 52:2761–2767, 2005.

Takada K, Arefayene M, Desta Z, et al: Cytochrome P450 pharmacogenetics as a predictor of toxicity and clinical response to pulse cyclophosphamide in lupus nephritis, Arthritis Rheum 50:2202–2210, 2004.

Touma Z, Gladman DD, Urowitz MB, et al: Mycophenylate mofetil for induction treatment of lupus nephritis: a systemic review and metaanalysis, J Rheumatol 38:69–78, 2011.

Vazquez SR, Rondina MT, Pendleton RC: Azathioprine-induced warfarin resistance, Ann Pharmacother 42:1118–1123, 2008.

Wilkes MR, Sereika SM, Fertig N, et al: Treatment of antisynthetase-associated interstitial lung disease with tacrolimus, Arthritis Rheum 52:2439–2446, 2005.

Winter JL: Plasma exchange: concepts, mechanisms, and an overview of the American Society of Apheresis guidelines, Hematology 7-12:2012, 2012.

Further Reading

www.rheumatology.org

BIOLOGIC AGENTS

Sterling G. West, MD

A cynic is someone who knows the cost of everything but the value of nothing.

—Anonymous

> **KEY POINTS**
>
> 1. Biologic agents differ in their effectiveness for controlling specific rheumatic diseases depending on which cytokine is driving the patient's inflammation.
> 2. Tumor necrosis factor inhibitors are more effective when combined with methotrexate.
> 3. Interleukin-1 inhibitors are most effective for Still's disease and the cryopyrinopathies.
> 4. Risk of hepatitis B reactivation and mycobacterial infections are increased in patients on biologics.
> 5. Live vaccines should not be given to patients on biologic agents.

1. **What biologic agents are currently available for use in the treatment of inflammatory rheumatic diseases?**
   With our increasing understanding of the pathogenesis of autoimmune rheumatic diseases, several biologic agents have been developed for treatment, especially for rheumatoid arthritis (RA), ankylosing spondylitis (AS), psoriatic arthritis (PsA), and systemic lupus erythematosus (SLE). These can be classified as follows:
   - Cytokine-targeted therapies.
     - Tumor necrosis factor (TNF)-α inhibitors: etanercept, infliximab, adalimumab, golimumab, certolizumab.
     - Interleukin (IL)-1 inhibitors: anakinra, rilonacept, canakinumab.
     - Anti-IL-6 receptor: tocilizumab.
     - Anti-IL-12/IL-23: ustekinumab.
     - Oral tyrosine kinase inhibitors: tofacitinib (Janus activated kinase [JAK] inhibitor).
   - B cell targeted therapies.
     - Rituximab (anti-CD20).
     - B cell growth factor inhibitors: belimumab (anti-Blys).
   - T cell targeted therapies.
     - Costimulatory molecule inhibitors: abatacept (anti-CD80/86).
   - Complement targeted therapies.
     - Eculizumab (anti-C5a/C5b-9).

2. **What nomenclature is used in naming the biologic agents?**
   - **-cept**: receptor drug which prevents a ligand from binding to its receptor (e.g., etanercept, abatacept, rilonacept).
   - **-ximab**: chimeric monoclonal antibody (e.g., infliximab, rituximab).
   - **-zumab**: humanized monoclonal antibody (e.g., certilizumab, tocilizumab, eculizumab).
   - **-mumab**: fully human monoclonal antibody (e.g., adalimumab, golimumab, belimumab, ustekinumab).
   - **-ra**: receptor antagonist (e.g., anakinra).
   - **-tinib**: inhibitor (e.g., tofacitinib).

3. **List the precautions that should be done before starting any biologic agents.**
   - Establish and record disease activity.
   - Screen for comorbidities: infection risk, HIV risk factors, hepatitis B/C risk factors, history of malignancy (lymphoma, melanoma, others), history of demyelinating disease, history of tuberculosis (TB), history of fungal exposure, hyperlipidemia, liver disease, pregnancy, medications.
   - Vaccination status: patients should receive inactivated influenza vaccine (seasonal) and age-appropriate pneumococcal, meningococcal, and *Haemophilus influenzae* B (Hib). Give herpes zoster vaccine (live) at least 2 to 4 weeks before biologic use.
   - Tests before use: complete blood count (CBC), creatinine, hepatic enzymes, lipids, C-reactive protein, hepatitis B and hepatitis C serologies, purified protein derivative (PPD) (or interferon gamma release assay), chest X-ray, HIV (if risk factors).

4. **What is the rationale behind the use of the biologics to inhibit cytokines in inflammatory diseases such as RA?**
TNF-α, IL-1, and IL-6 are key cytokines in the pathophysiology of inflammatory synovitis and destruction of bone and cartilage.
- **TNF-α** is initially expressed as a transmembrane molecule on the surface of macrophages. The extracellular portion is cleaved by TNF-α converting enzyme (TACE) to form a soluble molecule that circulates as a homotrimer. TNF-α (and TNF-β from T cells) binds to two receptors, TNF-RI (p55) and TNF-RII (p75), both of which are found on the surface of most cells. Binding of TNF-α to its receptor triggers a variety of intracellular signaling events, inducing production of prostaglandins and proinflammatory cytokines, endothelial cell expression of adhesion molecules that help recruit neutrophils and monocytes into the synovial fluid, and synoviocyte/chondrocyte production of matrix metalloproteinases (collagenase), which can destroy cartilage and bone.
- **IL-1** is a proinflammatory cytokine which exists in two forms, IL-1α and IL-1β, which are transcribed from closely related but distinct genes. IL-1α is in the cytosol and is membrane bound. IL-1β is secreted into the extracellular space after cleavage of pro-IL-1β by IL-1β converting enzyme (ICE, caspase 1). Thus, IL-1β is the predominant form that binds to the IL-1 receptor triggering intracellular signaling leading to a proinflammatory response, (which is synergistic to that induced by TNF-α), B cell activation and rheumatoid factor production, cartilage degradation by induction of synoviocyte/chondrocyte production of enzymes resulting in proteoglycan loss, and stimulation of osteoclasts causing bone resorption. Notably, cells producing IL-1 also produce IL-1Ra. However, in patients with inflammatory synovitis such as RA, the amount of IL-1Ra in the synovium is produced in insufficient amounts to neutralize the amount of locally produced IL-1.
- **IL-6** is critical for inflammatory and immune responses. It binds to its receptor, IL-6R, which is constitutively associated with glycoprotein 130 (gp130) on the cell membranes of hepatocytes and some leukocytes. Notably, binding of IL-6 to this *cell membrane bound IL-6R* on hepatocytes and leukocytes has an antiapoptotic/antiinflammatory effect. Additionally, there is a *soluble form of IL-6R* which can bind IL-6 and this complex can interact with gp130 on a wide variety of cells that are usually not affected by IL-6. This soluble IL-6/IL-6R complex is proinflammatory. IL-6 stimulates the development of T helper 17 (Th17) cells which produces IL-17, has a role in the activation of B cells and osteoclasts, helps recruit neutrophils, and acts synergistically with other cytokines to cause pannus formation.

5. **What biologic agents are currently available to inhibit TNF-α?**
Etanercept (Enbrel): a bioengineered molecule derived from Chinese hamster ovary cells which consist of a fusion protein created by linking the extracellular binding regions from two TNF-RII (p75) receptors to the Fc portion of human immunoglobulin G1 (IgG1). This molecule is a dimeric soluble TNF receptor that binds soluble TNF-α and lymphotoxin (TNF-β). Its half-life is 3 to 5 days.
Infliximab (Remicade): chimeric mouse–human monoclonal antibody composed of the constant regions of human IgG1 heavy and partial kappa light chain domains coupled to the variable region of a mouse light chain with high affinity for human TNF-α. Infliximab binds both soluble and cell bound TNF-α and thus has the ability to induce apoptosis of cells with TNF-α bound to its surface. It does not bind lymphotoxin. Its half-life is 8 to 9 days. Concomitant use of methotrexate (MTX) increases the amount of infliximab exposure by 30%.
Adalimumab (Humira): fully human IgG1κ monoclonal antibody that binds soluble and transmembrane forms of TNF-α. Its half-life is 10 to 13 days. Simultaneous use of MTX increases a patient's exposure to adalimumab by 30%.
Golimumab (Simponi): fully human IgG1κ monoclonal antibody that binds soluble and transmembrane forms of TNF-α. Median half-life is 14 days. Concomitant MTX use increases trough concentrations of golimumab by 30%.
Certilizumab pegol (Cimzia): Fab fragment of a recombinant, humanized anti-TNF monoclonal antibody that has been fused to a polyethylene glycol (PEG) moiety. Cannot bind to Fc receptors, fix complement, or cross placenta due to not having a functional Fc fragment. Its half-life is 14 days. The pegylation delays clearance and may help localize the molecule to acidic, inflammatory sites.

6. **How are TNF inhibitors supplied and used? What are their FDA indications in rheumatic diseases?**
- **Etanercept (Enbrel)**
  - Available formulations: single use 25-mg and 50-mg prefilled syringes; single use 50-mg SureClick autoinjector; single use vial with 25 mg of lyophilized powder for reconstitution.
  - Dosage: RA, PsA, AS: 25 mg subcutaneously (SC) twice a week or 50 mg SC once a week.
    - Skin psoriasis: 50 mg SC twice a week for first 12 weeks then once a week.
  - In RA, typically used in conjunction with MTX or another synthetic disease-modifying antirheumatic drug (DMARD). Not effective for uveitis in spondyloarthropathies. Should not be used if an patient with AS has uveitis or inflammatory bowel disease.
- **Infliximab (Remicade)**
  - Available formulations: single use vials of 100 mg.

- Dosage. RA: loading dose 3 mg/kg intravenous (IV) at weeks 0, 2, and 6; then every 8 weeks. Dose can be increased as high as 5 to 10 mg/kg every 4 to 8 weeks.
  - PsA, AS: loading dose 5 mg/kg IV at weeks 0, 2, and 6; then every 6 weeks. Dose can be increased as high as 5 to 10 mg/kg every 4 weeks.
  - Infusion takes 2 hours.
- In RA, typically used in conjunction with MTX or other synthetic DMARD to decrease development of human antichimeric antibodies (HACAs), which can neutralize/increase clearance of infliximab and/or cause infusion reactions. Concomitant DMARD (MTX) use not needed for spondyloarthropathies because HACAs are much less likely to occur.

PEARL: if a patient is not responding initially, increasing the frequency of infliximab infusions is more efficacious than increasing the dose. Rarely increase dose higher than 5 mg/kg every 4 weeks because of infection and malignancy concerns.

- **Adalimumab (Humira)**
  - Available formulations: single use 40-mg prefilled syringe; single use 40-mg autoinjector pen.
  - Dosage: RA, PsA, AS: 40 mg SC every other week.
  - Although approved for use as monotherapy, adalimumab works better in association with MTX in RA. Some patients who do not respond to every other week dosing may respond to weekly dosing, although this is unusual and expensive.
- **Golimumab (Simponi)**
  - Available formulation: single use 50-mg prefilled syringe; single use 50-mg SmartJect autoinjector; single use vials (50 mg/4 mL) for IV use.
  - Dosage: RA, PsA, AS: 50 mg SC once a month. **Simponi Aria**: an IV formulation (2 mg/kg at 0, 4, then every 8 weeks) is approved for RA.
  - Although SC formulation is prescribed as a once a month dose, some patients do not get a full month of benefit.
- **Certilizumab pegol (Cimzia)**
  - Available formulation: single use 200-mg prefilled syringe with specially designed grip.
  - Dosage: RA, PsA, AS: loading dose 400 mg (two syringes) SC at weeks 0, 2, and 4; then 200 mg every 2 weeks.
  - Owing to lack of functional Fc fragment, may be less injection site reactions and safer during pregnancy (does not cross placenta).

7. How effective are TNF inhibitors in inflammatory arthritis?

TNF inhibitors have an onset of action within days to weeks. Most patients will achieve their maximum improvement within 3 months, although some continue to improve with continued use. The following effects have been observed:
- Disease activity (RA, PsA MTX inadequate responders): 60% of patients achieve an ACR (American College of Rheumatology) 20; 40% an ACR 50; and 20% an ACR 70.
  - Psoriasis skin scores as measured by PASI (Psoriasis Area and Severity Index) improve more with infliximab than other TNF inhibitors.
- Disease activity (patients with AS): 60% of patients achieve an ASAS (Ankylosing Spondylitis Disease Activity Score) 20; 40% achieve an ASAS 40.
- Radiographic joint damage is inhibited in RA and PsA. Syndesmophyte formation is not inhibited in AS unless TNF inhibitors are started before they start to form. Once formed they may progress in spite of therapy over the first few years.
- Patients with inflammatory arthritis treated with TNF inhibitors have increased functionality, are more likely to stay employed, and have less cardiovascular mortality. This makes them cost effective with the number needed to treat being two at a cost of $30,000 to $50,000/QALY (quality-adjusted life year).
- The risk of a serious adverse event causing death from a TNF inhibitor is equivalent to the risk of getting into a serious car accident casing death.

8. What are some of the side effects observed with anti-TNF-α biologic agents? How can these toxicities be limited?

1. **Injection site and infusion reactions**
- *All injectable TNF inhibitors*: injection site reaction (up to 50% of patients) lasting 3 to 5 days. Some cause "bee sting" pain due to the preservative in the liquid. Treat with topical steroid or antihistamine. Rotate the injection sites. Usually reactions stop after 3 months of continued use. If problems persist, lyophilized etanercept or certilizumab pegol can be used which seem to have fewer injection site reactions.
- *Infliximab*: infusion reactions such as hypotension, headache (20%), nausea (15%), and dyspnea. Treat by stopping the infusion and restarting at a slower rate. If the patient has more than three drug allergies or has an infusion reaction, premedicate with Allegra (180 mg) 45 minutes before infusion; may also premedicate with aspirin (better than acetaminophen) and, if necessary, Solu-Cortef (100 to 125 mg IV).

2. **Infections**
- *Serious bacterial infections*: the overall prevalence of serious infections is 3% to 4% and overall relative risk is 2 to 3 times compared to DMARDs alone. However, when disease severity, comorbidities, and corticosteroid use are controlled for, the risk of serious infections may not be much higher than with other DMARDs. Infections tend to be pneumonias which occur more commonly within the first 6 months of use. TNF inhibitors should be stopped in all patients who develop a *febrile* infection, but do not need to be stopped for the "common cold." Patients with an open skin wound are most prone to develop cellulitis so stopping the TNF inhibitor until the wound is healed is prudent. TNF inhibitors should be avoided in patients with chronic ongoing infections such as osteomyelitis and bronchiectasis with recurrent pneumonias. The risk of infection is reduced if surgery is performed after waiting at least three half-lives from the last dose (9 days after etanercept; 4 to 5 weeks after infliximab and adalimumab; 6 weeks after golimumab or certilizumab).
- *Opportunistic infection (TB)*: TNF is important for granuloma formation and integrity. Therefore, all TNF inhibitors can cause reactivation of latent TB (risk increased 10×). Owing to long half-life and blood levels, infliximab may cause more of these infections than subcutaneous formulations. Patients who reactivate their TB typically do so within 6 to 12 months of starting a TNF inhibitor. In over 50% of cases the reactivation is at a site other than the lung (lymph nodes commonly). Therefore, all patients should be screened for risk factors for TB exposure and should be screened with a PPD or ex vivo testing for TB and chest radiograph before starting a TNF inhibitor. This should be repeated yearly in patients at risk for further TB exposure. Because patients are on immunosuppressants, a PPD ≥5 mm is considered positive even in patients who have received a Bacillus Calmette–Guérin (BCG) vaccine previously. The ex vivo interferon (IFN)-γ release assay (IGRA) may be a better screening test for TB than PPD, particularly in patients with a history of previous BCG vaccination which can cause a false-positive PPD. However, an indeterminant and/or false-negative IGRA can occur in patients on moderate doses of corticosteroids. Patients who have a positive TB screening test need TB prophylaxis with isoniazid (INH) (5 mg/kg) for 9 months. After 2 to 4 weeks of INH therapy the TNF inhibitor can be started. In patients with active TB, patients can start TNF inhibitors (if necessary) after 2 months of TB therapy.
- *Opportunistic infections (Hepatitis B/C)*: all TNF inhibitors increase the risk of *hepatitis B* reactivation. Patients with resolved hepatitis (HBsAg−, HBcAb+, undetectable viral load) have less than 2% risk of reactivation. As a result of this low rate, these patients can receive TNF inhibitors and have their symptoms, hepatic enzyme tests, and viral DNA loads checked periodically. Alternatively, patients with chronic and inactive hepatitis B (HBsAg+) should either not receive TNF inhibitors or must receive concomitant antiviral prophylaxis (lamivudine, other) starting 2 to 4 weeks before and continuing while on TNF inhibitors. Patients with *hepatitis C* can receive TNF agents without antiviral therapy but need hepatic enzyme and viral RNA load monitoring.
- *Opportunistic infections (other)*: TNF inhibitors increase risk of atypical mycobacterial infections, *Pneumocystis jiroveci*, *Listeria monocytogenes*, *Legionella*, Herpes zoster (shingles), and fungal infections. Patients with previous or current exposure to endemic fungi (*Histoplasmosis, Coccidioidomycosis*, others) need to be evaluated for these infections if they develop a febrile illness. Infliximab may be associated with increased risk of fungal infections compared to SC administered TNF inhibitors.

3. **Malignancy**
TNF is important for inducing apoptosis in tumor cells. However, it is unclear if TNF inhibitors increase the risk of malignancy, particularly lymphoma. Studies vary and state that the relative risk may (<5× relative risk) or may not be increased for lymphoma. However, most large studies report that it is not increased over the increased baseline risk of lymphoma associated with the underlying autoimmune disease being treated. Children treated with TNF inhibitors may have an increased lymphoma risk. Solid tumors are not increased. *Melanoma* and other skin cancers may be increased. Patients who develop a cancer (other than melanoma) while receiving a TNF inhibitor do not have worse histology, more widespread disease, or worse prognosis. Whether or not patients with active cancer or recently treated cancer can safely receive a TNF inhibitor is controversial, although it should not be used in patients with melanoma or lymphoma. Many experts recommend not starting these agents until a patient is cancer free for 5 years.

4. **Demyelinating syndromes**
Brain demyelination (multiple sclerosis-like), optic neuritis, Guillain–Barré syndrome, polyradiculopathy, and peripheral demyelinating neuropathy have been reported *rarely*. Most are reversible when the TNF inhibitor is stopped. Therefore, TNF inhibitors should not be given to patients with a history of multiple sclerosis or optic neuritis. Some experts recommend brain magnetic resonance imaging in patients with a strong family history of demyelinating disease to look for occult lesions. If silent lesions are present do not give the patient TNF inhibitors.

5. **Autoimmune phenomenon**
Between 10% and 50% of patients on TNF inhibitors will develop a positive antinuclear antibody, 10% to 15% develop anti-dsDNA antibodies (IgM isotype), and a small number (0.2% to 0.4%) develop drug-induced lupus (DIL). A few patients have developed antiphospholipid antibodies and antineutrophil cytoplasmic antibodies (ANCAs) that are rarely clinically significant. Patients who develop DIL have mild symptoms of arthritis, rash, and serositis that resolves with TNF inhibitor discontinuation. Small vessel leukocytoclastic vasculitis has rarely been reported. Infliximab is more likely to cause these autoimmune phenomena than other TNF inhibitors. Concomitant use of MTX does not lessen the frequency of these manifestations.

- *Antidrug antibodies*: over 20% of patients treated with infliximab will develop HACAs. Patients who develop HACAs may lose their response to infliximab (i.e., neutralizing antibodies) and/or experience more severe infusion reactions. Concomitant MTX therapy in RA patients (not spondyloarthropathy patients) is recommended to decrease the risk of developing HACAs. Less than 10% of patients receiving SC formulations of TNF inhibitors develop antidrug antibodies. This is decreased to less than 1% with concomitant MTX use. These antibodies are rarely neutralizing but may bind and increase the clearance making the TNF inhibitor less effective.

6. **Congestive heart failure**

Avoid TNF inhibitors (especially infliximab) in patients with class III or class IV congestive heart failure (CHF).

7. **Hematologic**

Neutropenia, thrombocytopenia, and pancytopenia have rarely been reported. Monitoring with periodic CBC (every 3 months) is recommended.

8. **Others**

Sarcoidosis, subacute cutaneous lupus-like rash, seizures, colonic perforations, increased liver enzymes >3-fold elevation (2% to 4%), severe hepatotoxicity (rare but most common with infliximab), and noninfectious pulmonary infiltrates have been reported.
- *Palmoplantar psoriasis*: less than 1% develop worsening psoriasis on palms and soles. Not prevented by using MTX. Etiology unknown but may be attributable to increased IFN-α production. Patients with SAPHO or pustular psoriasis are more likely to get this with infliximab.

9. **What diseases have been treated with TNF inhibitors?**
   - All TNF inhibitors are FDA-approved for treating RA patients who are inadequate responders to DMARDs (MTX).
   - All TNF inhibitors are FDA-approved for treating PsA. All except certolizumab are approved for AS therapy.
   - Etanercept and adalimumab are FDA-approved to treat polyarticular juvenile idiopathic arthritis (JIA).
   - All TNF inhibitors except etanercept and golimumab are FDA-approved to treat Crohn's disease. Infliximab, adalimumab, and golimumab are approved for ulcerative colitis.
   - Multiple other diseases have been treated off-label with success: uveitis (do not use etanercept), inflammatory bowel disease associated arthritis (do not use etanercept), reactive arthritis, Behçet's disease, TRAPS (use etanercept), sarcoidosis, relapsing polychondritis, Still's disease, pyoderma gangrenosum, SAPHO, hidradenitis suppurativa, polymyalgia rheumatica (?). Does not work in SLE, Sjögren's syndrome, ANCA-associated vasculitis, and giant cell arteritis.

10. **Can more than one TNF inhibitor be tried in a patient? Are there any useful switching "rules"?**

Most physicians and patients feel that at least a 50% overall clinical response is necessary to justify the cost and risk of using a TNF inhibitor. At least 50% of patients with RA, AS, or PsA may not achieve this response or will develop an intolerance to the first TNF inhibitor they are put on. Although controversial, most physicians will try a second TNF inhibitor. The effectiveness of switching TNF inhibitors and the "rules" for switching can be summarized as follows:
   - Patients who fail to respond to the first TNF inhibitor (primary failures) are less likely to get a good response to a second TNF inhibitor compared to patients who initially responded to a TNF inhibitor and then lose that response (secondary failures) or who had to stop the TNF inhibitor as a result of an adverse event (intolerance). Only 4% to 5% of primary failures will get a good response to a second TNF inhibitor compared to 27% to 30% of patients who had secondary failure/intolerance.
   - Patients who had an adverse event to their first TNF inhibitor are more likely (2 to 3 times) to develop an adverse event to a second TNF inhibitor.
   - To increase the chance of a response in a primary failure patient, choose a second TNF inhibitor which is a different molecule. For example, if the patient fails adalimumab (monoclonal antibody), put them on etanercept (soluble receptor) and vice versa. Some patients may respond well to certolizumab pegol which is a pegylated molecule even if they failed a TNF inhibitor that was a monoclonal antibody.
   - Patients who are secondary failures or have developed adverse events to a TNF inhibitor (especially infliximab) may have developed neutralizing antibodies, and switching to a second TNF inhibitor of any type can be beneficial.
   - If a patient has a primary failure to two TNF inhibitors, there is probably no benefit to try a third. There are some clinical trial data to suggest that patients who have failed two or more TNF inhibitors may still respond to certolizumab attributable to its unique formulation (controversial).

11. **What biologic agents are currently available to inhibit IL-1?**

Anakinra (Kineret): a recombinant, nonglycosylated form of the human IL-1 receptor antagonist (IL-1Ra). It blocks the biologic activity of IL-1 by competitively inhibiting IL-1 binding to the IL-1 type I receptor. The half-life is 4 to 6 hours.

Rilonacept (Arcalyst): dimeric fusion protein that incorporates in a single molecule the extracellular domains of both IL-1 receptor (IL-1R) and IL-1 receptor accessory protein (IL-1RAcP) fused to the Fc portion of an IgG1 molecule. Targets both IL-1α and IL-1β. Also known as IL-1 TRAP.

Canakinumab (Ilaris): human monoclonal antibody that specifically targets IL-1β.

12. **How are IL-1 inhibitors supplied and used? What are their indications and toxicities?**
    - **Anakinra (Kineret)**
      - Available formulation: single use vial of 100 mg.
      - Dosage: 100 mg SC daily.
      - Follow-up: CBC monthly for 3 months, then every 3 months.
      - Adverse reactions: serious infections (2%), neutropenia (3%).
        - Injection site reactions (70%): less likely if ice is placed on skin before injection. Treat with topical steroids.
      - Precautions: do not use in patients with active infection. Do not combine with other biologics.
      - FDA-approved indication: RA, neonatal onset multisystem inflammatory disease (NOMID).
      - Other diseases that it has been used with success: Still's disease, gout, familial Mediterranean fever, cryopyrin-associated periodic syndromes (CAPS).
      - Cost: $1500 per month.
    - **Rilonacept (Arcalyst)**
      - Available formulation: single use, glass vial containing 220 mg of lyophilized powder for reconstitution.
      - Dosage. Ages 12 to 17 dose: load with one dose 4.4 mg/kg (maximum 320 mg) followed by 2.2 mg/kg (maximum 160 mg) SC weekly.
      - Adult dose: load with one dose 320 mg followed by 160 mg SC weekly.
      - Follow-up: CBC periodically. Get lipid profile at 3 months.
      - Adverse reactions: injection site reaction (48%), infections (25%), serious infections (rare), other common symptoms.
      - Precautions: do not use in patients with active infection; warfarin interaction.
      - FDA-approved indication: CAPS (familial cold autoinflammatory syndrome [FCAS], Muckle–Wells syndrome [MWS]).
      - Other diseases that it has been used with success: gout, Still's disease, other cryopyrinopathies (CAPS).
      - Cost: $24,000 per month.
    - **Canakinumab (Ilaris)**
      - Available formulation: glass vial containing 180 mg of lyophilized powder for reconstitution.
      - Dosage. Patient weight 15 to 40 kg: 2 to 3 mg/kg SC every 8 weeks.
      - Patient weight >40 kg: 150 mg SC every 8 weeks.
      - Follow-up: CBC and hepatic enzymes periodically.
      - Adverse reactions: nasopharyngitis, diarrhea, vertigo (10%), headache, injection site reactions (9%), other common symptoms.
      - Precautions: do not use in patients with active infection; warfarin interaction.
      - FDA-approved indication: CAPS (FCAS, MWS), systemic JIA (Still's disease).
      - Other diseases that it has been used with success: gout, other cryopyrinopathies (CAPS).
      - Cost: $8000 per month.

13. **What biologic agent can inhibit IL-6? What are its uses and toxicities?**
    Tocilizumab (Actemra) is a humanized IgG1κ monoclonal antibody that binds to the soluble and membrane bound forms of the IL-6 receptor (IL-6R). This antibody inhibits IL-6 signaling of cells that constitutively express IL-6R as well as cells that bind the soluble form of IL-6R that interacts with gp130 on a wide variety of cells. Half-life is 8 to 14 days depending on dose. MTX does not help to increase the exposure to tocilizumab. It is controversial whether or not tocilizumab is more effective when used in combination with MTX.
    - Available formulation: 80 mg, 200 mg, 400 mg single use vials for IV administration; prefilled (1 mL) ready to use, single use syringe.
    - Dosage. RA: 4 mg/kg IV once every 4 weeks as a 60-minute infusion. Can increase to 8 mg/kg IV (not to exceed 800 mg) monthly if needed.
      - SC formulation: if >100 kg body weight 162 mg SC weekly; if <100 kg body weight 162 mg SC every other week. If not effective the dose can be increased to weekly.
    - Systemic JIA (Still's disease): patient weight <30 kg: use 12 mg/kg IV monthly; >30 kg: use 8 mg/kg IV monthly.
    - Tocilizumab can be used with or without MTX or another DMARD.
      - Monitoring: CBC (with differential) and hepatic enzymes monthly until stable dose, then every 1 to 2 months. Lipid panel every 1 to 2 months until stable dose, then every 6 months.
      - Adverse reactions: all adverse events more common on 8 mg/kg than 4 mg/kg dose.
    - Infusion reactions (8%): headaches, hypertension. Premedication usually not necessary. Serious reactions rare.
    - Infections: upper respiratory (8%), serious infections (3 to 5 events/100 patient years), Herpes zoster, opportunistic (rare).
    - Elevated hepatic enzymes: attributable to binding IL-6R on liver cells which blocks antiapoptotic effects of IL-6 on liver cells.
      - Enzymes between 1 and 3 times upper limit normal (ULN) (35% to 50% of patients): reduce tocilizumab dose and/or modify DMARD (MTX) dose.

- Enzymes >3 to 5 times ULN (5%): stop tocilizumab until enzymes <3 times ULN, then restart at lower dose and/or modify DMARD dose.
- Enzymes >5 times ULN (0.5% to 1.5%): discontinue tocilizumab.
- Neutropenia (29%): as a result of binding IL-6R on neutrophils.
  - Absolute neutrophil count (ANC) >1000/mm^3: continue tocilizumab.
  - ANC 500 to 1000/mm^3 (2% to 4% of patients): stop tocilizumab until ANC >1000/mm^3, then restart at lower dose.
  - ANC <500/mm^3 (0.4%): discontinue tocilizumab.
- Thrombocytopenia (8%): discontinue if <50,000/mm^3 (0.1%).
- Lipid elevations: mean increase low-density lipoprotein (LDL) was 10 to 20 mg/dL and mean high-density lipoprotein (HDL) increase was 3 to 5 mg/dL.
- Gastrointestinal perforations (0.26 events/100 patient years): IL-6 important for fibrotic healing and repair of gastrointestinal inflammation.
- Macrophage activation syndrome: seen in 3% of systemic JIA patients treated with tocilizumab.
- No increase in malignancy, CHF, or demyelinating disease noted. Patients with hepatitis B were excluded from trials and thus reactivation risk is unknown.
  - Precautions: do not use in patients with active infection, hepatic enzymes >1.5× upper limit, platelet count <100,000/mm^3, history of diverticulitis or other inflammatory bowel disease. Drug interactions include affecting blood levels of warfarin, cyclosporine, and theophylline. Lowers blood levels of omeprazole, simvastatin, and *birth control pills*. Advise patients about birth control.
  - FDA-approved indications: RA and systemic JIA (Still's disease).
  - Other diseases that it has been used with success: Castleman's disease, giant cell arteritis, Takayasu's arteritis, relapsing polychondritis, adult-onset Still's disease, SLE. Does not work for spondyloarthropathies.

14. What is ustekinumab (Stelara) and why is it effective in psoriatic arthritis?

Ustekinumab is a human IgG1κ monoclonal antibody that binds to the p40 subunit of both IL-12 and IL-23 preventing their binding to their shared cell surface receptor chain, IL-12β. The inhibition of IL-12 signaling abrogates Th1 response with reduction in TNF-α, IFN-γ, and IL-2 production. The inhibition of IL-23 signaling abrogates Th17 response with reduction in IL-6, IL-17, IL-21, IL-22, and TNF-α production. Th17 cells and IL-23 production by dendritic cells and keratinocytes are important in the pathogenesis of psoriasis. Half-life is 15 to 45 days.
- Available formulation: single use 45-mg and 90-mg prefilled syringes or vials.
- Dosage. psoriasis or PsA: patient ≤100 kg: 45 mg SC initially, followed by 45 mg in 4 weeks, then 45 mg every 12 weeks. Dosage for >100 kg: 90 mg SC initially, followed by 90 mg in 4 weeks, then 90 mg every 12 weeks.
- Monitoring: routine monitoring for other DMARDs (MTX).
- Adverse reactions: nasopharyngitis (10%), nonmelanoma skin cancers.
  - Serious infections (2% to 3%): IL-12/IL-23 are important for resistance against mycobacterial and salmonella infections. IL-17 is important for resistance against fungal infections.
- Precautions: do not use in patients with active infection. Do not combine with other biologics.
- FDA-approved indications: psoriasis and psoriatic arthritis.
- Cost: $28,000 to $56,000 per year depending on dose.

15. What is tofacitinib (Xeljanz)?

Tofacitinib is a novel oral DMARD which inhibits JAK. The JAK proteins are intracellular proteins that associate with and transduce signals from a number of cytokine and growth factor receptors. There are four JAKs that form various dimers with different pairings being associated with different cell surface receptors resulting in the production of a variety of inflammatory mediators. Tofacitinib acts on JAK1/JAK2 (important for IL-6 and IFN signaling), JAK1/JAK3 (important for T and B cell signaling), and JAK2/JAK2 (growth factor signaling) dimer pairs. As a result of JAK 3 inhibition, the production of IL-2, IL-4, IL-7, IL-9, IL-15, and IL-21, which are important in T and B cell activation and function, are decreased. Additionally, with JAK1 inhibition, IL-6 and IFN-γ production are attenuated. Finally IL-2-dependent differentiation of Th2 and Th17 cells is decreased. It is metabolized and eliminated primarily by the liver (70%) with the remainder excreted by the kidneys (30%). Half-life is short (3 hours).

16. How is tofacitinib supplied and used? What are its toxicities?
- **Tofacitinib (Xeljanz)**
  - FDA-approved indication: RA with inadequate response to MTX.
  - Available formulation: 5-mg tablet.
  - Dosage: 5 mg twice a day. Not affected by food. Dose should be decreased to 5 mg daily if severe liver or renal disease. Can be given alone or in combination with MTX. Avoid azathioprine.
  - Follow-up: CBC (with differential), creatinine, and hepatic enzymes monthly for 3 months, then every 3 months. Maximum effect on lipids occurs by 6 to 8 weeks, thus lipid panel should be done at that time.
  - Adverse reactions: common symptoms (4% to 5%) include nasopharyngitis, diarrhea, and headache.
    - Infections: any (20%), serious (2.7 events/100 patient years), opportunistic (0.3 events/100 patient years). Herpes zoster may be increased more than with other biologics and DMARDs.

- Hematologic: lymphopenia <500/mm³ (0.3%), ANC <1000/mm³ (0.07%), or hemoglobin drop >2 g/dL. Stop tofacitinib until counts recover, then restart at lower dose. Lymphopenia associated with higher infection rate.
- Hepatic enzyme elevations >3 × ULN (1.3%). Stop tofacitinib until enzymes improve, restart at lower dose.
- Lipid abnormalities: LDL increases 15% and HDL increases 10%.
- Creatinine increase >50% (2% of patients): etiology unknown. Discontinue tofacitinib.
- Malignancy: solid tumors (0.6 events/100 patient years) and lymphoma reported in tofacitinib group but not placebo-treated group.
- Gastrointestinal perforations: have been reported.
- Immunizations: decreases response to inactivated vaccines.
- Precautions: do not use in patients with active infection. Patients with hepatitis B and hepatitis C excluded from trials. Drug interactions include decreased effectiveness if used with rifampin. The tofacitinib dose needs to be decreased by half if the patient is put on ketoconazole/fluconazole.

17. What are B cell targeted therapies?

Rituximab (Rituxan): chimeric mouse–human IgG1κ monoclonal antibody directed against extracellular domain of CD20 antigen on B cells. B cells are eliminated by complement-mediated lysis, antibody-dependent cell mediated cytotoxicity, or apoptosis. All peripheral B cells are eliminated within days. Patients who fail to deplete their B cells respond less well. Notably, Ig levels are preserved due to preservation of plasma cells which lack the CD20 antigen on their cell membranes. Repeated infusions can cause decreased Ig levels (IgM > IgG > IgA). Half-life is 19 to 22 days.

Belimumab (Benlysta): fully human IgG1λ monoclonal antibody directed against B lymphocyte stimulator protein (BLyS)/B cell activating factor (BAFF). BLyS is the same as BAFF and promotes B cell survival, growth, and maturation by binding to three different B cell receptors. Inhibition of BLyS causes peripheral B cell counts to decrease by 40% to 50%. Ig levels usually not affected. Half-life is 11 to 14 days.

18. What are the indications and toxicities of rituximab (Rituxan)?

- FDA-approved rheumatologic indications: RA after MTX and anti-TNF failure; ANCA-associated vasculitis (granulomatosis with polyangiitis [GPA], microscopic polyangiitis [MPA]).
- Available formulation: single use vial of 100 mg and 500 mg.
- Dosage. RA: 1000 mg IV infusion repeated once 2 weeks later. Some physicians feel 500 mg dose is as effective as 1000 mg. Can be used with concomitant DMARDs (MTX).
  - ANCA-associated vasculitis: 375 mg/m² IV infusion once weekly for 4 weeks. Can also use RA dosage (1 g × 2).
- First infusion lasts 3 to 5 hours, subsequent infusions 2 to 3 hours. Patients are typically premedicated 30 minutes before each infusion with solumedrol 100 mg, acetaminophen 1000 mg, and an antihistamine to decrease chance of infusion reaction.
- Follow-up: CBC every 2 to 4 months to monitor for late-onset neutropenia.
- Adverse reactions:
  - *Infusion reaction* (10% to 35%): usually not severe if use premedication. Respond to stopping infusion until symptoms gone, then restart at slower rate. Stop infusion if patients start clearing their throat due to a scratchy feeling. Serious reactions (1%). Risk does not increase with subsequent infusions. May not need premedication with subsequent infusion if tolerated well.
  - *Infection:* any (35% or 78 events/100 patient years); serious (2% or 3 events/100 patient years); opportunistic (0.05/100 patient years, very low rate).
  - *Viral infections:* reactivation of resolved *hepatitis B* (HBsAg⁻, HBcAb⁺) occurs in 5% to 10%. Patients with chronic and inactive hepatitis B (HBsAg⁺) should either not receive rituximab or must receive concomitant antiviral prophylaxis (lamivudine, other) starting 2 to 4 weeks before and continuing while on rituximab and for 1 month after stopping. Patients with *hepatitis C* can receive rituximab without antiviral therapy but need hepatic enzyme and viral RNA load monitoring. The risk of JC *virus* infection resulting in progressive multifocal leukoencephalopathy (PML) may vary by disease being treated and previous immunosuppressive medications (1:25,000 RA patients, 1:4000 SLE patients compared to 1:200,000 in the general population). Owing to frequency of JC virus exposure (60% to 70%) and low rate of PML in RA patients treated with rituximab, it is not recommended to screen patients with antibody testing for previous JC virus exposure. Herpes zoster appears increased.
  - *Hypogammaglobulinemia:* only occurs in patients after multiple courses of rituximab therapy. IgG becomes low in 3.5% to 12% of patients, IgM low in 22% to 26%. Patients who develop low IgG more likely (2×) to get serious infection.
  - *Late-onset neutropenia:* occurs in 3% of patients with RA and up to 20% of SLE or ANCA-associated vasculitis patients treated. Occurs an average of 3 to 4 months post-therapy and is associated with increased infection risk (16%). Cause is unclear. Tends to recur with subsequent doses.
  - *Immunizations:* responses to killed vaccines are severely decreased if given after rituximab. Give 2-4 weeks before or 4 to 6 months post-rituximab infusion.

- *Other*: severe mucocutaneous reactions, hypertension/arrhythmias/myocardial infarction during infusions. Note that CHF, demyelinating disease, malignancy (except skin cancer), and mycobacterial infections were not increased over placebo. Rituximab may be used ahead of TNF inhibitors in patients with one of these conditions that makes TNF inhibitors contraindicated.
- Precautions: do not use in patients with active infection. Use pneumocystis jiroveci prophylaxis for patients with ANCA-associated vasculitis and lung disease.
- Other diseases that it has been used for: SLE, antiphospholipid antibody syndrome (APS), extraglandular Sjögren's syndrome, IgG4 disease, neuromyelitis optica spectrum disorder, idiopathic thrombocytopenic purpura, autoimmune hemolytic anemia, pemphigus vulgaris, Castleman's disease. Does not work in spondyloarthropathies.
- Cost: $14,200 total for two infusions of 1000 mg each not including infusion costs.

19. **When can/should rituximab be repeated? Can other immunosuppressive medications be used with it?**
Among RA patients, the response is variable. Patients who are seropositive (rheumatoid factor and/or anticyclic citrullinated peptide) are more likely to respond. All patients deplete their B cells so this does not need to be checked. B cell repopulation occurs at a mean of 8 months post-therapy. Patients who respond tend to by 4 to 6 months. The duration of response varies (median 30 weeks) and patients tend to relapse with reappearance of memory B cells (IgD$^+$CD27) and not naïve B cells. Retreatment is done when clinical symptoms recur and are not based on B cell counts; however, retreatment is not done sooner than 4 months after previous therapy. Recently, some physicians are giving one infusion of 1000 mg of rituximab every 6 months to maintain remission in responders to prevent relapse. Primary nonresponders usually do not respond to additional rituximab courses. These patients can be started on another biologic agent at 6 months after the initial course of two rituximab infusions even if B cells are still depleted without a significant increase in infection risk. Among ANCA-associated vasculitis patients, rituximab appears to be equivalent to cyclophosphamide. Patients can be treated with an RA dose schedule or lymphoma (4 weekly doses) schedule. All patients deplete their B cells. Patients relapse with recurrence of B cells at an average of 12 months. Patients can relapse before the reappearance of ANCA. Some physicians advocate giving 500 mg every 6 months to maintain remission and avoid relapse. In patients that relapse, a second course of rituximab is as effective as the first course. Rituximab is reportedly effective in GPA and MPA in patients who are ANCA negative.

20. **What are the indications, efficacy, and toxicities of belimumab (Benlysta)?**
    - FDA-approved indication: SLE. Does not work in RA.
    - Available formulation: single use vial containing 120 mg or 400 mg of lyophilized powder for reconstitution.
    - Dosage: loading dose of 10 mg/kg IV at 0, 2, and 4 weeks; maintenance 10 mg/kg IV every 4 weeks. Does not need premedication. Infusion takes 1 hour.
    - Follow-up: routine monitoring for SLE.
    - Efficacy: SLE patients who were not responding to standard therapy achieved primary endpoint in 43% to 58% of cases. Patients with severe renal and central nervous system disease were excluded from trials, thus these patients should not be primarily treated with belimumab. It seems to be most effective in patients with active serologies (low C3/C4, elevated anti-dsDNA antibody) and high BLyS levels (not available for testing). Manifestations that respond best are fatigue, rash, and arthritis. Hematologic abnormalities do not respond well.
    - Adverse reactions: infections, infusion reactions, serious infections, and malignancies were not increased over placebo rate.
        - Depression and suicide mildly increased over placebo rate.
        - Immunizations: response to killed/inactivated vaccines may be decreased.
    - Precautions: do not use in patients with active infection. Can be given with background immunosuppressive therapy.
    - Cost: $530/120-mg vial; $1770/400-mg vial. Monthly cost for 80 kg person: $3500 plus infusion costs.

21. **What T cell targeted therapies are available and how are they used?**
Abatacept (Orencia): a fully human fusion protein comprising the extracellular portion of CTLA4 and the Fc fragment of IgG1 (CTLA4Ig). Abatacept binds to CD80/CD86 on antigen-presenting cells (APCs) preventing these molecules from binding to their ligand, CD28, on T cells. This interferes with optimal T cell activation resulting in decreased production of proinflammatory cytokines. Notably, T cell activation is not completely inhibited because other interactions between APCs and T cells (ICAM-1:LFA-1; CD40:CD40L; LFA-3:CD-2) are not inhibited.
    - FDA-approved indication: RA and polyarticular JIA (>age 6 years, usually after TNF inhibitor) who are inadequate responders to DMARDs (MTX). Can use with DMARDs (MTX).
    - Available formulation: single use vial containing 250 mg of lyophilized powder for reconstitution for IV infusion; 125 mg/mL solution in a single dose prefilled glass syringe for SC administration.
    - Dosage. Intravenous dose is weight based (adults: 500 mg if <60 kg; 750 mg if 60 to 100 kg; 100 mg if >100 kg) (pediatrics: 10 mg/kg if <75 kg; same as adult dose if >75 kg). Loading dose at 0, 2, and 4 weeks, then every 4 weeks. Does not need premedication. Infusion takes 30 minutes.

- SC dose: one infusion of weight-based IV dose as above followed by 125 mg SC weekly. Some physicians do not give IV dose.
- Follow-up: routine monitoring for RA and DMARDs.
- Adverse reactions:
  - Infusion reactions: rare. Routine premedication not necessary.
  - Infections: routine similar to placebo. Serious infections (3%). Pneumonias increased in patients with chronic obstructive pulmonary disease. Opportunistic infections rare (0.01 to 0.05 events/100 patient years). Abatacept may be the safest biologic to use in patients at risk for TB.
  - Malignancy: standardized incidence rates for lung cancer, lymphoma, and other malignancies not increased over background rates of patients with RA who are not on biologics.
  - Immunizations: response to killed/inactivated vaccines may be decreased.
  - Others: headache. No increased rate of demyelinating disease, autoimmune phenomenon, CHF, hematologic abnormalities.
- Precautions: do not use in patients with active infection.
- Other diseases: used in PsA and SLE but unclear what subsets it works best for. Being tested in giant cell arteritis (GCA) and Takayasu's arteritis.

22. **How effective are biologics in RA?**
All biologics approved for RA work better in early disease. In patients who have an inadequate response to MTX, the rule of thumb is the 60-40-20 rate of response: 60% of patients with RA will achieve an ACR 20, 40% will achieve an ACR 50, and 20% will achieve an ACR 70. In patients who have an inadequate response to both MTX and TNF inhibitors, the response rate is approximately 10% less to another biologic, that is, 50-30-10 rate of response. All biologics have been shown to slow or prevent radiographic progression in RA.

23. **Can two biologics be used together?**
No, because of increased serious infection risk.

24. **Can live vaccines be given to patients on biologics?**
No. Patients should be given a live vaccine at least 4 weeks before starting a biologic therapy. If already on a biologic agent, the patients should stop the biologic at least 3 months before receiving the live vaccine. Others recommend that a live vaccine can be given if a patient has stopped the biologic for at least 3 to 5 times its half-life (2 to 30 days after tofacitinib; 9 to 15 days after etanercept; 4 to 6 weeks after infliximab and adalimumab; 6 to 10 weeks after golimumab, certilizumab, tocilizumab, or abatacept; 9 to 15 weeks after rituximab).

25. **Can biologic agents be given during pregnancy and breastfeeding?**
TNF inhibitors and ustekinumab are FDA Pregnancy Classification B medications. They can be used if clinically necessary for the mother's health. It should be noted that only 4% of the maternal blood level of etanercept is detected in the fetal circulation. Immunoglobulins do not cross placenta before 16 weeks of gestation, thus TNF inhibitors that are monoclonal antibodies should not cross the placenta until then. Recent data suggest that certilizumab pegol crosses the placenta less than other monoclonal antibodies because it does not have a functional Fc fragment attributable to the pegylation. Animal and observational data support that the congenital malformation rate is not more than the 3% risk in the general population. One report suggested that the VACTERL anomaly may be associated with TNF inhibitor use but this has not been confirmed. Importantly, infants born to mothers who have received monoclonal antibodies (especially infliximab) throughout pregnancy should not receive live vaccines until at least 6 months of age as a result of infliximab crossing the placenta and remaining in the infant's circulation for a prolonged period. Finally, only 4% of etanercept gets into breast milk, whereas very little of the monoclonal TNF inhibitors get into breast milk because IgG antibodies are not transferred from the maternal circulation to breast milk in high amounts.
All other biologic agents are FDA Pregnancy Classification C medications. They have not been studied sufficiently and therefore are not recommended to be used during pregnancy and probably not during breastfeeding. Rituximab has been reported to cause transient B cell depletion in the fetus and infant when given to the mother during pregnancy. The outcome of pregnancies of patients who receive any biologic agent during pregnancy should be reported to the Organization of Teratology Information Specialists (OTIS) registry at 1-866-626-6847.

26. **What are the relative *annual* costs for biologics used to treat RA?**
The relative *annual* costs for biologics used to treat RA are outlined in Table 85-1

27. **What are biosimilars?**
Biosimilars (also known as follow-on biologics) are biologics made by a different manufacturer from the original innovator of the biologic agent. The manufacturer does not have access to the originator's molecular clone or the exact fermentation and purification process. Therefore, concern about the safety and efficacy of biosimilars has been discussed. The Biologics Price Competition and Innovation Act was formally passed under the Patient Protection and Affordable Care Act in 2010. This gave 12 years of data exclusivity from the time of FDA approval to the innovator company. It also established a pathway for biosimilars to be approved by the FDA after this period of exclusivity. Some biologic agents used to treat RA will lose their exclusivity in

Table 85-1. The Relative Annual Costs for the Biologics Used to Treat Rheumatoid Arthritis.

BIOLOGIC	2010 WHOLESALE ACQUISITION COST (DOLLARS)	2013 BEST PRESCRIPTION PRICE (DOLLARS)
Etanercept (50 mg every week)	20,100	28,600
Adalimumab (40 mg every other week)	19,800	28,200
Infliximab (3 mg/kg every 8 weeks)	15,050	15,300
Golimumab (50 mg every month)	19,800	30,960
Certilizumab pegol (200 mg every other week)	21,200	27,300
Abatacept (125 mg every week)	22,000*	27,600
Abatacept (750 mg every month)	20,700	24,000
Tocilizumab (8 mg/kg every month)	25,500	37,600
Rituximab (1000 mg × 2 every 6 months)	22,150	28,400
Tofacitinib (5 mg twice a day)	24,660*	26,760

*These are annual costs. Note that wholesale acquisition costs (WACs) are from 2010, whereas best prescription prices are from 2013. Subcutaneous abatacept and tofacitinib were not available in 2010 and thus the WAC is 2012 pricing. WACs and prescription costs do not take into account discount pricing to federal entities (Medicare, Medicaid, VA, Tricare) or insurance prescription plans. Costs do not take into account intravenous administration costs. Costs are based on a 80-kg patient and doses are rounded up to use the entire vial.

2016/2017 at which time biosimilars will be introduced to the U.S. market. Biosimilars are already being used in some foreign markets with efficacy and safety similar to the original product. It is estimated that the cost of biosimilars will be 65% to 85% of the original product.

28. **What other biologic agents are being tested in trials which may help treat inflammatory rheumatic diseases?**
    - Cytokine-targeted therapies
        - Anti-IL-6 receptor: sarilumab; anti-IL-6: sirukumab, olokizumab.
        - Anti-IL-17A receptor: brodalumab; anti-IL-17A: secukinumab, ixekizumab.
        - Anti-IL-20: Nnc0109-0012.
        - IFN-α inhibitors: anti-IFN-α (sifalimumab); IFN-α kinoid.
        - Oral tyrosine kinase inhibitors: fostamatinib (SYK inhibitor), baricitinib (JAK inhibitor).
    - B cell targeted therapies
        - Anti-CD20: ofatumumab; ocrelizumab.
        - Anti-CD22: epratuzumab.
        - B cell stimulating factor inhibitors: atacicept (BLyS/BAFF, APRIL); tabalumab (anti-BAFF); blisibimod (fusion protein anti-BAFF).
    - Other molecules
        - Mavrilimumab (antigranulocyte macrophage colony stimulating factor [anti-GM-CSF] receptor α).
        - Chemokine inhibitor: CCX354-L2 (CCR1 inhibitor).

29. **What is eculizumab?**
    Eculizumab (Soliris) is a humanized IgG2/4κ monoclonal antibody that binds C5 to inhibit its cleavage to C5a and C5b preventing the generation of the terminal complement complex, C5b-9. It is approved for use to treat the complement-mediated thrombotic microangiopathy occurring in patients with atypical hemolytic uremic syndrome and to prevent the hemolysis that occurs in patients with paroxysmal nocturnal hemoglobinuria. Its most feared side effect is meningococcemia. It costs $450,000 to $600,000 annually for therapy.

BIBLIOGRAPHY

Aaltonen KJ, Virkki LM, Malmivarra A, et al: Systematic review and meta-analysis of the efficacy and safety of existing TNF blocking agents in treatment of rheumatoid arthritis, PLOS ONE 7:e30275, 2012.
Campbell L, Chen C, Bhagat SS, et al: Risk of adverse events including serious infections in rheumatoid arthritis patients treated with tocilizumab: a systematic literature review and meta-analysis of randomized controlled trials, Rheumatology 50:552–562, 2011.
Daien CI, Monnier A, Claudepierre P, et al: Sarcoid-like granulomatosis in patients treated with tumor necrosis factor blockers: 10 cases, Rheumatology 48:883–886, 2009.
Danila MJ, Patkar NM, Curtis JR, et al: Biologics and heart failure in rheumatoid arthritis: are we any wiser? Curr Opin Rheumatol 20:327–333, 2008.

Dao K, Cush JJ: A vaccination primer for rheumatologists, Drug Safety Quarterly 4, Jan, 2012.
Dedoglu F: Drug-induced autoimmunity, Curr Opin Rheumatol 2:547–551, 2009.
Engel P, Gomez-Puerta JA, Ramos-Casals M, et al: Therapeutic targeting of B cells for rheumatic autoimmune diseases, Pharmacol Rev 6:127–156, 2011.
Fleischmann R: Novel small-molecular therapeutics for rheumatoid arthritis, Curr Opin Rheumatol 24:335–341, 2012.
Fleischman R, Kremer J, Cush J, et al: Placebo-controlled trial of tofacitinib monotherapy in rheumatoid arthritis, N Engl J Med 367:495–507, 2012.
Geyer M, Muller-Ladner U: Actual status of antiinterleukin-1 therapies in rheumatic diseases, Curr Opin Rheumatol 22:246–251, 2010.
Kemper AR, Van Mater HA, Coeytaux RR, et al: Systematic review of disease-modifying antirheumatic drugs for juvenile idiopathic arthritis, BMC Pediatrics 12:29, 2012.
Kerbleski JF, Gottlieb AB: Dermatological complications and safety of anti-TNF treatments, Gut 58:1033–1039, 2009.
Lloyd S, Bujkiewicz S, Wailoo AJ, et al: The effectiveness of anti-TNF-α therapies when used sequentially in rheumatoid arthritis patients: a systematic review and meta-analysis, Rheumatology 49:2313–2321, 2010.
Lysandropoulos AP, Du Pasquier RA: Demyelination as a complication of new immunomodulatory treatment, Curr Opin Neurol 23:226–233, 2010.
Mariette X, Matucci-Cerinic M, Pavelka K, et al: Malignancies associated with tumor necrosis factor inhibitors in registries and prospective observational studies: a systematic review and meta-analysis, Ann Rheum Dis 70:1895–1904, 2011.
Mastroianni CM, Lichtner M, Del Borgo C, et al: Current trends in management of hepatitis B virus reactivation in the biologic therapy era, World J Gastroenterol 17:3881–3887, 2011.
Nam JL, Winthrop KL, van Vollenhoven RF, et al: Current evidence for the management of rheumatoid arthritis with biological disease-modifying antirheumatic drugs: a systematic literature review informing the EULAR recommendations for the management of RA, Ann Rheum Dis 69:976–986, 2010.
Ostenson M, Forger F: Treatment with biologics of pregnant patients with rheumatic diseases, Curr Opin Rheumatol 23:293–298, 2011.
Patkar NM, Teng GG, Curtis JR, et al: Association of infections and tuberculosis with antitumor necrosis factor alpha therapy, Curr Opin Rheumatol 20:320–326, 2008.
Ramos-Casals M, Brito-Zeron P, Munoz S, et al: A systematic review of the off-label use of biological therapies in systemic autoimmune diseases, Medicine 87:345–364, 2008.
Rubbert-Roth A, Finckh A: Treatment options in rheumatoid arthritis failing TNF inhibitor therapy: a critical review, Arthritis Res Ther 11(Suppl 1):51, 2009.
Salliot C, Finckh A, Katchamart W, et al: Indirect comparison of the efficacy of biologic antirheumatic agents in rheumatoid arthritis in patients with an inadequate response to conventional disease-modifying antirheumatic drugs or to an anti-tumor necrosis factor agent: a meta-analysis, Ann Rheum Dis 70:266–271, 2011.
Schiff M: Abatacept treatment for rheumatoid arthritis, Rheumatology 50:437–449, 2011.
Weger W: Current status and new developments in the treatment of psoriasis and psoriatic arthritis with biological agents, Br J Pharmacol 160:810–820, 2010.
Winthrop KL, Chang E, Yamashita S, et al: Nontuberculosis mycobacteria infections and anti-tumor necrosis factor-α therapy, Emerg Infect Dis 15:1556–1561, 2009.

FURTHER READING

www.rheumatology.org

HYPOURICEMIC AGENTS AND COLCHICINE

David R. Finger, MD

KEY POINTS
1. Urate-lowering therapy should maintain the serum uric acid level less than 6 mg/dL.
2. Allopurinol is the most convenient and cost-effective urate-lowering therapy.
3. Allopurinol should be started at a low dose and titrated up to effect.
4. Febuxostat is an alternative for patients who fail to respond to or tolerate allopurinol.
5. Pegloticase should not be used in patients with G6PD deficiency.

1. Identify the goals in the treatment of gout.
The first goal is safe and rapid treatment of acute gouty attacks to alleviate pain and to restore joint function. This is usually done with nonsteroidal antiinflammatory drugs (NSAIDs) or corticosteroids but colchicine can also be used. Once this is accomplished, the next goal is to prevent recurrent attacks and the future development of destructive arthropathy, tophi formation, and nephrolithiasis with hypouricemic therapy.

2. What is colchicine?
Colchicine, an alkaloid derivative from the plant *Colchicum autumnale*, has been used in the treatment of acute gout for nearly two centuries and for joint pain since the sixth century. It has long been believed that the clinical response of acute arthritis to colchicine was diagnostic for gout, although other inflammatory arthropathies such as familial Mediterranean fever, pseudogout, and acute sarcoid arthritis also respond. Garrod stated over a century ago that "colchicine possesses as specific a control over the gouty inflammation as cinchona barks over intermittent fever...We may sometimes diagnose gouty from any other sort of inflammation by noting the influence of colchicine on its progress."

3. When is colchicine therapy indicated? What are the correct dosages?
Colchicine (Colcrys) can be used in the treatment of acute gouty attacks and as prophylaxis against future attacks, especially when hypouricemic therapy is initiated. Colchicine is available orally in 0.6-mg tablets. Cost is over $5/pill or $160/month.

The average dose for **prophylaxis** is 0.6 mg once or twice daily if the patient has normal renal function. This completely prevents attacks or significantly lowers their frequency in 80% to 85% of patients followed long-term, with minimal toxicity. Prophylactic doses usually do not cause gastrointestinal (GI) side effects and should be continued until the patient is without symptoms of gout for several months.

For **acute attacks**, colchicine is most effective if given in the first few hours. A recent study showed that 1.2 mg followed in 1 hour by 0.6 mg provides similar efficacy with less toxicity compared with higher dose regimens.

The dose for colchicine must be reduced (or not used) in patients with severe renal insufficiency, severe hepatic disease, or on medications that are CYP 3A4 inhibitors (clarithromycin, erythromycin, ketoconazole, ritonavir, calcium channel blockers, others). Colchicine should be avoided (if possible) in patients on cyclosporine (P-glycoprotein inhibitor). Tacrolimus is less of a problem. Guidelines are listed in Table 86-1, but avoiding colchicine if possible is always the safer alternative.

4. Discuss the mechanism of action and pharmacokinetics of colchicine.
Colchicine has no effect on serum urate concentration or on urate metabolism. It functions as an antiinflammatory agent by inhibiting neutrophil chemotaxis through irreversible binding to tubulin dimers, preventing their assembly into microtubules. Colchicine also interferes with membrane-dependent functions of neutrophils, such as phagocytosis, and inhibits phospholipase A_2, which leads to lower levels of inflammatory prostaglandins and leukotrienes (LTB4). Colchicine is not bound to plasma proteins and is highly lipid-soluble, readily passing into all tissues. The half-life is 4 hours following oral administration. It can be detected in neutrophils up to 10 days after a single dose. It is hepatically metabolized and excreted principally in the bile, with 20% excreted unchanged in urine.

5. Describe the different manifestations of colchicine toxicity.
Most adverse effects of colchicine are dose and duration related. There are no antidotes to overdose and hemodialysis is ineffective. Potential side effects include:
- GI effects (diarrhea, nausea, vomiting, rarely malabsorption syndrome and hemorrhagic gastroenteritis).
- Bone marrow suppression (thrombocytopenia, leukopenia) – risk increased with chronic use and renal insufficiency.

Table 86-1. Correct Dosage for Colchicine Therapy		
	ACUTE ATTACK DOSE	**CHRONIC PROPHYLAXIS DOSE**
CYP 3A4 inhibitors	0.6 mg × 1, followed by 0.3 mg in 1 hour Do not repeat for 3 days	0.3 mg daily
Cyclosporine	0.6 mg × 1 Do not repeat for 3 days	0.3 mg every other day
On dialysis	0.6 mg × 1 Do not repeat for 2 weeks	0.3 mg twice a week
CrCl <30 mL/min	1.2 mg × 1, followed by 0.6 mg in 1 hour Do not repeat for 2 weeks	0.3 mg daily
CrCl <50 mL/min	1.2 mg × 1, followed by 0.6 mg in 1 hour	0.6 mg daily

CrCl, Creatinine clearance.

- Neuromyopathy (elevated creatine kinase, proximal weakness, peripheral neuropathy, lysosomal vacuoles on biopsy) – usually seen in patients on chronic colchicine who also have renal insufficiency. Patients on cyclosporine should not receive colchicine (if possible) because of risk of neuromyopathy.
- Alopecia.
- Oligospermia and amenorrhea – chronic use of colchicine.
- Central nervous system dysfunction.

6. What antihyperuricemic agents are available?

Antihyperuricemic agents include **uricosurics** (probenecid), which reduce the serum urate concentration by enhancing renal excretion of uric acid, **xanthine oxidase inhibitors** (allopurinol and febuxostat), which inhibit uric acid synthesis by inhibiting xanthine oxidase, the final enzyme involved in the production of uric acid, and **uricase** (pegloticase), which converts uric acid into allantoin. These agents should be initiated only after an acute attack of gout has resolved entirely.

The risk of acute gouty attacks following the initiation of antihyperuricemic therapy can be minimized by gradual dose increases and by prophylaxis with colchicine, NSAIDs, or low-dose prednisone. The decision to use uric acid-lowering therapy is a lifelong commitment, so it is essential that these agents are initiated only when they are truly indicated. Uricosurics can be safely used concomitantly with allopurinol in some patients with severe tophaceous gout.

7. Which patients with recurrent gouty arthritis are the best candidates for uricosuric therapy?

- Hyperuricemia secondary to underexcretion of uric acid (<800 mg of uric acid in a 24-hour urine collection, while on a regular diet).
- Age <60 years.
- Creatinine clearance >50 mL/min.
- No history of nephrolithiasis.
- Uric acid <9 mg/dL (uricosurics reduce urate levels an average of 33%).

8. Describe the renal handling of uric acid.

Uric acid is excreted primarily (66%) through the kidney. Up to one third is excreted through the GI tract. In cases of renal failure, GI excretion is increased. There are four components of renal excretion:
- Glomerular filtration: near complete excretion of urate.
- Proximal tubule reabsorption of urate in exchange for organic acids and monocarboxylates (lactate/pyruvate/acetoacetate/hydroxybutyrate): mediated by URAT1 and GLUT9 transporters.
- Tubular secretion of urate more distal to above mediated by ABCG2 and MRP4 transporters.
- Tubular reabsorption of urate a second time in exchange for dicarboxylates (oxalic acid/malonic acid/succinic acid): mediated by OAT4 and OAT10 transporters (Figure 86-1).

9. Identify some uricosuric agents and describe their mechanism of action.

Many drugs have uricosuric properties but only **probenecid** is used in the United States. Sulfinpyrazone and benzbromarone are available in other countries. Uricosuric agents are weak organic acids, such as uric acid, and they inhibit URAT1 and GLUT9 resulting in less tubular reabsorption of urate, which leads to increased urinary excretion of uric acid. Probenecid (1000 mg twice daily) is successful in lowering serum uric acid to <6.0 mg/dL in 70% of patients. Uricosurics work better when there is good urine alkalinization (pH >6.0) and flow (>1500 mL/day) to minimize the risk of uric acid nephropathy and nephrolithiasis.

There are several other drugs capable of lowering uric acid levels to a mild degree. These include: losartan, fenofibrate, atorvastatin, rosuvastatin, leflunomide, high-dose (>4 g/day) salicylates. These medications can be safely used in conjunction with other urate-lowering therapies.

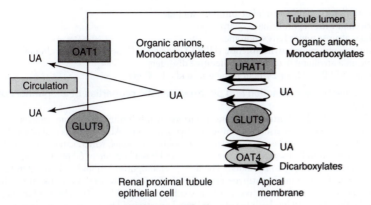

Figure 86-1. Renal handling of uric acid

PEARL: hypertension is common in patients with gout. Consider using a urate-lowering medication such as losartan to treat hypertension instead of hydrochlorothiazide, which raises uric acid levels.

10. **How is probenecid used? Are there any drug interactions?**
    - *Probenecid should never be started during the acute gout attack.* It can be started after the attack has completely resolved. If a patient is already on probenecid and experiences a gout attack the patient should not stop the probenecid. The half-life of probenecid is 6 to 12 hours so it is dosed twice a day. It is hepatically metabolized.
    - Probenecid is available in 500-mg tablets. It is also formulated as a combination tablet with colchicine (0.5 mg) (colbenemid). It is dosed initially at 500 mg twice daily but can be gradually increased up to 3 g daily (average dose 1 g/day) in two to three divided doses. Monthly cost (1000 mg twice a day: $60 to $70).
    - Probenecid has multiple possible drug interactions. Therefore, a thorough medication history needs to be taken and investigated before putting a patient on probenecid. Some examples of interactions: probenecid prolongs the half-life of multiple medications such as penicillin and other antibiotics, dapsone, methotrexate, indomethacin, and others by decreasing their renal excretion. It prolongs the metabolism of heparin.

11. **What are possible side effects of probenecid therapy?**
    Probenecid is generally well tolerated by >90% of patients and serious side effects only occur rarely (Box 86-1).

Box 86-1. Side Effects of Probenecid

Preventable
Acute gouty attacks
Urate nephropathy
Urate nephrolithiasis

Rare
Cytopenias
Anaphylaxis
Nephrotic syndrome

Relatively common
Nausea, loss of appetite (10%)
Dermatitis (5%)
Headache, flushing

---

12. **List the xanthine oxidase inhibitors available to inhibit uric acid synthesis?**
    - Allopurinol (Zyloprim).
    - Febuxostat (Uloric).

13. **What are the indications for using a xanthine oxidase inhibitor?**
    Indications in patients with recurrent gout include:
    1. Urate overproduction (uric acid >800 mg in 24-hour urine collection on a regular diet).
    2. Nephrolithiasis.
    3. Renal insufficiency (creatinine clearance <50 mL/min).
    4. Tophi (may take several months to resolve).
    5. Failure or intolerance of uricosuric agents.

Other indications for a xanthine oxidase inhibitor include:
1. Hyperuricemia with nephrolithiasis of any type.
2. Prophylaxis against tumor lysis syndrome.
3. Hypoxanthine phosphoribosyltransferase (HPRT) deficiency (Lesch–Nyhan syndrome).
4. Hyperuricemia attributable to myeloproliferative disorders.
5. Serum urate >12.0 mg/dL or 24-hour urine uric acid >1100 mg.

14. **Describe the mechanism of action and pharmacokinetic properties of allopurinol compared to febuxostat.**

    Allopurinol lowers blood and urine urate concentrations by inhibiting the enzyme, xanthine oxidase, thus leading to increases in the precursors, xanthine and hypoxanthine. Allopurinol is a hypoxanthine analog that is metabolized by xanthine oxidase to the active metabolite, *oxipurinol*, which can be measured to assess compliance. Allopurinol is well absorbed from the GI tract and has a half-life of 60 minutes, whereas oxipurinol has a much longer half-life (14 to 28 hours). The dosage of allopurinol should be lowered in the presence of renal insufficiency. The maximum antihyperuricemic effect is seen 7 to 14 days after starting allopurinol.

    Febuxostat is a potent and selective xanthine oxidase inhibitor. It is 50% absorbed through the GI tract, metabolized by the liver, and has both hepatic and renal excretion. The maximum antihyperuricemic effect is seen 5 to 7 days after starting febuxostat.

15. **How is allopurinol dosed? How is febuxostat dosed?**

    Allopurinol is available orally in 100- and 300-mg tablets, usually given in once-daily doses. To limit gout flares and toxicity, current guidelines recommend that allopurinol be started at 100 mg/day and increased by 100 mg every month. The average dose used is 300 mg/day but only 40% will achieve the desired urate level goal of <6 mg/dL. Therefore, an allopurinol dose of 4 mg/kg to as high as 600 mg/day may be necessary. One should investigate other correctable factors leading to hyperuricemia if it requires >300 mg/day to achieve adequate uric acid levels, although noncompliance and alcohol abuse are the most common causes. The dose should be reduced if possible in the presence of renal insufficiency because oxipurinol is renally excreted. Ideally, the dose should not exceed 200 mg/day when the glomerular filtration rate (GFR) is <60 mL/min, 100 mg/day when GFR is <30 mL/min, and 100 mg every other day when GFR is <15 mL/min. However, in 50% of patients the allopurinol dose will have to exceed these "renal doses" to achieve the desired uric acid goal. Monthly cost (300 mg/day): $4.

    Febuxostat is available as a 40-mg and 80-mg tablet, given as a once-daily dose. It is started at 40 mg/day and subsequently increased to 80 mg/day or 120 mg/day to achieve a goal uric acid of <6 mg/dL. Experience shows that 70% of patients with tophaceous gout can achieve these levels on 80 to 120 mg/day. Febuxostat is metabolized by the liver so there is no need to decrease the dose with GFR >30 mL/min. However, it should not be used in patients with severe hepatic disease. Both tablet doses cost the same: $200 per month.

    Neither allopurinol nor febuxostat should be started during an acute gout attack. Either one can be started after the attack is completely resolved. If a patient experiences a gout attack while receiving one of these drugs they should continue to take them throughout the attack.

16. **List the major toxicities of allopurinol.**

    The overall incidence of side effects is around 20%, but only 5% of all patients discontinue therapy as a result of drug toxicity (Box 86-2).

Box 86-2. The Major Toxicities of Allopurinol

Common (rarely serious)
Acute gouty arthritis
Maculopapular erythematous rash (3%) – risk is three times higher if on ampicillin/amoxicillin
Nausea
Diarrhea
Abnormal liver-associated enzymes (6%)
Headache
Cataracts

Uncommon (potentially serious)
Toxic epidermal necrolysis, exfoliative dermatitis
Allopurinol hypersensitivity syndrome (0.1% to 0.4%)
Bone marrow suppression
Hepatitis
Vasculitis
Peripheral neuropathy
Renal failure (interstitial nephritis)
Oxipurinol xanthine nephrolithiasis
Cataracts
Sarcoid-like reaction
Alopecia
Lymphadenopathy
Fever
Death

17. **What is the allopurinol hypersensitivity syndrome?**
The allopurinol hypersensitivity syndrome (AHS) occurs in 0.1% to 0.4% of patients. It is more common (5% to 10% of patients) in patients who have previously developed a maculopapular rash on allopurinol. Patients who develop this syndrome usually have associated renal insufficiency (75%) and are on diuretic therapy (50%). Recently, this syndrome has been reported to be associated with **HLA-B*5801**, which occurs with a frequency of up to 7% in all races. It is most common in Koreans, Han Chinese, and Thai patients. AHS typically occurs 2 to 4 weeks after initiating therapy, with significant morbidity and a mortality rate as high as 25%. Clinical manifestations of this syndrome include skin rash, fever, eosinophilia, hepatic necrosis, leukocytosis, and worsening renal function in most patients. Treatment includes high-dose steroids and hemodialysis (to remove oxipurinol).
PEARL: Some investigators recommend an allopurinol starting dose of no more than 1.5 mg per unit of estimated GFR to decrease the patient's risk for getting AHS (e.g., if GFR is 50 mL/min then the starting dose should be no more than 75 mg/day).

18. **An organ transplant patient with recurrent gouty arthritis and tophi is referred to you for treatment. His medications include prednisone, cyclosporine, and azathioprine. Laboratories include creatinine 1.8 mg/dL and uric acid 12 mg/dL. What precautions must be taken when prescribing medications for his tophaceous gout?**
Acute gout attacks:
- NSAIDs cannot be used, owing to renal insufficiency.
- Adrenocorticotropic hormone cannot be used, owing to lack of adrenal response as the patient is on chronic prednisone.
- Best therapy is oral, intramuscular, or intraarticular steroids.

Chronic suppression:
- Colchicine can be *dangerous in patients on cyclosporine*. Cyclosporine binds to the multidrug resistance (MDR-1)-related p-glycoprotein (P-gp) that is on the membrane of cells. This protein is an ATP-dependent efflux pump that transports drugs out of liver, renal, and intestinal cells. This transport system is important in hepatic and renal transport of colchicine. Cyclosporine is an inhibitor of MDR-mediated transport causing less colchicine excretion in urine and bile leading to higher colchicine blood levels. Patients most commonly develop a severe neuromyopathy. Tacrolimus is a weak P-gp inhibitor and thus is less likely to cause colchicine toxicity.

Hypouricemic therapy:
- Uricosuric medications are ineffective in patients with low creatinine clearance.
- Allopurinol and febuxostat inhibit xanthine oxidase, which also breaks down azathioprine. Consequently, azathioprine toxicity is magnified unless its dose is decreased 75%. Even with azathioprine dose reduction, neutropenia commonly occurs. Therefore, the safer option is to recommend the patient be switched from azathioprine to mycophenolate mofetil, which is not affected by allopurinol or febuxostat.
- Owing to renal insufficiency, allopurinol dose is adjusted to give 100 mg for each 30 mL/min of creatinine clearance. Febuxostat may be a safer choice because it is not renally excreted.
- Pegloticase may be considered to "debulk" his tophi.

19. **What drug interactions can occur with the xanthine oxidase inhibitors?**
- *Allopurinol:* azathioprine and 6-mercaptopurine, which are metabolized by xanthine oxidase, should not be given with allopurinol owing to risk of bone marrow suppression. Theophylline levels are also increased because it is also metabolized by xanthine oxidase. Ampicillin/amoxicillin increase the chance of developing an allopurinol rash. Thiazide diuretics reduce allopurinol excretion, increasing its toxicity. Allopurinol increases cyclophosphamide, warfarin, and cyclosporine levels.
- *Febuxostat:* because it inhibits xanthine oxidase, coadministration of febuxostat with azathioprine, 6-mercaptopurine, and theophylline should be avoided to limit toxicities.

20. **When should febuxostat be used instead of allopurinol?**
Febuxostat is 50 times more expensive than allopurinol. Therefore, it should be used in patients who have had severe allopurinol toxicity or who fail to respond to allopurinol. Use of desensitization protocols for allopurinol rashes is no longer recommended, especially in patients with the HLA-B*5801 allele.

21. **What is pegloticase?**
Unlike other mammals, humans do not have uricase to convert uric acid to the more soluble (5 to 10×) allantoin. Pegloticase is a recombinant mammalian uricase attached to polyethylene glycol (PEG). Owing to its cost, it is best used for the treatment of severe (tophi) or refractory (>3 attacks/year) gout patients who cannot lower their uric acid to <6 mg/dL with xanthine oxidase inhibitors. Some physicians use it as "induction" therapy to lower the uric acid load in patients with tophaceous gout. Notably, its pharmacokinetics is not affected by renal function.

22. **How is pegloticase administered? What precautions need to be taken?**
- Pegloticase (Krystexxa) is given as a 2-hour intravenous infusion of 8 mg every 2 weeks. Cost: $2300/infusion.
- All patients must be screened for G6PD deficiency before pegloticase administration. Do not use in patients with low G6PD enzyme activity.

- All patients should have a serum uric acid *before* each infusion after the initial dose. A uric acid level >6 mg/dL indicates there has been a loss of efficacy resulting from development of antipegloticase antibodies. Development of these antibodies is associated with infusion reactions including anaphylaxis (7%) and thus the infusion should not be given if the uric acid is not low.
- Patients who receive pegloticase should not be continued on other uric acid lowering medications. This is because use of these medications will keep the uric acid low and the physician will not be able to follow the uric acid level to determine if the patient has developed anti-PEG antibodies.
- All patients should receive premedication (fexofenadine 60 mg night before and before infusion, 1000 mg acetaminophen and Solu-Cortef 200 mg intravenous before infusion) to prevent mild/moderate infusion reactions, which occur in up to 25% of patients even when the uric acid is <6 mg/dL.
- Pegloticase profoundly lowers the uric acid level within 24 hours and increases the chance of gouty flares (80% of patients). Patients should receive prophylaxis against gout flares (colchicine, NSAIDs, or prednisone) starting 1 week before starting pegloticase.

23. **Identify the sites of action for drugs that are used to lower serum urate levels.**

    The sites of action for drugs that are used to lower serum urate levels are shown in Figure 86-2.

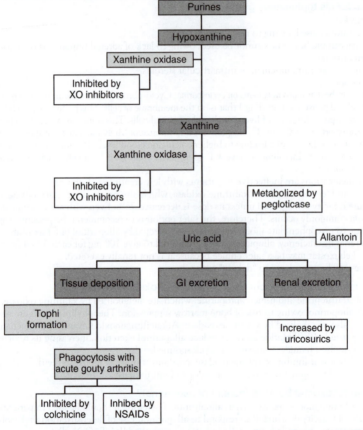

Figure 86-2. The sites of action for drugs that are used to lower serum urate levels. *GI*, Gastrointestinal; *NSAIDs*, nonsteroidal antiinflammatory drugs; *XO*, xanthine oxidase.

24. **Are any other drugs in development for gout therapy?**

    Lesinurad is a specific URAT1 inhibitor. Recent studies support its effectiveness when added to allopurinol. Others are in development.

BIBLIOGRAPHY

Becker MA, Schumacher HR, Espinoza LR, et al: The urate-lowering efficacy and safety of febuxostat in the treatment of the hyperuricemia of gout: the CONFIRMS trial, Arthritis Res Therapy 12:R63, 2010.

Becker MA, Schumacher HR, Wortmann RL, et al: Febuxostat compared with allopurinol in patients with hyperuricemia and gout, N Engl J Med 353:2450–2461, 2005.

Dalbeth N, Stamp L: Allopurinol dosing in renal impairment: walking the tightrope between adequate urate lowering and adverse events, Semin Dial 20:391–395, 2007.

Hung SI, Chung WH, Liou LB, et al: HLA-B*5801 allele as a genetic marker for severe cutaneous reactions caused by allopurinol, Proc Natl Acad Sci USA 102:4134–4139, 2005.

Khanna D, Khanna PP, Fitzgerald JD, et al: 2012 American College of Rheumatology Guidelines for management of gout. Part 2: therapy and antiinflammatory prophylaxis of acute gouty arthritis, Arthritis Care Res 64:1447–1461, 2012.

Simkin PA, Gardner GC: Colchicine use in cyclosporine treated transplant recipients: How little is too much? J Rheumatol 27:1334–1337, 2000.

Singer JZ, Wallace SL: The allopurinol hypersensitivity syndrome: unnecessary morbidity and mortality, Arthritis Rheum 29:82–87, 1986.

Stamp LK, O'Donnell JL, Zhang M, et al: Using allopurinol above the dose based on creatinine clearance is effective and safe in patients with chronic gout, including those with renal impairment, Arthritis Rheum 63:412–421, 2011.

Stamp LK, Taylor WJ, Jones PB, et al: Starting dose is a risk factor for allopurinol hypersensitivity syndrome: a proposed safe starting dose of allopurinol, Arthritis Rheum 64:2529–2536, 2012.

Sundy JS, Baraf HS, Yood RA, et al: Efficacy and tolerability of pegloticase for the treatment of chronic gout in patients refractory to conventional treatment: two randomized controlled trials, JAMA 306:711–720, 2011.

Suresh E, Das P: Recent advances in the management of gout, QJM 105:407–417, 2012.

Terkeltaub RA, Furst DE, Bennett K, et al: High versus low dosing of oral colchicine for early acute gout flare, Arthritis Rheum 62:1060–1068, 2010.

Terkeltaub RA, Furst DE, Digiacinto JL, et al: Novel evidence-based colchicine dose-reduction algorithm to predict and prevent colchicine toxicity in the presence of cytochrome P450 3A4/P-glycoprotein inhibitors, Arthritis Rheum 63:2226–2237, 2011.

Wason S, Digiacinto JL, Davis MW: Effect of cyclosporine on the pharmacokinetics of colchicine in healthy subject, Postgrad Med 124:189–196, 2012.

Further Reading

www.rheumatology.org

CHAPTER 87
BONE STRENGTHENING AGENTS
Michael T. McDermott, MD

KEY POINTS

1. Nonpharmacological measures that are effective for prevention and treatment of osteoporosis include adequate calcium and vitamin D nutrition, regular exercise, fall prevention, smoking cessation, and limitation of alcohol and caffeine intake.
2. Pharmacological therapy should be initiated in patients who have had a fragility fracture, a bone mineral density (BMD) T-score ≤ −2.5, or a FRAX-derived 10-year risk of ≥3% for hip fractures and ≥20% for other major osteoporosis fractures.
3. There are two primary categories of effective medications for treating osteoporosis: antiresorptive agents and anabolic agents.
4. Osteonecrosis of the jaw and atypical femoral fractures have been reported in some patients using antiresorptive therapies.
5. BMD loss during osteoporosis therapy is most often as a result of therapy nonadherence but affected patients should also be investigated for other causes of bone loss.
6. Bisphosphonates and teriparatide improve BMD and reduce fractures in patients with glucocorticoid-induced osteoporosis.

1. What nonpharmacological measures help to prevent and treat osteoporosis?

Adequate calcium intake (diet plus supplements)*: 1000 to 1200 mg/day, premenopausal women and men; 1200 to 1500 mg/day, postmenopausal women and men ≥ age 65 years.
Adequate vitamin D intake: 800 to 1200 international units/day.*,†
Regular exercise: aerobic and resistance.
Limitation of alcohol consumption to ≤2 drinks/day.
Limitation of caffeine consumption to ≤2 servings/day.
Smoking cessation.
Fall prevention.

*Taking more than the stated amounts of calcium and vitamin D is not recommended. Higher amounts may be associated with more kidney stones as well as more vascular calcifications, particularly in patients with renal insufficiency.
†Vitamin D3 and vitamin D2 are equivalent when taken on a chronic basis.

2. How can dietary calcium intake be accurately assessed?
The major bioavailable sources are dairy products and calcium-fortified fruit drinks. The following approximate calcium contents should be assigned for dairy product intake:

Milk/yogurt	300 mg/cup
Cheese	300 mg/oz
Fruit juice with calcium	300 mg/cup

In addition to calcium from dairy, add another 300 mg for the general nondairy diet for a reasonable estimate of total daily calcium intake.

3. How do you ensure adequate intake of calcium?
Low-fat dairy products are the *best* sources of calcium. Calcium supplements should be added when the desired goals cannot be reached with dietary sources. Calcium carbonate and calcium citrate are both well absorbed when taken with meals. Gastric acid is needed for normal calcium absorption; calcium carbonate absorption may be significantly reduced in patients who have achlorhydria or who use a proton pump inhibitor (PPI). Calcium citrate absorption is less likely to be affected by PPI use. Calcium citrate is also a better choice in patients with a history of kidney stones because citric acid is often low in the urine of stone formers.

4. What are the best ways to achieve adequate vitamin D intake?

There are two natural forms of vitamin D: cholecalciferol (D3) and ergocalciferol (D2). Fatty fish (D3) (400 international units/3.5 oz), fortified milk (400 international units/quart), and cereal products (50 international units/cup) are good dietary sources. Vitamin D2 and vitamin D3 supplements are available over the counter in multiple doses and 50,000 international units of vitamin D2 supplements can be given by prescription. Ten minutes of midday summer sunlight exposure to a fair-skinned person in a tank top and shorts not wearing sunscreen produces 10,000 international units of vitamin D3. Dark-skinned individuals and elderly get less production. However, many individuals wear sunscreen (SPF >8) which prevents vitamin D production by the skin. Therefore, oral vitamin D is necessary for most people. The optimal vitamin D intake is 800 to 1200 international units daily and should not exceed 4000 international units/day chronically.

5. How do you treat patients with vitamin D deficiency?

The goal serum 25-hydroxy vitamin D (25 OH vitamin D) level is 30 to 100 ng/mL. In general, 1000 units daily of vitamin D will raise the serum level by 6 to 10 ng/mL. I recommend the following:

25 OH D level	Management
20 to 30 ng/mL	2000 units of D3 daily
10 to 20 ng/mL	50,000 units of D2 weekly for 3 months, then 2000 units of D3 daily
<10 ng/mL	50,000 units of D2 twice weekly for 3 months, then 2000 units of D3 daily

Patients with malabsorption syndromes, bowel bypass surgery, and severe liver disease may require higher doses. Some may need to be treated with calcitriol. However, noncompliance is the most common reason that patients with persistently low vitamin D levels on therapy do not increase their levels.

6. When should pharmacological therapy be initiated for osteoporosis?

Pharmacological therapy should be advised for anyone who has any *one* of the following:
- History of vertebral or hip fragility fracture (also should include wrist and humerus).
- T-score < –2.5.
- The FRAX tool (Search Engine: FRAX), developed by the World Health Organization, is recommended for making treatment decisions in drug-naïve patients with osteopenia. Treatment is advised for those who have a 10-year risk of ≥3% for hip fracture or ≥20% for other major osteoporosis fractures.

7. Describe bone remodeling.

Bone remodeling is the process that removes old bone and replaces it with new bone. Osteoclasts attach to bone surfaces and secrete acid and enzymes that dissolve away underlying bone. Osteoblasts then migrate into these resorption pits and secrete osteoid, which becomes mineralized with calcium phosphate crystals (hydroxyapatite). Osteocytes serve as the mechanoreceptors that sense skeletal stress and send signals to orchestrate the process of bone remodeling in areas of bone that need renewal (Figure 87-1).

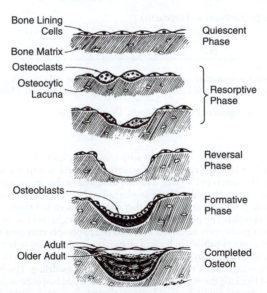

Figure 87-1. Bone remodeling. Osteoclasts resorb old bone, leaving an empty resorption pit. Osteoblasts then fill the pit by secreting osteoid, which is subsequently mineralized by calcium and phosphate from the extracellular fluid, forming new bone. (*From Peck WA, editor: Bone and mineral research annual 2, New York, 1984, Elsevier. Used with permission.*)

8. What are RANK, RANK-L, and osteoprotegerin?

RANK (receptor activator of nuclear factor κ) is a specific receptor on osteoclasts. RANK-L (RANK ligand) on osteoblasts binds to RANK to stimulate osteoclastic bone resorption. Osteoprotegerin (OPG) is a soluble decoy receptor produced by osteoblasts and bone marrow stromal cells that binds to RANK-L, preventing it from binding to RANK. Bone resorption is driven by RANK-L and inhibited by OPG.

9. How do the pharmacological agents for osteoporosis work?

Osteoporosis medications are classified into two main categories: antiresorptive agents and anabolic agents. Antiresorptive medications include the bisphosphonates, denosumab, raloxifene, calcitonin, and estrogens. Teriparatide is the only currently available anabolic agent.

10. What pharmacological agents are FDA-approved and how are they used?

Pharmacological agents that are FDA-approved and how are they used are outlined in Table 87-1.

Table 87-1. Pharmacological Agents That Are FDA-Approved

MECHANISM	ROUTE	DOSE	FREQUENCY
Antiresorptive agents			
Bisphosphonates			
Alendronate (Fosamax)*	Oral	10 mg	Daily
		70 mg	Weekly
Risedronate (Actonel)*	Oral	5 mg	Daily
		35 mg	Weekly
		150 mg	Monthly
Ibandronate (Boniva)	Oral	150 mg	Monthly
	IV	3 mg	Every 3 months
Zoledronic acid (Reclast)	IV	5 mg	Yearly
Nonbisphosphonates			
Denosumab (Prolia)	SC	60 mg	Every 6 months
Raloxifene (Evista)	Oral	60 mg	Daily
Calcitonin (Miacalcin)	Nasal	200 units	Daily
	SC†	100 units	Daily
Estrogen therapy (multiple preparations and regimens)			
Anabolic agents			
Teriparatide (Forteo)	SC†	20 μg	Daily

IV, Intravenous; SC, subcutaneous.
*Note that there is a Fosamax plus D preparation containing 70 mg of alendronate and either 2800 international units or 5600 international units of vitamin D3. There is also a 35-mg delayed release form of risedronate (Atelvia), which is given immediately after breakfast.
†Infusion times: IV ibandronate, 1 to 3 minutes; IV zoledronic acid, 15 to 30 minutes.

11. Explain how bisphosphonates are taken and why they work for osteoporosis?

The oral nitrogenous bisphosphonates are analogs of pyrophosphate and thus they avidly bind to bone. They have very poor intestinal absorption (<1%) that is further inhibited by the presence of food or medications in the gastrointestinal tract. Their major side effect is esophageal and gastrointestinal pain. To maximize intestinal absorption and to minimize gastrointestinal toxicity, they should be taken first thing each morning on an empty stomach with a full glass of water. The patient should then remain upright and take nothing by mouth for at least 30 to 60 minutes after medication ingestion. The absorbed bisphosphonate goes through the bloodstream and binds to bone with a terminal half-life in bone of up to 10 years. Approximately 50% to 60% of a dose does not bind to bone and is excreted unchanged in the urine. There are no drug interactions. Some of the bisphosphonate adsorbed to bone is ingested by the osteoclast during bone remodeling. The bisphosphonate acts on the osteoclast by binding and blocking the intracellular enzyme, farnesyl diphosphate synthase (FPPS), in the HMG CoA-reductase pathway (also known as the mevalonate pathway). Disruption of this pathway at the level of FPPS prevents the formation of two metabolites that are essential for connecting some small proteins (Ras, Rho, Rac) to the cell membrane, a process known as prenylation, which is important for proper subcellular protein trafficking. This interferes with lipid modification of the osteoclast cell membrane/cytoskeleton that is needed for maintaining the "ruffled border." This leads to osteoclast apoptosis causing significantly reduced bone resorption without affecting bone formation. As a result, bone formation temporarily exceeds resorption and bone mass increases. After approximately 24 months, bone formation declines to the level of resorption and bone mass stabilizes. Over this time, bone mass increases 4% to 8% in the spine and 3% to 6% in the hip. This is accompanied by a 33% to 68% relative risk reduction for incident vertebral fractures and a 40% to 50% reduction in hip fractures (not with ibandronate) depending upon the bisphosphonate that is studied. Zoledronic acid may be the most effective attributable to its antiresorptive potency, intravenous (IV) administration, and compliance.

12. **What precautions should be considered before prescribing bisphosphonates?**
    - Oral bisphosphonates are contraindicated in patients with esophageal problems (strictures, achalasia or severe dysmotility [scleroderma], varices), malabsorption, or inability to sit upright. These are indications for an IV formulation.
    - Oral bisphosphonates are contraindicated in patients with creatinine clearance (CrCl) <30 to 35 mL/min and IV bisphosphonates are contraindicated if CrCl <35 to 40 mL/min as a result of renal excretion. Patients with severe stage 3 chronic kidney disease (CrCl = 35 to 40 mL/min) who are receiving IV bisphosphonates should be taken off drugs affecting renal function if possible (nonsteroidal antiinflammatory drugs, diuretics), be well hydrated, and have slower infusion rates (ibandronate, 15 minutes; zoledronic acid, 60 minutes). IV ibandronate is probably safer than IV zoledronic acid because of less effect on renal tissue.
    - All invasive dental work should be performed before starting a bisphosphonate, if possible, to lessen future risk for osteonecrosis of the jaw.
    - Make sure 25 OH vitamin D is >20 (preferably 30) ng/mL before starting therapy.
    - IV bisphosphonates can cause a flu-like illness and bone pain lasting up to 2 to 3 days in 10% (ibandronate) to 30% (zoledronic acid) of patients. Premedication with acetaminophen will often prevent or lessen these symptoms.
    - Compliance is important. Failure to take a bisphosphonate at least 70% of the time significantly decreases its fracture protection.
    - BMD increase is less with low turnover and perimenopausal patients.
    - Fracture protection has not been proven in osteopenic patients, especially less than age 65 years. Use FRAX to determine need for therapy.
    - Bisphosphonates are contraindicated in patients who are pregnant or breastfeeding as a result of unknown effects on the developing skeleton. In the rare patient who requires a bisphosphonate and may want to get pregnant in the future, risedronate may be the safest to use attributable to more rapid clearance from the blood after it is stopped. However, risedronate should be stopped 6 months before getting pregnant.
    - Unusual side effects from bisphosphonates: ocular symptoms including uveitis, keratitis, optic neuritis, and orbital swelling have been reported.

13. **Is osteonecrosis of the jaw related to bisphosphonate therapy?**
    Osteonecrosis of the jaw (ONJ) presents as persistently exposed bone following an invasive dental procedure. It occurs most often (up to 10% risk) during high dose IV bisphosphonate therapy for multiple myeloma or bone metastases. ONJ has also been identified in some patients taking bisphosphonates for osteoporosis (0.3% risk). Good oral hygiene and regular dental care are the best preventive measures. Temporarily stopping bisphosphonates for invasive dental procedures (3 months before the procedure) is a common and reasonable practice but has not been shown to prevent ONJ. Some oral surgeons require a serum C-telopeptide to be in the normal range before they will do surgery.

14. **What about atypical femoral fractures with bisphosphonate use?**
    Atypical femoral fractures have been reported in some patients on long-term bisphosphonate therapy (>5 years). Any patient with unexplained thigh pain should be evaluated with a radiograph looking for a "bird beak" on the lateral aspect of the femoral shaft indicating a stress fracture (Figure 87-2). These fractures are frequently bilateral and may require femoral rods to stabilize. The risk appears low (1 in 2000 patients) but appears increased in active patients, those on corticosteroids, and those with very low bone turnover markers. Currently, no data exist regarding preventive measures. After 5 years of bisphosphonate use, many providers recommend a 1-year to 2-year drug holiday for osteopenic patients and a temporary switch to an anabolic or other nonbisphosphonate agent for those with previous fragility fractures or very low BMD. It is also recommended that after 3 years of zoledronic acid, treatment should be stopped for the next 3 years. A drug holiday decreases the risk for atypical fractures by 70%.

15. **Briefly discuss the issues regarding hormone replacement therapy.**
    The Women's Health Initiative (WHI) study report in 2002 confirmed the efficacy of estrogen replacement therapy (ERT) and hormone replacement therapy (HRT) for prevention of fractures but also confirmed a previously reported increased risk of breast cancer and cardiovascular events; following this report, the use of ERT and HRT significantly decreased. Currently, ERT (women without an intact uterus) and HRT (women with an intact uterus) are recommended mainly for limited use for up to 3 years to treat postmenopausal hot flashes.

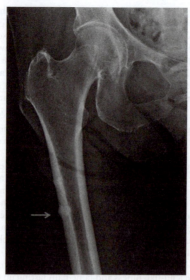

Figure 87-2. Atypical femoral fractures with bisphosphonate use.

16. **Discuss the use of selective estrogen receptor modulators in the management of osteoporosis.**
    Selective estrogen receptor modulators (SERMs) are agents that function as estrogen agonists in some tissues (bone) and estrogen antagonists in other tissues (breast). **Raloxifene (Evista)** is a SERM that has been shown to improve bone mass and to reduce spine fractures; it is FDA-approved for the treatment of postmenopausal osteoporosis. Raloxifene has also been shown to reduce the risk (76%) of developing invasive breast cancer. The dose is 60 mg every day. Side effects include hot flashes, leg cramps, and an increased risk of thromboembolic disease (especially in smokers) similar to that seen with HRT. Raloxifene increases BMD by 2% to 3% in both the spine and hip while reducing the relative risk of vertebral fractures by 31% to 49% without an effect on hip fracture reduction. An ideal patient to receive raloxifene is an osteoporotic patient with a personal or family history of breast cancer. It can also be used in osteoporotic patients with chronic kidney disease, although little data are available to support its efficacy in this patient group.

17. **What is denosumab and how does it work in osteoporosis?**
    Denosumab (Prolia) is a monoclonal antibody directed against RANK-L. This interferes with the ability of osteoblasts (and other cells with RANK-L on their surface) to bind to RANK and stimulate osteoclastic bone resorption. Denosumab is given in the clinic at a dose of 60 mg subcutaneously (SC) every 6 months. This medication is well tolerated, although there is a concern that infections could be increased because RANK-L is also on T helper cells and involved in dendritic cell activation. In trials, denosumab increased lumbar spine bone mass by 6.5% and hip mass by 3.5%. This was accompanied by a 68% reduction in vertebral and 40% reduction in hip fractures over 3 years. Because of lack of accumulation in bone, it is hoped that the incidence of ONJ and atypical femur fractures will be less, although both complications have been reported in patients on denosumab. Denosumab is cleared by the reticuloendothelial system and can therefore be used in osteoporotic patients with stage 4 chronic kidney disease (CrCl = 15 to 30 mL/min). Patients with chronic renal disease are most likely to get hypocalcemia with denosumab use and should be warned of this complication.

18. **How can parathyroid hormone be an anabolic agent for treating osteoporosis?**
    Persistently elevated serum parathyroid hormone (PTH) levels (primary hyperparathyroidism) promote osteoclastic bone resorption and bone loss. In contrast, intermittent daily pulses of exogenous PTH actually stimulate osteoblast differentiation, proliferation, and survival resulting in osteoid formation and increased bone mass. It also decreases the production of the bone inhibiting protein, sclerostin, from osteocytes.
    Teriparatide (forteo) is a 34 amino acid fragment of intact PTH that retains the ability to bind to and activate PTH receptors on osteoblasts and osteoblast precursors. It is self-administered daily at a 20-μg/day dose SC for 18 to 24 months. In trials, teriparatide increased lumbar spine bone mass by 9% to 13% and hip bone mass by 2.5% to 5% while decreasing the relative risk of new vertebral fractures by 65% and nonvertebral fractures by 50%. The most common side effects are similar to placebo and include headache, nausea, arthralgias, orthostasis, and flushing.

19. **What precautions should be considered before prescribing teriparatide?**
    - Teriparatide is contraindicated in patients at increased risk for osteosarcomas: Paget's disease, unexplained alkaline phosphatase elevation, children and young adults with open epiphyses, previous external beam or implant radiation therapy involving the skeleton.
        - In patients without contraindications, teriparatide does not cause an increased risk of osteosarcomas compared to the general population (1:250,000).
    - Use in patients with skeletal metastases and myeloma is contraindicated.
    - May cause hypercalcemia (digoxin toxicity, kidney stones) and hyperuricemia (gout).
    - Expensive. It is cost effective when used in patients at highest risk for osteoporotic fractures (T-score < −2.5 to −3.0 with history of fragility fracture; T-score ≤ −3.0) or in patients who develop a fragility fracture while on an oral bisphosphonate.
    - Teriparatide can help heal stress fractures (especially sacral, pelvic), nonunion fractures, and ONJ.
    - Teriparatide is usually not used concurrently with an antiresorptive agent as a result of blunting of the anabolic response. This is most applicable to patients who have previously received prolonged antiresorptive therapy before starting teriparatide. In patients who are started without previous exposure to antiresorptives, the simultaneous use of teriparatide and IV zoledronic acid may be better than either one alone.
    - A PTH level should be checked before use. If elevated, secondary causes (vitamin D deficiency) should be corrected to normalize the PTH level. The benefit of teriparatide in patients with persistent mild elevations of PTH is unclear but many experts feel it can still be effective. It can be used in patients with severe kidney disease but the effectiveness in these patients (who frequently have an elevated PTH) is unknown.
    - After treatment with teriparatide, an antiresorptive agent should be started to preserve the gains in bone mass.
    - After one 2-year course of teriparatide, a subsequent course in patients with severe osteoporosis is presently being studied (intermittent osteoanabolic therapy).

20. **Discuss the role of testosterone for the treatment of osteoporosis?**
    Men with osteoporosis and symptoms of hypogonadism may benefit from testosterone replacement therapy, especially if the level is <150 ng/dL. Testosterone can be administered intramuscularly (100 to 200 mg every 1 to 2 weeks) or as a transdermal patch (AndroDerm) or cream (Testim, AndroGel, Axiron, Fortesta). This therapy can increase bone mass but also increases risk of prostate cancer. Patients without improvement in hypogonadal symptoms should not continue because other therapies for osteoporosis are more beneficial.

21. **Outline an algorithm for the management of osteoporosis.**
    An algorithm for the management of osteoporosis is outlined in Figure 87-3.

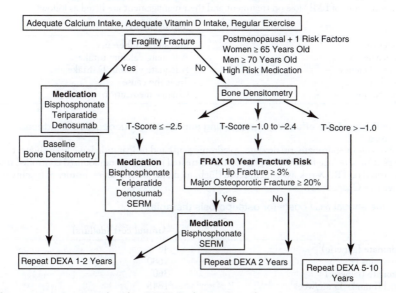

Figure 87-3. Osteoporosis management algorithm. *DEXA*, Dual-energy X-ray absorptiometry; *SERM*, selective estrogen receptor modulator.

22. **Have all of these medications been shown to prevent fractures?**
   All of the above FDA-approved medications have been demonstrated in randomized controlled trials to significantly reduce vertebral fractures in women with postmenopausal osteoporosis. Hip fractures have also been reduced by alendronate, risedronate, zoledronic acid, and denosumab. Nonvertebral fracture reduction has been reported with alendronate, risedronate, zoledronic acid, denosumab, and teriparatide.

23. **Are medication combinations more effective than single agents?**
   Combinations of antiresorptive agents increase bone mass more than single agents alone but fracture data are not yet available for such regimens. Furthermore, there are concerns that oversuppression of bone resorption may be harmful. Most combinations of anabolic and antiresorptive agents used concurrently have disappointingly shown no greater effects than single agents alone in patients who have previously received bisphosphonates; however, in drug-naïve patients the combination of teriparatide with zoledronic acid did show encouraging results. Studies investigating sequential rather than concurrent use of various agents are presently in progress.

24. **How should BMD be used to monitor the response to osteoporosis therapy?**
   BMD testing to monitor therapy responses is most often repeated after 2 years of treatment. The total hip BMD is the most accurate site to follow. To accurately interpret serial changes, the least significant change (LSC) for the specific instrument must be known. The LSC is a precision estimate that informs the user about the minimum BMD change that should be considered significant. Standard procedures for performing the LSC assessment are available on the International Society for Clinical Densitometry website, www.iscd.org.

25. **How do you interpret BMD changes in patients on osteoporosis medications?**

BMD change	Interpretation	Recommended action
Increase ≥ LSC	Good response	Continue therapy
No change or < LSC	Adequate response	Continue therapy
Decrease ≥ LSC	Treatment failure	Evaluate; consider therapy change

26. **What markers are available to assess bone remodeling and how are they used?**

Bone formation	Bone resorption
Serum alkaline phosphatase	Urine or serum N-telopeptides
Serum osteocalcin	Serum C-telopeptides

   Elevation of bone resorption biomarkers predicts future bone loss. A 30% reduction of these biomarkers after therapy is initiated verifies compliance and predicts an increase in bone mass. However, marked variability in biomarker measurement limits the utility of this tool.

27. **What do you do when BMD falls significantly during osteoporosis therapy?**
   The common causes of BMD loss on treatment and their management are listed as follows:

Cause	Management
Nonadherence	Encourage adherence
Calcium deficiency	Adequate calcium intake
Vitamin D deficiency	Adequate vitamin D intake
Secondary bone loss	Treat the cause
Treatment failure	Change medication

28. **Which medications are effective in preventing and treating glucocorticoid-induced osteoporosis?**
   Bisphosphonates (alendronate, risedronate, zoledronic acid) and teriparatide have been shown to significantly improve BMD and reduce fractures in glucocorticoid-treated patients in randomized controlled trials. They are instituted based on FRAX risk assessment score (high, medium, low), T-score, history of fragility fracture, and patient age (see Chapter 52).

29. **What are the annual *retail* costs for osteoporosis therapies?**

Drug	Annual cost (dollars)
• Alendronate (generic)	48
• Fosamax plus D	1680
• Risedronate (generic)	360
• Actonel (brand) 35 mg/week	1848
• Actonel (brand) 150 mg/month	2420
• Ibandronate (generic)	868

Drug	Annual cost (dollars)
• Boniva (brand)	2172
• Boniva (3 mg IV every 3 months)	2756 plus administration
• Reclast	1355 plus administration
• Evista	2160
• Prolia	2052 plus administration
• Forteo	15,600

30. **What new and emerging osteoporosis therapies are in development?**
    - Antiresorptive drugs
        - New SERMs: lasofoxifene, bazedoxifene, arzoxifene
        - Cathepsin K inhibitor: odanacatib
    - Osteoanabolic drugs
        - Teriparatide: transdermal, intranasal administration
        - Calcilytic (stimulates endogenous PTH release): ronacaleret
        - Sclerostin inhibitors: antisclerostin antibody (romosozumab)
        - Tryptophan hydroxylase 1 inhibitor: inhibit gut-derived serotonin

BIBLIOGRAPHY

Abrahamsen B, Eiken P, Eastell R: Subtrochanteric and diaphyseal femur fractures in patients treated with alendronate: a register-based national cohort study, J Bone Miner Res 24:1095–1102, 2009.

Andrews EB, Gilsenan AW, Midkiff K, et al: The US postmarketing surveillance study of adult osteosarcoma and teriparatide: study design and findings from the first 7 years, J Bone Miner Res 27:2429–2437, 2012.

Baron R, Hesse E: Update on bone anabolics in osteoporosis treatment: rationale, current status, and perspectives, J Clin Endocrinol Metab 97:311–325, 2012.

Black DM, Bauer DC, Schwartz AV, et al: Continuing bisphosphonate treatment for osteoporosis—For whom and how long? N Engl J Med 366:2051–2053, 2012.

Black DM, Cummings SR, Karpf DB, et al: Randomized trial of effect of alendronate on risk of fracture in women with existing vertebral fractures, Lancet 348:1535–1541, 1996.

Black DM, Delmas PD, Eastell R, et al: Once yearly zoledronic acid for treatment of postmenopausal osteoporosis, N Engl J Med 356:1809–1822, 2007.

Black DM, Schwartz AV, Ensrud KE, et al: Effects of continuing or stopping alendronate after 5 years of treatment: the Fracture Intervention Trial Long Term Extension (FLEX), a randomized trial, JAMA 296:2927–2938, 2006.

Bonnick S, Johnston CC, Kleerekoper M, et al: Importance of precision in bone density measurements, J Clin Densitom 4:1–6, 2001.

Chesnut CH, Silverman S, Andriano K, et al: A randomized trial of nasal spray salmon calcitonin in postmenopausal women with established osteoporosis: the Prevent Recurrence of Osteoporotic Fractures Study, Am J Med 109:267–276, 2000.

Cummings SR, San Martin J, McClung MR, et al: Denosumab for prevention of fractures in postmenopausal women with osteoporosis, N Engl J Med 361:756–764, 2009.

Dawson-Hughes B, Bischoff-Ferrari HA: Therapy of osteoporosis with calcium and vitamin D, J Bone Miner Res 22:V59–V63, 2007.

Delmas PD, Recker RR, Chesnut CH, et al: Daily and intermittent oral ibandronate normalize bone turnover and provide significant reduction in vertebral fracture risk: results from the BONE study, Osteoporosis Int 15:792–798, 2004.

Ettinger B, Black DM, Mitlak BH, et al: Reduction of vertebral fracture risk in postmenopausal women with osteoporosis treated with raloxifene, JAMA 282:637–645, 1999.

Fauvus MJ: Bisphosphonates for osteoporosis, N Engl J Med 363:2027–2035, 2010.

Goldstein SR, Duvernoy CS, Calaf J, et al: Raloxifene use in clinical practice: efficacy and safety, Menopause 16:413–421, 2009.

Grossman JM, Gordon R, Ranganath VK, et al: American College of Rheumatology 2010 recommendations for the prevention and treatment of glucocorticoid-induced osteoporosis, Arthritis Care Res 62:1515–1526, 2010.

Harris ST, Watts NB, Genant HK, et al: Effects of risedronate treatment on vertebral and nonvertebral fractures in women with postmenopausal osteoporosis. A randomized controlled trial, JAMA 282:1344–1352, 1999.

Hellstein JW, Adler RA, Edwards B, et al: Managing the care of patients receiving antiresorptive therapy for the prevention and treatment of osteoporosis: executive summary of recommendations from the American Dental Association Council on Scientific Affairs, J Am Dental Assoc 142:1243–1251, 2011.

Holick MF: Vitamin D deficiency, N Engl J Med 357:266–281, 2007.

Khosla S: Update on estrogens and the skeleton, J Clin Endocrinol Metab 95:3569–3577, 2010.

Khosla S, Burr D, Cauley J, et al: Bisphosphonate-associated osteonecrosis of the jaw: report of a task force of the American Society for Bone and Mineral Research, J Bone Miner Res 22:1479–1491, 2007.

Lewiecki EM: Nonresponders to osteoporosis therapy, J Clin Densitom 6:307–314, 2003.

Lewiecki EM: In the clinic. Osteoporosis, Ann Int Med 155:1–15, 2011.

Lyles KW, Colon-Emeric CS, Magaziner JS, et al: Zoledronic acid and clinical fractures and mortality after hip fracture, N Engl J Med 357:1799–1809, 2007.

McClung MR, Geusens P, Miller PD, et al: Effect of risedronate on the risk of hip fracture in elderly women, N Engl J Med 344:333–340, 2001.

McClung MR, Lewiecki EM, Cohen SB, et al: Denosumab in postmenopausal women with low bone mineral density, N Engl J Med 354:821–831, 2006.

Murad MH, Drake MT, Mullan RJ, et al: Comparative effectiveness of drug treatments to prevent fractures: a systemic review and network meta-analysis, J Clin Endocrinol Metab 97:1871–1880, 2012.

Neer RM, Arnaud CD, Zanchetta JR, et al: Effect of parathyroid hormone (1-34) on fractures and bone mineral density in postmenopausal women with osteoporosis, N Engl J Med 344:1434–1441, 2001.

Orwoll E, Ettinger M, Weiss S, et al: Alendronate for the treatment of osteoporosis in men, N Engl J Med 343:604–610, 2000.

Orwoll E, Scheele WH, Paul S, et al: The effect of teriparatide [human parathyroid hormone (1-34)] therapy on bone density in men with osteoporosis, J Bone Miner Res 18:9–17, 2003.

Rittmaster RS, Bolognese M, Ettinger MP, et al: Enhancement of bone mass in osteoporotic women with parathyroid hormone followed by alendronate, J Clin Endocrinol Metab 85:2129–2134, 2000.

Saag K, Zanchetta JR, Devogelaer JP, et al: Effects of teriparatide versus alendronate for treating glucocorticoid-induced osteoporosis: thirty-six month results of a randomized, double-blind, controlled trial, Arthritis Rheum 60:3346–3355, 2009.

Schilcher J, Michaelsson K, Aspenberg P: Bisphosphonate use and atypical fractures of the femoral shaft, N Engl J Med 364:1728–1737, 2011.

Shane E, Burr D, Ebeling PR, et al: Atypical subtrochanteric and diaphyseal femoral fractures: report of a task force of the American Society for Bone and Mineral Research, J Bone Miner Res 25:2267–2294, 2010.

Silva BC, Bilezikian JP: New approaches to the treatment of osteoporosis, Annu Rev Med 62:307–322, 2011.

Watts NB, Lewiecki EM, Bonnick SL, et al: Clinical value of monitoring BMD in patients treated with bisphosphonates for osteoporosis, J Bone Miner Res 24:1643–1646, 2009.

Weinstein RS: Clinical practice. Glucocorticoid-induced bone disease, N Engl J Med 365:62–70, 2011.

Woo SB, Hellstein JW, Kalmar JR: Systemic review: bisphosphonates and osteonecrosis of the jaws, Ann Intern Med 144:753–761, 2006.

Writing Group for the Women's Health Initiative Investigators: Risk and benefits of estrogen plus progestin in healthy postmenopausal women. Principal results from the Women's Health Initiative randomized controlled trial, JAMA 288:321–333, 2002.

Xiao Q, Murphy RA, Houston DK, et al: Dietary and supplemental calcium intake and cardiovascular disease mortality, JAMA Intern Med 173:639–646, 2013.

REHABILITATIVE TECHNIQUES

Venu Akuthota, MD

CHAPTER 88

> **KEY POINTS**
>
> 1. The major goal of rehabilitative techniques is to maximize function.
> 2. "ADEPTTS" is a useful mnemonic to screen for a patient's functional limitations.
> 3. A properly fitted cane used in the contralateral hand can unweight a diseased hip by 25%.
> 4. Physical modalities are used as an adjunct to facilitate active therapy.
> 5. Fatigue for more than 1 hour or soreness for more than 2 hours after exercise indicates too much exercise for a patient with arthritis.

1. **What are the goals of rehabilitation for patients with rheumatic disease?**
   The goals of rehabilitation are to:
   - Maintain or restore an individual's ability to function successfully in personal, family, and community life.
   - Maintain or improve range of motion (ROM).
   - Prevent or reduce contractures.
   - Increase strength and enhance endurance.
   - Improve a patient's overall feeling of well-being.
   - Self-management.

2. **Which functional areas may need to be assessed in a patient with a rheumatic disease?**
   - **Physical function assessment**
     - History: pain and fatigue (can use visual analog scales).
     - Physical examination.
       - Manual muscle strength testing.
       - ROM (can use goniometer).
       - Transfers and ambulation.
     - Ability to perform activities of daily living.
       - Recreational (avocational) or leisure activities.
       - Occupational (vocational) activities including job, housework, and schoolwork.
       - Sexual activities.
       - Sleep history.
   - **Psychological/cognitive functional assessment**
     - Affective function (depression, anxiety, mood).
     - Coping skills.
     - Cognitive function.
     - Compliance with treatment plan.
   - **Social function assessment** (family, friends, community)
     - Social support systems.
     - Interpersonal relationships.
     - Social integration.
     - Ability to fulfill social roles.
     - Socioeconomic/financial.

3. **A quick screen of the functional abilities of a patient with rheumatic disease should include which areas?**
   The most critical functional areas to be reviewed when time is limited can be remembered by using the mnemonic ADEPTTS—how well a patient "adapts" to his/her physical disability:
   A—Ambulation
   D—Dressing
   E—Eating
   P—Personal hygiene

T—Transfers
T—Toileting
S—Sleeping/Sexual activities

4. What healthcare personnel are available to help rehabilitate patients with rheumatic diseases? What rehabilitative techniques does each use?
Physical therapist (PT)—administers and instructs patients in the use of various therapeutic and pain-relieving techniques including heat, cold, traction, diathermy, electrical stimulation, therapeutic exercise, stretching, transfer skills, ambulation methods, and joint ROM/function/strength.
Occupational therapist (OT)—responsible for optimizing function by instruction in joint protection and energy conservation. In addition, OTs provide or fabricate adaptive equipment and splinting, especially for upper-extremity functional activities.
Podiatrist—evaluate and treat foot and ankle disorders, provide orthotics for foot problems.
Social workers and rehabilitation counselors—assist in the management of social, economic, and psychological problems that creates stress for each patient and family. This can include assistance in recreational activities as well as interpersonal and sexual relationships.
Psychotherapists—assist a patient with the psychological problems that arise from dealing with pain and loss of function.
Vocational counselors—can mobilize community resources to retrain and restore each patient to the workplace.
Arthritis rehabilitation nurses and patient educators—assist in instruction about the rheumatic disease and its therapy. Provide information, monitor compliance, and give emotional support to each patient and family.

EXERCISE AND REST

5. Name three forms of rest.
Rest in a person with arthritis may be done specifically to benefit an inflamed joint and to provide energy conservation.
Local rest is performed in a specific joint utilizing splinting techniques to reduce pain, inflammation, or to prevent contracture. However, disuse or excessive rest and inactivity must be avoided as a patient can lose up to 30% of muscle bulk and 5% to 10% of its strength within 1 week if a joint is immobilized.
Systemic rest is used for a period of up to 4 weeks if appropriate antiinflammatory medication and outpatient rehabilitation management are ineffective in alleviating the manifestations of systemic diseases such as rheumatoid arthritis or polymyositis. However, excessive rest must be avoided.
Short rest periods are becoming increasingly popular, particularly in patients with rheumatoid arthritis. These are a preventative and proactive means of managing inflammation and fatigue. The patient interrupts daily activities of longer than 30 continuous minutes to take short breaks.

6. How does exercise benefit a patient with arthritis?
Fatigue, weakness, and decreased stamina or endurance are common symptoms in patients with rheumatic disease. Disuse or excessive rest and inactivity can be a major cause of lost muscle strength. In addition, joint immobility can lead to contractures with loss of ROM. Therapeutic exercise can prevent or improve these problems.

7. Which factors need to be considered in prescribing an exercise program for a patient with a rheumatic disease?
- Stage of disease.
- Extent of inflammation and deformity.
- The patient's general medical condition.
- Types of activities a patient enjoys (to improve compliance).

8. Name three types of ROM exercise.
- **Passive ROM**—motion is performed by the therapist or mechanical device without help of a patient.
- **Active ROM**—a patient performs the movement.
- **Active-assisted ROM**—a patient moves the limb with the assistance of the therapist.

9. What is the minimum ROM of each joint that allows adequate function to perform activities of daily living?
The minimum ROM of each joint that allows adequate function to perform activities of daily living is outlined in Table 88-1.

10. What types of active exercise are used to increase muscle strength and endurance in a patient with arthritis?
- **Isometric training**: a static muscle contraction in which the muscle length does not change and the limb does not move through ROM. Two to six contractions of each muscle are recommended, with each contraction held for 3 to 6 seconds with 20- to 60-second rest periods between contractions. This form of exercise is particularly good to maintain or increase muscle bulk and strength without increasing joint inflammation in a patient with active arthritis.

Table 88-1. The Minimum ROM of Each Joint That Allows Adequate Function to Perform Activities of Daily Living

JOINT	ROM
TMJ	2.5 cm of jaw opening
Shoulder	Flexion 45°, abduction 90°, external rotation 20°
Elbow	Flexion 70°
Wrist	Dorsiflexion 5° to 10°, supination 10° to 15°
MCP	Flexion >30°
PIP	Flexion >30°
DIP	Flexion >30°
CMC	Internal rotation >30°
Hip	Extension 0° to flexion 30°
Knee	Neutral to 60° flexion
Ankle	Plantar flexion 20° to 10° of dorsiflexion

Adapted from Hicks JE: Exercise in patients with inflammatory arthritis and connective tissue disease, Rheum Dis Clin North Am 16:845, 1990.
CMC, Carpometacarpal joint; DIP, distal interphalangeal joint; MCP, metacarpophalangeal joint; PIP, proximal interphalangeal joint; ROM, range of motion; TMJ, temporomandibular joint.

- **Isotonic exercise**: a dynamic muscle contraction with movement through an arc of motion against a fixed resistance. It should be done when joint inflammation is under control. Isotonic training begins with 1- to 2-pound weights. Before increasing weight, patients should comfortably perform 12 repetitions.
- **Isokinetic exercise**: the rate of movement is held constant, but the force produced by the individual may vary through the arc of motion. This form of exercise is rarely used in rehabilitation of patients with arthritis.
- **Aerobic and aquatic exercise programs.**

11. **How does strength training differ from endurance training?**
    Strength is increased by isometric exercises and by isotonic exercises with increased resistance, resulting in fewer repetitions (7 to 10 repetitions). Endurance is increased by isotonic exercises with low resistance, enabling multiple repetitions (3 sets of 10 repetitions).

12. **In which aerobic activities can a patient with rheumatic disease participate to increase cardiovascular fitness?**
    Swimming, walking, stationary bicycling, elliptical training, and treadmill walking are recommended to increase cardiovascular fitness. The intensity should be sufficient to elevate the heart rate to 75% of maximum (220 − age) for 20 to 40 minutes.

13. **How often should a patient with arthritis exercise?**
    All patients with arthritis should perform stretching for 10 minutes and ROM exercises daily. A patient with active joint inflammation or those with Class III or Class IV functional capacity should also do isometric exercises and aquatic therapy for 30 minutes, 3 to 4 times a week. A patient whose disease is controlled and is functional Class I or Class II should do isotonic exercises and aerobic exercises for 30 minutes, 3 to 4 times a week. Particular attention should be given to strengthening the shoulder and knee musculature.

14. **How can a patient with arthritis determine if they have done too much exercise?**
    - Excessive pain during the exercise session.
    - Postexercise fatigue lasting >1 hour.
    - Postexercise soreness lasting >2 hours.
    - Increased joint pain or swelling the day following exercise.

15. **What precautions should be taken before advising a patient to perform isometric exercise training?**
    Isometric exercises, particularly of the upper extremities, increase systemic peripheral vascular resistance. These exercises are relatively contraindicated in patients with severe hypertension or a history of significant cardiovascular or cerebrovascular disease.

PHYSICAL MODALITIES

16. **Which physical modalities are available for the management of musculoskeletal pain?**
    The main purpose of physical modalities is to decrease pain so that a patient can participate in therapeutic exercises. Modalities available are:
    - Thermal agents
      - Superficial moist or dry heat.
      - Deep heat with ultrasound or diathermy.
      - Cryotherapy.
    - Electrotherapy
      - Transcutaneous electrical nerve stimulation.
      - Iontophoresis.
    - Traction

17. **How are superficial and deep heat used in the treatment of musculoskeletal problems?**
    Superficial heat includes moist heat delivered by hot packs, whirlpool, paraffin baths, or aqua therapy and dry heat delivered by fluidotherapy. This heat only penetrates tissue to a depth of 1 to 1.5 cm, and its effects last for 30 to 45 minutes.
    Deep heat is delivered by ultrasound or short-wave diathermy. Tissues at a depth of 3 to 6 cm can be heated to 41°C. The effect lasts for 30 to 45 minutes, during which time exercises should be done.

18. **What are some of the therapeutic effects of heat treatments?**
    By warming tissue, several effects occur simultaneously: increased tendon and joint capsule extensibility, reduction in muscle spasm, production of analgesia, increased tissue blood flow, and increased tissue metabolism. Superficial joints are typically easier to heat by techniques such as hot packs, paraffin wax, fluidotherapy, hydrotherapy, and radiant heat. Paraffin baths of the hands are often used in patients with rheumatoid arthritis and scleroderma to reduce pain and improve ROM. To restore function, heat, both superficial and deep, is used in conjunction with formal therapy and therapeutic exercise; this improves joint ROM by way of reduction in tendon and joint capsule tightness and reduction of contracture.

19. **What are the relative contraindications to treating with heat?**
    Tissue pain and damage commence with tissue temperatures of 113°F (45°C). Increased collagenolysis has been found to occur with increased intraarticular temperatures. Although there are potentially adverse implications for using heat in inflammatory conditions, such as rheumatoid arthritis, investigators have not found increased joint destruction to occur when heat is used.
    Because pain is a critical warning sign of tissue injury, desensitized areas or patients with a reduction in mental status are contraindications to the use of heat. Other common contraindications include bleeding diathesis, acute hemorrhage or trauma, atrophic or scarred skin, and malignancy. Also, heat applications to the gonads or to a fetus should be avoided. Areas with inadequate vascular supply should not be heated because of their inability to dissipate heat appropriately or to meet the increased metabolic demands caused by the increased temperature. Deep heat should not be used if metal is in the area being treated. **Erythema ab igne** is a localized, reticular, net-like rash which commonly occurs after chronic exposure to a heating pad or other heat sources. Care should be taken to avoid placing heat sources directly onto the skin and should be laid on, not under, the body.

20. **How is cryotherapy applied?**
    Cold application can be very specific, as in the use of vapocoolant sprays, localized massage, or locally applied cold pack. Or it can be very generally applied, as in ice-water immersion, refillable bladders, thermal blankets, or contrast baths. For subacute pain and spinal muscle spasm, it is typically applied as ice massage or cold packs. A simple inexpensive method is to apply a bag of frozen vegetables to the area or to freeze water in a paper cup and use it as an ice massage to an area. Cryotherapy is the treatment of choice following acute injury, particularly when combined with compression.

21. **Both superficial heat and cryotherapy reduce muscle spasm. How does the mechanism of cold differ from that of heat?**
    Cold has its effect directly on the muscle, the intrafusal fibers of the muscle spindle mechanism, and sensory wrappings of the muscle spindles. Heat primarily affects muscle spasm indirectly by slowing the firing rate of secondary afferents, increasing the firing rate of Golgi tendon organs, and decreasing the firing rate of efferent fibers to the muscle spindle (gamma fibers).

22. **What are iontophoresis and phonophoresis?**
    It is the use of direct current to induce topically applied medications to migrate into soft tissues and nerves up to 3 to 5 mm deep. Common topical medications applied include lidocaine gel, corticosteroid (usually dexamethasone) gel, and analgesics. This therapy has been used in tendonitis (especially Achilles tendonitis), bursitis, and neuritis. Phonophoresis is similar to iontophoresis except it uses ultrasound to "drive" medication more deeply.

23. When is traction useful for the management of cervical and lumbar spinal disorders?
Traction involves applying force in a manner to distract the cervical or lumbar vertebral bodies. This increases the intervertebral foraminal area, allowing more space for the exiting nerve root. Cervical traction is set up in a specific position with weight from 10 to 15 pounds or more. Cervical traction has limited evidence in the setting of cervical radicular pain. Supine cervical traction units, rather than "over the door" pulley system traction units, are considered to be safer and allow less cervical extension. Note that anything which causes more cervical extension reduces the size of the intervertebral foramina causing more radicular pain and thus should be avoided.

Lumbar traction is applied with a patient supine and both hips and knees flexed to 90 degrees. The traction is 40 to 80 pounds. There is limited evidence on the efficacy of lumbar traction with lumbar spine disorders. Both cervical and lumbar traction work best if applied 2 or 3 times a day until pain relief occurs. Failure to improve pain within 2 to 4 weeks and/or exacerbation of pain during traction are indications to stop this therapy.

ORTHOSES, JOINT PROTECTION, AND ASSISTIVE DEVICES

24. Why are splints and orthotics used in patients with arthritis?
Splints and orthotics are used in the treatment of inflammatory and degenerative arthritis to unweight joints, create stability in selected joints, decrease or increase joint motion, or support the joint in the position of maximal function. They can either be purchased over-the-counter or custom-formed to fit an individual patient.

25. Name the major factor in patient noncompliance in the use of splints and orthotics.
The cosmetic appearance of the splint is a major factor in nonuse. Fear of public attention to the device, including discrimination at work and in other environments, adds to a patient's unwillingness to use the device. Compliance with splints is increased when the splints significantly improve pain or function and when family or support groups reinforce the need to use the splint regularly. Cosmetic splints, particularly for the small digits of the hand, can be constructed with precious metals and semiprecious stones.

26. What are joint protection techniques?
Techniques for joint protection and energy conservation include task modification, environmental design/modification, and adaptation. By reducing mechanical stress, joint integrity is preserved and inflammation is reduced. Minimizing static positions while emphasizing proper posture reduces stress on individual joints. Joint protection includes maintaining ROM, unloading painful joints, and adequate rest periods throughout the day.

27. How can the use of adaptive devices and mobility aids benefit a patient with arthritis?
Assistive devices which substitute for deficient function help a patient with arthritis conserve energy, decrease stress on joints, relieve pain, and be more functionally independent. Adaptive devices for kitchen, bathroom, and self-care are readily available and listed in many patient manuals. Mobility aids include canes, crutches (axillary, forearm, platform), walkers (manual, wheeled), wheelchairs (manual, powered), and scooters. In patients with spinal stenosis, a rolling walker with a seat can be helpful in producing a relatively flexed lumbar spine walking posture as well as providing a seat when needed to relieve neurogenic claudication pain.

28. In which hand should a cane be placed to provide weight-bearing relief for a diseased hip?
The cane is placed in the hand of the contralateral arm. This creates a moment arm that counteracts a patient's weight and significantly reduces by 25% the amount of force applied to the hip joint. Placing the cane on the same side as the involved hip actually increases loading on the hip joint and potentially exacerbates the discomfort, pain, or joint dysfunction. Note that with walking, the stress across the hip joint is equal to 2 to 3 times body weight.

29. For an involved knee or ankle, which hand should hold the cane?
Below the level of the hip, ground reactive force to an individual joint is relieved most effectively when the cane is held on the ipsilateral side as the involved joint. This position can be advantageous for climbing and descending stairs but can be disruptive to the normal rhythm of gait because of the reversal of the natural swing of the arm. The patient may find that the cane works well when held in the contralateral hand during normal ambulation, but then can change it to the ipsilateral side for specific actions or activities requiring direct force on the ankle and knee. With walking, the normal stress across the knee is 3 to 4 times body weight, whereas stress across the ankle can be as high as 4 to 5 times body weight.

30. How can you tell if a cane or crutch has been properly fitted to a patient?
A properly fitted cane or crutch should reach 8 inches lateral to the front of the foot when a patient is standing and holding the cane or crutch handle with the elbow flexed 15 degrees to 30 degrees. This position permits stability on standing and an easy reach to the ground ahead during walking. A quicker but less precise way is to make sure the handle of the cane reaches the wrist crease when a patient is standing upright with their arms hanging down and the cane by the side of their leg.

31. **What are the documentation requirements required by the Centers for Medicare and Medicaid Services to justify reimbursement for a powered mobility device (power wheelchair, scooter)?**
    - There must be a documented in-person "face-to-face" visit for a mobility evaluation. The physician should label the visit and state that it was a "Mobility Examination." Information in the history and physical examination must be specific and objective.
    - Complete history relevant to a patient's mobility needs in the *home*. **A powered mobility device (PMD) will only be authorized to facilitate movement around the home and not outside the home.** In this part, discuss: (1) symptoms that limit ambulation; (2) medical diagnoses responsible for these symptoms; (3) list which mobility-related activities of daily living in the home are impaired as a result of mobility limitations (e.g., move from room to room, dressing, grooming, toileting, feeding, bathing); (4) medications and other treatments tried to treat ambulation problems; (5) how far and at what pace can a patient ambulate without stopping; (6) history of falls; (7) what ambulatory devices (cane, walker) have been tried and why are they not sufficient (e.g., unsteady gait with falls, desaturates to <88%, upper extremity and/or lower extremity strength of 2/5 or less, poor balance); (8) why a manual wheelchair cannot meet a patient's needs (e.g., upper extremity strength 1/5, grip strength of 2/5, hemiplegia 1/5 attributable to cerebrovascular accident, contractures of hands, decreased ROM of shoulders and elbows, pain level 8/10 in hands or shoulders); (9) state that a patient has the physical and mental capacity to use a PMD safely; (10) state that a patient is willing and motivated to use a PMD. In addition, if a physician wants a patient to have a power wheelchair and not a scooter they have to state why a scooter will not meet a patient's needs (e.g., cannot safely transfer in/out scooter, cannot operate tiller of scooter, lacks postural stability, upper extremity strength 1/5, home environment does not provide adequate maneuvering for scooter).
    - Physical assessment must include: (1) height and weight; (2) cardiopulmonary examination including oxygen saturation with exertion; (3) musculoskeletal examination including arm and leg strength (0 to 5/5) and joint range of motion; (4) neurologic examination including gait, balance, and coordination. A physician should document if they observed a patient ambulate.

32. **What are the seven elements which must be included in the written order for any PMD?**
    - Beneficiary's name.
    - Equipment ordered: PMD is sufficient.
    - Date of face-to-face mobility evaluation: order for PMD must be forwarded to the supplier within 45 days of this evaluation.
    - Pertinent diagnoses with ICD-9 codes relating to need for PMD.
      - Include patient's height and weight to help supplier select appropriate equipment.
    - Length of need in months: 99 = lifetime.
    - Physician's signature.
    - Date of physician's signature.

33. **Describe shoe characteristics that should be recommended to patients with foot pain/arthritis.**
    - High heels and pointy-toed shoes should be avoided. If such must be worn, should be for no longer than 3 hours a day 3 times a week.
    - Floppy loafers or other shoes (i.e., can fold shoe toe to touch heel) will hurt feet.
    - Tie lacing of several holes to secure foot and be able to loosen with foot swelling. If hand deformities prevent tying laces then consider Velcro closures.
    - Need wide, deep toe box so toes are not crowded. Leather should be soft with no rubbing from internal stitching.
    - Heel height should be around 1 inch.
    - Heel counter should be firm to prevent foot pronation or rolling.
    - Soft cushioned sole (crepe sole) serves as a shock absorber.
    - If significant bony foot deformity may need custom-made shoes.
    - Recommend that patient try on shoes and walk around store for 15 to 20 minutes before purchasing the shoes.

SPECIFIC DISEASE REHABILITATION

34. **Why should persons with osteoarthritis engage in physical activity including exercise?**
Physical activity can countervail the detrimental effects of aging on fitness, strength, cardiovascular endurance, and functional limitations. Patients should be reassured that regular activity or exercise does not increase the risk of osteoarthritis (OA). Generally, physical activity reduces the risk of chronic diseases (cardiovascular, stroke, hypertension, diabetes, obesity, some cancers, and depression) and falls in the elderly. Physical activity has also been shown to delay cognitive impairment and to improve sleep.

35. **What types of exercise are available for a patient with OA?**
The MOVE consensus group promotes physical activity as a low-cost therapeutic option for individuals with hip and knee OA. The consensus group particularly promotes aerobic exercise (brisk walking) and strength or resistance training because evidence shows improvements in pain and function, particularly in individuals with knee OA. However, one specific form of resistance training has not been shown to be superior to

another (i.e., high versus low resistance; isometric versus dynamic training). Aquatic exercise can also improve pain and function and is a particularly beneficial exercise to start with for obese patients or individuals with more severe disease. Balance training has also been proven to be effective, whereas electrical stimulation and manual therapy have not been shown to be helpful.

36. **What is the best method for a patient with knee arthritis to walk up and down the stairs?**
   Up to heaven, down to hell. A patient should lead with the leg having the good (heaven) knee as he goes up stairs because there is more force across the knee of the climbing leg. The patient should lead with the leg that has the bad (hell) knee when going down stairs because there is more force across the trailing leg which supports the decent. He can also lock his bad knee on the decent when he leads with it thus providing more stability. During both the ascent and descent of stairs, the cane (supporting body weight on it) advances when the arthritic limb is brought forward.

37. **Can patients with rheumatoid arthritis benefit from a regular exercise program?**
   Regular exercise can increase their functional levels, including endurance, activities of daily living, and mobility. Exercise programs must be adjusted specifically for the disease process. Adaptive equipment and gyms focused toward the disabled population can be particularly helpful. Patients with rheumatoid arthritis benefit from low-repetition, low-resistance isotonic exercises, frequently undertaken through short arcs as compared with the entire arc of motion. Upper extremity ergometers can be used for aerobic activity in patients with rheumatoid arthritis with significant lower limb joint involvement. The addition of swimming, bicycling, gardening, and other activities helps preserve and develop both type I and type II muscle fibers.

38. **What rehabilitative techniques can be used for some other rheumatic diseases?**
   - Ankylosing spondylitis—spinal extension and hip and shoulder ROM exercises. Deep breathing exercises. Swimming is the best aerobic exercise because it promotes spinal extension and shoulder ROM in a relatively humid setting.
   - Polymyositis/dermatomyositis—isometric exercises may be performed at least 3 times per week after inflammation is under control to maintain strength. However, patients should avoid overuse weakness by not exercising to the point of muscle fatigue. Daily ROM exercises are important to prevent contractures.
   - Steroid-induced myopathy—active isometric and isotonic exercise program may decrease the severity of steroid myopathy.
   - Systemic sclerosis—ROM exercises and splinting to decrease contractures. Finger flexion and extension exercises.
   - Complex regional pain syndrome (previously called reflex sympathetic dystrophy)—deafferential techniques and weightbearing exercises for upper or lower limbs are very important. ROM exercises must be part of any program. Intervention techniques, such as stellate ganglion blocks, lumbar sympathetic blocks, ketamine infusions, or spinal cord stimulators, may be used to facilitate exercise treatment of complex regional pain syndrome.

Bibliography

Ayan C, Martin V: Systemic lupus erythematosus and exercise, Lupus 16:5–9, 2007.
Braddom RL: Physical medicine and rehabilitation, ed 4, Philadelphia, 2011, Elsevier Saunders.
Brakke R, Singh J, Sullivan W: Physical therapy in persons with osteoarthritis, PM R 4(Suppl 5):S53–S58, 2012.
Callahan LF: Physical activity programs for chronic arthritis, Curr Opin Rheumatol 21:177–182, 2009.
Cameron MH: Physical agents in rehabilitation: from research to practice, ed 3, St. Louis, 2008, Elsevier Health Sciences.
Christie A, Jamtvedt G, Moe RH, et al: Effectiveness of nonpharmacological and nonsurgical interventions for patients with rheumatoid arthritis: an overview of systematic reviews, Phys Ther 87:1697–1715, 2007.
Dagfinrud H, Hagen KB, Kvien TK: Physiotherapy interventions for ankylosing spondylitis, Cochrane Database Syst Rev 1:CD002822, 2008.
Delisa JA, Gans BM: Rehabilitation medicine: principles and practice, ed 4, Philadelphia, 2005, Lippincott Williams & Wilkins.
Roddy E, Zhang W, Doherty M, et al: Evidence-based recommendations for the role of exercise in the management of osteoarthritis of the hip or knee – the MOVE consensus, Rheumatology 44:67–73, 2005.
Schonstein E, Kenny DT, Keating J, et al: Work conditioning, work hardening and functional restoration for workers with back and neck pain, Cochrane Database Syst Rev 1:CD001822, 2003.
Steultjens EEMJ, Dekker J, Bouter LM, et al: Occupational therapy for rheumatoid arthritis, Cochrane Database Syst Rev 1:CD003114, 2004.
van Baar ME, Assendelft WJ, Dekker J, et al: Evidence of exercise therapy in patients with osteoarthritis of the hip or knee: a systematic review of randomized clinical trials, Arthritis Rheum 42:1361–1369, 2009.
Vliet Vlieland TPM, de Buck PDM, van den Hout WB: Vocational rehabilitation programs for individuals with chronic arthritis, Curr Opin Rheumatol 21:183–188, 2009.
Youdas JW, Kotajarvi BJ, Padgett DJ, et al: Partial-weight bearing gait using conventional assistive devices, Arch Phys Med Rhabil 86:394–398, 2005.

Further Reading

www.aapmr.org

CHAPTER 89
SURGICAL TREATMENT AND RHEUMATIC DISEASES
Donald G. Eckhoff, MD, MS

KEY POINTS

1. Inability to walk more than one block or stand longer than 20 to 30 minutes as a result of pain are indications for total hip and total knee replacement.
2. Periprosthetic osteolysis attributable to a biologic response to particulate debris is the most common cause of implant loosening.
3. Arthroscopic debridement is most beneficial in patients with osteoarthritis with mechanical symptoms such as locking.
4. Lumbar spine surgery is most successful in patients with radicular symptoms confirmed by clinical examination, electromyography (EMG), and magnetic resonance imaging (MRI) findings who have failed conservative therapy.

1. What are the major indications for total joint replacement surgery in patients with arthritis?
Joint replacement is indicated when pain has failed to respond to nonoperative management and is limiting activities of daily living. Pain relief is the most attainable result of surgery. Restoration of motion and function are less predictable.

2. What medical factors require preoperative attention in patients undergoing total joint replacement?
All surgical candidates for orthopedic reconstructive procedures require a comprehensive history and physical examination to assess the overall general operative risks. Patients should be examined for carious teeth, skin ulcerations (especially around the feet), and symptoms of urinary tract infection or prostatism, because these could increase the risk of postoperative infections. Women should have a urine culture to rule out asymptomatic bacteriuria. If patients are receiving nonsteroidal antiinflammatory drugs (NSAIDs), these medications should be switched to a COX-2 specific NSAID or stopped several days (at least five half-lives) before surgery to prevent bleeding as a result of their antiplatelet effects. Holding at least one dose of methotrexate and a biologic should be strongly considered.

3. What other factors must be addressed preoperatively in patients with rheumatoid arthritis?
Cervical spine—an unstable cervical spine attributable to arthritic involvement places a patient at risk for catastrophic neurologic loss when the neck is manipulated during intubation. Preoperative lateral flexion and extension radiographs of the cervical spine are mandatory in patients with rheumatoid arthritis (RA), especially if they have neck symptoms or long-standing disease with peripheral deformities. An increased anterior atlanto-dens interval >3 mm indicates disruption of the transverse ligament. An anterior atlanto-dens interval >7 mm or posterior atlanto-dens interval of 14 mm or less suggests cervical spine instability.

Autologous blood transfusion—preoperative autologous blood donation should be discussed.

Temporomandibular arthritis (especially patients with juvenile idiopathic arthritis) and cricoarytenoid arthritis—may make intubations more difficult.

Immune status—infection rates are significantly higher in patients with RA, partly because of the disease process and partly because of the immunosuppressive drugs used to control it. Patients should be on the lowest corticosteroid dosage possible. It is recommended that methotrexate be withheld for the week of surgery and the week after surgery (**controversial**). At least one dose of a biologic should be held before surgery.

Nutritional status—patients with RA may be relatively malnourished, which predisposes them to infection. Patients with a total lymphocyte count >1500/mm^3 and albumin level >3.5 g/dL are less prone to infections.

Hypothalamic–pituitary–adrenal axis—patients on chronic corticosteroid therapy are unable to respond normally to surgical stress. They must receive increased corticosteroids (stress dose) immediately preoperatively, intraoperatively, and postoperatively.

Cardiovascular status—patients with RA are at risk for premature atherosclerosis (relative risk 1.5×). Attention should be given to anginal chest pain and bruits.

4. **Patients with RA frequently have multiple joints involved. What is the recommended sequence for reconstructive surgery?**
   - Lower-extremity surgery is done before upper-extremity surgery, because crutch use postoperatively would place excessive demands on any upper-extremity reconstructive surgery.
   - In the multiply involved lower-extremity, the hip is reconstructed before the knee to get the best possible alignment of the knee and relieve referred pain from the hip to the knee. However, in patients with normal knee alignment, foot and ankle surgery should be performed before hip and knee replacement to provide stability for lower-extremity rehabilitation. Ankle and hindfoot procedures are done before forefoot reconstruction.
   - In the upper extremity, the preferred order is controversial. Usually proximal joints, nerve, and tendon problems are addressed before the hand and wrist. The wrist is done before the hand joints to help with alignment. For the shoulder and elbow, the most symptomatic joint is usually done first.

5. **What additional intraoperative and postoperative medical procedures are done to prevent postoperative complications following total hip arthroplasty or total knee arthroplasty?**
   Intraoperative **prophylactic antibiotics** are given to decrease the chance of infection. For lower-extremity total joint replacement (hip, knee), compression stockings, early ambulation, and **anticoagulation** are done to prevent postoperative deep venous thrombosis. Deep venous thrombosis occurs in 50% to 60% of patients, pulmonary embolus in over 10% of patients, and fatal pulmonary embolus in 0% to 3% of patients if postoperative anticoagulation (1 to 6 weeks) is not done.

6. **What is Steel's rule of thirds?**
   At the level of the first cervical vertebra (C1), the anteroposterior diameter is divided into thirds, allowing one third for the dens, one third for the spinal cord, and one third for free space. Because there is significant free space at this level, small degrees of C1 to C2 subluxation (3 to 7 mm) usually do not compromise the cord. However, when the *anterior* atlanto-dens interval (measured from the posterior part of the anterior arch of C1 to the anterior aspect of odontoid) becomes >10 to 12 mm, all the atlantoaxial ligamentous complex has usually been destroyed, and the space available for the spinal cord is usually compromised. Likewise, when the *posterior* atlanto-dens interval (measured from posterior aspect of the odontoid to the anterior aspect of the posterior arch of C1) is <14 mm, the spinal cord is usually compressed. (See also Chapter 14.)

7. **When should the cervical spine (C1 to C2) be fused in patients with RA?**
   - Operative stabilization of the rheumatoid cervical spine is indicated in patients with the following structural abnormalities:
     - Have atlantoaxial subluxation with a posterior atlanto-dens interval of 14 mm or less.
     - Have atlantoaxial subluxation and at least 5 mm of basilar invagination.
     - Have subaxial subluxation and a sagittal diameter of the spinal canal of 14 mm or less.
   - Indications for surgical stabilization based on the presence of neurologic symptoms can be prognostically classified as follows:
     - Ranawat Class I: no neurologic deficits. Neurologic deterioration rarely (10%) occurs. Conservative and surgical outcomes are similar so patients should be treated conservatively with medical treatment of their RA. Ten-year survival rate is 75%.
     - Ranawat Class II: subjective weakness with hyperreflexia and/or dysesthesia. Neurologic deterioration will occur in 67% with conservative therapy. With surgery, 50% improve and 40% stabilize neurologically. Ten-year survival rate is 65%.
     - Ranawat Class IIIA: objective weakness and long tract signs but able to walk. Neurologic deterioration occurs in all with conservative therapy. With surgery, 55% improve and 35% stay the same. Ten-year survival rate is 50%.
     - Ranawat class IIIB: quadriparetic and unable to walk. Neurologic deterioration occurs in all with conservative therapy. With surgery, 60% improve. Ten-year survival rate is 30%.

8. **Give the potential intraoperative and postoperative complication rates following cervical spine fusion in a patient with RA.**
   - Postoperative mortality: 0% to 10%. Has been as high as 33% for patients with severe neurologic compromise.
   - Wound infections and dehiscence.
   - Nonunion rates: 0% to 50%. Average is 20%.
   - Late subaxial subluxation below previous fusion as a result of transfer of increased stresses.

9. **What surgical procedures are available for patients with RA with shoulder involvement?**
   Surgical procedures of the shoulder are performed predominantly for pain control. An increase in range of motion usually does not occur. Replacement arthroplasty can include the entire joint, termed **total shoulder arthroplasty**, or only the humeral head, termed **hemiarthroplasty**. The principal factor in choosing between the two is the status of the glenoid. For maximal functional use and stability of a total shoulder arthroplasty, soft-tissue tension from an intact rotator cuff plays an integral role. If the rotator cuff is not intact and cannot be repaired, then a constrained arthroplasty, *"reverse arthroplasty"* (ball on glenoid side), bipolar arthroplasty, or an oversized hemiarthroplasty is chosen.

10. **What are the surgical options for management of arthritis involving the elbow joint?**
    - **Inflammatory** arthritis not responsive to medical management, synovectomy will temporarily control the disease and reliably decrease pain, but it infrequently has any positive effect on joint motion. Open synovectomy may also include excision of the radial head if significantly involved. However, total elbow arthroplasty is preferred to radial head resection/synovectomy in most patients. Arthroscopy is used for diagnostic purposes, removal of loose bodies, and synovectomy for both biopsy and treatment purposes.
    - **Osteoarthritis**: the ulnohumeral articulation is predominantly affected, usually by osteophytes that develop on the coronoid process or olecranon. Surgically, these osteophytes are removed arthroscopically or through an open incision. When the articular cartilage is lost, the joint surface can be resurfaced with autologous tissue, fascia lata most commonly.
    - **Posttraumatic arthritis** involving the radiohumeral or proximal radioulnar joint, a radial head excision can be performed with predictably good results, as long as the medial collateral ligament of the elbow is intact.

    Total elbow arthroplasty is becoming the surgical option of choice for most arthritic conditions of the elbow. This is attributable to the increasing reliability of the current prostheses and the magnitude of functional improvement for a patient. Overall pain relief is 90% with long-term complications of 10%, most commonly loosening. Elbow arthrodesis should be a very last resort, because this procedure makes it impossible to position the hand for functional use. It is reserved for an end-stage arthritic elbow from previous septic arthritis and in patients when total elbow replacement is not feasible.

11. **How are the common problems of the wrist in RA managed surgically?**
    RA has a predilection for the small joints of the hand and wrist. The wrist is almost universally involved and usually presents predictable patterns of involvement and resultant deformities. The goal of medical management lies in control of the inflammatory synovitis to prevent destruction of bony and soft-tissue structures. When this fails, surgery can be used to remove inflammatory synovium or correct deformity.

    The *dorsal wrist* capsule and dorsal tendon sheath are commonly involved with synovitis and tenosynovitis that can lead to extensor tendon rupture. Prevention of tendon rupture is far better than tendon transfer and, therefore, if medical control is inadequate, early surgical synovectomy and tenosynovectomy are warranted. The term **Vaughn-Jackson syndrome** is applied when the extensor tendons of the ring and small finger have ruptured. Primary tendon repair is usually not possible, especially if the rupture occurred longer than a few days previously. Tendon transfer surgery is then required to restore function.

    On the *volar* aspect of the wrist, tenosynovitis of the flexor tendons can cause compression of the median nerve in the carpal canal, leading to carpal tunnel syndrome. It can also lead to rupture of the flexor pollicis longus tendon, leading to inadequate thumb flexion and resting hyperextension at the interphalangeal joint. This is the **Mannerfelt syndrome** and requires tendon transfer or arthrodesis of the interphalangeal joint of the thumb.

    The *distal radioulnar* joint is commonly involved by synovitis, which leads to laxity of this joint, osseous destruction of the ulnar head, and pain with forearm rotation. The ulnar head becomes dorsally prominent and adds to stress on the ulnar extensor tendons. This constellation of findings is called the **caput ulna syndrome**. Its surgical management entails aggressive synovectomy, ulnar head excision, capsulorrhaphy, and lateral tenodesis using a portion of the extensor carpal ulnaris tendon.

    When the *radiocarpal joint* is involved with advanced changes, total wrist arthroplasty (TWA) or wrist arthrodesis can be used to control pain and improve function in over 90% of patients. However, over 20% of patients receiving a TWA will need a revision.

12. **What are the surgical options for basilar thumb osteoarthritis?**
    The carpometacarpal joint of the thumb, also known as the trapeziometacarpal or basilar joint, is a saddle-shaped articulation with a high propensity for degenerative change. Surgical procedures include implant arthroplasty, tendon interposition arthroplasty, tendon suspension arthroplasty, and arthrodesis. Implants have a high rate of failure, and work continues on a better prosthetic design. Tendon interposition ("anchovy procedure") entails placing a wad of tendon into the cavity created by removal of some or all of the trapezium. Tendon suspension is similar, except after the trapezium is removed, a weave of tendon is created that supports the thumb metacarpal base like a sling. Both tendon procedures result in a 30% to 40% loss of pinch strength. Arthrodesis is probably the best procedure for longevity of the reconstruction, but it restricts metacarpal motion and requires very precise positioning or function will not be optimal.

13. **How is a mucous cyst and osteoarthritis of the distal interphalangeal joint managed?**
    Mucous cysts are commonly associated with osteoarthritis of the distal interphalangeal (DIP) joints of the fingers. They present as a clear mucin-filled cystic mass, usually between the DIP joint and the proximal aspect of the nail. Pathophysiologically, the mucous cyst results from chronic inflammation secondary to a dorsal osteophyte of the DIP joint. Therefore, appropriate evaluation includes an X-ray, and definitive management must be directed at removal of the osteophyte. If the DIP joint is significantly painful or unstable, fusion of the DIP joint in mild flexion becomes the treatment of choice.

14. **How are deformities of the proximal interphalangeal joints surgically managed in patients with RA?**
    Boutonnière deformities result from synovitis within the proximal interphalangeal (PIP) joints, causing extensor tendon elongation and rupture, and leading to progressive flexion contractures. During early stages, synovectomy may be helpful.
    Swan-neck deformities progress through four stages of deformity. During the first three stages, splinting, synovectomy, and surgical release of intrinsic muscle tightness and tendon adhesions are used. In the last stage, when the PIP joint is destroyed, surgical options include joint replacement or fusion.
    In patients with destroyed PIP joints, total joint replacement is preferred for PIPs involved in grasping (third, fourth, and fifth PIPs), whereas fusion is used more for PIPs involved in pinch (thumb IP, second PIP).

15. **Describe the results of metacarpophalangeal joint surgery in patients with RA.**
    Synovitis of the metacarpophalangeal (MCP) joints ultimately leads to joint destruction, MCP subluxation, and ulnar deviation of the fingers. There is little evidence that prophylactic synovectomy slows joint destruction, but it may postpone the need for joint replacement surgery when done early before X-ray changes. MCP arthroplasty is indicated when synovitis has resulted in cartilage destruction, decreased motion, pain, ulnar drift, deformity, and loss of function. MCP arthroplasties, irrespective of design, result in 50 to 60 degrees of motion which may decrease to 30 degrees over time. Postoperative splinting and hand rehabilitation are critical for optimal results. Arthrodesis is not done except for the thumb MCP joint. This is because the thumb needs strength for pinch, whereas motion is less important.

16. **Name several symptoms that are indications for joint replacement surgery in a patient with arthritis of the hip or knee.**
    - Inability to walk more than one block as a result of pain.
    - Inability to stand in one place for longer than 20 to 30 minutes as a result of pain.
    - Inability to obtain restful sleep resulting from pain when rolling over in bed at night.
    - Inability to climb stairs without a railing (fall risk).
    - Difficulty putting on pants, socks, and shoes.

17. **How do cemented, cementless, and hybrid prostheses differ?**
    The terms cemented and cementless refer to methods of fixation of total joint arthroplasty prostheses for the hip and knee. Most experience is with **cemented** prostheses where a self-curing acrylic cement, polymethylmethacrylate, is used to improve fixation between the prosthetic component and bone. Advances in cementing techniques and materials have led to improved longevity and fewer problems with aseptic loosening. Patients who receive cemented prostheses can be walking without crutches within a few days.
    Cementless prostheses include press fit and porous ingrowth prostheses. *Press fit* relies on a snug fit between prosthesis and bone without the use of cement. *Porous ingrowth* prostheses contain pores located on the proximal portion of the femoral component and acetabulum that allow ingrowth or ongrowth of bone. Hydroxyapatite or growth factors may be incorporated into the porous coating to stimulate bone ingrowth and better fixation. Overall, there is bone ingrowth into approximately 10% of the porous-coated surface. Patients receiving a cementless prosthesis are on crutches for up to 6 weeks postoperatively.
    Cemented stems and cementless acetabular components have demonstrated the best longevity. Consequently, many surgeons use a cementless acetabular component with a cemented femoral component. This is termed a **hybrid hip replacement**.

18. **Who should get a cemented arthroplasty and who should get a cementless prosthesis?**
    In the **hip**, this is an area of controversy. Conventional wisdom in the United States suggests that younger, active patients with good bone quality in whom intimate apposition of prosthesis to bone can be achieved intraoperatively are the best candidates for cementless total hip arthroplasty (THA). This is usually a patient <50 to 60 years old with osteoarthritis of the hip. Cemented prostheses remain the "gold standard" and preferred in patients with RA with poor bone stock, in the elderly with low activity levels, and in hybrid hip implants. Regardless of the prosthesis, over 90% of THA are pain-free and without complications 10 to 15 years postoperatively.
    In the **knee**, cemented implants (posterior cruciate retaining, posterior stabilized condylar, and total condylar prosthesis) demonstrate 90% to 95% satisfactory results at 5 to 10 years for both patients with RA and osteoarthritis. Cementless prostheses have not been successful as a result of poor bone ingrowth on the patella and tibial components. In the **hybrid knee replacement**, the cementless component is reserved for the femur, whereas tibia and patella components are cemented.

19. **What are the differences between minimally invasive and traditional/standard techniques for THA?**
    The *traditional/standard technique* for THA is a posterior lateral, direct lateral, or anterior approach with an incision that is 6 to 12 inches long. This technique provides good visualization for component placement. The posterior lateral approach and direct lateral approach have a longer recovery time resulting from splitting and dissection of hip musculature (gluteus maximus/external rotators or hip abductors). The posterior approach results in more risk for postoperative hip dislocation (1% to 2%). The anterior approach gains exposure to the hip without detachment of surrounding muscles. Recently, some surgeons have been performing a *limited*

incision technique where the incision is only 4 inches but the approaches are the same. It is unclear if there is any advantage to this technique other than cosmetic.

The *minimally invasive procedure technique* involves two small incisions (one anteriorly and one posteriorly) that are each only 1 to 2 inches in length. This technique does not split or detach surrounding musculature but requires special training, equipment, and fluoroscopy to perform. Patients undergoing this procedure have less blood loss and quicker recovery times compared with the standard THA procedure. Patients eligible for this procedure must be of normal weight and height, have normal hip anatomy, and can only receive a cementless prosthesis.

20. **How commonly does aseptic loosening occur?**
    In cemented THA done using inferior techniques, the rate of aseptic loosening requiring revision was 10% to 15% at 10 to 15 years of follow-up (1% per year). Radiographic loosening of the femoral prosthetic component was as high as 30% to 40%. With contemporary cement techniques there is now <3% loosening at 10 years, 5% at 15 years, and 10% at 20 years. These rates are comparable to the frequency of loosening in the best porous-coated cementless prostheses. Patients who are young (<age 50 years) and/or heavy (>200 lbs) have the highest incidence of loosening for both cemented and cementless methods.

21. **Why does aseptic loosening occur and what is periprosthetic osteolysis?**
    Osteolysis around prosthetic joints causing loosening of the components is the most important long-term complication of total hip and knee surgery. It is reported that between 30% and 70% of prosthetic components (both cemented and cementless) have evidence of periprosthetic osteolysis at 10 years post arthroplasty as evidenced by a radiolucent line >3 mm in thickness around the prosthesis. It is caused by polyethylene particles produced by wear at the articulating surfaces of the prosthesis. The particulate debris tracks down the side of the prosthesis where it is ingested by macrophages in the membrane lining the bone–cement or bone–implant interfaces. These macrophages produce prostaglandins and cytokines, such as interleukin-1 and tumor necrosis factor (TNF), which leads to osteoclast stimulation and endosteal bone resorption. Treatment has included bisphosphonates (downregulates macrophages and osteoclasts), indomethacin (decreases prostaglandin production), anti-TNF-α therapy, as well as revision surgery with bone grafting.

22. **What unique postoperative complication occurs in patients receiving cementless THA?**
    Mild to moderate **thigh pain** occurs in approximately 20% of patients receiving the porous-coated THA. This pain is attributable to a bony stress reaction occurring at the tip of the femoral stem. It usually does not require medication and resolves in 12 to 18 months.

23. **How is arthroscopy used in the management of knee osteoarthritis?**
    Arthroscopic debridement of the knee is indicated in patients with mechanical symptoms (e.g., locking) resulting from an internal derangement, such as a meniscal tear. Arthroscopic debridement and lavage may provide several months of lessened pain in *some* patients with more advanced degenerative arthritic changes (**controversial**).

24. **When should osteotomy about the knee be chosen over total knee replacement?**
    Osteotomy is appropriate in the young, active patient with unicompartmental arthritis. The **high tibial osteotomy** is the most commonly performed realignment procedure for the knee with degenerative changes limited to either the medial or lateral compartment. Involvement of the patellofemoral compartment, inflammatory arthritis, marked loss of motion, and instability are contraindications. This procedure is usually intended to relieve pain, preserve functional status, and delay the need for a total knee replacement. The most common complications include under correction and peroneal nerve injury.

25. **What are the indications for unicompartmental arthroplasty of the knee?**
    This is an area of some controversy, and many surgeons are opposed to unicompartmental arthroplasty. It is indicated in a patient with at least 90 degrees of flexion arc and arthritic involvement of only one compartment of the knee. It is contraindicated in inflammatory arthritis, obesity, young age, <90 degrees arc of motion, flexion contracture, fixed angular deformity, and involvement of the patellofemoral compartment. It is accomplished by resurfacing the femoral and tibial joint surface in the involved compartment. Revision to total knee replacement is possible, but this is technically more difficult and has higher complication and failure rates than primary arthroplasty.

26. **Discuss the problems that can occur with a revision THA/total knee arthroplasty.**
    Revision arthroplasties are technically more challenging than primary arthroplasty, and the outcome (longevity) of the revision is significantly shorter and attendant complications higher. One of the significant problems encountered during revision is loss of bone stock, irrespective of mode of fixation. Another problem is soft-tissue balance producing instability in the revised hip and altered mechanics in the revised knee.

27. **How frequently does infection complicate total hip and total knee replacements?**
    Early postoperative infection rates are typically <0.5% with use of perioperative antibiotics. Late infections (>1 year postoperatively) occur in 1% to 3% of patients with RA and fewer patients with osteoarthritis. A patient with a painful prosthesis or loosening and an elevated C-reactive protein should be evaluated for an infected prosthesis regardless of the absence of systemic symptoms such as fever.

28. **Should patients with total joint replacements receive prophylactic antibiotics before having dental work done?**
    Controversial. The American Academy of Orthopedic Surgeons (AAOS; orthopedists) and the American Dental Association (ADA; dentists) have recently issued a joint guideline stating there is insufficient evidence to recommend antibiotic prophylaxis for dental procedures in patients who have a history of total joint replacement. Some physicians disagree and use prophylactic antibiotics for at least the first 2 years postoperatively, especially in patients they consider immunosuppressed. The author uses amoxicillin, cephalexin, or cephadrine, 2000 mg orally 1 hour before the procedure. If allergic to penicillin, a patient should get clindamycin 600 mg orally 1 hour before the procedure.

29. **How is an infected joint prosthesis managed?**
    Early infections (<2 weeks' postoperatively) can be managed with antibiotics and open synovectomy, thorough debridement, and retention of the prosthesis. Multiple surgical debridements are often necessary.
    Late infections usually present with only pain but can present with obvious sepsis of the involved joint. Once the diagnosis is made, treatment is removal of prosthetic components, thorough debridement, and intravenous antibiotics for 6 weeks. If a low virulence organism is cultured, reimplantation with antibiotic-impregnated cement can be performed at 6 weeks. If gram-negative organisms are cultured, a longer duration of resection arthroplasty is required (up to 12 months) before reimplantation.

30. **Name the two most common etiologies of ankle arthritis. How are they managed surgically?**
    Posttraumatic arthritis and RA. The ankle joint very rarely develops osteoarthritis compared with the hip and knee, but when it does, it is most commonly related to posttraumatic changes. Fractures that result in minimal amounts (1 to 2 mm) of lateral talar subluxation will produce degenerative changes in a relatively short time because of decreased surface area contact and increased joint reactive forces.
    Regardless of the etiology, functional bracing (Arizona brace) should be pursued until a patient can no longer tolerate this form of management. Total ankle replacement arthroplasty has historically had a high failure rate from infection and prosthetic loosening and cannot be recommended as a procedure of choice. Ankle arthrodesis is currently the best salvage procedure for an end-stage arthritic ankle.

31. **Which joints are fused in a triple arthrodesis?**
    The subtalar, calcaneocuboid, and talonavicular joints. Both RA and juvenile idiopathic arthritis affect the subtalar and transtarsal joints. These joint involvements can be isolated or combined, and there has been a trend toward isolated arthrodesis of involved joints rather than triple arthrodesis when possible. Particularly common is isolated talonavicular joint destruction. If this presents in an adult with RA, then isolated fusion is recommended. Conversely, if the involvement occurs at a young age secondary to juvenile idiopathic arthritis, then the entire transtarsal joint (talonavicular, calcaneocuboid) should be arthrodesed because this will provide a longer-term satisfactory result. Isolated subtalar arthrodesis is commonly performed when the remaining articulations of the triple joint are uninvolved and supple. Triple arthrodesis requires similar precision in positioning as does ankle arthrodesis to maximize walking biomechanics. In general, insensate feet (usually secondary to diabetes) are a contraindication to bony fusion as a result of the high likelihood of skin ulceration and subsequent infection.

32. **What is hallux valgus and how is it evaluated for surgery?**
    Hallux valgus is the most common affliction of the normal adult foot. It is a condition where the large toe is deviated laterally with the first metatarsal head deviated medially causing bunion deformity. The hallux valgus angle is measured by a line drawn through the proximal phalanx of the large toe and through the first metatarsal. A normal angle is 0 to 15 degrees with moderate (>25 degrees) and severe (>35 degrees) deformities commonly occurring.
    The cause of hallux valgus can be attributable to heredity, especially in combination with a short big toe relative to the second toe (Greek foot). Other congenital causes include pes planovalgus (flat feet) and metatarsus primus varus. The intermetatarsal angle between the first and second metatarsals is measured by a line drawn through the first and second metatarsals. The intermetatarsal angle is normally 0 to 10 degrees, whereas angles >16 degrees are moderate and >21 degrees are severely deformed. The need for surgical correction is considered if the painful deformity interferes with a patient's lifestyle or ability to wear shoes and there is a failure of conservative management (wider toebox shoes). There are over 100 different operations for correction of hallux valgus. The choice depends on the surgeon's skill and how the deformity needs correction (i.e., proximal metatarsal wedge osteotomy if intermetatarsal angle too great, etc.). Implant arthroplasty does not provide reliable long-term results compared with arthrodesis (15 degrees valgus, 25 degrees dorsiflexion).

33. **What is a Clayton-Hoffman procedure?**
    A commonly performed salvage procedure for advanced rheumatoid forefoot deformity. The rheumatoid forefoot pattern of involvement usually includes degeneration and instability at the first metatarsophalangeal (MTP) joint, leading to hallux valgus and bunion deformity. The lesser toes are also involved with synovitis, leading to subluxation and eventual dislocation at the remaining MTP joints. This results in prominent metatarsal heads on the plantar surface and the development of intractable plantar keratoses. This progressive deformation commonly involves all the MTP joints to some degree.

The Clayton-Hoffman procedure entails resection of all the metatarsal heads through either a plantar or dorsal approach. Rarely, only two metatarsal joints will be involved, and the procedure can be performed only on the involved joints. However, it is not recommended to remove only one or three involved metatarsal heads. Fusion of the first MTP joint is often done concurrently with the Clayton-Hoffman procedure.

34. Differentiate between hammer toe, claw toe, and mallet toe.
Differences among hammer toe, claw toe, and mallet toe are outlined in Table 89-1

Table 89-1. Differences Among Hammer Toe, Claw Toe, and Mallet Toe

FLEXIBLE TOE DEFORMITY	MTP	JOINT POSITION PIP	DIP	SURGICAL MANAGEMENT
Hammer toe	Uninvolved, neutral	Flexion	Uninvolved, neutral	Flexible—flexor to extensor transfer Fixed—hemiresection arthroplasty excision of distal portion of proximal phalanx
Claw toe	Fixed, extension	Fixed, flexion	Uninvolved, neutral or flexion	Resection of both sides of the PIP joint; joint dorsal capsulotomy and extensor tenotomy, flexor to extensor transfer
Mallet toe	Uninvolved, neutral	Uninvolved, neutral	Fixed, flexion	Excision of middle phalanx and/or flexor tenotomy if flexible

DIP, Distal interphalangeal; *MTP*, metatarsophalangeal; *PIP*, proximal interphalangeal.

35. Discuss the indications for surgery in a patient with symptomatic disk herniation.
Overall, approximately 1% of patients with herniated disks eventually require surgery. Absolute indications include disk herniation causing cauda equina syndrome, progressive spinal stenosis, or marked muscular weakness and progressive neurologic deficit despite conservative management. Controversy arises over indications for surgery in patients with less severe symptoms and signs. Relative indications for laminectomy and disk removal include intolerable pain with sciatica symptoms unrelieved by nonsurgical treatment (including corticosteroid injections) and recurrent back pain and sciatica that fail to improve significantly so that a patient can participate in activities of daily living after 6 to 12 weeks of conservative nonsurgical therapy.

Overall, long-term relief of sciatica has been shown to be the same in operative versus nonoperative patients, although the operative patients achieve their degree of relief more rapidly. The best results from surgery are obtained in the emotionally stable patient who has unequivocal disk herniation documented by consistent symptoms, compatible physical examination and tension signs, abnormal EMG that confirms the physical examination, and an abnormal MRI of the spine or myelogram confirming the EMG. The most common cause for surgical failure is poor initial patient selection. Patients should be warned that surgery will help the radicular symptoms but may not help the back pain.

36. List and discuss some of the recent advances in lumbar spine surgery.
- Chronic (>1 year) low back pain with degenerative disk disease:
  - *Spinal fusion with bone graft*: this is most common surgery. Fusion can be done with or without instrumentation (plates, screws, cages) that serve as internal splints. Bone morphogenic proteins are frequently used to improve fusion. Unfortunately, there is little evidence that this improves pain more than conservative nonsurgical therapy.
  - *Lumbar artificial disk replacement*: theoretic advantage over fusion is that the prosthetic disk will help preserve range of motion and lessen the chance for progressive degeneration of disks above and below a fusion. There is little evidence that an artificial disk is any better than fusion. Patients who are candidates are less than 60 years of age, have disease limited to one disk space, and have no back deformities or neurologic deficits.
- Lumbar disk prolapse meeting criteria for surgery (see Question 35):
  - *Open diskectomy*: standard technique. Frequently involves a laminectomy.
  - *Microdiskectomy*: most common procedure performed. Smaller incision. Involves a hemilaminectomy and removal of disk material.
  - *Minimally invasive techniques to remove/vaporize the disk*: tubular or trocar diskectomy, percutaneous manual nucleotomy, laser diskectomy, endoscopic diskectomy, coblation nucleoplasty, disk DeKompressor, others. Smaller incisions and quicker recovery times.
- Spinal stenosis:
  - *Decompressive laminectomy*: most common surgery. Fusion with or without instrumentation is also done especially for multilevel laminectomy and for degenerative spondylolisthesis causing stenosis. Instrumentation and bone morphogenic proteins improve chance of fusion but not clinical outcomes.

- *Interspinous spacer implantation (X-STOP)*: titanium implant placed between two spinous processes. Patients who may be candidates for this procedure are over 50 years of age, have no spondylolisthesis, suffer from intermittent claudication/leg pain which is exacerbated by back extension and relieved by sitting forward, and have only one or at most two lumbar levels involved. Certain deformities and severe osteoporosis are contraindications.
- Spondylolysis and isthmic spondylolisthesis: spondylolysis, seen in 6% of the population, is a lytic defect of the pars interarticularis. Isthmic spondylolisthesis is much less common and is attributable to lytic defects in the pars interarticularis bilaterally with anterior subluxation occurring most commonly (90%) at L5 on S1. This differs from degenerative spondylolisthesis which occurs most commonly with L4 disk degeneration leading to posterior subluxation of L4 vertebrae causing spinal stenosis.
  - *Posterolateral fusion* is the procedure of choice for isthmic spondylolisthesis.

Bibliography

Beck RT, Illingworth KD, Saleh KJ: Review of periprosthetic osteolysis in total joint arthroplasty: an emphasis on host factors and future directions, J Orthop Res 30:541, 2012.

Berberi EF, Osmon DR, Carr A, et al: Dental procedures as risk factors for prosthetic hip or knee infection: a hospital-based prospective case-control study, Clin Infect Dis 50:8, 2010.

Cavaliere CM, Chung KC: A systematic review of total wrist arthroplasty compared with total wrist arthrodesis for rheumatoid arthritis, Plast Reconstr Surg 122:813, 2008.

Chou R, Baisden J, Carragee EJ, et al: Surgery for low back pain: a review of the evidence for an American Pain Society Clinical Practice Guideline, Spine (Phila Pa 1976) 34:1094, 2009.

Chou R, Loeser JD, Owens DK, et al: Interventional therapies, surgery, and interdisciplinary rehabilitation for low back pain: an evidence-based clinical practice guideline from the American Pain Society, Spine (Phila Pa 1976) 32:2403, 2007.

Falck-Ytter Y, Francis CW, Johanson NA, et al: Prevention of VTE in orthopedic surgery patients: antithrombotic therapy and prevention of thrombosis, 9th ed: American College of Chest Physicians Evidence-Based Clinical Practice Guidelines, Chest 141:e278S, 2012.

Farrow SJ, Kingsley GH, Scott DL: Interventions for foot disease in rheumatoid arthritis: a systematic review, Arthritis Rheum 53:593, 2005.

Ghattas L, Mascella F, Pomponio G: Hand surgery in rheumatoid arthritis: state of the art and suggestions for research, Rheumatology (Oxford) 44, 2005.

Goodman SM, Figgie MP, Mackenzie CR: Perioperative management of patients with connective tissue disease, HSS J 7:72, 2011.

Jacobs WC, van der Gaag NA, Kruyt MC, et al: Total disc replacement for chronic discogenic low back pain: a Cochrane review, Spine (Phila Pa 1976) 38:24, 2013.

Kirkley A, Birmingham TB, Litchfield RB, et al: A randomized trial of arthroscopic surgery for osteoarthritis of the knee, N Engl J Med 359:1097, 2008.

Mizra SK, Deyo RA: Systematic review of randomized trials comparing lumbar fusion surgery to nonoperative care for treatment of chronic back pain, Spine (Phila Pa 1976) 32:816, 2007.

Moran SL, Bishop AT: Clinical update: surgical management of rheumatoid hand, Lancet 370:372, 2007.

Pivec R, Johnson AJ, Mears SC, Mont MA: Hip arthroplasty, Lancet 380:1768, 2012.

Ravi B, Escott B, Shah PS, et al: A systematic review and meta-analysis comparing complications following total joint arthroplasty for rheumatoid arthritis versus for osteoarthritis, Arthritis Rheum 64:3839, 2012.

Wajon A, Ada L, Edmunds I: Surgery for thumb (trapeziometacarpal joint) osteoarthritis, Cochrane Database Syst Rev 2005. CD004631.

Weinstein JN, Lurie JD, Tosteson TD, et al: Surgical versus nonoperative treatment for lumbar dis herniation: four-year results for the Spine Patient Outcomes Research Trial (SPORT), Spine (Phila Pa 1976) 33:2789, 2008.

Wolfs JFC, Klopenburg M, Fehlings MG, et al: Neurologic outcome of surgical and conservative treatment of rheumatoid cervical spine subluxation: a systemic review, Arthritis Rheum 61:1743, 2009.

Further Reading

www.orthoinfo.aaos.org/main.cfm

CHAPTER 90: DISABILITY

Scott Vogelgesang, MD

> **KEY POINTS**
> 1. The Social Security Disability system only awards benefits for total disability.
> 2. A person with disabilities who receives Social Security Disability Insurance is eligible for Medicare after 24 months of disability.
> 3. A person with disabilities who receives Supplemental Security Income is immediately eligible for Medicaid in most states.
> 4. Workers' compensation is a state-based, no-fault insurance system that provides payments for medical care and lost income as a result of injury or illness caused by employment.

1. What options are available for an individual who can no longer perform his or her job satisfactorily because of a musculoskeletal problem?
- Adapt the workplace.
  - Obtain or modify special equipment or devices.
  - Modify work schedules.
  - Job restructuring.
- Consider switching jobs or reassignment to another position.
- Vocational rehabilitation (VR).
- Apply for disability benefits.

2. What is disability?
Disability can be defined **generally** as *not being able to do something because of an illness or injury*. Most often, disability refers to an **individual** economic loss (by not being able to work at a previously acceptable level) because of a physical or mental condition. In insurance policies, laws, and regulations, the word disability has a more specific definition and needs to be distinguished from two similar, yet specific, terms: **impairment** and **handicap**.

3. Give a specific definition of disability.
Disability is an alteration of an individual's capacity to meet personal, social, or occupational demands because of an impairment. It is the gap between what an individual can do and what an individual needs or wants to do. The degree of disability is affected by not only an individual's impairment, but also the economic and social aspects of that person's life (i.e., age, education, training). People with the same impairment do not necessarily have the same disability. Disability is assessed by nonmedical means.

4. Define impairment.
Impairment is a physical or mental **limitation to normal function** resulting from a disease process. Impairment is determined by a physician. An impairment does not necessarily mean that a person is disabled.

5. What is a handicap?
Handicap refers to the **social consequences** that relate to an impairment or disability. A handicap is present if an individual has:
1. An impairment or disability that substantially limits one or more of life's activities or prevents the fulfillment of a role that is normal for that individual;
2. Medical record of such an impairment;
3. Barriers to accomplishing life's tasks that can be overcome only by compensating in some way for the effects of the impairment. Such compensation involves factors such as crutches, wheelchairs, prostheses, or even the amount of time necessary to complete a task.

6. List the important factors contributing to work disability in patients with a chronic musculoskeletal disease.

Disease	*Work*
Type of musculoskeletal disease	Occupation
Disease severity	Job autonomy
Impairment severity	Work experience

Personal	Social
Age	Social support
Gender	Peer and social pressures for or against
Education/training	disability
Personality	

Most physicians concentrate on trying to alleviate the "disease" factors to decrease disability. The other factors may be just as important in determining whether a patient considers himself or herself disabled.

7. What state and federal programs are set up to deal with disability?
There are two major government programs that deal with a person's inability to work: **Social Security Disability** and **Worker's Compensation**. The Social Security Administration administers two programs that differ mainly in eligibility criteria: Social Security Disability Insurance (Title II) (SSDI, also called Disability Insurance Benefits) and Supplemental Security Income (Title XVI) (SSI). As of 2011, 9.8 million people (4.6% of the population aged 18 to 64 years) were receiving Social Security Disability (SSDI and SSI) benefits. The most common reason (30% of all claims) was for a musculoskeletal condition.

8. Who is eligible for Social Security Disability (SSDI) payments?
Any employee 18 to 64 years of age with an appropriate work history.
Dependent of a deceased person who was receiving SSDI (survivor SSDI benefits) includes:
Unmarried son or daughter disabled before age 22 years.
Spouse who is caring for a child who is <16 years.
Spouse who is ≥60 years of age.
Disabled widow or widower ≥50 years of age whose disability started within 7 years of spouse's death.
Disabled, divorced widow or widower ≥50 years of age. Must have been married at least 10 years.

9. Describe SSDI.
SSDI is a federally regulated program that was established in the 1950s. It is the largest disability insurance program in the world. In SSDI, employers and workers pay into a trust fund. Workers contribute through payroll taxes (Federal Insurance Contributions Act [FICA]) and receive benefits (based on lifetime earnings) if they meet certain listed criteria:
- Age: over 18 and less than 65 years.
- If over age 31 years, need 40 work credits with at least 20 of them earned in the past 10 years before year of disability onset. A person can only get 4 work credits a year which is met if that person earns over $4800 (in 2014) for that year and has paid FICA on that amount. Disabled worker's less than age 31 years have prorated criteria for work credit requirements.
- Unable to engage in any substantial gainful activity (SGA) by reason of any medically determinable physical or mental impairment which can be expected to result in death or which has lasted or can be expected to last for a continuous period of not less than 12 months. SGA is defined as unable to earn over $1070/month (in 2014).

A person can apply for SSDI immediately upon becoming disabled. The Social Security Administration tries to take into account individual variations in impairment, vocational, and educational backgrounds. SSDI considers only *global* disability, thus there are no partial awards. Disability payments can start 5 months after the date of disability onset. Persons may also qualify for Medicare to help cover medical expenses after receiving SSDI benefits for 24 months. A person with disabilities who cannot afford medical expenses during this 24-month waiting period can receive Medicaid if they qualify.

10. How much are SSDI benefits and how long can they be received? What are auxiliary benefits?
The monthly benefit varies and is based on a complex formula that looks at the average covered earnings over a period of years that a patient has paid into the social security system. In 2014, the amount can vary from $300 to $2600 a month with an average of $1148/month. A person on SSDI has a case review every 3 to 7 years to determine if they still qualify for disability. They can receive SSDI up to age 65 years at which time they receive their monthly retirement benefit payment. The following dependents of a worker with disabilities can receive auxiliary benefits which can be up to 50% of the monthly benefit that a worker with disabilities is receiving:
- Unmarried sons or daughters <18 years old (can be 18 years of age if attending high school).
- Unmarried son or daughter disabled before 22 years of age.
- Spouse ≥62 years.
- Spouse who is caring for a child who is disabled.
- Ex-spouse if previously married over 10 years, ≥62 years, and unmarried.

11. What is SSI?
Individuals not qualifying for SSDI because of a lack of work experience may be covered by another program, SSI. SSI pays monthly sums to financially needy people who are either >65 years of age or qualified persons of any age with documented disabilities. SSI requires an evaluation of assets, sometimes called a "means" test.

Usually, those who receive SSI are eligible to have some medical expenses covered by Medicaid and will be eligible for Supplemental Nutrition Assistance Program (SNAP, previously called food stamps). Disabled persons are eligible for SSI if they meet the following asset limits (means test):
- Individual has less than $2000 ($3000 if a couple) in liquid assets (bank account, stocks, bonds, etc.).
- Can have one vehicle for transportation.
- Can have a house that is a person's principal residence.
- Life insurance policies with combined face values less than or equal to $1500.
- Burial funds up to $1500 in a separate bank account.

12. How much are SSI benefits?
The monthly SSI payment is based on the federal benefit rate (FBR). In 2014, the FBR is $721/month for individuals and $1082/month for a couple who has one person with disabilities. In most states, there is a monthly state supplement ($10 to $200) added to the monthly SSI benefit payment. If a person with disabilities receives an SSDI benefit that is less than the FBR then he can also receive SSI in an amount that brings his monthly benefit up to the FBR. If a person with disabilities earns any income, half of whatever he earns over $85 is subtracted from the SSI monthly payment.

13. Describe the workers' compensation program.
Workers' compensation is primarily a state-based system, although there is also a program for federal employees under the auspices of the U.S. Department of Labor. Any worker who incurs an illness or sustains an injury during and because of employment is entitled to protection against financial loss. It is a "no-fault" insurance system that provides benefits to all workers who are covered and who meet criteria. It removes the necessity to sue the employer. The program is designed to pay medical expenses and a portion of lost income during the period of disability arising out of gainful employment. Workers' compensation deals effectively with work-related traumatic accidents but has more difficulty with occupational illnesses. Determining if an illness is related to a person's employment may be difficult but only has to exceed a 50% probability that it is related. Workers' compensation determines disability based on the "whole person concept." Unlike SSDI, it can award partial disability. The disability can be temporary or permanent and it can be partial or total. Disability payments can be a lump sum or structured payments over a period of time depending upon the state-based system.

14. What paperwork is necessary to apply for Social Security Disability?
Social Security number.
Birth certificate or other proof of age.
Names and addresses of doctors, hospitals, clinics, and institutions involved in medical care.
W2 forms or tax return from previous year.
Summary of work history for past 15 years.
Date employee stopped working.
Marital history (if spouse is applying).
Dates of military service.

15. For those who meet the eligibility criteria and assemble the required application items, the Social Security Administration then evaluates four major factors. Name them.
- **Inability to perform substantial gainful activity** (work). Gainful activity is defined as earnings that average > $1070/month (in 2014).
- **Work credits.** Workers >31 years must have contributed to the Social Security fund for 20 of the preceding 40 quarters. For younger workers, fewer years are required.
- **Severity and extent of impairment.** Objective evidence of a physical or mental impairment is required. Symptoms alone are never sufficient for a determination of disability. There must be corroborating physical, laboratory, and/or radiographic findings. The impairment must interfere with basic work-related activities.
- **Does the impairment meet or exceed listed criteria for disability for that impairment?** A patient's individual physician does not determine if a person is disabled. The Social Security Administration has a list of defined impairments under each body system. If a patient's disease meets the listed measurements of disease severity, then a patient is assumed to have a disabling impairment. These listings make the system more objective and uniform. If the impairment is severe but does not meet the criteria for disability, the Social Security Administration will determine if an individual can perform the work they did previously. If not, the Social Security Administration will try to determine if other work could be done based on medical condition(s), age, education, past work experience, and transferrable skills.

16. What is residual functional capacity? What is a functional capacity evaluation?
If an applicant's impairment fails to meet the listed criteria for automatic disability, a physician or vocational specialist employed by the Social Security Disability Determination Service must make a determination of an applicant's residual functional capacity (RFC). RFC is the degree to which an applicant has the

capacity for sustained performance of the physical requirements of certain levels of work. RFC is determined by a functional capacity evaluation (FCE). The FCE can be performed by appropriately trained physicians or therapists. This is a physical ability test that is specifically related to an individual's occupational requirements. Specific abilities and endurances are measured such as standing, sitting, crawling, lifting, bending, strength, flexibility, pushing, pulling, and climbing stairs. These abilities and endurances are quantified according to Department of Labor standards according to weight and frequency of the activity for five categories of work.

17. **Outline the physical requirements as defined by the Department of Labor for each of the five categories of work.**
    Sedentary work
      Sitting most of the time
      Occasional (up to one third of an 8-hour day) lifting of ≤10 lbs
      Occasional walking or standing
    Light work
      Lifting of ≤20 lbs
      Frequent (up to two thirds of an 8-hour day) lifting or carrying of ≤10 lbs
      Walking or standing to a significant degree
      Sitting with push/pull arm or leg controls
    Medium work
      Occasional lifting of 20 to 50 lbs
      Frequent lifting or carrying of 10 to 25 lbs
      Physical demands in excess of those for light work
    Heavy work
      Occasional lifting of 50 to 100 lbs
      Frequent lifting or carrying of 25 to 50 lbs
      Physical demands in excess of those for medium work
    Very heavy work
      Occasional lifting of >100 lbs
      Frequent lifting or carrying of >50 lbs
      Physical demands in excess of those for heavy work
    Other factors taken into account when determining a person's RFC are fatigue; ability to see, hear, and speak; adequate mental capacity; ability for social interaction with coworkers; and skills to adapt to changes in work routine.

18. **How does the Social Security Administration use the RFC in determining disability?**
    The disability examiner determines the physical demands of the work previously done by an applicant and judges whether an individual has the RFC to do such work. If not, the examiner considers whether an applicant's RFC, coupled with an individual's age, education, and previous work experience, makes it possible for an applicant to do any work. If not, an applicant can be declared disabled, even though his or her impairment did not meet listed disability criteria.

19. **How is an application for disability benefits evaluated? Can a decision be appealed?**
    An application to the Social Security Administration for disability benefits is first evaluated by a physician panel without a personal appearance by the applicant. A decision is supposed to be made within 90 days of filing the disability application; however, because of backlogs this may take up to a year. Consequently, a person should file for disability as soon as they become disabled. Approximately one third of applications are approved at this point. If denied, an individual has the option of appeal at many stages, whereas the Social Security Administration does not. After initially being denied, an individual may appeal within 60 days. They can have the application reviewed again by a separate physician panel. However, only approximately 10% to 15% of these appeals are granted benefits. A denial at this stage may be appealed to a third level, an administrative law judge, where a personal appearance may first take place. Approximately 50% to 60% of the cases appealed to administrative law judges are subsequently approved, making this application step very important. Applications denied by the administrative law judge can be appealed to the Social Security Appeals Council and ultimately to a U.S. District Court. Few of these cases (2%) are ultimately approved. Overall, approximately 40% to 50% of all applications to the Social Security Administration are ultimately approved.

20. **If an individual who is receiving disability benefits returns to work, will their benefits be stopped?**
    Disability recipients continue to receive full disability benefits for up to 9 months after returning to work. This 9-month period is called a trial work period. The 9 months need not be continuous, and only months count in which an individual earns >$770 (gross)/month or works >80 hours/month (in 2014). Disability benefits are reassessed after the trial work period. If it is decided that disability benefits are no longer needed, an individual receives three more monthly checks. Subsequently, benefits are paid for any month an individual is disabled and unable to perform substantial gainful activity (earn >$1070 in 2014 for up to 36 months after the trial work

Table 90-1. Activities of Daily Living

CATEGORIES	SPECIFIC ACTIVITIES
Self-care and personal hygiene	Bathing, dressing, brushing teeth, combing hair, eating, toileting
Communication	Writing, speaking, hearing
Ambulation, travel, and posture	Walking, climbing stairs, driving, riding, flying, sitting, standing, lying down
Movement	Lifting, grasping, tactile discrimination
Sleep, social activities, and sexual function	—

period ends. If disability payments end but an individual continues with impairment, the Medicare benefit can be continued for up to 39 months, even though a person is no longer receiving disability payments. If after returning to work a person subsequently finds they again cannot work at a level that earns the SGA minimum ($1070/month) attributable to their disability, then they can apply for expedited reinstatement of their disability benefits as long as they file within 5 years after their benefits ceased as a result of returning to work.

21. **What is Vocational Rehabilitation (VR)?**
    VR is a service provided for the Federal Rehabilitation Act of 1973. Funded by both state and federal governments, VR agencies assist people with disabilities to find and keep employment. Every state is required to have a VR program, although the range of services varies among states. Private VR agencies also provide a wide array of services to individuals with disabilities and injuries.
    Any person applying for disability is referred to and considered for VR. The participating agencies provide counseling, interest/skills evaluation, basic living expenses, education expenses, transportation costs, purchase of special equipment, job training, and placement. These agencies may also acquire services from other public programs. Not all VR services are provided free of charge, but in some cases, VR does pay for all expenses when an individual has very limited resources. Disability benefits may be continued while an individual receives VR services. Notably, refusal of VR services may stop disability benefits. If a person recovers while participating in VR services, disability benefits continue if the VR services are likely to enable a person to return to work.

22. **What is the role of a primary physician while a patient is applying for disability?**
    The primary physician may be asked to fulfill several roles:
    - Information source for a patient
    - Details of the disability insurance system
    - Options to be pursued if the request is denied
    - Information source for the agency by documenting the impairment
    - Previous health status
    - Objective evidence of impairment (physical findings, radiographs, laboratory abnormalities)
    - Progression of symptoms
    - Impact the impairment has on a patient's activities of daily living
    - Response to therapy
    - Patient advocate, supporting a patient during the process of application
    - Monitor of ongoing therapy
    - Independent validator of an impairment
    - Expert witness for litigation
    - Difficulties arise for both a physician and a patient when these roles become contradictory. A physician who tries to be an effective patient advocate and an impartial adjudicator at the same time may be risking a strain of the physician–patient relationship

23. **What are activities of daily living?**
    Usual activities that need to be assessed and documented when evaluating or documenting impairments. Over 60% of patients with chronic musculoskeletal disorders report some limitation with one or more of these activities of daily living (Table 90-1).

24. **Does the Americans with Disabilities Act of 1990 apply to musculoskeletal conditions?**
    Yes. This Act makes it unlawful to discriminate in employment against a qualified individual with a disability. It also outlaws discrimination against individuals with disabilities in state and local government services, public accommodations, transportation, and telecommunications. To be protected, one must have a "substantial" impairment (one that significantly limits or restricts a major life activity) and must be qualified to perform the essential functions or duties of a job with or without reasonable accommodation. Reasonable accommodations include modifying work schedules, equipment, or environment. An employer may deny providing reasonable accommodations for either financial hardship or business necessity.

Bibliography

American Medical Association: Guides to the evaluation of permanent impairment, ed 6, Chicago, 2007, American Medical Association.
Carey TS, Hadler NM: The role of the primary care physician in disability determination for Social Security Insurance and Worker's Compensation, Ann Intern Med 104:706, 1986.
Katz RT, Rondinelli RD: Impairment and disability rating in low back pain, Occup Med 13:213–230, 1998.
King PM, Tuckwell N, Barrett TE: A critical review of functional capacity evalutions, Phys Ther 78:852–866, 1998.
Michalopoulos C, Wittenburg D, Israel DA, Warren A: The effects of health care benefits on health care use and health: a randomized trial for disability insurance beneficiaries, Med Care 50:764, 2012.
Minnigerode LK: Social Security and the physician, Missouri Med 97:156–158, 2000.
Stewart AL, Painter PL: Issues in measuring physical functioning and disability in arthritis patients, Arthritis Care Res 10:395–405, 1997.
US Government Printing Office: Social security administration disability evaluation under social security, Washington, 2006, US Government Printing Office.

Further Reading

Department of Labor: http://www.dol.gov
Office of Administrative Law Judges: http://www.oalj.dol.gov
Social Security Administration: www.ssa.gov

XV
FINAL SECRETS

Repetition is the key to good pedagogy. Read this book again.
Thomas Brewer, MD
Senior resident who supervised the editor during his first month of internship
(July 1976)

COMPLEMENTARY AND ALTERNATIVE MEDICINE

Alan R. Erickson, MD

"I didn't say it was good for you," the king replied, "I said there was nothing like it."

—Lewis Carroll (1832-1898)
—Through the Looking Glass

KEY POINTS

1. Most patients with rheumatic disease are considering, have tried, or are presently using complementary and alternative medicine (CAM) therapies.
2. Some CAM therapies have proven but limited benefits for patients with certain rheumatic diseases.
3. Some CAM therapies can be harmful to patients undergoing surgery or taking particular medications.
4. Physicians should ask patients about CAM therapies and record them in the medical record.

1. What is the definition of complementary and alternative medicine?
The term "complementary and alternative medicine (CAM)" describes therapies that have not been proven scientifically to be beneficial. The World Health Organization CAM definition is: "A broad set of health care practices that are not part of the country's own tradition and are not integrated into the dominant health care system." This is not to be confused with quackery or fraud, which is a false claim made deliberately to promote a product or treatment.

2. Just how widely used are CAM remedies?
Over 130 unconventional modalities and more than 500 remedies to treat patients have been described. Various surveys show that 38% to 42% of patients with arthritis will use some form of CAM therapy (excluding prayer) during their lifetime. Notably, only 40% of patients using these remedies told their physician. It is estimated that patients with arthritis will spend over $3 billion annually on CAM remedies.

3. Who uses CAM and why?
There is no "typical patient profile" to predict who will be tempted by the promises of CAM remedies. Chronic pain is the primary reason for people with arthritis to adopt CAM. Despite our scientific advances toward the understanding and treatment of rheumatic diseases, many of our therapies are empirical. This, coupled with a lack of understanding by the lay public, psychosocial factors, and cultural practices, allows this huge market to succeed.

4. Why should physicians care if patients use CAM remedies?
Rheumatic diseases are confusing to both the medical community and lay public. CAM remedies often return to the patient a sense of understanding, responsibility, and hope. Unfortunately, not all CAM therapies are safe. Additionally, expenditures on CAM remedies can divert scarce healthcare resources.

5. List eight categories of CAM remedies.

Alternative medical systems

Holistic medicine	Homeopathy
Naturopathy	Indian traditional medicine (Ayurveda, Siddha)
Chinese traditional medicine	Anthroposophical medicine

Biologically based therapies

Diet therapies

Dong diet	Elimination diet
Low-fat diet	Macrobiotic diet
Unpasteurized milk	Vegetarian

Nutriceuticals

Glucosamine/chondroitin	Antioxidants
Cod liver oil	Amino acids

Fish oil (omega-3 fatty acids)
Propolis, royal jelly, bee pollen
Megavitamins and supplements

Green-lipped mussel
Cartilage (shark, bovine, chicken)
S-adenosyl-L-methionine (SAM-e)

Herbal and natural remedies

Devil's claw
Alfalfa
Garlic
Willow bark
Herbs rich in γ-linoleic acid (evening primrose oil, borage oil, blackcurrant seed oil)

Ginger, nettle, tumeric, wild yam, bromelain
Chinese herbs (corydalis, genetian, paeonia, scutellaria, *Tripterygium wilfordii* Hook F, and Ma-Huang)
Kelp, sarsaparilla, boswellia, meadowsweet

Body-based and manipulative therapies

Chiropractic	Rolfing
Massage	Reflexology
Osteopathy	Movement (Feldenkrais method, Alexander technique)

Mind–body interventions and spiritual medicine

Biofeedback	Meditation
Relaxation techniques	Guided imagery
Hypnotherapy	Prayer
Yoga, Tai Chi, Qi Gong	

Energy therapies

Magnets	Pulsed electric field
Reiki	Therapeutic (healing) touch
External qi gong	

Procedures

Acupuncture	Chelation
Colon cleansing	Hydrotherapy
Mineral baths	

Diagnostic tests

Cytotoxic testing	Hair analysis
Iridology	Kinesiology

Miscellaneous

Copper bracelets	Dimethyl sulfoxide (DMSO)
Snake oil	Venoms
Antimicrobials	Exercise
Leech therapy	

6. **Define holistic medicine, homeopathy, and naturopathy.**
   Holistic medicine holds that people should try to maintain a balance between their physical and emotional processes while seeking harmony with the environment. Disease occurs when this balance is disrupted. **Ayurveda** is an ancient Hindu variation of holistic medicine that uses meditation, breathing exercises, reciting mantras, yoga, and herbal medicines to restore balance of the three basic energy types called doshas within the body and with nature. Some Ayurveda herbs have been found to contain heavy metals (mercury, lead, arsenic) that may cause health problems.
   Homeopathy principles were set forth in the 1800s by German physician Samuel Hahnemann. They use dilute preparations of substances that cause the same symptoms the patient is experiencing to stimulate the body's natural defenses to fight disease.
   Naturopathy claims that disease is an imbalance in the body that results from the accumulation of waste products. Natural therapies are said to remove the body's "poisons."

7. **Is there any evidence that diet affects arthritis?**
   The subject of diet has attracted many claims of cures for patients with arthritis. This interest stems from various known facts. Autoimmune disease is a relatively current phenomenon and seems to correlate with our changing diet. In the Late Paleolithic Period, the human diet was rich in protein, as opposed to our current diet, which is rich in fat. This increase in dietary fat can affect the composition of cellular membrane fatty acids. These membrane fatty acids are the source of arachidonic acid-derived prostaglandins (PGs) and

leukotrienes (LTs), which contribute to inflammation. It has been noted that some patients with inflammatory arthritis may be deficient in zinc, selenium, and vitamins A and C, which are involved in the scavenging or inactivation of oxygen free radicals. Although no convincing scientific evidence indicates that diet causes or cures arthritis, there are observations that diet may modulate the immune system.

8. Can fatty acid ingestion alter our inflammatory response to rheumatic disease?
Yes. Fatty acids (FAs) are essential to the human diet, with omega-3 and omega-6 FAs being the two major groups. FAs are responsible for the composition of the phospholipids in cellular membranes, and thus these membranes can be altered by dietary intake of omega-3 or omega-6 FAs. Additionally, FAs are the precursors for LTs and PGs, the agents (among many) responsible for our inflammatory response. Omega-3 FAs are the precursors of PGE3 and LTB5, a less inflammatory PG and LT, compared with PGE2 and LTB4, which come from omega-6 FA.

9. How do fish oils and evening primrose oil affect rheumatic diseases?
It is known that ethnic cultures with diets rich in fish oils, which are primarily omega-3 FAs, tend to have less autoimmune disease. Omega-3 FA diets can reduce arachidonic acid levels by 33% and increase eicosapentaenoic acid levels in cellular membranes 20 times. This results in production of PGE3 and LTB5, which have less inflammatory potential than those agents made from omega-6 FA.

Evening primrose oil (also **borage seed oil** and **blackcurrant seed oil**) is rich in γ-linolenic acid (GLA), which is an omega-6 FA. In experimental animal models, excess dietary GLA results in more PG1 compounds (PGE1) and less LT production, leading to less inflammation. Some studies support that this therapy reduces inflammation in rheumatoid arthritis (RA).

10. What is the theory behind the use of antioxidants?
Antioxidants interfere with the production of free radicals, compounds with an unpaired free electron that takes electrons from others, potentially affecting the immune system or cell membranes. One well-known free radical is superoxide, which is formed using NADPH. Superoxide is both a reducing and oxidizing agent and can spontaneously undergo a reaction to form hydrogen peroxide and oxygen. Hydrogen peroxide can also react with superoxide to produce a hydroxyl radical (the most reactive of the oxygen products) or chloride ions to form hypochlorous acid (the active ingredient in chlorine bleach).

A variety of antioxidants exist—including vitamins A, C, D, and E and the trace elements copper, zinc, iron, and selenium—which scavenge free radicals and may protect cells against oxidation. To date, there is little evidence to support that this therapy is helpful in patients with arthritis.

11. The theory that arthritis is caused by an allergy to certain foods is the basis of several popular diets. What are the scientific studies to support this claim?
Several anecdotal reports have described certain foods causing or worsening arthritis. Many of these are single case reports (Table 91-1).

There have been animal models of chronic synovitis induced with dietary changes. Apparently, food antigens can cross the gastrointestinal barrier and circulate not only as food antigens but also as immune complexes. Fasting appears to decrease disease activity in patients with RA. The postulated mechanisms are a reduction in immune activity and a decrease in intestinal permeability potentially reducing arthrotropic bacterial exposure.

Table 91-1. Food Allergy

Rheumatoid arthritis	Dairy products Wheat and corn Beef Nightshade foods (tomatoes, potatoes, eggplant, peppers)
Behçet's disease	Black walnuts
Lupus in monkeys	Alfalfa (contains L-canavanine)
Palindromic rheumatism	Sodium nitrate

12. Propolis, royal jelly, and bee venom have been claimed to cure arthritis. What is the science behind these claims?
Propolis is a resin made by bees to seal the hives and is reportedly high in bioflavonoids. **Royal jelly** is a sticky substance secreted by the worker honeybees and fed to larvae; it is supposedly high in pantothenic acid. Both bioflavonoids and pantothenic acid are in the B-complex vitamin family, one of many vitamins said to cure and/or treat arthritis.

Bee venom has been said to cure arthritis in anecdotal reports. Patients receive the bee venom from bee stings or from a local injection in an affected joint. Adequate treatment of RA may require as many as 2000 or 3000 stings over the course of a year. Bee venom is rich in phospholipase and other antiinflammatory agents. As expected, these remedies may lead to serious allergic reactions. None of these agents has been shown scientifically to be useful.

13. A popular CAM remedy uses raisins and gin. What is the recipe and the origins?
Recipe
1. One box of golden raisins.
2. Cover the raisins with gin.
3. Let stand uncovered until the liquid disappears.
4. Eat 9 raisins per day.

Supposedly, as far back as biblical times the healing properties of juniper berries have been noted, and gin is made from juniper berries. Several of my patients with arthritis, both RA and osteoarthritis, have tried this remedy with mixed results. Some physicians think you should forget the raisins and just drink the gin!

14. Many patients with RA wear copper bracelets. Why?
Copper bracelets were used by the ancient Greeks for their healing powers. Copper salts have been used for the treatment of RA, achieving generally favorable responses, unfortunately along with significant side effects. Copper in bracelets is absorbed through the skin (turning the skin green) and is said to improve arthritis symptoms in some patients, perhaps by binding oxygen free radicals. Interestingly, D-penicillamine, a proven therapy for RA, binds copper, which would suggest that copper is not a useful therapy.

15. Why is there so much interest in using antimicrobials for the treatment of rheumatic disease?
For years it has been thought that arthritis, particularly RA, is caused by an infectious organism. Tetracycline was proposed for treating RA many years ago because it was thought that RA was caused by mycoplasmas. More recent research has shown that minocycline may be useful for RA, not because of its antimicrobial actions but because of its antiproliferative and antiinflammatory properties. Yesterday's unconventional remedy may be tomorrow's new therapy. Remember, most stomach ulcers are now known to be as a result of Helicobacter *pylori* infections, which was not known 30 to 40 years ago. The following is a list of antimicrobials used for the treatment of rheumatic diseases:

Metronidazole	Minocycline
Clotrimazole	Ceftriaxone
Rifampin	Ampicillin
Tetracycline	Sulfasalazine
Dapsone	Hydroxychloroquine
Clarithromycin	

16. Are herbal remedies used by patients with osteoarthritis and RA?
Yes. Herbal products have been referred to as the most commonly used and abused form of alternative therapies. Herbs are claimed to treat arthritis and other diseases, but are there truths to the claim? Yes. Data do point toward a potential for phytoantiinflammation, probably through effects on eicosanoid metabolism.
Osteoarthritis: randomized controlled trials (RCTs) have shown that **devil's claw** (*Harpagophytum procumbens*), **bromelain** (a pineapple extract), and **willow bark extract** are effective in reducing pain in patients with osteoarthritis. **Phytodolor** (golden rod, aspen leaf/bark, and ash bark) has been shown in RCTs to be as effective as nonsteroidal antiinflammatory drugs (NSAIDs) in treating osteoarthritis pain. **Nettle** (*Urtica dioica*) inhibits cyclooxygenase and lipoxygenase pathways as well as suppresses cytokine release. **Ginger** (*Zingiber officinale*) contains gingerol and shogaol that inhibits PG and LT production. Uncontrolled studies have shown benefit. Ginger can interact with antiplatelet and anticoagulant medications which may cause excess bleeding during surgery. **Avocado Soybean Unsaponifiables** (ASUs) are reported to slow progression of hip and knee osteoarthritis. ASUs contain plant sterols that are chondroprotective by their antiinflammatory and proanabolic effects on articular chondrocytes. **Green lipped mussels** (*Perna canaliculus*) contain omega-3 FAs, which are converted into less inflammatory mediators (PGE3, LTB5).
Rheumatoid arthritis: a herb commonly used in China is extract of **thunder god vine** (*Tripterygium wilfordii* Hook F). Its active compounds are celastrol and triptolide, which inhibit NF-κB and T cell proliferation, as well as production of proinflammatory cytokines to include interleukin-2 and γ-interferon. An RCT showed it was superior to sulfasalazine in treatment of RA. Side effects, however, were significant. **Cat's claw** (*Uncaria tomentosa*) and **tumeric** (*Curcuma longa*) contain immunomodulatory and antiinflammatory ingredients and have been shown in small RCTs to be moderately effective in RA. Tumeric is also used to treat osteoarthritis pain by depleting substance P from nerve root endings similar to capsaicin. **Tibetan Five Nectar Formula** medicated bath therapy is derived from five types of plants that are considered antiinflammatory. Studies in RA demonstrating benefit are of poor quality and cannot be critically evaluated.

17. What are some other herbs and dietary supplements our patients are commonly using?
- Black cohosh
  - Uses: treats hot flashes and moodiness at menopause.
- Cayenne

- Uses: contains the chemical capsaicin that gives hot cayenne peppers their heat. When applied as a skin cream, it can deplete substance P from nerve endings, thus decreasing pain. Used for postherpetic neuralgia and rubbed on single joint with arthritis.
- **Coenzyme Q-10**
  - Uses: relieves chronic fatigue, immune stimulant, heart failure, and relieves muscle pain related to statin use. Contains ubiquinone, which is a cofactor for metabolic pathways that generate ATP. Also a free radical scavenger and can act as an antioxidant.
  - Drug interactions: can decrease the effect of warfarin.
- **Echinacea**
  - Uses: stimulate immune system, upper respiratory infections.
  - Disease precautions: liver disease.
  - Drug interactions: chemotherapy drugs for cancer treatment, HIV drugs, anticoagulants, immunosuppressive drugs, drugs that may be toxic to the liver.
- **Feverfew**
  - Uses: migraine prophylaxis.
  - Disease precautions: pregnancy—uterine contraction causing abortion, ragweed allergy.
  - Drug interactions: anticoagulants, antiplatelet medications.
- **Garlic**
  - Uses: lower low-density lipoprotein cholesterol, platelet inhibition.
  - Disease precautions: surgery.
  - Drug interactions: anticoagulants, antiplatelet medications.
- **Ginkgo biloba**
  - Uses: treatment of dementia, vertigo, ringing in ears. Can inhibit platelets and increase blood flow.
  - Disease precautions: intracranial bleeding, gastrointestinal bleeding, seizures, surgery, peripheral vascular disease. Gingko has anticoagulant effects and decreases platelet aggregation. Can cause gastrointestinal upset.
  - Drug interactions: anticoagulants, antiplatelet medications, thiazide diuretics, tricyclic antidepressants, MAO inhibitors.
- **Ginseng**
  - Uses: to fight fatigue, improve performance, reduce stress. Can inhibit platelets.
  - Disease precautions: heart disease, diabetes, pregnancy/nursing, surgery.
  - Drug interactions: caffeine (using both may cause high blood pressure), antiplatelet medications, insulin (ginseng may lower blood sugar), anticoagulants, MAO inhibitors, loop diuretics.
- **Goldenseal**
  - Uses: it is not absorbed through the gastrointestinal tract. Used topically on canker sores.
- **Grape seed extract**
  - Uses: antioxidant similar to pycnogenol.
- **Green tea**
  - Uses: antioxidant, improve cardiovascular health.
  - Disease precautions: asthma, hypertension.
  - Drug interactions: decreases absorption of atropine, codeine, ephedrine, and asthma medications. Can cause hypertension.
- **Indian frankincense** (*Boswellia serrata*)
  - Uses: antiinflammatory by inhibiting LTs.
  - Disease precautions: none.
  - Drug interactions: none.
- **Kava kava** (*Piper methysticum*)
  - Uses: reduce anxiety and insomnia.
  - Disease precautions: persistent depression—increased risk of suicide, pregnancy/nursing, surgery (potentiates anesthesia), hepatotoxicity.
  - Drug interactions: alcohol, alprazolam, barbiturates, St. John's wort.
- **Ma-Huang** (*Ephedra sinica*)
  - Uses: for cough/bronchitis, as a stimulant, and for weight loss.
  - Disease precautions: anxiety and restlessness, high blood pressure, heart disease, glaucoma, prostate adenoma, cardiac arrhythmias, surgery (causes high blood pressure).
  - Drug interactions: caffeine, decongestants, digoxin, MAO inhibitors.
  - This is a dangerous herb.
- **Milk thistle**
  - Uses: as a liver protectant.
  - Disease precautions: none.
  - Drug interactions: phenothiazines.
- **Pycnogenol** (*Pinus pinaster*)
  - Uses: antioxidant because it is a bioflavonoid. Protects from heart disease and cancer.

- **Saw palmetto** (herbal catheter)
  - Uses: prostate and irritable bladder, stimulates libido.
  - Disease precautions: hormone-dependent cancer, pregnancy/nursing. Can cause diarrhea.
  - Drug interactions: hormone replacements, oral contraceptives, anticoagulants, finasteride.
- **St. John's wort** (*Hypericum perforatum*) (Nature's Prozac)
  - Uses: treatment of mild depression.
  - Disease precautions: can cause photosensitivity.
  - Drug precautions: MAO inhibitors (Nardil, Parnate), selective serotonin reuptake inhibitors (Prozac, Zoloft, Paxil) (mild serotonin syndrome), digoxin (decreases blood concentration), Ultram, oral contraceptives (decreased efficiency), photosensitizers (tetracycline, quinolones, Feldene), Dyazide, Bactrim, Septra, theophylline (decreased levels of theophylline), HIV protease inhibitors (decreased levels of Indinavir), cyclosporine (decreases levels of cyclosporine).
- **Valerian root** (Nature's Ambien)
  - Uses: insomnia.
  - Disease precautions: can cause hepatitis.
  - Drug interactions: increased sedation with alcohol and other sedating medications.
- **Wild yam**
  - Uses: natural source of DHEA. Cannot be utilized by the body.
- **Yucca** (Adam's needle)
  - Uses: contains saponin, which decreases abnormal fat content in blood and improves intestinal circulation. Claimed to have analgesic and antiinflammatory properties.
  - Disease precautions: current or previous gastrointestinal ulcers. These stimulate gastric acid.
- **Zinaxin**—ginger root extract called hydroxy-methoxy-phenyl-33 (HMP 33). *See* Ginger.

PEARL: there is no standardization of herbal medicine in the United States. Consequently, a patient has little idea of how much active herb they are getting in what they buy over the counter. Daily cost of most herbs ranges between $0.30 and $1.50 a day.

18. What CAM therapies have shown benefit in gout?
- **Cherry juice**—has phenolic compounds that are antiinflammatory and inhibit cyclooxygenase and nitric oxide production. In addition, it increases uric acid excretion by inhibiting proximal tubular reabsorption of uric acid.
- **Vitamin C**—at dose of 500 mg/day it lowers uric acid by being a competitive inhibitor of uric acid reabsorption at the proximal tubule of the kidney.

19. What CAM therapies have been shown to be beneficial for fibromyalgia?
No oral or topical CAM therapy has been proven to be beneficial. Randomized trials have shown Tai Chi, exercise, hydrotherapy, and thermal therapies to be beneficial.

20. What CAM therapies have been shown to be beneficial for Raynaud's phenomenon?
None. Notably, biofeedback has been shown not to be beneficial.

21. What is DMSO, methylsulfonylmethane, and SAM-e?
- **DMSO**—it is a byproduct of wood pulp processing. There is medical grade that is safe and an industrial grade that is used in paint thinner and antifreeze. DMSO can be used as a solvent to transport molecules across cell membranes such as the skin. DMSO taken internally or topically causes the person's breath to smell like garlic or oysters. DMSO is a prescription drug given by catheter to treat interstitial cystitis. Therefore, it cannot be sold over the counter. Patients getting it from vendors are taking industrial-grade DMSO, which is unsafe. There are reports supporting the ability of DMSO to relieve pain and reduce inflammation.
- **Methylsulfonylmethane (MSM)**—15% of DMSO is broken down to MSM. MSM does not cause an oyster–garlic smell. MSM is an organic sulfur compound which may contribute sulfur to the formation of connective tissue. Additionally, animal studies suggest it may be antiinflammatory, but there are no controlled scientific data to support its use. MSM became popular when the actor James Coburn said that it works for his RA. Usual dose is 1000 to 3000 mg twice a day.
- **SAM-e**—this is already formed in the body from methionine and ATP. SAM-e is a methyl accepting intermediate in homocysteine formation, which with the help of vitamin B12 will relinquish a methyl group to surrounding tissues (see Figure 56-1 in Chapter 56). SAM-e is then broken down to sulfate groups, which may help cartilage formation. SAM-e is equivalent to NSAIDs in therapy of osteoarthritis in controlled trials. Dose is 400 mg three times a day and costs $50 a month. Also used to treat depression.

22. Are there any herbs believed to be unsafe?
- **Carcinogens**—borage, calamus, coltsfoot, comfrey, life root, sassafras.
- **Hepatotoxicity**—chaparral, germander, life root, skullcap, Jin Bu Huan, comfrey, kava kava.
- **Other**—licorice (electrolyte imbalance), Ma Huang (hypertension, strokes, seizures), borage seed oil (seizures).

PEARL: stop all herbs for at least 24 hours before surgery, because many have an anticoagulant effect.

23. **What other CAMs have people tried?**
    - **Movement therapy**—Tai Chi has been shown to decrease falls in the elderly.
    - **Magnets**—static magnets cause a localized magnetic field. Theorized to interact with the nerve conduction of the body and reduce pain perception. Magnet strength ranges between 300 and 4000 G (refrigerator magnet is 60 G). Little data to support use of this expensive therapy. May help localized joint pain.
    - **Acupuncture**—theory is that good health is maintained by circulation of vital energy (known as Qi) in the body. Illness is attributable to disruption of this flow. In order to correct this disruption, insertion of needles at defined points along meridians causes discomfort that is necessary to elicit Qi. Actually, it has been shown that acupuncture causes endorphin and serotonin release, which can help pain. The best trials and/or metaanalyses show that acupuncture is better than sham therapy or education in relieving pain in patients with knee osteoarthritis, chronic back pain, and chronic neck pain. Improvement however is not prolonged so therapy must be continued. Acupuncture does not help pain more than standard therapy for acute low back pain.
    - **Shark cartilage**—reported to have antiinflammatory properties and to inhibit angiogenesis. No data to support its use. Because it may inhibit angiogenesis, it should not be used in pregnancy, children, or patients undergoing surgery or with coronary artery disease.

24. **Are manipulation techniques useful for the treatment of rheumatic diseases?**
    Yes. I recommend them regularly. Many patients with soft-tissue rheumatism respond positively to physical therapy and manipulation from chiropractors and osteopaths. Manipulation has been shown to decrease joint pain, although the mechanism of action is not well understood. I believe that if these modalities are used appropriately, it often leads to a decrease in the need for systemic antiinflammatories. They also give patients a sense of participation in their treatment program.

25. **How does one report a potentially unsafe CAM remedy?**
    The U.S. government publishes the Consumer Action Handbook that explains how to file a complaint. This handbook is available on line at www.gov/topics/consumer/consumer-action-handbook-online.shtml.

26. **In summary, how should CAM remedies be approached?**
    CAM remedies are widely used by patients with rheumatic diseases. Some are safe and harmless, and others can be deadly. Some remedies have therapeutic potential and may unlock the door to the next treatment for rheumatic disease; these deserve the attention of the medical community. I would encourage all healthcare providers to discuss their use with patients. There are several internet resources to get additional information. One of these is the National Center for Complementary and Alternative Medicine at www.nccam.nih.gov.

BIBLIOGRAPHY

Barnes PM, Bloom B, Nahin RL: Complementary and alternative medicine use among adults and children: United States, 2007, Natl Health Stat Report 12:1–23, 2008.
De Silva V, El-Metwally A, Ernst E, et al: Evidence for the efficacy of complementary and alternative medicines in the management of fibromyalgia: a systemic review, Rheumatology 49:1063–1068, 2010.
Ernst E: Complementary treatments in rheumatic diseases, Rheum Dis Clin North Am 34:455–467, 2008.
Ernst E: Herbal medicine in the treatment of rheumatic diseases, Rheum Dis Clin North Am 37:95–102, 2011.
Fouladbakhsh J: Complementary and alternative modalities to relieve osteoarthritis symptoms, Am J Nurs 112:S44–S51, 2012.
Gertner E, Marshall PS, Filandrinos D, Smith TM: Complications resulting from the use of Chinese herbal medications containing undeclared prescription drugs, Arthritis Rheum 38:614–617, 1995.
Goldbach Mansky R, Wilson M, Fleischmann R, et al: Comparison of Tripterygium wilfordii Hook F versus sulfasalazine in the treatment of rheumatoid arthritis, Ann Int Med 151:229–240, 2009.
Juraschek SP, Miller ER, Gelber AC: Effect of oral vitamin C supplementation on serum uric acid: a meta-analysis of randomized controlled trials, Arthritis Care Res 63:1295–1306, 2011.
Macfarlane GJ, El-Metwally A, De Silva V, et al: Evidence for the efficacy of complementary and alternative medicine in the management of rheumatoid arthritis: a systematic review, Rheumatology 50:1672–1683, 2011.
Malenfant D, Catton M, Pope JE: The efficacy of complementary and alternative medicine in the treatment of Raynaud's phenomenon: a literature review and meta-analysis, Rheumatology 48:791–795, 2009.
Michalsen A: The role of complementary and alternative medicine (CAM) in rheumatology – it's time for integrative medicine, J Rheumatol 40:547–549, 2013.
Rubenstein SM, van Middelkoop M, Kuijpers T, et al: A systematic review on the effectiveness of complementary and alternative medicine for chronic nonspecific low-back pain, Eur Spine J 19:1213–1228, 2010.
Tilley BC, Alarcón GS, Heyse SP, et al: Minocycline in rheumatoid arthritis: a 48-week, double-blind, placebo-controlled trial, Am Intern Med 122:81–89, 1995.
Quandt SA, Chen H, Grzywacz JG, et al: Use of complementary and alternative medicine by persons with arthritis: results of the national health interview survey, Arthritis Care Res 53:748–755, 2005.

FURTHER READING

www.nccam.nih.gov

CHAPTER 92: HISTORY, THE ARTS, AND RHEUMATIC DISEASES

Sterling G. West, MD and James S. Louie, MD

1. **What is the derivation of the word *rheuma*?**
   Rheuma is derived from the Greek term indicating "a substance which flows," a humor that originates in the brain and causes various ailments. Guillaume Baillou claimed that "what arthritis is in a joint is what rheumatism is in the whole body," raising the idea that arthritis is but one manifestation of systemic processes. In 1940, Bernard Comroe coined the term *rheumatologist*, and in 1949, Hollander used the term *rheumatology* in his textbook *Arthritis and Allied Conditions*.

2. **Who described and named rheumatoid arthritis?**
   Augustin-Jacob Landre-Beauvais (lahn-dray boh-vay) is credited with the first clinical description in 1800. He called it a variant of gout—"goutte asthenique primitif." Benjamin Brodie described the slow progression from a synovitis and bursa and tendon sheath involvement. A.B. Garrod (gair-roh) coined the term *rheumatoid arthritis* (RA) in 1858 and differentiated RA from gout in 1892.

3. **Which famous French painters were afflicted with RA?**
   Pierre Auguste Renoir (1841-1919), the popular French impressionist, developed a severe form of RA beginning around 1890. Despite his increasing disabilities, he continued to paint, supported his family, and devised his own exercises and adaptive equipment. By 1912, he was bedridden and unable to transfer. Just before his death, he developed vasculitis in his fingertips.
   Raoul Dufy (1877-1953), the talented Fauvist who explored "the miracle of imagination in color" in paintings, watercolors, ceramics, tapestries, and stage and mural designs, exhibited his first attack of RA at age 60 years. Within 13 years, when he became dependent on his crutches and wheelchair, he was invited to Boston to participate in one of the first drug studies that utilized different steroid preparations for the treatment of RA. He underwent a remarkable recovery, returned to his painting with vigor, but also suffered the consequences of the steroids, including a buttock abscess and a gastrointestinal bleed before his death.

4. **What other famous people had RA?**
   Performers who developed RA include Edith Piaf, the French chanteuse, motion picture actresses Rosalind Russell, Lucille Ball, and Kathleen Turner, and motion picture actors James Coburn and Jamie Farr. Other notables with RA include the cardiac surgeon Sir Christiaan Barnard, Los Angeles Dodgers' pitcher Sandy Koufax, and U.S. Presidents Thomas Jefferson, James Madison, and Theodore Roosevelt.

5. **Who is credited with the early descriptions of systemic lupus erythematosus?**
   1845—Ferdinand von Hebra described the butterfly rash on the nose and cheeks.
   1895—Sir William Osler described the systemic features under the name *exudative erythema*.
   1948—William Hargraves described the lupus erythematosus cell in bone marrow aspirates.
   1956—Peter Miescher described the absorption of the lupus erythematosus cell factor by cell nuclei.
   1958—George Friou described the method identifying antinuclear antibodies by labeling with fluorescent antihuman globulin.

6. **Name some famous people who had systemic lupus erythematosus.**
   - Southern authoress Flannery O'Connor.
   - Former Philippine President Ferdinand Marcos.
   - TV journalist Charles Kuralt; TV show host Nick Cannon.
   - Lucy Vodden—subject of Beatles' song *Lucy in the Sky with Diamonds*.
   - Singers: Seal, Toni Braxton, Lady Gaga.
   - Baseball player Tim Raines.

7. **Who is credited with the early descriptions of scleroderma?**
   ca. 400 BC—Hippocrates described "persons in whom the skin is stretched, parched and hard, the disease terminates without sweats."
   1842—English physician W.D. Chowne described a child with clinical features.
   1846—English physician James Startin described an adult with clinical features.
   1860—French clinician Elie Gintrac coined the term *sclerodermie*.
   1862—Maurice Raynaud described the vasospastic phenomenon of painful, cold-induced acrocyanosis.

1964—Richard Winterbauer, while a medical student, described the CRST syndrome of calcinosis, Raynaud phenomenon, sclerodactyly, and telangiectasia. The E for esophageal dysmotility was added subsequently (CREST).

8. **What famous Swiss painter and printmaker had scleroderma?**
Paul Klee (1879-1940), the complex and incredibly talented Swiss artist who completed more than 9000 works in diverse media, was stricken with scleroderma at age 56 years. His last paintings include "Ein Gestalter" (the Creator) as he recovered his desire and energy to paint; "Stern Visage," which described the skin changes; "Death and Fire," as he painted his requiem; and "Durchhalten" (Endure), a line drawing that described the dysphagia prompting his final admission to the sanitorium.

9. **Who is credited with the early descriptions of spondyloarthropathies?**
In 1691, the Irish physician Bernard Connor described a skeleton with ankylosing spondylitis. In 1818, the English physician Benjamin Brodie provided the first clinical description of a patient with ankylosing spondylitis and iritis. In the late 1890s, the Russian physician Vladimir von Bechterew, the German–Russian physician Adolf Strumpell, and the French physician Pierre Marie described the clinical features of ankylosing spondylitis before the development of severe deformities. In the early 1900s, the German physician Hans Reiter and the French physicians Noel Fiessinger and Emile Leroy described the clinical characteristics of reactive arthritis. The association with the class I gene, *HLA-B27*, is credited to the Americans Lee Schlosstein, Rodney Bluestone, and Paul Terasaki, and the English persons Derrick Brewerton, David James, Maeve Caffrey, and Anne Nicholls.

10. **Which famous personages had ankylosing spondylitis?**
    - Egyptian pharaoh Amenhotep II (1439–1413 BC).
    - Olympic gold medalist swimmer Bruce Furniss.
    - Cricket captain Mike Atherton.
    - Television emcee Ed Sullivan.
    - Renowned cellist Gregor Piatigorsky.
    - Motion picture actor Boris Karloff (All of the stiff walking in his Frankenstein role may not have been acting!).
    - Motley Crue's guitarist Mick Mars.

11. **Do any notable people have psoriasis or psoriatic arthritis?**
Psoriasis is a common disease with a strong hereditary predisposition. King Herod built his fortresses close to the Dead Sea so he could be close to the healing waters for his psoriasis and arthritis. Benjamin Franklin suffered with severe psoriasis. Fleet Admiral William "Bull" Halsey, Jr. could not command the Third Fleet during the WWII Battle of Midway due to a severe attack of psoriasis. Phil Mickelson, winner of the 2010 Masters and 2013 British Open, has been a spokesperson for the success of etanercept therapy. Performers Art Garfunkel (musician), Kathryn Hepburn (actress), LeAnn Rimes (singer), and Jerry Mathers *(Leave it to Beaver)* all had psoriasis and served as spokespersons for the disease. Famous villains with psoriasis include Russian dictator Joseph Stalin, and drug lord Pablo Escobar.

12. **What persons are credited with the early descriptions of gout?**
5th century BC—although gout was reported in medieval medicine as *gutta*, Latin for "a drop" of a poisonous noxa, Hippocrates first described the clinical features of gouty arthritis following dietary excesses in sexually active men and postmenopausal women.
Late 1600s—Thomas Sydenham described the clinical features, and Anton van Leeuwenhoek described the microscopic appearance of uric acid recovered from a tophus.
1814—John Want reported the effectiveness of colchicine in the treatment of 40 patients with gout.
1857—A.B. Garrod developed an assay that detected uric acid in hyperuricemic states, demonstrated uric acid in cartilage of those with gout, and formulated the current hypotheses that lead to gouty arthritis.
1961—Joseph Hollander and Daniel McCarty demonstrated monosodium urate in the synovial fluid cells of those with gout.
1964—Michael Lesch, as a medical student, wrote the clinical description of a patient with neurobehavioral changes for his mentor, William Nyhan, who described the complete deficiency of hypoxanthine-guanine phosphoribosyl transferase (HGPRT), the enzyme that catalyzes the salvage reactions of purines (Lesch–Nyhan syndrome).

13. **Which famous Flemish painter had gout?**
Peter Paul Rubens (1577-1640), the portrayer of Baroque, developed attacks of fevers and arthritis that put him to bed at age 49 years. Within 10 years, his attacks were continuous, and he had difficulty painting and ambulating. He died of "ague and the goutte" at age 63 years. Some interpret the stylistic paintings of the hands as deformities that resembled RA.

14. **Which American Presidents suffered from gout?**
James Buchanan (1791-1868) and Martin van Buren (1782-1862).

15. What was Beethoven's disease?
Ludwig von Beethoven (1770-1827) noted hearing loss at age 26 years, was "stone deaf" at age 49 years, and died at age 57 years. His deafness is popularly attributed to otosclerosis, or eighth nerve compression from Paget disease. More in-depth studies included records of attacks of rheumatism. A postmortem by Wagner and Rokitansky described "dense half-inch-thick cranial vault, shrunken auditory nerves, wasted limbs, with cutaneous petechiae, cirrhosis with ascites, a large spleen, and chalky deposits in the kidneys." These findings led to the differential diagnosis of meningovascular syphilis, sarcoidosis, and Whipple disease.

16. What were the rheumatic diseases in the Civil War era?
Medical records of the American Civil War recorded 160,000 cases of "acute rheumatism," mainly acute rheumatic fever, perhaps infectious arthritis or gout. More than 260,000 cases of "chronic rheumatism" were recorded, probably chronic rheumatic fever and reactive arthritis, of which 12,000 were discharged. The validity of these clinical diagnoses on the war front may temper some of these data, and more recent data of war-related rheumatic syndromes give a better perspective.

In 1863, General Robert E. Lee described paroxysms of chest pains radiating to the left shoulder and back, which was diagnosed as rheumatic pericarditis. He was given quinine. By 1870, because the pains occurred at rest, these attacks were probably advancing coronary atherosclerosis.

17. Which famous persons had their lives affected by rheumatic fever?
- Bobby Darin (singer)
- Andy Warhol (artist)
- Donald Sutherland (actor)
- Lou Costello (comedian)
- Robert Burns (Scottish poet)
- Amadeus Mozart (composer)
- Carson McCullers (writer)

18. Did Abraham Lincoln have a genetic disease?
The debate on whether the American President Abraham Lincoln had **Marfan syndrome**, the autosomal dominant disorder of connective tissue, reached national proportions when an advisory committee in the 1990s ruled against proposed molecular genetic testing of his tissue, which is preserved at the National Museum of Health and Medicine at the Armed Forces Institute of Pathology. Most geneticists do not feel he had the disease because of his excellent eye sight and normal vasculature throughout his 56 years of life.

19. What was Henri de Toulouse Lautrec's disease?
Henri de Toulouse Lautrec (1864-1901) developed growing pains at age 8 years, was hospitalized for rehabilitation at age 10 years, and fractured his femurs following minimal trauma at ages 14 and 15 years. The clinical geneticists Maroteaux and Lamy noted the parental consanguinity and short stature and proposed the diagnosis of pyknodysostosis, an autosomal recessive disease characterized by mutations of the *cathepsin K* gene on chromosome 1. This retrospective diagnosis has been disputed and other bone diseases proposed.

20. What musicians may have been "helped" by their proposed connective tissue disease?
Nicolo Paganini (1782-1840) of Genoa, Italy was a violin virtuoso who had a flair for the dramatic and ostentatious. Although he had extraordinary musical talent, he also had extraordinary manual dexterity and hypermobility believed to be due to Ehlers–Danlos syndrome or Marfan syndrome. This enabled him to play notes that most ordinary mortals could not.

Sergei Rachmaninov (1873-1943) was known to have hands so large that they "covered the keyboard like octopus tentacles." He was believed to have had Marfan syndrome.

21. What other celebrities have true connective tissue diseases?
- Marfan syndrome: Actor Vincent Schiavelli who starred in "One Flew over the Cuckoo's Nest" among others. The Olympic Silver Medalist in Women's Basketball, Flo Hymen, died of an aortic dissection and serves as a reminder that this disease can be lethal. Notably, the Olympic Gold Medalist in Swimming, Michael Phelps, does **not** have Marfan syndrome.
- Osteogenesis imperfecta: Actors Michael J. Anderson (*Carnivale*) and Atticus Shaffer (*The Middle*).

22. What is the purpose of recognizing "famous autoimmune" personalities?
Many patients who suffer from an autoimmune disease take comfort in knowing that they are not alone and that other people, both average and famous, are afflicted with their disease. It is particularly helpful when a famous person who has an autoimmune disease or a loved one with the disease becomes a spokesperson to raise awareness as well as funds for research and treatment. Some notable spokespersons for the disease they have:
- Sjögren's syndrome: tennis great Venus Williams.
- Sarcoidosis: basketball great, Bill Russell, comedian Bernie Mac, and football star Reggie White, before their deaths from the disease.

BIBLIOGRAPHY

Appelboom T, de Boelpaepe C, Ehrlich G, Famaey JP: Rubens and the question of antiquity of rheumatoid arthritis, JAMA 245:483–486, 1981.
Ball GV: The world and Flannery O'Connor. In Appelboom T, editor: Art, history and antiquity of rheumatic diseases, Brussels, 1987, Elsevier Librico.
Benedek T: History of the rheumatic diseases. In Schumacher HR, editor: Primer on the rheumatic diseases, ed 10, Atlanta, 1993, Arthritis Foundation.
Bollet AJ: Rheumatic diseases among Civil War troops, Arthritis Rheum 34:1197–1203, 1991.
Brewerton D, Caffrey M, Nicholls A: Ankylosing spondylitis and HLA-27, Lancet i:904–907, 1973.
Francke U, Furthmayr H: Marfan's syndrome and other disorders of fibrillin, N Engl J Med 330:1384–1385, 1995.
Frey J: What dwarfed Toulouse-Lautrec? Nature Genet 10:128–130, 1995.
Gelb BD, Shi GP, Chapman HA, Dresnick RJ: Pycnodysostosis, a lysosmal disease caused by cathepsin K deficiency, Science 273:1236–1238, 1996.
Homburger F, Bonner CD: The treatment of Raoul Dufy's arthritis, N Engl J Med 301:669–673, 1979.
Louie JS: Renoir—his art and his arthritis. In Appelboom T, editor: Art, history and antiquity of rheumatic diseases, Brussels, 1987, Elsevier Librico.
Mainwaring RD: The cardiac illness of General Robert E. Lee, Surg Gynecol Obstet 174:237–244, 1992.
Maroteaux P, Lamy M: The malady of Toulouse-Lautrec, JAMA 191:715–717, 1965.
Marx R: The health of the presidents, New York, 1960, G.P. Putnam's Sons.
Palferman TG: Beethoven: medicine, music, and myths, Int J Dermatol 33:664–671, 1994.
Parish LC: An historical approach to the nomenclature of rheumatoid arthritis, Arthritis Rheum 6:138–158, 1963.
Schlosstein L, Terasaki P, Bluestone R: High association of an HLA antigen, w27, with ankylosing spondylitis, N Engl J Med 288:704–706, 1973.
Sharma OP: Beethoven's illness: Whipple's disease rather than sarcoidosis? Int J Dermatol 87:283–286, 1994.
Shearer PD: The deafness of Beethoven: an audiologic and medical overview, Am J Otol 11:370–374, 1990.
Smith RD, Worthington JW: Paganini. The riddle and connective tissue, JAMA 199:820–824, 1967.
Young DAB: Rachmaninov and Marfan's syndrome, Br Med J 293:1624–1626, 1986.

INDEX

A

Aβ protein amyloidosis, 546
Abatacept (Orencia), 641
ABCDES mnemonic
  in assessing skeletal radiograph, 63
  for osteoarthritis, 382, 383f
  in perioperative evaluation of rheumatic disease, 96
  for radiologic features of reactive arthritis, 279
  for radiologic/pathologic changes in bacterial septic arthritis, 293t
Abdominal fat pad, 547
Abduction test, shoulder, 446
Abrasion surgery, as osteoarthritis therapy, 391
Abscess
  Brodie's, differentiated from sequestra, 299
  psoas, 270
Acetaminophen, 275, 389, 460
Acetylsalicylic acid (ASA), considerations of use of, 606
Aches, diffuse, differentiated from polyarthritis, 86
Achilles bursa, 468f
Achondroplasia, 413, 439
Acid maltase deficiency, 535t, 537f, 539
Acquired immunodeficiency syndrome (AIDS), rheumatic disease-related, 322
Acrocyanosis, 526
Acrodermatitis chronica atrophicans, 302
Acromegaly, 362, 362f, 387, 536t
  of hands, 362, 363f
  radiographic features of, 72
  rheumatologic syndromes and, 362
Acropachy, thyroid, 360, 361f
Acthar Gel, 616
Actin, 23
Action potential, 23
Activated partial thromboplastin time, lupus anticoagulant and, 180
Activities of daily living, 680, 680t
Acupuncture, 691
Acute calcium pyrophosphate crystal arthritis, 346, 348–349
Acute gouty arthritis, 339, 342–343, 343t
Adalimumab (Humira), 634
Adamantiades-Behçet's disease, 248
Adam's needle, 690
Addison's disease, 536t
A delta (δ) fibers, myelinated, 456
Adenosine triphosphate (ATP), 535–536, 536f
Adenovirus infection, 318
ADEPTTS mnemonic, for functional abilities assessment, 14, 661
Adhesin, 18
Adrenal gland
  glucocorticoid-related atrophy of, 615
  respond to surgery, 98

Adrenal insufficiency
  perioperative, exogenous corticosteroid-related, 99
  preoperative, 99
Adrenocorticotropic hormone (ACTH), 349, 615–616
Adson's maneuver/test, 45, 479–480
Adynamic bone disease, 571, 573
Agammaglobulinemia, X-linked
  rheumatologic manifestations of, 433, 433t
  therapy for, 435
Age, of patient, in differential diagnosis of monoarthritis, 83
Alarmins, 24
Albright's hereditary osteodystrophy, autosomal dominant, 362
Alcohol intake
  as hyperuricemia cause, 339t
  as osteonecrosis risk factor, 407
Alendronate, 654t
Alkaline phosphatase, in Paget's disease, 401
Alkaptonuria (ochronosis), 424, 428, 429f
Alkylating agent, for rheumatic diseases, 630
Allodynia, 484
Allopurinol, 344, 575, 648, 648b
Alopecia
  in Still's disease, 189
  in systemic lupus erythematosus, 120t, 123
Alphavirus infections, 317, 317t
Alport syndrome, 17t, 419
Aluminum, adverse renal effects of, 573
Alzheimer's disease, 543, 544t
Amaurosis fugax, 209
American College of Rheumatology, 625
American Committee for the Control of Rheumatism, 3
American Rheumatism Association (ARA), 3
Americans with Disabilities Act, 680
Aminoglycosides, 609t
Amitriptyline, 459
Amphiarthroses, 19
Amphotericin B, 311
Ampicillin, 688t
Amyloid, 543
Amyloid arthropathy, of renal failure, 574
Amyloid cardiomyopathy, 545
Amyloidosis, 543–548
  classification of, 544, 544t
  diagnosis of, 547
  dialysis-related, 546
  hepatic, 545
  hereditary, types of, 546
  in inflammatory bowel disease, 270
  malignancy associated with, 372t–373t
  primary, 544
  in rheumatoid arthritis, 115
  secondary, 545–546
  senile transthyretin, 546
  systemic AA, 545

Page numbers followed by *f* indicate figures; *t*, tables; *b*, boxes.

Amyloidosis (Continued)
  disorders associated with, 546
  treatment and prognosis of, 548
  systemic AL, 544
    epidemiology of, 544
    factors in, 547
    physical findings in patients with, 544
    symptoms in patients with, 544
    treatment for, 547
Amyotrophy, diabetic, 359
Anakinra, 637
  as pseudogout treatment, 349
  use in renal insufficiency patients, 575
Analgesia, 460
  nonsteroidal antiinflammatory drugs, 601
Andersen disease, 535t
Anemia
  of chronic disease, 56, 130–131
  Cooley's, 369
  hemolytic, 120t, 183
  iron deficiency, 56
  juvenile systemic connective tissue diseases-related, 527t
  mixed connective tissue disease-related, 168
  sickle cell, 367
    characteristic radiographic findings in, 369
    factors predisposing to, 369b
    hand-foot syndrome in, 367
    joint pain in, 368
    musculoskeletal infectious problem in, 369
Aneurysm
  abdominal visceral angiography of, 218
  aortic, genetic diseases in, 417
  coronary, 531–532
  mycotic, 203
Aneurysmal bone cyst (ABC), 505–506, 505f
Angiitis
  allergic. see Churg-Strauss syndrome
  amyloid β (Aβ)–related, 222
  cutaneous leukocytoclastic, 237
  frosted branch, 561
Angiocentric immunoproliferative lesions, 229t
Angiography
  of giant cell arteritis, 210
  of polyarteritis nodosa, 217–218, 218f
  of primary angiitis, 222
  of Takayasu arteritis, 213
  of vasculitis, 206, 206f
Angioid streaks, 418
Angiokeratomas, 422
Angiotensin-converting enzyme (ACE), 566
Angiotensin-converting enzyme (ACE) inhibitors, 152, 609t
Angiotensin II receptor antagonists, 146
ANK SPOND mnemonic, for ankylosing spondylitis, 263
Ankle
  examination of, 46–47
  primary osteoarthritis of, 388
Ankylosing spondylitis, 67, 68f, 103, 259–267, 667
  amyloidosis associated with, 546
  cervical spine involvement, 445t
  differentiated from diffuse idiopathic skeletal hyperostosis, 266
  early diagnosis of, 449–450
  in famous personages, 693
  natural course of, 266
  pathophysiology behind radiographic features in, 265
  physiotherapy used in, 267
  polyarticular symptoms of, 87
  radiographic features of, 71, 264, 280, 281t
  surgery indicated in, 267
  uveitis associated with, 556

Ankylosis
  reactive arthritis-related, 279
  septic arthritis-related, 293t
Antacids, 610t
Anterior cruciate ligament injury, 474
Anterior drawer sign, 474
Anterior interosseous nerve syndrome, 479
Anti-155/140 autoantibody, 162
Antibiotics
  prophylactic use of
    for acute rheumatic fever, 331, 332t
    for deep venous thrombosis, 669
    for prosthetic joint surgery, 100
    in total joint replacement patients, 673
  therapeutic uses of
    for acute rheumatic fever, 331, 332t
    for Lyme disease, 304–305
    for nongonococcal septic arthritis, 294, 295t
    for reactive arthritis, 282
    for Whipple's disease, 326–327
Antibodies
  classes of, 33
  in HBV infection, 314
  in immune and inflammatory response, 34
Antibodies to nerve growth factor, as osteoarthritis therapy, 391
Antibodies to ribonuclear protein, 53
Antibodies to SS-A/Ro, 52–53
Anticardiolipin antibodies (aCL abs), 179
Anticoagulation, in antiphospholipid antibody (aPLab)-positive patients, 10
Anticonvulsants
  as complex regional pain syndrome treatment, 487
  as fibromyalgia syndrome treatment, 460
Anti-cyclic citrullinated peptide antibodies, 54
Anticytoplasmic antibodies, autoimmune disease associated with, 52t
Anti-double-stranded (ds) DNA antibodies, in systemic lupus erythematosus, 120t, 127
Antigen-presenting cells (APCs), 28–29, 29t
Anti-glomerular basement membrane disease, 236t
Anti-β2GPI antibodies, 179, 181
  antigenic determinant for, 181
Antihistamines, as cause of dry eyes, 172
Antihistone antibodies
  drug-induced disease versus idiopathic SLE, 138
  in drug-induced lupus, 138
Antihyperuricemic agents, 646
Antiinflammatory agents, 487
Antimalarials
  use during breast feeding, 582
  effectiveness of, 620
  mechanism of action of, 619–620
  for psoriatic arthritis, 287
  use in renal insufficiency patients, 575
  as rheumatoid arthritis treatment, 619
  as sarcoidosis treatment, 569
  as systemic lupus erythematosus treatment, 620
Anti-MDA-5 (anti-CADM-140), 162
Anti-Mi-2 syndrome, 162
Antimicrobial peptides (AMPs), 24
Anti-MPO antibodies, sensitivity of, 228t
Anti-Müllerian hormone test, 580
Antineutrophil cytoplasmic antibodies (ANCAs)
  definition of, 55
  diseases associated with, 55
  in inflammatory bowel disease, 270
  in juvenile systemic connective tissue diseases, 527t
  perinuclear, 55
    in drug-induced lupus, 138

Antineutrophil cytoplasmic antibodies *(Continued)*
  in relapsing polychondritis, 256
  in vasculitis, 205, 224–235, 523
Antinuclear antibody (ANA)
  diseases associated with antibodies measured in, 52t
  in drug-induced lupus, 137
  drugs associated with, 138t
  in juvenile idiopathic arthritis, 519t–520t
  measurement of, 49
  in nonspecific arthralgias, 54
  pattern of, 51, 51b, 52f
  positive, 49
    medical conditions associated with, 50t
    in normal healthy individual, 50
    with polyarticular symptoms, 89
  as screening test for systemic lupus erythematosus, 51
  in systemic lupus erythematosus, 120t, 121, 522, 523t
  in systemic sclerosis, 141
  in uveitis, 558
Antiosteoporotic therapy, 487
Antioxidants, 687
Antiphosphatidylserine-dependent antibodies, 181
Antiphospholipid antibodies, 53f, 101, 103, 120t, 179
  associated with malignancy, 372t–373t
  in drug-induced lupus, 138
  elevated levels of
    noncerebral arterial thrombosis and, 186
    thrombosis caused by, 182
    treatment of, 185
  fetal losses in patients with, 186
  neoplasms associated with, 182
  pregnancy and, 580
  stability of, 181
Antiphospholipid antibody syndrome, 10, 179–188, 203, 580
  anticoagulation of patients with, 187
  clinical and laboratory manifestations of, 180
  International Consensus Classification Criteria for, 180
  parenteral anticoagulants for, 185
  perioperative management of, 103
  primary, 132, 180
  secondary, 180
  thrombotic manifestations in, 182
Anti-PR3, sensitivity of, 228t
Antiresorptive drugs, 659
Antirheumatic drugs, 575–576
Anti-signal recognition particle (SRP) syndrome, 161
Anti-Smith antibodies, in systemic lupus erythematosus, 120t
Antisynthetase syndrome, 161
Anti-tumor necrosis factor-α
  as ankylosing spondylitis treatment, 267
  for HIV infection, 323
  as rheumatic disease treatment, 101
  side effects of, 635
Antiviral (AV) agents, as mixed cryoglobulinemic vasculitis treatment, 244
Aortic arch syndrome, 212
Aortic insufficiency, 563
  relapsing polychondritis-related, 255
Aortitis, 209–210
  chronic lymphoplasmacytic, 215
  isolated, 214–215
Aphthosis, complex, 249
Apley's test, 44, 474
Apophysitis, medial, 472
Apoptosis
  differentiated from necrosis and autophagy, 35
  pathways lead to, 35
Apremilast, 251, 287, 625
Arachnodactyly, 417–418
Aristospan, as juvenile idiopathic arthritis treatment, 519

Aromatase inhibitors, 376
Arsenic, neuromuscular toxicity of, 93
Arterial rupture, in pseudoxanthoma elasticum, 418
Arteriography, 551
Arteritis
  coronary, in rheumatoid arthritis, 114t
  giant cell, 11, 194, 195t, 201–202, 208–212
    clinical presentations of, 208
    cranial involvement in, 209
    diagnosis of, from temporal artery biopsy, 211
    extracranial, 209
    histologic findings in, 210, 211f
    incidence of, 208
    mortality in, 212
    with "normal" ESR, 210
    pathogenesis of, 211
    standard treatment of, 211
    vascular distributions in, complications for, 209t
  Kawasaki disease-related, 530
  Takayasu, 206, 212–214
  of temporal artery, 211
Arthritis. *see also* Osteoarthritis; Rheumatoid arthritis
  acute rheumatic fever associated with, 330
  ankle, 673
  atrophic, classification of, 3
  in Behçet's disease, 250
  chronic villous, classification of, 3
  Cogan's syndrome-related, 563
  Crohn disease-related, 528
  crystal-induced, 83, 88
  crystalline, 4t
  degenerative
    radiographic features of, 65, 65f
    secondary causes of, 66, 66f
  dermatologic conditions of, 287
  diet effects on, 686
  as disability cause, 5
  of elbow, 44
  enteropathic, 88t–89t
  gonococcal, 87, 88t, 277, 278t, 516
  gouty. *see* Gout
  HIV infection-related, 320
  hypertrophic, classification of, 3
  infectious, 3, 88
  inflammatory, 11, 670
    assessment of, 41
    bowel diseases associated with, 268, 271
    chronic monoarticular, synovial biopsy for, 8
    multiple epiphyseal dysplasia-associated, 438
    radiographic features of, 63, 64f, 65
    synovial fluid WBC differential in diagnosing, 60
    TNF inhibitors in, 635
  intermittent, 592
  juvenile idiopathic. *see* Juvenile idiopathic arthritis (JIA)
  Kawasaki disease-related, 530
  Lyme disease-related, 301
  multicentric reticulohistiocytosis related, 594
  noninflammatory lumbar, 67
  ochronotic, treatment of, 428
  peripheral, 271t
    radiographic diagnosis of, 69, 70f
    polymyalgia rheumatica-related, 194
  poststreptococcal, 328–334, 516
  posttraumatic, 670
  pseudoseptic, 296, 348
  psoriatic, 103, 284, 287f
    asymmetric sacroiliac involvement in, 285
    axial involvement in, 285
    characteristics of, 12
    in children, 520

Arthritis (Continued)
    classic pattern of, 285
    classification criteria of, 285
    clinical features of, 285
    extraarticular features of, 286
    features associated with, 285
    laboratory test of, 286
    medications for, 287
    in notable people, 693
    polyarticular symptoms of, 88t
    prognosis of, 287
    radiographic features of, 72, 286
    skin involvement in, 284, 286
    treatment of, 10, 286
    uveitis associated with, 556
  pyogenic, associated with malignancy, 372t–373t
  radiographic evaluation of, 63
  reactive, 12, 88, 88t, 276–283. see also Reiter's syndrome.
    cutaneous lesions in, 277
    define, 276
    differential diagnosis of, 277
    distribution of, 280
    extraarticular manifestations associated with, 277
    HIV infection-related, 320
    infectious agents causing, 276
    laboratory investigations useful in, 278, 279t
    musculoskeletal manifestations of, 277
    nonpharmacologic management of, 281
    pharmacologic management of, 281
    poststreptococcal, 330
    prognosis of, 282
    radiographic features of, 71, 279
    refractory, 282
    symptoms of, 277
  of relapsing polychondritis, 255
  sarcoid, 82, 84t, 88t–89t, 568t
  septic, 348, 513–514
    in B-cell immunodeficiency, 433
    bacterial, 289–299
    in classic hereditary hemochromatosis, 425–426
    erythematosus joints in, 510
    factors predisposing, 291
    fungal, 310–311
    gonococcal, 291, 292t
    HIV infection-related, 322
    nongonococcal. see Nongonococcal septic arthritis
    organisms associated in, 292
    radiographic studies of, 293, 294t
  signs of, 9
  Sjögren's syndrome-related, 175
  spinal, 67, 68f, 68t, 268, 270, 271t
  Still's disease-related, 190
  surgical options for, 670
  in systemic lupus erythematosus, 125
  temporomandibular, 668
  theory of, 687
  total joint replacement surgery in patients with, 668
  tuberculous septic, 12
  viral, 89t, 313
  Whipple's disease-related, 325–326
Arthritis-dermatitis syndrome, 272
Arthritis rehabilitation nurses, healthcare personnel, 662
Arthritis robustus, 109
Arthrocentesis, 58–62, 101, 365. see also Synovial fluid analysis
    aseptic technique in, 58
    contraindications to, 58
    indications for, 83
    for polyarthritis evaluation, 90
    potential complications of, 59
Arthrodesis, triple, 673
Arthrography, 75
    magnetic resonance ((MR), 472
Arthropathy
    in acromegaly, 362
    apatite-associated, 354, 355f
    chronic hemophilic, treatment of, 367, 368b
    in classic hereditary hemochromatosis, 425–426
        clinical features of, 426
        radiographic abnormalities in, 426, 426f
    endocrine-associated, 357–364
    myxedematous, 360
    rotator cuff tear, 354, 355f
Arthroplasty
    of knee, 390, 672
    of metacarpophalangeal joints, 671
    total
        cemented, 671
        cementless, 671
        of elbow, 670
        of hip, 409, 669, 671
        of knee, 672
        of shoulder, 669
Arthroscopy
    complication rate for, 77
    invention of, 77
    of monoarthritis, 85
Ascending pain pathways, 456
Aseptic loosening, 672
Asherson's syndrome, 183–184
Aspergillus fumigatus, 311
Aspiration
    abdominal fat pad, 13
    of joints, 7, 514
Aspirin
    cardiovascular effects of, 605
    development of, 601
    use during breast feeding, 582
    use during pregnancy, 582
    as hyperuricemia cause, 339t
    as Kawasaki disease treatment, 531–532
    preoperative discontinuation of, 98
Assistive devices, 665–666
Asthma, 603–604
Atherosclerosis, in rheumatoid arthritis, 115
Atlanto-axial (C1-C2) instability, 97, 98f
Atypical femoral fractures, bisphosphonate for, 655, 656f
Autoantibodies
    drug-induced, development of, 10
    in HCV infection, 314
    in HIV infection-associated rheumatic syndromes, 320
    in systemic lupus erythematosus, 129, 578
Autoantigens, 36
Autoimmune disease
    anticytoplasmic antibodies associated with, 52t
    differentiated from autoinflammatory disease, 38
    eye and ear, 555–564
    famous people with, 694
    female/male ratio of, 5t
    immunoablative therapy for, 632
    inflammatory bowel disease-related, 274
    mixed cryoglobulinemia and, 242
    pathogenesis of, 37
    prevalence of, 4
    stages of, 37
    in women, 4
Autoimmune/inflammatory syndrome induced by adjuvants (ASIA syndrome), 597

INDEX

Autoimmune phenomena
  anti-TNF-α biologic agents and, 636
  PID syndromes associated with, 433, 435
Autoimmune syndromes, 596
Autoimmunity, 36–38
  definition of, 37
  overview of, 24–38
Autoinflammatory syndrome, 13
Autologous blood transfusion, rheumatoid arthritis of, 668
Autophagy, differentiated from apoptosis and necrosis, 35
Axon, 78
Axonotmesis, 79
Ayurveda, 686
Azathioprine, 627
  as Behçet's disease treatment, 251
  as connective tissue disease treatment, 376t
  use during pregnancy and lactation, 583
  use in renal insufficiency patients, 575
  as juvenile systemic lupus erythematosus treatment, 524
  mechanism of action and metabolism of, 627, 628f
  organ transplantation, 649
  as rheumatic disease treatment, 628
  as sarcoidosis treatment, 569
  as systemic lupus erythematosus treatment, 132

B

Babesiosis, 305
Back, arthritis of, radiographic diagnosis of, 69, 70f
Back pain, 7
  approach for patient with, 443–451
  category of, historical symptoms of, 447t
  in children, 13, 513
  as disability cause, 5
  inflammatory, 11
  prevalence of, 4t
  primary care office visits for, 4
  tests for, 451
  tests/treatments not to be done in patients with, 8
Baker's cyst, 468
Balanitis, circinate, 277
Barium enema, in systemic sclerosis, 148f
Barnard, Sir Christiaan, 692
Basic calcium phosphate (BCP), 347, 352–356
  deposition of, 352
  diseases associated with, 352
  inflammatory synovitis, 354
  in joints, 354, 354f
  and osteoarthritis, 355
B cells, 31
  function, laboratory tests for, 430, 431t
  stimulation of, to produce humoral antibody response, 32
B-cell immunodeficiency syndromes, 430, 433
B cell targeted therapies, 640
Becker dystrophy, 541
Beethoven, Ludwig von, 694
Beethoven's disease, 694
Bee venom, 687
Behçet, Hulusi, 251
Behçet's disease, 248–251
  clinical symptoms of, 249
  common laboratory findings in, 250
  cutaneous manifestations of, 250
  food allergy-associated, 687t
  major causes of mortality in, 251
  neurologic manifestations of, 250
  pathogenesis of, 251
  therapies for, 251
  uveitis associated with, 557, 557t

Beighton score, for joint laxity and hypermobility, 414
Belimumab, 134, 640–641
Bell's palsy, 302
Benign hypermobility syndrome, 87
Benign joint hypermobility syndrome (BJHS), Brighton diagnostic criteria for, 415
Benzbromarone, 646
Benzodiazepines, as cause of dry eyes, 172
Beta-blocker, 609t
Betamethasone, 614t
Biologic agents, 633–644
  half-lives of selective, 102t
  use in renal insufficiency patients, 575
  nomenclature of, 633
  precautions of, 633
  relative annual cost for, 642, 643t
  used together, 642
Biopsy
  for amyloidosis evaluation, 547
  brain, of primary angiitis, 222
  liver, 622
  lung, in interstitial lung disease, 149
  of minor salivary gland, 174
  of muscle, 159, 159f, 541, 541t
  in osteoarticular TB, 308
  of polyarteritis nodosa, 217
  renal, 125, 127, 127t, 217
  synovial, 76–77, 76b
    of complex regional pain syndrome, 486
    of monoarthritis, 85
    techniques in, advantages and disadvantages of, 77t
  of temporal artery, 210–211, 211f
  for vasculitis diagnosis, 206
Biosimilars, 642
Birdshot retinochoroidopathy, 557
Bisphosphonates, 575, 654, 658
  atypical femoral fractures, 655, 656f
  as osteonecrosis cause, 407
  as Paget's disease treatment, 403, 403t
  precautions for, 655
Black cohosh, 688
Blackcurrant seed oil, 687
Blastomyces dermatitidis, 311
Blau syndrome, 591
Bleeding diatheses, as arthrocentesis contraindication, 58
Bleomycin, 376
Blepharitis, 172
Blindness, 250
Blood cultures, in monoarthritis, 83
Blood tests, in septic arthritis, 293
Bluestone, Rodney, 693
Bone
  infections of, fungal, 310
  metabolic disease of, 393–399
  Paget's disease of, 400–404
  in tuberculosis, 307
  types and composition of, 21
Bone deformities, in Paget's disease, 400
Bone demineralization, in reactive arthritis, 279
Bone diseases
  in HIV infection, 323
  mycobacterial and fungal joint, 307–312
Bone lesions, radiographic features of, 497–506, 498f–499f, 498t
Bone marrow edema, 387
Bone marrow edema syndrome, 409
Bone mass, low, 395
Bone mineral densitometry, 394, 394f, 397b, 613

Bone mineral density
  causes of low, 395
  measurement of, 393
  for response to osteoporosis, 658, 658t
Bone pain, in Paget's disease, 400–401
Bone remodeling, 653, 653f, 658
Bone resorption, 401, 654
Bone scan, 74
  of monoarthritis, 85
  of Paget's disease, 401
  of pediatric joint pain, 510
  radiation exposure during, 75
  radionuclide, of osteonecrosis, 407–408
  of septic arthritis, 294t
  three phase, 74, 74t
    for complex regional pain syndrome, 485
Bone strengthening agents, 652–660
Bony reactivity, in reactive arthritis, 279
Borage seed oil, 687
Borrelia burgdorferi, 300, 305. see also Lyme disease
Boswellia serrata, 689
Botulinum toxin A, for osteoarthritis, 390
Bouchard, Charles-Joseph, 384
Bouchard's nodes, 383, 384f
Boutonniere deformity, 110, 110f, 671
Boxer's knuckle, injury to, 475
Brancher enzyme deficiency, 535t, 537f
Breastfeeding, biologic agents use during, 583, 642
Brewerton, Derrick, 693
Brittle bone disease, 413
Brodie, Benjamin, 693
Brodie's abscess, 73
Bronchiolitis obliterans (BO), 114
Brown tumors, 361, 572, 572f
Brucellosis, 312
Bruits, subclavian, 11
Buchanan, James, 693
Budapest criteria, for complex regional pain syndrome, 483
Budd-Chiari syndrome, 182
Buerger disease. see Thromboangiitis obliterans
Bunion deformity, 673
Bursa, 21
  amount of glucocorticoid injected in, 618t
Bursae, infection in, 299
Bursitis, 289–299, 452
  anserine, 467
  definition of, 462
  olecranon, 44, 466, 466f
  osteoarticular TB-related, 307
  preadventitial Achilles, 47
  prepatellar, 46, 467
  primary care office visits for, 4
  retrocalcaneal, 47, 468
  septic, 299
  subacromial, 464
  trochanteric, 46, 467

C

Caffeine, drug interactions of, 610t
Calcaneal spurs. see Heel spurs
Calcific deposits, in pseudoxanthoma elasticum, 418
Calcification
  of disc space, 71
  dystrophic, 596
  of soft tissue, 574, 595
  subcutaneous, 159
  synovial sarcoma-related, 495
  of vertebral disc, 72

Calcinosis, 146
Calcitonin, 403, 654t
Calcitriol, 653
Calcium
  dietary intake of, 652, 652t
  for osteoporosis prevention, 652
Calcium carbonate, 652
Calcium channel blockers, 146, 552–553
Calcium citrate, 652
Calcium hydroxyapatite, 347, 352
Calcium oxalate crystals, 355
Calcium pyrophosphate deposition (CPPD) disease, 12, 346–351
  asymptomatic, 346
  chondrocalcinosis and, 347
  clinical presentations associated with, 346
  joint involvement in, 88t
  laboratory studies for, 350
  pathogenesis of, 347, 347f
  polarized light microscopy for, 348
  polyarticular arthritis symptoms of, 87
  predisposing factors of, 346
  radiographic features of, 72, 350
  and rheumatoid arthritis, 349
Calcium pyrophosphate dihydrate, 346
Calcium pyrophosphate dihydrate crystals, in pseudogout, 352
Calcium pyrophosphate dihydrate deposition disease, 574
Calvé's disease, 405
Cam impingement, 387, 388f
Canakinumab (Ilaris), 637
Canale-Smith syndrome, 597
Cancer
  dermatomyositis/polymyositis-associated, 160, 373
  as low back pain cause, 447
  rheumatoid arthritis-related, 117
  Sjögren's syndrome-related, 176
Candida skin test, 431
Candida species, 311
Cane, 665
CAN'T LEAP mnemonic, for hyperuricemia, 339t
Capsaicin, 689
Capsulitis, adhesive, 359
Carbohydrate metabolism, during muscle work, 537, 537f
Carcinogens, 690
Carcinoid syndrome, 536t
Cardiac disorders, in granulomatosis with polyangiitis, 227
Cardiopulmonary testing, in systemic sclerosis, 147
Cardiovascular disease
  glucocorticoid-related, 613
  rheumatic diseases-related, 96
  rheumatoid arthritis-related, 668
Carditis
  and acute rheumatic fever, 331
  rheumatic, 330
Carnitine deficiency syndrome, 535t, 539
Carpal tunnel syndrome, 43, 81, 81t, 477–478, 478f
  and diabetes mellitus, 359
  treatment options for, 478
Carroll, Lewis, 685
Cartilage
  in arthritis, 279
  function, structure, and composition of, 19, 20f
  hyaline, 19
  matrix turnover of, 20
  in relapsing polychondritis, 257
  shark, 691
  zones of, 20
Cartilage transplant, for osteoarthritis, 391
Cataracts, relapsing polychondritis-related, 255

Catastrophic antiphospholipid syndrome (CAPS), 183–184, 184t, 187
Cauda equina syndrome, 449, 674
Causalgia, 483
Cayenne, 688–689
Cefixime, 298t
Ceftriaxone, 298t, 688t
Celecoxib, 98, 606
Celiac disease, 271–272
Cellcept. *see* Mycophenolate mofetil
Cellular immunity, 32
Cellulitis, 58, 74t
Central nervous system (CNS) disorders
  fibromyalgia syndrome-related, 457
  granulomatosis with polyangiitis in, 227
  Lyme disease and, 302
  in systemic lupus erythematosus, 129
Cerebellar ataxia, 250
Cerebral arterial clot, treatment of, 185
Cerebrovascular disease, 95, 95b
Certilizumab Pegol (Cimzia), 634
Cervical spine
  nerve root compression assessment of, 446
  nerve root lesions of, 446t
  range of motion assessment of, 445–446
  rheumatoid arthritis of, 97, 445t, 668–669
Cervical traction, 665
Cervical whiplash syndrome, 445
Cevimeline, 177
C fibers, 456
Charcot arthropathy, radiographic features of, 72
Charcot joints, 357, 358f
Cheiroarthropathy, diabetic, 357, 358f
Cherry juice, as CAM therapy, 690
Chest expansion, for ankylosing spondylitis assessment, 262
Chest pain, Raynaud's phenomenon-related, 551
Children
  acute osteomyelitis in, 299
  acute rheumatic fever in, 330
  differential diagnosis of monoarthritis in, 83
  erythema chronicum migrans treatment in, 302
  Henoch-Schönlein purpura in, 524
  joint pain in, 507–515
  Kawasaki disease in, 524
  rubella infections in, 316
  septic arthritis in, 292, 292t, 295
  systemic connective tissue diseases in, 522–529
Chlorambucil, 559, 583
Chloroquine, 569
  use during pregnancy, 582
  as retinopathy cause, 620
Chlorpromazine, 182
Cholecalciferol, 397
Cholestasis, 604
Cholesterol crystals, 355
Cholesterol emboli syndrome, 203
Cholestyramine, 610t
Chondritis
  auricular, 254
  nasal, 254, 255f
Chondroadherin, 18
Chondroblastoma, 500, 501f
Chondrocalcinosis, 71, 347, 348f, 574
  in arthropathy of HHC, 426
  and calcium pyrophosphate crystal deposition, 347
  and primary hyperparathyroidism, 361
Chondrocytes, 19–20
Chondrodysplasia, 17t
Chondroitin sulfate, as osteoarthritis treatment, 389
Chondroma, 495

Chondromalacia, 513t
Chondromalacia patellae, 473
Chondromatosis, synovial, 84t, 85, 494, 494f
Chondrosarcoma, synovial, 496
Chorea, Sydenham, 331
Chowne, W.D, 692
Chromogenic factor X, 187
Chronic atypical neutrophilic dermatosis with lipodystrophy and elevated temperature (CANDLE) syndrome, 591
Chronic infantile neurologic, cutaneous, and articular syndrome (CINCA), 590
CHRONIC mnemonic, for diseases associated with rheumatoid factor production, 54
Chronic pain syndrome, peripheral and central sensitization in, 456
Chronic recurrent multifocal osteomyelitis (CRMO), 591
Chronic regional pain syndrome, 359
Churg-Strauss syndrome, 232–234
Cimetidine, 610t
Citrullinated protein antigens, antibodies directed against, 54
Civil War era, rheumatic diseases in, 694
Clarithromycin, 688t
Claudication, 220, 545
Clavicle distal end, "penciling" of, 69
Claw toe deformity, 674t
Clayton-Hoffman procedure, 673
CLOT mnemonic, associated with elevated antiphospholipid antibodies, 182
Clotrimazole, 688t
Clubbing, of fingers, 270, 373, 374f
Coccidioides immitis, 311
Codman's triangle, 499, 499f
Coenzyme Q-1O, 689
Cogan's syndrome, 252, 563–564
Colchicine, 344, 645
  dosage for, 646t
  use in renal insufficiency patients, 575
  indication to, 645
  manifestations of toxicity, 645
  mechanism of action of, 645
  oral, as Behçet's disease treatment, 251
  as pseudogout treatment, 349
Cold agglutinin disease, 246
Cold exposure, as Raynaud's phenomenon precipitant, 551
Colitis
  collagenous, 270–271, 272t
  lymphocytic, 272t
  microscopic, 270–271
  ulcerative, 234
Collagen, 16–18
  abnormality in synthesis of, 414
  classes of, 16
  degradation, enzymes for, 18
  diseases caused by mutations, 17t
  fibril-forming (interstitial), synthesis of, 17–18, 18f
  structural features of, 16, 17f
  tissue distribution of, 17t
  types of, 16, 17t
Collagen vascular disease
  differentiated from connective tissue disease, 4
  Hashimoto's thyroiditis and, 360
Collagenases, 18
Collectins, 25
Common variable immunodeficiency (CVID)
  rheumatologic manifestations of, 434, 434b
  therapy for, 435
Complement, 55
  in active inflammation, 55
  components of, 56
  conditions associated with hereditary deficiency of, 56t

Complement (*Continued*)
  diseases associated with decreased levels of, 55
  low serum level of, polyarticular diseases associated with, 90
  role of, in immune response, 34, 34f
  in systemic lupus erythematosus, 120t
Complement-deficient states, homozygous
  infectious, 432
  rheumatologic, 435
Complement system, activation of, 35
Complementary and alternative medicine (CAM), 683–691
  definition of, 685
  remedies, 685
    approach for, 691
    categories of, 685, 685t–686t
    physicians care for, 685
    unsafe, 691
Complete blood count (CBC)
  glucocorticoids and, 613
  in monoarthritis, 83
  for suspected vasculitis evaluation, 205
Complex regional pain syndrome (CRPS), 483–490
  inciting factors for, 484t
  pathophysiology of, 486
  precipitating factors for, 484
  predisposing factors for, 484t
  prevalence of, 484
  prognosis for, 488
  radiographic findings in, 485, 486f
  scintigraphic findings in, 485
  signs and symptoms of, 483
  stages of, 485
  synonyms for, 484
  therapy for, 487
  trauma-related, 485
  treatment of, 486
Computed tomography (CT)
  comparison with magnetic resonance imaging, 72
  dual-energy, 73
    of gout, 340
  for herniated lumbar disk evaluation, 450t
  of osteonecrosis, 407–408
  radiation exposure during, 75
  of septic arthritis, 294t
  single-photon emission, 74
  thoracic high-resolution, for systemic sclerosis evaluation, 148
Computed tomography myelogram
  for herniated disk evaluation, 450
  for low back pain evaluation, 449
Congenital heart block (CHB), 524
Congestive heart failure
  anti-TNF-α biologic agents and, 637
  in classic HHC, 425–426
Conjunctivitis, 250, 530–531
Connective tissue, macromolecular "building blocks" of, 16
Connective tissue diseases, 10
  in celebrities, 694
  differentiated from collagen vascular disease, 4
  dystrophic calcification associated with, 596
  heritable, 411–419
    barrier, 419
    characteristics of, 413
    classification of, 413
    compressive, 418
    tensile, 413–418
  malignancies associated with, 375t
  mixed, 10, 166–169
    in children, 522
    clinical manifestations of, 166, 167t

Connective tissue diseases (*Continued*)
  course and prognosis of, 168
  diagnosis of, 166
  gastrointestinal manifestations of, 167
  laboratory findings in, 168, 169t
  nervous system manifestations of, 168
  pulmonary manifestations of, 167, 168t
  in musicians, 694
  patient history for, 41
  prevalence of, 4t
  systemic, juvenile, 522–529
  undifferentiated, 166, 169–170, 170t
Connor, Bernard, 693
Contractures, of finger, 357–358
Control points, of fibromyalgia, 453
Coombs test, direct, 120t
Copper accumulation, in Wilson disease, 427–428
Copper bracelets, as rheumatoid arthritis remedy, 688
Core decompression, of femoral head, 408–409
Cori-Forbes disease, 535t
Cornea verticillata, 422
Corneal dystrophy, 17t
Coronary artery disease, in systemic lupus erythematosus, 135
Corticosteroids
  as ankylosing spondylitis treatment, 267
  as dermatomyositis/polymyositis treatment, 163
  use during breast feeding, 582
  use during pregnancy, 582
  as giant cell arteritis treatment, 211–212
  glucocorticoids properties of, 614, 614t
  use in renal insufficiency patients, 575
  as juvenile systemic lupus erythematosus treatment, 526
  as osteoarthritis treatment, 390
  as osteonecrosis risk factor, 407
  perioperative regimens for, 100t
  as polyarteritis nodosa treatment, 219
  "pulse," 631
  as reactive arthritis treatment, 282
  as relapsing polychondritis treatment, 257
  as sarcoidosis treatment, 569
  as systemic lupus erythematosus treatment, 131–132
  as Takayasu arteritis treatment, 213
  as uveitis treatment, 559
Cortisol, 92, 614
Cortisone, 614t
Costochondritis, 593
Costoclavicular maneuver, 479–480
Cosyntropin stimulation test, 99
Coumadin, 58, 186–187
Coxsackievirus infection, 318
Crain's disease, 384–385
Cranial nerve palsies, in Behçet's disease, 250
C-reactive protein (CRP), 49, 133, 293
Creatine kinase
  as dermatomyositis/polymyositis marker, 159
  serum, causes of elevation of, 94
Crepitus, 42, 382
Crescent sign, 407, 408f
CREST syndrome, 143, 169
Cricoarytenoid (CA) disease, 98
Crohn's disease, 268, 269f, 528
Crossed-straight leg test, 448
Crowned dens syndrome, 353
Cryofibrinogens, 245
Cryoglobulinemia, 241–247
  articular manifestations of, 244
  cause of, 12
  clinical and laboratory features of, 242, 243f
  clinical manifestations of, 243, 243t, 245
  diagnosis of, 245

Cryoglobulinemia *(Continued)*
  HCV-associated, treatment of, 246f
  malignancy associated with, 372t–373t
  mixed, 11, 242
    cutaneous manifestations in, 243
    hepatitis C infection and, 242
    pathogenicity of, 242
    renal finding for, 243
  neurologic manifestations of, 243
  treatment of, 246
  type I, 242
Cryoglobulins, 241
Cryopyrin-associated periodic syndromes (CAPS), 590
Cryotherapy, 664
Cryptococcus neoformans, 310
Crystal deposition diseases, 82b, 347, 350, 574
Crystalline diseases, 352–356
C-SPINE mnemonic, for cervical spine disease evaluation, 97
Cubital tunnel syndrome, 81, 479
Cushing's disease, 536t
Cushing's syndrome, 362–363
  iatrogenic, 363
Cutaneous pustular lesions, musculoskeletal symptoms associated with, 287
Cutis laxa, 418
Cyanosis, Raynaud's phenomenon-related, 145
Cyclobenzaprine (Flexeril), 460
Cyclooxygenase-1/2 (COX-1/2) inhibitors, 602, 603t
Cyclooxygenase-3 (COX-3), 603
Cyclooxygenase pathway, 27
Cyclophosphamide, 629
  action and metabolism of, 629
  as connective tissue disease treatment, 376t
  contraindications to, 583
  use in dialysis patients, 576
  as juvenile systemic lupus erythematosus treatment, 524
  as lupus nephritis treatment, 128
  protocols for using monthly IV, 128
  use in renal insufficiency patients, 575
  as rheumatic disease treatment, 629
  toxicities of, 629
  as uveitis treatment, 559
Cyclosporine, 344
  adverse effects of, 574
    gout, 574–575
    toxicities, 630
  as connective tissue disease treatment, 376t
  use during pregnancy and lactation, 583
  as hyperuricemia cause, 339t
  organ transplantation, 649
  use in renal insufficiency patients, 575
  as rheumatic disease treatment, 630
  as uveitis treatment, 559
Cyst, of bone, 572f
Cystathionine β-synthase deficiency, in homocystinuria, 420
Cysteine, 420
Cystic fibrosis, 596
Cytotoxic drugs
  as lupus nephritis treatment, 129
  as polyarteritis nodosa treatment, 219
  as systemic AL amyloidosis treatment, 547
Cytotoxic T lymphocytes (CTLs), activation of, 35

D

Dactylitis, 277, 307–308
  sickle cell, 367–368
Danazol, 131
Dapsone, 251, 257, 575, 624, 688t
Deafness, in Ludwig von Beethoven, 694

Debrancher enzyme deficiency, 535t, 537f
Deep Koebner phenomenon, in psoriatic arthritis, 284
Deep venous thrombosis (DVT) prophylaxis, options for, in patients undergoing joint replacement procedures, 101
Deficiency of IL-1 receptor antagonist (DIRA), 591
Deficiency of IL-36 receptor antagonist (DITRA), 591
Degenerative disc disease. *see* Osteoarthritis
Degenerative joint disease, radiographic features of, 72
Demyelinating syndromes, anti-TNF-α biologic agents and, 636
Dendritic cells, 26
Dengue fever, 317
Denosumab, 654t, 656
Depression, 129, 456
Dermatomyositis. *see also* Polymyositis
  amyopathic, 160
  cancer-associated, 373
  characteristic rash of, 159
  dermatologic manifestations of, 159
  diagnostic criteria of, 158
  epidemiologic features of, 158
  extraarticular organ involvement in, 89t
  extramuscular/extradermatologic manifestations of, 160
  juvenile
    in children, 526
    chronic sequelae in patients with, 526
  laboratory abnormalities of, 161
  malignancy associated with, 10, 372t–373t
  mimics of, 159
  prognosis of, 163
  Raynaud phenomenon-associated, 89
  rehabilitative techniques for, 667
  treatment of, 162
Desipramine, 177
Dexamethasone, 614t
Diabetes mellitus, 357–360, 546
  carpal tunnel syndrome and, 359
  in classic HHC, 425–426
  rheumatologic syndromes and, 357
Diabetic stiff hand syndrome, 12
Dialysis patients
  amyloidosis in, 546
  anti-rheumatic drug therapy in, 575
  destructive spondyloarthropathy in, 574
Diarthroses (synovial joints), 19
Diclofenac, 604
Diet, effect on arthritis, 686
Diffuse idiopathic skeletal hyperostosis (DISH), 266, 360, 385, 445t
  radiographic findings in, 386, 386f
Diffuse infiltrative lymphocytosis syndrome (DILS), 321
  differentiated from Sjögren's syndrome, 322t
DiGeorge syndrome, 431
Digoxin, 609t
Dilute Russell viper venom test (dRVVT), 180–181
Dimethyl sulfoxide (DMSO), 690
Disability, 676
  benefits, application for, 679
  fibromyalgia-related, 461
Discitis, in children, 513
Disease-modifying antirheumatic drugs (DMARDs), 101, 102t, 619
  combinations of, 623
  use during pregnancy and lactation, 582–583
  nonbiologic, 619
Disk herniation, 674
Diskogenic, cervical spondylosis, 445
Disseminated gonococcal infection (DGI), 296
  arthritic symptoms developing in, 296
  cultures and Gram stains in, 297, 298t
  evaluation for, 12

Disseminated gonococcal infection *(Continued)*
  host factors enhancing susceptibility in, 296–297
  laboratory test in, 298
  symptoms associated with, 297, 297f
  treatment of, 298, 298t
Down syndrome, 544t
Doxycycline, 298t, 302
Drug abuse
  intranasal, 229t
  and septic arthritis, 295
Dual energy x-ray absorptiometry (DXA), 393–395
Duchenne dystrophy, 541
Dufy, Raoul, 692
Dupuytren's contracture, 359
Dwarfism, 439
Dysferlinopathies, 541
Dysplasias, 437
  of bone and joint, 437–442
  as cause of secondary osteoarthritis, 386
  diaphyseal, 439
  epiphyseal, 438
  fibrous, 502–503, 504f
  metaphyseal, 17t, 439
  multiple epiphyseal, 17t
  spondyloepiphyseal, 17t
Dystonia, treatment for, 487

E

Eales' disease, 561
Ear
  autoimmune disorders of, 563–564
  chondritis of, 254
Eaton-Lambert syndrome, 92
Echinacea, 689
Echocardiography, 545
Echovirus infection, 318
Eclampsia, 578
Ectopia lentis, 420
  in Marfan syndrome, 417
Eculizumab (Soliris), 643
Ehlers-Danlos syndrome (EDS), 17t, 218, 694
  benign joint hypermobility syndrome and, 416
  clinical manifestations of, 414, 415f
  types of
    arthrochalasia, 415
    classic, 414–415
    dermatosparaxis, 415
    hypermobile, 415
    kyphoscoliosis, 415
    vascular, 415
Eicosanoid pathway, 27f
Elastases, 18
Elastin, 18
Elbow
  arthritis of, 44
  soft tissue nodules in, 69
Elbow pain, nonarticular, 465
Elderly patients
  amyloidosis in, 546
  giant cell arteritis in, 208
  nonsteroidal antiinflammatory drug use by, 609
Electrodiagnostic tests, 78, 477
Electrolyte disorders, 536t
Electromyography, 78–81, 539
  clinical indications for, 78
  findings for normal and denervated muscles, 80t
  findings for normal muscle and myopathic disorders, 80t
  of herniated lumbar disk, 450t
  of low back pain, 450

Electrophoresis, serum protein, 49
EMPD mnemonic, for osteochondrodysplasia classification, 437, 437f
Enchondroma, 502, 503f
Enchondromatosis, 502
Endocarditis, bacterial, extraarticular organ involvement in, 89t
Endocrine diseases, rheumatologic manifestations associated with, 357
Endocrinopathy, occult, signs/symptoms of, 357
Endothelial adhesion molecules, 26t
Enteropathy, gluten sensitive, 271
Enterovirus infection, 318
Enthesis, 262
Enthesitis, 11, 277, 452, 468
  Achilles, 468, 468f
Enthesopathy, 67, 452
Entrapment neuropathies, 477–482
Enzyme-linked immunosorbent assay (ELISA), 303, 305
Eosinophilia, in eosinophilic fasciitis, 156
Eosinophilic granulomatosis with polyangiitis (EGPA). *see also* Churg-Strauss syndrome
  clinical features of, 232t
  clinical phases of, 232
  diagnosis of, 233
  drugs for, 233
  histopathologic findings in, 233
  laboratory abnormalities in, 233
  organ involvement in, 233t
  treatment of, 233
Eosinophilic-myalgia syndrome (EMS), 155
Eosinophilic synovitis, 593
Ephedra sinica, 689
Epicondylitis, 465
  lateral, 43, 465, 472
  medial, 465, 472
Epidermolysis bullosa, 419
Epidermolysis bullosa dystrophica, 17t
Epiphyseal ossification, 438
Episcleritis, 559–561
Epitope spreading, 38
Epstein-Barr virus (EBV) infection, 528
Erdheim-Chester disease, 595
Ergocalciferol, 397
Erosions, in reactive arthritis, 280
Erythema
  in children, 510
    Kawasaki disease-related, 530
    periarticular, gout-related, 339
    Raynaud's phenomenon-related, 145
Erythema ab igne, 664
Erythema chronicum migrans (ECM), 301f, 302
Erythema elevatum diutinum (EED), 236t, 239
Erythema marginatum, 331, 516, 517f
Erythema nodosa, 85
Erythema nodosum, 248, 566
Erythema nodosum leprosum, 310
Erythrocyte sedimentation rate (ESR), 48–49
  elevated
    evaluation of, 48
    in polymyalgia rheumatica, 194
  extremely high or extremely low, causes of, 48
  in giant cell arteritis, 210
  in monoarthritis, 84
  in systemic lupus erythematosus, 133
Erythromelalgia, 372t–373t, 595
Esophageal dysmotility, in systemic sclerosis, 147
Estrogen
  exogenous, in systemic lupus erythematosus, 133
  therapy, FDA-approved, 654t

Estrogen replacement therapy (ERT), 655
Etanercept (Enbrel), 634
Ethambutol, 308–309, 339t
Evening primrose oil, 687
Ewing sarcoma, 512–513
Exercise, 662–663
  aerobic, 663
  benefit of, 662
  factors to be considered in prescribing, 662
  as fibromyalgia syndrome therapy, 459
  isokinetic, 663
  isometric, 662
  isotonic, 663
  for low back pain therapy, 450
  as osteoarthritis therapy, 389
  range of motion (ROM), 662
  Williams', 450
Exostoses, 501
  hereditary, multiple, 502
Eye, anatomy of, 555f
Eye disorders
  autoimmune, 555–559
  in granulomatosis with polyangiitis, 227
  sarcoidosis-related, 566

F

^{18}F-Fluorodeoxyglucose (FDG)-PET scans, 210
FABER mnemonic, for sacroiliitis diagnosis, 449
Fabry disease, 421
Facet joint pain, 445
Facial nerve palsy, 566, 567t
Falls, risk factors for, 396
Familial autoinflammatory syndromes (FAS), 586–591, 587t
Familial cold autoinflammatory syndrome (FCAS), 590
Familial Hibernian fever, 589
Familial Mediterranean fever (FMF), 545–546, 548, 588–589
Farber disease, 421
Fasciculation potential, 79
Fasciitis
  eosinophilic, 155–156
    diagnosis of, 156
    hematologic abnormalities associated with, 156
    laboratory and radiographic abnormalities in, 155
    malignancy associated with, 375t
    stages of, 155
    therapies for, 156
  palmar, 12, 372t–373t, 375
  plantar, 47, 270, 468–469
Fascioscapulohumeral dystrophy, 541
Fatigability, 92
Fatigue
  common systemic causes of, 91b
  inflammatory arthritis-related, 42t
  neuromuscular disease-related, 91
  Sjögren's syndrome-related, 177
Fatty acids, 537, 687
Fatty acid transport defects, 535t
Febuxostat, 275, 344, 648–649
  dosage of, 648
Federal benefit rate (FBR), 678
Federal Rehabilitation Act, 680
Felty's syndrome, 115
Femoral head, osteonecrosis of, 405, 409t
Femoral nerve lesion, 81t
Femoral nerve stretch test, 448
Femoroacetabular impingement (FAI), 9, 387, 388f
Ferritin
  elevated serum, in Still's disease, 190
  as Still's disease indicator, 517–518

Fever
  and acute rheumatic fever, 331
  differential diagnosis of, 597
  familial Mediterranean fever-related, 545–546, 548, 588
  juvenile idiopathic arthritis-related, 517, 517f
  Kawasaki disease-related, 530
  in monoarthritis, 83
  in rheumatoid arthritis, 113
  Still's disease-related, 189
  of unknown origin, 208, 517
Feverfew, 689
Fibrillation potential, 79
Fibrillins, 18
Fibroma, nonossifying, 502, 503f
Fibromyalgia, 13, 422, 452–461, 690
  cervical spine involvement, 445t
  in children, 512t
  Lyme disease-related, 305
  polyarticular symptoms of, 87
  prevalence of, 4t
  primary, 13
  primary care office visits for, 4
  prognosis for, 461
Fibromyalgia syndrome (FMS)
  analgesia therapy for, 458
  brain imaging in, 457
  central pain sensitivity syndromes associated with, 453
  control points of, 453
  definition of, 452
  descending analgesia pathway in, 457, 458f
  diagnostic criteria for, 454
  differentiated from widespread arthritis, 454
  education programs for, 458–459
  evaluation of, 455
  impact on patient and society, 461
  medications for
    FDA-approved, 459
    side effects of, 460
  predisposing factor of, 456
  prevalence of, 454
  psychological disorders associated with, 455
  symptoms of, 453
  tender points in, 452, 453f, 454
  triggering factors for, 455
Fibronectin, 18
Fibrosis
  idiopathic retroperitoneal, 214
  pulmonary, 114
Fibrous cortical defect, 502
Fibroxanthoma, 493, 502
Fibula grafting, vascularized, 408–409
Finkelstein's maneuver/test, 43, 466
Fish oils, 687
Five factor score (FFS), 233
Flattened pinch sign, 479
Flavocoxid (Limbrel), 609
Flexor retinaculum, 468f
Focal neural entrapment, 79
Fondaparinux (synthetic heparin), 101
Food allergy, as arthritis cause, 687t
Foot
  diseases associated with radiographic changes in, 69
  examination of, 47
  flat, 469
  Reiter's syndrome of, 280f
Foot-drop, painless, 481
Forearm-based thumb spica splint, 466
Forearm ischemic test, 540
Forestier's disease, 360, 385
Fracture Risk Assessment (FRAX) tool, 396

Fractures
  as chronic osteomyelitis cause, 299
  fragility, 393
  as hemarthrosis cause, 12
  humeral, nonsteroidal antiinflammatory drugs and, 607
  osteoporotic, 393
  in Paget's disease, 400
  stress, 475
  vertebral, 395
Freiberg's disease, 405
Friou, George, 692
Fructose-1-phosphate aldolase deficiency, 338
Functional capacity evaluation, 678
Fungal infections, 84t, 85
Fungi, as septic arthritis cause, 310, 311t
Furniss, Bruce, 693
F-wave, 80

G

Gabapentin, 460
Gadolinium, as contrast agent in MRI, 72
Gaenslen's sign, 449
Gaenslen's test, 262, 263f
Gait, abnormal, 47
Gallbladder hydrops, 531
GAMED mnemonic, for immunoglobulin classification, 33
Gamekeeper's thumb, injury to, 475
Gangrene, 220
Gardner's syndrome, 500
Garlic, 689
Garrod, A.B., 693
Gastric antral venous ectasia ("GAVE"), 147
Gastritis, nonsteroidal antiinflammatory drug-induced, 604
Gastroduodenal ulcer disease, nonsteroidal antiinflammatory drug-induced, 604
Gastrointestinal disorders
  enteropathic arthritides-related, 268–272
  systemic sclerosis-related, 146
Gaucher's disease, 386
  skeletal manifestations of, 422
  type I, 421
Gelatinases, 20–21
Gender, role in psoriatic arthritis, 284
"Geologic" time, in chronic polyarthritis diagnosis, 90
Gerber lift-off test, 472
Gerber push with force test, 463
Ghent criteria, for diagnosing Marfan syndrome, 416
Giant cell tumor (GCT), 504–505, 505f
Gin, as arthritis treatment, 688
Ginkgo biloba, 689
Ginseng, 689
Gintrac, Elie, 692
Glenohumeral joint, in shoulder pain, 44
Glomerulonephritis
  focal necrotizing, and polyarteritis nodosa, 217
  focal proliferative, 126
  granulomatosis with polyangiitis-related, 225
  relapsing polychondritis-related, 256
  systemic lupus erythematosus-related, 127
Glucocorticoids (GCs). *see also* Corticosteroids
  adverse consequences of, 615
  antiinflammatory effects of, 612
  basic measures of, 616
  characteristics of, 617
  clinical baseline for, 613
  in combination with anesthetic, 617
  dosage scheduling of, 613, 614t
  excessive, 362
  factors affecting efficacy of, 614

Glucocorticoids (Continued)
  grouped, in terms of biologic activity, 614, 614t
  indications to, 612, 616
  injection into joint, bursa, or tendon sheath, 617, 617t
  method(s) of administration of, 613
  mineralocorticoid properties of, 615t
  as osteoporosis cause, 396
  as polymyalgia rheumatica treatment, 195
  problems and sequelae of, 618
  as rheumatic disease treatment, 613, 613t
  systemic and injectable, 612–618
  tapering schedule for, 616
Glucosamine sulfate, as osteoarthritis treatment, 389
Glucose-6-phosphatase deficiency, 338
Glucose intolerance, glucocorticoids and, 613
Glucose metabolism defects, 538
Gluteus medius, weakness of, 45
Glycogen metabolism, 535t, 538
Glycogen storage diseases, 535
β2-Glycoprotein I (β2GPI), 181
Glycosaminoglycan, 18
Goldenseal, 689
Golfer's elbow, 472
Golimumab (Simponi), 634
Gonococcal infection, disseminated, 296
Gonorrhea, arthritis associated with, 297
Goodpasture disease, 228
Gorlin sign, 414
Gottron's papules, 159, 526
Gout, 335–345
  acute attack of, 339
  alcohol consumption associated with, 339
  CAM therapies for, 690
  chronic, radiographic features of, 66, 67f
  classification of, 3
  conditions associated with, 341
  cyclosporine-related, 574–575
  diagnosis of, 340, 340f
  early descriptions of, 693
  famous people with, 693
  gender differences in, 337, 342
  intercritical, 339
  management of, 340
  in men, 12
  monoarticular, 82b, 83
  perioperative, 102
  polyarticular, 87t–89t
  postoperative, 103
  prevalence and epidemiology of, 337
  primary care office visits for, 4
  radiographic features of, 72, 340, 341f
  renal disease-related, 574
  renal transport of uric acid in, 342
  secondary, malignancy associated with, 372t–373t
  sickle cell disease-related, 369
  stages of, 339
  synovial fluid findings in, 61t
  tophaceous, 102, 339, 344, 649
  treatment of, 645, 647f
  urate crystal of, 61f
Gower maneuver, 526
Gower's sign, 93
Granuloma
  eosinophilic, 506, 506f
  noncaseating, sarcoidosis-related, 565
Granuloma annulare, 114
Granulomatosis, lymphomatoid, associated with malignancy, 372t–373t

Granulomatosis with polyangiitis (GPA), 11, 225–231.
  see also Wegener's granulomatosis
  clinical association between, 227
  definition of, 225
  differential diagnosis of, 228
  epidemiology of, 227
  kidney manifestation in, 226
  kidney transplant in, 231
  lower respiratory tract involvement in, 226
  natural history of, 228
  organ involvement in, 233t
  organ systems affected by, 227
  tests for, 228
  treatment of, 229
  upper and lower respiratory tracts affected by, 226
Granulomatous angiitis of central nervous system (GACNS), 222
Grape seed extract, 689
Groin, pain, in hip joint pathology, 45
Group A streptococci (GAS), 328, 330
  as acute rheumatic fever cause, 330
"Growing pains," 510, 512t

H

Hallux valgus, 673
Hammer toe deformity, 674t
Hand
  arthritis of, 110
  diseases associated with radiographic changes in, 69
  mechanic's, 159
  sports-related injuries of, 475
Hand-Christian-Schüller disease, 506
Hand-foot syndrome, 367–368
Hand rash, for systemic lupus erythematosus diagnosis, 124f
Handicap, 676
Hargraves, William, 692
Hashimoto's thyroiditis, and collagen vascular disease, 360
Hawkins-Kennedy test, 463
Headaches
  in Behçet's disease, 250
  migraine, 183
  mixed connective tissue disease-related, 168
  relapsing polychondritis-related, 256
Hearing loss, 209, 562–563
Heart block, congenital, 579
Heart disease, with systemic sclerosis, 151
Heat, therapeutic effects of, 664
Heberden, William, 383–384
Heberden's nodes, 383, 384f
Heel fat pad atrophy, 469
Heel pain, 47, 468
"Heel-rise" sign, 469
Heel spurs, 71, 469
Heerfordt's syndrome, 567
Heliotrope (lilac-colored) rash, 159
HELLP syndrome, 183–184, 578
Hemangiomas, 495
Hemarthrosis, 83, 365
  causes of, 60, 366b
  identification of, 365
  recurrent, long-term consequences of, 367
  septic arthritis coexisting with, 367b
  in warfarin therapy, 366
Hematologic diseases, arthropathies associated with, 365–370
Hematopoietic stem cell transplantation (HSCT), in systemic sclerosis, 153
Hemiarthroplasty, 669
Hemiplegia, 250

Hemochromatosis, 386
  calcium pyrophosphate dihydrate deposition disease-related, 347
  extraarticular organ involvement in, 89t
  hereditary, 424
    classic/HFE-related, 424–426
    diagnosis of, 426
    ferroportin-related, 425
    iron homeostasis in, 424
    juvenile type of, 425
    transferrin-receptor 2-related, 425
    treatment plan for, 427
  polyarticular symptoms of, 87, 88t
  radiographic features of, 72
Hemoglobin SC disease, 369
Hemoglobinopathies, 369
Hemophilia, 366
  acute hemarthrosis in, 366
  radiographic findings of, 367, 368f
Henri de Toulouse Lautrec's disease, 694
Heparin, 101, 185
  low molecular weight, 101
Heparinization, with prolonged aPTT, 185
Hepatitis
  lupoid, 273
  nonsteroidal antiinflammatory drugs and, 604
  type I autoimmune, 273t
Hepatitis A infection, 313–314
  rheumatic manifestations of, 313
Hepatitis B infection, 313–314
Hepatitis B surface antigen
  in polyarteritis nodosa, 216
  in vasculitis, 205
Hepatitis B vaccination, 314
Hepatitis C antibodies, 205
Hepatitis C infection, 242, 314–315
Hepatobiliary diseases, 273–275
  antirheumatic medications in, 274
  rheumatic manifestations of, 268–275
Hepatolenticular degeneration. see Wilson disease
Hepatomegaly, 425–426, 566
Herbal remedies, 688
Herbs, hepatotoxicity, 690
Herniated disk, lumbar, 450
Herpetovirus infection, 318
Hexagonal phase phospholipid neutralization assay (STACLOT-LA), 181
HFE gene, 424–425
Highly active antiretroviral therapy (HAART), 319, 319b
Hip
  in ankylosing spondylitis, 263
  arthroplasty of, 409, 669, 671
  congenital dislocation/dysplasia of, 440, 441f
  congenital dislocation of, 386
  fractures of, 393
  osteoarthritis of, 9, 390
  osteonecrosis of, 132
  snapping, 473
Hip girdle, diffuse aches and pains of, 94
Hip pain, 45
  in children, 513
Hip pointer, 472
Hippocrates, 693
Hirudin, 101
Histiocytosis X, 506
Histoplasma capsulatum, 310
History, in rheumatic disease assessment, 39–47
Hitchhiker thumb, 110
HLA-A29, birdshot retinochoroidopathy-associated, 557

HLA-B27, 11
 in ankylosing spondylitis, 264
 in inflammatory arthritis, 270
 in inflammatory bowel disease, 270t
 reactive arthritis/Reiter's syndrome associated with, 276, 281
 uveitis-associated, 556, 556t
HLA-B38, psoriatic arthritis associated, 284
HLA-B39, psoriatic arthritis associated, 284
Hodgkin's lymphoma, 546t
Holistic medicine, 686
Hollander, Joseph, 693
Holster-sign rash, 159
Homeopathy, 686
Homocystinuria, 417
Homocystinurias, 420
 affecting connective tissue, 420
 clinical manifestations of, 420
 diagnosis of, 420
 metabolic pathway of homocysteine, 421f
 treatment of, 421, 421f
Hormone replacement therapy (HRT), 133, 579–580
"Housemaid's knee," 467
H-reflex, 80
Hughes-Stovin syndrome, 250
Hughes syndrome, 180
Human immunodeficiency virus (HIV) infection
 as juvenile connective tissue disease mimic, 528
 psoriatic arthritis associated with, 286
 reactive arthritis associated with, 282
 rheumatic manifestations of, 319, 319b
 rheumatic syndromes of, 319–324
Human leukocyte antigens (HLAs), 29
 differentiated from major histocompatibility complex, 30t
 peptide antigen-binding site of, 30, 31f
Human parvovirus (HPV) B19 infection, 316–317
Human T lymphotropic virus type I (HTLV-1), 323
Humoral immunity, 31
 negative regulation of, 36
Hunter syndrome, 422
Hurler syndrome, 422
Hyaluronic acid, 19–20
Hybrid hip replacement, 671
Hybrid knee replacement, 671
Hydralazine, 137–138, 182, 234, 609t
 as lupus cause, 137
Hydrarthrosis, intermittent, 592
 laboratory studies and joint radiographs of, 592
Hydrocortisone, 99, 614t
Hydroxyapatite, 653
Hydroxyapatite arthropathy, 574
Hydroxyapatite pseudopodagra, 353, 353f
Hydroxychloroquine, 92, 524, 569, 688t
 as connective tissue disease treatment, 376t
 as systemic lupus erythematosus treatment, during pregnancy, 577
 use during pregnancy, 582
Hyman, Flo, 416–417
Hyper-IgM immunodeficiency syndrome, 435
Hyper immunoglobulin D syndrome (HIDS), 589
 genetic mutation associated with, 590
 laboratory abnormalities in, 589
 treatment and prognosis of, 590
 triggers for acute attacks in, 589
Hyperabduction maneuver, 479–480
Hyperaldosteronism, 536t
Hypercoagulable states, 181
Hypergammaglobulinemia, 244
Hypericum perforatum, 690
Hyperlipoproteinemia, familial, 363

Hyperparathyroidism, 536t
 calcium pyrophosphate dihydrate deposition disease-related, 347
 primary, 574
  chondrocalcinosis and, 361
  rheumatic syndrome associated with, 361
  skeletal ramification of, 361, 362f
 radiographic features of, 72
 secondary, 571–572, 572f
 tertiary, 573
Hyperpathia, 484
Hyperphosphatemia, 572
Hypersensitivity syndrome, to allopurinol, 649
Hypertension
 glucocorticoids and, 613
 pulmonary, 167–168
  gold standard test for, 150
  symptoms and signs of, 149
  systemic sclerosis-related, 149
  therapies for, 151
  types of, 149
Hyperthyroidism, 536t
 myopathies of, 361t
 rheumatic problems occurring in, 360
  medication causing, 361
Hyperuricemia, 337
 acquired causes of, 339
 alcohol consumption associated with, 339
 asymptomatic, 339
  treatment for, 343
 conditions associated with, 341
 drugs causing, 339t
 management of, 340
 pathogenic process for, development of, 338
 renal disease associated with, 342
 renal transport of uric acid in, 342
 symptomatic, treatment for, 344
Hypocomplementemia, 244
Hypocomplementemic urticarial vasculitis syndrome (HUVS), 239
Hypogonadism, in classic hereditary hemochromatosis, 425–426
Hypomagnesemia, 536t
Hypophosphatasia, 398, 439
 calcium pyrophosphate dihydrate deposition disease-related, 347
Hypopyon, 250
Hypothalamic-pituitary-adrenal axis, 668
 glucocorticoid-related suppression of, 613
Hypothyroidism, 12, 438, 536t
Hypouricemic agents, 645–651
Hypoxanthine-guanine phosphoribosyltransferase (HGPRT), deficiency of, 338

I

Ibandronate, 654t
Ibuprofen, 606
IdentRA test, 56–57
IgA deficiency, selective
 autoantibodies seen in, 434
 autoimmune diseases associated with, 434t
 rheumatologic manifestations of, 434
 therapy for, 435
IgG4-related systemic disease, 215
Iliotibial band friction syndrome, 473
Iliotibial band syndrome, 467
Immune complex formation, malignancy associated with, 374
Immune-mediated inner ear disease (IMIED), 562–563

Immune reconstitution inflammatory syndrome
(IRIS), 322, 327
Immune response, 36
causing immunopathology, 36
overview of, 24–38
Immune status, rheumatoid arthritis of, 668
Immune system
cellular, 431
effects of glucocorticoids in, 612
humoral, 430
innate, 9
Immunity
adaptive, 28–36
categories of, 25t
innate, 24–28
Immunoablative therapy, for autoimmune disease, 632
Immunodeficiency syndromes, primary, 430–436
aseptic arthritis in, 435
autoimmune phenomena associated with, 433, 435
components of immune system involved in, 430
Immunoglobulins
in cryoglobulinemia, 241
structure of, 33
Immunoglobulin A (IgA), 34
Immunoglobulin D (IgD), 34
Immunoglobulin E (IgE), 34
Immunoglobulin G (IgG), 33
Immunoglobulin M (IgM), 34
Immunosuppressive agents, 623, 627–632
as Behçet's disease treatment, 251
as connective tissue disease treatment, 376t
as dermatomyositis/polymyositis treatment, 163
as septic arthritis cause, 295
use in surgical patients, 668
as uveitis treatment, 559
Impairment, 676
Impingement sign, 387, 464
Inborn errors of metabolism, affecting connective tissue, 420–423
Indian frankincense, 689
Indirect immunofluorescence (IIF) technique, 49
Indirect immunofluorescence test, 121, 121f
Indium-111 scan, of septic arthritis, 294t
Indomethacin, 349, 601
children using, 604
Induction therapy, in granulomatosis with polyangiitis, 229–230
Infections
anti-TNF-α biologic agents and, 636
granulomatous, 229t
of prosthetic joints, 295
in rheumatic disease, 96
in small-vessel vasculitides, 236t
susceptibility to, in classic HHC, 425–426
in total hip and total knee replacements, 672
uveitis associated with, 557
Infectious diseases, antiphospholipid antibodies in, 182
Inflammasome, 588, 588f
Inflammation
cardinal signs of, 27, 41
fascial, in eosinophilic fasciitis, 156
overview of, 24–38
Inflammatory bowel disease, 234
idiopathic
clinical and radiographic characteristics of, 269
frequency of HLA-B27 in, 270t
inflammatory peripheral arthritis associated with, 268, 269t
Inflammatory mediators, 27t
Inflammatory response, 28

Infliximab (Remicade), 634
Infraspinatus isolation test, 463
Injuries, prevention of, 476
Insulinoma, 544t, 546
Interferon-α, 376
as Behçet's disease treatment, 251
in drug-induced lupus, 139
Interleukin-1 (IL-1), in familial Mediterranean fever, 588
Interleukin-1β (IL-1β), in pathogenesis of familial
autoinflammatory syndromes, 588, 588f
Interleukin (IL)-1 inhibitors, 634
biologic agents available to, 637
indications and toxicities of, 638
Interleukin (IL)-6 inhibitors, 634, 638
Intersection syndrome, 466
Interstitial lung disease (ILD), 148
drugs of choice for, 149
treatment of, 148
Intravenous gammaglobulin
as immunomodulator in rheumatic diseases, 631
as rheumatic disease treatment, 631
side effects of, 631
Intravenous immunoglobulin (IVIG)
as dermatomyositis/polymyositis treatment, 163
for Kawasaki disease, 532
Iontophoresis, 664
Iritis, 555
Iron, normal homeostasis of, 424, 425f
Iron deficiency anemia, 56
Isoniazid, 138, 308–309
Ixodes scapularis, 300, 305

J

Jarisch-Herxheimer reaction, 327
Jefferson, Thomas, 692
Jersey finger, injury to, 475
Jobe test, 463
Joint count, 43t
Joint effusions, noninflammatory (group 1), causes of, 60
Joint pain
cause of, joint fluid for, 511t
in children, 507–515
diurnal variation in, 510
evaluation of, 42
organic *versus* nonorganic, 509, 509t
in Paget's disease, 400
Joint replacement surgery, 14
Joints
amount of glucocorticoid injected in, 618t
aspiration of, 348, 514
benign and malignant tumors of, 491–496
biopsy with closed-biopsy needle, 76
classification of, 19
diarthrodial (synovial), 19
lubrication of, 20
frequent injections of glucocorticoids in, 617
fungal infections of, 310
in gout, 339
increased mobility of, 414
infections of, 82, 115
in inflammatory arthritis, 41
malignant diseases-related, 496
neuropathic, radiographic features of, 72
in nongonococcal septic arthritis, 291
palpation of, 42
protection of, 665–666
in psoriatic arthritis, 285, 285t
septic, in monoarthritis, 82
"stressing" of, 42

Joints (*Continued*)
  synovitis of, 41
  in tuberculosis, 307
  volume of glucocorticoids injected into, 617, 617t
JONES mnemonic, for acute rheumatic fever, 328
Jumper's knee, 473
Juvenile idiopathic arthritis (JIA), 13, 103, 438, 445t, 510, 516–521
  migrating *versus* summating patterns of, 516
  oligoarticular, demographics and clinical characteristics of, 518
  pharmacologic treatment for, 519–520
  radiographic features of, 71
  rashes associated with, 516
  special education services for, 521
  systemic, 517
    complication in, 518
    demographic and clinical characteristics of, 516
    differential diagnosis for, 518
    therapy for, 518
  types of, 516
  uveitis associated with, 556

K

Karloff, Boris, 693
Kava kava, 689
Kawasaki disease (KD), 13, 524, 530–532
  causes of, 531
  diagnostic criteria for, 530
  diagnostic test for, 531
  epidemiologic and clinical factors associated with, 531
  epidemiologic facts about, 530
  treatment for, 531, 532t
Kayser-Fleischer rings, in Wilson disease, 427
Kelley-Seegmiller syndrome, 338
Kellgren's syndrome, 385
Keratitis, 564
Keratoconjunctivitis, sarcoidosis-related, 567t
Keratoconjunctivitis sicca (KCS), 171
Keratoderma blennorrhagicum, 277
Kienböck's disease, 405
Kikuchi's disease, 189, 595
Kineret. *see* Anakinra
Kinky hair syndrome. *see* Menkes disease
Klee, Paul, 693
Knee
  anatomy of, 467f
  arthritis of, 46, 109b
    method for patient with, 667
  effusion of, 46
  inflammation of, 9
  osteoarthritis of, 9, 390
  spontaneous osteonecrosis of, 407
  swelling of, 46
  unstable, 46
Knee injury, "terrible triad" of, 474
Knee pain, anterior, 473, 473t
Knobloch syndrome, 17t
Knuckle, knuckle, dimple, knuckle sign, 362
Knuckle cracking, as osteoarthritis cause, 387
Koebner phenomenon, 189–190
Köhler's disease, 405

L

Laboratory evaluation, 48–57
Laboratory tests, for rheumatic disease evaluation, 7
Lachman test, 46, 474
Lactate dehydrogenase deficiency, 535t, 537f

Lady Gaga, 692
Laminin, 18
Landre-Beauvais, Augustin-Jacob, 692
Langerhans cell histiocytosis, 506
Large granular lymphocyte (LGL) syndrome, 115
Lasegue's sign, 448
Lasix (furosemide), as hyperuricemia cause, 339t
Lateral femoral cutaneous nerve, anatomy of, 480f
Latex, "allergic" to, precautions in patients, 58
Lead, neuromuscular toxicity of, 93
Lectins, 25
Lee, Robert E., 694
Leflunomide
  as connective tissue disease treatment, 376t
  contraindications to, 583
  dosing and side effects of, 622
  hepatotoxicity of, 623
  mechanism of action of, 623
  precautions and monitoring of, 623
  as rheumatoid arthritis treatment, 622–623
Leg-length discrepancy, 45–46, 511
Leg pain, cancer-related, 519
Legg-Calvé-Perthes disease, 386, 405
Lepirudin, 101
Leprosy, 310, 546t
Lesch, Michael, 693
Lesch-Nyhan syndrome, 338, 693
Lesinurad, as gout treatment, 650
Letterer-Siwe disease, 506
Leukemia, 371, 512–513, 519
Leukocytosis, 83, 293, 527t
Leukopenia, 131, 527t
Leukotrienes
  formation of, 27
  in inflammation, 28
Levamisole-cut cocaine, as ANCA-associated vasculitis cause, 234
Lhermitte's sign, 446
Lidocaine, "allergic" to, precautions in patients, 58
Ligaments
  differentiated from tendons, 21
  overuse injuries of, 471
Limb, tender and swollen, differential diagnosis of, 485
Limb-girdle muscular dystrophy, 541
Limited joint mobility syndrome, 357, 358f
Lincoln, Abraham, 416–417, 694
Lipid droplets, in synovial fluid, 355
Lipid metabolism, during muscle work, 537, 538f
Lipid metabolism disorders, 535t, 537, 539
Lipoma, of joints, 494
Lipoma arborescens, of joints, 494
Lipoxygenase pathway, 27
Lissamine green, 172–173
Lithium, 609t
Little Leaguer's elbow, 472
Live vaccines, 642
Livedo reticularis, 182, 204f
Liver dysfunction, 538f
Liver function tests, asymptomatic abnormal, in classic HHC, 425–426
Local corticosteroid creams, as Behçet's disease treatment, 251
Localized scleroderma syndromes, characteristics of, 154
Löffler syndrome, 232
Lofgren's syndrome, 567
Low back pain
  in ankylosing spondylitis, 262t
  categories of, 446
  evaluation of, 446
  mechanical

Low back pain *(Continued)*
  exercise for, 450
  pain generators of, 447
  prognosis of, 450
  strategy for recovery in, 450
  red flag signs and symptoms of, 448–449
Low-fat dietary products, 652
Lower serum urate levels, 650f
Lubricin, 20
Lucent defect, 73
Lucio phenomenon, 310
Lumbar spinal disorders, and cervical, 665
Lumbar spine
  herniated disk of, 450
  nerve root lesions of, 448t
  stenosis of, 449
  surgery in, 14, 674
Lumbar traction, 665
Lung disease, in systemic sclerosis, 148
Lupus anticoagulant, 132, 179, 181
Lupus erythematosus. *see also* Systemic lupus erythematosus (SLE)
  cutaneous
    acute, 120t, 122–123
    chronic, 120t
    subacute, 123–124, 139
  discoid, 123, 375t
  drug induced, 137–140
    genetic risk factors in, 139
    pathogenetic mechanisms causing, 139
    treatment of, 139
  in monkeys, food allergy-associated, 687t
  neonatal, 579
  neuropsychiatric, 129
Lupus erythematosus (LE) cell, 49
Lupus-like syndrome, malignancy associated with, 372t–373t
Lupus profundus, 123
Lyme disease, 12, 300–306
  arthritis associated with, 82b, 85, 88
  clinical manifestations of
    in second stage, 302
    in third stage, 302
  diagnostic tests for, 303
  as distinct clinical entity, 300
  etiology of, 300
  false-positive serologic test for, 303
  geographic distribution and seasonal occurrence of, 300
  as juvenile connective tissue disease mimic, 528
  laboratory abnormalities of, 304
  organ systems involvement in, 301
  prevention of, 304
  stages of, 302
  treatment of, 304
  typical rash of, 301
Lyme test, false-negative, 303
Lymphadenopathy
  generalized, 597
  in rheumatoid arthritis, 113
Lymphocytes, 31
Lymphoma, 176, 372
Lysosomal storage disease, 421

M

MacKenzie's exercises, 450
Macrophage activation syndrome (MAS), 192, 518
Macrophages, 26
Madison, James, 692
Madurella species, 311
Maffucci's syndrome, 502

MAGIC syndrome, 251, 256
Magnesium, 350
Magnetic resonance imaging (MRI), 72
  of cervical spine, 112f
  comparison with computed tomography, 72
  of complex regional pain syndrome, 486
  of fibromyalgia syndrome, 457
  for herniated lumbar disk, 450, 450t
  for low back pain evaluation, 449
  for metabolic myopathy evaluation, 540
  of monoarthritis, 85
  of muscle, 159, 160f
  of osteonecrosis, 407, 408f
  of septic arthritis, 294t
  of sportsman's hernia, 473
  T1-weighted *vs.* T2-weighted images in, 72, 60t
  of Takayasu arteritis, 213
  time of repetition (TR) parameter in, 72
  time to echo (TE) in, 72
Magnets, as pain therapy, 691
MAIN mnemonic, associated with increased antiphospholipid antibodies, 182
Major histocompatibility complex (MHC), 29, 29f
  antigen-binding site of, 30
  in autoimmunity, 38
  differences between class I and class II molecules, 30t
Malabsorption, 147
Malar rash, 122, 124f
Malaria, 300
Malignancy
  anti-TNF-α biologic agents and, 636
  causing musculoskeletal symptoms, 371
  paraneoplastic syndromes associated with, 372t–373t
  rheumatic disorders and, 371
Mallet finger, injury to, 475
Mallet toe deformity, 674t
Manipulation techniques, 691
Mannan-binding lectin (MBL), 25
Mannerfelt syndrome, 670
Mannkopf's test, 451
Manual labor metacarpal arthropathy syndrome, 387
Marble bone disease, 399
Marco Polo, Silk Route of, 248
Marcos, Ferdinand, 692
Marfan syndrome, 694
  genetic defect in, 416
  manifestations of
    nonmusculoskeletal, 417
    phenotype and skeletal, 416
  nonasthenic, 417
  revised Ghent criteria for diagnosing, 416
  treatment of, 418
Marfanoid hypermobility syndrome, 417
Marie, Pierre, 693
Marie-Strümpell's disease, 261
Maroteaux-Lamy syndrome, 422
Matrix metalloproteinase (MMP) group, 18
McArdle's disease, 538, 538f
McCarty, Daniel, 693
McCune-Albright syndrome, 502–503
McMurray's maneuver/test, 85, 474
Medial collateral ligament tear, complete, 474
Medial tibial stress syndrome, 475
Melanoma, 546t
Melanoma, malignant, 496
Melorheostosis, 439, 439f
Meltzer's triad, 11
Ménière's disease, 562
Meningitis, 222
Meningococcemia, 298

Meningoencephalitis, in Behçet's disease, 250
Meniscus, tears of, 474
Menkes disease, 421
Meralgia paresthetica, 46, 480
Mercury, neuromuscular toxicity of, 93
Metabolic disease
   of bone, 393–399
   myopathies, 533–542
Metabolism, inborn errors of, affecting connective tissue, 420–423
Metacarpal index, of arachnodactyly, 417
Metacarpophalangeal (MCP) joints
   arthritis of, 268–269
   synovitis of, 671
Metastases, to joints, 496
Methimazole, 234, 361
Methotrexate (MTX), 101, 609t
   as connective tissue disease treatment, 376t
   contraindications to, 583
   dose and toxicities of, 621
   immunologic effects of, 622
   as juvenile idiopathic arthritis treatment, 519–520
   precautions and monitoring for, 621
   preoperative use of, 668
   rationale and value of testing for, 622
   use in renal insufficiency patients, 575
   as rheumatoid arthritis treatment, 116, 621
   use in rheumatologic conditions, 622
   as sarcoidosis treatment, 569
   as uveitis treatment, 559
Methylprednisolone, 257, 527, 614t
Methylsulfonylmethane (MSM), 690
Metoclopramide, 610t
Metronidazole, 688t
Mevalonate pathway, 654–655
Microfracture surgery, as osteoarthritis therapy, 391
Microscopy
   nailfold capillary, 551, 552f
   polarized, in synovial fluid analysis, 59, 348
Microvascular and microangiopathic antiphospholipid-associated syndrome (MAPS), 183
Miescher, Peter, 692
Milk thistle, 689
Milwaukee shoulder syndrome, 354, 355f
Mini-Mental status examination, 613
Minocycline, 139, 234, 688t
Mitchell, Silas, 484
Mixed disease, 571
Modafinil (Provigil), 460
Molecular mimicry, 38
   in HLA-B27, 264
Monoarthritis, 82–85
   acute, 367
   in children, 511b
   chronic, 84, 84t
   diseases with, 82b
Monoarticular arthritis. *see* Monoarthritis
Monocytes, 26
Mononeuritis multiplex, 94, 203, 227, 567t
Monosodium urate (MSU), deposition of, in gout, 337
Moraxella infections, as discitis cause, 513
Morning stiffness, 41, 42t, 88
Morphea, 141, 154–155
Morquio syndrome, 422
Motor disorder, and complex regional pain syndrome, 485
Motor neuron, 78
Motor unit, 78
Motor unit action potentials (MUAPs), 79
Motor weakness. *see also* Muscle weakness
   dermatomyositis/polymyositis-related, 158

Movement disorder, and complex regional pain syndrome, 485
Movement therapy, 691
Muckle-Wells syndrome (MWS), 590
Mucopolysaccharidoses (MPS), 19, 421
   musculoskeletal manifestations of, 422
Mucous cyst, of distal interphalangeal joint, 670
Mulder click, 481
Multiple epiphyseal dysplasia (MED), 438
Multiple sclerosis, uveitis associated with, 557
Mumps virus infection, 317
Muscle abnormalities, systemic sclerosis-related, 153
Muscle diseases
   enzymes elevated in, 94t
   HIV infection-related, 321
   inflammatory, 158–165
Muscle fibers, 23, 78
Muscle infarction, diabetic, 359
Muscle spasm, 664
Muscle-tendon junction, acute injury to, 471
Muscle weakness, 91
   amyloidosis-related, 545
   grading of, 93, 93t
   neuromuscular disorders-related, 91, 92b, 94
   temporal pattern of, 92
Muscles
   contraction and relaxation of, 23, 536f
   in human body, 23
   morphology of, 23
Muscular dystrophies, 541
Muscular dystrophy syndrome, 92t
Musculoskeletal disease
   chronic, important factors contributing to work disability in patients with, 676, 676t–677t
   economic impact of, 5
   morbidity and mortality of, 5, 5b
Musculoskeletal disorders
   classification of, 3
   familial hyperlipoproteinemia associated with, 363
   in general population, 4
   neoplasms-related, in pediatric patients, 512
   prevalence of, 4t
   primary care office visits for, 4
   regional, 462–470
Musculoskeletal syndromes, malignancy associated with, 371
Musculoskeletal system
   anatomy and physiology of, 16–23
   components of, 16
   functions of, 16
   granulomatosis with polyangiitis in, 227
Musicians, connective tissue diseases in, 694
Myalgia
   Cogan's syndrome-related, 563
   statins and, 10
   in Still's disease, 190t
Myasthenia gravis, 92
Mycobacteria, atypical
   musculoskeletal problems caused by, 309
   osteoarticular infections of, treatment of, 309
Mycobacterial infection, 84t, 85
   prevention of, 310
Mycobacterium avium-intracellulare, 309
Mycobacterium kansasii, 309
Mycobacterium leprae, 310
Mycobacterium marinum, 309
Mycobacterium tuberculosis (MTB) infection, 307
Mycophenolate mofetil, 628
   as connective tissue disease treatment, 376t
   contraindications to, 583
   mechanism of action of, 628

Mycophenolate mofetil *(Continued)*
  use in renal insufficiency patients, 575
  as rheumatic disease treatment, 628
Myelodysplastic syndrome, relapsing polychondritis-related, 256–257
Myelography, of herniated lumbar disk, 450t
Myelopathy, cervical, 447t
Myfortic (mycophenolic acid, MPA), 628
Myoadenylate deaminase deficiency, 535t, 536, 540
Myocardial infarction (MI), 605
Myocarditis, 114t
Myofascial pain, 445
Myofilaments, 23
Myopathy, 9
  congenital, 542
  critical illness, 94
  electromyographic findings in, 80t
  excessive glucocorticoids and, 363
  hyperthyroid, 360, 361t
  idiopathic inflammatory, 158, 163b, 361t
  metabolic, 13, 533–542, 536t
  mitochondrial, 535t, 539
  as muscle weakness/pain cause, 92
  necrotizing autoimmune, 162
  noninflammatory necrotizing, 321
  steroid-induced, 10, 667
    separating from polymyositis, 164
  systemic sclerosis-related, 153
  zidovudine, 321
Myophosphorylase deficiency, 535t, 537–538, 537f
Myositis
  autoantibodies in, 161, 161t
  idiopathic inflammatory, muscle biopsies of, 162
  inflammatory, 10, 13
    during pregnancy, 581
  sarcoidosis-related, 567t
  sporadic inclusion body, 164
  unspecified, 162
Myotonic dystrophies, 541–542
Myxoma, atrial, 203, 218

N
Nail changes, 286
Nailfold capillary abnormalities, 145, 159
Nailfold capillary microscopy, 552f
Naltrexone, 461
Narcotic analgesics, as osteoarthritis treatment, 389
Narcotics, use in renal insufficiency patients, 575
Natural killer (NK) cells, 26
  activation of, 35
Naturopathy, 686
Neck pain
  approach for patient with, 443–451
  bony differentiated from muscular, 445
  causes of, 445
  in children, 13, 513
  prevalence of, 4t
Necrosis
  avascular, 82b, 84t, 85, 323, 369. *see also* Osteonecrosis.
    radiographic features of, 72
  differentiated from apoptosis and autophagy, 35
  digital, malignancy associated with, 372t–373t
  fibrinoid, 217
  in small-vessel vasculitides, 236
Neer test, 463
Neisseria gonorrhoeae, 296
Neisseria meningitidis infection, as septic arthritis cause, 298
Neonatal lupus erythematosus (NLE), 524, 579

Neonatal-onset multisystem inflammatory disease (NOMID), 590
Neoplasia
  erythematosus joints in, 510
  as joint pain cause, 511
Neoplasms, amyloidosis associated with, 546t
Neoplastic disease, dermatomyositis/polymyositis associated with, 160
Neoplastic syndrome, 229t
Nephritic syndrome, in cryoglobulinemia, 243
Nephritis, lupus, 125
  diffuse, 126
  membranous, 126–127
  mesangial proliferative, 126
  minimal mesangial, 126
  during pregnancy, 578
  renal biopsy for, 125, 126t
  serological tests for, 127
  severe, 127–128
Nephrogenic systemic fibrosis (NSF), 156
Nephrolithiasis, uric acid, 342
Nephropathy, urate/uric acid, 342
Nephrotic syndrome, 545
Nerve conduction studies (NCS), 78–81, 450
Nerve conduction velocity, 80
Nerve root compression, as muscle weakness/pain cause, 92
Neuralgia, trigeminal, mixed connective tissue disease-related, 168
Neurapraxia, 79
Neuroblastoma, 512, 519
Neurofibromatosis, 218
Neurological disorders
  systemic lupus erythematosus-related, 120t
  Whipple's disease associated with, 326
Neuroma, Morton's, 481
Neuromuscular disease, 91–95
  tests for evaluation of, 94b, 95t
  toxins in, 92
Neuromuscular junction, 78
Neuromuscular lesions, cardinal symptoms of, 91
Neuromyopathy, 344
Neuropathy, 9
  autonomic, amyloidosis-related, 545
  axonal, 80–81
  demyelinating, 80–81
  entrapment, 115
  peripheral, 80, 545
  peripheral, as muscle weakness/pain cause, 92
Neuroplasticity, 457
Neurotmesis, 79
Neutrophils, 25–26
  function, measurement of, 432
"Niche" therapies, 460
Nicotinic acid, as hyperuricemia cause, 339t
Night pain, inflammatory arthritis-related, 41
Noble test, 473
Nodules
  Aschoff, 331
  of elbow, 69
  rheumatoid, 113, 114t
  subcutaneous, 44b, 204
    acute rheumatic fever-related, 331
Nongonococcal septic arthritis, 291, 292t
  bacteria responsible for, 292
  clinical manifestations of, 291
  laboratory tests of, 293t
  poor outcome in, 295
  prognosis of, 294
  treatment of, 294
Nonhereditary periodic arthritis syndrome, 592

Nonsteroidal antiinflammatory drugs (NSAIDs), 99t, 476, 599–611
  as acute calcific periarthritis treatment, 353
  adverse reactions to, 606
  as ankylosing spondylitis treatment, 266
  beneficial effects of, 601
  cardiovascular effects of, 605
  cardiovascular risk of, 606
  considerations of use of, 606
  drug-drug interactions of, 609, 609t–610t
  use during breast feeding, 582
  use during pregnancy, 582
  efficacy studies of, 603
  factors affecting the choice of, 603, 603b
  as fibromyalgia treatment, 460
  first used of, 601
  formulations of, 607
  future uses for, 607–608
  gastrointestinal side effects of, 604
  half-lives of, 607, 608t
  hepatotoxicity of, 604
  hypersensitivity reaction to, 603
  as juvenile connective tissue disease treatment, 524
  as juvenile idiopathic arthritis treatment, 519
  mechanism of action of, 602
  for mild renal compromise, 605
  nephrotoxic, 605
  nonprostaglandin mediated effect of, 602
  as osteoarthritis treatment, 389–390
  as Paget's disease treatment, 403
  as pediatric arthritis treatment, 514t
  as polymyalgia rheumatica treatment, 195
  preoperative discontinuation of, 98
  preoperative use of, 668
  properties of, 601
  as pseudogout treatment, 349
  as reactive arthritis treatment, 281
  use in renal insufficiency patients, 575
  structural classification of, 602
  as systemic lupus erythematosus treatment, during pregnancy, 577
Nontuberculous (atypical) mycobacteria (NTM), conditions predisposing to, 309
Nucleic acid amplification tests (NAATs), 308
Nutritional status, in patients with rheumatoid arthritis, 668
Nyhan, William, 693

O

Ober test, 46, 473
Obesity, as osteoarthritis risk factor, 384
Obstructive sleep apnea, 13
Occiput-to-wall test, 262
Occupational injuries, 471–476
Occupational therapist (OT), 662
Ochronosis, 72, 347, 386
O'Connor, Flannery, 692
O'Donoghue's maneuver, 451
Ollier's disease, 502
Oral contraceptives, combined, 579
Oral nitrogenous bisphosphonates, 654–655
Organ transplant patients, gout in, 344, 649
Organophosphates, neuromuscular toxicity of, 92
Orthoses, 665–666
Orthotics, 665
Ortolani's sign, 440
Osgood-Schlatter disease, 513t, 521
Osler, William, 601, 692
Ossicles of ear, 115
Ossification of posterior longitudinal ligament (OPLL), 71

Osteitis, chronic recurrent multifocal, 288
Osteitis condensans ilii, 266, 266f
Osteitis fibrosa cystica, 361, 571
Osteoadherin, 18
Osteoanabolic drugs, 659
Osteoarthritis, 9, 379–392, 670
  basic calcium phosphate and, 355
  basilar thumb, 670
  cervical spine involvement, 445t
  classification of, 383
  clinical features of, 382
  development of, 381
  differentiated from rheumatoid arthritis, 44t
  of distal interphalangeal joint, 670
  erosive (inflammatory), 384, 385f
  femoroacetabular impingement and, 387
  generalized, 385
  joint distribution of, 110f
  joint replacement for, 390
  knee, arthroplasty used in, 672
  laboratory features in, 382
  medical treatment for, 389
  monoarticular, 82b
  natural history of, 391
  nonpharmacologic interventions for, 388
  occupational factors in, 475
  pain associated with, 20
  pathologic features of, 381
  polyarticular, 87, 88t
  prevalence of, 4t
  primary care office visits for, 4
  primary (idiopathic), 382
    differentiated from secondary, 386
    epidemiologic features of, 383
    sites of joint involvement in, 66
  pseudo, 346
  radiographic features of, 112t
  risk factors for, 384
  secondary, causes of, 386
  therapies for, 390
  treatments not to be done in patients with, 8
Osteoarthropathy, hypertrophic, 72, 323, 373, 374f
  associated with malignancy, 372t–373t
Osteoblasts, 21, 653
Osteochondritis, vertebral, 440, 440f
Osteochondrodysplasias, 437
Osteochondroma, 501, 502f
Osteochondrosis, juvenile, 438
Osteoclasts, 21, 399
Osteodystrophy, renal, 571
Osteogenesis imperfecta, 17t, 413, 439
Osteolysis
  diabetic, 358
  periprosthetic, 672
Osteoma, 500, 500f
  osteoid, 495, 500, 501f
Osteomalacia, 397, 439, 571
  clinical manifestations of, 397
  major causes of, 397b
  oncogenic, 372t–373t, 398
  treatment of, 398t
Osteomyelitis, 289–299
  acute
    differentiated from chronic, 299
    radiographic abnormality in, 73, 73f
  amyloidosis-related, 546t
  fungal, 310
  in osteoarticular TB, 307–308
  sickle cell disease-related, 369, 370b
  three phase bone scan of, 74t

Osteonecrosis, 323, 360, 363, 387, 405–410
  bilateral, 408
  clinical conditions associated with, 406b
  clinical features of, 406
  definition of, 405
  epidemiologic features of, 406
  etiology of, 405
  femoral head, in sickle cell disease, 369
  of hip, 132
  idiopathic, cause of, 407
  of jaw, 655
  management of
    medical, 408
    surgical, 408
  medications associated with, 407
  pathogenesis and resulting symptoms of, 405
  prevention of, 409
  role of radiographs in diagnosis of, 407
  skeletal regions predisposed to, 405
  spontaneous, of knee, 407
  spontaneous syndromes of, 405
Osteopenia
  diffuse, 361
  generalized, in HHC, 426
  periarticular, 63, 279
Osteopetrosis, 399
Osteophyte, differentiated from syndesmophyte, 69t
Osteophytosis, 67
Osteoporosis, 12
  definition of, 393
  diagnosis of, 394
  glucocorticoids-related, 396, 613
    treatment of, 397
  in HIV infection, 323
  inflammatory bowel disease-related, 270
  management algorithm of, 657f
  medications for, 396
  in men, 396
  nonpharmacological measures for, 652
  outline algorithm for management of, 657
  pharmacological therapy for, 396, 653
  prednisone-related, 518
  prevalence of, 4t
  in rheumatoid arthritis, 115
  risk factors for, 395
  therapy, annual retail cost for, 658
"Osteoporosis circumscripta," 401
Osteoprotegerin (OPG), 21, 654
Osteotomy, in total knee replacement, 672
Ovarian carcinoma, 375
Overlap syndromes, 153, 166, 169
Overuse injuries, 471
  occupational, 475
  principles of treatment to, 476, 476t
Oxalosis, secondary, 574

P

Pachydermoperiostosis, 440
Paganini, Nicolo, 694
Paget's disease
  abnormal laboratory tests in, 401
  clinical features of, 400
  complications of, 401
  definition of, 400
  diagnosis of, 401
  differential diagnosis of, 402
  genetic, 400
  incidence of, 400
  indications to treat, 402

Paget's disease (Continued)
  malignancy associated with, 375t
  onset of, 400
  phases of, 402
  radiographic and scintigraphic findings in, 401, 402f
  skeletal involvement in, 400
  treatment for, 403
Pain
  diffuse, differentiated from polyarthritis, 86
  neuromuscular disorders-related, 91–92, 95t
  osteoarthritis-related, 20, 387
  in osteonecrosis, 406
  in Paget's disease, 403
Pain amplification syndromes, of childhood, 512
PAIN mnemonic, for inflammatory bowel diseases, 269
Painful articular syndrome, 320
Pallor, Raynaud's phenomenon-related, 145
Palmar fibromatosis, 375
Pancreatic cancer, 11
Panner's disease, 405
Panniculitis, 372t–373t, 596
Pannus, 110
Panuveitis, 557
Papular mucinosis. see Scleromyxedema
Paralysis, hypokalemic periodic, 92
Paramethasone, 614t
Paraneoplastic syndromes, polyarthritis, 87
Paraparesis, 250
Parasitic infection, as osteoarticular problem cause, 312
Parathyroid disease, 361–362
Parathyroid hormone, 572, 656
  as myopathy marker, 92
Parotid gland, enlargement, differential diagnosis of, 174
Pars planitis, 557
Partial thromboplastin time (PTT)
  effect on lupus anticoagulant on, 132
  in monoarthritis, 83
Parvovirus infection, 12, 316–317, 528
Patellofemoral compression test, 46
Patellofemoral syndrome, 473
Pathergy, in Behçet's disease, 248
Pathogen-associated molecular patterns (PAMPs), 24
Patient educators, healthcare personnel, 662
Patrick's test, 45, 262, 449
Pattern-recognition receptors (PRRs)
  intracellular, 25
  linked to phagocytosis, 25
  other cells exhibiting, 26
Pediatric autoimmune neuropsychiatric disorders associated with streptococci (PANDAS), 331
Pegloticase, 344, 649
Pelvic compression test, 262, 449
Pelvis, sacroiliitis of, 281f
Pemberton, R., 3
"Pencil-in-cup" deformity, 72
D-penicillamine, 688
  responsible for neuromuscular symptoms, 92
Penicillamine chelation therapy, as Wilson disease treatment, 428
Pentraxins, 25
Peptic ulcers, 604
Periaortitis, chronic, 214–215
Periarthritis
  acute calcific, 353
  diabetic, of shoulder, 359
Pericarditis, 114, 114t
Perifascicular atrophy, of muscle fibers, 162
Periodic fever syndromes, 588–590
Periodic fever with aphthous stomatitis, pharyngitis, and adenitis syndrome (PFAPA), 591

Peripheral nerve disorders, 78, 81t
Peripheral nervous system
  in granulomatosis with polyangiitis, 227
  nerve conduction studies of, 80
Peroneal nerve palsy, 81t, 481
Pes anserine bursa, 46
Pes planus, 387
  acquired, 469
Phagocytes, 25–26
Phagocytic cell, dysfunction of, 431–432
Phagocytosis, pattern-recognition receptors (PRRs) linked to, 25
Phalen's test, 43, 478
Phenothiazines, 182
Phenoxybenzamine, 553
Phenylbutazone, 601
Phenytoin, 182, 609t
Philadelphia finger, 354
Phlegm, 3
Phonophoresis, 664
Phosphate, 653f
Phosphocitrate, 350
Phosphofructokinase deficiency, 535t, 537f, 538
Phosphoglycerate kinase deficiency, 535t, 537f
Phosphoribosylpyrophosphate (PRPP) synthetase, 338
Phosphorylase b kinase deficiency, 535t, 537f
Photophobia, 42, 556
Photosensitivity, 42
Physical examination
  of carpal tunnel syndrome, 478
  of neuromuscular symptoms, 93t
  for rheumatic disease evaluation, 7, 39–47
Physical modalities, 664–665
Physical therapist (PT), healthcare personnel, 662
Physical therapy
  for complex regional pain syndrome, 486
  for fibromyalgia syndrome, 459
  for soft tissue rheumatism, 691
Physician, primary, role of, 680
Piaf, Edith, 692
"Piano key" ulnar head, 110
Piatigorsky, Gregor, 693
Pilocarpine, 177
Pincer impingement, 387
Pinus pinaster, 689
Piper methysticum, 689
Piriformis syndrome, 480
Pivot shift test, 474
Plasma exchange, for rheumatic diseases, 631
Platyspondyly, 438
Pleural disease, 114
Pleuritis, 130
Plexopathy, 78
Pneumonia, cryptogenic organizing, 114
Pneumonitis, nonspecific interstitial, 114
Podagra, 339, 344
Podiatrist, healthcare personnel, 662
Polyangiitis, microscopic, 11, 201–202, 231–232
Polyarteritis nodosa (PAN), 201f, 208–212, 211f, 231
  cause of, 214
  in children, 524
  clinical features of, 212, 231t
  cutaneous, 211
  malignancy associated with, 372t–373t
  prevalence and manifestations of, 209t
  prognosis for, 210
Polyarthralgia, 86
Polyarthritis, 86–90
  acute, diseases with, 87t
  carcinomatous, 372t–373t, 374

Polyarthritis *(Continued)*
  in children, 511b
  chronic, diseases with, 87b
  extraarticular manifestations of, 9
  joint involvement patterns in, 86–87
  migratory, 332
  paraneoplastic, 87
  symmetric, 108, 310
Polyarticular arthritis. *see* Polyarthritis
Polyarticular diseases, with monoarticular onset, 82
Polychondritis, 11
  relapsing, 253–258, 254f, 254t, 560, 560t, 562–563
    audiovestibular damage in, 255
    dermatologic manifestations in, 256
    neurologic manifestation of, 256
    prognosis of, 257
Polymodal receptor, 456
Polymyalgia rheumatica, 11, 193–198
  cervical spine involvement in, 445t
  core criteria of, 193
  course of, 196
  definition of, 193
  diagnosis of, 195
  differential diagnosis of, 195t
  etiopathogenesis of, 194
  extraarticular organ involvement in, 89t
  giant cell arteritis-related, 194, 195t, 208
  laboratory abnormalities in, 194
  malignancy associated with, 372t–373t
  physical examination of, 194
  polyarticular symptoms of, 87
  prevalence of, 4t
  source of symptoms of, 194
  stiffness and pain of, 193
  temporal artery biopsy in, 195
  treatment plan for, 196
Polymyositis, 361t
  cervical spine involvement in, 445t
  diagnostic criteria of, 158
  differentiated from inclusion body myositis, 164, 164t
  epidemiologic features of, 158
  extraarticular organ involvement in, 89t
  extramuscular/extradermatologic manifestations of, 160
  HIV infection-related, 321
  juvenile dermatomyositis differentiated from, 526
  laboratory abnormalities of, 161
  malignancy associated with, 372t–373t, 375t
  occurrence of cancer in, 373
  prognosis of, 163
  Raynaud phenomenon-associated, 89
  rehabilitative techniques for, 667
  treatment of, 162
Polyneuropathy, 81, 94
Polyostotic sclerosing histiocytosis. *see* Erdheim-Chester disease
Pompe disease, 539
Poncet disease, 308
Positive sharp wave potential, 79
Positron emission tomography (PET), 74
Postinjection flare, after glucocorticoid injection, 618
Posttreatment Lyme disease syndrome (PLDS), 305
Pott disease, 307
Pouchitis, 270, 272t
Povidone-iodine, "allergic" to, precautions in patients, 58
Powered mobility device (PMD), 666
PQRST mnemonic, for low back pain evaluation, 446
PRAGMATIC mnemonic, for carpal tunnel syndrome, 478
"Prayer sign," 357–358, 358f
Prazosin, 609t
Prednisolone, 349, 614t

Prednisone, 613, 614t
  adverse effects of, in children, 518
  as Cogan's syndrome treatment, 564
  dosage levels of, 363, 615
  as giant cell arteritis treatment, 11, 211
  as lupus nephritis treatment, 129, 578
  in organ transplantation, 649
  as osteonecrosis risk factor, 407
  as polymyalgia rheumatica treatment, 11, 195–196
  as systemic lupus erythematosus treatment, 132
    during pregnancy, 577–578
  as Takayasu arteritis treatment, 213
Preeclampsia, 578
Pregnancy
  antiphospholipid antibodies during, 184
  biologic agents use during, 583, 642
  erythema chronicum migrans treatment during, 302
  Food and Drug Administration categories during, 581
  mycophenolate mofetil precaution during, 628
  nonsteroidal antiinflammatory drugs and, 607
  rheumatic diseases and, 577
  systemic lupus erythematosus during, 577
  toxemia of, 578
Preiser's disease, 405
Preoperative assessment, of rheumatic disease patients, 96
PRICES mnemonic, for tendinitis and overuse injuries treatment, 476, 476t
Primary angiitis of central nervous system, 221–222
  atypical, 222
Primary biliary cirrhosis (PBC)
  common autoimmune diseases associated with, 274
  versus rheumatoid arthritis, 274t
Primary immunodeficiency (PID) syndromes, rheumatologic manifestations of, 430–436
Primary vasculitis syndromes, 229t
PRIME BONE PAIN mnemonic, for joint pain diagnosis, 509
Probenecid, 350, 610t, 646–647
  use in renal insufficiency patients, 575
  side effects of, 647b
Procainamide, 138, 182
  as lupus cause, 139
Procalcitonin, 293
PROMISSE (Predictors of pRegnancy Outcome: bioMarkers In antiphospholipid antibody Syndrome and Systemic lupus Erythematosus) trial, 577–578
Pronator teres syndrome, 81t, 479
Prophylactic therapy, in granulomatosis with polyangiitis, 230
Propolis, 687
Proptosis, 567t
Propylthiouracil, 234, 361
Prostaglandins, 553, 604
  formation of, 27
  in inflammation, 28
Prostheses
  cemented, 671
  cementless, 671
  porous ingrowth, 671
Prosthetic joints, infections of, 100
  incidence/risk factors of, 295
  management of, 673
  organisms causing, 295
  separated from aseptic loosening, 296
  treatment of, 296
Protease inhibitors, as osteonecrosis cause, 407
Proteoglycans, 18–19
Prothrombin, serum, in monoarthritis, 83
Prothrombin time (PT)
  lupus anticoagulant and, 180
  prolonged, 181
Pseudobulbar palsy, 250

Pseudogout, 346
  acute, 349
  calcium pyrophosphate dihydrate crystals in, 61f, 352
  monoarticular, 82b, 83
  synovial fluid findings in, 61t
Pseudohypoparathyroidism, type Ia, 362
Pseudosepsis, of joint, 60
Pseudovasculitis syndromes, 229t
Pseudoxanthoma elasticum, 218, 418
Psoriasis, 284, 286. *see also* Arthritis; psoriatic
  examination of, 284
  HIV infection-related, 321
  in notable people, 693
  relationship between arthritis and, 284
Psychiatric disorders
  functional, fibromyalgia-related, 455
  organic, fibromyalgia-related, 456
Psychological therapy, 487
Psychotherapists, healthcare personnel, 662
Pulmonary function tests (PFTs), for systemic sclerosis evaluation, 148
Pulmonary renal syndrome, 228, 229t, 232
Pulseless disease, 212
Purine metabolism disorders, 535t, 540
Purine nucleotide cycle, 536, 537f
Purpura
  acute thrombotic thrombocytopenic, 131
  amyloidosis-related, 544–545
  cryoglobulinemia-related, 243
  Henoch-Schönlein, 201–202, 236t, 238, 516, 517f
    in children, 524
    clinical manifestations of, 525t
    diagnosis of, 525
    prognostic factors in, 525t
    signs and symptoms associated with, 524
    skin biopsy in, 11
    treatment of, 525
  vasculitis-related, 237
Pyarthrosis, 60
Pycnogenol, 689
Pyelonephritis, amyloidosis associated with, 546t
Pyknodysostosis, 694
Pyoderma gangrenosum, 114, 596
Pyogenic sterile arthritis, pyoderma gangrenosum, and acne syndrome (PAPA), 590–591
Pyomyositis, 322
Pyrazinamide, 308–309, 339t
Pyrophosphate arthropathy, 346, 350

Q

Quinidine, 182
Quotidian fever, 189

R

Rachmaninov, Sergei, 694
Radial nerve entrapment, 480
Radial nerve palsy, 81t
Radiation exposure, during radiographic procedures, 75
Radiculopathy
  cervical, 446, 447t
  peripheral, 78
Radiographic evaluation
  of bone lesions, 497–506, 498f–499f, 498t
  of hyperparathyroidism, 572
  of pediatric joint pain, 510
Radiographic procedures, in musculoskeletal imaging of joint, relative costs of, 75

Radiographs
  in chronic arthritis, 90
  in monoarthritis, 83
  in septic arthritis, 293
Radioulnar joint, arthritis of, 69
Ragged red fiber, 539
Raines, Tim, 692
Raisins, as CAM remedy, 688
Raloxifene, 654t, 656
Range of motion, minimum required to perform activities of daily living, 663t
RANKL/RANK/OPG signaling pathway, 21, 22f
Rat bite erosions, 340
Raynaud, Maurice, 692
Raynaud's disease, 10, 526
Raynaud's phenomenon, 549–554, 690
  in children, 526, 527t
  as CREST component, 143
  diagnosis of, 42
  ischemic crisis in, 553
  pathophysiology of, 550
  polyarticular conditions associated with, 89
  primary, 549
    differentiated from secondary, 550
  prognosis for patients with, 553
  secondary, 549, 549t
  systemic sclerosis-related, 145
  treatment of, 552–553
  triphasic color response of, 550, 550f
Rayos, 616
Reactive hemophagocytic syndrome, 192
Receptor activator of nuclear factor κ (RANK), 654
Recurrent fever syndromes, 586
Reflex sympathetic dystrophy, 359, 483
Regional myofascial pain syndrome, 452
Rehabilitation, 666–667
  as dermatomyositis/polymyositis treatment, 163
Rehabilitation counselors, 662
Rehabilitative techniques, 661–667
Reiter, Hans, 693
Reiter's cells, 279
Reiter's syndrome, 276
  HIV infection-related, 320
  polyarticular symptoms of, 88
  radiographic features of, 71
Remission therapy, in granulomatosis with polyangiitis, 230
Renal cell carcinoma, 546t
Renal diseases
  crystal deposition diseases associated with, 574
  hyperuricemia associated with, 342
  relapsing polychondritis-related, 256
Renal disorders, systemic lupus erythematosus-related, 120t
Renal failure
  amyloid arthropathy of, 574
  chronic, secondary hyperparathyroidism associated with, 571
  systemic sclerosis-related, 152
Renal insufficiency, 575, 605, 648
Renal osteodystrophy, 571
Renal transplantation, 574
Renoir, Pierre Auguste, 692
Repetitive stimulation studies, 78
Repository corticotropin injection (H.P. Acthar gel), as dermatomyositis/polymyositis treatment, 163
Residual functional capacity, 678
Residual functional capacity, for determining disability, 679
Rest, 662–663
  forms of, 662
  as pseudogout treatment, 349
  effect on rheumatic disorder symptoms, 42t

Reticulohistiocytosis, multicentric, 594
  cutaneous manifestations of, 594
  disorders associated with, 594
  histologic findings of, 594
  malignancy associated with, 372t–373t
  treatment of, 594
Retinopathy, antimalarial drugs-related, 620
Reversible cerebral vasoconstriction syndrome (RCVS), 222
Rheuma, 3, 692
Rheumatic diseases
  cardiac disease in, 9
  cardiovascular risk in, 96
  categories of, 3
  cervical spine disease in, 96
  classification and health impact of, 1–6
  "cleared" for surgery, 96
  complementary and alternative medicine (CAM) therapies for, 15
  in dialysis patients, 571–576
  economic impact of, 5
  functional areas, 661
  goals of rehabilitation for patients with, 661
  history, arts and, 692–695
  inflammatory
    biologic agents for, 633, 643
    differentiated from mechanical (degenerative), 42t
  laboratory tests for, 96, 97t
  medications for, 14
  monthly cost of medications in, 625, 626t
  morbidity and mortality of, 5, 5b
  neuromuscular disease and, 91
  perioperative management of, 96–104
  plasma exchange for, 632
  rehabilitative techniques for, 667
  risk for perioperative complications, 97
  surgical treatment in, 668–675
  systemic, 9, 88
  tests/treatments not be done in adult with, 8
  tests/treatments not be done in pediatric patients with, 8
  time, cost, and success rate of drug for, 625
  uveitis associated with, 557, 557t
Rheumatic disorders
  classification of, 3
  in general population, 4
  malignancy-associated, 371–378
  prevalence of, 4t
  primary care office visits for, 4
  small vessel vasculitis-related, 236t
Rheumatic fever
  acute, 328–334
    antibodies in, 329
    in children, 528
    clinical and laboratory criteria of, 329
    diagnosis of, 328, 329b
    erythema marginatum associated with, 516
    extraarticular organ involvement in, 89t
    history of, 329
    host factors contributing to, 330
    impact of, 333
    Jones criteria for, 328
    manifestations of, 331
    polyarticular symptoms of, 88
    prophylaxis, 331, 332t
    sequela of, 331
    studies on, 328
    treatment of, 331, 332t
  erythematosus joints in, 510
  famous persons affected with, 694

Rheumatic syndromes
  cyclosporine for, 630
  of HIV infection, 319–324
  malignancy associated with, 371
  and pancreatic disease, 272–273
Rheumatism
  fibroblastic, 594
  palindromic, 592
    clinical features of, 592
    course of, 593
    food allergy-associated, 687t
    laboratory studies and joint radiographs of, 593
    treatment of, 593
  postchemotherapy, 376
  soft tissue, 452
Rheumatoid arthritis, 9, 105–118
  amyloidosis associated with, 546
  biologic agents for, 642
  calcium pyrophosphate deposition disease-related, 349
  cervical spine involvement in, 112, 445t
  classification criteria for, 108b
  clinical features of, 278t
  common problems of wrist with, 670
  definition of, 107
  diagnosis of, 108
  differentiated from osteoarthritis, 44t
  disease-modifying antirheumatic drug for, 619
  entrapment neuropathies associated with, 477
  epidemiologic characteristics of, 109
  exercise for, 667
  extraarticular manifestations of, 113, 113t
  extraarticular organ involvement in, 89t
  factors addressed in patients with, 668
  famous people with, 692
  of feet, 111
  fibromyalgia syndrome associated with, 454–455
  first clinical description of, 692
  food allergy-associated, 687t
  goals for treatment of, 115
  of hand, 110
  initial treatment of, 116
  insidious onset of, 109
  instruments used for disease activity measurement, 116, 116t
  joint involvement in, 109b, 110f
  juvenile, laboratory abnormalities in, 527t
  laboratory findings in, 113
  laryngeal manifestations of, 115
  long-term prognosis for, 116
  malignancy associated with, 375t
  mixed cryoglobulinemia, 242
  monoarticular, 82
  mortality in, 116
  palindromic arthritis-related, 593
  palindromic (episodic) pattern in, 109
  polyarteritis nodosa-related, 219
  polyarticular symptoms of, 87, 88t
  polymyalgia rheumatica-related, 195
  during pregnancy, 581
  prevalence of, 4t
  prognosis of, 287
  radiographic features of, 71, 111, 111f
  relapsing polychondritis-related, 256
  rheumatoid factor in, 54, 113
  sarcoidosis associated with, 569
  scleritis associated with, 559, 560t
  septic joint associated with, 295
  sequence for reconstructive surgery for, 669
  seronegative, 10, 117
  seropositive, 10

Rheumatoid arthritis (Continued)
  surgical management of, 673
  synovial biopsy in, 76
  synovial fluid analysis of, 111
  treatment goal for, 10
Rheumatoid factors, 54
  causes of positive, 54
  in children, 520, 520t
  in juvenile systemic connective tissue diseases, 523
  polyarticular symptoms of, 89–90
  in rheumatoid arthritis, 54, 113
  in Sjögren's syndrome, 176
Rheumatoid nodulosis, 109
Rheumatologist, origin of term, 3
Rheumatology, 7–15
  definition of, 3
  "do nots" in, 8
  origin of term, 692
  PID syndromes in, 430
  rehabilitative techniques in, 14
  roots of, 3
Rickets, 439
  causes of, 397, 398t
  clinical manifestations of, 397–398
  treatment for, 398t
Rifampin, 308–309, 688t
Right-heart catheterization (RHC)
  in pulmonary arterial hypertension, 150–151
  in scleroderma, 151t
Rilonacept (Arcalyst), 637
Risedronate, 654t
Rituximab, 131, 640
  as dermatomyositis/polymyositis treatment, 163
  indications and toxicities of, 640
  as mixed cryoglobulinemic vasculitis treatment, 244–245
  repetition of, 641
  as systemic lupus erythematosus treatment, 134
Rodnan skin score, modified, 144–145
Rofecoxib, 605
Roosevelt, Theodore, 692
Ropinirole (Requip), 460
Rose Bengal test, 173f
Rotator cuff
  impingement of, 462
  tears of, 464
  tests for isolation of, 463
Royal jelly, 687
RS3PE (remitting seronegative symmetrical synovitis with pitting edema) syndrome, 117, 372t–373t
Rubella, 315–316
  laboratory abnormalities of, 316
  natural
    clinical course of, 315
    joint manifestation associated with, 315
    pathogenesis of, 315
  vaccine, 316
Rubens, Peter Paul, 693
Rubor, Raynaud's phenomenon-related, 550
Rugger-jersey spine, 572, 573f
Runners, tendon injuries in, 475
Runner's knee, 473
Russell, Rosalind, 692

S

Sacroiliac joints
  radiographic abnormalities of, 266
  radiographic view used for, 265f, 266
  tenderness of, 262

Sacroiliitis
  ankylosing spondylitis-related, 261
  diagnostic tests for, 449
  inflammatory bowel disease-related, treatment of, 271t
  monoarthritis-related, 85
  psoriatic arthritis related, 284
  radiographic features of, 71
  Whipple's disease associated with, 325
Saddle nose deformity, 255f
S-adenosyl-l-methionine (SAM-e), 690
Salicylates, 601
  nonacetylated, 605
Salivary gland, enlargement, differential diagnosis of, 174
Salmonella infections, 369
Salsalate, as osteoarthritis treatment, 389
Salvage therapy, in granulomatosis with polyangiitis, 230–231
SAPHO syndrome, 288
Sarcoglycanopathy, 541
Sarcoidosis, 13
  biopsy in, 566
  clinical manifestations of, 566
  clinical presentation of, 565
  definition of, 565
  early-onset, 591
  evaluation of a patient with, 566
  immunopathologic features of, 565
  malignancy associated with, 372t–373t
  osseous changes occur in patients with, 568, 568f
  prognostic factors in, 569
  respiratory tract manifestations of, 565
  rheumatic manifestations of, 567t
  rheumatic syndromes associated with, 565–570
  treatment for, 569
  uveitis associated with, 557
Sarcolemma, 23
Sarcoma
  clear cell, 496
  Ewing, 512–513
  osteogenic, 401
  synovial, 495, 496b
Saturday night palsy, 480
Saw palmetto, 690
Scadding staging system, 566, 566t
Scalp tenderness, and giant cell arteritis, 209
Scarlet fever, differentiated from Kawasaki disease, 531
Scedosporium species, 311
Scheuermann's disease, 440, 513
Schirmer's test, 172, 173f
Schlosstein, Lee, 693
Schmidt's triad, 11
Schober's test, 262, 263f, 448
Sciatica, 448, 480–481
Scleredema, 155
Scleritis, 559–561, 560t
Sclerodactyly, 152f
Scleroderma
  in children, 527
  classification of, 141, 142f
  clinical characteristics of, 154
  diabetes-associated rheumatologic syndrome and, 360
  early description of, 692
  in famous Swiss painter and printmaker, 693
  linear, 154–155
  malignancy associated with, 372t–373t
  mimics of, 154–157
  PAH in, 149, 150t
  prevalence of, 4t
  radiographic features of, 72
  skin type and autoantibody profile of, 143
  suspicion of, 10
Scleroderma renal crisis (SRC), 151–152
Scleromalacia perforans, 559
Scleromyxedema, 155
Sclerosis, systemic, 103, 141–153, 667
  American College of Rheumatology/European League against Rheumatism (ACR/EULAR) classification criteria for, 144t
  bone and articular involvement in, 152, 152f
  causes of, 143
  classification criteria of, 144t
  CREST syndrome associated with, 143
  definition of, 141
  diffuse cutaneous, 141, 142f
  extraarticular organ involvement in, 89t
  gastrointestinal (GI) manifestations of, 146
  limited cutaneous, 141, 142f
  malignancy associated with, 375t
  mortality in, 144
  organ system involvement in, 144t
  during pregnancy, 581
  Raynaud phenomenon-associated with, 89
  Raynaud's phenomenon associated with, 145
  small and large bowel involvement, 147
  specific autoantibodies of, 143t
  treatments of, 143
Scotomata, 556
Seal, 692
"SECRET" mnemonic, for polymyalgia rheumatica, 193
Segmental arterial mediolysis (SAM), 218
Seizures, 183
  in Behçet's disease, 250
  in giant cell arteritis, 209
  relapsing polychondritis-related, 256
Selective estrogen receptor modulators (SERMs), 656
Selective serotonin reuptake inhibitors (SSRIs), 460
Self-antigens, tolerance to, 37
Sensory nerve action potentials (SNAPs), 81
Septic joint, surgical drainage for, 294
Sequestra, differentiated from Brodie's abscess, 299
Serositis, 120t
Serotonin-norepinephrine reuptake inhibitors (SNRIs), 459
Serum CPK MB band, and myocardial involvement, 161
Shawl-sign rash, 159
Shepherd's crook deformity, 502–503
Shin splint, 475
Shoes and socks sign, 451
Shoulder
  anatomy of, 464f
  in ankylosing spondylitis, 263
  calcification in, 353
  diseases associated with radiographic changes in, 69
  "frozen" (periarthritis), 359, 465
  with rheumatic diseases involvement, 669
Shoulder girdle, diffuse aches and pains of, 94
Shoulder-hand syndrome, 375, 485
  and frozen shoulder, 359
Shoulder impingement syndrome, 45, 462, 463f
  clinical presentation of, 463
  stages of, 463
  treatment of, 464
Shoulder pain, 462–463, 471
"Shrinking lung syndrome," 130
Sialography, 173
Sialometry, 173
Sickle cell anemia, 367
Sillence classification, of osteogenesis imperfecta, 414
Sinusitis, 567t
Sirolimus (Rapamune), 630
Sit-up test, 451
Sjögren, Henrich, 171

Sjögren's syndrome, 10, 13, 103, 115, 171–178
  American College of Rheumatology classification criteria for, 176
  antibodies in, 523
  differential diagnosis of, in children, 524
  differentiated from diffuse infiltrative lymphocytosis syndrome, 322t
  exocrine glands involved in, 174
  malignancy associated with, 375t
  as overlap syndrome, 169
  primary, 171
    arthritis of, 175
    extraglandular manifestations of, 174–175
    initial manifestations of, 171
    laboratory and autoantibody findings in, 175
    pathology and pathogenesis of, 172, 172f
  in relapsing polychondritis, 256–257
  rheumatoid factor in, 113
  sarcoidosis associated with, 569
  secondary, 171
  uveitis associated with, 558
Skin disorders
  in granulomatosis with polyangiitis, 227
  scleroderma associated with, 154
Skin fragility, in Ehlers-Danlos syndrome, 414
Skin lesions, for acute/chronic polyarthritis diagnosis, 88
Skin pigmentation, in classic HHC, 425–426
Skin thickening, 144–145, 145f
Skull, "salt and pepper," 72, 572
Sleep disorders, fibromyalgia syndrome-related, 454
Slit-lamp screening, in juvenile idiopathic arthritis, 519, 519t
Slocumb's syndrome, 363
Slump test, 448
Smoking, 146, 221, 620
Snapping hip, 467, 473
Social Security Disability Insurance (SSDI), 677–678
Social workers, 662
Sodium retention, corticosteroid related, 615
Sodium valproate, 609t
Soft tissue
  calcification of, 574
  swelling of, 73, 280
Soft tissue rheumatism, 4t, 7, 452
Somatosensory evoked potentials, 78
SONK (spontaneous osteonecrosis of the knee), 407
Speed's test, 45, 465
Spider digits. *see* Arachnodactyly
Spinal cord lesions, as muscle weakness/pain cause, 92
Spine
  arthritis of, 270
  radiographic changes in, 71
  "rugger-jersey," 572, 573f
  tuberculosis of, 307
Splenectomy, 131
Splenomegaly, 190t, 566
Splints, 665
Spondylitis, 449
  inflammatory bowel disease-related, treatment of, 271t
  psoriatic arthritis-related, 284
  reactive arthritis-related, 277
  Whipple's disease associated with, 325
Spondyloarthritis, axial, 261b
Spondyloarthropathies, 76, 449
  in children, 519t
  in dialysis patients, 574
  early descriptions of, 693
  monoarticular, 84t, 85
  pregnancy and, 581
  prevalence of, 4t
  sarcoidosis associated with, 569

Spondyloarthropathies (Continued)
  seronegative, scleritis associated with, 560t
  undifferentiated, 282
    in HIV infection with arthritis, 321
Spondyloepiphyseal dysplasia (SED), 413, 438, 438f
Spondyloepiphyseal dysplasia tarda, 438
Spondylolisthesis, 449, 513
Spondylolysis, 449, 513
Spondylosis, 449
  cervical, 445
Sporothrix schenckii, 311
Sports medicine, 471–476
Sportsman's hernia, 473
Sprains, 471
  of ankle, low and high, 474
  cervical, 445
Spurling's maneuver, 446
St. John's wort, 690
St. Vitus' dance, 331
Staphylococcus aureus infections, 513
  as septic arthritis cause, 292
Starch particles, 355
Startin, James, 692
Statin therapy, associated with myopathy, 162
Steel's rule of thirds, 669
Steinberg sign, of arachnodactyly, 417, 417f
Stem cells, autologous mesenchymal, 408–409
Stem cell transplantation
  hematopoietic, 632
  as osteoarthritis therapy, 391
Steroid crystals, 355
Steroid withdrawal syndrome, 363
Steroids
  as Kawasaki disease treatment, 532
  stress-dose, 99
Stickler syndrome, 17t, 418
Stiff hand syndrome, diabetic, 357, 358f
Stiff-person syndrome, 597
Still's disease, 10, 517
  adult-onset, 189–192
    clinical course and prognosis of, 192
    laboratory features of, 190, 191t
    manifestations of, 189
    rash associated with, 189
    signs and symptoms seen in, 189, 190t
    treatment of, 191
"Still's" rash, 516
Stinger (burner) injury, 472
Stomach, "watermelon," 147
Stomatitis, aphthous, 249, 249t
Storage/deposition diseases, 424–429
Straight-leg raise test, 448
  distracted, 451
Strain, 471
Strength training, *vs.* endurance training, 663
Streptococcus pyogenes, 330
Streptozyme test, 329
Stroke, 95, 182
Stromelysins, 20–21
Strontium ranelate, for osteoarthritis, 391
Strumpell, Adolf, 693
STWL (swelling, tenderness, warmth, and limitation) system, for recording degree of arthritic involvement of joint, 42
Subclavian artery, irregular tapering and narrowing of left, in Takayasu arteritis, 206f
Subperiosteal resorption, of phalanges, 362f
Sudeck's atrophy, 485

Sulfasalazine, 688t
  as ankylosing spondylitis treatment, 266–267
  as connective tissue disease treatment, 376t
  use during pregnancy and lactation, 582
  as inflammatory peripheral arthritis treatment, 271t
  as liver disease treatment, 275
  metabolism and mechanism of action (MOA) of, 621
  use in renal insufficiency patients, 575
  as rheumatic disease treatment, 621
  as rheumatoid arthritis treatment, 620
Sulfinpyrazone, 646
Sulfonylurea, 609t
Sullivan, Ed, 693
Superantigens, 38
Superior labrum anterior-to-posterior (SLAP) lesion, 472
Supplemental Security Income (SSI), 677–678
Suprascapular nerve entrapment, 480
Suprascapular nerve lesion, 81t
Surgical treatment, of rheumatic diseases, 668–675
Susac's syndrome, 223, 561
Swan-neck deformities, 69, 110, 110f, 125f, 671
Sweet's syndrome, 372t–373t, 374
Swelling
  fusiform, in rheumatoid arthritis, 110
  gout-related, 339
  of joints, in children, 514–515
  of soft tissue, 73, 280
Swimmer's knee, 473
Sydenham, Thomas, 693
Sympathetic blocks, 487
Sympatholytic agents, 553
Symptom severity (SS) scale score, 454
Synarthrosis, 19
Syndesmophytes, 71, 265, 279, 280f
  differentiated from osteophyte, 69t
Synovectomy, 670
Synovial fluid, 59
  bloody, 365
  classification of, 60t
  crystals and particles in, 61, 352, 352b, 355, 356f
  group 2 (inflammatory), rheumatic disorders for, 60b
  physical characteristics of, 19
  viscosity of, 19
  white blood cell count in, 59
Synovial fluid analysis, 8, 58–62
  of amyloid arthropathy of renal failure, 574
  in children, 514
  "dry tap" in, 59
  of fungal septic arthritis, 310
  of gout, 340
  Gram stain and culture in, 59
  indications for, 83
  of monoarthritis, 85
  of nongonococcal septic arthritis, 293
  of osteoarticular TB, 308
  of pigmented villonodular synovitis, 493
  for polyarthritis evaluation, 90
  of polymyalgia rheumatica, 194
  of pseudogout, 348
  of reactive arthritis, 278
  of rheumatoid arthritis, 111
  time frame of, 59
  total leukocyte count and differential in, 59
  in Whipple's disease, 326
Synovial joint, "bare areas" of, 64, 64f
Synovial tissue, obtaining of, 77t
Synovioma, 84t, 85
  giant cell, benign, 493

Synovitis
  elective surgery for, 97
  eosinophilic, 593
  foreign body, 82b, 84t, 593–594
  of hip, 513
  inflammatory, basic calcium phosphate and, 354
  in joint, 41
  localized nodular, 493
  pigmented villonodular, 82b, 84t, 493
    radiographic findings of, 493
  RS3PE syndrome-related, 117
  in systemic lupus erythematosus, 120t
  three phase bone scan of, 74t
Synovium
  benign and malignant tumors of, 491–496
  biopsies of, 76–77
  microanatomy of, 19
  in septic arthritis, 291
Syphilis, 298, 558
Systemic antirheumatic drugs, 619–626
Systemic lupus erythematosus (SLE), 10, 13, 103, 119–136
  activity indices used in, 134
  antinuclear antibody-negative, 50
  antiphospholipid antibodies in, 180
  autoantibodies in, 122t
  biological therapies of, 134
  in children, 522
  classification criteria for, 119
  clinical manifestations of, 522, 523t
  common causes of death in patients with, 135
  diagnosis of, 119
  estrogens, 133
  extraarticular organ involvement in, 89t
  famous people with, 692
  fibromyalgia syndrome associated with, 454
  gastrointestinal tract, 130
  heart involvement in, 130
  idiopathic, 137
  importance of heredity in development of, 119
  laboratory hallmark of, 121
  lung involvement in, 130
  malignancy associated with, 375t
  mixed cryoglobulinemia-related, 242
  mucocutaneous lesions associated with, 122–123
  as overlap syndrome, 169
  pediatric, 522
  polyarticular symptoms of, 86, 87t
  pregnancy during, 577–578
  prevalence of, 4t
  radiographic features of, 72
  rashes associated with, 124f
  Raynaud phenomenon-associated with, 89
  relapsing polychondritis-related, 256–257
  sarcoidosis associated with, 569
  scleritis associated with, 560t
  stem cell transplantation in, 135
  Systemic Lupus International Collaborating Clinics criteria used in, 119, 119t
  treatment of, 132–133
  versus type I autoimmune hepatitis and, 273t
Systemic Lupus International Collaborating Clinics/American College of Rheumatology Damage Index, 134
Systemic sclerosis sine scleroderma, 142

T

Tacrolimus, 163, 251, 344, 576, 630
Talc particles, 355
Tardy ulnar nerve palsy, 479
Tarsal tunnel syndrome, 481

Tarui's disease, 535t, 538, 538f
Taxanes, 376
T-cell immunodeficiency, primary, organisms responsible for infections in, 431
T cell targeted therapies, 641
T cells, 31
   CD4+, activation of, 32, 32f
   function, laboratory tests for, 431, 432t
   and MHC HLA molecules, 30–31
Telangiectasia, 146
N-telopeptide, urinary, 401
Temporal artery
   abnormalities of, 209
   biopsy of, 210–211, 211f
   duplex ultrasound of, 210
Temporomandibular arthritis, 668
Tender points, 43t, 452, 453f, 454
Tendinitis, 452
   Achilles, 468
   bicipital, 464
   calcific, treatment of, 353
   definition of, 462
   patellar (jumper's knee), 473
   posterior tibial, 469
   primary care office visits for, 4
   principles of treatment to, 476, 476t
   rotator cuff/supraspinatus, test for, 45
Tendinopathy
   definition of, 462
   gluteus medius, 467
Tendinosis, definition of, 462
Tendon friction rubs, 152
Tendon reflexes, grading of, 93t
Tendon sheath
   amount of glucocorticoid injected in, 618t
   frequent injections of glucocorticoids in, 617
   giant cell tumor of, 493
   tenosynovial giant cell tumor of, localized, 493
Tendonitis
   Achilles, 47
   posterior tibialis, 47
Tendonitis, subscapularis, 472
Tendons
   Achilles, 468f
      rupture of, 475
   differentiated from ligament, 21
   overuse injuries of, 471
Tennis elbow. *see* Epicondylitis; lateral
Tenosynovial giant cell tumor (TGCT)
   histologic characteristics of, 494
   treatment for, 494
Tenosynovitis, 88, 452
   definition of, 462
   De Quervain's, 43, 466
   flexor, 359
   gonococcal arthritis-related, 297
   in osteoarticular TB, 307
Tension test, upper limb, 446
Terasaki, Paul, 693
Teriparatide, 576, 657
Testosterone, 657
Tetracycline, 251, 688, 688t
Thalassemia, sickle-β, 369
Thalidomide, 251, 624
Thallium, neuromuscular toxicity of, 93
Thenar atrophy, in carpal tunnel syndrome, 43
Thermography, 486
Thiazides, as hyperuricemia cause, 339t
Thiemann's disease, 405
Thompson test, 468

Thoracic outlet syndrome, 45, 479
Thromboangiitis obliterans, 220–221
   angiogram of, 221f
   clinical features of, 220
   diagnosis of, 220
   differential diagnosis of, 221
   etiology of, 220
   treatment of, 221
Thromboaortopathy, occlusive, 212
Thrombocytopenia, 120t, 183–184
Thromboembolism, 420
Thrombopoietin receptor agonists, 131
Thrombosis, 182
   cardiac arterial, treatment of, 186
   in patient with aPL abs, risk of, 182–183
   treatment for, 185
Thumb sign, of arachnodactyly, 417, 417f
Thyroid cancer, medullary, 544t
Thyroid disease, 360–361
Thyroiditis, Hashimoto's, 360
Thyroxine, as myopathy marker, 92
Tibial nerve, posterior, 468f, 481f
Tibial tendon, posterior, 468f
   dysfunction/rupture of, 469
Tick, as *Borrelia burgdorferi* vector, 300
Tietze's syndrome, 593
Tinel's sign, 478, 481
Tinel's test, 43
Tocilizumab (Actemra), 638
Toes, deformities of, 674t
Tofacitinib (Xeljanz), 639
Tolerance
   definition of, 36
   innate or acquired, 36
Toll-like receptors (TLRs), 25
"Too many toes" sign, 469
Tophi, 341
Total hemolytic complement assay, 432–433
Touraine-Solente-Golé syndrome, 440
Tourniquet test, 481
Toxemia, of pregnancy, 578, 579t
Toxic oil syndrome, 155
Toxoplasmosis, uveitis associated with, 557
Tracheostomy, in relapsing polychondritis, 257
Tramadol, 460, 576
Transcranial direct current stimulation, 461
Transthyretin, amino acid variants of, 543–544, 546
TRAP mnemonic, for rheumatologic syndrome of hypothyroidism, 360
Trazodone (Desyrel), 460
Trendelenburg's test, positive, 45
Triamcinolone, 614t
Triamcinolone acetonide, as pseudogout treatment, 349
Triamcinolone hexacetonide
   as juvenile idiopathic arthritis treatment, 519
   as pseudogout treatment, 349
Triangular fibrocartilage complex, of wrist, chondrocalcinosis of, 348f
Tricyclic antidepressants (TCAs), 459, 460t
Trigger points, 43t
Tropheryma whipplei, 325
T-tubule system, 23
Tuberculin skin test, 613
Tuberculosis (TB)
   amyloidosis associated with, 546t
   bone/joint involvement in, 307
   osteoarticular, 307
      diagnosis of, 308
      peripheral joint involvement in, 307–308
      radiographic features of, 308

Tuberculosis (*Continued*)
    signs and symptoms of, 307
    spine involvement in, 307–308, 309f
    treatment of, 308
    uveitis associated with, 556–557
Tumor necrosis factor-α antagonists, as Behçet's disease treatment, 251
Tumor necrosis factor-α inhibitors, 634
    biologic agents available as, 634
    diseases treated with, 637
    in drug-induced lupus, 139
    FDA indications in rheumatic diseases of, 634
    injection site, 635
    switching "rules" in, 637
Tumor necrosis factor α receptor autoinflammatory periodic syndrome (TRAPS), 589
Tumor necrosis factor blockers, as connective tissue disease treatment, 376t
Tumor necrosis factor inhibitors
    malignancies associated with, 376
    as rheumatoid arthritis treatment, 116
Tumors, of joints and synovium, 491–496, 495f
"Turf toe," 475

U

Ulcers
    aphthous, in Behçet's disease, 249
    corneal, 250
    digital, 146
    duodenal, 604
    genital, 249
    of leg, 244
    nasal, 123
    oral, 120t, 123
    "punched-out," 204f
Ulnar deviation deformities, 69, 110
Ulnar nerve, anatomy of, 479f
Ulnar nerve entrapment syndromes, 479
Ulnar tunnel syndrome, 479
Ultrasound
    of gout, 340, 341f
    of musculoskeletal disorders, 74
    radiation exposure during, 75
    of sportsman's hernia, 473
Unicameral (simple) bone cyst (UBC), 503–504, 504f
Upper respiratory tract, affected clinically by GPA, 225, 226f
Uremia, 536t
Uric acid, 337
    in cold environment, 12
    crystals, detection in synovial fluid, 61, 61f
    in gout, 12, 337–338, 338f
    in monoarthritis, 84
    renal handling of, 646
    renal transport of, 342
Uricase, 337
Uricosuric agents, 646
Urine, red-wine-colored, as metabolic myopathy indicator, 540
Urine collection, for gout, 338
U1-RNP, 168
Urticaria, 313
Urticarial lesions, 11
    in small-vessel vasculitides, 237
Ustekinumab (Stelara), 639
Uveitis, 13, 555–559
    anterior, 556
    causes of, 558t
    intermediate, 556
    juvenile idiopathic arthritis-related, 519, 519t

Uveitis (*Continued*)
    Kawasaki disease-related, 530
    masquerade syndromes of, 557
    posterior, 556
    sarcoidosis-related, 567t
    treatment principles of, 559

V

Vaccination, immunosuppressive agents as contraindication to, 623
Vacuum disc sign, 71, 428
Valerian root, 690
Valsalva maneuver, in sciatica, 448
Valvulitis, relapsing polychondritis-related, 256t
van Buren, Martin, 693
Vasculitis, 11
    angiographic features of, 206, 206f
    antineutrophil cytoplasmic antibody-associated, 224–235
        atypical, 224
        clinical association of, 227
        cytoplasmic, 224, 225f
        diseases of, 234
        major autoantigens of, 224
        perinuclear, 224, 225f
        primary, 224
        tests used to detect, 224
    of central nervous system, 11
    in children, 524
    cryoglobulinemic, 201–202, 236t, 242
        mixed, 244
    definition of, 201
    diagnosis of, approach to, 203
    disorders that can mimic, 203
    drug-induced ANCA-associated, 234
    evaluation of, 205
    extraarticular organ involvement in, 89t
    focal and segmental transmural necrotizing, polyarteritis nodosa and, 217
    histologic features of, 201, 201f
    HIV infection-related, 322
    hypersensitivity, 202t, 236, 236t
    IgA, 236t, 238
    immune mechanism of, 201
    in inflammatory bowel disease, 270
    juvenile dermatomyositis-related, 526
    laboratory tests for, 204
    large-vessel, 203, 208–215
    leukocytoclastic, 12, 114, 236, 374
    medium-vessel, 114, 203, 216–223
    mimics of, 203
    necrotizing, 201f, 236, 372t–373t
    nomenclature for, 202t
    noninvasive tests to determine vessel involvement in, 206
    as paraneoplastic syndrome, 374
    pregnancy and, 581
    primary central nervous system, 524
    Raynaud phenomenon-associated with, 89
    "refractory," 11
    relapsing polychondritis-related, 256–257
    retinal, 250, 561–562
    in rheumatoid arthritis, 114
    sarcoidosis-related, 566
    skin lesions in, 204, 204f
    small arteriolar, 114
    small-vessel, 203
        causes of, 236
        diagnosis of, 238
        due to immune complex deposition, 236, 236t
        immune-complex-mediated, 236–240

Vasculitis (Continued)
  laboratory and radiographic tests for, 237
  malignancy in, 236t
  manifestation in, 237, 237f
  mimicking diseases of, 237
  skin involvement in, 237
  treatment of, 238
suspected, approach for patients with, 199–207
systemic, 314
  forms of, 524
  scleritis associated with, 560
in systemic lupus erythematosus, 125
Takayasu's arteritis, 524
treatment of, approach to, 206
types of, 203, 204t
urticarial, 236t, 239, 243
vascular consequences of, 201
Vasodilators
  direct, 553
  indirect, 553
Vasomotor instability, 484
Vasospasm, as Raynaud's phenomenon cause, 550–551
Vaughn-Jackson syndrome, 670
Vectra-DA test, 56
Venereal Disease Research Laboratory (VDRL) test, false positive, 179
Venlafaxine (Effexor), 459
Vertebra plana, 506
Vertigo, in giant cell arteritis, 209
Vestibuloauditory dysfunction, 563
Vibration, as Raynaud's phenomenon cause, 549, 551
Viral infections, as discitis cause, 513
Virchow, Rudolph, 543
Viscosupplementation, 390
Vision blurring, 209, 556
Visual loss, in giant cell arteritis, 209
Vitamin C, 488
  as CAM therapy, 690
Vitamin D
  intake of, 653
  metabolism and action of, 397
  to prevent and treat osteoporosis, 652
Vitamin D deficiency, 397, 536t, 653, 653t
Vitamin E deficiency, 536t
VITAMINS ABCDE mnemonic, for renal osteodystrophy, 571
Vocational counselors, healthcare personnel, 662
Vocational rehabilitation (VR), 680
Vodden, Lucy, 692
Vogt-Koyanagi-Harada (VKH) disease, 557
von Bechterew, Vladimir, 693
von Bechterew's disease, 261
von Gierke glycogen storage disease, 338
von Hebra, Ferdinand, 692
V-sign rash, 159

W

"Waddell's sign," 451
Walker-Murdoch sign, of arachnodactyly, 417
Want, John, 693
Warfarin, 58, 101, 188, 366, 609t
Wasting syndrome, HIV-related, 321
Water, as articular cartilage component, 20
"Weaver's bottom," 467
Weber-Christian syndrome, 596
Wegener's granulomatosis
  anti-neutrophil cytoplasmic antibodies in, 55
  in children, 523
  scleritis associated with, 560
Western blot analysis, 303

Whipple's disease, 325–327
  arthrocentesis and synovial biopsies for, results from, 326
  clinical presentation of, 325
  diagnosis of, 326
  etiology of, 326
  immunologic defects in, 326
  presentation of, 326
  relapses of, 327
  therapy for, 326
WHIPPLES DISEASE mnemonic, for Whipple's disease, 325t
White blood cell counts
  in synovial fluid, "wet drop" examination of, 59
  in systemic lupus erythematosus, 133
  in Whipple's disease, 326
Wide dynamic range (WDR) neurons, 456
Widespread pain index (WPI), 454
Wild yam, 690
Williams' exercises, 450
Wilson disease
  calcium pyrophosphate dihydrate deposition disease-related, 347
  clinical presentations of, 427
  diagnosis of, 427
  genetic mutation in, 427
  musculoskeletal manifestations of, 427
  pattern of inheritance for, 424
  treatment of, 428
Windup, 457
Winterbauer, Richard, 693
Wnt/β-catenin signaling pathway, 21, 22f
Work, categories of, physical requirements for, 679
Workers' Compensation program, 678
Wrist
  rheumatoid arthritis of, 109b, 670
  triangular fibrocartilage complex of, 348f
Wrist hyperflexion and abduction of the thumb (WHAT) test, 466
Wrist sign, of arachnodactyly, 417

X

Xanthine oxidase inhibitors, 647
  drug interactions occur with, 649
  indications for using, 647
Xanthomatoid papules, in pseudoxanthoma elasticum, 418
Xerophthalmia
  Sjögren's syndrome-related, 172
  treatment of, 176
Xerostomia
  complications of, 176–177
  Sjögren's syndrome-related, 173–174
X-rays
  chest, 558
    in glucocorticoids use, 613
    for sarcoidosis evaluation, 566
  for low back pain evaluation, 449
  radiation exposure during, 75

Y

Yamaguchi classification criteria, 191–192
Yergason's maneuver, 45, 465
Young adults, in reactive arthritis, 277
Yucca, 690

Z

Zidovudine, 92
Zinaxin, 690
Zoledronic acid, 654t
Zone-Quick Diagnostic Threads method, 172